D1558457

TOURO COLLEGE LIBRARY
Bay Shore Campus

Chassin's Operative Strategy
in General Surgery

Third Edition

Springer
New York
Berlin
Heidelberg
Barcelona
Hong Kong
London
Milan
Paris
Singapore
Tokyo

Carol E.H. Scott-Conner, MD, PhD

Professor and Head, Department of Surgery
University of Iowa Hospitals and Clinics
Iowa City, Iowa

Chassin's Operative Strategy in General Surgery
An Expositive Atlas

Third Edition

Illustrations by Caspar Henselmann

With 1065 Illustrations

WITHDRAWN
TOURO COLLEGE LIBRARY
Bay Shore Campus

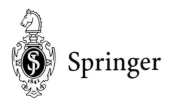 Springer

Carol E.H. Scott-Conner, MD, PhD
Department of Surgery
University of Iowa Hospitals and Clinics
200 Hawkins Drive, #1516 JCP
Iowa City, IA 52242-1086
USA
carol-scott-conner@uiowa.edu

BS

Library of Congress Cataloging-in-Publication Data
Scott-Conner, Carol E.H.
    Chassin's operative strategy in general surgery : an expositive atlas / Carol E.H.
    Scott-Conner.—3rd ed.
        p. cm.
    Includes bibliographical references and index.
    ISBN 0-387-95204-7 (hc : alk. paper)
    1. Anatomy, Surgical and topographical—Atlases.   2. Surgery, Operative—Atlases.
    I. Title.
    QM531 .S42 2001
    617′.91—dc21   2001020044

Printed on acid-free paper.

© 2002, 1994, 1984 (vol. 2), 1980 (vol. 1) Springer-Verlag New York, Inc.
All rights reserved. This work may not be translated or copied in whole or in part without the written permission of
the publisher (Springer-Verlag New York, Inc., 175 Fifth Avenue, New York, NY 10010, USA), except for brief ex-
cerpts in connection with reviews or scholarly analysis. Use in connection with any form of information storage and
retrieval, electronic adaptation, computer software, or by similar or dissimilar methodology now known or hereafter
developed is forbidden.
The use of general descriptive names, trade names, trademarks, etc., in this publication, even if the former are not especially identified, is not to be taken as a sign that such names, as understood by the Trade Marks and Merchandise
Marks Act, may accordingly be used freely by anyone.
While the advice and information in this book are believed to be true and accurate at the date of going to press, neither the authors nor the editors nor the publisher can accept any legal responsibility for any errors or omissions that
may be made. The publisher makes no warranty, express or implied, with respect to the material contained herein.

Production coordinated by WordCrafters Editorial Services, Inc., and managed by Lesley Poliner; manufacturing
supervised by Joe Quatela.
Typeset by Matrix Publishing Services, Inc., York, PA.
Printed and bound by Maple-Vail Book Manufacturing Group, York, PA.
Printed in the United States of America.

9 8 7 6 5 4 3 2 1

ISBN 0-387-95204-7   SPIN 10790788

Springer-Verlag   New York Berlin Heidelberg
A member of BertelsmannSpringer Science+Business Media GmbH

4/14/03

To Harry

       Carol E.H. Scott-Conner

To Charlotte

Jameson L. Chassin

Preface to the Third Edition

The year was 1979. I was a fourth year surgical resident at New York University, sent for a two-month rotation to the (then) Booth Memorial Medical Center. Many university programs have a similar rotation: residents are sent to an outlying affiliated hospital for a couple of months of intensive bread-and-butter surgery and an experience of what life is like in the real world of private practice. Jim Chassin, his associates Jim Turner and Kenny Rifkind, and the Booth Memorial residents welcomed me and shared their busy surgical practice with me. My notes from the time indicate I scrubbed on a wide variety of cases, many with Jim Chassin. The procedures were the very operations described in this text, and I hear his voice coaching me as I read his words.

Surgical staplers were just coming into common use that year. My university program had not yet adopted these devices, reasoning that residents need to learn how to suture before using staplers. Thus it was from Jim Chassin that I learned how to do a low anterior resection with a circular stapled anastomosis. He reinforced his instructions with copies of the typed manuscripts of the relevant chapters from a book he was writing, complete with rough sketches by his artist. When the first volume of the first edition of Chassin's *Operative Strategy in General Surgery* came out, I bought it, and literally wore out my copy. The second volume followed in due course, and eventually a second edition. I recommended the book to untold numbers of residents.

It was thus with a sense of the circle coming around to full closure that I undertook the editorship of this third edition. Searching through my files, I found original manuscript copies with my handwritten notes from that 1979 rotation. I can only hope that in bringing this classic up to date I have remained true to the intent of the author. Eight years have passed since the second edition. Much has changed, much remains the same. Eight new technical chapters for new procedures have been added. New authors, each an expert in his/her own field, have been recruited to write 13 "concepts" chapters. These chapters introduce each section to put the technical chapters that follow into perspective. New references have been added. Caspar Henselmann, the gifted illustrator of the first two editions, created hundreds of new illustrations specifically for this edition.

The purpose of this volume remains, as it was so eloquently stated by Frank C. Spencer, MD, in the Foreword to the First Edition, to serve "all clinical surgeons, both those in training and those in surgical practice" by "specifically discussing the conceptual basis of the operation as well as the strategy that will help the surgeon avoid common pitfalls . . . the operative technique is then described step by step." *No procedure has been deleted.* No surgeon who has relied on the second edition need keep a dogeared copy of that volume out of concern that technical material has been cut. Think of this third edition as the edition for the current awkward state of surgical evolution: where some, but not all, abdominal operations can be performed through laparoscopic approaches; where most, but not all, ulcers can be managed medically; where sentinel node biopsy is still being validated; and where most, but not all, subphrenic abscesses are drained percutaneously.

As an academic surgeon, I am struck by how frequently a resident will comment "I've never even seen one of these" when we embark upon certain formerly-common operations, such as an open common bile duct exploration. For this new generation of surgeons, I've included all the procedures that were in the second edition. Those that are rarely used are labeled *Legacy material*, for that is what this book is—the legacy of a master surgeon: an extraordinary surgeon and a kind and gentle man I have been privileged to scrub with and to have as a friend. I hope that you will still hear his voice speaking through these pages.

This work could not have been completed without the wise counsel of Laura Gillan, Caspar Henselmann, and Jameson Chassin. Katherine Carolan and Lana Slagle at the University of Iowa, and Liz Corra provided invaluable help during the editing phase. The library at the Marine Biological Laboratory in Woods Hole, Massachusetts, provided a refuge and quiet working space for me as it has for generations of scholars. Finally, my patients, students, residents, and coworkers continue to teach and inspire me.

Carol E.H. Scott-Conner, MD, PhD
Iowa City, Iowa
2001

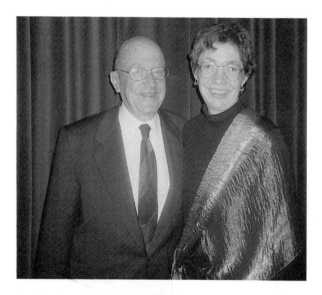

Dr. Jameson L. Chassin and Dr. Carol E.H. Scott-Conner at the Chassin Surgical Society Dinner, April 4, 2000, at the Harvard Club, New York, New York, where Dr. Scott-Conner gave the guest lecture, "Women in American Surgery."

Foreword to the Third Edition

Eight years have passed since the publication of the second edition of this atlas. During that period, I retired from the practice of surgery and from the chairmanship of the Department of Surgery at the New York Hospital Medical Center of Queens, concluding an exciting and stimulating run of 34 years, the highlight of which was teaching several generations of residents the intellectual and technical details of surgery. A vital component of this program was the atlas *Operative Strategy in General Surgery*, the first edition of which was published in 1980. The success of this work was due in large part to the fact that it was based on my day-to-day learning and teaching in the operating room. Having retired from the operating room, I felt that I could not produce a quality, up-to-date product for the third edition of this work. Fortunately, we were able to recruit an outstanding surgeon-teacher to edit the third edition.

Dr. Carol Scott-Conner, whom I taught when she was a resident in 1980, has the intellect, teaching skills, and drive to have functioned as an author, surgeon, teacher, and Head of the Department of Surgery at the University of Iowa. In editing this volume, she has reviewed each chapter to make sure that the text and references are up to date. Although the previous editions were the work of a single author (me), it is a fact that surgery and medical science have advanced so rapidly that it is no longer feasible for a single author to write a comprehensive surgical text like this one. Consequently, 13 prominent surgeons have each contributed a chapter that reviews and analyzes recent advances in the fields of the contributor's special expertise. Eight new operations have been added, most of which are laparoscopic procedures. In addition, 77 operations from my last edition, having proven themselves worthy by the test of time, are included in this volume, together with the meticulous operating room illustrations by Caspar Henselmann. Many of these procedures are complex, such as esophagectomy, total colectomy with ileoanal pouch, and pancreatoduodenectomy. Special attention has been paid to emphasize in the drawings the detailed teaching points that will make these operations safe for the patient.

I hope that our combined efforts have produced an atlas that you will find useful.

Jameson L. Chassin, MD
Professor of Clinical Surgery
New York University School of Medicine
New York, New York
2001

Foreword to the First Edition

This surgical atlas should be of great value to all clinical surgeons, both those in training and those in surgical practice, and Dr. Chassin is superbly qualified to author this work. During more than three decades as a member of the faculty of the New York University School of Medicine, he has taught countless residents many aspects of the art of surgical technique. One measure of Dr. Chassin's unusual teaching ability is that he is both Professor of Clinical Surgery at New York University and Director of Surgery at Booth Memorial Hospital where our fourth-year surgical residents have rotated regularly for the past 12 years. Booth Memorial is the only hospital outside the New York University Medical Center to which New York University residents rotate. This simple fact well underlines Dr. Chassin's remarkable capability for teaching.

When a surgical complication develops after an operation, two or three possibilities should be considered. First, of course, was the diagnosis correct? If it was, then the cause of the complication is usually either an inadequate operative technique or a flawed concept underlying the selection of the operative procedure. When the surgical technique seems faultless, a postoperative complication would strongly indicate that the concept was erroneous, albeit cherished perhaps for decades.

Unlike any other atlas on operative technique, this book specifically discusses the conceptual basis of the operation as well as the strategy that will help the surgeon avoid common pitfalls. The operative technique is then described step by step.

I am confident that in the years ahead this atlas will be regarded as one of the major contributions to our literature of surgical technique.

Frank C. Spencer, MD
George David Stewart Professor and Chairman
Department of Surgery
New York University School of Medicine
New York, New York
1980

Contents

Contributors

Samir S. Awad, MD
Department of Surgery
Baylor College of Medicine
Houston, TX 77030, USA

Claudia L. Corwin, MD
Department of Surgery
The University of Iowa Hospitals and Clinics
Iowa City, IA 52242-1086, USA

Daniel T. Dempsey, MD
Department of Surgery
University of Pennsylvania Medical Center
Philadelphia, PA 19104, USA

Stephen B. Edge, MD
Roswell Park Cancer Institute
Department of Surgery
State University of New York at Buffalo
Buffalo, New York 14263, USA

Michael B. Edye, MD
Department of Surgery
New York University School of Medicine
New York, NY 10016, USA

Alison Estabrook, MD
Division of Breast Surgery
St. Lukes-Roosevelt Hospital
New York, NY 10019, USA

Robert J. Fitzgibbons, Jr., MD
Department of Surgery
Creighton University School of Medicine
Omaha, NE 68131, USA

John F. Gibbs, MD
Roswell Park Cancer Institute
Department of Surgery
State University of New York at Buffalo
Buffalo, New York 14263, USA

Thomas H. Gouge, MD
Department of Surgery
New York University School of Medicine
New York, NY 10016, USA

Nelson J. Gurll, MD
Department of Surgery
The University of Iowa Hospitals and Clinics
Iowa City, IA 52242-1086, USA

Amber A. Guth, MD
Department of Surgery
New York University School of Medicine
New York, NY 10016, USA

Daniel P. Guyton, MD
Department of Surgery
Northeastern Ohio Universities College of Medicine
Akron General Medical Center
Akron, Ohio 44307, USA

Jade Hiromoto, MD
Department of Surgery
San Francisco VA Medical Center
University of California, San Francisco
San Francisco, CA 94121-1598, USA

Jamal J. Hoballah, MD
Department of Surgery
The University of Iowa Hospitals and Clinics
Iowa City, IA 52242-1086, USA

Muhammed Ashraf Memon, MD
Department of Transplant Surgery
St. Louis University Hospital
St. Louis, MO 63110, USA

Amanda M. Metcalf, MD
Department of Surgery
The University of Iowa Hospitals and Clinics
Iowa City, IA 52240-1086, USA

Fabrizio Michelassi, MD
Department of Surgery
The University of Chicago
The Pritzker School of Medicine
Chicago, IL 60637-1463, USA

Michael W. Mulholland, MD, PhD
Department of Surgery
University of Michigan
Ann Arbor, MI 48109-0331, USA

William H. Nealon, MD
Department of Surgery
University of Texas Medical Branch
Galveston, TX 77550, USA

Jeffrey A. Norton, MD
Department of Surgery
San Francisco VA Medical Center
University of California, San Francisco
San Francisco, CA 94121-1598, USA

H. Leon Pachter, MD
Department of Surgery
New York University School of Medicine
New York, NY 10016, USA

Danny M. Takanishi, MD
Department of Surgery
The University of Chicago
The Pritzker School of Medicine
Chicago, IL 60637-1463, USA

Part I
General Principles

1 Concepts and Strategies of Surgery

DEVELOPING A CONCEPT

Successful surgery requires study, advance planning, clear thinking, and technical skill. Brilliant execution of the wrong operation at the wrong time can only lead to disaster. To achieve consistently good results for each surgical condition the surgeon must develop a concept that combines analysis of the literature, study of the disordered physiology, and comprehension of the hypothesis underlying the contemplated operation.

To develop a concept properly a surgeon must:

Know the normal and pathologic physiology and anatomy.

Explore the relative merits of alternative operations and treatment options.

Analyze the operation selected for the problem at hand: Are there *valid data* to demonstrate that it can accomplish the desired goal? Is the mortality rate for the procedure such that the benefit outweighs the risk? Are there alternative treatments that may offer lower morbidity and potential mortality?

Reflect on personal experience with complications and deaths following the operation selected. This information is more relevant than are the results that may be reported from some renowned medical center, where one surgeon may have developed expertise in a particular operation. Superior results under such circumstances obviously do not indicate that less experienced surgeons are as successful.

Review postoperative complications and poor results. When a complication or a death occurs, analyze the case carefully and attempt to make an objective appraisal of what went wrong. Was there poor judgment regarding the choice of operation? Was the diagnosis inaccurate? Was the assessment of the risk incorrect? Was there an error of technique? Did the surgeon lack the technical expertise required to undertake the procedure?

Keep records of mortality and morbidity for each operation. Frequent analysis of results increases the database of the surgeon's own experience. Knowledge the surgeon gains leads to self-renewal and improved performance: Without it the surgeon learns nothing from experience.

Persist in a lifetime study of the published literature in basic science and clinical surgery. Only in this way could one become aware that the trauma of surgery induces the release of inflammatory mediators that make the patient feel weak and ill after surgery; that long abdominal incisions, large retractors, and rough surgical technique produce more mediators; that gentle dissection and minimally invasive techniques with 5- or 10-mm incisions and "retraction" by 15 mm Hg CO_2 reduce the mediator cascade and minimize postoperative pain and malaise. These scientific advances support the development of laparoscopic surgery.

ESTABLISHING STRATEGY

Establishing an *operative strategy*—advance planning of the technical steps of the operation—is vital to the safety and efficiency of complex surgical procedures. The operative strategy is what the surgeon ponders the night before the operation: What are the major steps of the procedure? How should it be modified for this particular case? Where are the potential pitfalls? How can they be avoided? In some ways this exercise is similar to the visualization employed by highly skilled athletes. The thesis of this book is that by creating a strategy the surgeon can reduce the incidence of operative misadventures and postoperative complications.

Anticipating and analyzing potential problems and danger points before an operation leads to success more surely than does frenzied activity in the operating room after the surgeon and patient are in deep trouble. Anticipation enhances the surgeon's capacity for prompt decision making in the operating room.

MAKING THE OPERATION EASY

The main goal of any successful operative strategy is to make the operation easy. The main goal of this book is to show how to develop such strategy. Easy operations are safe operations. A prime requirement for making an operation simple is good exposure with excellent light. Strategy also means planning the sequence of an operation to expose vital structures clearly early during the dissection to avoid damaging them.

Even more important is to *do the easy steps of any operation first*. This practice often makes the next step easy. If the surgeon continues to do easy steps, there may never be any difficult steps with which to contend. Another aid to making an operation easy is for the surgeon to adopt the proper foot and body position for each surgical maneuver (see Chapter 2).

The reputation for being a rapid operator is highly prized by some surgeons. More important than speed, however, are accuracy and delicacy of technique, especially when good anesthesia and patient support technology are available. Nevertheless, time should not be wasted. A reduction in operating time is not achieved merely by performing rapid hand motions. An operation can be expedited without sacrificing safety only when thoughtful advance planning, anticipation, and alert recognition of anatomic landmarks are combined with efficiency of execution. Together, they eliminate wasted motion and wasted time.

The surgeon in difficulty should stop cutting and start thinking. Why is the step difficult? Poor exposure? Bad light? Bloody field? The good surgeon makes operations look easy because of good operative strategy, rarely needing to resort to spectacular maneuvers to extricate the patient from danger.

The surgeon in real trouble should call for help from a senior colleague. Situations such as hemorrhage from the vena cava or laceration of the common bile duct are best managed with the calming influence of an experienced consultant who is not burdened by the guilt and anxiety of having caused the complication.

The chapters that follow in Part I discuss in detail the general principles that underlie successful open and laparoscopic surgery. Subsequent sections work through the anatomic regions and operations that are the familiar terrain of the general surgeon. A "concepts" chapter introduces each section. The technical chapters that then follow deal with specific surgical procedures. No procedure, however rarely used, has been omitted. These uncommon procedures are labeled "legacy" material. In each technical chapter, a discussion of the concept underlying the operation and the operative strategy precedes the description of each operative technique.

2 Mechanical Basics of Operative Technique

Rare is the novice who has the inborn talent to accomplish all the mechanical manipulations of surgery with no more thought or analysis than the natural athlete gives to hitting a ball. Most surgeons in training can gain much from analyzing such basics of surgery as foot position, hand and arm motion, and efficient use of instruments.

When considering the mechanics discussed here, remember that underlying all aspects of surgical technique are the fundamental principles articulated by Halsted, who emphasized that the surgeon must minimize trauma to tissues by using gentle technique. Halsted also stressed the importance of maintaining hemostasis and asepsis.

This text has been written from the vantage point of the right-handed surgeon. Left-handed surgeons should of course reverse the instructions where appropriate.

IMPORTANCE OF SURGEON'S FOOT AND BODY POSITION

A comfortable, relaxed stance enables the surgeon to spend hours at the operating table without back or neck strain and the accompanying muscle tremors. It is particularly important to keep the shoulders and elbows relaxed. The novice surgeon commonly tenses and elevates the shoulders and elbows. A relaxed posture is facilitated by dropping the operating table a few inches.

When deciding which side of the operating table is the "surgeon's side," consider which side allows you to most easily use you right arm and hand to reach into the area of pathology. For every activity involving the use of hands and arms, there is a body stance that allows the greatest efficiency of execution. For example, the right-handed professional who uses a baseball bat, tennis racket, wood chisel, or golf club places the left foot forward and the right foot 30–50 cm to the rear; the right arm and hand motion are then directed toward the left foot. Similarly, for the greatest efficiency when suturing, the surgeon assumes a body position such that the point of the needle is aimed toward the left foot. This is termed "forehand suturing." It allows the shoulder, arm, and wrist to occupy positions that are free of strain and permits the surgeon to perceive proprioceptive sensations as the needle moves through the tissues. Only in this way can the surgeon "feel" the depth of the suture bite. Combining this proprioceptive sense with visual monitoring of the depth of the needle bite is the best way to ensure consistency when suturing. Because accurate placement of sutures through the submucosa is one of the most important factors during construction of an intestinal anastomosis, the surgeon must make every effort to perfect this skill.

Forehand suturing maneuvers use the powerful biceps to move the hand from a pronated to a supinated position in a natural rolling motion. Backhand maneuvers require the surgeon to begin from a supinated position and roll backward to return to a pronated position. With practice this action becomes smooth but is not as easy or natural as forehand suturing. Whenever possible, establish your position relative to the field to allow forehand suturing. When placing a running suture, begin at the farthest aspect of the suture line and sew toward yourself.

Figure 2–1 illustrates the proper foot position of the surgeon inserting Lembert sutures during construction of an anastomosis situated at right angles to the long axis of the body. To insert sutures backhand, the needle is directed toward the surgeon's right foot. If only a few backhand sutures are needed, it is not necessary to change position. If an entire row of sutures requires backhand suturing, however, consider reversing your position relative to the surgical field so the row may be placed in the more natural forehand manner.

Some maneuvers require a backhand motion. For instance, cutting by scalpel is properly performed with a backhand motion directed toward the surgeon's right foot (**Fig. 2–2**). Similarly, when electrocautery is used as a cutting instrument, it is commonly drawn toward the right foot in a manner analogous to using a scalpel. In contrast, when using scissors the point of the scissors should be directed toward the surgeon's *left* foot. The proper foot position for inserting Lembert sutures in an

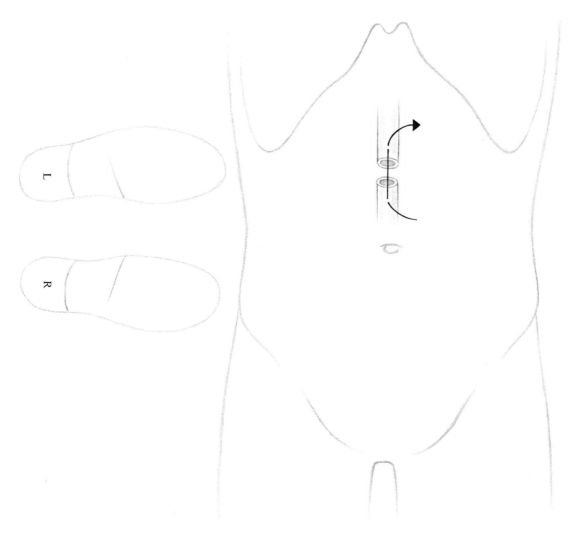

Fig. 2-1

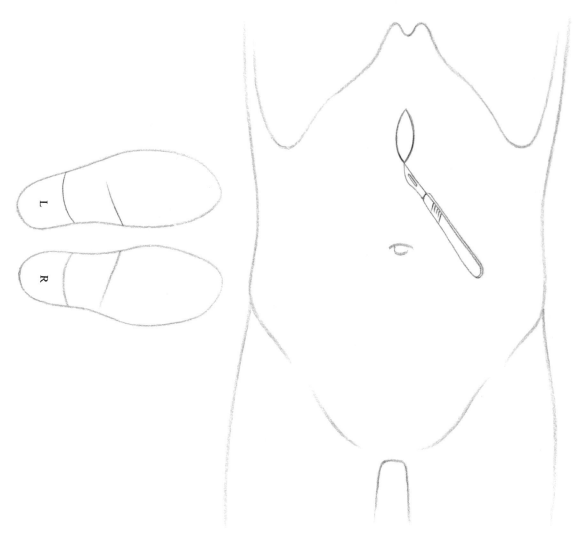

Fig. 2-2

anastomosis oriented in a line parallel to the long axis of the body is shown in **Figure 2–3**.

Some surgeons do not have a highly developed proprioceptive sense when they use the backhand suture. Therefore whenever feasible they should avoid this maneuver for seromuscular suturing, which is almost always possible if the surgeon re-arranges the direction of the anastomosis or assumes a body stance that permits optimal forehand sutur-ing. This is sometimes termed "reversing the field." Consider reversing the field whenever you find your-self in a mechanically awkward situation.

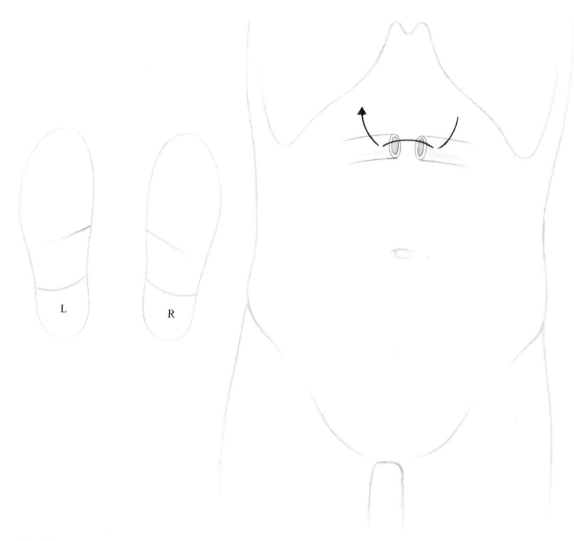

Fig. 2-3

The method of changing body position so all sutures can be placed with a forehand motion is illustrated in **Figure 2–4**, which shows Cushing sutures being inserted into an esophagogastric anastomosis, with the surgeon standing on the left side of the patient. When the needle is passed through the gastric wall from the patient's left to right, the surgeon's left foot is planted close to the operating table along the *left* side of the patient's abdomen. The surgeon's right foot is placed more laterally. When the suture

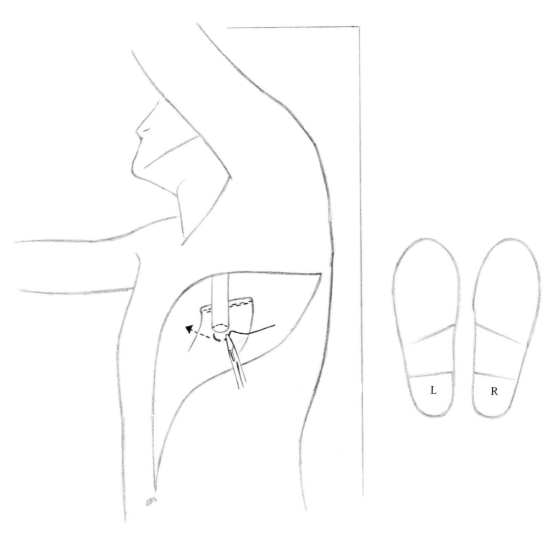

Fig. 2-4

is passed from the patient's right to left, on the posterior aspect of the esophageal wall, the surgeon's right foot is placed alongside the operating table. The surgeon's body faces the patient's feet, and the

surgeon's left foot is somewhat lateral to the right foot **(Fig. 2–5)**. This positioning directs the point of the needle toward the surgeon's left foot at all times.

A similar change in body stance is illustrated in

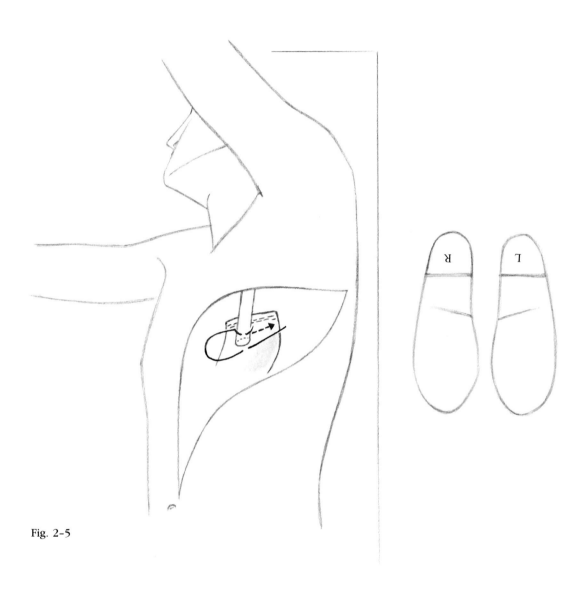

Fig. 2-5

Figures 2–6 and 2–7, where Cushing sutures are being inserted into a low-lying colorectal anastomosis. Of course, if the surgeon chose to use the Lembert-type suture for an esophagogastrostomy or a coloproctostomy, a single stance would be efficient for the entire anastomosis.

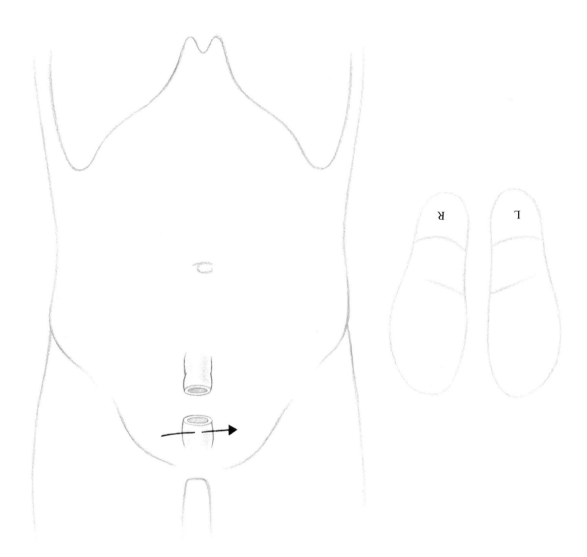

Fig. 2-6

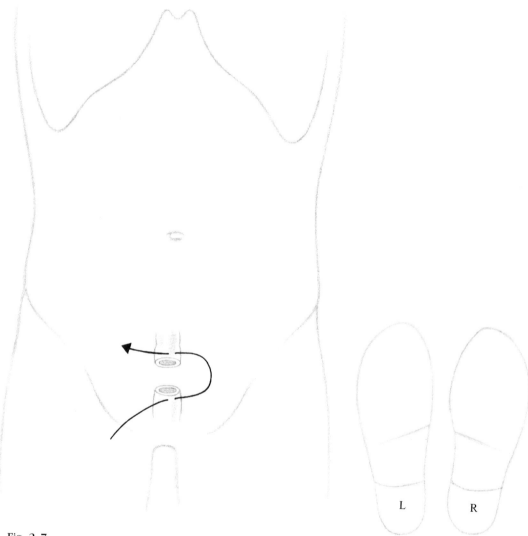

Fig. 2-7

Figures 2–8 and 2–9 illustrate insertion of Lembert sutures for the final layer of a gastrojejunal anastomosis, showing the foot position of the surgeon, who is standing on the patient's right side, compared with a position on the patient's left side.

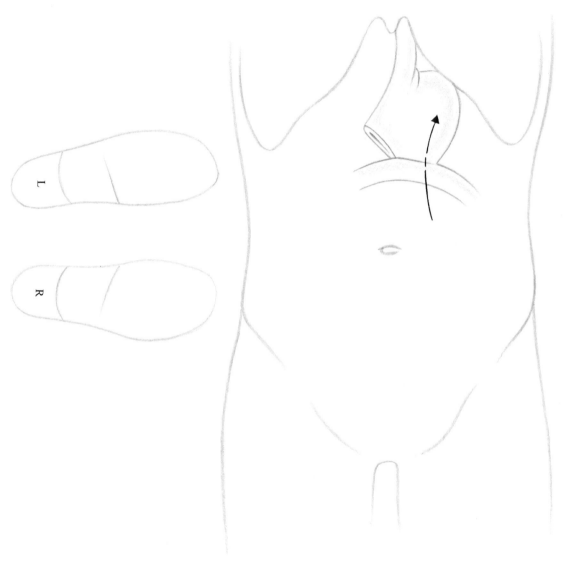

Fig. 2-8

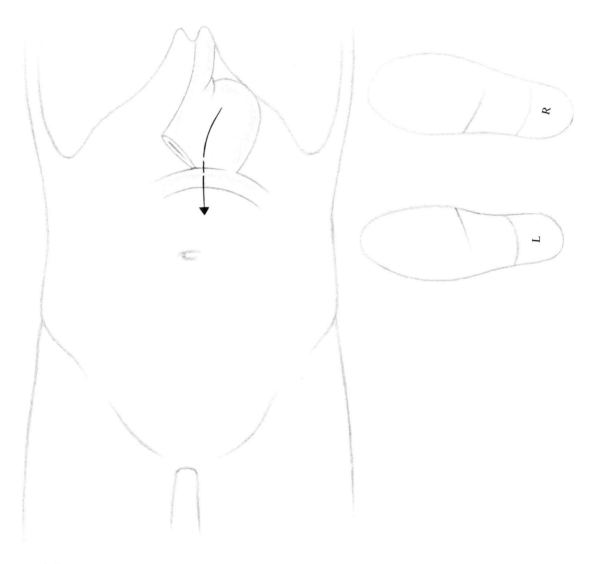

Fig. 2-9

Figure 2–10 illustrates closure of an upper vertical midline abdominal incision. **Figure 2–11** shows a lower midline incision with the surgeon standing at the patient's right side.

Although it is true that some surgeons are able to accomplish effective suturing despite awkward or strained body and hand positions, it must be emphasized that during surgery, as in athletics, good form is an essential ingredient for producing consistently superior performance.

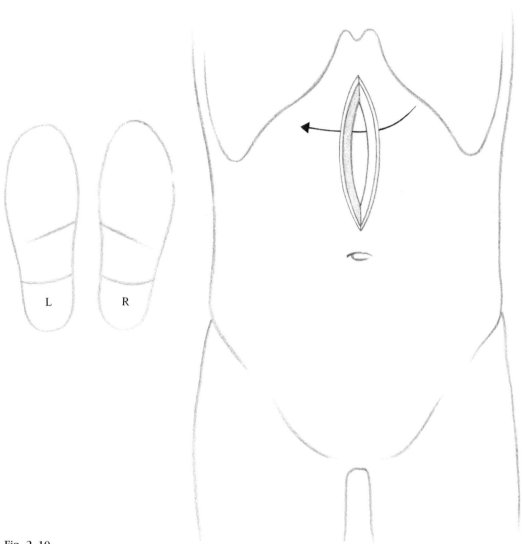

Fig. 2-10

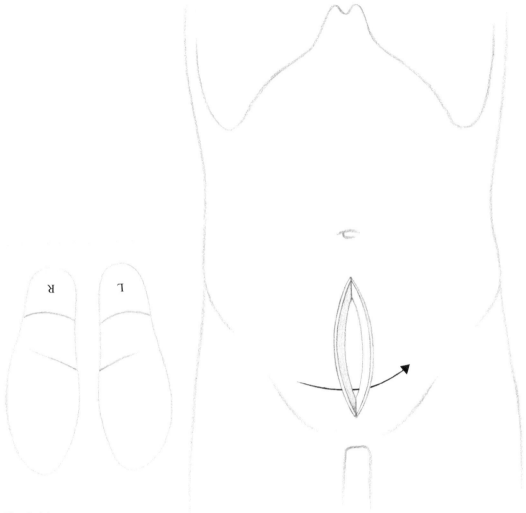

Fig. 2-11

USE OF INSTRUMENTS

With rare exceptions, all surgical instruments used for soft tissue dissection should be held with fingertip pressure rather than in a tight, vise-like grip. A loose grip is essential if the surgeon is to perceive proprioceptive sensations as the instrument is applied to the tissue. A relaxed grip also helps avoid fatigue, which contributes to muscle tremors. This requirement applies whether the instrument used is a scalpel, forceps, needle-holder, or scissors.

Scalpel

When making the initial scalpel incision in the skin, the surgeon can minimize tissue trauma by using a bold stroke through the skin and subcutaneous fat. It requires a firm grip. In most other situations, how-

ever, the scalpel should be held gently between the thumb on one side of the handle and the other fingers on the opposite side. Long, deliberate strokes with the scalpel are preferred. Generally, cutting is best done with the belly of the scalpel blade, as it enables the surgeon to control the depth of the incision by feel as well as by vision. The scalpel is a particularly effective instrument when broad surface areas are to be dissected, as during radical mastectomy or inguinal lymphadenectomy.

In such situations as an attempt to define the fascial ring surrounding an incisional hernia, the surgeon can clear overlying adherent fat rapidly from broad areas of fascia using a scalpel. The efficiency of knife dissection is greatly enhanced when the tissues being incised are kept in a state of tension, which can be brought about by traction between the surgeon's left hand and countertraction by the first assistant.

The surgeon must always be alert to the nuances of anatomy revealed by each scalpel stroke, especially if a structure appears in an unexpected location. This is not possible if the surgeon is in the habit of making rapid, choppy strokes with the scalpel, like a woodpecker. Rapid, frenzied motions do not afford sufficient time for the surgeon's brain to register and analyze the observations made during the dissection. Nor do they allow sufficient time for feedback to control the hand motions. Slow, definitive, long sweeping strokes with the scalpel make the most rapid progress and yet allow enough time to permit activation of cerebral control mechanisms and prevent unnecessary damage.

Metzenbaum Scissors

The round-tipped Metzenbaum scissors are valuable because they serve a number of essential functions. Closed, they are an excellent tool for dissection. They may be inserted behind adhesions or ligaments to elevate and delineate planes of dissection before dividing them. Properly held, with the fourth finger and thumb in the two rings and the index finger and middle finger extended along the handle, this instrument serves as an extension of the hand when detecting sensations and provides the surgeon with information concerning the density, pliability, and thickness of the tissue being dissected. As with other instruments, this proprioceptive function is enhanced if the hand grasps the instrument gently.

Electrocautery as a Cutting Device

Some surgeons prefer to use electrocautery, set for the "cutting" current, for such maneuvers as elevating skin flaps during mastectomy or incising subcutaneous fat. Transecting fat with a cutting current makes hemostasis only partially effective but minimizes tissue trauma. If the current is set for "coagulation," considerable heat may be generated, causing the fat to boil. Excessive tissue trauma contributes to postoperative wound infection.

On the other hand, transection of muscle bellies (e.g., during a subcostal or thoracic incision) may be accomplished efficiently when the electrocautery is set for "coagulation" or "blend" current. This setting provides good hemostasis and appears not to injure the patient significantly. Occasionally, the peritoneum and ligaments in the paracolic gutters are somewhat vascular secondary to inflammation. Electrocautery can be used here to divide these normally "avascular" structures.

In many areas, such as the neck, breast, and abdominal wall, it is feasible to cut with electrocautery, now set for "cutting," without causing excessive bleeding. To divide a small blood vessel, change the switch from "cutting" to "coagulation" and occlude the isolated blood vessel by electrocautery. Carefully performed, this sequence of dissection seems not to be damaging. If the incidence of wound infections, hematoma, or local edema is increased using this technique, the surgeon is overcoagulating the tissues and not isolating the blood vessels effectively.

Forceps

Care must be taken to avoid unnecessary trauma when applying forceps to body tissues. As with other instruments, hold the forceps gently. It is surprising how little force need be applied when holding the bowel with forceps while inserting a suture. If the imprint of the forceps appears on the wall of the bowel after the forceps have been removed, it is a clear warning that excessive force was applied when grasping the tissue.

With the goal of avoiding unnecessary trauma, when selecting forceps recognize immediately that "smooth" and "mouse-toothed" forceps are contraindicated when handling delicate tissue. Applied to the bowel, smooth forceps require excessive compression to avoid slipping. In this situation DeBakey-type forceps do not require excessive compression to prevent tissue from slipping from the forceps' jaws. For more delicate dissection, the Brown-Adson-type forceps are even more suitable. This instrument contains many tiny interdigitating teeth, which allow the surgeon to hold delicate tissues with minimal force.

Needle-Holder

Match the size and weight of the needle-holder to the size of the needle and suture. For example, do not use a delicate needle-holder to manipulate the heavy needle and suture used for fascial closure. Similarly, a heavy needle-holder is too cumbersome to allow accurate suturing of bowel or blood vessels. Ideally, needle-holders are paired so the scrub assistant is loading one with a suture while the surgeon is suturing.

It should be obvious that a curved needle must be inserted with a circular motion to avoid a tear at the site of the needle's point of entry into the tissue. It requires a rotatory motion of the surgeon's wrist, which in turn is aided by proper body stance and relaxed shoulder and elbow positions. Stability is enhanced if the elbow can be kept close to the body. Many novices tend to ignore the need for this rotatory wrist motion, especially when the suture line is in a poorly accessible anatomic location. They tend to insert a curved needle with a purely horizontal motion of the needle-holder, causing a small laceration at the entrance hole.

Using the same hand grip throughout the suturing sequence enhances the surgeon's capacity to detect proprioceptive impulses from the needle-holder. It is difficult to sense the depth of the needle bite accurately if the surgeon's fingers are sometimes in the rings of the instrument's handle and at other times are not. For gastrointestinal suturing, where proprioception is of great importance, we prefer a grip with the thumb in one ring and the ring finger in the other, steadying the handle with the extended index and middle fingers.

With practice, a delicate needle-holder may be palmed, that is, manipulated, opened, and closed without placing the thumb or ring finger through the rings. It requires facility and practice and should not be attempted by the novice, who is apt to find it necessary to put the thumb and finger into the rings to open and close the needle-holder after palming the needle-holder to place the stitch. This sequence is awkward, increases tissue trauma, and significantly slows suture placement.

Although most suturing is accomplished using a needle-holder with a straight shaft, some situations require a needle-holder whose shaft is angled or curved (e.g., for low colorectal and some esophagogastric anastomoses). In both instances, inserting the suture with a smooth rotatory motion may not be possible unless a curved needle-holder such as the Stratte or Finochietto is used (see Fig. G–18).

Hemostat

Ideally, a hemostat is applied to a vessel just behind the point of bleeding, and the bite of tissue is no larger than the diameter of the vessel. Obtaining hemostasis may *seem* to take less time if large bites of tissue are grasped by large hemostats than if small, accurate bites are taken. On the other hand, with small bites *many* bleeding points can be rapidly controlled by electrocautery rather than ligature, a technique that is especially helpful during such operations as those for radical mastectomy.

The choice between straight- and curve-tipped hemostats is a matter of personal preference, as either may be applied with equal accuracy. Curve-tipped hemostats make it somewhat easier to bring a ligature around the back and tip of the clamp for tying. The manner in which the curved hemostat is applied differs depending on whether the vessel is to be cauterized or tied. The hemostat should be applied points down and then lifted clear of all adjacent tissue to cauterize the vessel. It should be applied points up if the vessel is to be tied.

Whenever possible, small Halsted or Crile hemostats should be employed. For deeper vessels (e.g., the cystic artery), Adson clamps provide more handle length combined with delicate jaws. Hemostats vary in the length of the serrated segment. Some are fully serrated, whereas others are serrated only at the distal portion. Only the serrated portion of the clamp grasps tissue.

Occasionally it is more efficient to use a single, large Kelly hemostat to grasp a large pedicle containing a number of vascular branches than to cause additional bleeding by dissecting each small branch away from the pedicle. An example is ligation of the left gastric artery–coronary vein pedicle along the lesser curvature of the stomach during gastric resection. A right-angled Mixter clamp is useful for obtaining hemostasis in the thoracic cavity and when dividing the vascular tissue around the lower rectum during the course of anterior resection.

In all cases the preferred hand grip for holding hemostats is identical with that for holding the needle-holder and scissors. When the hemostat has a curved tip, the instrument should be held so the tip curves in the same direction in which the surgeon's fingers flex.

3 Incision, Exposure, Closure

ACHIEVING EXPOSURE

Many dangerous surgical mishaps occur because the operative exposure is inadequate. The *first step* toward obtaining good exposure is a well planned incision of sufficient length. The *second step* during abdominal surgery requires that the intestines be packed away from the area of operation. If a dissection requires exposure of a large portion of the abdominal cavity, such as for left hemicolectomy or excision of an abdominal aortic aneurysm, it may be necessary to exteriorize the small intestine for the duration of the dissection. The *third step* is retraction of the wound edges, which is accomplished by having an assistant apply a Richardson retractor to the abdominal wall and deep retractors, such as the Harrington retractor, to deeper structures. In some situations, a mechanical self-retaining retractor, such as the Balfour or the Thompson, may be inserted to separate the lips of a long abdominal incision. For thoracotomy and thoracoabdominal incisions, a Finochietto retractor is excellent for separating the ribs.

One disadvantage of using a mechanical self-retaining retractor in the abdomen is that it may inflict trauma if intense pressure is exerted against the rectus muscles. This pressure can be lessened by using long incisions and padding the musculature with moist gauze pads. A second potential disadvantage when deep blades are used to retract intraabdominal viscera is distortion of normal anatomy, which may make it difficult for the surgeon to identify vi-

tal structures. If the field is difficult to interpret, consider removing any fixed deep blades and reassessing the exposure.

Fixed retractors vary from the simple "chain" retractor to fancy systems such as the Omni. The *"chain" retractor* (**Fig. 3–1**) is an inexpensive improvisation that permits insertion of a retractor blade underneath the lower end of the sternum or underneath either costal margin. The retractor is attached to an ordinary link chain, which can be purchased in a hardware store. The anesthesiologist attaches a curved steel post borrowed from the gynecologic lithotomy stirrup set to the side rail at the head of the operating table. When the post is adjusted to the proper height, the chain is fixed to a snap at the tip. By rotating the post in the proper direction, the lower end of the sternum and the thoracic cage can be retracted forcefully cephalad and anteriorly to elevate the sternum by as much as 8–10 cm.

This device is ideal for operations around the lower esophagus, such as hiatus hernia repair. It does not require purchase of new instruments other than 25–30 cm of chain. It may be installed when necessary without preparation, even during an operation. It is also helpful for liberating the splenic flexure of the colon. Here the device is placed on the left side of the operating table, and the retractor is positioned to draw the left costal margin to the left, cephalad, and anteriorly, significantly improving exposure. Whenever exposure for operations on the biliary tract is difficult, applying the "chain" retractor to the right costal margin can be of benefit.

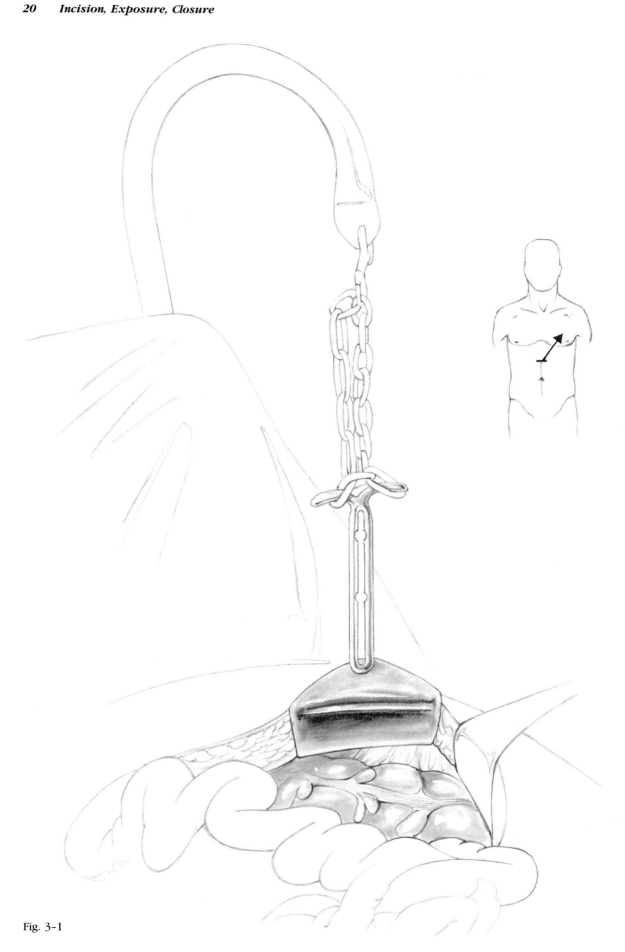

Fig. 3-1

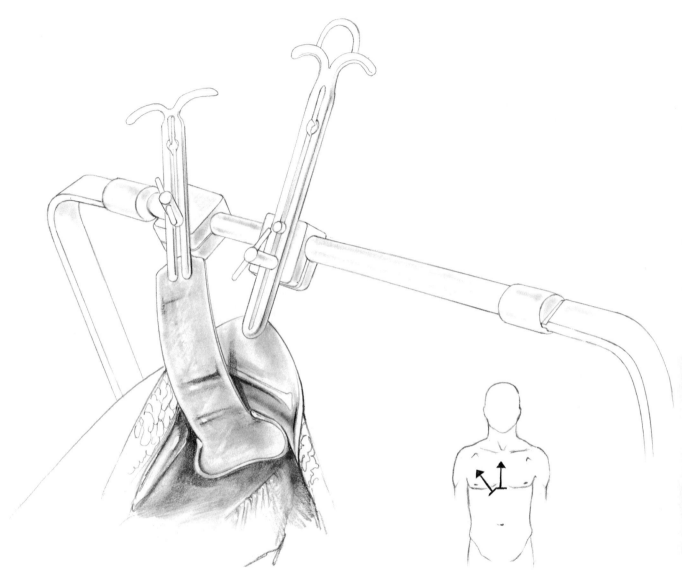

Fig. 3–2

A slightly more complex retractor that attaches to the operating table to improve upper abdominal exposure is the *Upper Hand retractor* (**Fig. 3–2**). This device is a steel bridge that is attached to both sides of the operating table and passes across the patient at the mid-sternal level. Its height is set at 4–10 cm above the sternum, depending on the type of retraction desired. Two retractor blades can be attached to the steel bridge, one of which may be used to elevate the lower sternum in a manner similar to the "chain" retractor. A second blade may be attached to the bridge to retract the liver for biliary tract surgery; this method sometimes eliminates the need for a second assistant.

A variety of more complex self-retaining retractors are available, and the particular one chosen depends on personal preference and availability. The Thompson (see Fig. G–26) or Omni retractors attach to the operating table and have a large variety of components for retraction. These devices are more flexible during operation than is the Upper Hand retractor.

The primary aim of all fixed retractors is not to reduce the number of assistants in the operating room but to provide better and more stable exposure.

INCISIONS FOR ABDOMINAL SURGERY

Although many surgeons have long believed that transverse incisions are stronger and have a lower incidence of dehiscence than midline incisions, this belief is false (see following section). Some think that the upper transverse incision interferes less with respiration than does the upper midline incision. Clinically, this does not appear to be important. A long, vertical *midline incision* gives excellent exposure for all parts of the abdomen. It also provides flexibility, as extensions in either direction are simple to execute. Reoperation for other pathology is simpler if the previous operation was performed through a midline incision rather than a paramedian incision.

Splenectomy, splenic flexure resection, hiatus hernia repair, vagotomy, pancreatectomy, and biliary tract surgery are easily done with the aid of the "chain" or more sophisticated retractors. Whenever exposure in the upper abdomen by this technique is inadequate, it is a simple matter to extend the midline incision via median sternotomy or into a right or left *thoracoabdominal approach*. Yet another advantage of midline incisions is the speed with which they can be opened and closed.

Despite these advantages, we often use a *subcostal approach* for open cholecystectomy because a short incision provides direct exposure of the gallbladder bed. If the gallbladder has already been removed and a secondary common duct exploration is necessary or a pancreaticoduodenectomy is contemplated, a midline incision extending 6–8 cm below the umbilicus provides excellent exposure and is preferred.

For the usual appendectomy, the traditional *McBurney incision* affords reasonable exposure, a strong abdominal wall, and a good cosmetic result. Accomplishing the same exposure with a vertical incision would require either a long midline or a paramedian incision or an incision along the lateral border of the rectus muscle, which might transect two intercostal nerves and produce some degree of abdominal weakness.

AVOIDING WOUND DEHISCENCE AND HERNIA

Wound dehiscence spans a spectrum from catastrophic evisceration through occult dehiscence. Major wound disruption is associated with significant postoperative mortality; and even minor degrees of occult dehiscence may result in a postoperative incisional hernia.

The major causes of wound disruption are as follows:

Inadequate strength of suture material, resulting in breakage.

Suture material that dissolves before adequate healing has occurred (e.g., catgut)

Knots becoming untied, especially with some monofilaments (e.g., nylon and Prolene)

Sutures tearing through tissue

All these causes except the last are self-explanatory; suture tears are poorly understood by most surgeons. A stitch tears tissue if it is tied too tightly or encompasses too little tissue. Although it is true that in some patients there appears to be diminution in the strength of the tissue and its resistance to tearing, especially in the aged and extremely depleted individuals, this does not explain the fact that many wound disruptions occur in healthy patients. The sutures must hold throughout the initial phase of wound healing, which lasts several weeks and involves softening of the collagen around the wound edges.

When the incision is disrupted following an uncomplicated cholecystectomy in a healthy, middle-aged patient with good muscular development, there must be a mechanical explanation. Often the surgeon has closed the wound with multiple small stitches of fine suture material. Under these circumstances, a healthy sneeze by a muscular individual tears the sutures out of the fascia and peritoneum because the muscle pull exceeds the combined suture–tissue strength.

If the problem, then, is to maintain tissue approximation during a sneeze or abdominal distension for a period of time sufficient for even the depleted patient to heal, what is the best technique to use? We now have adequate data to identify the principles that must be observed if the rate of dehiscence is to be reduced to less than 1%, especially in the poor-risk patient. Adequate bits of tissue must be included in each suture; the sutures must be placed neither too close nor too far apart; and they must be tied securely in a manner that approximates but does not strangulate the tissue. For general abdominal wound closure we prefer the interrupted Smead-Jones closure technique with a monofilament suture, described below.

Many surgeons believe that a patient who is at increased risk of wound dehiscence by virtue of malnutrition, chronic steroid therapy, or chronic obstructive pulmonary disease should have an abdominal incision closed with "retention sutures" that go through the skin and the entire abdominal wall. If retention sutures are used they should be considered an adjunct to good closure rather than a substitute for it. Suture bridges protect the skin, and retention sutures tied loosely do not cut through the fascia. Retention sutures should be used only when delayed healing is anticipated and should be left in place until healing is complete, which often is signaled by

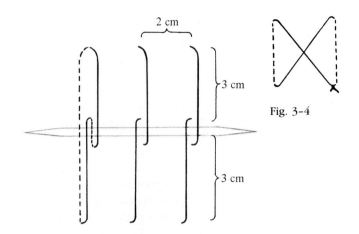

Fig. 3-4

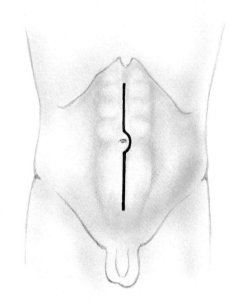

Fig. 3-5

the previously snug retention sutures becoming loose as the wound contracts. A properly placed Smead-Jones suture creates a row of internal retention sutures by taking bites through the fascia and muscle layers but avoiding the skin **(Figs. 3–3, 3–4)**. Although this text describes the interrupted Smead-Jones technique, some have used a similar running suture technique with great success.

OPERATIVE TECHNIQUE FOR A MIDLINE INCISION

Making the Incision

Hold a large gauze pad in the left hand and apply lateral traction on the skin; the first assistant does the same on the opposite side of the incision. Use the scalpel with a firm sweep along the course of the incision **(Fig. 3–5)**. The initial stroke should go well into the subcutaneous fat. Then reapply the gauze pads to provide lateral traction against the subcutaneous fat; use the belly of the scalpel blade to carry the incision down to the linea alba, making as few knife strokes as possible. The linea alba can be identified in the upper abdomen by observing the decussation of fascial fibers. It can be confirmed by palpating the tip of the xiphoid, which indicates the midline.

The former custom of discarding the scalpel used for the skin incision (in the belief that it incurred bacterial contamination) is not supported by data or logic and is no longer observed. Because subcutaneous fat seems to be the body tissue most susceptible to infection, every effort should be made to minimize trauma to this layer. Use as few hemostats and ligatures as possible; most bleeding points stop spontaneously in a few minutes. Subcutaneous bleeders should be electrocoagulated accurately and with minimal trauma.

Continuing lateral traction with gauze pads, divide the linea alba with the scalpel. If the incision is to be continued around and below the umbilicus, leave a 5- to 8-mm patch of linea alba attached to the umbilicus to permit purchase by a suture during closure. Otherwise, a gap between sutures may appear at the umbilicus, leading to an incisional hernia.

Open the peritoneum to the left of the falciform ligament. Virtually no blood vessels are encountered when the peritoneum is opened close to its attachment to the undersurface of the left rectus muscle. Elevate the peritoneum between two forceps and incise it just above and to the left of the umbilicus. Using Metzenbaum scissors, continue this incision in a cephalad direction until the upper pole of the incision is reached. If bleeding points are encountered here, electrocoagulate them.

So as not to cut the bladder, be certain when opening the peritoneum in the lower abdomen to identify the prevesical fat and bladder. As the peritoneum approaches the prevesical region, the preperitoneal fat cannot be separated from the peritoneum and becomes somewhat thickened and more vascular. If there is any question about the location of the upper margin of the bladder, note that the balloon of the indwelling Foley catheter can be milked in a cephalad direction. It is easy to identify the upper extremity of the bladder this way. It is not necessary to open the peritoneum into prevesical fat, as it does not improve exposure. However, opening the fascial layer down to and beyond the pyra-

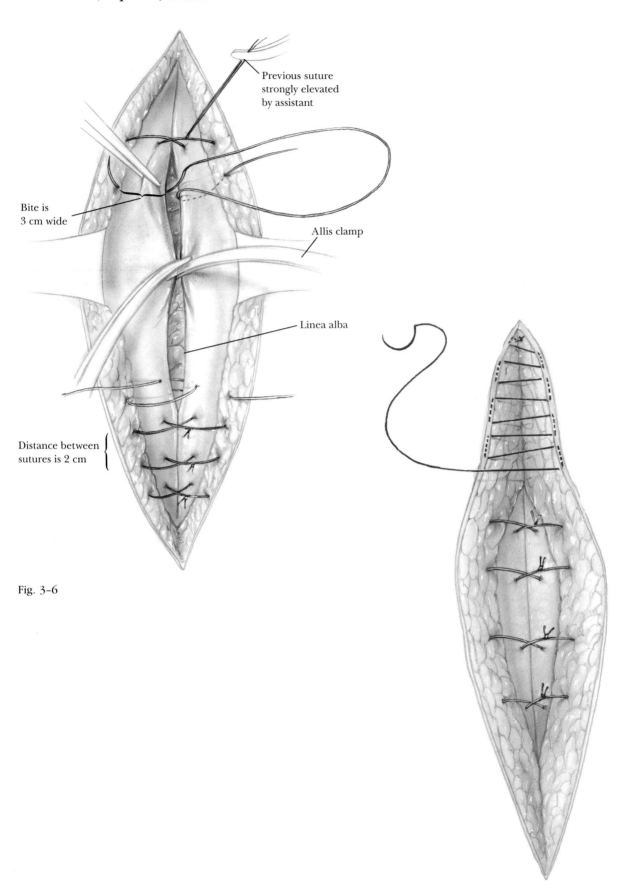

Previous suture
strongly elevated
by assistant

Bite is
3 cm wide

Allis clamp

Linea alba

Distance between
sutures is 2 cm

Fig. 3-6

Fig. 3-7

midalis muscles to the pubis does indeed improve exposure for low-lying pelvic pathology.

Closure of Midline Incision by Modified Smead-Jones Technique

In the upper abdomen it is unnecessary to include the peritoneum or falciform ligament in the suture. Below the umbilicus there is no distinct linea alba, and the rectus muscle belly is exposed. In this region include the peritoneum in the stitch.

Apply Allis clamps to the linea alba at the midpoint of the incision, one clamp on each side. Below the umbilicus the Allis clamps should include a bite of peritoneum and of anterior fascia. With no. 1 polydioxanone suture (PDS), encompass 3 cm of tissue on each side of the linea alba; then take a small bite of the linea alba, about 5 mm in width, on each side. This results in a small loop within a large loop **(Fig. 3–6)**. The purpose of the small loop is simply to orient the linea alba so it remains in apposition rather than one side moving on top of the other. Place the small loop 5–10 mm below the main body of the suture to help eliminate the gap between adjacent sutures. Insert the next suture no more than 2 cm below the first. Large, curved Ferguson needles are used for this procedure.

Tie the sutures with at least four square throws. *Avoid excessive tension*. When half of the incision has been closed, start at the other end and approach the midpoint with successive sutures (Fig. 3–6). Do not tie the last few stitches, leaving enough space to insert the remaining stitch under direct vision. In no case should the surgeon insert a stitch without seeing the point of the needle at all times. Tie all the remaining sutures **(Fig. 3–7)**. Close the skin with interrupted 4-0 nylon vertical mattress sutures, a continuous subcuticular suture of 4-0 polyglycolic (PG), or staples.

Other special incisions such as the *McBurney* (see Chapter 40), *subcostal* (see Chapter 66), and *Pfannenstiel* (see Chapter 56) incisions are found elsewhere in this volume where the operations most commonly performed through these exposures are introduced.

REFERENCES

Ellis H, Bucknall TE, Cox PJ. Abdominal incisions and their closure. Curr Probl Surg 1985;22(4):1.

Goligher JC, Irgin TT, Johnston D, et al. A controlled clinical trial of three methods of closure of laparotomy wounds. Br J Surg 1975;62:823.

Jacobs HB. Skin knife-deep knife: the ritual and practice of skin incisions. Ann Surg 1974;179:102.

Jenkins TPN. The burst abdominal wound: a mechanical approach. Br J Surg 1976;63:873.

Jones TE, Newell ET Jr, Brubaker RE, et al. The use of alloy steel wire in the closure of abdominal wounds. Surg Gynecol Obstet 1941;72:1056.

Lumsden AB, Colborn GL, Sreeram S, Skandalakis LJ. The surgical anatomy and technique of the thoracoabdominal incision. Surg Clin North Am 1993;73:633.

Masterson BJ. Selection of incisions for gynecologic procedures. Surg Clin North Am 1991;71:1041.

Wind GG, Rich NM. Laparotomy. In: Principles of Surgical Technique. Baltimore, Urban & Schwarzenberg, 1987, pp 177-200.

4 Dissecting and Suturing

ART OF DISSECTING PLANES

Of all the skills involved in the craft of surgery, perhaps the single most important is the discovery, delineation, and separation of anatomic planes. When this is skillfully accomplished, there is scant blood loss and tissue trauma is minimal. The delicacy and speed with which dissection is accomplished can mark the difference between the master surgeon and the tyro.

Of all the instruments available to expedite the discovery and delineation of tissue planes, none is better than the surgeon's *left index finger*. [References here are again to right-handed surgeons.] This digit is insinuated behind the lateral duodenal ligament during performance of the Kocher maneuver, behind the renocolic ligament during colon resection, and behind the gastrophrenic ligament during a gastric fundoplication. These structures can then be rapidly divided, as the underlying left index finger is visible through the transparent tissue. Dissection of all these structures by other techniques not only is more time-consuming, it is frequently more traumatic and produces more blood loss.

To identify adhesions between the bowel and peritoneum, pass the left index finger behind the adhesion. This maneuver produces gentle traction on the tissue to be incised. If the finger is visible through the adhesion it can aid dissection.

If there is insufficient space for inserting the surgeon's left index finger, often *Metzenbaum scissors*, with blades closed, can serve the same function when inserted underneath an adhesion for delineation and division. This maneuver is also useful when incising adventitia of the auxiliary vein during a mastectomy. To do this, the closed Metzenbaum scissors are inserted between the adventitia and the vein itself, they are then withdrawn, the blades are opened, and one blade is inserted underneath the adventitia. Finally, the jaws of the scissors are closed, and the tissue is divided. This maneuver is repeated until the entire adventitia anterior to the vein has been divided.

In many situations a closed blunt-tipped right-angle *Mixter clamp* may be used the same way as Metzenbaum scissors for dissecting and delineating anatomic structures. Identification and skeletonization of the inferior mesenteric artery or the cystic artery and delineation of the circular muscle of the esophagus during cardiomyotomy are some uses to which this instrument can be put.

The *scalpel* is the instrument of choice when developing a plane that is not a natural one, such as when elevating skin flaps over the breast. When the scalpel is held at a 45° angle to the direction of the incision **(Fig. 4–1)**, it is useful for clearing fascia of overlying fat.

More important, when the surgeon must cope with advanced pathologic changes involving dense scar tissue, such as may exist when elevating the posterior wall of the duodenum in the vicinity of a penetrating duodenal ulcer, the scalpel is the only instrument that can divide the dense scar accurately until the natural plane of cleavage between the duodenum and pancreas is reached, beyond the diseased tissue.

The *peanut sponge* (Kutner dissector), a small, 1.5 cm gauze sponge grasped in a long hemostat, is an appropriate device for separating fat and areolar tissue from anatomic structures. It should not be used to tear tissues while making a plane. After the peritoneum overlying the cystic duct and artery has been incised, the peanut sponge can separate peritoneum and fat from the underlying duct and artery. It is similarly useful for elevating a thyroid lobe from its capsule. After sharp dissection has exposed the major arteries during the course of a colon resection, the peanut sponge can be used to skeletonize the vessels and sweep the lymphatic and areolar tissue toward the specimen.

A folded 10 × 10 cm *gauze square* grasped in a sponge holder has occasional application for sweeping perirenal fat from the posterior aspect of the peritoneum during lumbar sympathectomy. It is useful also for separating the posterior wall of the stomach from peripancreatic filmy peritoneal attachments. Because use of a large sponge does not permit anatomic precision, small veins may be torn during this type of gross dissection; therefore the sponge's applicability is limited to avascular planes.

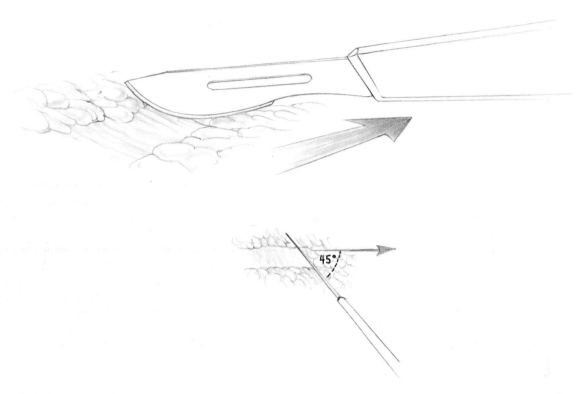

Fig. 4-1

The surgeon who wants to perform accurate dissections is greatly aided by a *talent for quickly recognizing tissues and structures* as they are revealed by the scalpel or scissors. A truly alert surgeon can promptly evaluate the structural characteristics of a nerve, blood vessel, ureter, or common bile duct, so each is identifiable at a glance, even before the structure is thoroughly exposed. An intimate knowledge of anatomy is required for the surgeon to know *exactly where each structure will appear* even before it has been revealed by dissection.

SEWING TECHNIQUE

Use of a Needle-Holder

Smooth rotary wrist action and the surgeon's awareness of what it feels like when a needle penetrates the submucosa of the bowel are important when suturing with a typical half-circle needle on a needle-holder (see Chapter 2).

Selection of Needle

The needle selected for any use should have the least possible thickness commensurate with adequate strength to achieve its purpose. Tapered-point needles are used to insert sutures into soft tissue such as the fascia, fat, or gastrointestinal viscera. Cutting needles are used for the skin and occasionally for tough fibrous tissue such as breast. Use of a too delicate needle risks bending or breaking the needle. More often such damage is due to failure to follow the curve of the needle as it passes through the tissue or placing the needle too far back on the needle-holder.

Size of Bite

The width of the tissue enclosed in the typical seromuscular suture varies between 4 and 6 mm, depending on the thickness and consistency of the tissue involved. Hypertrophied gastric wall requires a larger bite than the normally thin colon. As discussed in Chapter 3, our version of the Smead-Jones closure includes a bite of abdominal wall 3 cm wide. Thus the size of the bite must be matched to the purpose of the suture, the size of the suture, and the amount of force the suture line must withstand.

Distance between Sutures

The distance between bites for a typical approximation of the seromuscular layer with interrupted Lembert sutures is 5 mm. When continuous mucosal or other sutures are used, the width of the bites and the distance apart should be approximately the same as those specified for interrupted stitches.

After one layer of sutures has been inserted, the surgeon should use the forceps to test tentatively the optimal degree of inversion that permits the second layer to be inserted without tension (see Figs. 29–23a, 29–23b).

Size of Suture Material

As there must never be any tension on an anastomosis in the gastrointestinal tract, it is not necessary to use suture material heavier than 4-0 or 3-0. Failure to heal often is due to a stitch tearing through the tissue; it is almost never due to a broken suture. When two layers of sutures are used for an anastomosis in the gastrointestinal (GI) tract, the inner layer should be 5-0 or 4-0 PG. This layer provides immediate, accurate approximation of the mucosa and, in some instances, hemostasis.

When taking large bites of tissue with considerable tensile strength, such as with the Smead-Jones closure of the abdominal wall, heavier suture material is indicated. Here, 1-0 PDS is suitable. Obviously, the size of the suture material must be proportional to the strength of the tissues into which it is inserted and to the strain it must sustain.

Continuous versus Interrupted Sutures

End-to-end anastomosis of the GI tract should be done with interrupted seromuscular sutures to avoid the possibility that the purse-string effect of the continuous stitch would narrow the lumen. A continuous suture is permissible in the mucosal layer if it is inserted with care to avoid narrowing. When an anastomosis is large, as with gastrojejunostomy, the use of two continuous layers of PG appears safe.

How Tight the Knot?

If the knot on a suture approximating the seromuscular coats of two segments of intestine is tied so tightly it causes ischemic necrosis, an anastomotic leak may follow. This is especially likely if the stitch has been placed erroneously through the entire wall of the bowel into the lumen. Because considerable edema follows construction of an anastomosis, knots should be tied with tension sufficient only to provide apposition of the two seromuscular coats. Caution must be exercised when tying suture material such as silk or Prolene, which are slippery enough that each knot may have the effect of a noose that is repeatedly tightened with the tying of each addi-

tional knot. Nylon sutures also exhibit excessive slippage; even when the first knot has been applied with proper tension, each succeeding knot often produces further constriction. When nylon sutures in the skin have been tied with too much tension, marked edema, redness, and cross-hatching can be seen at the site of each stitch. The same ill effects occur when intestinal sutures are made too tight, but the result is not visible to the surgeon.

Catching Both Walls of Intestine with One Pass of the Needle-Holder

Most surgeons who insert seromuscular sutures to approximate two segments of intestine were taught to insert the Lembert suture through the intestine on one side of the anastomosis. They then pick up the needle with the needle-holder to take another Lembert stitch in the opposite wall of the bowel. Occasionally, under ideal conditions it is possible to pass a needle of proper length through one side of the intestine and then, without removing the needle-holder, pass the needle through the opposite wall before pulling the thread through. The danger associated with this shortcut is that one may traumatize the entrance wound made on the side of the intestine through which the needle was first inserted. This problem can occur as the surgeon moves the needle and the intestinal wall in a lateral direction to bring it closer to the opposing intestine, thereby making a small tear at the entrance hole **(Fig. 4–2)**. With proper technique this shortcut can be accomplished without undue trauma. After the needle has been passed through the first segment of intestine, the surgeon should avoid any *lateral* move-

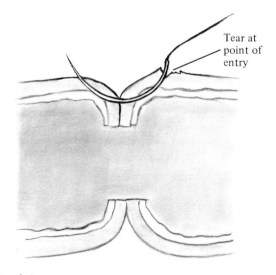

Tear at point of entry

Fig. 4–2

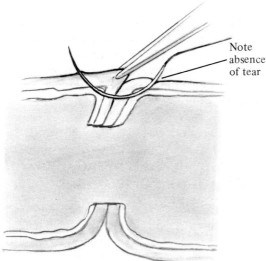

Fig. 4-3

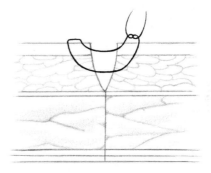

Fig. 4-5

ment of the needle-holder. Instead, the surgeon *gently* picks up the opposing segment of intestine with a forceps and brings this portion of bowel to the needle. Then, with a purely *rotatory* motion of the wrist, the surgeon allows the needle to penetrate the second side (**Fig. 4-3**). If the surgeon is conscious of the need to avoid trauma and uses a rotatory maneuver, there are situations in which this technique is acceptable and efficient.

Types of Stitch

Simple Everting Skin Stitch

Eversion of the edges is desired when closing skin. Consequently, the wrist should be pronated and the needle inserted so the deeper portion of the bite is slightly wider than the superficial portion (**Fig. 4-4**). When this stitch is tied, the edges are everted (**Fig. 4-5**).

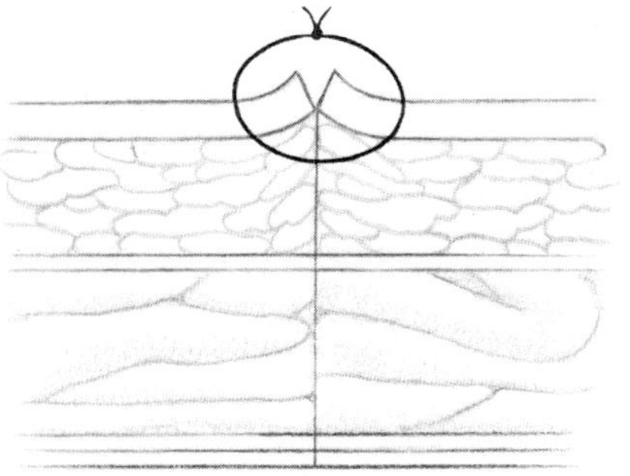

Vertical Mattress (Stewart) Stitch

With the classic Stewart method of skin suturing, eversion is guaranteed by the nature of the vertical mattress stitch (**Figs. 4-6, 4-7**). Neither of these two types of skin suture should be tied with excessive tension if cross-hatching is to be avoided.

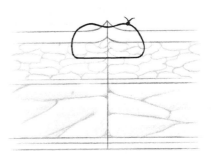

Fig. 4-6

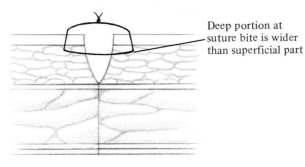

Deep portion at suture bite is wider than superficial part

Fig. 4-4

Fig. 4-7

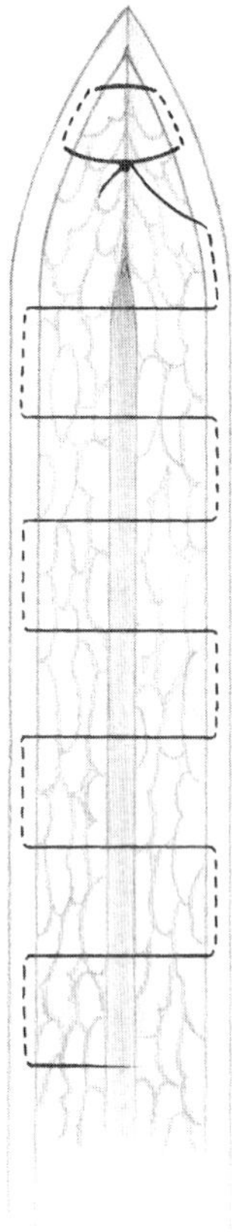

Fig. 4-8

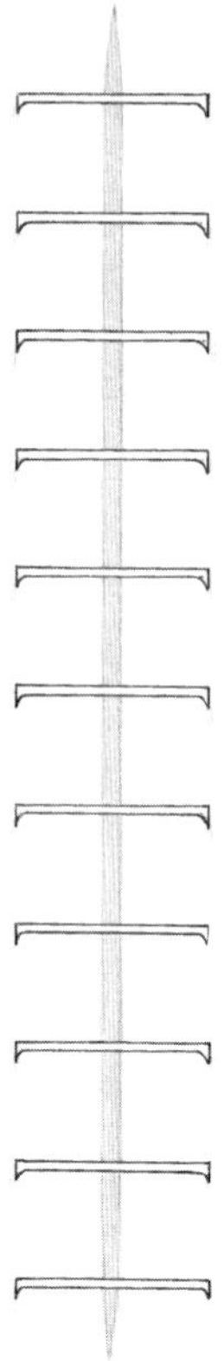

Fig. 4-9

Continuous Subcuticular Stitch

For the continuous subcuticular stitch, 4-0 PG may be employed on an atraumatic, curved, cutting needle. With practice the surgeon may insert it rapidly and obtain a good cosmetic result **(Fig. 4–8)**. Because it is absorbable there are no sutures to remove postoperatively. If preferred, continuous 3-0 nylon may be used, with lead shot or an external knot fixing the stitch at its points of origin and termination. This stitch should not be removed for 10-14 days following the operation. If the nylon stitch is longer than 7-8 cm, it may break during removal.

Skin Staples

Skin staples can be applied with force just sufficient to achieve approximation without producing crosshatching of the skin. They allow good cosmetic results. Depending on the thickness of the skin and the underlying structures, staples may be placed 5-10 mm apart **(Fig. 4–9)**. Align the skin edges to produce good apposition with slight eversion. When working with a less skilled assistant, it is preferable for the surgeon to align the edges and allow the assistant to place the staples.

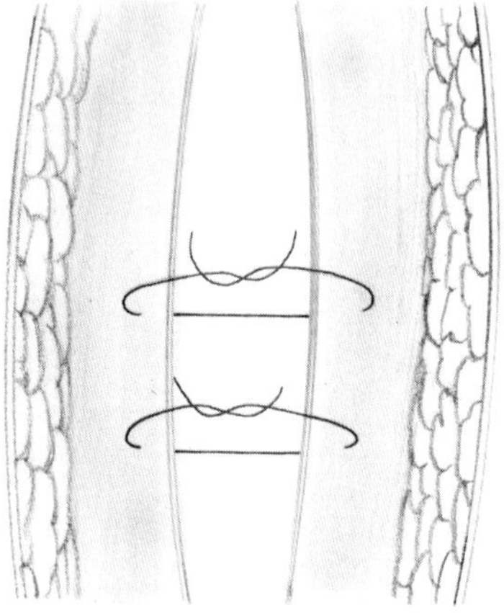

Fig. 4-10

Simple Interrupted Fascial Stitch

The McBurney and other special incisions may be closed by simple interrupted fascial sutures. These sutures are placed so they include 8-10 mm of tissue with each bite, as shown in **Figure 4–10**. Except for use in the McBurney and Pfannenstiel incisions, this abdominal wall closure should be considered obsolete.

Continuous Simple Over-and-Over Stitch

Figure 4–11 illustrates the simple over-and-over continuous stitch frequently used for closure of the peritoneum. It is sometimes applied to the mucosal layer of bowel anastomoses as well.

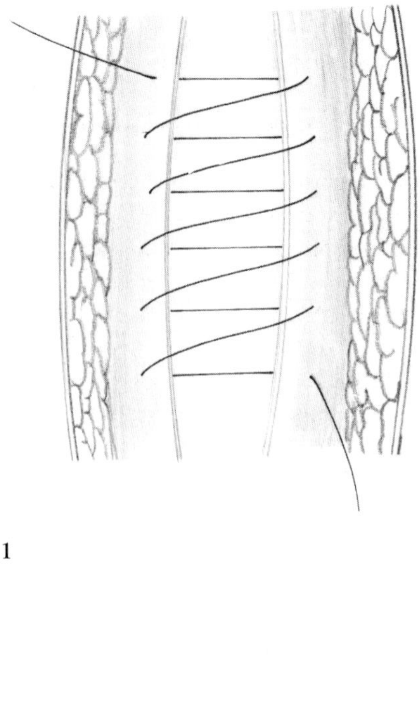

Fig. 4-11

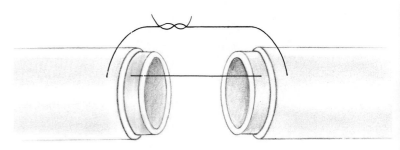

Fig. 4-13

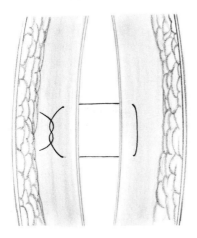

Fig. 4-12

Horizontal Mattress Stitch

The mattress suture is occasionally used to close fascia and sometimes for ventral hernia repair (**Fig. 4–12**). It can also serve as a hemostatic stitch.

Smead-Jones Stitch

The Smead-Jones stitch is well suited for closure of major abdominal incisions. It is, in essence, a buried "retention" suture, as it encompasses all layers of the abdominal wall, except the skin, in its large loop. The large loop is followed by a small loop, which catches only 4-5 mm of linea alba on each side. The purpose of this small loop is to orient the abdominal wall in perfect apposition. It is described in detail in Chapter 3.

Hemostatic Figure-of-Eight Stitch

The classic hemostatic figure-of-eight stitch is used for occlusion of a bleeding vessel that has retracted into muscle or similar tissue. It is illustrated in Figure 3-4.

Single-Layer Bowel Anastomosis

Bowel anastomoses employing one layer of sutures have become acceptable. An effective method for accomplishing inversion and approximation simultaneously is use of the seromucosal stitch (**Fig. 4–13**), which is an inverting stitch that catches the seromuscular and submucosal layers and a small amount of mucosa. When properly applied, it produces slight inversion of the mucosal layer and approximation. It is not necessary to pass this stitch deeper than the submucosal layer.

If it is passed into the lumen before emerging from the mucosal layer, it is identical with that described

by Gambee, whose technique was at one time applied to one-layer closure of the Heinecke-Mikulicz pyloroplasty. Used in an interrupted or a continuous fashion, it is an excellent alternative to the Connell stitch for inversion of the anterior mucosal layer of a two-layer bowel anastomosis. When used for construction of a single-layer intestinal anastomosis, it should of course be done only in interrupted fashion.

Lembert Stitch

Perhaps the most widely used technique for approximating the seromuscular layer of a bowel or gastric anastomosis is the Lembert stitch (**Fig. 4–14**). This stitch catches about 5 mm of tissue, including a bite of submucosa, and emerges 1-2 mm proximal to the cut edge of the serosa. It also has been used for one-layer intestinal anastomoses. Under proper circumstances it may be applied in a continuous fashion.

Cushing Stitch

The Cushing stitch is similar to the Lembert stitch, except it is inserted parallel to and 2-4 mm from the cut edge of the bowel. It should catch about 5 mm of the bowel, including the submucosa. It is especially applicable to seromuscular approximation for anastomoses in poorly accessible locations, such as the low colorectal anastomosis. The interrupted

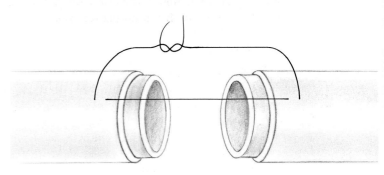

Fig. 4-14

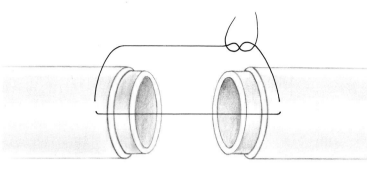

Fig. 4-15a

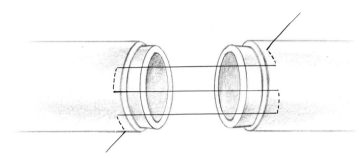

Fig. 4-15b

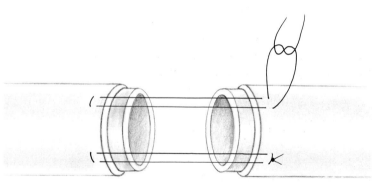

Fig. 4-16

Cushing technique is illustrated in **Figure 4–15a**. When used as a continuous stitch **(Fig. 4–15b)** the Cushing is a good alternative to the Connell stitch for inverting the anterior mucosal layer of an anastomosis. The main difference between the Connell stitch (see Fig. 4-18, below) and a continuous Cushing suture is that the former penetrates the lumen of the bowel, whereas the latter passes only to the depth of the submucosal layer. The continuous Cushing suture is also much easier and more efficient to accomplish than the Connell stitch.

Halsted Stitch

The Halsted stitch **(Fig. 4–16)** provides excellent seromuscular approximation in a bowel anastomosis. It shares with the Cushing stitch the danger that when tied with excessive tension it causes strangulation of a larger bite of tissue than does the Lembert suture.

Continuous Locked Stitch

Figure 4–17 illustrates approximation of the posterior mucosal layer of a bowel anastomosis with a continuous locked stitch. This stitch ensures hemostasis and approximation. When hemostasis is not a problem, some surgeons prefer to close this layer with a simple over-and-over continuous stitch (Fig. 4-11).

Connell Stitch

The Connell suture was originally described as a technique for performing a single-layer end-to-end anastomosis of the bowel. This suture has been used for many decades as the method for inverting the anterior mucosal layer of a *two-layer* bowel anastomosis. The stitch goes from the serosa through all layers of intestine into the lumen **(Fig. 4–18)**, comes out through all the layers on the same side, and passes over to the opposite segment of the bowel, where the same sequence takes place.

Because it forms a loop on the mucosa the Connell stitch is slightly hemostatic, but one should not

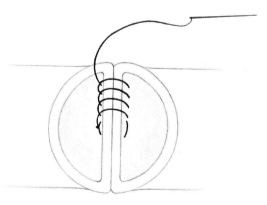

Fig. 4-17

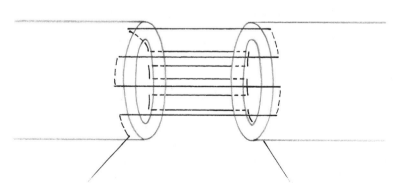

Fig. 4-18

depend entirely on it for that purpose. The suture is placed loosely to avoid purse-stringing the anastomosis and hence is inadequate to produce hemostasis for small arterial bleeders. As the bowel is inverted, intraluminal bleeding does not remain visible to the surgeon and may go undetected. This is particularly common with the stomach, which has a rich submucosal blood supply. Rather than rely on the Connell stitch, individually ligate the bleeding points or secure them with electrocautery.

TECHNIQUE OF SUCCESSIVE BISECTION

The technique we named "successive bisection" ensures consistently accurate intestinal anastomoses, especially when the diameters of the two segments are not identical. As illustrated in **Figure 4–19**, the first stitch is inserted at the antimesenteric border and the second at the mesenteric border. The third is then inserted at a point that exactly bisects the entire layer. The fourth stitch bisects the distance between the first and third stitches. This pattern is then repeated until the anastomotic layer is complete **(Fig. 4–20)**.

Intestinal Anastomoses

One Layer or Two?

Although abundant data confirm that an intestinal anastomosis can be performed safely with one or two layers of sutures, to our knowledge there is no consistent body of randomized data conclusively demonstrating the superiority of one or the other in humans. It is obvious that the one-layer anastomosis does not turn in as much intestine and consequently has a larger lumen than the two-layer anastomosis. However, in the absence of postoperative leakage, obstruction at the anastomotic site is rare except perhaps when the esophagus is involved. It seems reasonable, though, to assume that if the seromuscular layer sutured by the surgeon suffers from some minor imperfection the mucosal sutures may compensate for the imperfection and prevent leakage. Although we have had good results with one-layer techniques, we recommend that each surgeon master the standard two-layer technique before considering the other.

End-to-End or End-to-Side Technique?

In most situations, the end-to-end technique is satisfactory for joining two segments of bowel. If there is some disparity in diameter, a *Cheatle slit* is performed on the antimesenteric border of the narrower segment of intestine to enable the two diameters to match each other **(Figs. 4–21, 4–22)**. If

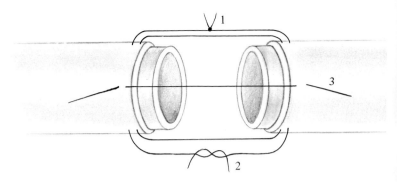

Fig. 4-19

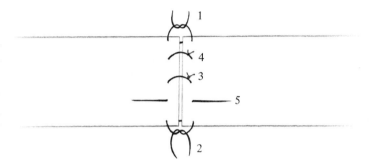

Fig. 4-20

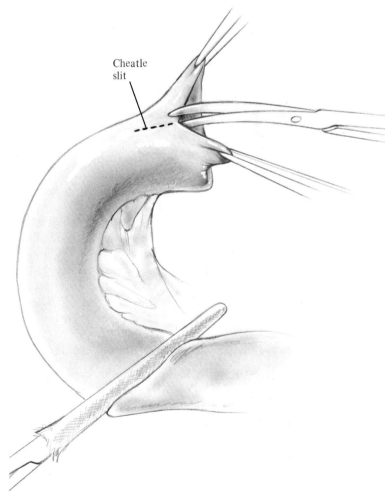

Cheatle slit

Fig. 4-21

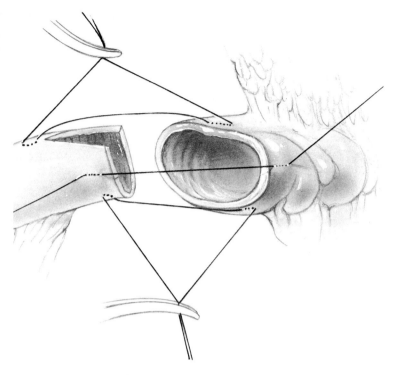

Fig. 4-22

there is a large disparity in the two diameters (>1.5–2.0 cm) the end-to-side anastomosis has advantages, provided the anastomosis is not constructed in a manner that permits a blind loop to develop. If the end-to-side anastomosis is placed within 1 cm of the closed end of the intestine, the blind-loop syndrome does not occur. Stapled closure of the end segment is rapid and efficient.

There are two instances in which the end-to-side anastomosis is clearly superior to the end-to-end procedure. We have reported that for the esophagogastric anastomosis following esophagogastrectomy the incidence of leakage, postoperative stenosis, and mortality is distinctly less with the end-to-side technique. This is probably true also for an esophagojejunal anastomosis. The second instance is the low colorectal anastomosis. With this procedure the ampulla of the rectum is often much larger in diameter than the descending colon.

Sutured or Stapled Anastomosis?

The question of whether to use sutures or staples for anastomoses is less frequently asked as techniques for gastrointestinal stapling (see Chapter 5) have become standardized. When done by surgeons whose techniques are sophisticated, stapling and suturing can achieve equally good results.

Some anastomoses are naturally easier to suture (e.g., choledochojejunostomy), whereas others are more rapidly and easily stapled. For example, a side-to-side functional end-to-end anastomosis is an easy way to create an ileocolonic anastomosis after right hemicolectomy because it eliminates the problems previously described for joining bowel of varying size.

SUTURE MATERIAL

Absorbable Sutures

Plain Catgut

Plain catgut is not commonly used during modern surgery. Although its rapidity of absorption might seem to be an advantage, this rapidity is the result of an intense inflammatory reaction that produces enzymes to digest the organic material. Plain catgut is acceptable for ligating bleeding points in the subcutaneous tissues and not for much else. Electrocautery has largely rendered that application unnecessary.

Chromic Catgut

Chromic catgut has the advantage of a smooth surface, which permits it to be drawn through delicate tissues with minimal friction. It thus may be good for splenorrhaphy or hepatorrhaphy. Moisten the chromic catgut with saline and allow it to soften for a few seconds before inserting the suture. Chromic catgut generally retains its strength for about a week and is suitable only when such rapid absorption is desirable. It is completely contraindicated in the vicinity of the pancreas, where proteolytic enzymes produce premature absorption, or for closure of abdominal incisions and hernia repair, where it does not hold the tissues long enough for adequate healing to occur.

Chromic catgut is useful for approximating the mucosal layer during two-layer anastomosis of the bowel. For this purpose, size 4-0 is suitable. Bear in mind that wound infection increases the rapidity of catgut digestion.

Chromic catgut swells slightly as it absorbs water after contact with tissue, with the knots becoming more secure. It is used for some endoscopic pretied suture-ligatures for this reason.

Polyglycolic Synthetics

Polyglycolic synthetic sutures (PG), such as Dexon or Vicryl, are far superior to catgut because the rate at which they are absorbed is much slower. About

20% of the tensile strength remains even after 15 days. Digestion of the PG sutures is by hydrolysis. Consequently, the proteolytic enzymes in an area of infection have no effect on the rate of absorption of the sutures. Also, the inflammatory reaction they incite is mild compared to that seen with catgut. The chief drawback is that their surface is somewhat rougher than that of catgut, which may traumatize tissues slightly when the PG suture material is drawn through the wall of the intestine. This characteristic also *makes tying secure knots somewhat more difficult* than with catgut. However, these factors appear to be minor disadvantages, and these products have made catgut an obsolete suture material for many purposes.

Nonabsorbable Sutures

Natural Nonabsorbable Sutures

Natural nonabsorbable sutures, such as silk and cotton, have enjoyed a long period of popularity among surgeons the world over. They have the advantage of easy handling and secure knot tying. Once the knots are set, slippage is rare. On the other hand, they produce more inflammatory reaction in tissue than do the monofilament materials (stainless steel, Prolene) or even the braided synthetics. Silk and cotton, although classified as nonabsorbable, disintegrate in the tissues over a long period of time, whereas the synthetic materials appear to be truly nonabsorbable. Despite these disadvantages, silk and cotton have maintained worldwide popularity mainly because of their ease of handling and surgeons' long familiarity with them. Because there are no clear-cut data at this time demonstrating that anastomoses performed with synthetic suture material have fewer complications than those performed with silk or cotton, it is not yet necessary for surgeons to abandon the natural nonabsorbables sutures if they can handle them with greater skill.

With the exception of the monofilaments, a major disadvantage of nonabsorbable sutures is the formation of chronic draining sinuses and suture granulomas. This problem is especially marked when material larger than size 3-0 is used in the anterior abdominal fascia or subcutaneous tissue. For this reason many surgeons do not use nonabsorbable sutures above the fascia.

Synthetic Nonabsorbable Braided Sutures

Synthetic braided sutures include those made of Dacron polyester, such as Mersilene, Ticron (Dacron coated with silicone), Tevdek (Dacron coated with Teflon), and Ethibond (Dacron with butilated coating). Braided nylon (Surgilon or Nurolon) is popular in the United Kingdom. All these braided synthetic materials require four or five knots for secure closure, compared to the three required of silk and cotton.

Synthetic Nonabsorbable Monofilaments

Monofilament synthetics such as nylon and Prolene are so slippery that as many as six or seven knots may be required. They and monofilament stainless steel are the least reactive of all the products available. For this reason, 2-0 or 0 Prolene has been used by some surgeons for the Smead-Jones abdominal closure in the hope of eliminating suture sinuses. Because of the large number of knots, this hope has not been realized, but there are fewer sinuses than when nonabsorbable braided materials are used. Prolene size 4-0 on atraumatic needles has been used for the seromuscular layer of intestinal anastomoses. Both Prolene and various braided polyester sutures have achieved great popularity for vascular surgery.

Monofilament Stainless Steel Wire

Monofilament stainless steel wire has many of the characteristics of an ideal suture material, but it is difficult to tie. Also, when used for closure of the abdominal wall, patients have occasionally complained of pain at the site of a knot or of a broken suture. True suture sinuses and suture granulomas have been rare when monofilament stainless steel has been used: no more than 1 in 300 cases. Size 5-0 monofilament wire has been used for single-layer esophagogastric and colon anastomoses. Three square throws are adequate for a secure knot with this material. Stainless steel has largely been supplanted by the synthetic monofilament sutures but is still used for closing median sternotomy incisions and for other highly selected applications.

KNOT-TYING TECHNIQUE

The "three-point technique" for tying knots is important when ligating blood vessels. The surgeon's left hand grasping one end of the ligature, the vessel being ligated, and the surgeon's right hand grasping the opposite end of the ligature are positioned in a straight line, as illustrated in **Fig-**

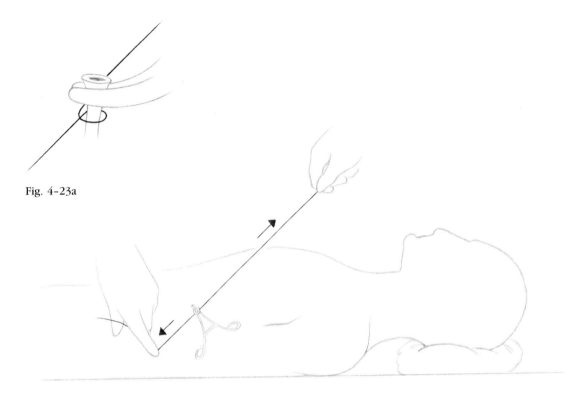

Fig. 4–23a

Fig. 4–23b

ure 4–23a and Figure 4–23b. If this is not the case, as the surgeon's hands draw apart when tightening the knot they exert traction against the vessel. When tying deep bleeding points, this traction tears the vessel at the point of ligature and exacerbates bleeding. When tying a deep structure, such as the cystic artery, the surgeon's left index finger should draw the deep end of the ligature deep to the artery so the left index finger, the cystic artery, and the surgeon's right hand always form a straight line.

When using silk, three square throws provide adequate security. With PG sutures, four throws are necessary. With the various coated polyester sutures, four or five knots must be tied. When using the synthetic materials, many prefer the "surgeon's knot" (Fig. 4–24) as a first throw.

For heavy monofilament suture material such as 0 or 1 Prolene, we have used modified fisherman's 3-1-2 knot: First, make a triple throw "surgeon's knot" (Fig. 4–25a), and then square it with a single throw (Fig. 4–25b). Complete the knot with the usual double throw "surgeon's knot" (Fig. 4–25c). This knot seems to hold without slipping.

When tying a knot in a deep or poorly accessible location, it is vital that the two-hand tying technique be used. For superficial bleeding points in the skin and subcutaneous tissues, one- or two-hand knots are efficacious.

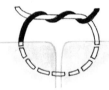

Fig. 4–24

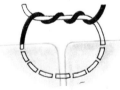

Fig. 4–25a

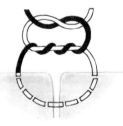

Fig. 4–25b

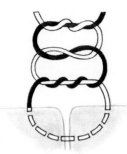

Fig. 4-25c

REFERENCES

Chassin JL. Esophagogastrectomy: data favoring end-to-side anastomosis. Ann Surg 1978;188:22.

Connell ME. An experimental contribution looking to an improved technique in enterorrhaphy whereby the number of knots is reduced to two or even one. Med Record 1982;42:335.

Wind GG, Rich NM. Surgical knots and suture materials. In: Principles of Surgical Technique. Baltimore, Urban & Schwarzenberg, 1987, pp 41-52.

5 Surgical Stapling

Principles and Precautions

TO STAPLE OR TO SEW?

Surgical staplers facilitate gastrointestinal surgery by rapidly closing or anastomosing bowel. Some anastomoses (e.g., choledochojejunostomy) are best done by hand. For other purposes, such as joining colon to a rectal remnant after a low anterior resection, stapling is easier and faster, or it creates a more consistent anastomosis in an inaccessible location. For most procedures, however, the choice is up to the surgeon. The advantages and disadvantages of various techniques are pointed out throughout this volume in the appropriate chapters.

Stapled anastomoses, when constructed with proper technique, are no better and no worse than those done with sutures. Stapling has the disadvantage of increased expense but the advantage of speed: A stapled anastomosis can generally be completed within 2–5 minutes, which is a significant benefit in the poor-risk patient who is critically ill and who may be undergoing an emergency operation. Even with the availability of skilled anesthesiologists expert in the physiologic support of desperately ill patients, there is indubitably an advantage to completing the operation speedily.

Stapled anastomoses cannot be expected to succeed under conditions that would make construction of a sutured anastomosis dangerous. There is no evidence that staples are safer than sutures, for instance, in the presence of advanced peritonitis or poor tissue perfusion.

Whereas sutures can be inserted and tied to appropriate tension to approximate but not strangulate a wide range of tissue thicknesses, staplers are much less tolerant. The stapler must be matched to the task and the tissue thickness (see below). In some situations (e.g., stricturoplasty for Crohn disease) the bowel may be too thick and diseased to staple accurately.

There are occasional, though rare, instances in which the exposure does not allow enough room to insert a stapling instrument into a body cavity. If this is the case, do not apply traction to the tissues to bring them within stapler range.

CHARACTERISTICS OF STAPLES

Modern gastrointestinal staplers are designed to preserve the viability of the tissues distal to the staple line. This is analogous to the "approximate but do not strangulate" principle used when a bowel anastomosis is hand-sewn. **Figure 5–1a and Figure 5–1b** shows how two common staples sizes are designed to enter the tissue straight and then bend into a B configuration. This allows blood to flow through the staple line. If staple size and tissue thickness are appropriately matched, one sees blood oozing through the staple line. Occasionally a figure-of-eight suture of fine PDS must be inserted to stop a small bleeder, particularly when the stomach is being stapled. This technique is contraindicated if the tissues are so thick compression by the stapling device is likely to produce necrosis. On the other hand, if the tissues are so thin the staples cannot provide a firm approximation, bleeding and anastomotic leakage may occur.

There is some leeway when approximating tissues of varying thickness. Two standard staple sizes are available for the standard linear stapler. The 3.5 mm staple is 3.5 mm in leg length and 4.0 mm wide across the base. The 4.8 mm staple also is 4.0 mm wide across the base, but its leg length is 4.8 mm. The 3.5 mm stapler achieves a closed size of 1.5 mm, and the 4.8 mm stapler closes to 2 mm. For some staplers the smaller (3.5 mm) cartridge is blue and the larger (4.8 mm) cartridge is green; hence the mnemonic "little boy blue and the jolly green giant." As a general rule, the 3.5 mm cartridge is appropriate for most tasks. The 4.8 mm cartridge is used for thicker tissues, such as stomach. Some stapling devices are continuously variable within this range, and the thickness may be tested with a gauge and then dialed in. Become

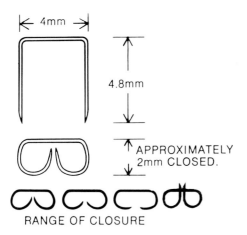

RANGE OF CLOSURE

Fig. 5-1a

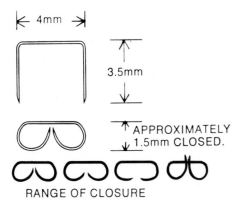

RANGE OF CLOSURE

Fig. 5-1b

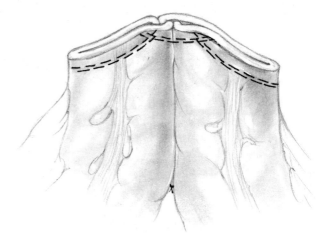

Fig. 5-2

familiar with the particular stapling devices used in your operating room and learn their operating characteristics.

The endoscopic linear cutting stapler compresses tissues to a thickness of approximately 1.75 mm.

STAPLING IN INVERSION

The circular stapler and the linear cutting stapler create inverted staple lines that mimic the equivalent hand-sutured anastomosis. In many situations, both inverted and everted staple lines are created, as illustrated by the completed functional end-to-end anastomosis shown in **Figure 5–2**. Here a linear cutting stapler was used to create the first (inverting) staple line, which brought the two segments of colon into side-to-side alignment. A single stitch at the apex of this suture line helps provide mechanical stability. Three applications of a linear stapler have been used to close the open ends of bowel in an everting fashion.

STAPLING IN EVERSION

Everted staple lines are commonly created when the linear stapler is used to complete an anastomosis or to close the end of a piece of bowel. Even when tissues are stapled in eversion, with mucosa facing mucosa, satisfactory healing takes place. This is in contrast to sutured everting anastomoses, which are generally weaker than inverting anastomoses.

STAPLING DEVICES USED FOR GASTROINTESTINAL TRACT ANASTOMOSIS

Linear Stapling Devices

The 55 mm linear stapler applies a doubled staggered row of staples approximately 55 mm long; similarly, the 90 mm linear stapler applies a doubled staggered row about 90 mm long. There is also a 30 mm stapler that is occasionally useful for extremely short suture lines.

Each device may be used with 3.5- or 4.8-mm staples, according to the principles described above. These devices are used to approximate the walls of the stomach or intestine in an everting fashion. They find application in closure of the duodenal stump, the gastric pouch during gastrectomy, and the end of the colon when a side-to-end coloproctostomy is performed.

Linear staplers use an aligning pin to ensure that the stapler cartridge meets the anvil accurately. This limits the length of bowel that can be stapled to a length that can be contained between the closed end of the device and the pin. For this reason it is

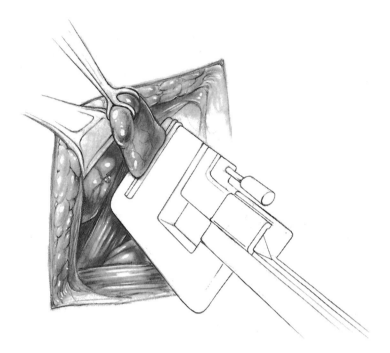

Fig. 5-3

easier to use a cutting linear stapler (described below) when a long staple line must be produced. **Figure 5–3** shows a linear stapler being used to close a Zenker's diverticulum prior to excision. Note that the tissue to be stapled is comfortably centered between the closed end of the stapler and the pin, and that the stapler is longer than the desired staple line.

Linear Cutting Stapling Device

The linear cutting stapling device creates a stapled anastomosis with the tissues in inversion. It applies two double staggered rows of staples while the knife in its assembly divides the tissue between the two double rows. It is used for side-to-side anastomoses

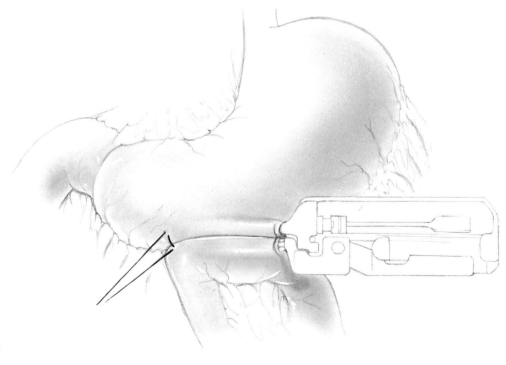

Fig. 5-4

(e.g., with gastrojejunostomy) and "functional end-to-end" anastomoses. It may also be used to divide the bowel prior to anastomosis. **Figure 5–4** shows a linear cutting stapling device being used to join the stomach to the jejunum during a gastrojejunostomy.

Circular Stapling Device

The circular stapling device utilizes a circular anvil, a circular staple cartridge, and a circular knife to produce a double staggered row of staples that approximate two tubular structures in inversion while the knife cuts the tissue just inside the staple line. This creates an end-to-end anastomosis with a lumen ranging from 12 to 24 mm depending on the size of the device. The smaller sizes are rarely used. This stapler compresses tissues to a thickness of approximately 2.0 mm. Some circular stapling devices allow the surgeon to adjust the thickness within a range of 1.0–2.5 mm. When the device is inserted through the anal canal, it is ideally suited for a low colorectal anastomosis **(Fig. 5–5)**. The circular stapler has also been used successfully for esophageal and gastroduodenal anastomoses.

CAUSES OF FAILURE FOLLOWING STAPLED ANASTOMOSIS

Quality of the Tissues

The blood supply of the bowel to be anastomosed must be vigorous when staples are used, just as it must be for suturing. *Bowel that is not fit for suturing is not suitable for stapling.* Do not let the ease of inserting staples impair good judgment about the adequacy of tissue perfusion in the vicinity of any staple line. Always think of the blood supply.

When the linear cutting stapler is used to anastomose the jejunum to the back wall of a gastric pouch (see Fig. 29–44), at least 2.0–2.5 cm of gastric wall should be left between the linear cutting staple line and the closed end of the gastric pouch. This avoids a narrow ischemic strip of stomach and anastomotic failure.

Excessive compression of thickened tissues (e.g., gastric wall hypertrophied by chronic obstruction to a thickness of 6–8 mm) may produce a linear tear in the serosa adjacent to the stapling device. Seeing this, the surgeon should invert the staple line with a layer of seromuscular Lembert sutures; otherwise the staple line should be excised and the closure accomplished entirely with sutures. Although tissue thickness rarely is a contraindication to the use of staples, failure by the surgeon to identify those cases in which the tissues are unsuitable for reliance on stapling may lead to serious complications.

Linear tension that exerts a distracting force against a sutured anastomosis certainly is detrimental. This tension is even more undesirable in the stapled anastomosis. One should assume that the fine wire in the staples tends to cut through tissues more readily than sutures, producing a leaking anastomosis. Reinforce points of expected tension (e.g., apex of a linear cutting staple line) with sutures.

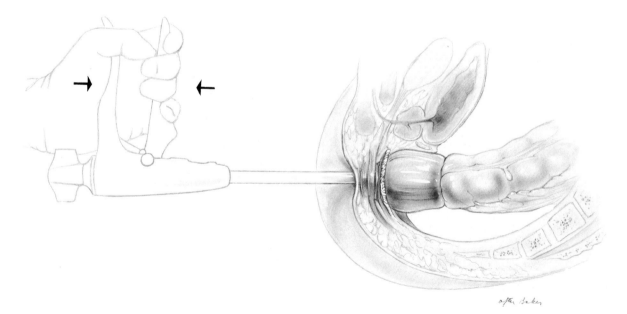

Fig. 5-5

Instrument Failure

The linear cutting stapling instrument may be misaligned, especially if it has been dropped on a ceramic floor and the two forks of the instrument diverge instead of remaining parallel. In this case the increased distance between the cartridge and the anvil prevents the staples at the distal end of the instrument from closing properly. As a precaution, *check the staple formation following completion of each anastomosis*. In addition, when a reusable stapling device is used frequently, it should be test-fired once a month on a latex drain or a sheet of plastic to verify proper B formation (Fig. 5–1).

Partial failure of the knife assembly in the linear cutting stapling instrument occurs on rare occasions. When this happens the scalpel fails to make a complete incision between the two double rows of staples. If it is not detected by careful inspection, the resulting anastomosis has an extremely narrow lumen.

Complete failure of the staple cartridge to discharge staples has been known to happen. An inattentive surgeon may not notice it, as pressure alone may hold the bowel walls in apposition temporarily. A cartridge also fails to discharge staples if it has been spent and not replaced by a fresh cartridge before *each* application of the instrument.

Failure to wipe the excess spent staples from the anvil before inserting a fresh cartridge may result in poor apposition and difficult cutting. Check it before applying the stapler.

Human Error/Judgment

Do not place a staple line so it includes the mesentery of the bowel, as it may result in bleeding or intramural hematoma formation. Similarly, do not include mesenteric fat between the seromuscular layers of an anastomosis. Whenever the linear cutting stapling device is used on the gastric wall, carefully inspect the staple line for gastric bleeding. Transfix bleeding points with absorbable sutures. Occasionally an entire staple line in the stomach bleeds excessively. If it does, oversew the entire line with absorbable sutures inserted in the lumen of the stomach. Although it is preferable to insert sutures superficial to the staple line, there may not be sufficient tissue beyond the staples to accomplish it. On such occasions we have not had complications when 4-0 PG atraumatic sutures were inserted in the lumen of a linear cutting stapled anastomosis and were passed deep to the staples. These sutures must be tied with excessive tension. We have not observed significant bleeding following stapling in organs other than stomach. Minor bleeding may be controlled by cautious use of electrocautery.

When an excessive amount of tissue is bunched up in the crotch of the linear cutting stapler, firing the knife assembly may fail to incise the bowel between the two double rows of staples because the knife blade cannot penetrate the compressed tissue. As a result there is narrowing or absence of an anastomotic lumen. Every linear cutting staple line must be inspected for completeness and hemostasis upon removing the instrument. If the incision between the staple lines has not been made by the stapler knife assembly, it should be accomplished with straight scissors. Although this type of stapler failure is rare, its possibility should not be overlooked.

Multiple Allis clamps should be applied to the walls of the intestine included in a linear staple line. This prevents the bowel from retracting from the jaws of the instrument as the tissue is being compressed. If the tissue should retract from the jaws of the instrument, obviously the stapled closure would fail.

If an anastomosis constructed by the stapling technique has a lumen that is too small, the lumen probably cannot dilate following the passage of stool or food as much as it would if interrupted sutures had been used. If a stapled stoma is made too small, the two staggered rows of staples may keep it that way permanently after the anastomosis has been constructed. Consequently, more attention should be paid to the size of the lumen when constructing a stapled anastomosis than when constructing one by sutures.

Avoid making a false intramural passage when inserting the forks of the cutting linear stapler into stab wounds of the intestine or stomach, as it would prevent formation of a proper anastomosis. Place each fork accurately in the lumen of the intestine or stomach.

The segments of bowel should be in a relaxed position when a stapling device is applied to them. If excessive tension is applied while the stapler is being fired, the tissue may be too thin for proper purchase by the staples.

SPECIAL PRECAUTIONS

After completing a stapled anastomosis, always inspect the entire circumference meticulously to ascertain that each staple has been formed into an adequate B. Test the lumen by invaginating the bowel wall with the index finger. Any point at which two or more staple lines cross should be carefully checked for possible leakage. Inspect the serosa for possible cracks or tears. If there is any doubt about the integrity of a stapled anastomosis, oversew it with a layer of interrupted or continuous seromuscular Lembert sutures of 4-0 atrau-

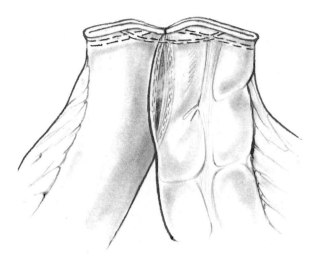

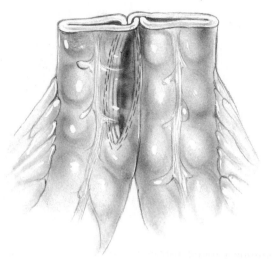

Fig. 5-6

Fig. 5-7

matic PG. Although the need to oversew the staple line occurs in no more than 1–2% of cases managed by a surgeon experienced in performing stapled anastomoses, oversewing can be an essential step in preventing leaks in some situations.

During the last step of a functional end-to-end anastomosis, the defect is closed with a linear stapling device. If the first two stapling lines **(Fig. 5–6)** are kept in perfect apposition during this maneuver, six rows of staples can be seen to come together at one point after the linear stapler is fired. We believe that such a point is weak and permits development of an anastomotic leak because the presence of many staples and excess tissue in one spot results in failure to close properly. Occasionally this situation is seen in the operating room when carefully inspecting the completed anastomosis. To prevent this weak point we have modified our technique by deliberately avoiding perfect apposition of the first two staple lines to achieve more security **(Fig. 5–7)**. A better way to avoid this problem is to use our modification of the functional end-to-end anastomosis, as illustrated in Figures 44–35 through 44–38.

The many possible technical pitfalls of stapled low colorectal anastomoses are described in Chapter 45. Inserting the circular stapler anvil into the colon or esophagus is a problem when the lumen is too narrow to accommodate the anvil's diameter. The problem may result from muscle spasm or use of a cartridge that is too large. Forceful dilatation may tear the coat of the colon or dilate the bowel to the point where it is too thin to hold staples firmly. The smallest available cartridges may result in an inadequate stoma size and should be used with care.

REFERENCES

Chassin JL, Rifkind KM, Turner JW. Errors and pitfalls in stapling gastrointestinal tract anastomoses. Surg Clin North Am 1984;64:441.

Steichen FM, Ravitch MM. Contemporary stapling instruments and basic mechanical suture techniques. Surg Clin North Am 1984;64:425.

Turner JW, Chassin JL. The ideal gastrointestinal anastomosis: staplers. In: Schein M, Wise L (eds) Crucial Controversies in Surgery. Basel, Karger Landes, 1997.

6 Control of Bleeding

TECHNIQUES FOR ACHIEVING HEMOSTASIS

Hemostat and Ligature

A hemostat of the proper length and design is a suitable instrument for occluding most bleeding vessels, followed by a ligature of a size compatible with the diameter of the vessel. As demanded by the situation, hemostats the size of a Halsted, Crile, Adson, Kelly, or Mixter may be indicated (see Glossary).

Polyglycolic (PG) ties are useful for most routine ligatures. Silk provides greater security when tying major vessels, such as the left gastric or inferior mesenteric artery. When the mesentery of the sigmoid colon is being divided during treatment of perforated diverticulitis, use 2-0 PG to ligate the vessels. If the splenic artery is being divided and ligated during resection of a pseudocyst of the pancreas, use a 2-0 ligature of Prolene.

Ligature-Passer

When ligating large vessels such as the inferior mesenteric, ileocolic, or left gastric artery, it is convenient to pass a blunt-tipped right-angle Mixter clamp behind the vessel. The blunt tip of the clamp separates the adventitia of the artery from the surrounding tissue. Preferably, at least 1.5 cm of vessel is dissected free. When this has been done, use a ligature-passer, which consists of a long hemostat holding the 2-0 silk ligature, to feed the thread into the jaws of the open Mixter clamp. Then draw the ligature behind the vessel and tie it. Pass the Mixter clamp behind the vessel again, feed a second ligature into its jaws, and ligate the distal portion of the vessel. Divide the vessel, leaving a 1 cm stump distal to the proximal tie and about 0.5 cm on the specimen side. Leaving a long stump of vessel distal to a single tie of 2-0 silk prevents the ligature from slipping off, even when it is subjected to the continuous pounding of arterial pulse waves.

Suture-Ligature

Two simple ligatures of 2-0 silk placed about 3 mm apart, with a free 1 cm stump distal to the ligatures, ensure hemostasis when ligating the large arteries encountered during gastrointestinal surgery. If there is not a sufficient length of artery to meet these conditions, a 2-0 silk ligature supplemented by insertion of a transfixion suture-ligature that pierces the center of the artery 3 mm distal to the simple ligature is almost as good as a free 1 cm arterial stump. Pass the suture part of the way through the vessel wall rather than completely transfixing it. This maneuver avoids bleeding through the needle hole.

Another type of suture-ligature is used in tissue into which a vessel has retracted. This problem may occur on the surface of the pancreas, where attempts to grasp a retracted vessel with hemostats can be much more traumatic than a small figure-of-eight suture of atraumatic 4-0 silk. The same figure-of-eight suture-ligature technique is valuable when a vessel has retracted into a mesentery thickened by obesity or Crohn's disease.

Hemostatic Clips

Metallic hemostatic clips offer a secure, expedient method for obtaining hemostasis, provided the technique is properly applied. These clips are useful *only* when the *entire circumference* of a vessel is visible, preferably *before* the vessel has been lacerated. Applying a clip inaccurately often results in incomplete occlusion of the vessel and continued bleeding, following which the presence of the metal clip obstructs any hemostat or suture-ligature in the same area. Attempts to remove the clip from a thin-walled vein may increase the rate of bleeding.

When clips are applied in an area where subsequent steps in the operation require blunt dissection or vigorous retraction, such as when performing a Kocher maneuver, the subsequent surgical maneuvers often dislodge the clips and lacerate the vessels, producing annoying hemorrhage. Hemostatic clips may similarly interfere with application of a stapling device.

It is futile to apply multiple clips in the general area from which blood is oozing in the hope it will somehow catch the bleeder. Again it must be emphasized that applying a clip is counterproductive unless a bleeding vessel can be clearly visualized.

In the absence of these contraindications, hemostatic clips speed dissection and allow secure control of bleeding vessels. An example is in the mediastinum during esophageal dissection or in the retroperitoneal area during colon resection.

Electrocautery

With electrocautery a locally high current density is passed through the target tissues to achieve rapid tissue heating. Monopolar cautery devices allow the surgeon to cut or cauterize with a blade-like tip. The return current path is through a large grounding electrode placed on the patient's thigh or back. Two types of current are supplied by most electrocautery generators: cutting and coagulating. Cutting current is continuous-wave, high-frequency, relatively low-voltage current. It produces rapid tissue heating, which allows the blade of the cautery to cut through tissue like a scalpel. There is minimal hemostatic effect. Coagulating current is pulsed-waveform, low-frequency, high-voltage current that heats tissues slowly. The resulting protein coagulation seals small vessels.

Cautery is most effectively employed by grasping the bleeding vessel with forceps or a hemostat, elevating it slightly above surrounding tissue, and then touching the cautery blade to the instrument. The resulting coaptive coagulation seals the front and back wall of the collapsed vessel together. Small punctate bleeders may be secured by touching them directly with the tip of the cautery.

Bipolar cautery units generally have a forceps-like configuration that facilitates use of coaptive coagulation. It is less useful, however, for cutting.

Electrocautery is a valuable, rapid means to achieve hemostasis, provided certain contraindications are observed. Vessels that have an external diameter of more than 2–3 mm should not be electrocauterized. As with hemostatic clips, any tissue that will subsequently be subjected to blunt dissection or retraction may not be suitable for electrocautery, as the friction often wipes away the coagulum, causing bleeding to resume. Fat does not conduct electricity well, and extensive use of cautery in fatty tissues may result in excessive tissue destruction. Similarly, when many subcutaneous bleeding points are subjected to electrocoagulation, the extensive tissue insult may contribute to wound infection.

Ultrasonic Shears

Ultrasonic shears were initially introduced for minimal access surgery but are now available with shorter shanks for use during open surgery. These devices use ultrasound to heat and coagulate tissue in a coapted position. The tissue is then cut with the device or with scissors. Slightly larger vessels (e.g., short gastric vessels or vessels in the lateral rectal pedicles) may be secured with this device rather than with coaptive coagulation using electrocautery.

Physicochemical Methods

Gauze Pack

Physical application of a large, moist gauze pad has been employed for decades to control diffuse venous oozing. It enhances the clotting mechanism because pressure slows down the loss of blood, and the interstices of the gauze help form a framework for the deposition of fibrin. Unfortunately, after the gauze pack is removed bleeding sometimes resumes. Packing has been lifesaving after major hepatic trauma or for persistent pelvic bleeding during abdominoperineal resection, particularly when the patient has become cold or developed a coagulopathy. Packs may be left in and removed after 24 hours when the patient is stable and all hemostatic parameters have returned to normal.

Topical Hemostatic Agents

A variety of topical hemostatic agents are available in powder, sheet, and woven form. They vary in chemical formulation, but most are collagen or cellulose derivatives and act as a matrix and stimulant for clot formation; thus the patient must be able to form clot for these agents to work. It is wise to remember the old axiom that *topical agents work best in a dry field*. In other words, these agents are adjuncts that help stop oozing but do not substitute for definitive hemostasis of individual bleeding vessels.

Topical agents may be applied in a thin layer to an oozing surface, such as liver or spleen from which the capsule has been avulsed. An overlying gauze pad is then placed and pressure applied. When the pack is removed 10–15 minutes later, the topical hemostatic agent remains adherent to the surface, preventing disruption of the coagulum that is forming underneath. Choice of an agent is dictated in part by the physical geometry of the bleeding site (powders are best for irregular surfaces), availability, and surgeon preference.

Avitene (microfibrillar collagen) comes in powdered form to be sprinkled on a bleeding surface, or it can be applied with clean, dry forceps. Any moisture on instruments or gloves that come into contact with Avitene causes the Avitene to stick to the moist instrument rather than to the bleeding surface. If blood oozes through the layer of Avitene, another layer should be applied and pressure exerted over it. When flat surfaces of a denuded spleen or gallbladder bed are oozing, oxidized cellulose seems to be as effective as Avitene at one-twentieth the cost.

Avitene is better for irregular surfaces because it is a powder. Microfibrillar collagen and oxidized cellulose are valuable when some portion of the splenic capsule has been avulsed during a vagotomy or splenic flexure mobilization.

Fibrin Sealant

Fibrin sealant is a hemostatic agent that mimics the final stage of blood coagulation. Fibrinogen and thrombin are combined at the bleeding site in the presence of calcium and in appropriate concentrations to produce an artificial coagulum. There is no current consensus on the usefulness of this agent in general surgical practice, although it is an area of active investigation.

CONTROL OF HEMORRHAGE

Temporary Control

During the course of operating, the equanimity of the surgeon is jarred occasionally by a sudden hemorrhage caused by inadvertent laceration of a large blood vessel. One should have in mind a sequence of steps to execute in such an event, aimed at temporary control of the bleeding in preparation for definitive steps later. The sequence should go something like the following.

1. *Finger pressure*. The simplest step, especially useful for controlling bleeding from an artery, is simple application of a fingertip to the bleeding point. In the case of a large vein, such as the axillary vein or vena cava, pinching the laceration between the thumb and index finger is sometimes effective. Notify the anesthesiologist that you are dealing with bleeding. Ascertain that the patient is fully resuscitated, that large-bore intravenous catheters are in place, and that blood and blood products are available.

2. *Elevation of the structure by placing the hand behind it*. If step 1 is not applicable, sometimes the left hand can be placed behind a structure such as the hepatoduodenal ligament to control bleeding from the cystic artery or the pancreas or behind the portal vein for bleeding in that area. This maneuver may bring temporary control.

3. *Compression by hand pressure or gauze-pad pressure*. Large lacerations of the liver may be temporarily controlled by compressing the liver between two hands while the patient is being resuscitated. Massive venous bleeding from the presacral space can be controlled by applying a large gauze pad.

4. *Satinsky clamp*. When direct pressure is not effective, a partially occluding Satinsky-type vascular clamp may be used to control the laceration of a large vessel.

5. *Proximal and distal control*. Sometimes even temporary control of hemorrhage is impossible without proximal and distal occlusion of the vessel, in some cases involving the aorta or vena cava. Preferably, vascular clamps are used; but in their absence umbilical tape is a satisfactory temporary substitute. The aorta may even be clamped or occluded by pressure in a suprarenal position for 15–20 minutes if no other means of hemostasis is effective. This safe period may be lengthened if iced sterile saline is poured over the kidneys to reduce their metabolic requirements.

Definitive Control

Once hemorrhage has been temporarily controlled, the surgeon reassesses the strategic situation. The field is cleared of all instruments and hemostats not relevant to the major problem at hand. If additional exposure is needed, plans are outlined immediately to accomplish this by extending the incision or repositioning gauze pads or retractors. Optimal light and suction lines are put in place, and arrangements are made with the blood bank for adequate support of the patient. Additional personnel are recruited as necessary.

Assign someone to be "bookkeeper." This individual's only duty is to keep track of the volume of blood lost and the rate at which it is replaced, reporting this information to the operating surgeon at frequent intervals. Otherwise, the surgeon and anesthesiologist may become so involved with the task at hand they make inadequate provision for resuscitating the patient.

After all these steps have been completed and the patient's condition has stabilized, the surgeon can convert the measures for temporary control of hemorrhage to maneuvers to ensure permanent control. This step generally involves applying a partially occluding Satinsky-type clamp to the vessel or achieving proximal and distal control with vascular clamps, so the laceration can be sutured in a definitive fashion with a continuous suture of atraumatic Tevdek or Prolene. No surgeon should undertake to perform major surgery unless trained and experienced in suturing large arteries and veins.

REFERENCES

Holcomb JB, Pusateri AE, Hess JR, et al. Implications of new dry fibrin sealant technology for trauma surgery. Surg Clin North Am 1997;77:943.

Jackson MR, Alving BM. Fibrin sealant in preclinical and clinical studies. Curr Opin Hematol 1999;6:415.

7 Management of the Contaminated Operation

Claudia L. Corwin

Infectious complications following surgery remain a major cause of morbidity and mortality in the surgical patient. Bacteria are commonly present during surgical procedures, and the balance between bacterial presence and host defense is of critical importance. The degree of bacterial inoculum is thought to correlate with the risk of developing postoperative infection. Traditionally, surgical wounds have been classified according to the predicted degree of bacterial contamination. Surgical management of "classes" of surgical wounds has evolved using this classification (Table 7–1).

Management of the contaminated operation presents the greatest clinical challenge. Postoperative complications may manifest with a wide range of sequelae, including subcutaneous wound infections, fasciitis, and abscess formation (e.g., intraabdominal, intrathoracic). Management should be directed toward minimizing the bacterial inoculum, addressing the patient's additional risk factors for infection and augmenting the patient's host defenses. This chapter reviews current methods employed to manage the contaminated operation, including well established practices and more modern approaches.

PREOPERATIVE CONSIDERATIONS

Risk Assessment

When considering the possibility of any type of complication in the surgical patient, one must formulate a "risk assessment" for the development of a particular complication. Although it seems intuitively obvious, accurate risk assessment or stratification is difficult to achieve. The Centers for Disease Control (CDC) has devised a predictive index for the development of nosocomial wound infection through the Study on the Efficacy of Nosocomial Infection Control project (SENIC score) [1]. This index is based on a score of 0 or 1 for the following four factors: an abdominal operation, operating time more than 2 hours, a contaminated operation, and a patient who has three or more diagnoses at the time of discharge (exclusive of wound infection). A second risk index developed by the CDC is the Nosocomial Surveillance System (NISS). This risk index consists of scoring each operation by counting the number of risk factors present, including the American Society of Anesthesiologists' (ASA) preoperative assessment score, a contaminated operation, and the length of the operation [2]. Data from the NISS indicates infection rates of 2.1%, 3.3%, 6.4%, and 7.1% for clean, clean-contaminated, contaminated, and dirty-infected cases, respectively [3]. Although neither of these indices is a perfect predictor, these large-scale efforts by the CDC have translated into better patient stratification than that based on traditional wound classification alone.

Adequate Resuscitation of the Patient

Maximizing tissue perfusion and oxygen supply form the cornerstone of successful preoperative resuscitation. Two important components of resuscitation are (1) restitution of adequate circulatory volume and (2) avoidance of peripheral vasoconstriction. Successful cardiopulmonary resuscitation ultimately results in a higher PO_2 in injured tissue, which in turn results in increased bacterial resistance, collagen synthesis, and epithelialization [4].

Peripheral vasoconstriction is a clinically important contributor to poor oxygen supply in wounded tissue. Mediators of vasoconstriction include blood volume deficits, cold temperatures, smoking (nicotine), and certain medications. Some surgeons actively seek to enhance tissue perfusion and arterial PO_2 through the use of vasodilating antihypertensive drugs (clonidine patches) in adequately volume-resuscitated and normothermic patients [5]. Perioperative hypothermia has been shown possibly to delay healing and predispose surgical patients to wound infections [6]. Clearly, volume resuscitation, avoidance of peripheral vasoconstriction, and maintenance of normothermia are supportive measures appropriate for patient management from the preoperative through the postoperative periods.

Table 7-1. Classification of Surgical Wounds by Degree of Contamination

Definition	Example
Clean wound	Hernia repair, breast biopsy
Nontraumatic	
No inflammation	
No break in aseptic technique	
GI, respiratory, or GU tract not entered	
Clean-contaminated wound	Elective colon resection
Nontraumatic	
No inflammation	
Minor breaks in aseptic technique	
GI, respiratory, or GU tracts entered with minimal spillage	
or with prior decolonization	
Contaminated wound[a]	Emergent colon resection for diverticular abscess
Traumatic	
Inflammation or gross purulence	
Major break in aseptic technique	
GI, respiratory, or GU tract entered with gross spillage	

GI, gastrointestinal; GU, genitourinary.
[a]Older classifications include a fourth category called "dirty," which is now included in the "contaminated" cases category.
Adapted from Drebin JA. Surgical wound infection. In: Cameron JL (ed). Current Surgical Therapy, 6th ed. St. Louis, Mosby, 1998, p 1079; and Chassin JL. Management of the contaminated operation. In: Operative Strategy in General Surgery, 2nd ed. New York, Springer-Verlag, 1994, p 3.

Perioperative Parenteral Antibiotics

The use of perioperative antibiotics, an excellent method to increase a host's resistance to infection, has been studied widely [7]. Much of the research has focused on the efficacy of prophylactic antibiotic use for clean or clean-contaminated surgical cases. Data suggest that antibiotics administered within at least 2 hours [8] but ideally within 30 minutes [9] prior to clean or clean-contaminated surgery is most effective in preventing wound infections. The perioperative use of antibiotics for contaminated cases is much less controversial and is considered therapeutic rather than prophylactic. Certainly, if one is able to predict that an operation is likely to be contaminated, the concept of "prophylactic" antibiotic coverage is irrelevant. Nonetheless, it is worthwhile to review the basic principles of antibiotic use for cases in which the surgeon anticipates contamination, including some elective and many urgent/emergent abdominal operations.

Contaminated abdominal wounds often involve the gastrointestinal tract. Procedures that involve gastrointestinal pathology place the patient at relatively high risk for postoperative intraabdominal or wound infection. Thus perioperative antibiotics are recommended for most operations that involve the gastrointestinal (GT) tract. The number of organisms and proportion of anaerobic organisms increase along the GI tract. Colorectal operations place the patient at the highest risk for infectious complications. When preparing a patient for an exploratory laparotomy, and anticipating colorectal pathology, therapy is directed toward anaerobic and gram-negative organisms. Metronidazole is a good choice for anaerobic coverage, as it has relatively few side effects. To complete the coverage, metronidazole combined with an aminoglycoside, quinolone, or a second- or third-generation cephalosporin is indicated. If an operation lasts beyond the half-life of the antibiotic, additional doses are administered during the operation.

For the operation that proves to be contaminated, the issue of postoperative antibiotics is a controversial issue. No data have confirmed that extended postoperative antibiotic coverage prevents postoperative intraabdominal abscess formation. The guidelines regarding the duration of postoperative antibiotic coverage for the contaminated operation are vague at best, regardless of the situation (i.e., peritonitis due to nontraumatic bowel perforation, traumatic bowel injury with fecal leakage). In general, the consensus is to minimize the length of postoperative coverage as much as possible, especially with concerns increasing about cost containment and the emergence of resistant organisms [10].

Mechanical and Antibiotic Bowel Preparation

Mechanical bowel preparation for many gastrointestinal operations continues to be a mainstay of preoperative preparation. This prophylactic measure may not be relevant to the emergent setting when a patient is known preoperatively to have a bowel perforation and likely gross contamination; but it is important for those more elective cases where contamination is anticipated to occur during the course of the operation. Various bowel preparation strategies have been employed, but all preparation methods share certain common elements. Fecal bulk is reduced by oral polyethylene glycol or magnesium citrate, as well as by enema administration; this phase is considered the "mechanical" portion of bowel preparation. The goal is a clear effluent. The addition of intraluminal (oral) antibiotics has been shown to decrease the incidence of infection. A well accepted oral regimen consists of erythromycin base (1 g) and neomycin (1 g), administered at 1 p.m., 2 p.m., and 11 p.m. the day before surgery. The use of preoperative parenteral antibiotics in addition to the oral antibiotics is a more controversial issue [11]. Many, but not all, surgeons believe that there is an additive effect to using oral and parenteral antibiotics. Thus many general surgeons administer a single dose of preoperative parenteral antibiotics within 30 minutes of the surgery. A second-generation cephalosporin is a good choice, especially for lower-risk, elective procedures.

INTRAOPERATIVE CONSIDERATIONS

Supporting the Patient/Continuing Resuscitation

Resuscitative measures must continue in the operating room, as intraoperative support is an important factor in augmenting host defense against infection. Hypothermia during abdominal surgery has been associated with an increase in surgical wound infections. In animals it has been shown to cause intraoperative and postoperative vasoconstriction with a resultant decrease in subcutaneous tissue oxygen tension. Decreased oxygen tension, in turn, results in decreased microbial defense and impaired immune function. Thus attention has been directed to the effect of perioperative normothermia versus hypothermia and the incidence of surgical wound infection. A double-blind randomized study in humans undergoing elective colorectal surgery showed that patients who were normothermic during surgery experienced wound infections one-third as often as patients who were hypothermic during surgery [12]. Methods to achieve and maintain normothermia include forced air warming at 40°C, conductive warming using a full-length circulating water mattress at 40°C, and warmed intravenous fluids. Various studies have supported using one method versus another [13], but one should make the best practical use of whatever equipment is available and not hesitate to use more than one method when necessary.

Surgical Technique: Does the Surgeon Make a Difference?

Studies have shown that when infection rates of individual surgeons are followed and the surgeons are provided with feedback regarding these data, their postoperative infection rates are reduced. Meticulous surgical technique is an important principle that affects postoperative results, including the incidence of postoperative infections. Sharp dissection, gentle tissue manipulation, and adequate hemostasis have often been cited as important factors that constitute proper surgical technique. Although there are historical data that attempt to compare resistance of surgical wounds to infection based on the use of a steel knife versus electrocautery [14], few data support one technique or the other. Some attention has also been given to the use of proper suture usage. The guiding message in this regard should be to limit suture use to a necessary minimum, avoiding undue tissue tension and strangulation.

Localizing Contamination

Although it is not possible to eliminate local peritoneal contamination during operations on the biliary or gastrointestinal tract, one can concentrate on completely identifying and localizing the spill and on minimizing the bacterial insult to the abdominal cavity and subcutaneous tissue. Therefore a contaminated operation is best served by a generous incision. Adequate exposure with proper retraction is essential for conducting appropriate exploration of the contaminated field. Many surgeons drape off (isolate) the wound by applying wet towels or gauze to the subcutaneous tissue, but it does not create a good barrier to microbes. Historically, a *wound protector* has been used, which is a ring drape device that consists of an impermeable plastic sheath to protect the wound and the subcutaneous fat from contamination. The wound protector is not a stock item in many operating rooms today, although it may still be available in some hospitals and used by some surgeons [15].

Subtle behaviors in the operating room may play a role in minimizing infectious complications. Upon conclusion of the contaminated segment of the operation, wound drapes, the surgeon's gloves and gowns, and the instruments should all be changed.

Wound Irrigation

Adequate intraoperative irrigation of the wound minimizes the bacterial inoculum and has been shown to decrease postoperative infection. It has long been customary to pour several liters of saline into the contaminated cavity during the contaminated portion of an operation and just prior to closing, although specific practices vary widely among surgeons. Frequent irrigation with 200 ml of saline followed by aspiration is a rationale approach to washing out bacteria spilled into the field. One should take caution not to let the irrigation fluid spill over onto subcutaneous tissues. Experimental models have shown that the most important factor that determines wound infection during contaminated surgery is the number of bacteria present at the wound margins at the end of the operation [16]. The effect of operative field irrigation on the incidence of deep wound/abscess formation is less clear.

The use of antibiotic agents in the irrigating solution is more controversial, although many surgeons routinely irrigate with antibiotic saline solutions. Irrigants have contained such antibiotics as a cephalosporin, an aminoglycoside, neomycin, and metronidazole. In addition to decreasing the bacterial inoculum, wound irrigation rinses the operative field of tissue debris and blood clots, which may be relevant to prevention of postoperative infection.

Other Topical Antibiotic Methods

Local antibiotic therapy has received relatively little attention in the United States, with most of the available literature arising from European study groups. The application of local antibiotic therapy has the advantage of providing high concentrations of antibiotic to a well defined area. On the other hand, once the wound is closed, it is not simple to reduce or remove the source of antibiotic.

Local antibiotic therapy has been supplied in the form of undiluted parenteral antibiotic powder, antibiotic beads, and antibiotic collagen sponges. The latter two methods are most popular and usually involve the use of gentamicin. Gentamicin-containing collagen sponges appear to be most practical, as the collagen dissolves and does not require removal. The sponges are usually in the form of sheets and therefore can be used to cover large areas more accurately than the beads. Local antibiotic therapy has been utilized for orthopedic procedures, pilonidal surgery, colorectal procedures, and cardiovascular and vascular surgery.

POSTOPERATIVE CONSIDERATIONS

Wound Closure

Primary wound closure during contaminated operations has been associated with a nearly 40% wound sepsis rate [17]. Thus healing by secondary intention has been the tradition when dealing with wounds of highly contaminated operations. It is well accepted practice to leave the skin and subcutaneous tissue open after such operations to allow drainage. The main goal of such management is to prevent potentially devastating complications, such as fasciitis.

Delayed primary closure, within 4–6 postoperative days, results in fewer wound infections than primary closure after contaminated operations. Many surgeons believe that attempted delayed primary closure is a reasonable "compromise" between healing by secondary intention and primary closure. When successful, delayed primary closure avoids large wounds that require labor-intensive, potentially expensive care.

Wound Dressings

Wound dressings are a means to protect the wound and a mechanism for absorbing wound drainage. Wounds that are to heal by secondary intention or delayed primary closure require a wound dressing. Wet gauze should be applied to the subcutaneous tissue, covered with a dry pad, and then covered with occlusive tape. These dressings must be changed at least twice a day. To create a wet to dry dressing, the gauze is removed from the wound without soaking the gauze prior to removal. The wet to dry dressing mechanically helps debride the subcutaneous tissue of any debris that collects between dressing changes. On occasion, contaminated and infected abdominal operations require marsupialization, leaving the abdominal cavity open. In these cases dressing changes using sterile technique and optimal exposure must often take place in the operating room. They can also take place, with care, in the intensive care setting.

REFERENCES

1. Haley RW, Culver DH, Morgan WM, et al. Identifying patients at high risk of surgical wound infection: a simple multivariate index of patient susceptibility and wound contamination. Am J Epidemiol 1985;121:206.

2. Culver DH, Horan TC, Gaynes RP, et al. Surgical wound infection rates by wound class, operative procedure and patient risk index. Am J Med 1991; 91(suppl 3B):152S.

3. Culver DH, Horan TC, Gaynes RP, et al. Surgical wound infection rates by wound class, operative procedure and patient risk index. Am J Med 1991;(suppl 3B):152S.

4. Hunt TK, Hopf HW. Wound healing and wound infection. Surg Clin North Am 1997;77:587.

5. Hunt TK, Hopf HW. Wound healing and wound infection. Surg Clin North Am 1997;77:587.

6. Kurz A, Sessler D, Lenhardt R. Perioperative nor-

mothermia to reduce the incidence of surgical-wound infection and shorten hospitalization. N Engl J Med 1996;334:1209.

7. Kaiser AB. Antimicrobial prophylaxis in surgery. N Engl J Med 1986;315:1129.

8. Classin DC, Evans RS, Pestotnik SL, et al. The timing of prophylactic administration of antibiotics and the risk of surgical-wound infection. N Engl J Med 1992; 326:281.

9. Woods RK, Patchen Dellinger E. Current guidelines for antibiotic prophylaxis of surgical wounds. Am Fam Pract 1998;57:2731.

10. Fisher JE. The status of anti-infectives in surgery [roundtable discussion]. Am J Surg 1996;172(suppl 6A): 49s.

11. Fisher JE. The status of anti-infectives in surgery [roundtable discussion]. Am J Surg 1996;172(suppl 6A): 49s.

12. Kurz A, Sessler DI, Lenhardt R. Perioperative nor-

mothermia to reduce the incidence of surgical-wound infection and shorten hospitalization. N Engl J Med 1996;334:1209.

13. Kurz A, Kurz M, Poeschl G, et al. Forced-air warming maintains intraoperative normothermia better than circulating-water mattresses. Anesth Analg 1993;77:89.

14. Madder JE, Edlich RF, Custer JR, et al. Studies in the management of the contaminated wound. Am J Surg 1970;119:222.

15. Krukowski SH, Matheson NA. The management of peritoneal and parietal contamination in abdominal surgery. Br J Surg 1983;70:440.

16. Badia JM, Torres JP, Tue C, et al. Saline wound irrigation reduces the postoperative infection rate in guinea pigs. J Surg Res 1996;63:457.

17. Meissner K, Meisner G. Primary open wound management after emergency laparotomies for conditions associated with bacterial contamination. Am J Surg 1984;148:613.

8 Mechanical Basics of Laparoscopic Surgery

Flawless and smooth completion of laparoscopic surgical procedures requires complete understanding of equipment, techniques, and regional anatomy. This chapter details some of the basic principles common to all laparoscopic surgical procedures. It should be read and thoroughly understood as a background to the technical chapters that deal with specific surgical procedures.

EQUIPMENT AND SUPPLIES

A few minutes of thought and planning may save a lot of time once the operation begins. Ascertain that all needed equipment is present and in working order and that the room is properly set up *before* scrubbing. For most laparoscopic equipment and supplies there is a choice of manufacturers. Apparently similar devices frequently have subtle points of difference when compared to other brands. Thus it is crucial for surgeons to be familiar with the particular brands in use in their own hospitals.

A troubleshooting guide, such as the one produced by the Society of American Gastrointestinal Endoscopic Surgeons (SAGES) facilitates finding and fixing problems with the insufflator, the light source, the video equipment, cautery, suction, and other complex devices. Such a chart may be laminated and affixed to the laparoscopy cart for ready reference. This is particularly important when laparoscopy is performed during the evening or night shift (e.g., for acute appendicitis) with personnel who may not be familiar with the equipment and its setup.

ROOM SETUP

The patient position and details of the room setup vary depending on the procedure to be performed. Laparoscopic surgery is extremely dependent on optimum patient and equipment position. Whereas during an *open* procedure the surgeon is free to move from side to side and vary his or her stance even from moment to moment to assume the ergonomically best position, the *laparoscopic* surgeon is limited by port placement. Think of the laparoscope as the surgeon's eyes, and the two operating ports as the left and right hands. Although it is indeed possible to switch the laparoscope from one port to another, poorly positioned port sites limit visibility and access.

Plan the room setup so the surgeon can stand facing the quadrant containing the anticipated pathology. For example, laparoscopic cholecystectomy is comfortably performed by a surgeon standing to the patient's left, facing a monitor positioned at the patient's right shoulder (**Fig. 8–1**). Surgery around the esophageal hiatus is best performed with the patient in a modified lithotomy position, the surgeon standing behind the patient's legs, and the monitor at the left shoulder or head of the bed (**Fig. 8–2**). Even a relatively minor detail such as whether the arms are tucked at the side or placed out on arm boards becomes significant. In the technical chapters dealing

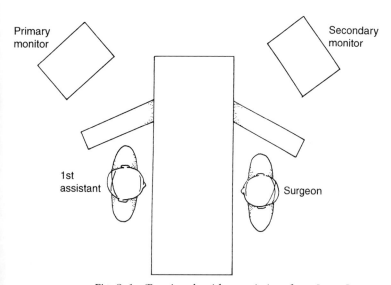

Fig. 8–1. (Reprinted, with permission, from Scott-Conner CEH (ed) The SAGES Manual: Fundamentals of Laparoscopy and GI Endoscopy. New York: Springer-Verlag, 1999.)

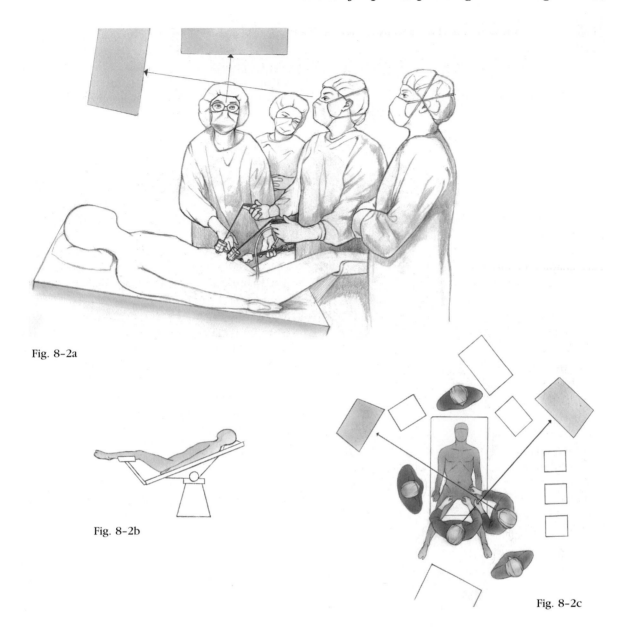

Fig. 8–2a

Fig. 8–2b

Fig. 8–2c

with specific laparoscopic procedures, the important points relevant to each operation are explained. For now, suffice it to say that no detail is unimportant.

CHOICE OF LAPAROSCOPE: STRAIGHT VERSUS ANGLED?

A straight (0°) laparoscope is easy to use and may be adequate for basic laparoscopic procedures in which the scope is easily brought to an en face view from a standard umbilical port site. The angled laparoscope allows the surgeon to view a structure from several viewpoints through a single trocar site and thus provides good flexibility. For some laparoscopic procedures, such as laparoscopic choledochotomy, Nissen fundoplication, and inguinal hernia repair, an angled laparoscope is virtually a necessity. Most commonly, laparoscopes with 30° or 45° angles are used.

The commonest error with an angled laparoscope is to point the angle *away* from the area of interest rather than *toward* it. It is easy for the neophyte camera holder to become confused unless a simple principle is kept in mind: Always remember that the angle of the laparoscope points away from the point of entry of the light handle **(Fig. 8–3)**. Instruct the camera handler to hold the laparoscope cradled in the hand with the light cord between the thumb and forefinger. This comfortable and stable grip allows the camera holder easily to angle the scope to one side or the other by pronating or supinating the wrist. If this causes the horizon to tilt noticeably, compensate by rotating the camera on the scope, if necessary.

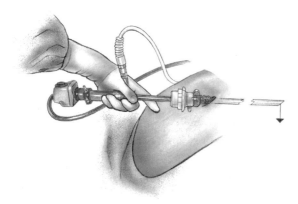

Fig. 8-3a

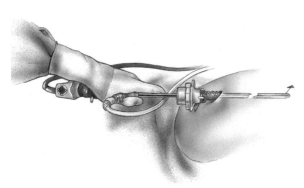

Fig. 8-3b

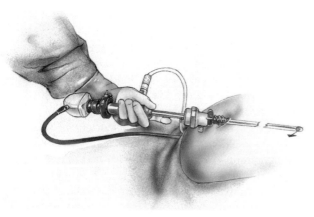

Fig. 8-3c

Many experienced laparoscopic surgeons use an angled laparoscope (usually a 30° scope) as their standard scope. Become accustomed to an angled laparoscope by using it for laparoscopic cholecystectomy and note how it facilitates visualization of both sides of critical structures.

CHOICE OF INITIAL PUNCTURE SITE

When planning trocar sites, particularly the initial puncture site, examine the abdomen for masses and scars from previous surgery and plan the location of the probable operative field. Think in terms of relative distance rather than fixed landmarks.

The umbilicus is a common site for primary entry and placement of the initial trocar. Use this site unless you have a specific reason to prefer an alternate position. Because the umbilicus represents the point where fascia and skin are adherent, entry is easy. The resulting scar is easily hidden in the skin creases around the umbilicus or is incorporated in a midline incision if conversion is required. The position of the umbilicus relative to the costal margin and symphysis pubis varies from one individual to another, particularly with increasing amounts of abdominal fat. Therefore when considering this initial entry site for a particular patient, take note of how high or low the umbilicus is situated.

In the patient with a normally placed umbilicus, an infraumbilical "smile" incision works well for laparoscopic cholecystectomy. An obese patient with a low-lying umbilicus may require a supraumbilical "frown" incision or possibly a midline or right paramedian entry site placed even higher.

Alternate puncture sites include the subcostal region. Here the costal arch provides counterpressure against which the Veress needle is easily passed into the abdomen. Subcostal entry sites are particularly useful for laparoscopic procedures done with the patient in the lateral position (e.g., laparoscopic splenectomy) or in the extremely obese patient.

PATIENT PREPARATION

An orogastric or nasogastric tube should be passed after induction of anesthesia to decompress the stomach. This maneuver minimizes the chance of inadvertent injury and significantly facilitates visualization. For laparoscopic procedures in the lower abdomen, catheter drainage of the bladder is needed. Monitoring devices should include end-tidal CO_2 measurement and pulse oximetry.

CREATING PNEUMOPERITONEUM

Closed Technique with Veress Needle

Begin with the operating table at a comfortable height for working on the anterior abdominal wall. Place the patient in 10°–15° Trendelenburg position. Estimate the distance between the abdominal wall and the abdominal aorta by palpating the aorta. In a thin patient this distance may be only 3 cm. Make a 1 cm incision at the chosen entry site and deepen the incision to expose the anterior rectus fascia. This is most easily done by spreading with a hemostat. The incision must be large enough to accept the 10/11 mm trocar if a 10 mm laparoscope is being used. It is better to err on the side of slightly larger, as a small incision causes the trocar sheath to catch at the skin level.

Expose the fascia for a distance of about 10 mm in a vertical direction. If the subcutaneous fat is thick and it is difficult to visualize the fascia, apply a Kocher clamp to the underside of the umbilicus and pull up. The umbilicus is adherent to the fascia, and this traction pulls the fascia into view. Then apply a Kocher clamp to the lower margin of the exposed fascia and elevate the clamp in an anterior direction to increase the distance between the abdominal wall and the great vessels.

Now grasp the Veress needle between thumb and forefinger **(Fig. 8–4)**, and hold it like a dart. After the tip of the needle has been inserted into the abdominal wall, place one drop of saline in the hub of the needle. Aim the needle roughly in the direction of the sacral promontory. As the needle passes through the abdominal wall, one should feel a pop as it passes through the fascia and another when it penetrates the peritoneum **(Fig. 8–5)**. At this point, the drop of saline in the hub should be drawn into

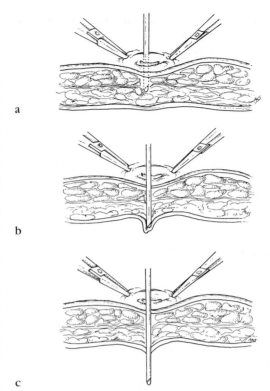

a

b

c

Fig. 8-5 a. Veress needle inserted at umbilicus (sagittal view; the blunt tip retracts as it encounters the fascia of the linea alba. b. As the sharp edge of the needle traverses the fascia, the blunt tip springs forward into the preperitoneal space and then retracts a second time as it encounters the peritoneum. c. Blunt tip springs forward as Veress needle passes across the peritoneum to enter the abdominal cavity. (Reprinted, with permission, from Scott-Conner CEH (ed) The SAGES Manual: Fundamentals of Laparoscopy and GI Endoscopy. New York: Springer-Verlag, 1999.)

the peritoneal cavity owing to the negative pressure that exists in the peritoneal cavity with traction upward on the abdominal wall. Confirm this by placing another drop of saline in the hub of the needle and then elevating the abdominal wall to create more negative pressure. If the drop of fluid is not drawn into the peritoneal cavity, readjust the position of the needle. If this move is unsuccessful, withdraw the needle and reinsert it. When the needle appears to be in the proper position, perform a confirmatory test by attaching a syringe containing 10 ml of saline in the hub of the needle and inject the saline into the abdominal cavity. Then attempt to aspirate the fluid. If the needle is in the peritoneal cavity, no fluid is aspirated. If turbid fluid is aspirated, suspect that the needle has entered bowel. If blood returns, remove the needle and promptly insert a Hasson cannula as described below and insert the laparoscope to inspect the abdominal cavity for vascular injury.

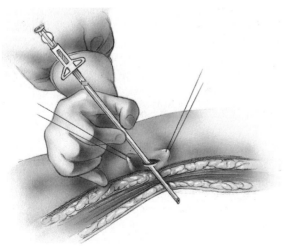

Fig. 8-4

Assuming that the Veress needle has entered the abdominal cavity uneventfully, attach the tube leading to the CO_2 insufflator. Begin at low flow or regulate the inflow to a rate of 1 liter per minute. The initial reading in the gauge measuring intraabdominal pressure should be 5–10 mm Hg if the needle is in the free peritoneal cavity. After 3–4 liters of gas has been injected into the peritoneal cavity, percuss the four quadrants of the abdomen to confirm that the gas is being evenly distributed. This confirms proper needle placement. Increase the flow rate until the intraabdominal pressure has reached 15 mm Hg. At this stage, remove the Veress needle and insert the trocar-cannula into the previous umbilical incision. Direct this device in the direction of the sacral promontory and exert gradual pressure with no sudden motions until it has penetrated the abdominal cavity. Then connect the insufflation device to the cannula and continue insufflation to maintain the desired intraabdominal pressure. This initial cannula should have a diameter of 10–11 mm for the standard 10 mm laparoscope.

Open Technique with Hasson Cannula

The Hasson cannula is designed to be inserted under direct vision through a mini-laparotomy incision. It is thus the method of choice in the previously operated abdomen when a scar encroaches on the proposed insufflation site. Some surgeons use this method preferentially for all cases.

Make a vertical 2- to 3-cm incision in the umbilicus and adjacent subumbilical area with a scalpel. Then identify the rectus fascia in the midline. Make a scalpel incision through the fascial layer and identify the peritoneum. Insert the index finger and carefully explore the undersurface of the fascia for adherent bowel. Open the peritoneum under direct vision with a scalpel. The commonest error is to make the incision too small. The peritoneal incision should comfortably admit the surgeon's index finger, and the skin incision should allow easy visualization of the peritoneum. After visual and finger exploration ascertains that the abdominal cavity has been entered,

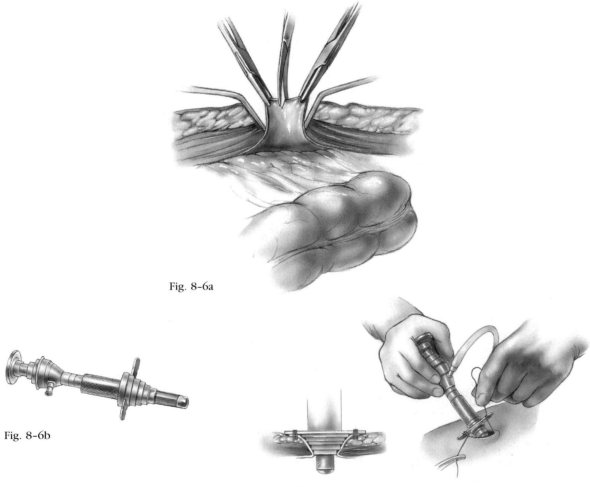

Fig. 8-6a

Fig. 8-6b

Fig. 8-6c

insert the Hasson cannula under direct vision **(Fig. 8–6)**. This cannula has an adjustable olive-shaped obturator that partially enters the small incision. Insert a heavy PG suture, one on the left and another through the fascia on the right aspect of the incision. These sutures are used to anchor the cannula and at the end of the procedure to close the incision.

Attach each suture to the respective wing of the Hasson cannula, which firmly anchors the olive obturator in the incision and prevents loss of pneumoperitoneum. After this step has been accomplished, insufflate CO_2 as previously described. When the pressure reaches 12–15 mm Hg, the telescope is inserted and the operation can begin.

Occasionally there is difficulty or uncertainty about inserting the initial trocar-cannula into the abdomen. In such cases do not hesitate to abandon the blind steps of inserting the Veress needle or the trocar-cannula and to switch to an open "mini-laparotomy" for insertion of a Hasson cannula.

MANAGEMENT OF HYPOTENSION DURING LAPAROSCOPY

When the patient deteriorates after induction of pneumoperitoneum, the safest immediate response is to withdraw any instruments into the trocars and release the pneumoperitoneum while seeking the cause of the problem. Among the possible causes are the following.

Interference with venous return. The increased intraabdominal pressure is not always tolerated, especially in frail, elderly patients. Compounding the problem are the frequent use of reverse Trendelenburg position and relative hypovolemia due to bowel preparation or overnight fasting prior to surgery. Often the procedure can resume if additional volume is infused and the insufflator is set at a lower pressure. Some patients do not tolerate pneumoperitoneum, and the procedure must then be converted to an open laparotomy.

Hypercapnia. Cardiac dysrhythmias may be induced by CO_2 pneumoperitoneum, which may produce hypercapnia and occasionally hypoxia. A sudden increase in the end-tidal CO_2 level may indicate subcutaneous emphysema, preperitoneal trapping of CO_2, or injection of CO_2 into the liver by incorrect positioning of the Veress needle. Subcutaneous emphysema may be the result of an excessively high intraabdominal pressure. Extraperitoneal CO_2 insufflation may progress to pneumomediastinum and subcutaneous emphysema. After checking all of these possibilities, the anesthesiologist can generally maintain the patient with hyperventilation. Gas embolus is rare if aspiration is performed before CO_2 is insufflated.

Tension pneumothorax. This should be suspected if unexpected hypotension occurs during the operation. It is particularly apt to occur during laparoscopic surgery in the vicinity of the esophageal hiatus.

Intraabdominal or retroperitoneal bleeding. Bleeding related to trocar insertion is another cause of hypotension, and should be suspected when no other cause is found. A quick survey of the abdomen with the laparoscope is indicated. Look for hematomas, especially arising in the retroperitoneum. If the laparoscopic search is not adequate, do not hesitate to make an emergency midline laparotomy incision, leaving all of the instruments and trocars in place. Explore the retroperitoneal area for damage to the great vessels, including the aorta, vena cava, and iliac vessels.

SECONDARY TROCAR PLACEMENT

Place secondary trocars in accordance with the triangle rule: Think of the laparoscope (the surgeon's eyes) as being at the apex of an inverted isoceles triangle with the primary and secondary operating ports as the left and right hands, as shown in **Figure 8–7** for performance of laparoscopic Nissen

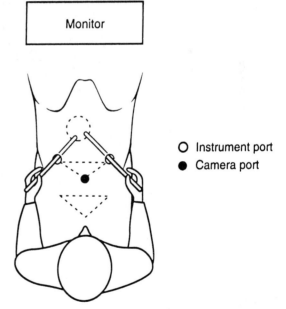

Fig. 8-7 Position of the surgeon for visual path coaxial alignment. Note the triangulation of camera and operating ports, which corresponds to the triangulation of the surgeon's eyes and two hands. The surgeon, target tissue, suture line, and monitor are aligned. (Reprinted, with permission, from Scott-Conner CEH (ed) The SAGES Manual: Fundamentals of Laparoscopy and GI Endoscopy. New York: Springer-Verlag, 1999.)

fundoplication. Proper placement of these operating ports is crucial. For that reason inspect the abdomen with the laparoscope and, if necessary, insert one of the ports that will be used for retraction before placing the operating ports. For example, when setting up ports for a laparoscopic cholecystectomy, place the most lateral retracting port first. Then grasp the fundus of the gallbladder and try lifting it to get a feeling for the degree of mobility of the gallbladder and liver. Finally, place the two operating ports.

Adopt a two-handed technique early in your laparoscopic career. This is the only way to become proficient with the maneuvers needed for laparoscopic suturing and knot-tying. Instruments placed through the primary and secondary operating ports should intersect at the operative field at an angle of 60°–90°. If you are uncertain, try out a contemplated trocar site by passing a long spinal needle through the insufflated abdominal wall into the field under direct vision and observe the position and angle at which it enters the operative field.

Additional trocars are frequently placed to allow retraction and assistance. Trocar diagrams given in textbooks, including this one, are just guidelines as each case is slightly different. If you are having difficulty, consider whether inserting another trocar for additional retraction or to substitute for an ill-placed port might help. It is generally necessary to leave the original trocar in place to avoid loss of the pneumoperitoneum.

ERGONOMIC CONSIDERATIONS

Once the ports have been placed, adjust the operating table and dim the overhead lights. The optimum table position allows the hands to be held at approximately elbow height with instruments in the trocars. Because laparoscopic instruments are longer than conventional instruments, it is generally necessary to lower the table. Adjust the position of the operating table to allow gravity to displace viscera (reverse Trendelenburg for upper abdominal surgery, Trendelenburg for lower abdominal surgery with the operative side rotated up). If lowering the table has made it impossible to position the patient optimally, raise the table and stand on a platform to compensate.

LAPAROSCOPIC DISSECTION AND HEMOSTASIS

Because even a small amount of bleeding absorbs light and obscures visualization, laparoscopic dissection places strong emphasis on careful hemostasis. For basic procedures such as laparoscopic cholecystectomy, monopolar hook cautery works well. The blunt back-side of the hook may be used, cold, as a blunt dissector, and the hook then used to elevate, cauterize, and divide small structures. The back-side of the hook may be used with cautery as a spatula cautery tip. The tip of the suction irrigator is also a useful dissecting tool. Curved "Maryland" dissectors, endoscopic right-angle clamps, and a variety of blunt graspers are used to stabilize and dissect in a manner analogous to that used for open surgery (Fig. G–41).

For more extensive surgery an ultrasonic scalpel or shears allows better hemostasis with less threat of damage to adjacent structures than cautery. Heat is generated by ultrasonic vibration of an active blade. Because this device works best when the active blade is placed against well supported tissues, it is most commonly used with a slightly curved grasping tip. The tissue to be divided is grasped and gently compressed as the shears are activated. With the correct combination of ultrasonic power and compression, the tissue within the shears is first coagulated and then cut. A lower power setting, or less pressure on the tissue, produces more coagulation and slower cutting. Higher power and greater compression produce a cutting effect. The cutting speed is inversely proportional to the effectiveness of hemostasis. This instrument greatly facilitates advanced procedures such as Nissen fundoplication where sizable vessels (the short gastrics) must be divided.

LAPAROSCOPIC SUTURING

Laparoscopic procedures that require suturing are considered advanced procedures; yet the ability to place one or two sutures may enable the laparoscopic surgeon to avoid conversion to open surgery if a minor mishap occurs during basic laparoscopic procedures such as laparoscopic appendectomy. Every laparoscopic surgeon should have basic lap-aroscopic suturing and knot-tying skills. Practice suturing in a box trainer until you are facile.

Port placement is crucial for successful laparoscopic suturing. As previously mentioned, the primary and secondary ports should bring instrument tips together at an angle of 60°–90° in the field. These ports should generally be at least 6 inches apart at the skin to avoid "dueling trocars," a situation where two trocars rub against and over or under each other at every movement.

Knots may be tied intracorporeally in a manner

analogous to that used during open surgery or extracorporeally. Intracorporeal tying has the broadest range of applications and is briefly described here. For intracorporeal tying, the entire needle and suture are passed into the abdomen. The suture is cut short (generally around 10 cm): just long enough to be able to produce the loops required for intracorporeal knotting but short enough that the tail can be easily manipulated. Generally a pliable braided material such as silk or PG is used. The size of the suture must be appropriate to the intended purpose; for instance, during laparoscopic Nissen fundoplication a heavier suture must be used to approximate the diaphragmatic crura than is used to anchor the fundoplication. Sutures for laparoscopic applications are ideally either dark or brightly fluorescent (rather than beige) to facilitate easy visualization.

Interrupted suturing requires that the laparoscopic surgeon be able to place a stitch accurately, pass it through tissue, and securely tie a knot. Tactile feedback is limited, and only visual cues are available. Two needle-holders, each capable of securely grasping and holding a needle, are used. Needle-holders with curved tips facilitate manipulation in the limited laparoscopic field. Load the needle forehand in the right-hand needle driver. Pass the needle through the tissue with a scooping motion. Following the curve of the needle requires a different set of motions than the simple supination used during open surgery. Watch the needle pass through the tissue and adjust your hand motions to pass it in a smooth, atraumatic fashion.

Grasp the needle with the left-hand needle-holder and release the right. Pull the needle through the tissue with the left-hand needle-holder.

Intracorporeal knots are placed and tied by the familiar "instrument tying" method used during open surgery. The sequence of movements to create the first throw of a square knot is shown in **Figure 8–8**. The second throw is shown in **Figure 8–9**.

Continuous suturing is more rapid because only two knots are needed. Applications are limited, however.

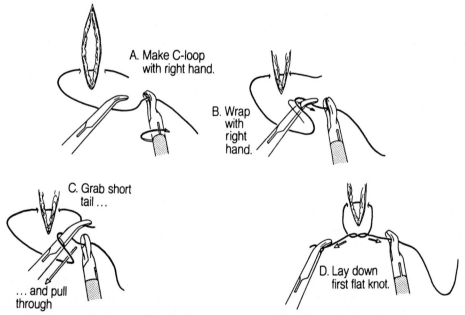

Fig. 8–8 **Square and surgeon's knot. Overhand Flat Knot.** (Reprinted with permission, from Scott-Conner CEH (ed) The SAGES Manual: Fundamentals of Laparoscopy and GI Endoscopy. New York: Springer-Verlag, 1999.)

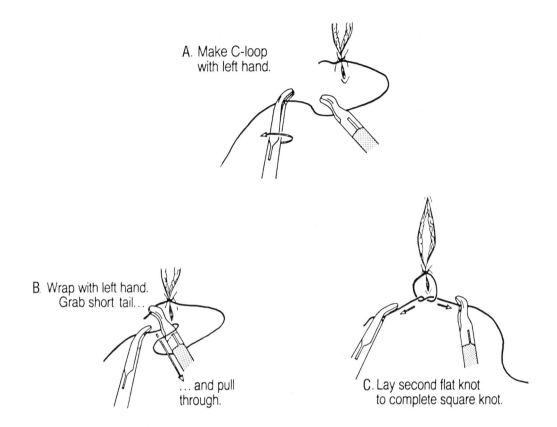

A. Make C-loop
with left hand.

B. Wrap with left hand.
Grab short tail...

...and pull
through.

C. Lay second flat knot
to complete square knot.

Fig. 8-9 **Second opposing flat knot.** (Reprinted with permission, from Scott-Conner CEH (ed) The SAGES Manual: Fundamentals of Laparoscopy and GI Endoscopy. New York: Springer-Verlag, 1999.)

USING A PRETIED SUTURE LIGATURE

Pretied endoscopic suture ligatures are available and useful for simple applications (e.g., ligating a cystic duct if the clip closure appears tenuous). They are commonly loaded with chromic catgut because this material swells slightly as it absorbs water, rendering the knot even more secure. Pretied ligatures are best used to secure the stump of a structure that has already been divided or to ligate the base of an appendix. They are not applicable to the problem of applying a tie in continuity because you must be able to pass the loop over the structure to be ligated.

To use a pretied endoscopic ligature, pass it into the field and slowly advance the loop. As the loop comes into contact with tissue, it absorbs water and softens, becoming limp and therefore much more difficult to handle. Avoid this problem by keeping the loop away from tissue until you are ready to close it. Pass a grasper through another port and pass it *through the loop* of the pretied ligature **(Fig. 8–10)**. Ignore the loop and grasp the stump of the struc-

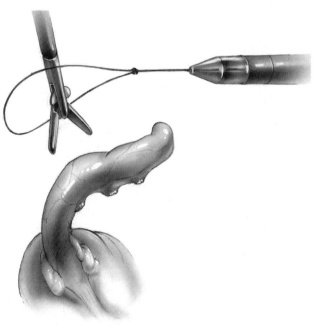

Fig. 8-10

ture to be ligated **(Fig. 8–11)**. Then slide the loop down the grasper until it encircles the stump. The loop is quite large, and drawing up on the tail to make the loop slightly smaller may facilitate this maneuver. Shorten the loop with care, as it is not possible to enlarge the loop again. Once the stump is surrounded, place the tip of the knot-pusher against the base exactly where you want the knot to sit. Slowly tighten the loop while maintaining slight tension on the stump with the grasper **(Fig. 8–12)**. Withdraw the knot pusher through the trocar and pass endoscopic scissors down to cut the ligature. As with all monofilament sutures, leave a tail of about 2 mm for security. Withdraw the grasper and inspect the ligated stump for security.

LAPAROSCOPIC STAPLING

Laparoscopic stapling may be performed intra- or extracorporeally with the same staplers used during open surgery. Purely intracorporeal stapling is possible using an endoscopic linear cutting stapler that passes through a 12 mm port. This stapler may be used to secure the base of an appendix; then, loaded with smaller staples, it may be fired across the mesentery. It fires two triple rows of staples and cuts between them. The device is illustrated and its use described in Chapter 41.

CLOSING TROCAR SITES

Any port site larger than 5 mm must be sutured closed to prevent hernia formation. Special suture passers are available to facilitate passing a suture through the skin incision at the trocar site and thence through all the layers of the abdominal wall and back out under direct vision. The suture is then tied at the level of the fascia to close the trocar site securely. These sutures are especially useful in obese patients.

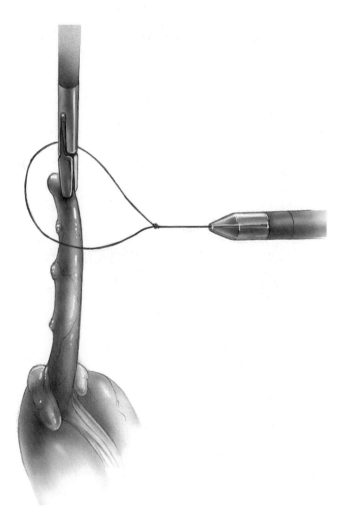

Fig. 8–11

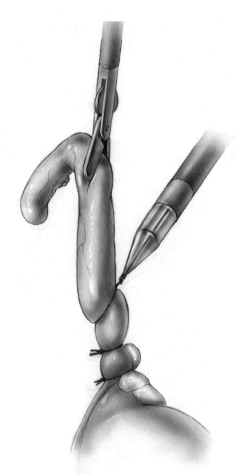

Fig. 8–12

TROUBLE-SHOOTING EQUIPMENT

Many hours of frustration can be avoided if laparoscopic surgeons take the time to become thoroughly familiar with the specific equipment in use in their particular operating suite. Adopt a standardized terminology for all the individual instruments you use so it is easy for the scrub person to pass you the specific grasper you need. Know where supplies and equipment are kept. A trouble-shooting chart, such as that developed by SAGES, should be easily accessible.

LOSS OF WORKING SPACE

If visualization is difficult and the working space seems to be collapsing, feel the abdominal wall and check the pressure reading on the insufflator. If the abdominal wall is tense and flat and the insufflator pressure readings are normal or high, the problem is likely to be inadequate muscle relaxation. Instruct the anesthesiologist to correct the situation.

Conversely, a loose, limp, flaccid abdominal wall and low insufflator pressures mean inadequate CO_2. This may be due to an empty cannister, a dislodged insufflator line, or leaks in the system.

AVOIDING COMPLICATIONS

Although each procedure has its unique complications, there are a set of problems shared by all laparoscopic operations. They are briefly considered here.

Hypercarbia from absorption of CO_2 gas is prevented by hyperventilation and vigilance on the part of the anesthesiologist. An occasional patient does not tolerate the physiologic stress of pneumoperitoneum, and conversion to open surgery may be needed.

Gas embolus is signaled by a sudden jump in end-tidal CO_2 followed by a rapid fall as cardiac output goes to zero. This rare complication is avoided by aspirating to check for blood before insufflating CO_2 through the Veress needle and employing special precautions during procedures (e.g., hepatic resection) where venous sinusoids are cut.

Bleeding from the abdominal wall is a common, annoying complication of trocar site placement. Blood may run down the instruments or laparoscope to obscure the view during surgery or cause hematoma or hemoperitoneum after surgery is complete. Avoid this situation by making the lower abdominal trocar sites lateral to the border of the rectus sheath (to avoid the inferior epigastric vessels), by avoiding umbilical puncture sites in cirrhotic patients (to avoid entering the dilated veins of a caput medusae), and by inspecting trocar sites as the last step before withdrawing the laparoscope. Generally such bleeding can be controlled by sutures through the abdominal wall.

Visceral or vascular injury during Veress needle or trocar placement is avoided by following the guidelines for Veress needle placement outlined in the previous sections. Place secondary trocars under direct vision. If visceral or vascular injury is suspected, leave the Veress needle or trocar in situ as you convert to a formal laparotomy. This may tamponade any bleeding and greatly facilitates finding the site of injury.

REFERENCES

Cuschieri A, Szabo Z. Tissue Approximation in Endoscopic Surgery. Oxford, Isis Medical Media, 1995.

Green FL, Taylor NC. Operating room configuration. In: Laparoscopic Surgery. Philadelphia, Saunders, 1994, pp 34–41.

Ponsky JF. Complications of Endoscopic and Laparoscopic Surgery: Prevention and Management. Boston, Little Brown, 1997.

SAGES Laparoscopy Troubleshooting Guide (http://www.sages.org/).

Scott-Conner CEH. The SAGES Manual: Fundamentals of Laparoscopy and GI Endoscopy. New York, Springer-Verlag, 1999.

9 Rational Use of Drains

PURPOSE OF DRAINS

Drains permit purulent material, blood, serum, lymph, bile, pancreatic juice, and intestinal contents to escape from the body. They form a walled-off passageway that leads from the source of infection or fluid buildup to the outside. This passageway, or tract, must persist for a period long enough to ensure complete evacuation of the collection, collapse of the cavity, and ultimately healing from the inside out.

In the presence of a discrete abscess, the need for and purpose of a drain is obvious and not controversial, as its therapeutic benefits are clear. In most other situations the drain acts as a prophylactic instrument to prevent accumulation of undesirable products. Because it is a foreign body, the drain also has the paradoxical effect of potentiating infection. When and how a drain should be used for prophylactic purposes has long been a source of controversy. Controlled trials have significantly decreased the indications for "prophylactic" drainage; some are cited in the references at the end of the chapter.

PROS AND CONS OF VARIOUS DRAINS

Latex (Penrose) Drain

The Penrose drain is a soft latex drain of various dimensions. It has the shape of a flattened cylinder and is made of a thin, radiopaque sheet of rubber. It has the advantage of being inexpensive. It is also successful in encouraging fibrosis, so it forms a well established tract within 8–10 days.

It has many disadvantages as well. Ideally, the drain is placed to create a dependent tract through which fluid may escape by gravity. If the surgeon does not take pains to bring the drain out in a straight line, without wrinkles, stagnant pools of serum accumulate around the wrinkled areas of the drain. After the drain is removed, the patient may have a 24-hour increase in temperature of as much as 1°C. More fundamentally, the passive latex drain does not empty a cavity; it simply permits secretions to overflow from the abdomen to the outside. It is not particularly effective in evacuating oozing blood before

a clot forms. There is no method by which the depth of the wound can be irrigated with this type of drain as there is when a tube or sump type is used.

Finally, the most important objection to the latex drain arises from the fact that it requires a 1- to 2-cm stab wound in the abdominal wall, which permits retrograde passage of pathogenic bacteria down into the drain tract. It also creates a sizable fascial opening that may be the site of subsequent hernia formation.

Polyethylene or Rubber Tube Drain

Both polyethylene and rubber tube drains establish tracts to the outside, as they are mildly irritating and stimulate adhesion formation. They effectively evacuate air and serum from the pleural cavity and bile from the common bile duct. Drainage tract infection following the use of tube drains is rare for the reasons discussed below.

Among the disadvantages of rubber and polyethylene tubes is that they become clogged with clotted serum or blood unless they are large. Large tubes, however, are unsuitable for placement deep in the abdominal cavity for a period of more than a few days, as there is considerable danger of erosion through an adjacent segment of intestine, resulting in an intestinal fistula.

Silicone Tube Drain

Silicone or Silastic tubes are less reactive than are other types of drain. They are less prone to become plugged as a result of clotting serum. Because of the soft texture of silicone, erosion into the intestine is uncommon.

A disadvantage of silicon drains is their lack of reactivity; hence there is minimal fibrous tract formation. This lesson was learned when Silastic T-tubes were (briefly) used in the common bile duct, and their removal often resulted in bile peritonitis because a firm fibrous channel had not been established between the bile duct and the outside.

Sump Suction Drains

Generally constructed of silicone or polyethylene tubing, sump drains must be attached to a source of continuous suction. They effectively evacuate blood and serum, especially if suction is instituted in the operating room so the blood is evacuated before it clots. Instillation of an antibiotic solution also is feasible when indicated. If used regularly, fluid instillation prevents obstruction of the drain due to coagulation of serum or secretions. Drainage tract infections with sumps are uncommon even though unsterile, bacteria-laden air is drawn into the depths of the patient's wound by the continuous suction. Filters are available to minimize this problem. A major disadvantage of sump drains is the requirement that the patient be attached permanently to a suction device, thereby impairing mobility.

Closed-Suction Drain

The closed-suction drain consists of one or two multiperforated silicone or polyethylene catheters attached to a sterile plastic container, the source of continuous suction. It is a closed system; and the catheters are brought out through puncture wounds. These drains have replaced other drains for most applications. Patient mobility is unimpaired, as the plastic container is easily attached to the patient's attire. The depths of the wound can be irrigated with an antibiotic solution by disconnecting the catheter from the suction device and instilling the medication with a sterile syringe.

Closed-suction drains are commonly used in a clean field, such as at axillary node dissection sites to prevent seroma formation. They should be removed as soon as possible to prevent bacterial entry.

Some closed-suction drains contain multiple perforations. In time, tissues are sucked into the fenestrations, and tissue ingrowth may even occur. This makes removal difficult (occasionally to the point of requiring relaparotomy), and most surgeons are reluctant to leave a fenestrated closed-suction drain in the abdomen for more than 10 days. Fluted suction drains are also available and avoid this potential complication.

GAUZE PACKING

When a gauze pack is inserted into an abscess cavity and is brought to the outside, the gauze, in effect, serves as a drain. Unless the packing is changed frequently, this system has the disadvantage of potentiating sepsis by providing a foreign body that protects bacteria from phagocytosis. Management of pancreatic abscesses by marsupialization and packing is an example of this technique. Daily dressing changes keep the packing fresh.

PREVENTION OF DRAINAGE TRACT INFECTION

Retrograde transit of bacteria from the patient's skin down into the drainage tract is a source of postoperative sepsis and may even follow clean operations. When a polyethylene sump or a silicone closed-suction catheter is brought through a puncture wound of the skin, it is easy to suture it in place and minimize or eliminate the to-and-fro motion that encourages bacteria to migrate down the drain tract. On the other hand, when a latex drain is brought out through a 1- to 2-cm stab wound in the abdominal wall, there is no possibility of eliminating the to-and-fro motion of the drain or retrograde passage of bacteria into the drainage tract. Consequently, when latex or gauze drains are required for an established abscess, the surgeon must accept the added risk of retrograde contamination with bacteria despite sterile technique when dressings are changed.

MANAGEMENT OF INTRAPERITONEAL SEPSIS

When managing intraperitoneal sepsis a distinction must be made between an isolated abscess (e.g., around the appendix) and multiple abscesses involving the intestines accompanied by generalized peritonitis. With the latter type of sepsis, the presence of fibrin and necrotic tissue prevents adequate phagocytosis and perpetuates sepsis.

When an abscess has developed rigid walls that do not collapse after evacuation of pus, large drains must be inserted to establish a reliable tract to the outside. Sometimes a rigid abscess cavity requires 2–5 weeks to fill with granulation tissue. It is not safe to remove the drains until injecting the abscess with an aqueous iodinated contrast medium has produced a radiograph demonstrating that the cavity is no longer significantly larger in diameter than the drainage tract. If this is not done, the abscess may rapidly recur. For rigid-walled abscesses of this type, several large latex drains should be inserted together with one or two sump drains. Some surgeons place an additional straight 10F catheter for intermittent instillation of dilute antibiotic solution. At least one drain is left in place until the sinogram shows that the abscess cavity has essentially disappeared. Care should be taken that none of the rigid drains comes into contact with the intestine or stomach, as intestinal fistulas can be a serious complication.

PERCUTANEOUS DRAINAGE OF ABDOMINAL ABSCESSES WITH COMPUTED TOMOGRAPHY OR ULTRASOUND GUIDANCE

Treatment of abdominal abscesses underwent a revolutionary change during the 1990s owing to the demonstrated efficacy of percutaneous drainage by the interventional radiologist. In the case of most abdominal abscesses, the skilled radiologist can find a safe route along which to insert a drainage catheter that evacuates the pus without a need to perform laparotomy for drainage. This technology is especially welcome in the critically ill patient who may not tolerate a major operation.

OTHER INDICATIONS AND METHODS OF DRAINAGE

Abscess

For abscesses of the extremities, trunk, or perirectal area, the important step is to unroof the abscess by making a cruciate incision so the tract does not close before all the pus has been evacuated. An unroofing procedure is adequate for superficial abscesses, and any type of temporary drain is sufficient. When the danger exists that the superficial portion of the tract might close before deep healing takes place, insertion of gauze packing is indicated. The packing is then changed often enough to keep it from blocking the egress of pus.

Blood and Serum

The presence of blood, serum, or fibrin in a perfectly sterile area is not dangerous to the patient, although the operative field is never completely sterile following any major operation. For this reason, postoperative puddles of blood or serum in combination with even a small number of bacteria can result in abscess formation because the red blood cell impairs antibacterial defenses. With the low colorectal anastomosis, accumulated serum or blood in the presacral space, together with secondary infection and abscess formation, may result in anastomotic breakdown. For these reasons, strenuous efforts should be exerted to eliminate bleeding during any abdominal operation. If these efforts must be supplemented by some type of drainage, the ideal method is to insert one or two multiperforated Silastic drains, which are brought out through puncture wounds in the abdominal wall and attached to a closed suction system.

Closed suction drainage is extremely effective following radical mastectomy or regional lymph node dissections of the neck, axilla, or groin. Small-diameter tubing is acceptable. This technique has also been employed successfully following abdominoperineal proctectomy with primary closure of the perineal floor and skin.

Bile

Because bile has an extremely low surface tension, it tends to leak through tiny defects in anastomoses or through needle holes. It is essentially harmless if a passageway to the outside is established. A sump drain or closed suction system works well for this purpose. Silastic tubes are contraindicated whenever formation of a fibrous tract to the outside for the bile is desirable, especially with use of a T-tube in the common bile duct, as previously noted.

Pancreatic Secretions

It is not dangerous for pure pancreatic juice to drain into the abdominal cavity, as is evident in patients who have pancreatic ascites or a fistula. If the pancreatic secretion is activated by the presence of bile, duodenal contents, or pus, however, trypsinogen is converted to trypsin and the adjacent tissues are subjected to a raging inflammatory reaction. Recently constructed adjacent anastomoses may be digested and destroyed. Eventually, hemorrhage from retroperitoneal blood vessels ensues.

Consequently, it is important to evacuate bile and pancreatic secretions completely, especially after pancreaticoduodenectomy. This is accomplished by inserting a long plastic catheter into the pancreatic duct in the tail of the pancreas. The catheter is brought through the segment of jejunum to which the duct is anastomosed. Then it is brought through a jejunostomy opening to an outside drainage bag. Unless the tube is accidentally displaced, it conveys all pancreatic secretions from the abdominal cavity. In addition, a suction catheter is inserted in the vicinity of the anastomosis, between the tail of the pancreas and the jejunum. Many surgeons routinely drain pancreatic staple lines or suture lines (e.g., after distal pancreatectomy or pancreaticojejunostomy) with closed suction drains.

Anastomosis

It makes little sense to place a drain down to a gastrointestinal anastomosis simply because the surgeon has some doubt about its integrity. If anastomotic breakdown occurs, the presence of a drain may not prevent generalized peritonitis. If the surgeon believes there is significant risk of anastomotic failure, the anastomosis should be taken apart and done over, or else both ends should be exteriorized and reconnected at a second-stage operation. The surgeon must not fall into the trap of fuzzy thinking, which would permit acceptance of an anastomosis that might be less than adequate, rather than reconstructing the anastomosis or eliminating it from this stage of the operation.

When treating Crohn's disease accompanied by extensive cellulitis, some surgeons believe the inflamed areas should be drained. In reality, cellulitis or contamination, such as might follow a perforated duodenal ulcer, do not benefit from drainage. It is well established that the peritoneal cavity as a whole cannot be drained.

If complete hemostasis cannot be achieved in the vicinity of an anastomosis, there may be some merit to inserting a silicone closed-suction drain for a few days, provided it does not come into direct contact with the suture line.

REFERENCES

Deitch E. Placement and use of drains. In: Tools of the Trade and Rules of the Road. A Practical Guide. Philadelphia, Lippincott-Raven, 1997, pp 91–102.

Dellinger EP, Steer M, Weinstein M, Kirshenbaum G. Adverse reactions following T-tube removal. World J Surg 1982;6:610.

Gillmore D, McSwain NE, Browder IW. Hepatic trauma: to drain or not to drain? J Trauma 1987;27:898.

Hoffman J, Shokouh-Amiri MH, Damm P, et al. A prospective, controlled study of prophylactic drainage after colonic anastomoses. Dis Colon Rectum 1987;24:259.

Malangoni MA, Dillon LD, Klamer TW, et al. Factors influencing the risk of early and late serious infection in adults after splenectomy for trauma. Surgery 1984;96:775.

Maul KI, Daugherty ME, Shearer GR, et al. Cholecystectomy: to drain or not to drain; a randomized prospective study of 200 patients. J Surg Res 1978;24:259.

Robinson JO. Surgical drainage: an historical perspective. Br J Surg 1986;73:422.

Vansonnenberg E, D'Agostino HB, Casola G, Halasz NA, et al. Percutaneous abscess drainage: current concepts. Radiology 1991;181:617.

Part II
Esophagus

10 Concepts in Esophageal Surgery

Thomas H. Gouge

Advances in diagnostic studies, perioperative management, and the techniques of esophageal surgery have greatly reduced mortality, morbidity, and length of hospital stay. Multidisciplinary approaches have even begun to improve the long-term results of treatment for esophageal malignancy. Long-term survival following resection of a carcinoma of the esophagus is usually limited to patients without regional spread whose tumors are confined to the wall of the esophagus. Successful esophageal surgery still requires knowledge of the anatomy and physiology of the esophagus and attention to the details of the operative technique.

CARCINOMA OF THE CARDIA REGION

Resection of lesions of the distal esophagus and gastric cardia with esophagogastric anastomosis is no longer an operation with high mortality, significant complications, and intractable reflux esophagitis. Resection with an overall mortality of 2% should be routine, and anastomotic leakage should be a rare event today. Operation without an intensive care unit stay, with early ambulation, return to oral intake within 48 hours, and hospitalizations of 1 week are achievable even for patients over age 70. Continuing epidural analgesia with patient control after surgery has been an important advance. Although return of normal appetite and meal volume is slow, most patients have no dietary restrictions after the early narrowing of the anastomosis due to edema has resolved.

Important concepts are resection with adequate margins of normal esophagus and stomach, resection of the fibroareolar tissue around the tumor to ensure local circumferential margins, and adequate lymphadenectomy for adequate staging. The stomach must be well mobilized with preserved vascularity and esophagogastric continuity restored with an end-to-side anastomosis. The gastroepiploic arcade must be carefully preserved and the esophageal hiatus widened to prevent a tourniquet effect with obstruction to venous outflow. Properly performed, esophagogastrectomy is a safe operation with good symptomatic and nutritional results.

If a tumor extends into the stomach a significant distance along the lesser curvature or into the fundus, a significant proximal gastrectomy is necessary for adequate tumor margin. If resection of more than 50% of the stomach is required for tumor margins or if the anastomosis is less than 10 cm from the pylorus, a total gastrectomy with roux-Y esophagojejunostomy gives a much more satisfactory result. Intraabdominal esophagogastric anastomoses near the pylorus permit too small a gastric remnant to construct a satisfactory end-to-side anastomosis. Such end-to-end anastomoses have a higher leak rate and severe problems with uncontrolled bile reflux esophagitis.

Laparotomy with right thoracotomy can be used for lesions at any level of the thoracic esophagus, and transhiatal esophagectomy is an option for lesions in the distal 10 cm of the esophagus. I continue to prefer a left thoracoabdominal approach with the patient in the lateral position for tumors whose proximal extent on computed tomography (CT) are clearly below the carina. One-stage mobilization and anastomosis shortens the operating time, provides superb exposure to both esophagus and stomach, and decreases blood loss. Although the upper extent of the tumor should be known with accuracy with CT imaging, the need for additional proximal length can easily be addressed. The surgeon can simply mobilize the esophagus from under the aortic arch and make the anastomosis as high in the pleural space as necessary.

CARCINOMA OF THE MIDDLE AND UPPER ESOPHAGUS

The operation of choice for lesions in the mid-thoracic esophagus is subtotal resection by right thoracotomy following full mobilization of the stomach through a midline laparotomy. I routinely place a feeding jejunostomy as part of the abdominal phase.

The anastomosis should be constructed with an end-to-side technique at the apex of the right chest or in the neck. A stapled anastomosis at the apex of the chest usually provides at least as much esophageal margin as a cervical anastomosis. The same considerations of blood supply and lack of tension apply. Good vascularity ensured by preservation of the gastroepiploic arcade, enlargement of the hiatus to prevent compression, and wide mobilization of the stomach and duodenum to eliminate tension are essential to a satisfactory anastomosis. With appropriate preparation the laparotomy and subsequent right thoracotomy approach can be done safely with resultant good digestive function and little or no reflux problems. The tumor must be staged as completely as possible prior to operation to ensure resectability because the surgeon cannot assess local fixation until after completion of the abdominal mobilization if the thoracic phase is done second. Bronchoscopy and endoscopic ultrasonography are the most accurate studies to determine the extent of invasion for these tumors. Doing the thoracic mobilization first has the advantage of evaluating the local condition early in the operation but adds substantially to the operating time.

I prefer dissection under direct vision through a posterolateral thoracotomy for these lesions even though the same thing can be accomplished by the transhiatal approach. The use of video-assisted surgery may prove to be a good alternative. I use a transhiatal approach only for mid-esophageal lesions that were clearly confined to the wall of the esophagus to avoid injury to major vessels and the trachea. Wide resection around the esophagus is not as feasible in the mid and upper esophagus as it is in the lower third and cardia because of the adjacent respiratory and vascular structures.

My preference has been for a high intrathoracic anastomosis when the location of the tumor permits rather than using a cervical anastomosis on principle. Anastomosis in the neck has a higher leak rate than intrathoracic anastomosis. As the incidence of anastomotic failure in the intrathoracic anastomoses has been reduced to a rarity, the previous arguments about safety have lost their force. Cervical leaks do not necessarily remain localized. If it does not drain anteriorly, a cervical leak can track down and cause thoracic mediastinitis. Cervical leaks, however, often cause strictures that require dilation and can be difficult to manage. The amount of esophagus resected with an anastomosis in the neck is minimally (if any) longer than for an anastomosis at the apex of the thorax. Cervical anastomosis has improved neither local recurrence nor long-term survival.

UNRESECTABLE CARCINOMA

Patients whose lesions appear locally unresectable on initial evaluation by CT scan or ultrasonography should be treated with radiation and chemotherapy and then reevaluated for surgical treatment after completing the course of neoadjuvant therapy. For patients with significant invasion beyond the esophageal wall, a multimodality approach with radiation and chemotherapy has the potential to reduce significantly or even eliminate the tumor mass. Resection may be feasible for palliation or even with curative intent after such neoadjuvant treatment.

Tumors that invade the aorta or the tracheobronchial tree must be approached with extreme caution. It is doubtful that heroic measures can prove more beneficial than a palliative approach, and the chance of creating an unsalvageable situation is great.

Distant metastases are not a contraindication to palliative resection of a locally resectable tumor. The patient's condition and the potential benefit must be carefully weighed when deciding whether to resect for palliation. A suitable patient is one whose tumor has caused obstruction or bleeding and who can easily withstand the operation. For such a patient, the ability to swallow can significantly enhance the quality of life. A palliative resection can be accomplished during a short hospitalization in appropriately selected patients.

Although it is feasible to interpose a colon segment between the proximal esophagus and the stomach for palliation of obstruction caused by an unresectable carcinoma, the operation has a high mortality rate and provides poor palliation for the short expected survival of such patients. The development of new techniques including endoscopic treatment with dilators, lasers, and stents provides a much more acceptable means of palliation.

CARCINOMA OF THE ESOPHAGUS: TRANSHIATAL OR TRANSTHORACIC APPROACH

Each approach to resection of esophageal cancers has had strong proponents. Each also has advantages and disadvantages, and no series has demonstrated a clear superiority of one over the others. Although the left-sided approach I favor for distal lesions has been widely accepted, some have reported excessive mortality and leak rates. We have not had this experience, and others have also noted exceedingly low mortality and complication rates. Akiyama [1], Ellis et al. [2], and Mathiesen et al. [3] have reported the same experience we have had with complications and mortality, both in the 2% range or lower. With a large experience, Orringer et al.'s [4] results with transhiatal resections are similar.

Each operative approach requires knowledge of the anatomy, appropriate staging and preparation of the patient, a well orchestrated team approach in the operating room and afterward with meticulous and delicate surgical technique, careful anesthetic technique and monitoring, and devoted postoperative care to achieve comparable results.

REPLACING OR BYPASSING THE ESOPHAGUS: STOMACH, COLON, OR JEJUNUM

The stomach is the closest we have to the ideal esophageal replacement. When fully mobilized and based on the gastroepiploic arcades, the apex of the stomach reaches the nasopharynx. When the stomach is stretched out to reach the neck, it becomes a tubular organ of modest diameter, with the fundus at its apex and the site of the gastroesophageal junction one-third of the way down the lesser curvature side. Its arterial supply and venous drainage are reliable and difficult to compromise even if the lesser curvature arcades are divided to gain length. The stomach is thick-walled and resistant to trauma when passed up to the neck by any route. Restoration of continuity to the esophagus or pharynx is straightforward and requires only a single anastomosis.

Although end-to-side anastomosis and creation of a partial antireflux "fundoplication" by wrapping or "inkwelling" the anastomosis help decrease the amount of reflux, all patients with esophagogastrostomies have abnormal gastroesophageal reflux. Significantly symptomatic reflux, however, is seen primarily with low anastomoses and rarely with cervical anastomoses. Deprived of vagal innervation, the stomach acts as a passive conduit, but its function is usually satisfactory. High anastomoses (in the neck or apex of the pleural space) help minimize the amount of reflux. I believe this improvement is on a purely mechanical basis. The complete vagotomy that occurs as part of an esophageal resection makes acid secretion minimal. Bile is the main culprit. A long, thin gastric tube helps minimize pooling in the intrathoracic stomach and facilitate emptying, thereby decreasing the amount of bile reflux. When the stomach is available I have used it and reserved intestinal interposition for special circumstances. I have not had the opportunity to use the gastric tube technique described by Gavrilu [5] and Heimlich [6] and prefer other techniques in adults.

The use of the jejunum or colon to replace a resected segment of esophagus preserves a functioning stomach intact. Although less used today than previously, colon or jejunal interposition is an essential technique if the stomach is diseased or was previously resected. Most of the benign strictures formerly treated by short segment colon interposition are now managed without resection. The colon is easily mobilized and can be supported on one of several major vascular pedicles and the marginal arcades. The transverse and descending colon based on the ascending branches of the left colic artery in isoperistaltic position is the appropriate size and length for substernal or intrathoracic interposition. The arterial supply is reliable and the venous pedicle short and less prone to kinking or twisting. Although sufficient length of colon can usually be achieved to reach the neck, use of the colon presents some special problems. The colon serves as a passive conduit and does not have effective peristalsis. Gastrocolic reflux occurs routinely, and the refluxate is slowly cleared; but the reflux is seldom symptomatic. The transit time for a bolus of food to pass into the stomach is invariably slow but variably symptomatic. Benign or malignant disease of the colon may preclude its use; and the mesenteric vascular arcade is variable, especially on the right. The interposed colon is also subject to venous infarction by trauma to the colon mesentery or compression at the hiatus.

The jejunum retains effective peristalsis when used to replace a segment of the esophagus. Short segment jejunal interposition has been used effectively as a salvage operation to prevent reflux when multiple direct operations on the gastroesophageal junction for reflux esophagitis have failed. The shape of the jejunal mesentery limits the length of the interposition that can be achieved with a conventional technique. Without special techniques, the jejunum does not reach above the inferior pulmonary vein. Some of the limitations of jejunal interpositions have been solved by microvascular techniques, which allow either free transfer of jejunum to replace segments of the pharynx or proximal esophagus or interruption of the mesentery with a second proximal vascular anastomosis.

Even without microvascular techniques, the major objection to using jejunum or colon as an esophageal substitute has been the time involved in the additional dissection and the three required anastomoses. Mobilizing the bowel with careful preservation of both arterial and venous circulation can be difficult and time-consuming. Although experienced surgeons have reported excellent results with both colon and jejunum, higher mortality and morbidity rates are the rule. The higher complication rate for interposition operations likely reflects both the additional surgery required and the more complicated nature of the patients who require such an approach. When approaching a patient who needs an intestinal interposition, the surgeon must know as much as possible about the condition of the bowel and its vascular supply. Endoscopy, contrast studies, and vascular studies by angiography or magnetic resonance imaging (MRI) should be performed and the bowel prepared both mechanically and with antibiotics in every case. The surgeon must have alternatives well thought out if the originally selected segment of bowel is not usable or the adequacy of the blood supply is questionable.

Effective complete vagotomy is likely after any esophageal resection. Although it may not be necessary in more than one-third of cases, I routinely do a pyloromyotomy to facilitate gastric emptying. It is a simple maneuver if the patient does not have scarring from a chronic duodenal ulcer. I have not found it harmful, and it avoids the need for balloon dilation or reoperation. Although a matter of judgment, a pyloromyotomy or other drainage procedure should be done any time the pyloroduodenal segment is within the hiatus when the stomach is pulled up because reoperation in this area is extremely difficult.

HIATUS HERNIA AND REFLUX DISEASE

With the exception of traumatic diaphragmatic rupture, virtually all acquired diaphragmatic hernias enter the chest through the esophageal hiatus. Parahiatal hernia occurs but is a rare finding of no particular significance. On the other hand, it is essential for a surgeon to understand the difference between a sliding and a paraesophageal hiatus hernia and to differentiate them from posttraumatic hernias caused by blunt or penetrating trauma.

A sliding hiatus hernia may be thought of as a disease of the esophagus whose significance depends on the severity of associated gastroesophageal reflux and its consequences. A sliding hiatus hernia is sliding both in the anatomic sense (one wall of the hernia is made up of the visceral peritoneum covering the herniated stomach) and in the direction it herniates (the gastroesophageal junction migrates cephalad along the axis of the esophagus): hence the synonym axial hiatus hernia. The hiatus hernia must be reduced and the hiatus repaired as part of the operation to control reflux.

A paraesophageal hernia, also known as a rolling hiatus hernia, is best conceived as a disease of the diaphragm. In this case the gastroesophageal junction is in its normal position, and the stomach with the attached greater omentum and transverse colon herniates into the posterior mediastinum through an anterior widening of the hiatus. This hernia has a true sac of parietal peritoneum. The problems associated with paraesophageal hernias are the same as those with any abdominal wall hernia with the additional special problems of having the acid-secreting stomach involved. Patients with paraesophageal hernia are more often older and frequently have kyphoscoliosis. They usually do not have significant reflux but often have abnormal esophageal peristalsis. Many are entirely asymptomatic, and the diagnosis is suggested by the presence of a mediastinal air-fluid level on chest radiography. Unlike sliding hernias, all patients who have a significant paraesophageal hernia should undergo repair to avoid the mechanical complications of the hernia unless they are unfit candidates for general anesthesia. All symptomatic patients require surgical repair because this disease is caused by a mechanical problem for which there is no medical therapy. The essentials of the operation are reduction of the stomach and repair of the hiatus. Patients who do not have reflux do not benefit from an antireflux operation.

Complicating the matter is the combined hernia with features of both paraesophageal hernia and sliding hernia with reflux. These hernias are usually large and symptomatic. They should be repaired anatomically and to control reflux. They require an anatomic repair *and* an antireflux procedure.

A posttraumatic hernia may involve any injured portion of the diaphragm. Deceleration injuries from blunt trauma usually involve the apex of the left hemidiaphragm. These hernias are usually large and are detected soon after injury from a fall or motor vehicle accident. Posttraumatic hernias involving penetrating trauma, on the other hand, can be small and miss initial detection. Any atypical diaphragmatic hernia that appears to arise away from the hiatus should raise the suspicion of previous injury. Because these hernias do not have sacs, the abdominal contents are adherent to intrathoracic structures if time has passed between the time of injury and the time of repair. Consequently, all such hernias should be approached through the abdomen if repaired at the time of the injury and through the chest if operated late. Immediately after the trauma, the concern should be for the abdominal viscera; reduction should be a simple matter of traction. Late recognition of injury leads to incarceration of the viscera in the chest. The primary risk under these circumstances is injury to both the viscera and the lung.

The abdominal contents are adherent to the edges of the diaphragmatic hernia, the lung, and the pleura and can much more safely be freed via the thoracic approach.

Complicated Paraesophageal Hiatus Hernia: Obstruction, Gastric Volvulus, and Strangulation

The patient with a large paraesophageal hernia may have a large portion of the stomach in the chest. As more and more stomach herniates, the fixed ends at the pylorus and the esophagogastric junction come close together, and volvulus becomes likely with intermittent obstruction. More complete volvulus leads to the rare but lethal complication of strangulation with necrosis and perforation. Much more commonly patients develop gastric ulcer with bleeding or obstruction with pain. An incarcerated hernia usually causes severe substernal or epigastric pain, often with an inability to vomit because of obstruction at the esophagogastric junction. All patients with these symptoms should have surgery as soon as the diagnosis has been confirmed with a chest radiograph and contrast esophagram unless the obstruction can be relieved. It may be hazardous to insert a nasogastric tube for the same reason the patients cannot vomit. If the patient is vomiting a tube can be passed safely, but in either case it should be inserted carefully with the distances measured out prior to insertion. Endoscopy or fluoroscopy should be used if there is any resistance to avoid perforation.

Surgical repair of a paraesophageal hernia should include resection of the sac, closure of the hiatus, and fixation of the anterior wall of the stomach in the abdomen if the esophagogastric junction is in normal position. The esophagogastric junction should be reduced and fixed in the abdomen if it has migrated cephalad.

Sliding Hiatus Hernia

The presence of a sliding hiatus hernia is not an indication for operation. An asymptomatic patient with a sliding hernia who has normal sphincter pressures and no significant reflux cannot be made better by medical or surgical therapy. The patient without a hiatus hernia who has significant reflux and esophagitis may be greatly improved by medical therapy or operation. It is generally agreed that medical management is the treatment of choice for patients who have symptomatic reflux with minimal esophagitis. Surgery is most clearly indicated for patients with reflux that causes significant esophagitis

and its complications of ulceration and stricture. Patients whose symptoms are completely relieved or greatly improved by modern medical management are also excellent candidates for surgery if their symptoms recur after the withdrawal of therapy (as is likely but not certain). Patients whose reflux symptoms cannot be controlled even by escalating doses of proton pump inhibitors should be carefully evaluated prior to operation to exclude other causes for their symptoms. Atypical symptoms not clearly related to reflux episodes are rarely improved by antireflux operations. The use of antireflux surgery for patients with Barrett's esophagus (columnar-lined esophagus with intestinal metaplasia) is an unresolved issue at this time. Although Barrett's esophagus is clearly a premalignant lesion, it is less clear that it can be eliminated by antireflux surgery. Comparisons of medical and surgical treatment in controlled studies have proven the superiority of surgical control of reflux during every era of medical treatment: antacids, H_2-blockers, and proton pump inhibitors [7]. Surgical control of reflux also has the advantage of controlling all the refluxate—duodenal as well as gastric—whereas medical therapy at best reduces only the amount of acid refluxed.

The minimal preoperative evaluation of a patient with gastroesophageal reflux disease (GERD) and classic symptoms should include esophagoscopy with biopsy to confirm the presence of esophagitis and a barium contrast foregut study. A timed esophageal pH study confirms the relation of symptoms to episodes of acid reflux. Manometry is useful for defining any abnormalities of sphincter location and pressure. It is also essential to position the pH probe at the proper place. Manometry can define the strength and regularity of the contractions of the body of the esophagus and can exclude defined motility disorders such as achalasia. It is not clear, however, how the surgeon can use manometric information to modify antireflux surgery. I have been able to plan antireflux surgery much more effectively by looking at the results of a standard barium meal, which clearly demonstrates the size and reducibility of the sliding hiatus hernia, the amount of shortening, and the effectiveness of peristalsis in the body of the esophagus.

Minimally invasive approaches can clearly replicate open antireflux surgery, and the short-term results with laparoscopy are excellent, although significant additional time must pass before long-term results are confirmed. At present, patients with early-stage disease seem best suited for minimally invasive surgery. With the availability of effective acid reduction, fewer patients have peptic stricture, severe ulceration, or dramatic shortening of the esophagus.

I continue to recommend open operations to patients with peptic stricture, nonreducing hernias, or an esophagus shortened enough that the gastroesophageal junction never returns to the abdomen. Further advances in laparoscopy will likely make minimally invasive surgery available to increasing numbers of patients with reflux disease.

Antireflux Operations

The multiple operations developed to prevent gastroesophageal reflux were developed empirically and only later validated. They have in common the principles of successful antireflux surgery, which seek to reproduce normal reflux control.

1. Reduce the gastroesophageal junction into the abdomen to restore the intraabdominal segment of esophagus
2. Narrow the esophageal hiatus posteriorly to increase the intraabdominal length of esophagus and prevent the development of an iatrogenic paraesophageal hernia
3. Restore the lower esophageal sphincter mechanism by creating a high pressure zone in the distal esophagus with a fundoplication

They differ in the degree of fundoplication, the method of fixation, and the approach required. Although known by the name of one or more of a technique's primary developers, it is preferable for the surgeon to define the operation by what is done than by the use of an eponym, as the current operation may little resemble the original description.

A complete (360°) fundoplication done by either the abdominal or thoracic approach is termed a Nissen-type operation [8]. Lesser degrees of anterior fundoplication follow the models of Hill [9], Watson et al. [10], or Dor et al. [11], which can only be done by the abdominal approach, or that of Belsey [12], which can only be done by the thoracic approach. Partial posterior fundoplication is termed a Toupet [13] procedure. It can be done effectively only through the abdomen. All these operations have been done by minimally invasive and open techniques.

Personal preference aside, the more complete the fundoplication, the more complete is control of reflux. The advantages of greater reflux control are offset by the more numerous postfundoplication symptoms created by the complete fundoplication. Fundoplications are associated with a reduced gastric reservoir and more rapid emptying of the stomach in addition to the abolition of both physiologic and pathologic reflux. The patient experiences postfundoplication symptoms as a result of these changes. Most patients have symptoms of early satiety, diarrhea, and increased flatus, which are usually mild and resolve over weeks to months. Some patients have a sensation of upper abdominal pressure or fullness, called the gas bloat syndrome. These symptoms are related to the changes created by the fundoplication and the habit of frequent swallowing or aerophagia common to refluxers. As the reflux resolves, so too do the postfundoplication symptoms.

The inevitable results of surgery to control reflux must be distinguished from the consequences of surgery done incorrectly. Dysphagia and the inability to belch or vomit are often listed as postfundoplication symptoms. I believe they are most often the result of too long or too tight a fundoplication and are rarely seen with appropriate narrowing of the hiatal opening, full mobilization of the fundus with division of both the short gastric vessels and posterior gastropancreatic folds, and a floppy fundoplication. Whichever operation is chosen, the fundoplication should be kept to the physiologic length and too tight a closure of the hiatus is avoided to minimize the undesirable effects of the antireflux surgery. The most reproducible operation with the best combination of durability and reflux control is the complete, loose (floppy) fundoplication done with posterior crural closure and complete mobilization of the fundus.

Benign Reflux Stricture

The most important step when dealing with a stricture in a patient with reflux is to be certain that the stricture is benign. Most carcinomas of the cardia present with symptoms of obstruction. The possibility of Barrett's esophagus with malignancy must be considered especially in white men over age 50 who have a long history of heartburn. If carcinoma can be excluded, the patient should undergo aggressive medical treatment with proton pump inhibitors and at least 40F sequential dilation prior to surgery. Almost all strictures regress with this treatment, and surgery is then greatly simplified. All patients who are good candidates for operation should undergo this initial treatment followed by antireflux surgery. Strictures that do not respond to acid reduction therapy and that cannot be dilated preoperatively with available techniques have a substantial chance of being malignant. When operating for such lesions, the surgeon must be prepared to resect the stricture, as for carcinoma. If the strictured esophagus splits open during aggressive dilation, resection is the only option. Some strictures that appear resistant to dilation dilate readily at operation with the esophagus mobilized. In my experience, all strictures not dilatable in the operating room or that split during operative dilation proved to be malignant.

The approach used when operating for stricture depends on the level of the stricture and the degree of esophageal shortening. In most cases with sliding hiatus hernia the shortening is more apparent than real, and I would approach those cases by laparotomy. Mobilization through the hiatus allows the surgeon to have the stricture under vision and in hand when dilators of increasing size are passed through the mouth to dilate the stricture. After dilation, an ample length of intraabdominal esophagus can ordinarily be restored. In the unusual case where mobilization does not allow reduction of the esophagogastric junction into the abdomen without tension, an esophageal lengthening procedure such as the standard Collis gastroplasty [14] or the uncut Collis gastroplasty described by Demos [15] can be used.

With long-standing reflux and columnar-lined esophagus, the stricture may be in the mid-esophagus and the shortening real. Such cases are best approached by thoracotomy with plans for an esophageal lengthening procedure. The surgeon must always be prepared to resect the esophagus under these circumstances. The bowel should be prepared to allow for colon or jejunal interposition as well as gastric advancement in all cases when an esophageal lengthening operation is done. Dilation is safest when it can be done with the esophagus completely mobilized using soft, tapered, mercury-filled, rubber (Maloney) bougies. With the stricture in hand, the surgeon can see and feel the stricture and dilator and can then guide the dilator precisely into the stricture and assess the pressure required to achieve dilation. Only when the esophagus is pliable and easily reducible after mobilization should transthoracic fundoplication alone be done. All other patients should have a Collis gastroplasty combined with fundoplication.

Intrathoracic fundoplication is a potentially dangerous condition. Incomplete intrathoracic fundoplications do not prevent reflux. A complete intrathoracic fundoplication is an incarcerated paraesophageal hernia and has all the associated complications of that condition including ulceration and perforation. The intraabdominal segment of tubular esophagus should be restored in all cases, and the fundoplication should always be comfortably in the abdomen. Patients with these complications have advanced reflux disease and should always be treated with a complete, short, loose (Nissen) fundoplication to control their reflux.

Failed Antireflux Operation

Secondary operations for reflux are a challenge at best and are associated with increased mortality and failure rates. After abdominal operation, the decisions to reoperate and by what technique can be dif-

ficult. Following thoracic antireflux surgery an abdominal approach may provide relatively easy access for successful fundoplication provided the esophagus is not significantly shortened or adherent to the mediastinum. Likewise, following abdominal antireflux operations a transthoracic approach has the advantage of going through a previously unoperated body cavity. In general this plan has merit, but the surgeon must be prepared to use the alternative approach of a thoracoabdominal operation or another type of surgery when dealing with this clinical problem. For the abdominal surgeon the secondary approach should be a diversion procedure [16]. Distal gastrectomy and Roux-en-Y gastrojejunostomy prevents reflux of either acid or bile into the esophagus if the defunctionalized limb is 40–50 cm long. This operation usually provides relief of symptoms at minimal surgical risk. Especially in poor risk patients, it has much to recommend it over extensive operations, such as thoracoabdominal reoperation with resection and interposition. If a resection has been done previously, a complete vagotomy can be correctly assumed. Even if vagal trunks remain, an adequate distal gastrectomy prevents marginal ulcer formation. The possibility of delayed gastric emptying following the Roux-en-Y reconstruction is a concern that has been overstated. An individualized decision based on the situation and the surgeon's expertise should be used because of the complex nature of the disease and the understandable lack of consensus among experts.

PHARYNGOESOPHAGEAL DIVERTICULUM

Normal swallowing is an elegant, complex series of events coordinated by the swallowing center in the medulla. In the peristaltic sequence, both the upper and lower esophageal sphincters must relax to ensure proper timing to allow the bolus to pass. The upper esophageal sphincter—the cricopharyngeus muscle and the adjacent upper cervical esophagus—and the lower esophageal high pressure zone are physiologic sphincters. They are in a state of contraction in the resting state and then relax on stimulation. A pharyngoesophageal (Zenker's) diverticulum develops in the posterior midline just above the cricopharyngeus muscle. The pathophysiology appears to be a lack of coordination in the relaxation of the upper sphincter with a resultant false diverticulum through the weak area of the distal pharyngeal constrictor. Whatever the cause, Zenker's diverticulum is a progressive disorder with no known medical treatment that should be corrected by surgery when diagnosed. The operation is simple and straightforward with the use of surgical staplers. The diverticulum almost always projects toward the left, so it is best approached through a left cervical incision. Although the operation can be performed under local anesthesia, it is far better done under general anesthesia to control the airway and allow intubation of the esophagus. It is well tolerated in elderly, poor risk patients who characteristically have this disease.

The size of the diverticulum is not predictive of the severity of the patient's symptomatology. Small diverticula can be associated with severe dysphagia. Both that and the average length of the upper sphincter of >3 cm make combining myotomy and diverticulectomy the only logical operation for both the more common Zenker's diverticula, which are easily diagnosed radiographically, and those rare patients with dysphagia caused by upper esophageal sphincter disorders and so-called cricopharyngeal achalasia, which are related to neurologic dysfunction and which must be manometrically proven.

PERFORATIONS AND ANASTOMOTIC LEAKS

"Conservative" Management

Untreated, esophageal perforations are uniformly fatal. Expectant or nonoperative management of esophageal perforations is hardly "conservative." Although nonoperative treatment has a place in highly selected situations such as small perforations of the pharynx from endoscopy and clinically insignificant anastomotic leaks, its use must be confined to those settings in which the leak is proven to be small, contained or adequately drained, and minimally symptomatic with no sign of systemic sepsis. The posterior mediastinum has no compartments and poor defenses against the spread of infection. Perforation of the cervical esophagus can track through the mediastinum and into the retroperitoneum. A radiographically "small" thoracic perforation can cause a fulminant mediastinitis and lead to hydropneumothorax and empyema. Any pleural air or fluid is a contraindication to continued expectant management.

The essentials for treating perforations are as follows:

1. Early identification of the perforation
2. Accurate localization of the site of perforation
3. Control of the airway and pulmonary decompression
4. Adequate drainage of the leak
5. Broad-spectrum antibiotic coverage
6. Supportive care

7. Operation for débridement and closure of the perforation whenever it is appropriate and possible

Adequate drainage can be accomplished surgically or by radiographically guided intervention. Adequate drainage implies that the drain goes to the site of the perforation and completely controls the leakage. Débridement of devitalized mediastinal tissues and decortication of the pleural space are necessary to restore pulmonary function and treat the infection.

The mixture of digestive enzymes and foreign material characteristic of traumatic and postemetic perforations creates a fertile ground for microbial growth. Antibiotic therapy should cover aerobic and anaerobic bacteria and yeasts. Although proximal perforations contain mouth organisms generally sensitive to penicillin, the bacterial flora quickly changes to resemble that in the colon, so an antibiotic regimen suitable for a colon perforation should be used. The esophagus also contains large numbers of yeast, especially *Candida* species, which are more of a problem the longer the perforation is untreated.

Supportive care must include enteral or parenteral nutritional support. A feeding jejunostomy should be done in most cases.

Surgical Repair

Suture or stapled repair alone is unwise unless the perforation occurs during operation, occurs in normal tissue, and can be immediately repaired. Even under those circumstances, buttress of the repair with viable tissue is a logical approach. For all other circumstances, the surgeon should always buttress the repair with viable tissue and provide adequate drainage [17]. Parietal pleura, intercostal muscle, pericardium, diaphragm, and stomach have all been used successfully, and the choice depends on location and available tissue. Successful repair can still be achieved more than 48 hours after perforation with a buttress of viable tissue so long as the esophagus was normal prior to perforation and there is no distal obstruction [18]. Proximal and distal tube decompression are useful adjuncts but are not substitutes for an adequate repair.

When the esophagus is abnormal, resection is the best treatment. The resection can be done by a cervical approach combined with an abdominal and transhiatal or a transthoracic approach. The most effective proximal esophageal diversion is total thoracic esophagectomy with end-cervical esophagostomy. Primary anastomosis is usually unwise in this setting. The esophagogastric junction should be closed and the stomach decompressed with a gastrostomy. Reconstruction with stomach or colon can follow at an appropriate interval. In the special case of perforation following balloon dilation for achalasia, a complete myotomy of the distal sphincter must be done along with the buttressed repair.

ESOPHAGEAL PERFORATION AT VARIOUS ANATOMIC LEVELS

Cervical Esophagus

The cervical esophagus may be perforated during endoscopy, during endotracheal intubation, by swallowing a foreign body, or by external trauma. Although endoscopic perforations of the pharynx can almost be managed with antibiotics and usually do not need drainage, cervical perforations below the cricopharyngeal sphincter are a much more serious matter. The esophageal perforation in this location may be several centimeters long, and prompt surgical exploration should be the rule. Exploration of this area is a simple procedure, and adequate drainage prevents spread of the contamination into the thoracic mediastinum. All patients who are febrile or have tenderness or swelling in the neck should undergo exploration and drainage of the retropharyngeal space. All cervical esophageal perforations should be repaired. Repair of pharyngeal perforations is usually neither feasible nor necessary.

Thoracic Esophagus

Perforation by Instrumentation: Dilator or Endoscope

Pain, crepitation, fever, leukocytosis, mediastinal emphysema, and pneumothorax or hydropneumothorax are evidence of esophageal perforation following instrumentation as under other circumstances, but these findings develop gradually over 12–24 hours. When selecting the proper treatment for a patient with an iatrogenic perforation diagnosed within a few hours of the event, remember that the patient may look quite well during the first few hours only to collapse hours later with fulminating mediastinitis. Water-soluble contrast can define the presence and location of a perforation in almost all cases, but the study cannot accurately define the size of the perforation or the extent of spread of contamination in the mediastinum. If the signs and symptoms suggest a perforation but the contrast study is negative, CT or barium should be used to confirm the absence of perforation. Flexible endoscopy has only a limited role. Although normal esophageal mucosa excludes perforation, if a perforation is present insufflation can lead to tension pneumothorax. Therefore flexible endoscopy should be used only after decompressive thoracostomy or negative contrast studies.

All patients with instrumental perforation should be treated by exploration and drainage. Closed-tube thoracostomy is ineffective as definitive therapy. Buttressed repair or resection should be done depending on the pathology of the esophagus. Obstruction of the esophagus must be relieved if treatment is to be successful.

Barotrauma: Boerhaave Syndrome and External Pressure

Postemetic perforations of the thoracic esophagus are dangerous because they occur in a patient with a full stomach. Vomiting against a closed glottis floods the mediastinum with food, microbes, and digestive secretions. Rapidly developing, fulminant mediastinitis is the result, and patients often present late for medical care. Diagnosis is often further delayed because esophageal perforation is not considered. A missed diagnosis is common after the patient presents for emergency care. Mediastinal emphysema on the chest radiograph is diagnostic and should lead to a water-soluble contrast study to confirm the diagnosis and location even though the site of perforation is almost always in the distal esophagus with extension into the left pleura with Boerhaave syndrome. With a blast injury from external pressure, the perforation may be anywhere in the esophagus. In the absence of trauma, hydropneumothorax is diagnostic of esophageal perforation.

After resuscitation, chest decompression, and control of the airway, thoracotomy for decortication, repair of the esophagus with a parietal pleural flap, and adequate drainage is almost always successful even if the delay to operation is more than 24 hours. Although primary closure without leak is not achieved in every case, the fistula can be well controlled by the flap and drainage; and spontaneous closure occurs within weeks [19]. After completion of the thoracic phase, a separate laparotomy to place a gastrostomy and jejunostomy should be done in all patients.

ANASTOMOTIC LEAKS

Patients who develop a leak following a cervical anastomosis respond well to drainage so long as the interposition is viable, especially if drainage was established at surgery. Although an anastomotic stricture may develop secondary to the leak, systemic or mediastinal sepsis is unusual and recovery is expected. These strictures usually respond to sequential dilations.

Anastomotic failure following intrathoracic anastomosis is a far more serious occurrence. Although most patients survive, their hospitalizations are usually long and complicated. Without prompt, adequate treatment, death from sepsis and organ failure is probable. I believe that virtually all anastomotic leaks result from technical errors at operation. They are present but not clinically apparent early when the defect could be corrected by reoperation. The best time to check for leakage is in the operating room. In addition to inspection of the anastomosis, insufflation through the nasogastric tube distends the stomach and reveals gross defects in a stapled or sutured anastomosis. In the past, we conducted studies at 5–7 days, if at all, before allowing oral intake. For the past several years I have been doing contrast studies on all patients on the first postoperative day. The study is done first with a small amount of water-soluble contrast and then with barium if the first part of the swallow shows no leak. If the study is normal, patients are allowed liquids immediately. If the study is equivocal, a CT scan is obtained to look for extraluminal contrast. If none is seen, I leave the chest tube in place to maintain the seal of the lung around the anastomosis and withhold oral intake until a repeat study is normal. If a leak is demonstrated, the patient can be returned to the operating room for repair with a viable tissue buttress and wide drainage before extensive tissue reaction and infection limit the chance of success. Even if the leak is not completely sealed, the resulting lateral fistula is well controlled and closes spontaneously. If a jejunostomy was not done at the original operation, it should be done at this time.

If a leak is recognized late, reoperation should be done as soon as the patient can be prepared for anesthesia. Débridement, decortication, and closure can be attempted if the defect is small; but the realistic goal is creation of a controlled fistula and control of sepsis. Antibacterial and antifungal therapy is essential under these circumstances. Enteral feeding by jejunostomy is a necessary part of management.

Nonoperative treatment is a tenable plan only if strict criteria are met [18]. The leak must be an insignificant radiographic finding. It must be a small, localized sinus that drains completely back into the lumen and does not involve the pleural space. The presence of pneumothorax or significant effusion mandates exploration, as does any sign of systemic toxicity. CT scanning is essential to confirm that the sinus is behaving like a diverticulum, which would promptly resolve by itself. Broad-spectrum antibiotics and parenteral or enteral nutrition by jejunos-

tomy should be used until healing is confirmed by a contrast study. Oral intake should await proof that no leak is present.

In the catastrophic situation of complete anastomotic dehiscence or necrosis of the interposition, the source of sepsis must be completely eliminated to avoid death from multiple organ failure. All nonviable tissue must be débrided. Decortication and wide pleural drainage help the antibacterial and antifungal therapy clear the sepsis. The anastomosis should be resected and the esophagus exteriorized as an end-esophagostomy. The stomach should be returned to the abdomen, closed, and drained with a gastrostomy. Reconstruction usually requires colon interposition and can be done at an appropriate time.

Occult perforation is a problem during esophageal surgery, especially with minimally invasive approaches. Hence testing for leaks should be done in the operating room and on the first postoperative day in all patients who undergo resection, myotomy, and fundoplication.

ACHALASIA

Achalasia, an acquired disease of unknown etiology, is characterized by denervation pathology. The ganglion cells of the myenteric plexus are lost, and the patient develops a hypertonic, nonrelaxing distal esophageal sphincter with an aperistaltic body of the esophagus that progressively dilates and then elongates. In the long term, patients with achalasia have an increased risk of epidermoid carcinoma. Their nutrition is usually well preserved, and patients typically present with a long history of eating slowly and dysphagia to liquids more than solids that is not progressive. All treatment modalities rely on ablation of the lower esophageal sphincter mechanism to allow more normal but passive emptying of the esophagus. In all cases, the striated muscle proximal to the esophagus retains its normal size and contraction. The methodologies available today include temporary paralysis of the muscle of the sphincter with botulinum toxin, disruption of the muscle by balloon dilation, and surgical myotomy. Botulinum injection has had a predictably transient effect. The only difference between surgical and balloon myotomy is that the modified Heller myotomy is more controlled and more effective than the balloon procedure. The availability of minimally invasive surgical approaches has largely rendered balloon myotomy irrelevant. Because of the possibility of perforation, all patients with balloon disruption of the sphincter should have surgical backup, and all should have follow-up contrast studies as soon as possible to exclude perforation.

All patients should be studied with radiography, manometry, and endoscopy to confirm the diagnosis and to exclude other causes of pseudoachalasia in even the most typical cases. When the diagnostic combination of an aperistaltic body of the esophagus with a nonrelaxing distal sphincter is present, the surgeon must chose among the available surgical approaches. The sphincter can be approached to perform a myotomy from the left chest or from the abdomen. The surgeon may use either a minimally invasive or open technique with or without an antireflux fundoplication. Although a complete myotomy can be done by any of the approaches, only a myotomy done by an expert through a left thoracotomy can be done accurately enough to complete the myotomy and not have an unacceptable amount of reflux [20]. Approached through the left chest, the pattern of vessels that mark the cephalad margin of the stomach can be identified as the lower limit of the sphincter and of the myotomy without disrupting the anatomy of the cardia. This anatomic landmark cannot be visualized adequately by thoracoscopy or through the abdomen. The most important principle is to complete the division of the sphincter. To do so by any of the other approaches, the myotomy must be carried down well onto the stomach, and the operation must include a partial circumference fundoplication to minimize reflux. At present, a laparoscopic myotomy with anterior, partial fundoplication is the operation most acceptable to patients and physicians and most easily done by many surgeons. The integrity of the mucosa must be ensured in the operating room and should be confirmed by a contrast study within 24 hours to identify incomplete myotomy and exclude perforation.

The morbidity associated with laparotomy is little different than that seen with laparoscopy for myotomy and fundoplication. The surgeon must exercise good judgment when choosing the approach best suited to the individual patient. Extensive previous abdominal surgery may make a laparotomy or thoracic approach a better choice for such a patient. Reoperative surgery for achalasia can be challenging. For patients with failed operations for achalasia and for end-stage disease with sigmoidization of the esophagus, resection with gastric interposition and esophagogastrostomy in the neck or at the apex of the right thorax is an effective, durable option.

OTHER MOTILITY DISORDERS

Diverse motility disorders of the esophagus—diffuse esophageal spasm, corkscrew esophagus, nutcracker esophagus, and others—have been described. They are poorly understood disorders of the body of the esophagus that do not affect the distal sphincter. The various diseases can be diagnosed and distinguished from achalasia and reflux by motility and pH studies. In the past, there has been enthusiasm for surgical procedures such as long myotomy of the body of the esophagus, but the results are mediocre at best. Although there may be a place for long myotomy in carefully selected patients who have failed medical therapy, almost all these patients should be treated pharmacologically.

REFERENCES

1. Akiyama H. Surgery for Cancer of the Esophagus. Baltimore, Williams & Wilkins, 1980.
2. Ellis FH Jr, Gibb SP, Watkins E Jr. Esophagogastrectomy: a safe, widely applicable, and expeditious form of palliation for patients with carcinoma of the esophagus and cardia. Ann Surg 1983;198:531.
3. Mathiesen DJ, Grillo HC, Wilkins EW, et al. Transthoracic esophagectomy: a safe approach to carcinoma of the esophagus. Ann Thorac Surg 1988;45:137.
4. Orringer MB, Marshall B, Stirling MC. Transhiatal esophagectomy for benign and malignant disease. J Thorac Cardiovasc Surg 1993;105:265.
5. Gavrilu D. Report on the procedure of reconstruction of the esophagus by gastric tube. Int Abstr Surg 1965;121:655.
6. Heimlich HJ. Esophagoplasty with reversed gastric tube: review of 53 cases. Am J Surg 1972;123:80.
7. Spechler SJ, Veterans Administration Reflux Disease Study Group. Comparison of medical and surgical therapy for complicated gastroesophageal reflux disease in veterans. N Engl J Med 1992;326:786.
8. Donahue PE, Samuelson S, Nyhus LM, Bombeck CT. The floppy Nissen fundoplication: effective long term control of pathologic reflux. Arch Surg 1985;120:663.
9. Hill LD. An effective operation for hiatal hernia: an eight year appraisal. Ann Surg 1967;166:681.
10. Watson A, Jenkinson LR, Ball CS, Barlow AP, Norris TL. A more physiological alternative to total fundoplication for the surgical correction of resistant gastroesophageal reflux. Br J Surg 1991;78:1088.
11. Dor J, Humbert P, Paoli JM, et al. Traitement du reflus per la technique de Helle-Nissen modifiee. Presse Med 1967;75:2563.
12. Belsey R. Hiatal herniorrhaphy. In: Malt R (ed) Surgical Techniques Illustrated, vol 1, no. 2. Boston, Little Brown, 1976, p 5.
13. Toupet A. Technique d'oesophagogastroplastie avec phrenogastropexie appliquee dans la cure radicale des hernia hiatales et comme complement de l'operation de Heller dans les cardiospasms. Mem Acad Chir (Paris) 1963;89:374.
14. Pearson FG, Langer B, Henderson RD. Gastroplasty and Belsey hiatus hernia repair. J Thorac Cardiovasc Surg 1971;61:50.

15. Demos NJ. Stapled, uncut gastroplasty for hiatal hernia: 12 year follow-up. Ann Thorac Surg 1984;38:393.

16. Fekete F, Pateron D. What is the place of antrectomy with Roux-en-Y in the treatment of reflux disease? Experience with 83 total duodenal diversions. World J Surg 1992;16:349.

17. Richardson JD, Martin LF, Borzotta AP, Polk HC. Unifying concepts in the treatment of esophageal leaks. Am J Surg 1985;149:157.

18. Cameron JL, Kieffer RF, Hendrix TR, Mehigan DG, Baker RR. Selective nonoperative treatment of contained intrathoracic esophageal disruptions. Ann Thorac Surg 1979;27:404.

19. Gouge TH, DePan HJ, Spencer FC. Experience with the Grillo pleural wrap procedure in 18 patients with perforation of the thoracic esophagus. Ann Surg 1989;209:612.

20. Ellis FH Jr, Watkins E Jr, Gibb SP, Heatley GJ: Ten to 20 year clinical results after short esophagomyotomy without an antireflux procedure (modified Heller operation) for esophageal achalasia. Eur J Cardiothorac Surg 1992;6:86.

11 Esophagectomy

Right Thoracotomy and Laparotomy

INDICATIONS

Carcinoma of the esophagus

PREOPERATIVE PREPARATION

Institute nutritional rehabilitation by parenteral alimentation or nasogastric tube feeding in patients who have lost more than 10 lb.

Perform preoperative esophagoscopy and biopsy.

Use computed tomography (CT) and other staging studies, including preoperative bronchoscopy, to detect invasion of the tracheobronchial tree.

Improve oral and dental hygiene, if necessary.

Insist on smoking cessation.

Conduct pulmonary function studies.

Preoperative chemotherapy and radiation therapy is appropriate in selected cases.

Pass a nasogastric tube before operation.

Administer perioperative antibiotics.

PITFALLS AND DANGER POINTS

Hemorrhage from aorta

Perforation of trachea or bronchus

Anastomotic leak

Anastomotic stenosis

Inadvertent interruption of gastroepiploic arcade on greater curvature of the stomach

OPERATIVE STRATEGY

The right chest allows access to the upper esophagus with resection of associated lymphatic tissue. The stomach must be fully mobilized during the abdominal phase of the operation. With care to preserve the arterial supply and venous drainage, the stomach can be extended as far as the cervical esophagus. Anastomosis in the neck allows the greatest margin of safety if anastomotic leakage occurs.

Critical errors such as attempting to resect a tumor that has invaded adjacent structures (aorta, bronchus, trachea) can be avoided by accurate preoperative staging. Anastomotic leakage and postoperative stenosis may be minimized by adopting several techniques. Maintain the blood supply to the stomach by meticulous attention to the gastroepiploic arcade. *The esophageal hiatus must be enlarged sufficiently to prevent any element of venous compression, as obstruction of the venous circulation is as detrimental as arterial ischemia.* The end-to-side esophagogastric anastomosis described here has markedly reduced the incidence of anastomotic leaks in our experience (see Chapter 12).

Because the submucosal spread of esophageal carcinoma has been observed by microscopy to extend a considerable distance cephalad from the visible carcinoma, remove a 10 cm margin of apparently normal esophagus with the specimen. Check the upper limit of the specimen by frozen section examination. Ease of access to the proximal esophagus is one of the major advantages of this operative approach.

OPERATIVE TECHNIQUE

Incision and Position

Use a small sandbag to elevate the patient's right side 30°, with the right arm abducted and suspended from the "ether screen" cephalad to the surgical field. Turn the patient's head to the left in case the right cervical region has to be exposed for the esophagogastric anastomosis. Prepare the right neck, right hemithorax, and abdomen. Rotate the operating table slightly so the abdomen is parallel with the floor. After induction of one-lung endotracheal anesthesia, perform a midline upper abdominal

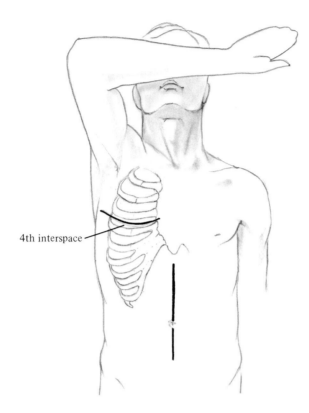

4th interspace

Fig. 11-1

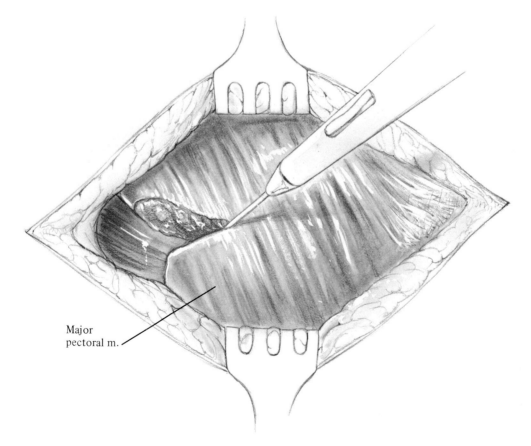

Major
pectoral m.

Fig. 11-2

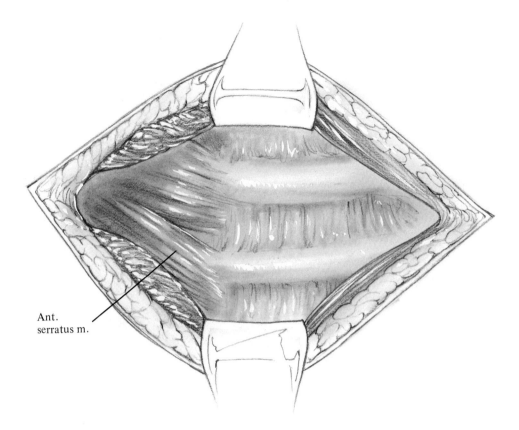

Ant.
serratus m.

Fig. 11-3

incision for preliminary exploration of the liver and lower esophagus to help determine if resection should be attempted.

Then, in men, make an incision along the course of the fourth intercostal space from the sternum to the posterior axillary line **(Fig. 11–1)**. In women, make the skin incision in the inframammary fold. Incise the pectoral and anterior serratus muscles with electrocautery along the fourth interspace **(Figs. 11–2, 11–3)**. Similarly incise the intercostal muscles along the upper border of the fifth rib. Identify the internal mammary artery near the sternal margin, doubly ligate it, and divide it. Enter the pleura of the fourth intercostal space and then divide the cartilaginous portion of the fourth rib near its articulation with the sternum **(Fig. 11–4)**. Clamp the

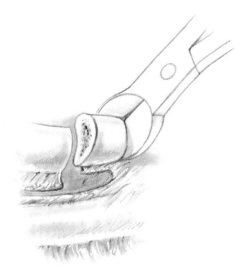

Fig. 11-4

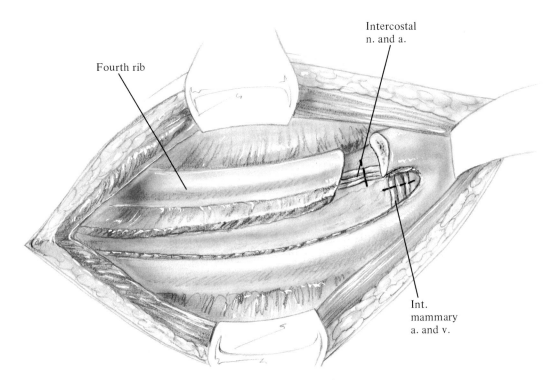

Fourth rib

Intercostal
n. and a.

Int.
mammary
a. and v.

Fig. 11-5

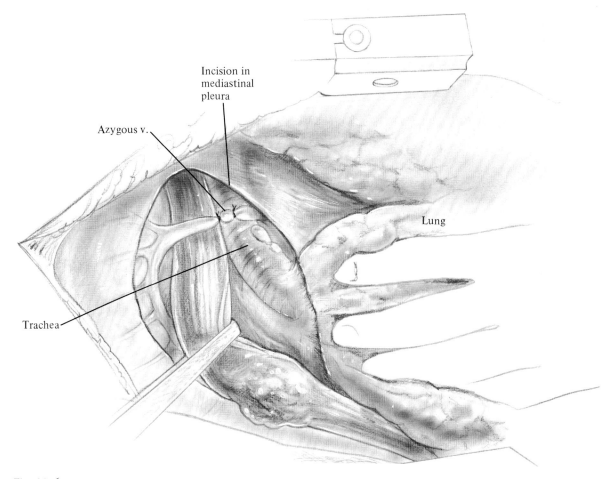

Incision in
mediastinal
pleura

Azygous v.

Lung

Trachea

Fig. 11-6

neurovascular bundle, divide it, and ligate with 2-0 silk **(Fig. 11–5)**.

Insert a Finochietto retractor over gauze pads and separate the ribs. If an additional costal cartilage requires division for adequate exposure, do not hesitate to perform this maneuver. Retract the lung anteriorly, cover it with gauze pads, and hold it with Harrington refractors.

Some surgeons prefer a posterolateral thoracotomy incision from the region of the paraspinal muscles to the sternum through the fourth or fifth interspace, but we have found the above exposure to be satisfactory. Using the anterior incision permits placing the patient in a position that is convenient for operating in the abdomen, the thorax, and even the neck, as necessary.

Mobilization of Esophagus

Make an incision in the mediastinal pleura, exposing the esophagus. Identify the azygous vein. Skeletonize, divide, and ligate it with 2-0 silk **(Fig. 11–6)**. Encircle the esophagus with the index finger at a point away from the tumor. The dissection reveals several small arterial branches to the esophagus. Divide each branch between hemostatic clips. Wherever the pericardium or pleura is adherent to the tumor, excise patches of these structures and leave them attached to the specimen. Include adjacent mediastinal lymph nodes in the specimen. Dissect the esophagus from the apex of the chest to the diaphragmatic hiatus; this maneuver requires division of the proximal vagal trunks. To minimize spillage of tumor cells, ligate the lumen of the esophagus proximal and distal to the tumor, utilizing narrow umbilical tapes or a 55 mm linear surgical stapler.

Remove the Harrington retractors and gauze pads, permitting the right lung to expand. Cover the thoracic incision with a sterile towel.

Mobilization of Stomach

Expose the abdominal incision. Use a Thompson retractor to elevate the sternum. Elevate the left lobe of the liver in a cephalad direction with the Weinberg blade of the Thompson retractor and incise the peritoneum overlying the abdominal esophagus. Circumferentially mobilize the lower esophagus. Transect the vagal trunks and surrounding phrenoesophageal ligaments **(Figs. 11–7, 11–8, 11–9)**. The cephalad portion of the gastrohepatic ligament, generally containing an accessory left hepatic artery, should be doubly clamped, divided, and ligated with

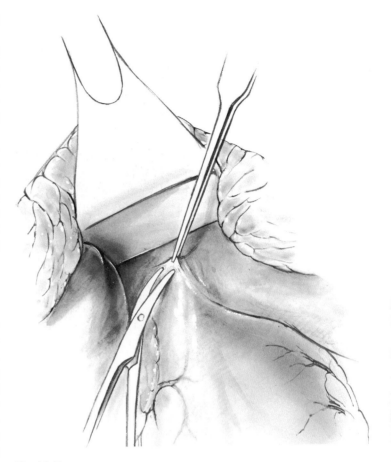

Fig. 11-7

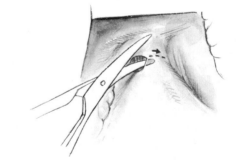

Fig. 11-8

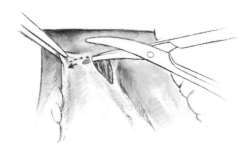

Fig. 11-9

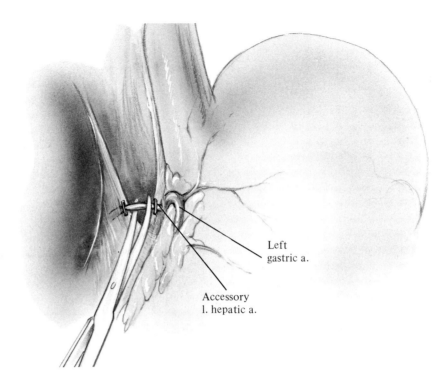

Left
gastric a.

Accessory
l. hepatic a.

Fig. 11–10

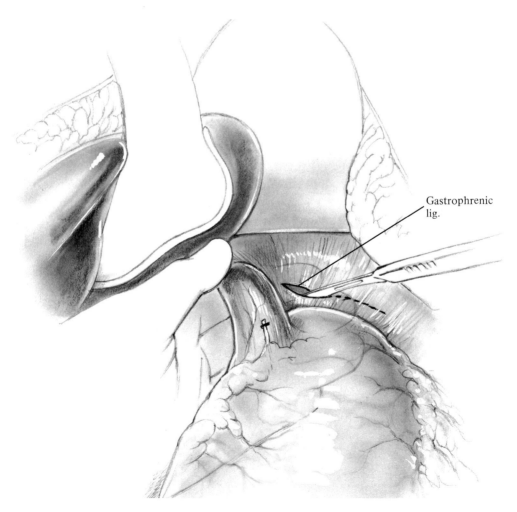

Gastrophrenic
lig.

Fig. 11–11

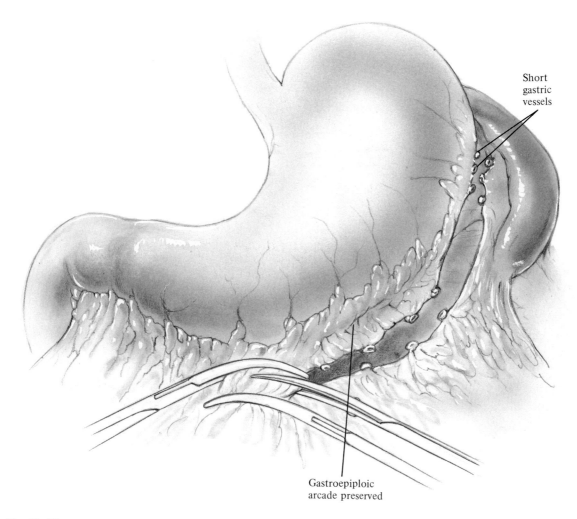

Short
gastric
vessels

Gastroepiploic
arcade preserved

Fig. 11-12a

2-0 silk or Hemoclips **(Fig. 11–10)**. Insert the left
hand behind the esophagus and cardia of the stomach, elevate the gastrophrenic ligaments on the index finger, and transect them **(Fig. 11–11)**. This dissection leads to the cephalad short gastric vessel;
divide it between clamps and ligate it, along with
the remaining short gastric vessels. The spleen need
not be removed.

Divide and ligate the *left* gastroepiploic artery, but
perform the remainder of the dissection *outside the
gastroepiploic arcade, which must be kept intact
and free of trauma*. This is accomplished by dividing the greater omentum serially between Kelly
clamps, leaving 3-5 cm of omentum attached to
the arcade as a margin of safety. Discontinue this
dissection 6-8 cm proximal to the pylorus **(Fig.
11–12)**.

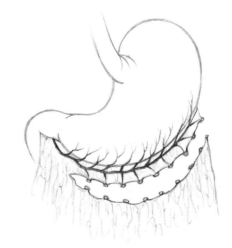

Fig. 11-12b

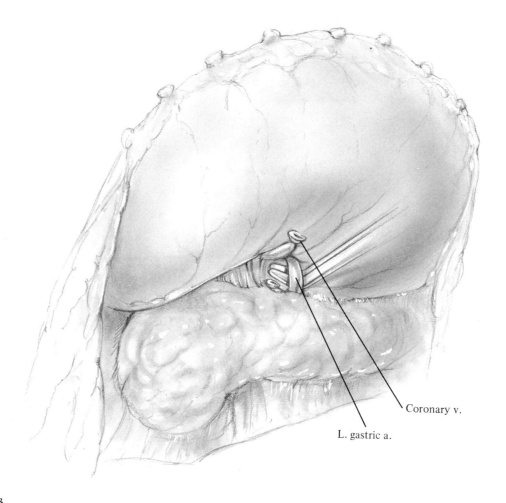

Coronary v.

L. gastric a.

Fig. 11-13

With the greater curvature of the stomach elevated, use palpation to identify the origin of the left gastric artery at the celiac axis. The coronary vein is situated just caudal to the artery. Clear it and encircle it with a Mixter clamp. Then divide it between 2-0 silk ligatures. Skeletonize the left gastric artery **(Fig. 11–13)** so two 2-0 ligatures can be placed on the proximal portion of the artery and one on the specimen side. Transect the vessel and follow with an extensive Kocher maneuver.

Kocher Maneuver

Make an incision in the peritoneum lateral to the proximal duodenum **(Fig. 11–14)**. Insert the left index finger behind the peritoneum and compress this tissue between fingertip and thumb, pushing retroperitoneal blood vessels and fat away. Incise the peritoneum on the index finger with scissors until the third portion of the duodenum is reached. Note that dividing the peritoneum alone is not sufficient to release the duodenum from its posterior attachments.

There remains a ligamentous structure connecting the posterior duodenum to the region of Gerota's fascia. This ligamentous structure is easily delineated by inserting the left index finger behind the pan-

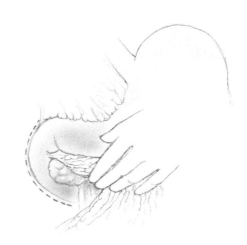

Fig. 11-14

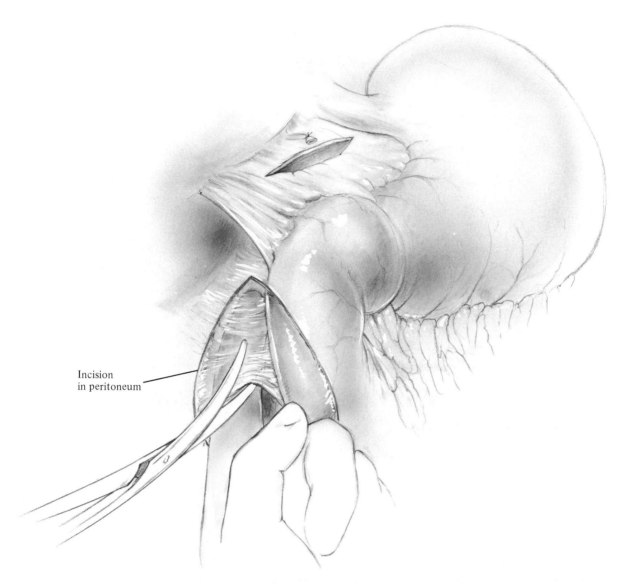

Incision
in peritoneum

Fig. 11-15

creas. Move the finger laterally, exposing a lateral duodenal "ligament" behind the descending duodenum. Again, pinch the tissue between fingertip and thumb, which leaves vascular and fatty tissue behind, allowing this ligamentous structure to be divided. Incise it with Metzenbaum scissors **(Fig. 11–15)**. Repeat this maneuver, going around the second and third portions of duodenum (behind the hepatic flexure); this leads to the point at which the superior mesenteric vein crosses over the duodenum. *Be careful*, as excessive traction with the index finger may tear this vessel.

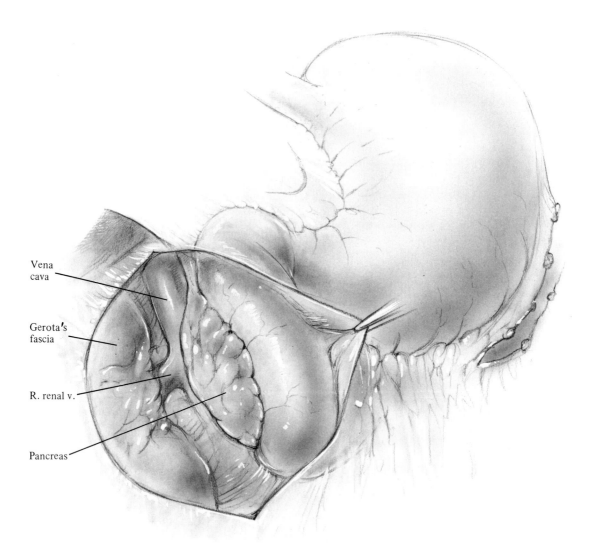

Vena
cava

Gerota's
fascia

R. renal v.

Pancreas

Fig. 11-16

For esophagogastric resection the Kocher maneuver need not be continued much beyond the
junction of the second and third portions of the duodenum. At this point the left hand is easily passed
behind the head of the pancreas, which should be
elevated from the renal capsule, vena cava, and aorta
(Fig. 11–16). This permits the pyloroduodenal segment to be placed high in the abdomen, 8-10 cm
from the esophageal hiatus, which in turn permits
the gastric fundus to reach the thoracic apex, or
neck, without tension.

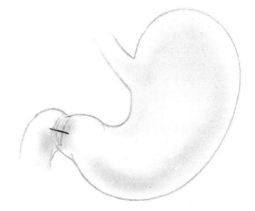

Fig. 11-17

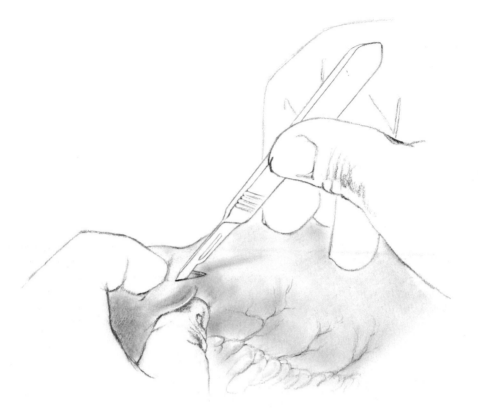

Fig. 11-18

Pyloromyotomy

Although in 80% of patients satisfactory results may
be obtained without it, pyloromyotomy is generally
performed at this point to prevent secondary operations for excessive gastric stasis due to vagotomy.
Pyloromyotomy is accomplished by making a 1.5-
to 2.0-cm incision across the anterior surface of
the pyloric sphincter muscle **(Figs. 11–17, 11–18,
11–19)**. This maneuver is more difficult in an adult
(who has only the normal thickness of muscle) than
in an infant who suffers hypertrophic pyloric stenosis. Frequently, sharp dissection with a no. 15 scalpel
blade must be done through most of the circular
muscle. Separate the muscle fibers with a hemostat
until the mucosa bulges out. This procedure may be
expedited by invaginating the anterior gastric wall
into the pyloric sphincter with the index finger to
divide the few remaining circular muscle fibers.
Exercise care not to perforate the mucosa, which is
prone to such injury at the duodenal end of the incision.

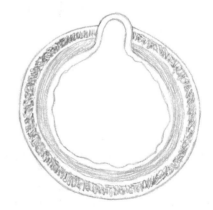

Fig. 11-19

Advancement of Stomach into Right Chest

Divide the right crux of the diaphragm transversely using electrocautery **(Fig. 11–20)** and further dilate the esophageal hiatus manually. Advance the stomach into the right hemithorax, which should again be exposed by expanding the Finochietto retractor. There must be *no constriction of the veins* in the vascular pedicle of the stomach at the hiatus. Suture the wall of stomach to the margins of the hiatus by means of interrupted 3-0 silk or Tevdek sutures spaced 2 cm apart to avoid postoperative herniation of bowel into the chest.

With the right lung collapsed, expose the esophagogastric junction in the right chest. When the esophageal carcinoma is located in the middle or upper esophagus, it is not necessary to remove the lesser curvature of the stomach and the celiac lymph nodes.

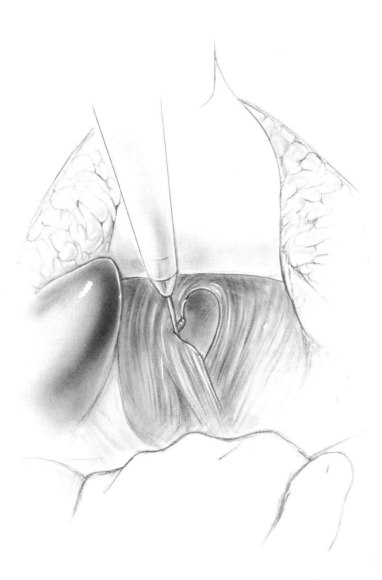

Fig. 11-20

After clearing the areolar tissue and the fat pad from the region of the esophagocardiac junction, apply a 55/4.8 mm linear stapler to the gastric side of this junction and fire the staples. Apply an Allen clamp to the esophagus, which should be transected flush with the stapler. Place a rubber glove over the divided esophagus and fix it in place with a narrow tape ligature. Lightly electrocoagulate the everted gastric mucosa and remove the stapling device **(Fig. 11–21)**. It is not necessary to invert this stapled closure with a layer of sutures. The fundus of the stomach should now reach the apex of the thorax without tension. Take care to avoid twisting the stomach and its vascular pedicle.

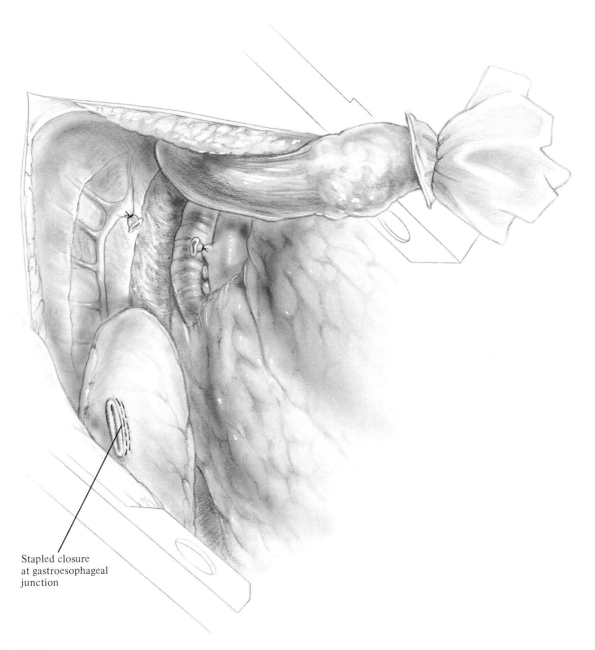

Stapled closure
at gastroesophageal
junction

Fig. 11-21

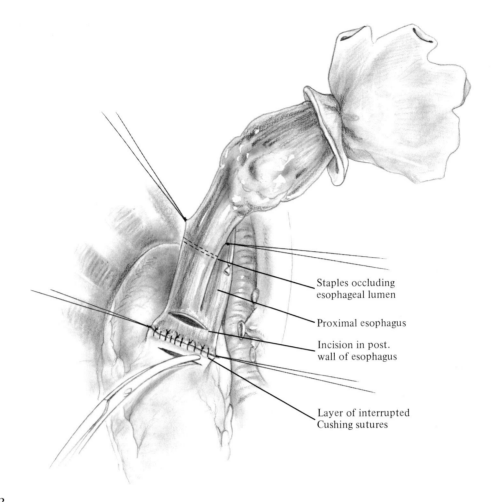

Staples occluding
esophageal lumen

Proximal esophagus

Incision in post.
wall of esophagus

Layer of interrupted
Cushing sutures

Fig. 11-22

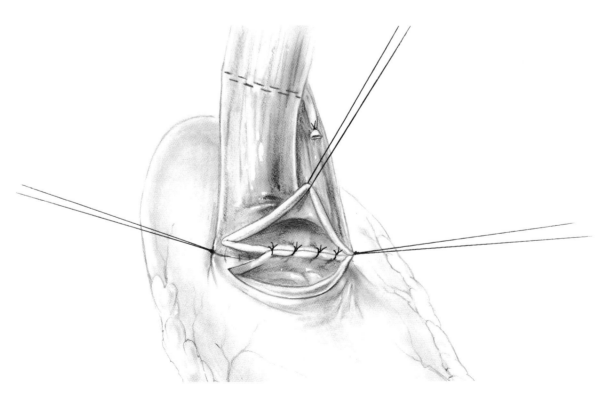

Fig. 11-23

Esophagogastric Anastomosis

Select a point on the proximal esophagus 10 cm above the tumor for the anastomosis. Before removing the specimen, insert the posterior layer of sutures to attach the posterior esophagus to the anterior seromuscular layer of the stomach at a point 6–7 cm from the cephalad end of the fundus **(Fig. 11–22)**. The posterior layer should consist of about five interrupted atraumatic 4-0 silk Cushing sutures. Each bite should be 5 mm in width and deep enough to catch submucosa. The Stratte needle-holder (see Glossary) may facilitate suture placement.

Transect the posterior wall of the esophagus with a scalpel at a point 6 mm beyond the first line of sutures. One can be certain that the esophageal mucosa has been transected when the nasogastric tube appears in the esophageal lumen. Now make a transverse incision in the stomach and control the bleeding points. This incision should be slightly longer than the diameter of the esophagus (Fig. 11-22).

Approximate the posterior mucosal layer by means of interrupted or continuous 5-0 atraumatic PG sutures, with the knots tied inside the lumen **(Fig. 11–23)**. Then pass the nasogastric tube from the proximal esophagus through the anastomosis into the stomach.

Detach the specimen by dividing the anterior wall of the esophagus with scissors in such fashion as to leave the anterior wall of the esophagus 1 cm longer than the posterior wall **(Fig. 11–24)**. This maneuver enlarges the stoma if the incision in the stomach is large enough to match that of the elliptical esophageal lumen.

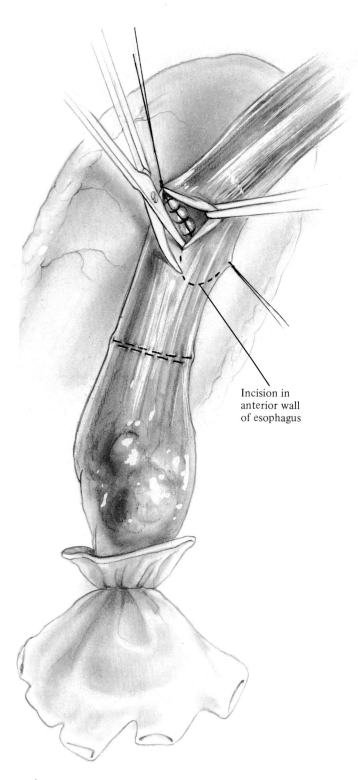

Incision in anterior wall of esophagus

Fig. 11-24

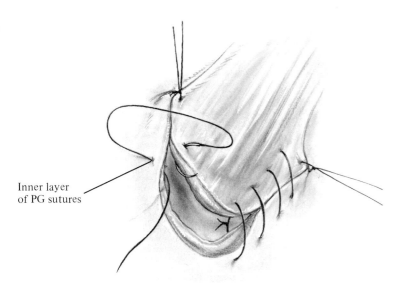

Inner layer
of PG sutures

Fig. 11-25

Execute the anterior mucosal layer by means of interrupted sutures of 5-0 PG, with the knots tied inside the lumen thus inverting the mucosa **(Fig. 11–25)**. Accomplish the second anterior layer by means of interrupted Cushing sutures of 4-0 silk **(Fig. 11–26)**. Tie these sutures gently to approximate but not strangulate the tissue.

At this point some surgeons perform a Nissen fundoplication, which can be done if there is enough loose gastric wall to permit a wraparound without constricting the esophagus. Otherwise, a partial fundoplication may be accomplished by inserting several sutures between the outer walls of the esophagus and adjacent stomach. We have observed that even if fundoplication is not performed few patients develop reflux esophagitis following this operation so long as end-to-side esophagogastric anastomosis has been accomplished 6 cm or more below the cephalad margin of the gastric remnant.

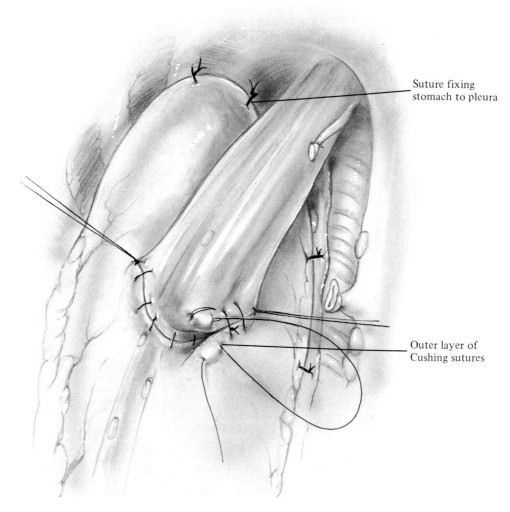

Suture fixing
stomach to pleura

Outer layer of
Cushing sutures

Fig. 11-26

Surgeons who lack wide experience with this anastomosis might find it wise to inflate the gastric pouch to test the anastomosis for leakage. A solution of methylene blue is injected into the nasogastric tube by the anesthesiologist for this purpose.

As a final, essential step in this operation, tension on the anastomosis is prevented by tacking the fundus of the stomach to the prevertebral fascia and mediastinal pleura at the apex of the thorax. Use interrupted sutures of 3-0 silk or Tevdek for this purpose (Fig. 11–26). These sutures must not penetrate the lumen of the stomach, lest a gastropleural fistula result.

As soon as the specimen has been removed, examine the proximal end of the esophagus by frozen section to see if there has been submucosal extension of the cancer. If the pathologist detects tumor cells in the esophageal margin, more esophagus should be resected.

Stapled Esophagogastric Anastomosis

Stapling techniques for this anastomosis are described in Chapter 12.

Cervical Esophagogastric Anastomosis

When treating carcinoma of the mid-esophagus it is often necessary to resect the entire thoracic esophagus to obtain a sufficient margin of normal tissue above the tumor. This requires esophagogastric reconstruction in the neck.

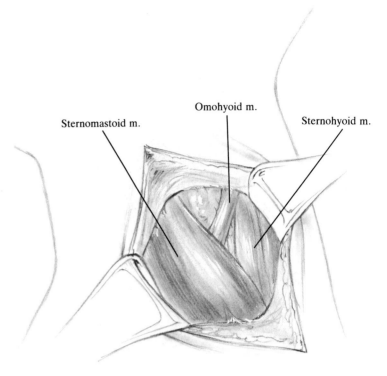

Fig. 11-28

With the patient's head turned slightly to the left, make an oblique incision along the anterior border of the right sternomastoid muscle **(Fig. 11–27)**. Carry the incision through the platysma. Identify **(Fig. 11–28)** and transect the omohyoid muscle. Retract the sternomastoid muscle and carotid sheath laterally and retract the prethyroid muscles medially, exposing the thyroid gland **(Fig. 11–29)**. The mid-

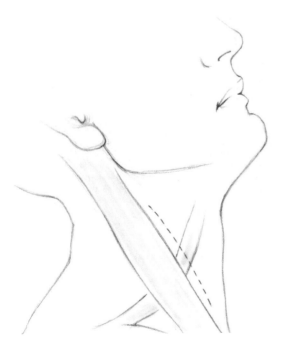

Fig. 11-27

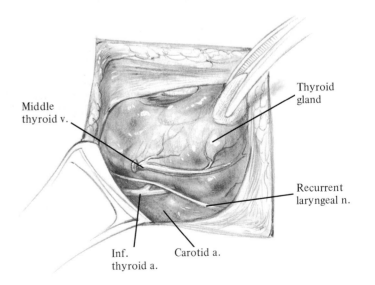

Fig. 11-29

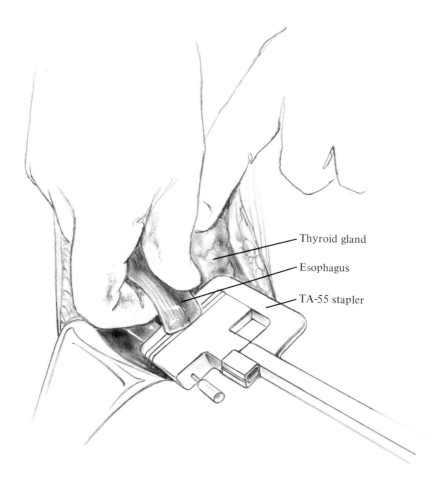

Thyroid gland

Esophagus

TA-55 stapler

Fig. 11-30

dle thyroid vein, when present, should be doubly ligated and divided. Put traction on the areolar tissue between the gland and the carotid sheath by upward and medial displacement of the thyroid. Excessive traction applied to the thyroid or larynx may injure the contralateral recurrent laryngeal nerve. Identify and skeletonize the inferior thyroid artery, which crosses the lower third of the surgical field in a transverse direction, by a Metzenbaum dissection toward the prevertebral fascia. Dissect it toward the thyroid gland until the recurrent laryngeal nerve can be seen. Then dissect the nerve upward to achieve thorough exposure, so it can be preserved (Fig. 11-29).

At this point the tracheoesophageal groove is seen, and the cervical esophagus can be encircled by the surgeon's index finger, which should be passed between the esophagus and the prevertebral fascia and then between the esophagus and trachea. The finger should stay close to the esophageal wall; otherwise the *left* recurrent laryngeal nerve may be avulsed during this dissection. Although the inferior thyroid artery generally must be ligated and divided before the esophagus is mobilized, in some cases its course is low enough in the neck so it can be preserved.

Because the thoracic esophagus has been dissected up to the thoracic inlet, it is a simple matter to transect the esophagus low in the neck. When the proper point of transection of the esophagus has been selected, apply a 55 mm linear stapler to the specimen side **(Fig. 11–30)** and transect the esophagus flush with the stapler. Remove the specimen through the thoracic incision.

Now pass the fundus of the stomach (which has already been passed into the thorax) through the

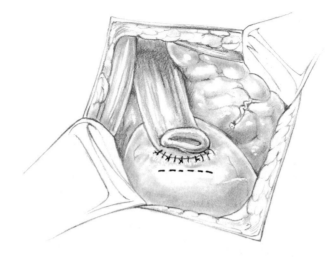

Fig. 11-31

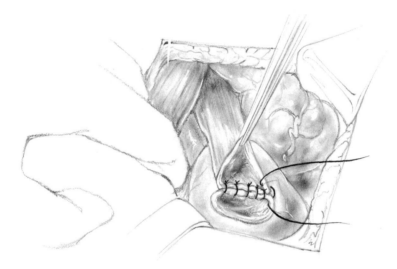

Fig. 11-32

thoracic inlet into the cervical region. The fundus should reach the hypopharynx without tension. Anchor it to the prevertebral fascia with several 3-0 silk sutures. Then construct an end-to-side anastomosis by the same technique described above **(Figs. 11-25, 11-26, 11–31, 11–32)**.

Lavage the operative site with an antibiotic solution and initiate wound closure by inserting a layer of interrupted 4-0 PG sutures, approximating the anterior border of the sternomastoid to the prethyroid strap muscles. Several similar sutures may be used loosely to approximate the platysma. Close the skin, generally by means of a continuous 4-0 PG subcuticular suture, leaving sufficient space to bring a latex drain out from the prevertebral region through the lower pole of the incision.

TOURO COLLEGE LIBRARY

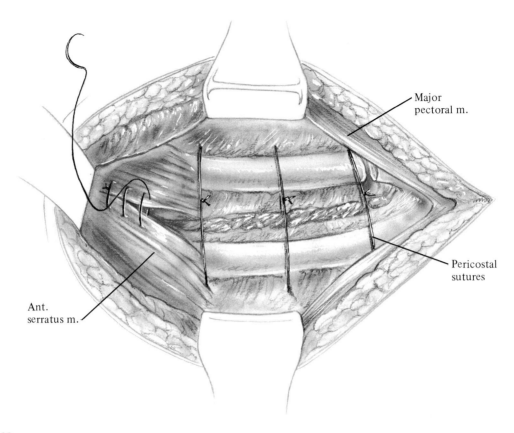

Major
pectoral m.

Pericostal
sutures

Ant.
serratus m.

Fig. 11-33

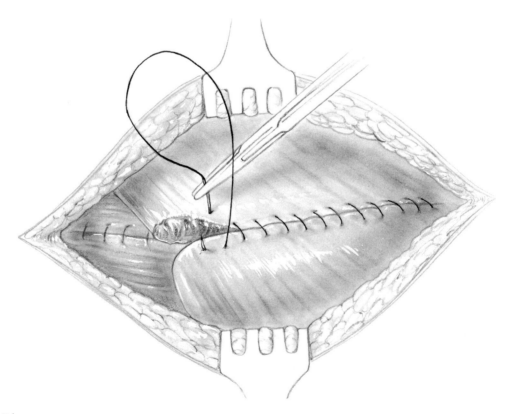

Fig. 11-34

Closure

Insert a 36F chest tube through a stab wound in the ninth intercostal space, and use 4-0 absorbable sutures to secure the catheter to the posterior pleura in the upper thorax. After thoroughly irrigating the thoracic and abdominal cavities with an antibiotic solution, approximate the ribs with four or five interrupted pericostal sutures of no. 1 PDS and approximate the serratus and pectoral muscles in layers by means of continuous 2-0 atraumatic PG **(Figs. 11–33, 11–34).** Close the skin with continuous 3-0 nylon or subcuticular 4-0 PG. Consider inserting a needle-catheter feeding jejunostomy. Close the abdominal wall in the usual fashion by means of interrupted no. 1 PDS sutures.

POSTOPERATIVE CARE

Keep the nasogastric tube on low suction for 4-5 days. Permit nothing by mouth until a contrast study has demonstrated integrity of the anastomosis.

Obtain an esophagram with water-soluble contrast followed by thin barium on the seventh postoperative day. If no leak is demonstrated, the patient is given a liquid diet, which is advanced to a full diet within 3-5 days.

Attach the chest tube to underwater suction drainage for 4-5 days. Follow the routine steps for managing a postoperative thoracotomy patient, including frequent determinations of arterial blood gases and pH. Tracheal suction is used with caution to avoid possible trauma to the anastomosis. Ventilatory support is employed when necessary. Continue prophylactic antibiotics until removal of the chest tube. Use the needle-catheter jejunostomy for enteral alimentation beginning promptly after surgery.

COMPLICATIONS

Anastomotic leaks. Anastomotic leaks constitute by far the most important complication of this operation, but they are *preventable if proper surgical technique is used.* Although minor contained leaks may be treated nonoperatively, most leaks require operative drainage, diversion, repair, or a combination of these maneuvers (see Chapter 23).

Abscesses. A subphrenic or subhepatic abscess may follow an operation for an ulcerated malignancy be-

cause a necrotic gastric tumor often harbors virulent organisms. The incidence of this complication can be reduced by administering prophylactic antibiotics before and during the operation. Treatment is by computed tomography (CT)-directed or surgical drainage.

Pulmonary problems. Pulmonary complications were common in the past, but their incidence has been minimized by proper postoperative pulmonary care. Adequate pain control may require epidural analgesia.

Cardiac arrhythmias. Cardiac failure and arrhythmia are not uncommon in patients who are in their seventh or eighth decade of life. Generally, with careful monitoring and early detection these complications can be easily managed. Hemodynamic monitoring may be helpful.

Stenosis. In the absence of recurrent mediastinal cancer, stenosis of the anastomosis has not occurred in any of the cases Chassin managed and reported. When this complication does occur, repeated passage of Maloney bougies may reverse the condition.

REFERENCES

Bates BA, Detterbeck FC, Bernard SA, et al. Concurrent radiation therapy and chemotherapy followed by esophagectomy for localized esophageal carcinoma. J Clin Oncol 1996;14:156.

Chassin, JL. Esophagogastrectomy: data favoring end-to-side anastomosis. Ann Surg 1978;188:22.

Chu KM, Law SY, Fok M, Wong J. A prospective randomized comparison of transhiatal and transthoracic resection for lower-third esophageal carcinoma. Am J Surg 1997;174:320.

Lee RB, Miller JI. Esophagectomy for cancer. Surg Clin North Am 1997;77:1169.

Lerut T, Coosemans W, De Leyn P et al. Treatment of esophageal carcinoma. Chest 1999;116(suppl):463S.

Skandalakis JE, Ellis H. Embryologic and anatomic basis of esophageal surgery. Surg Clin North Am 2000;80:85.

Skinner DB, Little AG, Ferson MK, Soriano A. Selection of operation for esophageal cancer based on staging. Ann Surg 1986;204:391.

Stark SP, Romberg MS, Pierce GE, et al. Transhiatal versus transthoracic esophagectomy for adenocarcinoma of the distal esophagus and cardia. Am J Surg 1996;172:478.

Sugarbaker DJ, Jaklitsch MT, Liptay MJ. Thoracoscopic staging and surgical therapy for esophageal cancer. Chest 1995;107(suppl):218S.

12 Esophagogastrectomy
Left Thoracoabdominal Approach

INDICATIONS

Carcinoma of the distal esophagus or proximal stomach

Distal esophageal stricture

PREOPERATIVE PREPARATION

See Chapter 11.

PITFALLS AND DANGER POINTS

Anastomotic failure.

Ischemia of gastric pouch. Pay meticulous attention to preserving the entire arcade of the right gastroepiploic artery and vein along the greater curvature of the stomach.

Hemorrhage. Occasionally, the left gastric artery is embedded in tumor via invasion from metastatic lymph nodes. Unless this vessel can be identified, transecting the artery through the tumor may produce hemorrhage that is difficult to control.

Pancreas. Trauma to the tail of the pancreas may cause a pancreatic fistula or acute hemorrhagic pancreatitis.

Sepsis. Some malignancies in the proximal portion of the stomach are ulcerated and bulky with areas of necrosis that contain virulent bacteria. These bacteria may produce postoperative subhepatic or subphrenic abscesses via operative contamination even without anastomotic leakage. Both enteral and parenteral antibiotics that cover colon flora should be used.

Inadequate cancer operation. Because gastric and esophageal malignancies can spread submucosally for some distance without being visible, frozen section studies of both proximal and distal margins of the excision are helpful.

Paralysis of the diaphragm. The diaphragm should be divided around the periphery to preserve phrenic innervation and prevent paralysis.

OPERATIVE STRATEGY

Objectives of Esophagogastrectomy

With operations done for cure, the objective is wide removal of the primary tumor, along with a 6- to 10-cm margin of normal esophagus in a proximal direction and a 6 cm margin of normal stomach below. Even if the stomach is not involved, when the tumor is situated low in the esophagus the proximal lesser curvature of the stomach should be included to remove the left gastric artery at its origin and the celiac lymph nodes. Splenectomy and removal of the lymph nodes at the splenic hilus may be required for large lesions of the proximal stomach and fundus. Any suspicious nodes along the superior border of the pancreas should also be removed.

Thoracoabdominal Incision with Preservation of Phrenic Nerve Function

When gastric cancer encroaches on the gastroesophageal junction, operations done by abdominal incision exclusively are contraindicated for several reasons. In the first place, this anastomosis frequently requires the surgeon's hand and the needle-holder to be in an awkward position and may result in leakage. Furthermore, the abdominal incision makes it difficult to perform wide excision of possible areas of invasion of the distal esophagus. We have seen some upper gastric lesions that extended into the esophagus as far as 10 cm.

The left thoracoabdominal incision, we have found, is both safe and efficacious. It is easy to divide all the muscles of the thoracic cage rapidly by electrocautery. Even patients in their eighties have tolerated this incision well when given adequate postoperative support. Epidural anesthesia minimizes pain and allows early mobilization.

Positioning the patient in the full lateral position with an incision through the fifth or sixth intercostal space gives wide exposure to the mediastinum, left pleural space, and left upper quadrant of the abdomen.

The diaphragm should *not* be incised radially from the costal margin to the esophageal hiatus because it would transect the phrenic nerve and paralyze the left diaphragm. Many patients who require gastric surgery for cancer are aged and have limited pulmonary reserve; moreover, because atelectasis is a common postoperative complication, it is better to make a circumferential incision in the periphery of the diaphragm to preserve phrenic and intercostal nerve function and normal diaphragmatic motion.

Postoperative pain at the site of the divided costal margin is allegedly common following a thoracoabdominal incision. In our experience proper resuturing of the costal margin with monofilament steel wire results in solid healing of this area. Neither pain nor costochondritis has been a problem.

Anastomotic Leakage

Delicacy and precision of anastomotic technique and adequate exposure are important for preventing anastomotic leaks. If a gastric or lower esophageal lesion has spread up the lower esophagus for a distance of more than 6–8 cm, the esophagogastric anastomosis should not be constructed high up under the aortic arch, as it is a hazardous technique. Instead, 1 cm posterior segments of two additional ribs are resected if necessary to give more proximal exposure, and the esophagus is liberated behind the arch of the aorta and passed out to an intrapleural, supraaortic position. This exposure permits the anastomosis to be done in a manner less traumatic to the tissues than an anastomosis constructed high up under the aortic arch. Otherwise, the surgeon's hand and wrist are situated in an awkward position, which makes smooth manipulation of instruments difficult. Jerky suturing motions produce small tears in the esophagus, especially in the posterior layer, where access is difficult.

End-to-End versus End-to-Side Anastomosis

We showed that the end-to-end esophagogastric anastomosis carries with it a much higher rate of leakage and a higher mortality rate than the end-to-side variety (Chassin 1978). Explanations for the increased complication rate following end-to-end esophagogastrostomy are not difficult to find.

1. It is necessary to close a portion of the end of the stomach because of the disparity between the lumen of the stomach and that of the esophagus. This increases the technical difficulty of doing the end-to-end anastomosis **(Fig. 12–1a,b)**.
2. The blood supply of the gastric pouch at its proximal margin is inferior to that at the site of the end-to-side anastomosis.
3. Inserting the posterior layer of esophagogastric sutures may be difficult. Traction must be applied to the esophagus to improve exposure, and the surgeon's hand and the needle-holder may have to assume positions that are awkward for efficient, atraumatic suturing, which produces imperfections in the suture line.
4. As seen in **Figure 12–2a**, protection from posterior leakage is achieved in the end-to-side cases by the buttress effect of a 6- to 7-cm segment of

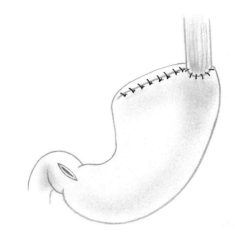

Fig. 12-1a

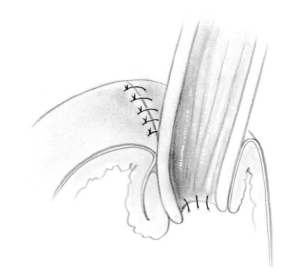

Fig. 12-1b

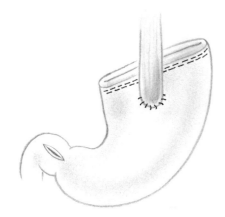

Fig. 12–2a

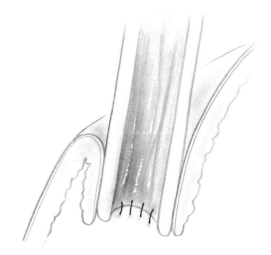

Fig. 12–2b

gastric wall behind the esophagus. In end-to-end operations, however, there is no second line of defense against technical error.

5. Although the anterior layer of the end-to-end or the end-to-side esophagogastrostomy is much easier to construct without technical defects than the posterior layer, even here the end-to-side version offers advantages. **Figure 12–2b** illustrates how the anterior wall of the esophagus invaginates into the stomach for additional protection. If this were attempted with an end-to-end anastomosis, the large inverted cuff would produce stenosis at the stoma (Fig. 12–1b).

Additional protection against leakage from the anterior aspect of the end-to-side anastomosis can be achieved by performing a Nissen fundoplication around the anastomosis. This also helps prevent postoperative gastroesophageal reflux, but it requires the presence of a large gastric pouch and cannot be performed, unless modified, when the proximal stomach has been resected.

Avoiding Postoperative Reflux Esophagitis

Another serious drawback of an end-to-end esophagogastric anastomosis is the occurrence of reflux esophagitis in patients who achieve long-term survival. It can be avoided by implanting the end of the esophagus end-to-side into the stomach at least 6 cm beyond the proximal margin of the gastric pouch. This type of construction functions as a valve, probably because air in the gastric pouch behind the distal esophagus and above the esophagogastric anastomosis compresses the overlying esophagus. This is fortunate, as there is rarely enough remaining stomach to fashion an adequate "fundoplication" when the gastric fundus has been resected.

When the anastomosis is performed by the stapling method, the anastomosis should still be a comfortable distance from the proximal end of the gastric interposition for the same reason as elaborated for the sutured anastomosis.

Efficacy of Stapling Techniques for the Esophagogastric Anastomosis

We have developed a stapling technique for end-to-side esophagogastrostomy that can be done swiftly with an extremely low leak rate (Chassin 1978). After a long, sometimes complicated dissection, an accurate anastomosis that takes only 2–3 minutes of operating time constitutes a welcome epilogue, especially when treating poor-risk patients. Whereas 28 mm and 31 mm circular stapling cartridges produce a good anastomosis, use of the 25 mm cartridge results in a high incidence of anastomotic postoperative strictures requiring dilatation.

Postoperative Sepsis

To prevent postoperative sepsis, meticulously avoid spillage of the gastric content, which can contaminate the subhepatic or subcutaneous space. Any instruments that come into contact with the lumen of the stomach or esophagus should be treated as dirty and the area walled off wherever possible. During the operation intravenous antibiotics that cover a spectrum from lower mouth to skin to enteric organisms should be given at appropriate intervals to ensure that body fluid and tissue levels are maintained.

OPERATIVE TECHNIQUE

Incision and Position

Endobronchial (double-lumen) one-lung anesthesia permits atraumatic collapse of the left lung during the esophageal dissection. It is far preferable to advancing an endotracheal tube down the right mainstream bronchus.

With the aid of sandbags and wide adhesive tape across the patient's hips and left shoulder, elevate the patient's left side to a 60°-90° angle. Place the right arm straight on an arm board. Pad the patient's left arm and suspend it in a forward position **(Fig. 12–3)**.

Begin the incision at the umbilicus and continue it up the midline about halfway to the xiphoid, or use an oblique incision parallel to the right costal margin midway between the xiphoid and umbilicus. Explore the abdomen. The presence of metastasis of moderate degree to the celiac lymph nodes or to the liver does not constitute a contraindication to resection.

Redirect the incision to cross the costal margin into the sixth intercostal space and continue to it the region of the erector spinae muscle near the tip of the scapula. After the skin incision has been completed, use the coagulating current to divide the latissimus dorsi muscle in as caudal a location as possible **(Fig. 12–4)**. The index fingers of both the surgeon and first assistant should be inserted side by side underneath the latissimus muscle while the electrocautery divides

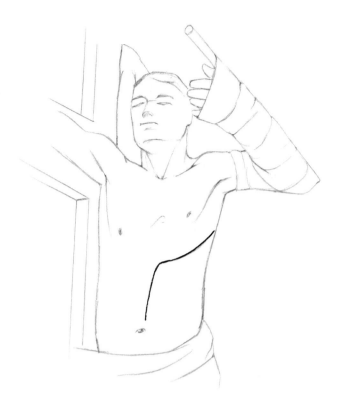

Fig. 12-3

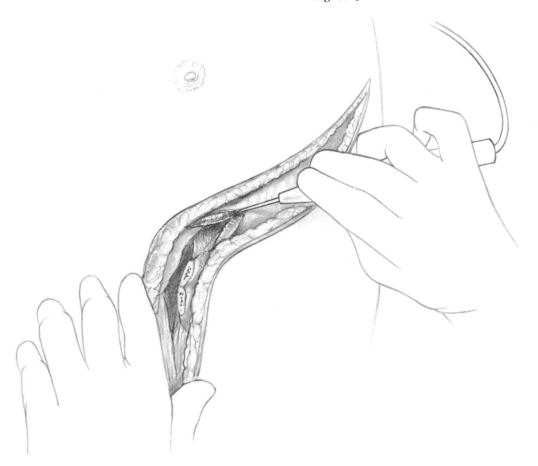

Fig. 12-4

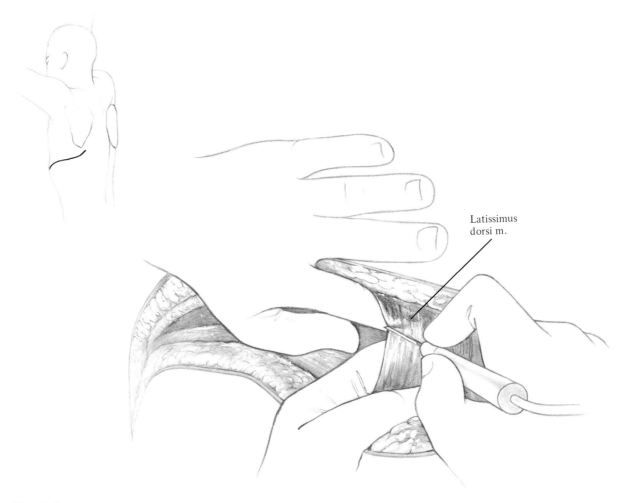

Latissimus
dorsi m.

Fig. 12-5

the muscle **(Fig. 12–5)**. Divide the anterior serratus muscle in a similar fashion. The rhomboid muscles medial to the scapula need not be divided unless a supraaortic dissection proves necessary.

Next retract the scapula in a cephalad direction and count down the interspaces from the first rib to confirm the location of the sixth interspace. Divide the intercostal musculature by electrocautery along the superior surface of the seventh rib and enter the pleura **(Fig. 12–6)**. Divide the costal margin where it is a wide plate with a scalpel, heavy scissors, or rib cutter. Divide the internal mammary artery, deep and slightly lateral to the costal margin, ligate or electrocoagulate it **(Fig. 12–7)**.

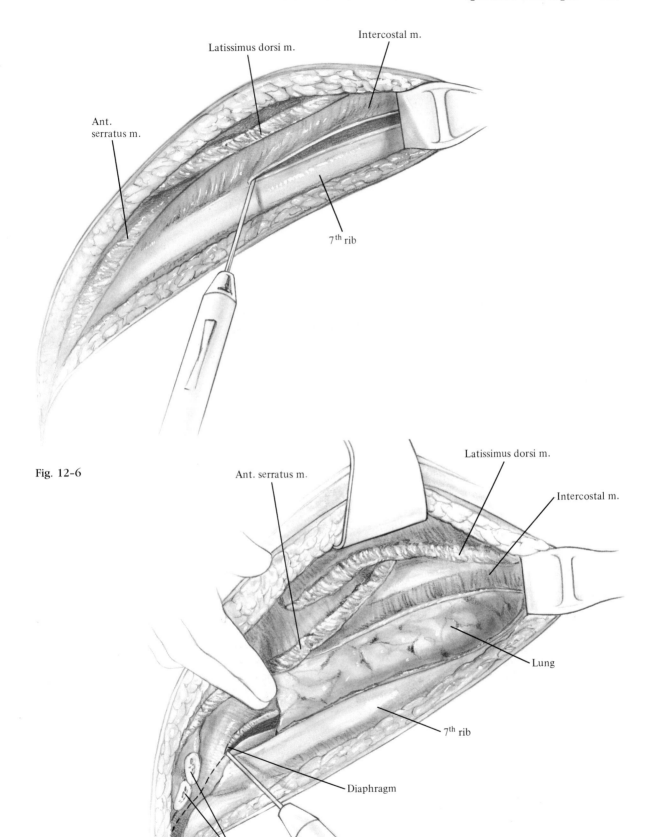

Fig. 12-6

Fig. 12-7

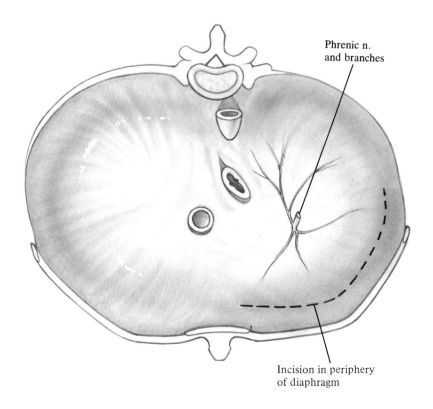

Phrenic n.
and branches

Incision in periphery
of diaphragm

Fig. 12-8

Incise the diaphragm in a circumferential fashion **(Figs.** 12-7, **12–8)** along a line 3-4 cm from its insertion into the rib cage. Use electrocautery for this incision, which should extend laterally about 15 cm from the divided costal margin. Spread the intercostal incision by inserting a mechanical retractor. Use of a multiarm retraction system without a mechanical advantage allows retraction of the lung, diaphragm, and liver for both the thoracic and abdominal phases of the operation, and it avoids fracturing the ribs.

Liberation of Esophagus

Divide the inferior pulmonary ligament with electrocautery or long Metzenbaum scissors, progressing in a cephalad direction until the inferior pulmonary vein has been reached. Collapse the lung, cover it with moist gauze pads, and retract it in a cephalad and anterior direction with Harrington retractors.

Incise the mediastinal pleura from the aorta to the hiatus, beginning at a point above the tumor **(Fig. 12–9)**. Encircle the esophagus first with the index finger and then with a latex drain **(Fig. 12–10)**. Divide the vagus nerves as they approach the esophagus from the hilus of the lung. Dissect the tumor and the attached vagus nerves away from the mediastinal structures. If the pleura of the right thoracic cavity or pericardium has been invaded by tumor, include it in the resection. Dissection of the esophagus should free this organ from the arch of the aorta down to the hiatus, including all the periesophageal areolar tissue. Generally, only two or three arterial branches of the descending aorta join the esophagus. They should be occluded by hemostatic clips and divided. Use an umbilical tape ligature or a 55/3.5 mm linear stapler to occlude the lumen of the proximal esophagus (above the tumor) to prevent cephalad migration of tumor cells **(Fig. 12–11)**. The esophagus may be divided at

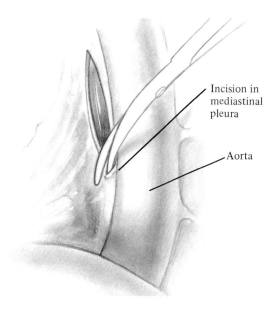

Incision in
mediastinal
pleura

Aorta

Fig. 12-9

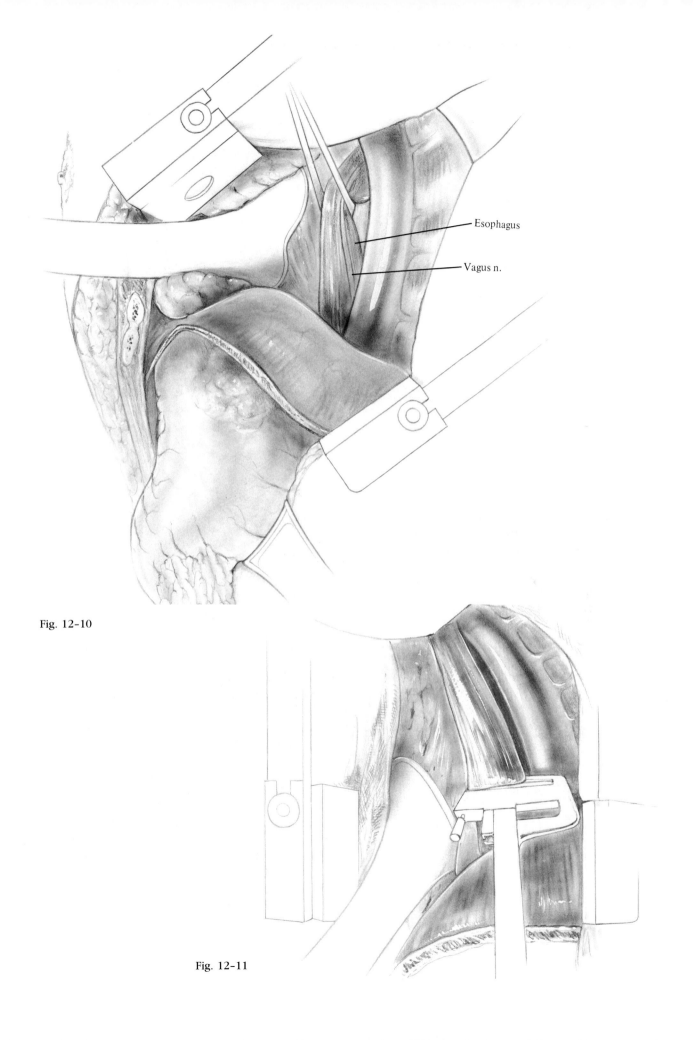

Esophagus

Vagus n.

Fig. 12-10

Fig. 12-11

this time and reflected into the abdomen once hiatal mobilization is complete, or it may be delayed until the stomach is mobilized.

Splenectomy

If the proximity of the carcinoma makes splenectomy necessary, retract the spleen medially and divide the lienophrenic ligament **(Fig. 12–12)**. Gently elevate the spleen and the tail of the pancreas from the retroperitoneal tissues by finger dissection. Divide the lienocolic ligament. Identify the splenic artery and vein on the posterior surface of the splenic hilus. Each should be divided and ligated with 2-0 silk. It may be convenient to remove the spleen as a separate specimen after dividing each of the short gastric vessels. Do this on the anterior aspect of the stomach to visualize the greater curvature accurately, thereby avoiding any possibility of trauma to the stomach. If splenectomy is not necessary, enter the lesser sac through the avascular space above the left gastroepiploic vessels and individually control and divide the short gastric vessels.

Gastric Mobilization

The gastroepiploic arcade along the greater curvature of the stomach *must be preserved with compulsive attention to detail*, as the inadvertent occlusion of this vessel in a clamp or ligature results in ischemia of the gastric pouch and anastomotic leakage. Working from above down, divide the left gastroepiploic vessels and open the lesser sac to identify the gastroepiploic arcades from both front and back. Be sure always to *leave 3-5 cm of redundant omentum attached* to the vascular arcade. Identify the plane separating the colon mesentery from the gastroepiploic arcade. Continue the dissection to a point 6–8 cm cephalad to the pylorus **(Figs. 12–13a, 12–13b)**. The greater curvature now should be elevated. Complete posterior mobilization of the stomach by incising the avascular attachments that connect the back wall of the stomach to the posterior parietal peritoneum overlying the pancreas (gastropancreatic folds) and continue the dissection to the pylorus. Carefully preserve the subpyloric vessels (right gastroepiploic and right gastric).

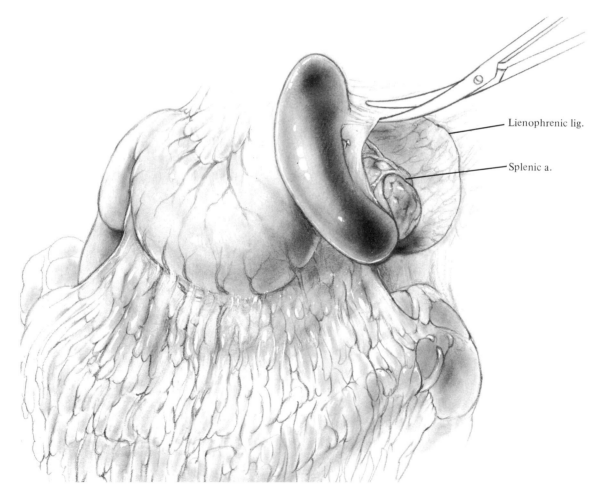

Lienophrenic lig.

Splenic a.

Fig. 12-12

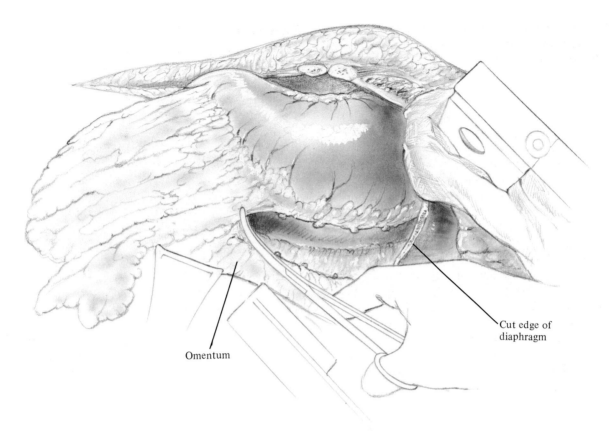

Omentum

Cut edge of
diaphragm

Fig. 12–13a

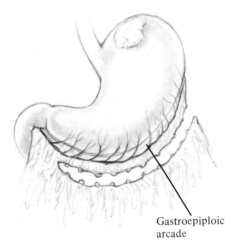

Gastroepiploic
arcade

Fig. 12–13b

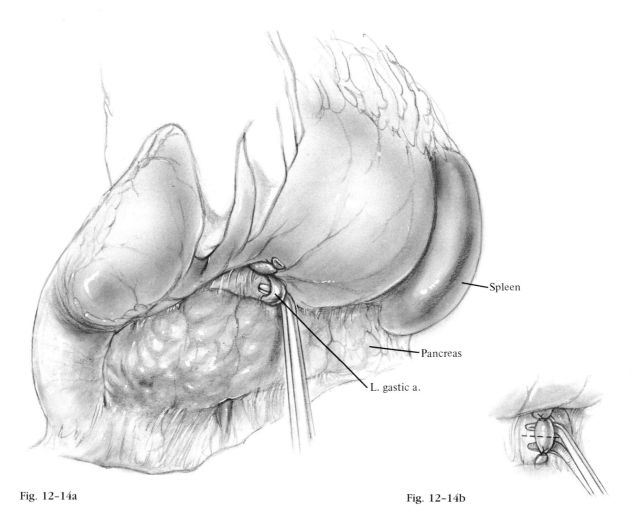

Spleen

Pancreas

L. gastic a.

Fig. 12-14a   Fig. 12-14b

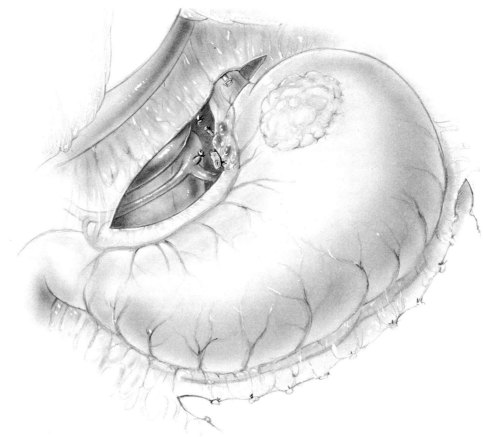

Fig. 12-15

Identify the celiac axis by palpating the origins of the splenic, hepatic, and left gastric arteries. Dissect lymphatic and areolar tissues away from the celiac axis toward the specimen. Skeletonize the coronary vein and divide and ligate it with 2-0 silk. Immediately cephalad to this structure is the left gastric artery, which should be doubly ligated with 2-0 silk and divided **(Figs. 12–14a, 12–14b)**. Incise the gastrohepatic ligament near its attachment to the liver **(Fig. 12–15)**. An accessory left hepatic artery generally can be found in the cephalad portion of the gastrohepatic ligament. Divide the artery and ligate it with 2-0 silk; then divide the remainder of the ligament and the peritoneum overlying the esophagus.

Hiatal Dissection

A gastrophrenic ligament attaches the posterior aspect of the gastric fundus to the posterior diaphragm. Divide the ligament using the left index finger as a guide. If tumor has encroached on the hiatus, leave crural musculature attached to the tumor and divide it from the surrounding diaphragm with electrocautery. This may require division and ligature of the inferior phrenic artery. Divide the vagus nerves just below the hiatus **(Fig. 12–16)** and divide the phrenoesophageal ligaments; this frees the esophagus and stomach from the arch of the aorta down to the duodenum.

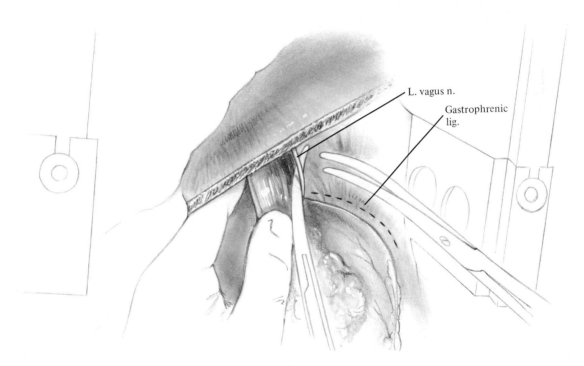

L. vagus n.

Gastrophrenic lig.

Fig. 12–16

Fig. 12-17

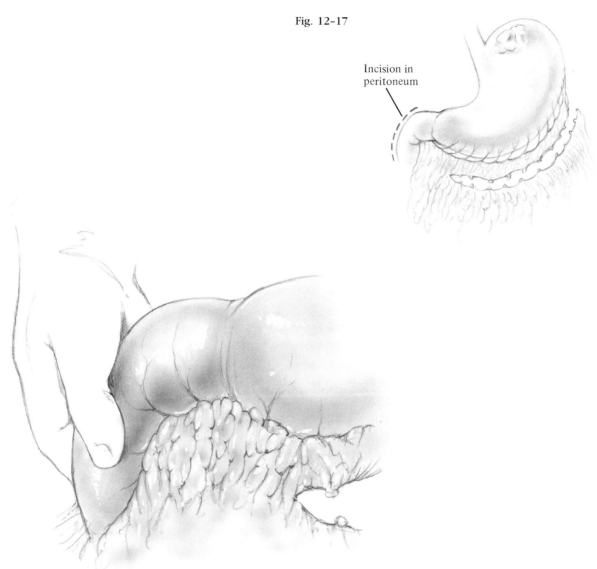

Incision in
peritoneum

Fig. 12-18

Kocher Maneuver

To achieve maximum upward mobility of the gastric pouch, divide the avascular lateral duodenal ligament and pass a hand behind the duodenum and the head of the pancreas **(Figs. 12–17, 12–18)**. If necessary, continue this Kocher maneuver along the duodenum as far distally as the superior mesenteric vein (see Figs. 11-15, 11-16). Additional freedom of the mobilized stomach can be achieved by dividing the attachments of the greater omentum to the duodenum beyond the right gastroepiploic vessels.

Pyloromyotomy

Perform a pyloromyotomy as described in Chapter 11 (see Figs. 11-17 to 11-19).

Transection of Stomach and Esophagus

To treat a primary tumor of the lower esophagus, apply either a long linear cutting stapler or a 90 mm linear stapler (loaded with 4.8 mm staples) in an oblique fashion to remove the stump of the left gastric artery, the celiac lymph nodes on the lesser curvature of the stomach, and 5-6 cm of the greater curvature.

To treat lesions of the proximal stomach, which is the operation illustrated in **Figures 12–19a**, and **12–19b**, apply the stapler so 5-6 cm of normal stomach distal to the lesion is removed. *Ascertain that the nasogastric tube has been withdrawn*, and divide the stomach with a long linear cutting stapler or with

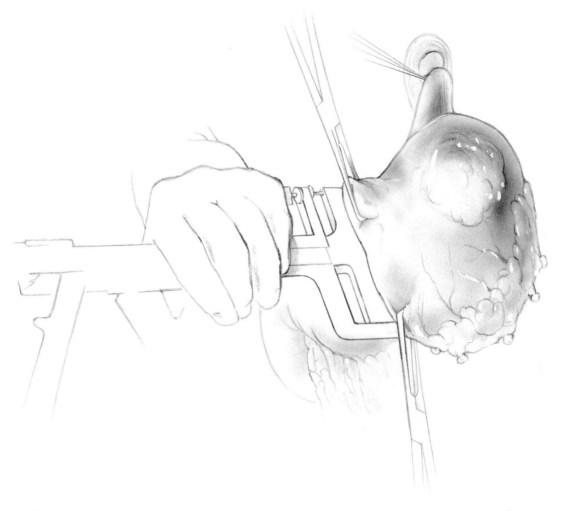

Fig. 12-19a

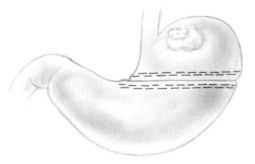

Fig. 12-19b

two 90 mm linear staplers applied in a parallel fashion. Make an incision with the scalpel flush with the stapler attached to the residual gastric pouch. If two 90 mm linear staplers are not available, the first stapler should be applied to the stomach, fired, and then reapplied 1 cm lower on the gastric wall. The transection should be made flush with the stapler on the gastric pouch. Control individual bleeding vessels with electrocautery after removing the device. This staple line should be oversewn with fine inverting sutures. The gastric wall is of variable thickness, and we have seen isolated leakage from this staple line when it was not reinforced. If multiple applications of the cutting stapler were required, a running 4-0 polypropylene Lembert suture conveniently reinforces the staple line without excess inversion.

In a previous step the esophageal lumen proximal to the tumor was occluded with a row of staples (Fig. 12-11). If the esophagus has not yet been divided, transect it now 8–10 cm proximal to the tumor and remove the specimen **(Fig. 12–20)**. Submit the proximal and distal margins of the specimen to frozen section examination. Clean the lumen of the proximal esophagus with a suction device **(Fig. 12–21)**.

Enlargement of Hiatus

Enlarging the hiatus is rarely necessary if the crura have been skeletonized as described by division of the phrenoesophageal ligament. If the hiatus appears tight, make a transverse incision by electrocautery in the left branch of the crux **(Fig. 12–22)**. The incision should be of sufficient magnitude to allow the gastric pouch to pass into the mediastinum *without constriction* of its venous circulation.

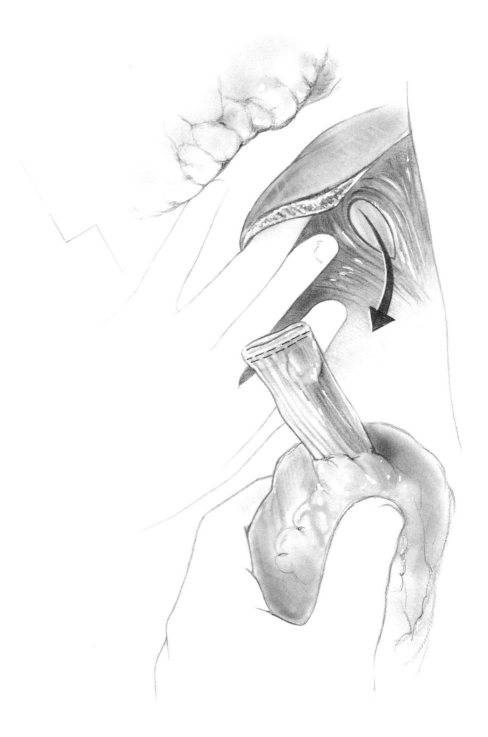

Fig. 12-20

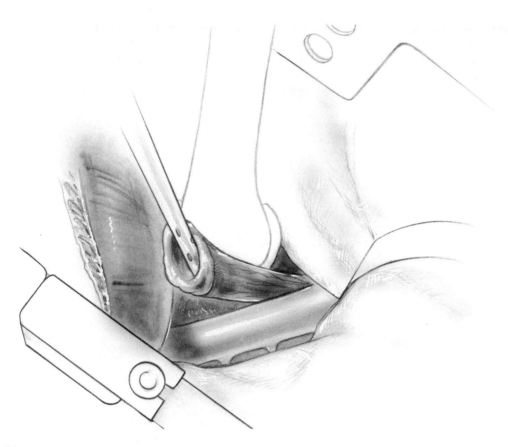

Fig. 12-21

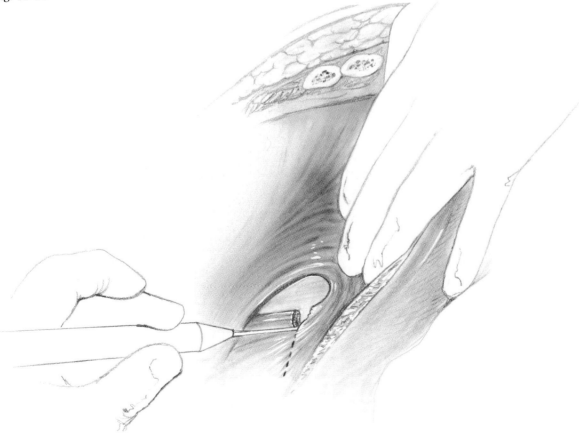

Fig. 12-22

Enlargement of Thoracic Incision If Supraaortic Anastomosis Is Necessary

A properly fashioned end-to-side esophagogastric anastomosis requires the presence of 6–8 cm of esophagus below the aortic arch. If there is not 6–8 cm of esophagus below the aortic arch, the surgeon should not hesitate to enlarge the thoracic incision so the esophagus can be passed behind the arch into a supraaortic position. This makes the anastomosis far simpler and safer to perform and requires only a few minutes to accomplish.

Move to a position on the left side of the patient. Extend the skin incision up from the tip of the scapula in a cephalad direction between the scapula and the spine. With electrocautery divide the rhomboid and trapezium muscles medial to the scapula. Retract the scapula in a cephalad direction and free the erector spinal muscle from the necks of the sixth and fifth ribs. Free a short (1 cm) segment of the sixth (and often of the fifth) rib of its surrounding periosteum and excise it **(Fig. 12–23)**. Divide and ligate or electrocoagulate the intercostal nerves with their accompanying vessels **(Fig. 12–24)**. Reinsert the Finochietto or other mechanical retractor **(Fig. 12–25)**. If the exposure is still inadequate, a segment of the fourth rib may also be excised, but this is rarely necessary.

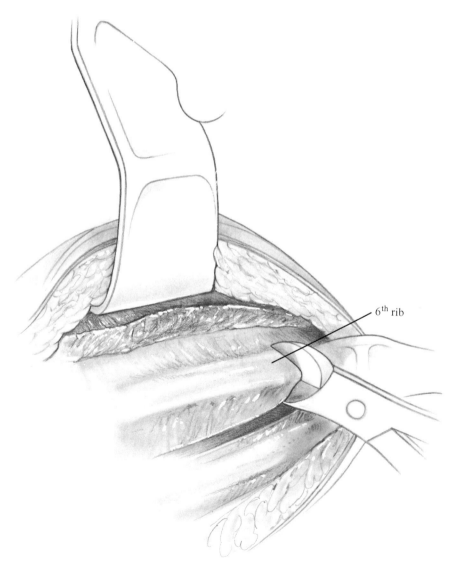

6th rib

Fig. 12-23

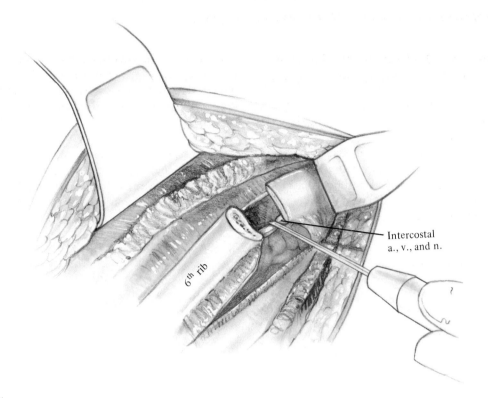

Intercostal
a., v., and n.

6th rib

Fig. 12-24

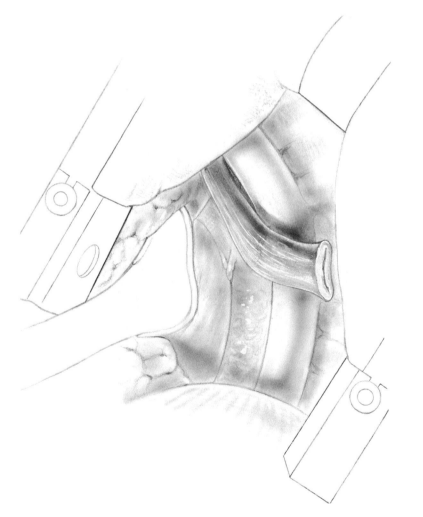

Fig. 12-25

Enter the space between the anterior wall of the esophagus and the aortic arch with the index finger **(Figs. 12–26a, 12–26b, 12–26c)**. There are no vascular attachments in this area. The index finger emerges cephalad to the aortic arch behind the mediastinal pleura. Incise the mediastinal pleura on the index finger, making a window extending along the anterior surface of the esophagus up to the thoracic inlet. Now dissect the esophagus free of all its attachments to the mediastinum in the vicinity of the aortic arch. Avoid damage to the left recurrent laryngeal nerve, the thoracic duct, and the left vagus nerve located medial to the esophagus above the aortic arch. One or two vessels may have to be divided between hemostatic clips.

Deliver the esophagus from behind the aortic arch up through the window in the pleura between the left carotid and subclavian arteries **(Fig. 12–27)**. If the space between the carotid and subclavian arteries is narrow, bring the esophagus out through a pleural incision lateral to the subclavian artery.

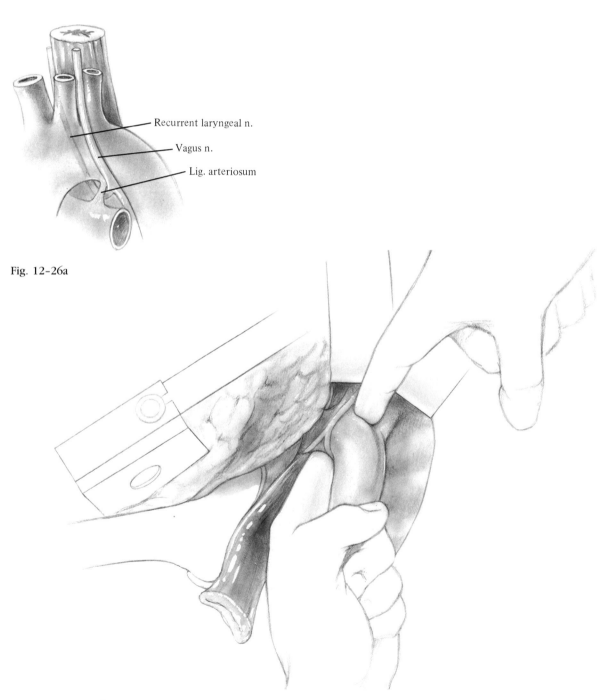

— Recurrent laryngeal n.

— Vagus n.

— Lig. arteriosum

Fig. 12–26a

Fig. 12–26b

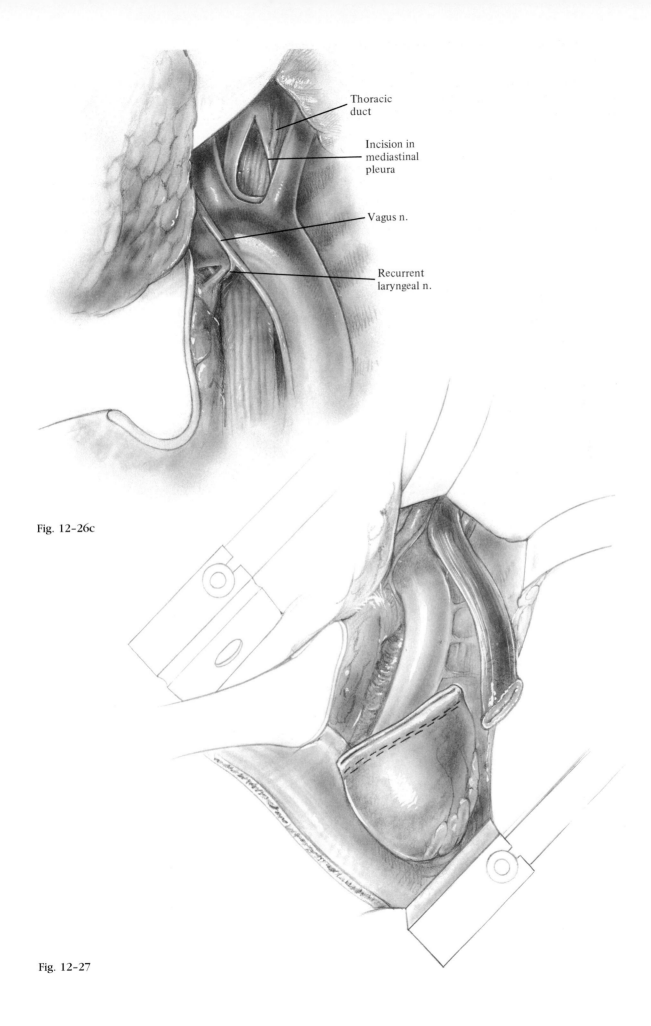

Thoracic
duct

Incision in
mediastinal
pleura

Vagus n.

Recurrent
laryngeal n.

Fig. 12-26c

Fig. 12-27

The esophagogastric anastomosis, as described below, should be constructed in a position lateral and anterior to the aortic arch. Exposure for the anastomosis in this location is excellent. Bring the esophagus down over the anterior wall of the stomach for a sutured anastomosis. An overlap of 6–7 cm is desirable. If the esophageal dissection has been carried out without undue trauma, the esophageal segment has an excellent blood supply even though its distal 10 cm has been liberated from its bed in the mediastinum. The anastomosis can readily be performed as high as the apex of the thorax by this method, and a level of resection comparable to that achieved by adding a cervical incision can often be used. Use of the circular stapling technique to perform the anastomosis high in the chest is an excellent alternative to sutured intrathoracic or cervical anastomosis. For this technique the stomach is placed in front of the esophagus for the end-to-side anastomosis.

Esophagogastric Anastomosis, Suture Technique

The technique for sutured esophagogastric anastomosis is described and illustrated in Chapter 11.

Esophagogastric Anastomosis, Stapling Technique (Surgical Legacy Technique)

In 1978 Chassin described a linear stapling technique for esophagogastric anastomosis. Although circular staplers are more commonly used currently, this method is still occasionally useful and applica-

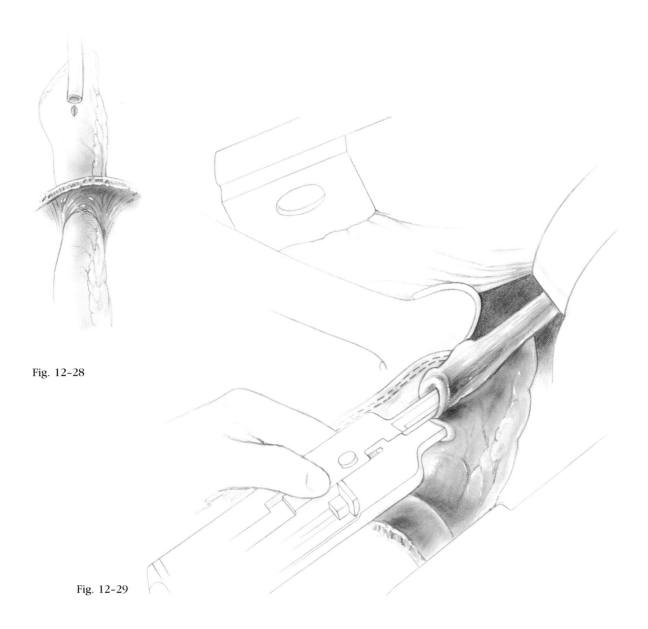

Fig. 12-28

Fig. 12-29

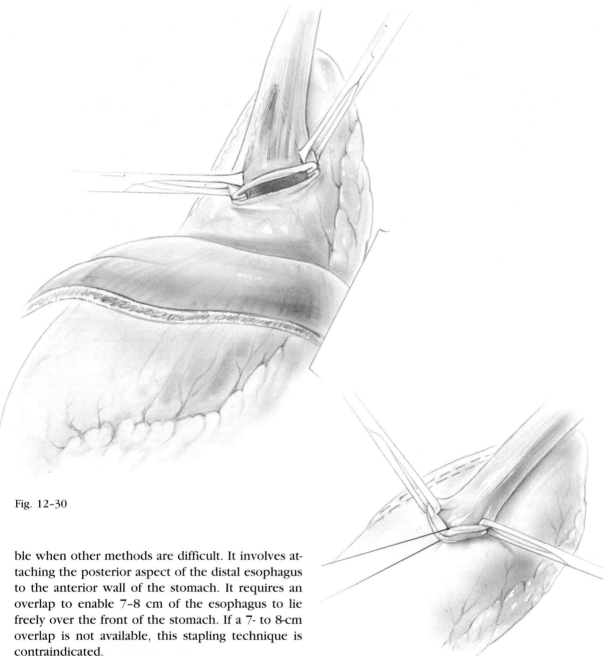

Fig. 12-30

ble when other methods are difficult. It involves attaching the posterior aspect of the distal esophagus to the anterior wall of the stomach. It requires an overlap to enable 7-8 cm of the esophagus to lie freely over the front of the stomach. If a 7- to 8-cm overlap is not available, this stapling technique is contraindicated.

Make a stab wound, 1.5 cm long, on the anterior wall of the gastric pouch at a point 7-8 cm from the cephalad margin of the stomach **(Fig. 12–28)**. Insert one fork of the cutting linear stapler through the stab wound into the stomach and the other fork into the open end of the overlying esophagus **(Fig. 12–29)**. Insert the stapling device to a depth of 3.5-4.0 cm. Fire and remove the stapling device. This step leaves both the end of the esophagus and a large opening in the stomach unclosed **(Fig. 12–30)**. The posterior layer of the anastomosis has already been accomplished by the stapling device. Complete the anastomosis in an everting fashion by triangulation with two applications of the 55 mm

Fig. 12-31

linear stapler. To facilitate this step, insert a 4-0 temporary guy suture through the full thickness of the anterior esophageal wall at its midpoint, carry the suture through the center of the remaining opening in the gastric wall **(Fig. 12–31)**, and tie the suture. Apply Allis clamps to approximate the everted walls of the esophagus and stomach. Apply the first Allis clamp just behind termination of the first staple line on the medial side. Hold the suture and the Allis clamps so the linear stapler can be applied just underneath the clamps and the suture **(Fig. 12–32)**. Tighten and fire the stapling device. Excise the esophageal and gastric tissues flush with the stapling device with Mayo scissors. Leave the guy suture intact.

Use an identical procedure to approximate the lateral side of the esophagogastric defect. Apply additional Allis clamps. Then place the 55 mm linear stapling device into position deep to the Allis clamps and the previously placed guy suture. Close and fire

the stapler and remove the redundant tissue with Mayo scissors **(Fig. 12–33)**. It is essential that a small portion of the lateral termination of the stapled anastomosis be included in the final linear staple line. Include the guy suture also in this last application of the linear stapler. These measures eliminate any possibility of leaving a gap between the various staple lines. Test the integrity of the anastomosis by inserting a sterile solution of methylene blue through the nasogastric tube into the gastric pouch. The appearance of the completed stapled anastomosis is shown in **Figure 12–34**.

Whether a Nissen fundoplication is to be constructed following this anastomosis depends on the judgment of the surgeon and the availability of loose gastric wall. In some cases partial fundoplication can be done.

Esophagogastric Anastomosis Performed by Circular Stapling Technique

The circular stapling technique is especially suitable for patients in whom the lumen of the esophagus is large enough to admit a 28- or 31-mm circular stapling device. The esophageal lumen can be measured by attempting to insert sizers (which come in 25, 28, and 31 mm sizes). It is dangerous to stretch the esophagus with these sizers, because it can result in one or more longitudinal tears of the mucosa and submu-

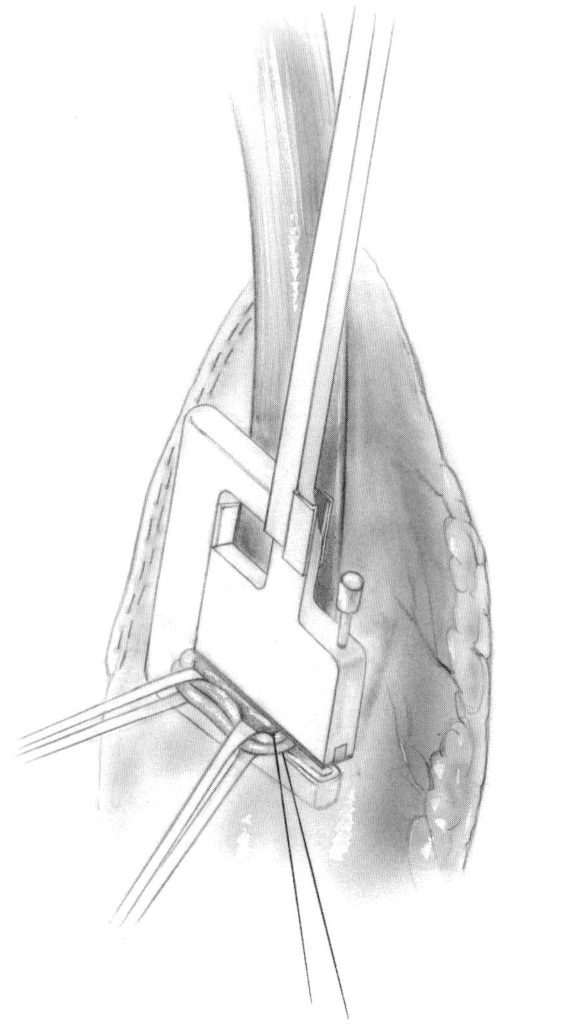

Fig. 12-32

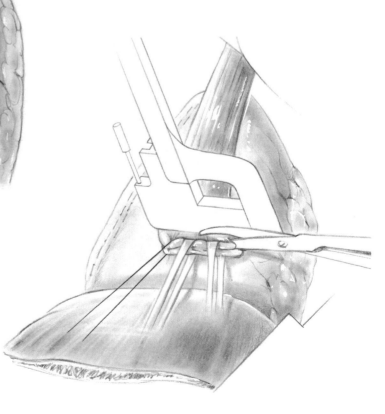

Fig. 12-33

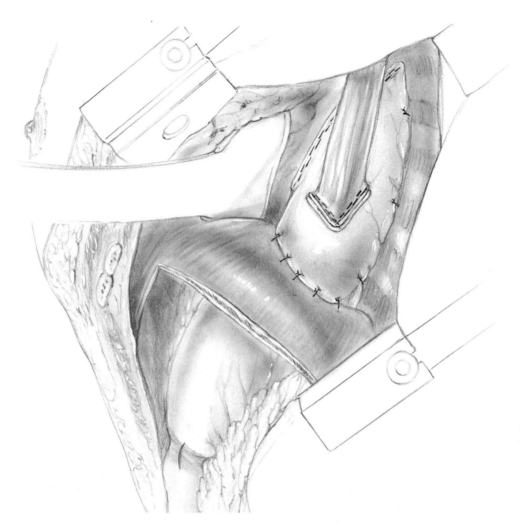

Fig. 12-34

cosa. Gentle dilatation with a Foley catheter balloon is the safest way to achieve lumen of adequate size for anastomosis. Use a 16F Foley catheter with a 5 cc balloon attached to a 20 cc syringe filled with saline. Insert the Foley catheter well above the site for anastomosis and inflate the balloon in 2.5 cc increments. Withdraw the inflated balloon slowly after each inflation. A 28 mm circular staple can almost always be inserted with ease (use the largest size that can be inserted easily). Place four long Allis clamps or guy sutures equidistant around the circumference of the esophagus to maintain a wide lumen and minimize difficulty with insertion of the stapler head.

If a tear is detected, resect an additional segment of the esophagus to remove the laceration. If the tear is not detected and a stapled anastomosis is constructed, postoperative leakage is a potentially dangerous complication.

Next, insert the 25 mm sizer and then the 28 mm sizer. If the 28 mm sizer passes easily, the circular stapling technique is a good one. If only the 25 mm sizer can be inserted, there is danger of postoperative stenosis when this size staple cartridge is used. Although this type of stenosis frequently responds well to postoperative dilatation, we prefer to utilize the alternative technique described above (Fig. 12-28 to 12-34), which corrects for the narrow esophagus without requiring postoperative dilatation. Use a purse-string suture to tighten the esophagus around the shaft of the stapler. After inserting a 28- or 31-mm sizer, place one or two purse-string sutures of 0 or 2-0 Prolene, making certain to include the mucosa and the muscularis in each bite.

The anastomosis can be done to the anterior or posterior wall of the stomach. We generally prefer to use the posterior wall if the anastomosis is high in the chest, as it allows an easy anterior hemifundoplication.

Make a 3 cm linear incision somewhere in the antrum of the gastric pouch utilizing electrocautery.

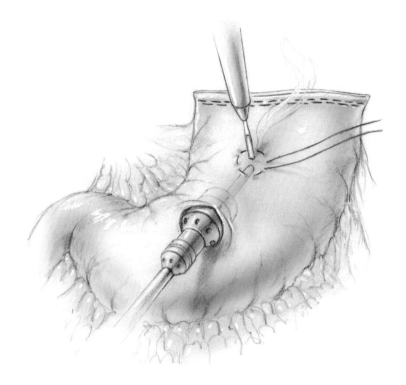

Fig. 12–35

Through this opening in the anterior wall of the gastric pouch, insert the cartridge of a circular stapling device after having removed the anvil.

Then choose a point 5–6 cm from the proximal cut end of the gastric pouch and use the spike of the stapler to puncture it. Advance the shaft as far as it will go and then insert a small purse-string suture of 2-0 Prolene around the shaft. Alternatively, place the purse-string suture first; then make a stab wound in the middle of it **(Fig. 12–35)** and permit the shaft of the circular stapler to emerge from the stab wound. Tie the purse-string suture around the shaft. Remove the spike. Gently insert the anvil of the device into the open end of the esophagus. Draw the esophagus down over the anvil. When this has been accomplished, tie the purse-string suture around the instrument's shaft, fixing the esophagus in position **(Fig. 12–36)**. Ensure that there is no axial rotation of the stomach. Now attach the anvil to the shaft of the device and approximate the anvil to the cartridge of the circular stapling device by turning the wing-nut in a clockwise direction to the indicated tightness. Be certain that the purse-string suture fits snugly around the shaft and that it does not catch on grooves in the shaft. After this has been accomplished, fire the stapling device.

Now rotate the wing-nut the appropriate number of turns in a counterclockwise direction, gently disengage the anvil from the newly created anastomo-

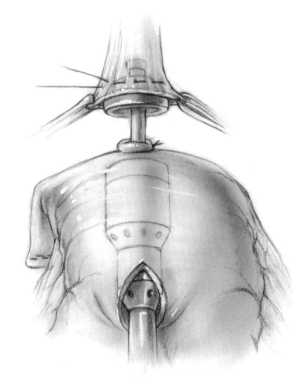

Fig. 12–36

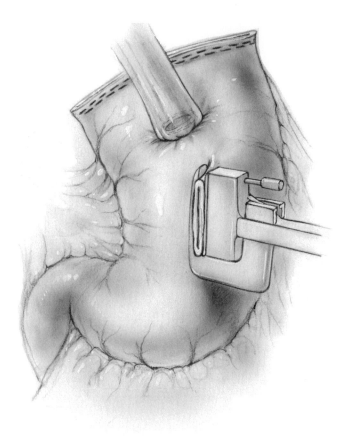

Fig. 12-37

sis, and remove the entire device from the gastric pouch. Carefully inspect the newly constructed circular anastomosis between the open end of the esophagus and the gastric pouch to see that all the staples have fired and that the anastomosis is intact. Confirm this by inserting the index finger through the previously made gastrotomy incision and pass the finger into the esophagus, confirming the presence of an open lumen. Now apply Allis clamps to the gastrotomy incision on the anterior wall of the gastric pouch. Apply a linear stapling device for thick tissue (4.8 mm) and fire. Excise any redundant gastric tissue, remove the stapler, and lightly electrocoagulate bleeding vessels. Carefully inspect the staple line to be sure all of the staples have closed. Many surgeons oversew the gastrotomy incision with a layer of continuous or interrupted Lembert sutures of a nonabsorbable nature, although this step may not be essential if 4.8 mm staples are used (**Fig. 12–37**). Do not convert the linear gastrotomy to a transverse closure as you would for a pyloroplasty because it increases tension on the suture line.

Muehreke and Donnelly reported four leaks from stapled gastrotomies in 195 patients undergoing esophageal resection using circular stapling instruments. A possible explanation for failure of the stapled gastrotomy closure to heal properly is the use of a 3.5 mm staple. In a stomach of normal thickness, using a small staple can produce a line of necrosis. We prefer that a 4.8 mm staple be used when closing the stomach. These authors found that there was a reduction in the leak rate from their gastrotomy closures if they oversewed the gastrotomy staple line with a continuous noninverting layer of 3-0 Mersilene. We have used a 4-0 polypropylene running, inverting seromuscular suture to cover the staple line and have seen leaks only when this step was omitted.

Stabilizing the Gastric Pouch

To prevent any gravity-induced tension on the anastomosis, the apex of the gastric pouch should be sutured to the mediastinal pleura or the prevertebral fascia with 2-0 or 3-0 nonabsorbable sutures. The gastric pouch should then be fixed to the enlarged diaphragmatic hiatus with interrupted 2-0 or 3-0 nonabsorbable sutures, which attach the gastric wall to the margins of the hiatus (Fig. 12–34). These sutures

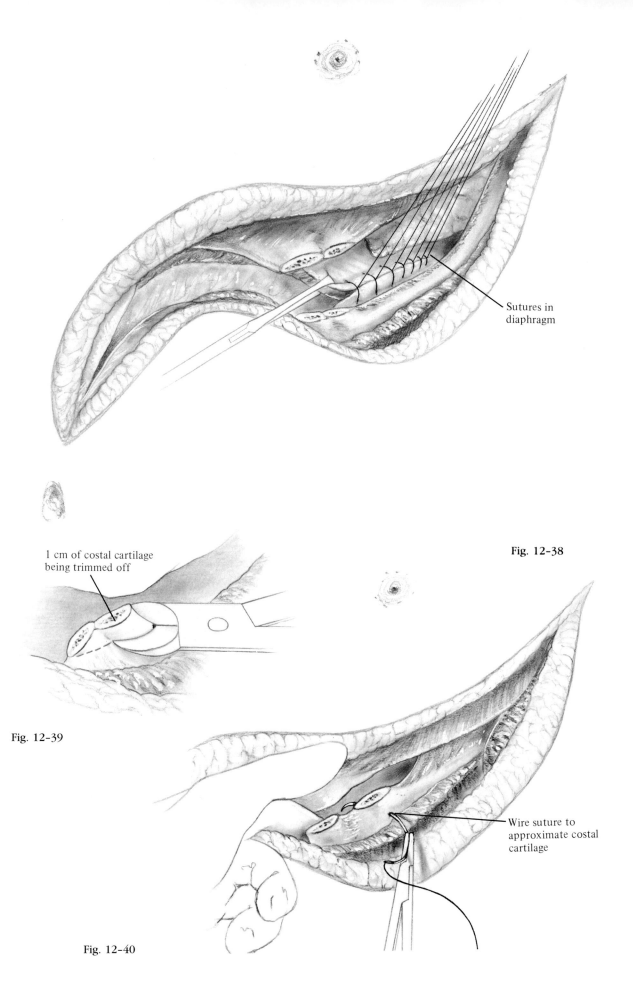

Sutures in diaphragm

Fig. 12-38

1 cm of costal cartilage being trimmed off

Fig. 12-39

Wire suture to approximate costal cartilage

Fig. 12-40

should be 2 cm apart and should not penetrate the gastric mucosa lest they induce a gastropleural fistula. Consider performing a jejunostomy for immediate postoperative enteral alimentation.

Closure

Irrigate the thoracic and abdominal cavities and close the incision in the diaphragm with interrupted sutures of 2-0 Tevdek or a running suture of 0 monofilament **(Fig. 12–38)**. In either case, take fairly large (1 cm) bites, as dehiscence of this suture line can have serious consequences, such as herniation of small intestine into the chest. Do not try to complete this closure until the costal margin has been approximated to avoid tearing the diaphragm.

Excise approximately 1 cm of cartilage from the costal margin to improve apposition **(Fig. 12–39)**. Close the incision in the costal margin with one or two sutures of monofilament stainless steel wire **(Fig. 12–40)**. Either 2-0 or no. 5 wire may be used. Insert four or five pericostal sutures of no. 1 PDS to approximate the ribs **(Fig. 12–41)**. Bring a 30F chest tube through the ninth intercostal space in the anterior axillary line and carry it up to the level of the anastomosis. Place it under direct vision. If it does not sit comfortably, suture it to the parietal pleura posterior to the aorta using fine absorbable sutures.

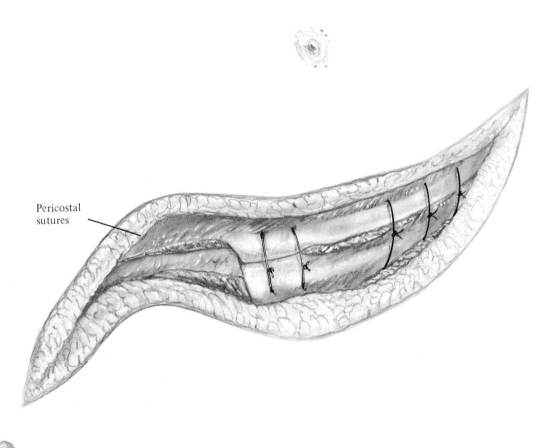

Pericostal sutures

Fig. 12–41

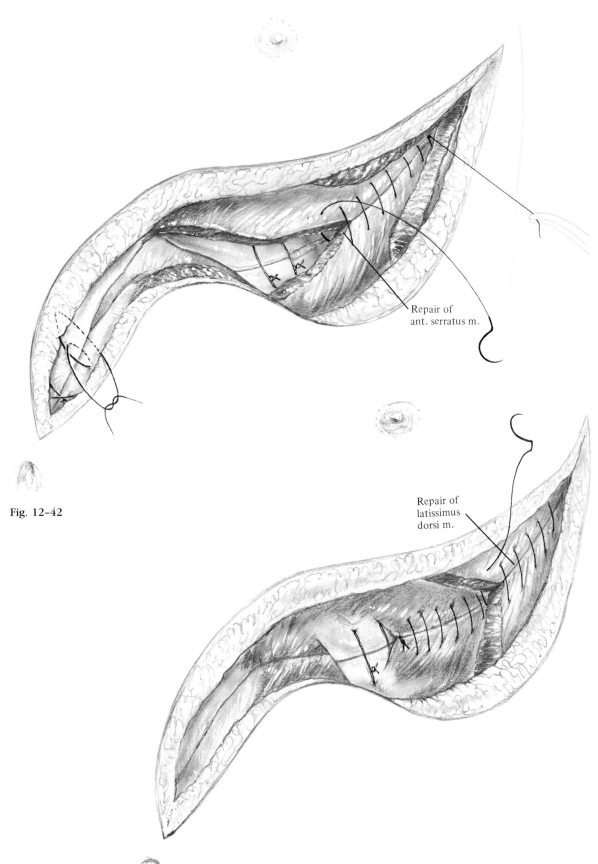

Repair of
ant. serratus m.

Fig. 12-42

Repair of
latissimus
dorsi m.

Fig. 12-43

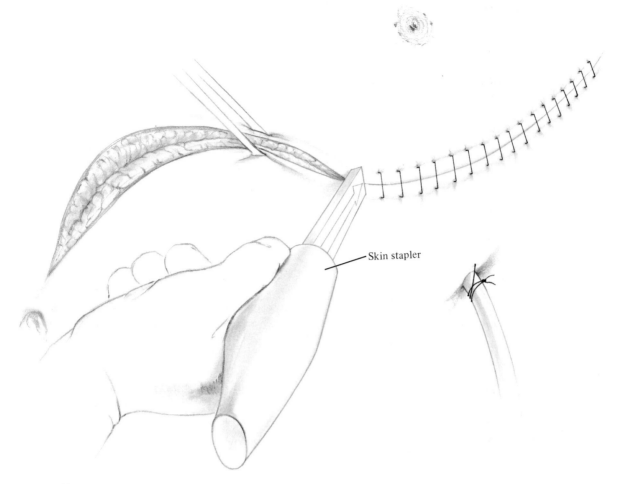

Fig. 12-44

Inflate the lung to eliminate any atelectatic patches. If a significant number of air leaks from the lung are noted, pass a second chest catheter anterior to the lung up to the apex of the thorax. Tie the pericostal sutures and the final diaphragm sutures and close the muscles in two layers with a continuous 2-0 or 0 PG atraumatic synthetic absorbable suture in each **(Figs. 12–42, 12–43)**.

Close the abdominal portion of the incision with interrupted no. 1 PDS Smead-Jones sutures as described in Chapter 3. The diaphragm is continuous with the endoabdominal fascia, and separate closure of this layer to meet the diaphragmatic closure facilitates closure of both diaphragm and abdominal wall. Use staples or a subcuticular suture to close the skin **(Fig. 12–44)**. No drains should be needed in the abdominal cavity.

POSTOPERATIVE CARE

See Chapter 11.

COMPLICATIONS

See Chapter 11.

REFERENCES

Chassin JL. Esophagogastrectomy: data favoring end-to-side anastomosis. Ann Surg 1978;188:22.

Chassin JL. Stapling technic for esophagogastrostomy after esophagogastric resection. Am J Surg 1978;136:399.

Ellis FH, Heatley GJ, Krasna MJ, Williamson WA, Balogh K. Esophagogastrectomy for carcinoma of the esophagus and cardia: a comparison of findings and results after standard resection in three consecutive eight-year intervals with improved staging criteria. J Thorac Cardiovasc Surg 1997;113:836.

Fisher RD, Brawley RK, Kieffer RF. Esophagogastrostomy in the treatment of carcinoma of the distal two-thirds of the esophagus. Ann Thorac Surg 1972;14:658.

Humphrey EW. Stapling techniques in esophageal replacement. Surg Clin North Am 1984;64:499.

Krasna MJ. Advances in the staging of esophageal carcinoma. Chest 1998;113:107S.

Muehrcke DD, Donnelly RJ. Complications after esophagogastrectomy using stapling instruments. Ann Thorac Surg 1989;48:257.

Skandalakis JE, Ellis H. Embryologic and anatomic basis of esophageal surgery. Surg Clin North Am 2000;80:85.

Steichen FM. Varieties of stapled anastomoses of the esophagus. Surg Clin North Am 1984;64:481.

13 Transhiatal Esophagectomy

INDICATIONS

Carcinoma of the esophagus

Esophageal stricture

PREOPERATIVE PREPARATION

See Chapter 11.

Prepare for possible massive blood loss during the blunt phase of the thoracic dissection.

Prepare a single-lumen endotracheal tube, not cut short.

Consider hemodynamic monitoring.

PITFALLS AND DANGER POINTS

Excessive bleeding

Laceration of membranous trachea

Injury to spleen

Hypotension during mediastinal dissection due to compression of the heart

Trauma to thoracic duct; chylothorax

Traction injury or laceration of the recurrent laryngeal nerve

Bowel herniation through a too large diaphragmatic hiatus

Undetected pneumothorax

Ischemia or trauma to tip of gastric tube in the neck inducing necrosis and sepsis

Anastomotic leak

Inadvertent laceration of right gastroepiploic artery

OPERATIVE STRATEGY

Although a large portion of this operation is accomplished by blunt dissection, there are five areas where dissection must be performed with consummate delicacy to avoid devastating complications.

1. *Membranous trachea.* A small linear laceration of the membranous trachea can be repaired by suturing. However, if a patch of the membranous trachea is avulsed while dissecting an esophageal cancer that has invaded the trachea, adequate repair may be impossible. In the absence of a malignancy in the area of the trachea, dissection of the esophagus away from the trachea should not be difficult if carried out in a gentle manner.
2. *Right gastroepiploic artery.* While dissecting the omentum away from the gastroepiploic artery, continually keep in mind that this vessel constitutes the major blood supply to the tip of the gastric tube to be constructed. In many areas this vessel is covered by omental fat so its exact location is not obvious to the naked eye. Consequently, when dividing the omentum, leave a few centimeters of omentum attached to the artery, as inadvertent division of this vessel makes the stomach useless as an esophaeal substitute.
3. *Gastric tip.* Be aware that the gastroepiploic artery does not continue to the tip of the gastric tube. Beyond the termination of this artery the blood supply to the gastric tip consists of intramural circulation. Although this circulation is *normally* adequate to sustain the healing process of the gastroesophageal anastomosis in the neck, *unnecessary trauma* to this area can threaten this precarious anastomosis. Consequently, be aware throughout the operation that this tissue must be protected from rough handling. Even inserting a suture between the gastric tip and the prevertebral fascia in the neck has been reported to have caused focal necrosis of the stomach and a gastric fistula with vertebral osteomyelitis. If an anchoring stitch is considered necessary, use 5-0 PG suture material, do not place the suture too deeply, and do not tie a tight knot.
4. *Recurrent laryngeal nerve.* Aside from hoarseness, damage to the left recurrent laryngeal nerve during the cervical dissection can also result in swallowing difficulty and aspiration. Use the assistant's index finger rather than a rigid instrument to retract the trachea and the thyroid gland.

5. *Azygos vein*. Laceration or avulsion of the azygos vein results in massive hemorrhage that in most cases requires right thoracotomy for control. Avoid this by careful preoperative staging and careful dissection at the point where the azygous vein crosses the esophagus.

OPERATIVE TECHNIQUE

Place the patient in a supine position on the operating table and insert bilateral intravenous catheters and one intraarterial catheter, which permits continuous monitoring of the patient's blood pressure. Both arms are padded and aligned alongside the body. If a central venous pressure or a Swan-Ganz catheter is to be used, insert it into the right internal jugular vein, as the left side of the neck is preserved for the esophagogastric anastomosis. Request that the anesthesiologist use a standard endotracheal tube of standard length that has not been shortened. If the membranous trachea is inadvertently lacerated, the anesthesiologist can then advance the tip of the endotracheal tube into the left main bronchus. After the balloon is inflated, this maneuver enables the anesthesiologist to control the patient's respiration while repair of the laceration is attempted. Place a small blanket roll under the upper thorax to keep the neck extended.

Turn the head to the right. Attach a self-retaining Thompson, Omni, or similar retractor to the operating table for later use (see Glossary).

Abdomen

Make a midline incision from the xyphoid to a point a few centimeters distal to the umbilicus, and enter the abdominal cavity. Check the stomach carefully to ascertain that it is indeed suitable for the development of a gastric tube that reaches up into the neck. Check the celiac lymph nodes for metastases. Liberate the left lobe of the liver by incising the triangular ligament. Expose the spleen and divide any adhesions that involve the capsule of the spleen, so the short gastric and left gastroepiploic vessels are easily identified. Insert the Weinberg blade of the Thompson retractor underneath the sternum and retract the liver in a cephalad direction, exposing the esophageal hiatus. Thereupon free the lower esophagus and divide the gastrophrenic ligament as described in Figures 11-7 to 11-11. Encircle the esophagus with the index finger and then with a 2 cm wide Penrose drain. Divide the right and left vagus nerves. Apply caudad traction to the esophagus via the Penrose drain and free up the lower esophagus by blunt dissection. If the tumor can be reached by digital palpation, ascertain that it is not fixed to the aorta or vertebral column. If it is fixed, transhiatal esophagectomy without thoracotomy is contraindicated. If not, expose the gastric cardia and then carefully divide and ligate each of the short gastric vessels as well as the left gastroepiploic artery.

Divide the greater omentum serially between Kelly clamps leaving 3–5 cm of omentum attached to the right gastroepiploic arcade to avoid injury to the gastroepiploic artery. Remember that this vessel will be the main blood supply to the gastric conduit (see Figs. 11-12a,b).

Elevate the greater curvature of the stomach in a cephalad direction and identify the origin of the left gastric artery. Divide and ligate it as described in Figure 11-13 and then perform an extensive Kocher maneuver (see Figs. 11-14 to 11-16). Perform a pyloromyotomy (see Figs. 11-17 to 11-19). Cover the abdominal incision with sterile towels and start the neck operation.

Cervical Dissection

Expose and mobilize the cervical esophagus as described in Chapter 11. Encircle the esophagus with a Penrose drain and apply cephalad traction. Use the index finger with the volar aspect of the fingers facing the esophagus to dissect the esophagus away gently from the overlying trachea and the posterior prevertebral fascia. With this dissection, the index finger can reach down almost to the carina of the trachea.

Transhiatal Dissection

Wear a headlamp for this phase of the operation. Adjust the Thompson retractor to elevate the sternum and liver. Enlarge the hiatal opening by incising the diaphragm with electrocautery in an anterior direction through the middle of the central tendon, dividing and ligating the transverse phrenic vein during this step. Dissect the central tendon away from the pericardium. If necessary, insert a flat malleable retractor behind the heart and elevate gently. Push the right and left diaphragmatic plurae laterally to improve exposure. Palpate the esophagus and the tumor. Determine that they are flexible and mobile, and that there are no points of tumor invasion that would make resection without thoracotomy inadvisable. Before embarking on further dissection, pass a 28F Argyle Saratoga suction catheter into the neck incision and then down into the lower mediastinum to facilitate evacuation of blood from the surgical field.

Despite the limited exposure allowed by the transhiatal approach, the transhiatal esophagectomy is neither a blind nor a crude operation. Dissection of the esophagus from the diaphragm to the arch of the aorta is performed under direct vision. Exposure can be enhanced by inserting long, narrow retractors along the lateral aspects of the hiatal aperture. Many of the vascular attachments to the esophagus can be divided and occluded by hemostatic clips or ligatures. When dissecting the esophagus in the mediastinum, make no special effort to excise any pleura or lymph nodes. The strategy of the operation is to separate the surrounding anatomy from the esophageal tube as efficiently as possible. When dissecting the esophagus along its posterior surface, keep the hand flat against the vertebral column. Orringer et al. stated that entry into one or both pleural cavities occurs in 75% of patients during this operation. After the esophagus has been removed from the mediastinum, and before the stomach is brought into the chest, examine the pleura visually and by palpation. If a tear has occurred, insert an appropriate chest tube to prevent a postoperative tension pneumothorax.

After the lower esophagus has been mobilized, insert a small sponge on a long sponge-holder ("sponge on a stick") along the prevertebral fascia in the neck behind the esophagus while the other hand is placed behind the esophagus in the mediastinum **(Fig. 13–1)**. When the sponge-stick meets the hand, the posterior dissection of the esophagus has been completed. Try not to compress the heart unduly with the hand in the prevertebral space. Remind the anesthesiologist to monitor the arterial pressure carefully during this dissection. Now remove the sponge-stick from the neck. With the assistant exerting traction in a caudal direction on the Penrose drain encircling the esophagogastric junction, place the hand, palm down, on the anterior surface of the esophagus and with finger dissection free the esophagus from overlying pericardium and carina. With the other hand insert one or two fingers, volar surface down, over the anterior face of the esophagus in the neck while cephalad traction is being applied to the Penrose drain encircling the cervical esophagus. Working with both hands simultaneously, disrupt the filmy attachments between the esophagus and the membranous trachea-left main stem bronchus. After this has been accomplished, there remain lateral attachments to be disrupted before the esophagus is freed. Again retract the upper esophagus in a cephalad direction and separate the esophagus from these attachments until the upper 8 cm of thoracic esophagus is freed circumferentially. Now insert the hand into the hiatus and slide upward along the anterior esophagus behind the trachea until the circumferentially freed upper esophagus is contacted. Trap the esophagus against the vertebral column between the index and middle fingers. Then with a down-

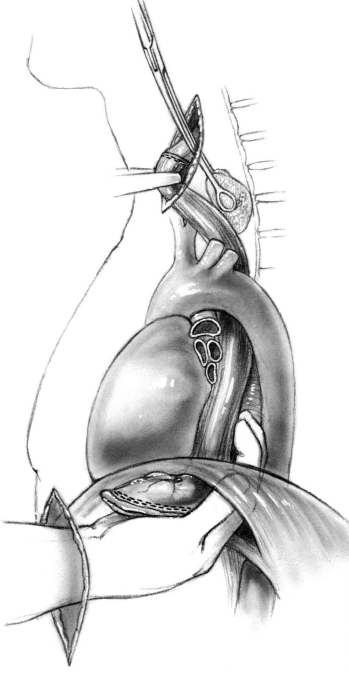

Fig. 13-1

ward raking motion, avulse the lateral attachments until the esophagus has been completely mobilized.

Deliver 7–8 cm of thoracic esophagus into the neck and transect the esophagus with a linear cutting surgical stapler. This maneuver provides a few centimeters of extra esophagus, allowing the option of selecting the best length when the anastomosis is performed.

Suture a long 2 cm wide Penrose drain to the distal end of the divided esophagus. Apply a hemostat to the proximal end of the drain in the neck. Draw the

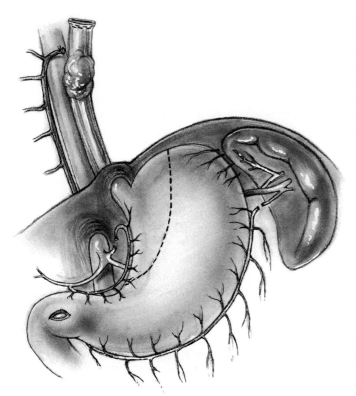

Fig. 13-2

about 6–8 cm width of cardia intact at the gastric tip **(Fig. 13–3)**. Remember that with each application of the stapler a small portion of the previous staple line must be included. Now invert the entire staple line by means of a continuous 4-0 Prolene Lembert suture. Remove the identifying hemostat from the previously positioned Penrose drain that was brought down from the neck into the mediastinum. Suture this Penrose

thoracic esophagus down into the abdomen. Then cut the drain and apply a hemostat to the proximal cut end in the abdomen. This drain with its two identifying hemostats is later used to draw the stomach up through the posterior mediastinum into the neck.

Insert two narrow retractors into the mediastinum and retract laterally. Inspect the mediastinum for any laceration of the pleura. If a laceration is encountered, insert a 32F chest tube into the chest cavity on the side of the laceration, in the mid-axillary line. Then insert moist gauze packing into the mediastinum to help achieve hemostasis while the stomach is being prepared.

Exteriorize the stomach and attached esophagus by spreading it out along the patient's anterior chest wall. Because the blood supply to the lesser curvature subsequent to ligation of the left gastric artery is poor (Akiyama), the lesser curvature is excised, converting the stomach into a tubular structure **(Fig. 13–2)**. Manually stretch the proximal tip of the cardia in a cephalad direction. Observe the esophagogastric junction and note where the second or third branch down of the left gastric artery enters the lesser curvature. At this point, apply the linear cutting stapler and aim it in a cephalad direction toward the cardia. While continuing to apply cephalad traction on the cardia, fire the stapler. Sequentially reapply and fire the stapler until the lesser curvature has been amputated, leaving

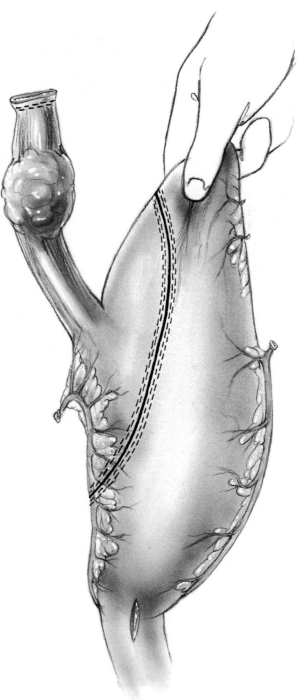

Fig. 13-3

drain to the most cephalad point of the gastric cardia using 3-0 silk sutures. Leave a 4- to 5-cm tail on the medial suture to identify the lesser curvature side of the gastric tube. Place gentle cephalad traction on the proximal end of the Penrose drain that remains in the cervical incision while using the right hand to maneuver the gastric tip gently through the hiatus and into the posterior mediastinum until the stomach has been manipulated into the neck. To avoid the possibility of gastric torsion, be certain that the staple line along the lesser curvature is located to the patient's right and the greater curvature to the patient's left. The long-tailed suture at the junction of the Penrose drain and the gastric cardia identify the medial aspect of the gastric tube. Confirm the absence of torsion by inserting the right hand through the hiatus and palpating the anterior surface of the stomach up to the aortic arch and with the left hand from the cervical approach. With both hands, deliver the gastric tip up to the apex of the cervical incision. Insert several sutures of 5-0 Vicryl to attach the gastric fundus to the fascia of the longus colli muscles on both sides of the neck. Do not take deep bites of stomach or tie the sutures so tight that necrosis of the gastric wall occurs.

Return to the abdomen and close the incision in the diaphragm with interrupted 2-0 silk sutures but do not constrict the newly formed hiatus to the point where it obstructs venous return from the gastric tube. Leave about three fingers' space between the diaphragm and the stomach. Then insert enough interrupted 3-0 silk sutures between the muscle surrounding the hiatus and the stomach to prevent the possibility of bowel herniating through the newly formed diaphragmatic hiatus. Cover the pyloromyotomy with omentum. Perform a feeding needle catheter jejunostomy in the proximal jejunum. Close the abdominal incision and then return to the neck to perform the esophagogastric anastomosis.

To avoid any tension whatsoever on the anastomosis, divide the cervical esophagus at a point where it can easily reach the clavicle. When dividing the esophagus, cut the anterior flap of esophagus so it is at least 1 cm longer than the posterior flap, as illustrated in Figure 11-24. This maneuver converts the anastomotic suture line into an ellipse instead of a circle and should result in a larger stoma. Now reflect the esophagus in a cephalad position above the cervical incision. The uppermost gastric cardia has already been sutured to the neck muscles as high as is comfortable in the cervical incision. Using Babcock forceps, gently elevate the anterior wall of the stomach from behind the clavicle to a more superficial and superior location in the neck. The anastomosis between the end of the esophagus and the anterior wall of the stomach should be located 3–5 cm down from the apex of the gastric tube and above the level of the clavicle. Bring the esophagus back into the neck so it rests on the anterior wall of the gastric tube. Make an incision in the anterior wall of the gastric tube in a vertical direction, the length being appropriate to the diameter of the elliptical esophageal orifice, which is approximately 2.5 cm.

Be certain that the esophagus and stomach are positioned such that there is no tension on the suture line. Using 4-0 PG or PDS insert the first stitch in the mucosa 4 mm from the cut end. This stitch passes through the muscle layer of the esophagus and then enters the cephalad margin of the gastric incision 4 mm above the incision, entering the lumen of the stomach. When tying these sutures, make the knot just tight enough to afford approximation, not strangulation. Place the second stitch through the left lateral wall of the esophagus into the lumen, again catching at least 4 mm of mucosa, and bring the stitch into the stomach and out the center of the left lateral wall of the stomach. Do not tie this stitch; rather, clamp it in a hemostat and place the third stitch in the same fashion in the right lateral margin of the esophagus and stomach. Ask the assistant to apply hemostats to stitches 2 and 3 and then to apply lateral traction to separate the two stitches. This maneuver lines up the esophagus and stomach so closing the posterior layer is simple. Insert interrupted sutures about 4 mm apart from each other. When the knots are tied the mucosa will automatically have been inverted into the lumen. Cut the tails of all the sutures in the posterior anastomosis but retain the hemostats on stitches 2 and 3. Maintain lateral traction on these two stitches and begin the anterior anastomosis by inserting the first stitch at 12 o'clock at the midpoint of the inferior esophagus. Bring this stitch into the lumen of the stomach and bring it out of the stomach at 6 o'clock. Apply a hemostat to this stitch, which serves as an anchor. Now close the anterior layer by inserting Lembert sutures and then invert the tissues as the knots are being tied. These knots remain outside the lumen **(Fig. 13–4)**. We frequently use the technique of successive bisection (see Figs. 4-19, 4-20). After the anastomosis is completed, ask the anesthesiologist to pass a nasogastric tube and guide it through the anastomosis into the gastric pouch.

Closure

Close the cervical incision in layers with interrupted 4-0 PG after inserting a 1.5 cm latex drain to a point near the anastomosis. Consider a needle catheter jejunostomy. Close the abdominal cavity without drainage using the modified Smead-Jones closure de-

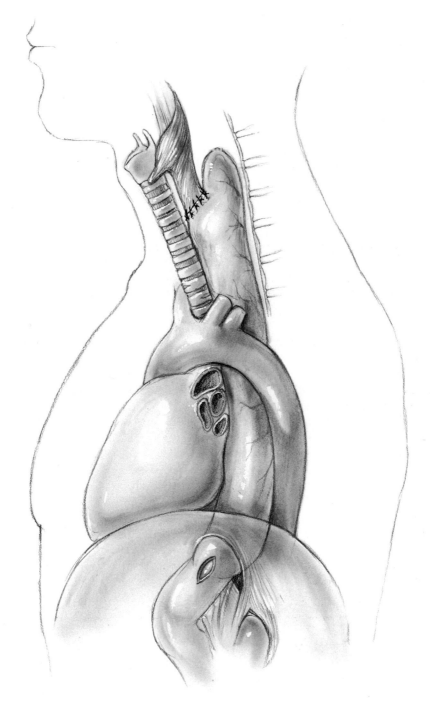

Fig. 13-4

scribed in Chapter 3 and no. 1 PDS sutures. Close the skin with interrupted fine nylon, subcuticular continuous 4-0 PG, or staples

POSTOPERATIVE CARE

Continue nasogastric suction for 4-5 days. Maintain the chest catheter on some type of underwater drainage for 4-5 days or until the volume of drainage becomes insignificant. Leave the cervical drain in place 7-10 days.

COMPLICATIONS

Anastomotic leak. This is seen especially in cases of anastomoses involving the cervical esophagus.

Stricture of the cervical anastomosis. This occurs especially after leaks.

Intestinal obstruction. Obstruction is due to adhesions.

Trauma to recurrent laryngeal nerve. The nerve is traumatized during dissection of the cervical esophagus.

Pneumothorax and intraoperative or postoperative hemorrhage. Insert a large drainage tube into the right or left hemithorax (or both) if a pneumothorax has been produced by the transhiatal dissection. Inspection of the mediastinum reveals most gaps in the mediastinal pleura.

Chylothorax. Chylothorax may follow transhiatal esophagectomy. It should be suspected whenever the chest tube drainage exceeds 800 ml per day after the third postoperative day. The diagnosis can be confirmed by administering cream via the jejunostomy catheter and observing an opalescent tinge to the pleural drainage. Early recognition, exploration, and transthoracic ligation may hasten resolution when compared with traditional conservative management.

Leaking thoracic duct. To identify the leaking thoracic duct at reoperation, Orringer et al. injected cream into the jejunostomy feeding tube at a rate of 60–90 ml/hr for 4–6 hours prior to reoperation for duct ligation. A limited fifth-interspace posterolateral thoracotomy under one-lung anesthesia was the approach these authors employed for the reoperation.

REFERENCES

Akiyama H. Surgery for carcinoma for the esophagus. Curr Probl Surg 1980;17:56.

Bolton JS, Fuhrman GM, Richardson WS. Esophageal resection for cancer. Surg Clin North Am 1998;78:773.

Chu KM, Law SY, Fok M, Wong J. A prospective randomized comparison of transhiatal and transthoracic resection for lower-third esophageal carcinoma. Am J Surg 1997;21:320.

Gluch L, Smith RC, Bambach CP, Brown AR. Comparison of outcomes following transhiatal or Ivor Lewis esophagectomy for esophageal carcinoma. World J Surg 1999;23:271.

Orringer MB, Stirling MC. Cervical esophagogastric anastomosis for benign disease: functional results. J Thorac Cardiovasc Surg 1988;96:887.

Orringer MB, Bluett M, Deeb GM. Aggressive treatment of chylothorax complicating transhiatal esophagectomy without thoracotomy. Surgery 1988;104:720.

Orringer MB, Marshall B, Iannettoni MD. Eliminating the cervical esophagogastric anastomotic leak with a side-to-side stapled anastomosis. J Thorac Cardiovasc Surg 2000;119:277.

Orringer MB, Marshall B, Iannettoni MD. Transhiatal esophagectomy: clinical experience and refinements. Ann Surg 1999;230:392.

Pinotti HW, Cecconello I, De Oliveira MA. Transhiatal esophagectomy for esophageal cancer. Semin Surg Oncol 1997;13:253.

Rindani R, Martin CJ, Cox MR. Transhiatal versus Ivor-Lewis oesophagectomy: is there a difference? Aust NZ J Surg 1999;69:187.

Stark SP, Romberg MS, Pierce GE, et al. Transhiatal versus transthoracic esophagectomy for adenocarcinoma of the distal esophagus and cardia. Am J Surg 1996;172:478.

Swanstrom LL, Hansen P. Laparoscopic total esophagectomy. Arch Surg 1997;132:943.

14 Operations to Replace or Bypass the Esophagus

Colon or Jejunum Interposition

INDICATIONS

Esophageal stricture or perforation

PREOPERATIVE PREPARATION

Nutritional rehabilitation, if needed

Perioperative antibiotics

Preoperative assessment of colon or jejunum by contrast studies, colonoscopy, and arteriography (if necessary)

Routine bowel preparation

OPERATIVE STRATEGY

Resect the damaged esophagus and replace it with a conduit whenever possible. When this is not feasible, a bypass leaving the damaged esophagus in situ is occasionally warranted. Patients who have an irreversible stricture due to peptic esophagitis require esophageal resection. Esophagectomy is also performed on patients who have undergone failed operations for neuromotor esophageal disorders or who have had diversion-exclusion operations (see Chapter 23) for esophageal perforations or anastomotic leakage. Orringer and Orringer (1983) did not open the chest in most of these patients but instead performed transhiatal esophagectomy from the abdominal and cervical approaches.

The colon is a versatile conduit that is applicable to most situations unless the patient has had a previous colon resection. Sufficient length can be obtained to perform a cervical anastomosis if necessary. Jejunum provides a better size match than colon but is considerably more difficult to use owing to the small size of the vessels. It has been used for cervical reconstructions using microsurgical free flap techniques.

The conduit must be carefully developed to preserve the blood supply, positioned in an isoperistaltic fashion without kinking or twisting, and the gastrointestinal continuity restored. These complex operations require thorough preoperative planning and must be individualized.

OPERATIVE TECHNIQUE

Incision and Resection of Esophagus

The choice of incision is determined by whether, and how much, esophagus is to be resected. Transhiatal esophagectomy is an option that obviates the need for a thoracic incision (see Chapter 13).

We prefer a sixth interspace left thoracoabdominal incision for most of these esophagectomies (see Figs. 12-3 to 12-8). Close the gastroesophageal junction in an area relatively free of disease using a 55- or 90-mm linear stapler on the stomach side. Close the esophageal end with another application of the stapling device. Dissect the esophagus out of the mediastinum. If the esophagus is markedly fibrotic, this dissection may require a scalpel. After the esophagus has been freed to the arch of the aorta, dissect the esophagus from underneath the arch of the aorta, as illustrated in Figure 12-26. Temporarily leave the esophagus in its bed until the colon has been liberated.

Long Segment Colon Interposition: Colon Dissection

The initial step for preparing a long colon segment is to liberate the hepatic flexure and the transverse and descending colon. If necessary, extend the thoracoabdominal incision below the umbilicus. Dissect the omentum away from the transverse colon and its mesentery, as illustrated in Figures 33-3, 33-4, 44-3, and 44-8.

With this accomplished, inspect the blood supply of the left and transverse colon. Preserving the left colic artery in most cases permits transection of the middle colic vessels close to the point of origin and yields a segment of colon that could include a good portion of the descending colon as well as the entire transverse colon if it should be necessary. We have not encountered any cases where the "marginal artery" did not continue unimpeded from the left colon around to the transverse colon. However, verify this by careful palpation of the marginal artery and transillumination of the mesentery. Apply bulldog vascular clamps along the marginal artery at the points selected for division

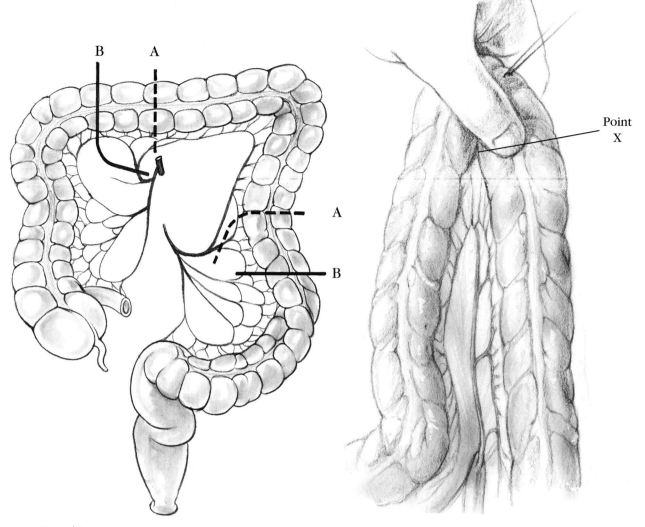

Fig. 14-1a

Fig. 14-1b

Point X

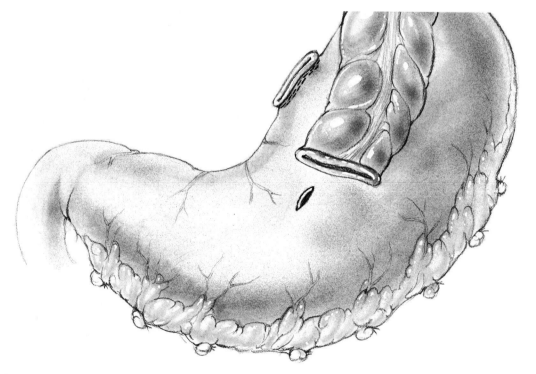

Fig. 14-2

and check the adequacy of the pulse in the vessels being retained to supply the transplanted segment.

To ensure a vigorous blood supply to the proximal portion of the transverse colon, with sufficient length to reach the cervical region, ligate and divide the middle colic artery at a point well proximal to its bifurcation (along line A rather than line B in **Figure 14–1a**). This allows the blood flow from the left colic artery to enter the left branch of the middle colic artery and to continue along the right branch to nourish the right portion of the transverse colon. For this reason it is critical that this division and ligature of the middle colic artery and vein be done with great care.

Estimating the Length of Colon Required to Reach the Neck

After the omentum has been dissected off the colon and after both the left and right colon segments have been freed from the posterior abdominal wall, grasp the splenic flexure at the point of termination of the left colic artery and draw this segment of colon in a cephalad direction toward the sternum. Then measure the distance from this point (point X in **Fig. 14–1b**) on the sternum to the neck. This distance approximates the amount of colon required going in a proximal direction from the termination of the left colic artery. Add about 4-5 cm to the estimate and insert a marking stitch in the right transverse colon at this point. In most cases the point marked is at the right of the middle colic vessels, indicating that division of the origin of the middle colic artery and vein is required.

Transect the colon at the proximal margin of the segment selected for transplantation. Restore continuity to the colon by performing a stapled anastomosis as illustrated in Figures 44-35 to 44-38. Close the proximal (right) margin of the colon transplant (temporarily) with a 55 mm linear stapler and leave the distal end of the colon segment open.

Cologastrostomy

Elevate the stomach with its attached omentum away from the pancreas. Divide the avascular attachments between the peritoneum overlying the pancreas and the back wall of the stomach. Also incise the avascular portion of the gastrohepatic omentum; then draw the colon transplant with its mesentery in an isoperistaltic direction through the retrogastric plane and through the opening in the gastrohepatic omentum. Be certain not to twist the mesentery. Verify that the colon does indeed reach the cervical esophagus without tension.

Prepare to anastomose the open end of the distal colon transplant to a point on the stomach approximately one-third the distance down from the fundus to the pylorus. The anastomosis may be made on the anterior or posterior side of the stomach. As illustrated in **Figure 14–2**, make a 1.5 cm vertical incision in the stomach about one-third of the way down from the fundus; then insert the cutting linear stapler—one fork in the stab wound of the stomach and one in the open lumen of the colon—to a depth of 3 cm and lock it **(Fig. 14–3)**. Fire the

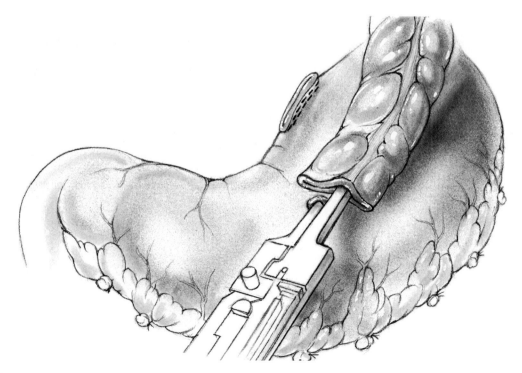

Fig. 14-3

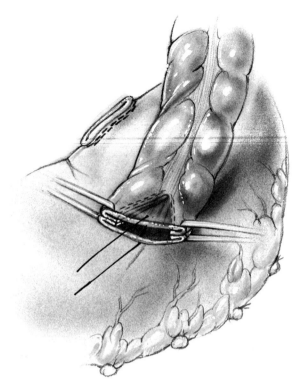

Fig. 14-4

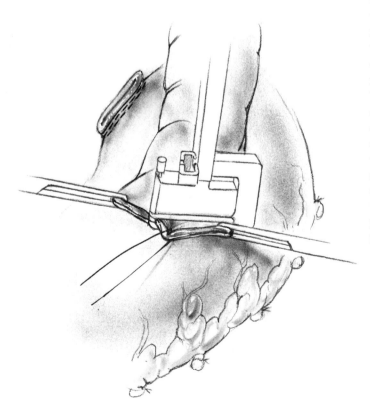

Fig. 14-5

stapler and remove it. Inspect the staple line for bleeding. Then apply Allis clamps to the left and right terminations of this staple line. Place a guy suture through the midpoint of the stab wound of the stomach as illustrated in **Figure 14–4**. Close the remaining defect by two applications of the 55 mm linear stapler. First, apply the stapler just deep to the Allis clamp and the guy suture to close the left half of the gap. After firing the stapling device **(Fig. 14–5)**, excise the surplus tissue but preserve the guy suture. Lightly electrocoagulate the everted mucosa and remove the stapling device. Then reapply the stapler in similar fashion to close the remaining defect. Be sure to place the stapler deep to the Allis clamp and the guy suture. After firing the stapling device, cut away the surplus tissue and lightly electrocoagulate the mucosa. This creates a fairly large anastomosis between the stomach and colon, as illustrated in **Figure 14–6**.

DeMeester et al. pointed out that it is possible to divide the descending colon as it comes behind the stomach without simultaneously dividing the marginal artery of the descending colon. If the marginal artery is not divided, it provides an added avenue of blood flow to the colon that has been transplanted into the neck. By carefully transecting the colon behind the stomach and then dividing and ligating the end branches of the marginal artery close to the colon for a distance of about 4 cm, sufficient colon will have been liberated that a cologastric anastomosis can be constructed to the posterior wall of the stomach, and the distal segment of descending colon can be anastomosed to the remaining hepatic flexure. If the anastomosis is made at the junction between the upper third and the lower two-thirds of the stomach, it seems not to matter whether the cologastrostomy is constructed on the posterior wall or the anterior wall of the stomach. However, if one wishes to preserve the marginal artery of the descending colon, it is necessary to place the cologastrostomy on the posterior wall of the stomach **(Fig. 14–7a)**. The posterior cologastric anastomosis may be constructed by suturing (as illustrated here) or by stapling (as described in Figs. 14-3 to 14-6). In

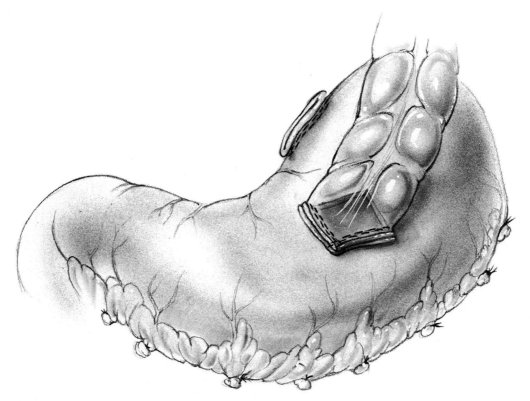

Fig. 14-6

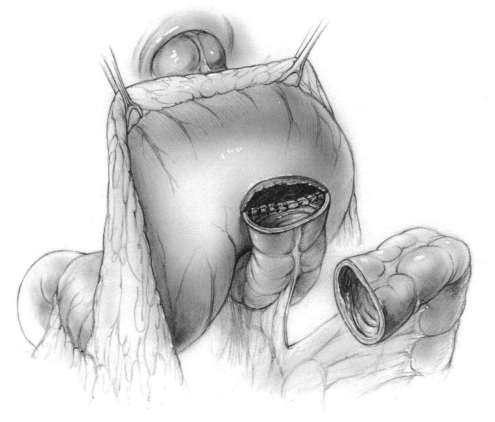

Fig. 14-7a

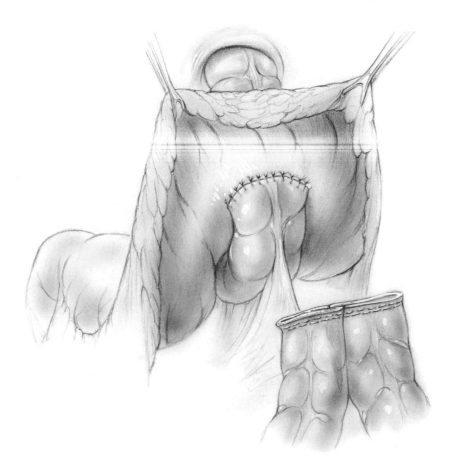

Fig. 14-7b

this manner the colocolostomy can also be performed close by, preserving the marginal artery (**Fig. 14-7b).**

Pyloromyotomy

In most conditions for which a thoracic esophagectomy is being performed, the vagus nerves are destroyed, which impairs gastric emptying to a fairly severe degree in about 20% of cases. To prevent this complication, a pyloromyotomy may be performed by the technique illustrated in Figures 11-17 to 11-19.

Advancing the Colon Segment to the Neck

Be certain to enlarge the diaphragmatic hiatus (see Fig. 11-20) sufficiently that the veins in the colon mesentery are not compressed by the muscles of the hiatus. The most direct route to the neck follows the course of the original esophageal bed in the posterior mediastinum. Place several studies between the proximal end of the colon transplant and the distal end of the esophagus; then draw the colon up into the neck by withdrawing the esophagus into the neck. This brings the colon into the posterior mediastinum behind the arch of the aorta and into the neck posterior to the trachea. If there is no constriction in the chest along this route, the sternum and clavicle at the root of the neck are also not likely to compress the colon. On the other hand, if a substernal tunnel is selected for passing the colon up to the neck, it is generally necessary to resect the head of one clavicle and a 2 cm width of adjacent sternal manubrium to be certain there is no obstruction at that point.

A good alternative method for transporting the colon up to the neck is to pass a 36F rubber catheter from the neck down into the abdominal cavity. Obtain a sterile plastic sheath such as a laser drape and suture the end of this plastic cylinder to the termination of the rubber catheter. Insert the proximal end of the colon into this plastic sheath and suture it lightly to the red rubber catheter. By withdrawing the catheter through the thoracic cavity into the neck, the colon with its delicate blood supply can be delivered into the neck without trauma.

Verify that the tube of colon from the neck to the abdominal cavity lies in a straight line and there is no surplus of colon in the chest. Leaving redundant colon in the thorax may produce a functional obstruction to the passage of food. Then suture the colon to the muscle of the diaphragmatic hiatus with interrupted sutures of atraumatic 4-0 Tevdek at intervals of about 2 cm around half the circumference of the colon. This helps maintain a direct passageway from the neck into the abdomen. Be sure not to pass the needle deep to the submucosa of the colon, as colonic leaks have been reported to result from this error.

Dissecting the Cervical Esophagus

Change the position of the patient's left hand, which is suspended from the ether screen. Bring the left hand laterally and place it along the left side of the patient. Turn the head slightly to the right and make an incision along the anterior border of the left sternomastoid muscle; continue the dissection as described in Figures 11-27 to 11-30. Be careful not to damage the left or the right recurrent laryngeal nerve. After dissecting the esophagus free down into the superior mediastinum, extract the thoracic esophagus by applying gentle traction in the neck. In this way the thoracic esophagus and the attached colon interposition segment may be drawn gently into the neck. Divide the distal cervical esophagus and remove the thoracic esophagus. Inspect the end of the colon. There should be a good pulse in the marginal artery. Cyanosis indicates venous obstruction, which must be corrected. Draw the closed stapled end of the colon transplant to a point about 6-7 cm above the cut end of the esophagus and, taking care not to penetrate the lumen of the colon, su-

ture the colon to the prevertebral fascia with several interrupted 4-0 silk sutures.

Esophagocolonic Anastomosis

Perform an end-to-side esophagocolonic anastomosis at a point about 4 cm below the proximal end of the colon using a technique similar to that described in Figures 11-22 to 11-26 and by using interrupted 4-0 silk Cushing sutures for the outer layer and 5-0 PG or PDS for the mucosal layer. Before closing the anterior portion of the anastomosis, ask the anesthesiologist to pass a nasogastric tube into the esophagus and guide this tube through the anastomosis into the colon.

Retrosternal Passage of Colon Transplant

When the posterior mediastinum is not a suitable pathway for the colon or if the esophagus has not been removed, make a retrosternal tunnel to pass the colon up to the neck. If the left lobe of the liver is large or if it appears to be exerting pressure on the posterior aspect of the colon transplant, liberate the left lobe by dividing the triangular ligament. This permits the left lobe to fall in a posterior direction and thereby relieves this pressure. If the xiphoid process curves posteriorly and impinges on the colon, resect the xiphoid.

Enter the plane just posterior to the periosteum of the sternum. Start the dissection with Metzenbaum scissors; then insert one or two fingers of the right hand. Finally, pass the entire hand just deep to the sternum up to the suprasternal notch. This is generally an avascular plane. Orient the colon segment so the mesentery enters from the patient's left side. Resect the medial 3-4 cm of clavicle using a Gigli saw. Then rongeur away about 2 cm of adjacent sternal manubrium to be certain the aperture at the root of the neck is sufficiently large to avoid any venous obstruction in the mesentery. Pass a long sponge-holder into the retrosternal tunnel from the neck down into the abdomen and suture the proximal end of the colon segment to the tip of the sponge-holder. Gently pass the colon into the substernal tunnel while simultaneously drawing the sutures in a cephalad direction.

There may be fewer symptoms after resection of the clavicular head if it is performed on the side

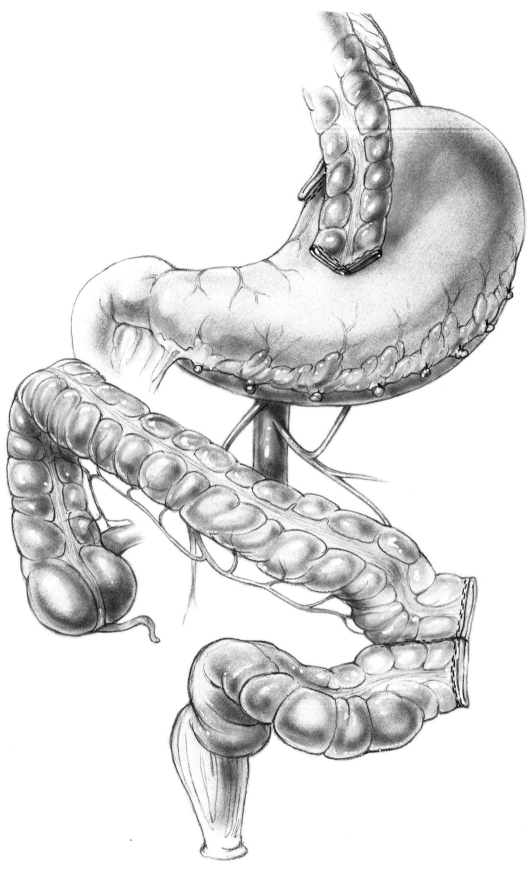

Fig. 14-8

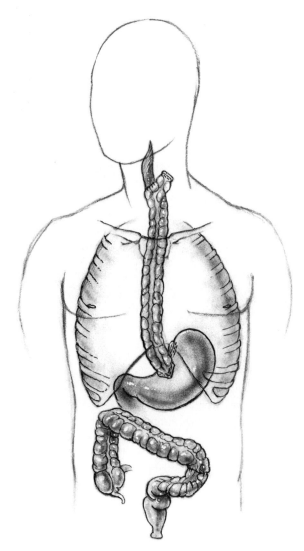

Fig. 14-9

even in the operating room, without rupturing the esophagus. If there is no significant amount of disease above the level of the inferior pulmonary ligament, resect the diseased esophagus down to the esophagogastric junction and replace the missing esophagus with a short isoperistaltic segment of colon to extend from the divided esophagus to a point about one-third the distance between the fundus and the pylorus of the stomach. For a short segment operation it is not necessary to divide the middle colic artery, and only the distal portion of the transverse colon and the splenic flexure need be employed. Otherwise, the operation is much the same as described above. The cologastric anastomosis is identical. The esophagocolonic anastomosis may be sutured in an end-to-end fashion, an end-to-side fashion, or even by a stapling technique. The latter involves inserting a proper circular stapling cartridge (generally 28 or 25 mm) into the open proximal end of the colonic segment. The anastomosis is made between the end of the esophagus and the side of the colon by the usual circular stapling technique. Then, after disengaging the instrument, explore the anastomosis visually and manually with a finger through the open end of the colon. If the exploration appears satisfactory, close the opening in the colon about 1 cm away from the circular stapled anastomosis using a 55/3.5 mm linear stapler. Excise the redundant tissue and remove the stapler.

Jejunum Interposition

Incision and Mobilization

Although Polk advocated mobilizing the esophagogastric junction through an upper midline abdominal incision, we prefer the left sixth interspace thoracoabdominal incision with a vertical midline abdominal component. This is because the jejunal interposition operation is performed primarily in patients who have had multiple failed previous operations for reflux esophagitis. The Collis-Nissen gastroplasty combined with dilatation of the esophageal stricture suffices in most patients. This leaves a few of the most advanced cases that require a colon (short-segment) or jejunum interposition.

The combined thoracoabdominal incision provides superb exposure and makes this operation as safe as possible. It should be emphasized that creating a jejunal segment is much more difficult than the short-segment colon interposition. When performing the thoracoabdominal incision, incise the diaphragm with electrocautery in a circumferential fashion, as depicted in Figure 12-8.

Dissect the left lobe of the liver carefully away from the anterior wall of the stomach; in doing so,

opposite the dominant hand. Once it has been ascertained that the circulation to the colon segment is good, perform the esophagocolonic anastomosis as above. The final appearance of the colon interposition is depicted in **Figures 14-8** and **14-9**.

Closure

Close the cervical incision in layers with interrupted 4-0 PG sutures. Insert one or two drains in the general vicinity of the anastomosis and leave them in place 7-10 days. Close the skin in the usual fashion. Close the thoracoabdominal incision as illustrated in Figures 12-35 to 12-41.

Colon Interposition, Short Segment

In rare cases of benign peptic stricture of the lower esophagus, it is impossible to dilate the stricture,

approach the dissection from the lesser curvature aspect of the stomach. At the same time, incise the gastrohepatic omentum by proceeding up toward the hiatus. This may require division of the accessory left hepatic artery, provided it has not been done at a previous operation (see Fig. 17-4). It may also be difficult to free the upper stomach from its posterior attachments to the pancreas. Careful dissection with good exposure from the thoracoabdominal incision should make it possible to preserve the spleen from irreparable injury. At the conclusion of this dissection, the upper portion of the stomach and lower esophagus should be free. Freeing the esophagus in the upper abdomen may be expedited by first dissecting the esophagus out of its bed in the lower mediastinum.

Resection of Diseased Esophagus

After the esophagus has been freed from its fibrotic attachments in the mediastinum and upper stomach, select a point near the esophagogastric junction for resection. If the upper stomach has been perforated during this dissection and the perforation can be included in the specimen, do so. If the upper stomach is not excessively thickened, apply a 55 or 90 mm linear stapling device with 4.8 mm staples and fire it. Transect the esophagogastric junction just above the stapling device. Lightly electrocoagulate the everted mucosa and remove the stapler. Deliver the transected esophagus into the chest and select the point of transection on the esophagus above the stricture. A mild degree of mucosal inflammation in the esophagus is acceptable at the point of transection. Remove the specimen.

If the point of division of the esophagus is not higher than the inferior pulmonary vein, jejunal interposition is a good method for establishing continuity. If the esophagus must be transected at a higher level, use a short segment of colon for the interposition or remove the remainder of the thoracic esophagus and reestablish continuity by means of a long-segment colon interposition from the neck to the stomach or by bringing the stomach up into the neck for this purpose, as described below. The graft of jejunum may be lengthened safely if its circulation can be boosted by creating microvascular anastomoses from a thoracic artery and vein to the upper end of the graft.

Mobilizing the Jejunum Graft

Because the vascular anatomy of the proximal jejunum varies somewhat from patient to patient, it is necessary to individualize the dissection according to the conditions encountered. First, try to stretch the proximal jejunum in a cephalad direction to determine where the greatest mobility is located. Be certain to leave intact at least the first major jejunal artery to the proximal jejunum. The average length of the jejunal segment to be transplanted varies between 12 and 20 cm, and the pedicle should consist of at least one major arcade vessel with careful preservation of the veins. Most jejunal grafts fail not because of poor arterial circulation but because the veins have been injured or compressed at some point. Follow the principles illustrated in Figure 34-4 and try to preserve a vascular pedicle containing two arcade vessels with their veins intact. When dividing an arcade vessel, be sure to place the point of transection sufficiently proximal to a bifurcation so the continuity of the "marginal" artery and vein is not interrupted. Divide and temporarily close the jejunum proximally and distally with a linear cutting stapler, preserving a segment measuring 15-20 cm for interposition.

Make an incision in the transverse mesocolon through its avascular portion just to the left of the middle colic vessels. Carefully pass the jejunal graft together with its vascular pedicle through this incision into the previously dissected lesser sac behind the stomach. Be absolutely certain the incision in the mesentery does not constrict the veins of the vascular pedicle. Also be careful not to twist the pedicle. Pass the proximal portion of the jejunal segment through the hiatus into the chest. Be certain that the hiatus is large enough that it does not compress the veins in the vascular pedicle.

Esophagojejunostomy

Establish an end-to-side esophagojejunal anastomosis on the antimesenteric border of the jejunum beginning about 1 cm distal to the staple line on the proximal closed end of the jejunal segment. A technique similar to that described in Figures 34-5 to 34-15 using 4-0 atraumatic interrupted silk Cushing or Lembert sutures for the outer layer and interrupted or continuous 5-0 Vicryl for the mucosal layer may be employed. Pass the nasogastric tube through this anastomosis down to the lower end of the jejunal graft. It is also possible to perform a stapled esophagojejunostomy by the technique described in Figures 34-16 to 34-21.

Jejunogastrostomy

Place the jejunogastric anastomosis 5-7 cm below the proximal margin of the stomach in an area of stomach that is relatively free of fibrosis and that permits the vascular pedicle to be free of tension. This may be done by the same suture technique as mentioned

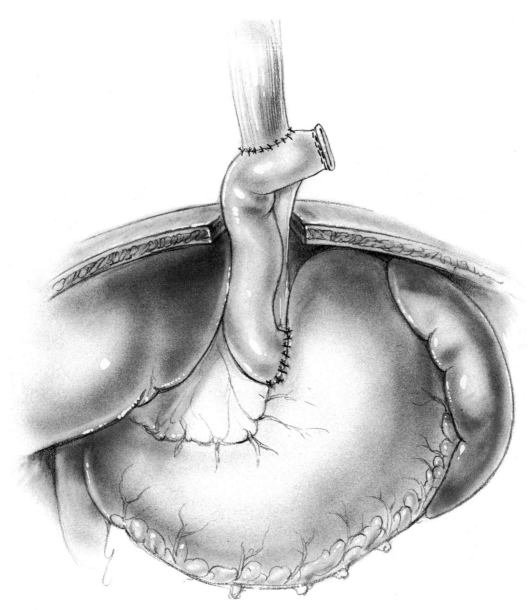

Fig. 14-10

above (see Figs. 34-5 to 34-15), but if there is sufficient length of jejunum it may also be performed by a stapled anastomosis similar to that described in Figures 14-2 to 14-6. The appearance of the completed anastomosis is shown in **Figure 14–10**.

Jejunojejunostomy

Reestablish the continuity of the jejunum by creating a functional end-to-end anastomosis using the stapling technique described in Figures 37-12 to 37-16. Then carefully resuture the defect in the jejunal mesentery without compressing the vascular pedicle jejunal graft.

Use interrupted 4-0 Tevdek sutures to approximate the diaphragmatic hiatus to the seromuscular wall of the jejunum to avoid herniation of bowel through the hiatus. Be certain not to compress the vascular pedicle.

Gastrostomy; Pyloromyotomy

Although the nasogastric tube has been passed through the jejunal graft into the stomach to maintain the position of the graft, there is a risk that the nasogastric tube may be inadvertently removed before the patient's gastrointestinal tract has resumed function. For this reason, perform a Stamm gastrostomy as described in Figures 32-1 to 32-5 and remove the nasogastric tube.

Most surgeons advocate performing a pyloromyotomy or pyloroplasty during this type of operation because it is assumed that the vagus nerves have been interrupted during the course of dissecting a heavily scarred esophagus out of the mediastinum. Polk stated that this step may not be necessary.

Closure

Repair the diaphragm and close the thoracoabdominal incision as illustrated in Figures 12-38 to 12-44 after inserting a chest tube. No abdominal drains are utilized.

REFERENCES

Belsey R. Reconstruction of the esophagus with the left colon. J Thorac Cardiovasc Surg 1965;49:33.

Curet-Scott M, Ferguson MK, Little AG, et al. Colon interposition of benign esophageal disease. Surgery 1987; 102:568.

DeMeester TR, Johansson K-E, Franze I, et al. Indications, surgical technique, and long-term functional results of colon interposition and bypass. Ann Surg 1988;208:460.

Furst H, Hartl WH, Lohe F, Schildberg FW. Colon interposition for esophageal replacement: an alternative technique based on the use of the right colon. Ann Surg 2000;231:173.

Loinaz C, Altorki NK. Pitfalls and complications of colon interposition. Chest Surg Clin North Am 1997;7:533.

Moylan JP Jr, Bell JW, Cantrell JR, Merendino KA. The jejunal interposition operation: a follow-up on seventeen patients followed 10–17 years. Ann Surg 1970;172: 205.

Orringer MB, Orringer JS. Esophagectomy without thoracotomy: a dangerous operation? J Thorac Cardiovasc Surg 1983;85:72.

Polk HC Jr. Jejunal interposition for reflux esophagitis and esophageal stricture unresponsive to valvuloplasty. World J Surg 1980;4:741.

Thomas P, Fuentes P, Giudicelli R, Reboud E. Colon interposition for esophageal replacement: current indications and long-term function. Ann Thorac Surg 1997; 64:757.

Wilkins EW Jr. Long-segment colon substitute for the esophagus. Ann Surg 1980;192:722.

15 Transabdominal Nissen Fundoplication

INDICATIONS

Gastroesophageal reflux (see Chapter 10), especially in patients in whom laparoscopic Nissen fundoplication is not applicable

PREOPERATIVE PREPARATION

Esophagogastroduodenoscopy with brushing and biopsies of any abnormal mucosa

Esophageal manometry or pH studies in selected patients

PITFALLS AND DANGER POINTS

Inadequate mobilization of gastric fundus and abdominal esophagus

Injury to spleen or to vagus nerves

Fundoplication wrap too tight or too long

Inadequate fundoplication suturing

Undiagnosed esophageal motility disorders, such as achalasia, diffuse spasm, aperistalsis, or scleroderma

Hiatal closure too tight, causing esophageal obstruction

Hiatal closure too loose, permitting postoperative paraesophageal herniation

Injury to left hepatic vein or vena cava when incising triangular ligament to liberate left lobe of liver

OPERATIVE STRATEGY

Mobilizing the Gastric Fundus

To perform a hiatus hernia repair efficiently, the lower 5–7 cm of the esophagus and the entire gastric fundus from the gastroesophageal junction down to the upper short gastric vessel must be completely mobilized from all attachments to the diaphragm and the posterior abdominal wall. Identify the gastrophrenic ligament by passing the left

hand behind the stomach so the fingertips can identify this avascular ligament, which attaches the greater curvature to the diaphragm. The ligament extends from the gastroesophageal junction down to the first short gastric vessel. It is simple to divide once it has been stretched by the surgeon's left hand behind the stomach. Although in a few cases no short gastric vessels must be divided, there should be no hesitation to divide one to three proximal short gastric vessels to create a loose fundoplication.

On the lesser curvature aspect of the gastroesophageal junction, it is necessary to divide the proximal portion of the gastrohepatic ligament. This ligament often contains an accessory left hepatic artery arising from the left gastric artery and going to the left lobe of the liver and the hepatic branch of the left vagus nerve. Division of the accessory left hepatic artery has, in our experience, not proved harmful. Do not divide the left gastric artery itself. Preserving the left gastric artery and the hepatic branch of the vagus nerve helps prevent the fundoplication from slipping in a caudal direction. The lower esophagus is freed by incising the overlying peritoneum and phrenoesophageal ligaments; continue this incision in a semicircular fashion so the muscular margins of the diaphragmatic crura are exposed down to the median arcuate ligament. During all of this mobilization, look for the major branches of the anterior and posterior vagus nerves and preserve them.

Preventing Splenic Injury

Splenic trauma is a common but preventable complication of the Nissen operation. With use of the Thompson or Upper Hand retractor there is no reason for any retractor to come into contact with the spleen. The mechanism of splenic injury is usually traction on the body of the stomach toward the patient's right, which avulses that portion of the splenic capsule attached to the omentum or to the gastrosplenic ligament. Early during the operation, make it a point to look at the anterior surface of the spleen. Note where the omentum may be adherent to the splenic capsule. If necessary, divide these attachments under direct vision. Otherwise, simply apply a moist gauze pad over the spleen and avoid lateral traction on the stomach. Traction on the gastroesophageal junction in a caudal direction along the *lesser* curve of the stomach generally does not cause injury to the spleen.

If a portion of the splenic capsule has been avulsed, it can almost always be managed by applying topical hemostatic agents followed by 10 minutes of pressure. Other splenic injuries can be repaired by suturing with 2-0 chromic catgut (see Chapter 85). Extensive disruption of the spleen at its hilus may necessitate splenectomy.

Avoiding Postoperative Dysphagia

Probably secondary to local edema, transient mild dysphagia is common during the first 2–3 weeks following operation, although some patients have difficulty swallowing for many months after a hiatus hernia operation. There are several possible causes for this dysphagia. First, it is possible to make the fundoplication wrap so tight or so wide that permanent dysphagia ensues (see below). Second, the defect in the hiatus may be sutured so tightly the hiatus impinges on the lumen of the esophagus and prevents passage of food. With an 18F nasogastric tube in place, after the crural sutures have been tied to repair the defect in the hiatus it should still be possible to insert an index finger without difficulty between the esophagus and the margins of the hiatus. There is no virtue in closing the hiatus snugly around the esophagus. A final cause of dysphagia in patients who have experienced this symptom as a preoperative complaint is the presence of an esophageal motility disorder such as achalasia or aperistalsis. Patients who present to the surgeon with reflux esophagitis and who also complain of dysphagia should undergo preoperative esophageal manometry to rule out motility disorders that may require surgery in addition to the antireflux procedure or instead of it.

How Tight Should the Fundoplication Be?

The Nissen operation produces a high pressure zone in the lower esophagus by transmitted gastric pressure in the wrap, rather than by the tightness of the wrap itself. An excessively tight wrap causes dysphagia and the gas bloat syndrome. Therefore the fundoplication should be made loose, rather than

tight enough to constrict the esophagus. Many surgeons use an indwelling esophageal bougie to avoid creating a wrap that is too tight. Regardless of whether the indwelling bougie is used, it is possible to judge the tightness of the wrap by applying Babcock clamps to each side of the gastric fundus and tentatively bringing them together in front of the esophagus. This mimics the effect of the sutures. The surgeon should be able to pass one or two fingers between the wrap and the esophagus without difficulty with an 18F nasogastric tube in place. Otherwise readjust the fundoplication so it is loose enough for this maneuver to be accomplished.

How Long Should the Fundoplication Be?

Another cause of postoperative dysphagia is making the fundoplication wrap too long. For the usual Nissen operation, do not wrap more than 2–3 cm of esophagus. A shorter wrap may be appropriate when esophageal dysmotility and gastroesophageal reflux coexist (e.g., when a fundoplication is added to a myotomy).

Avoiding Fundoplication Suture Line Disruption

Polk and others have noted that an important cause of failure after Nissen fundoplication has been disruption of the plication because the sutures broke. For this reason, use 2-0 sutures. Generally, the sutures that were found to have broken were silk. We have used 2-0 Tevdek because it retains its tensile strength for many years, whereas silk gradually degenerates in the tissues. It is also important not to pass the suture into the lumen of the stomach or esophagus. If this error is committed, tying the suture too tight causes strangulation and possibly leakage. Some insurance against the latter complication is to turn in the major fundoplication sutures with a layer of continuous 4-0 Prolene seromuscular Lembert sutures.

Failure to Bring the Esophagogastric Junction into the Abdomen

If it is not possible to mobilize the esophagogastric junction from the mediastinum and bring it into the abdomen while performing transabdominal repair of a hiatus hernia, it is likely that esophageal fibrosis has produced shortening. Such a situation can generally be suspected prior to operation when the lower esophagus is strictured. In our opinion, these patients require a transthoracic Collis-Nissen operation (see Chapter 18). Although it is possible to perform a Collis-Nissen procedure in the abdomen, it is difficult. If it cannot be accomplished transabdominally, it is necessary to open the chest through a separate incision or through a thoracoabdominal extension to perform the Collis-Nissen operation.

Keeping the Fundoplication from Slipping

Various methods have been advocated to keep the fundoplication from sliding in a caudal direction, where it constricts the middle of the stomach instead of the esophagus and produces an "hourglass" stomach with partial obstruction. The most important means of preventing this caudal displacement of the wrap is to include the wall of the esophagus in each of the fundoplication sutures. Also, catch the wall of the stomach just below the gastroesophageal junction within the lowermost suture. This suture anchors the lower portion of the wrap (see Fig. 15-10, below).

OPERATIVE TECHNIQUE

Incision

Elevate the head of the operating table 10°–15°. Make a midline incision beginning at the xiphoid

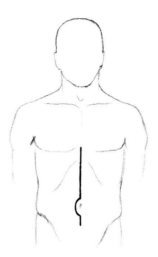

Fig. 15-1

and continue about 2–3 cm beyond the umbilicus **(Fig. 15–1)**. Explore the abdomen. Insert a Thompson or Upper Hand retractor to elevate the lower portion of the sternum. Reduce the hiatus hernia by traction along the anterior wall of the stomach. Look at the anterior surface of the spleen to determine whether there are omental adhesions to the capsule that may result in the capsule avulsing later during the operation. Place a moist gauze pad over the spleen. In most cases it is not necessary to free the left lobe of the liver; simply elevate the left lobe with a Weinberg retractor to expose the diaphragmatic hiatus.

Mobilizing the Esophagus and Gastric Fundus

Make a transverse incision in the peritoneum overlying the abdominal esophagus **(Fig. 15–2)** and continue this incision into the peritoneum overlying the right margin of the crus. Then divide the peritoneum overlying the left margin of the diaphragmatic hiatus. Separate the hiatal musculature from the esophagus using a peanut dissector until *most of the circumference of the esophagus has been exposed.*

Then pass the index finger *gently* behind the esophagus and encircle it with a latex drain **(Fig. 15–3)**. Enclose both the right and left vagus nerves in the latex drain and divide all the phrenoesophageal attachments behind the esophagus. If the right (posterior) vagus trunk courses at a distance from the esophagus, it is easier to dissect the nerve away from the upper stomach and to exclude the right vagus from the fundoplication wrap. Some exclude both vagus trunks from the wrap, but we prefer to include them inside the loose wrap. Before the com-

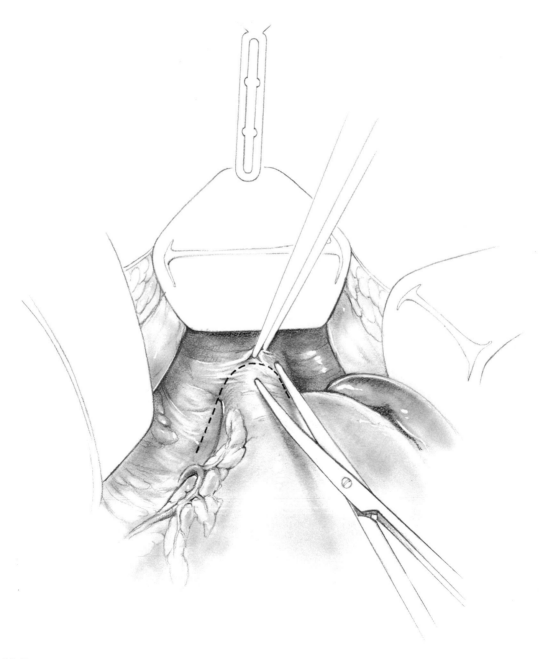

Fig. 15-2

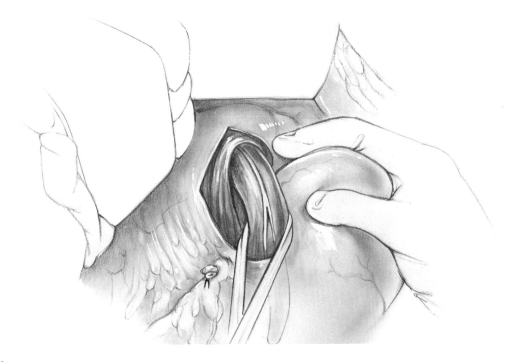

Fig. 15-3

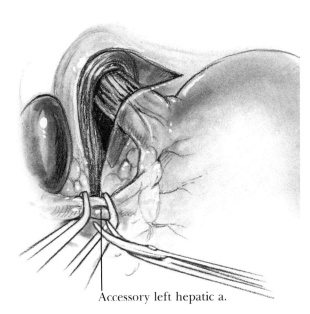

Accessory left hepatic a.

Fig. 15-4

plete circumference of the hiatus can be visualized, it is necessary to divide not only the phreno-esophageal ligaments but also the cephalad portion of the gastrohepatic ligament, which often contains an accessory left hepatic artery that may be divided **(Fig. 15–4)**. The exposure at the conclusion of this maneuver is seen in **Figure 15–5**. Now pass the left

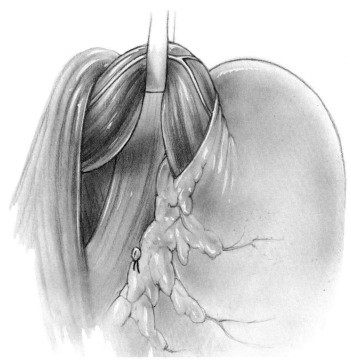

Fig. 15-5

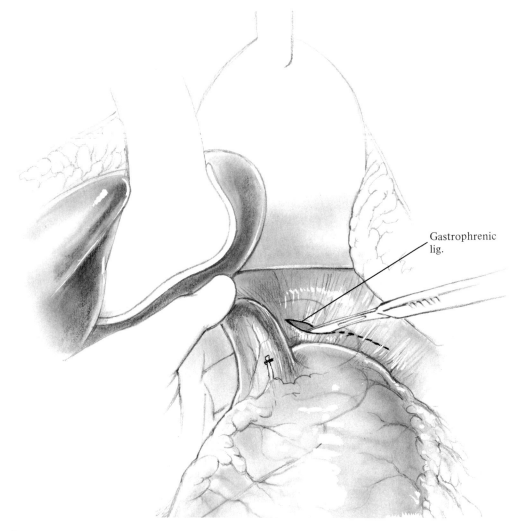

Gastrophrenic lig.

Fig. 15–6

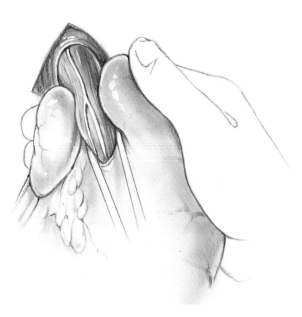

Fig. 15–6

hand behind the esophagus and behind the gastric fundus to identify the gastrophrenic ligament and divide it carefully down to the proximal short gastric vessel (**Fig. 15–6**).

While the assistant is placing traction on the latex drain to draw the esophagus in a caudal direction, pass the right hand to deliver the gastric fundus behind the esophagus (**Fig. 15–7**). Apply Babcock clamps to the two points on the stomach where the first fundoplication suture will be inserted and bring these two Babcock clamps together tentatively to assess whether the fundus has been mobilized sufficiently to accomplish the fundoplication without tension. **Figure 15–8**, a cross-sectional view, demonstrates how the gastric fundus surrounds the lower esophagus and the vagus nerves.

Generally, there is inadequate mobility of the gastric fundus unless one divides the proximal one to three short gastric vessels. Ligate each with 2-0 silk.

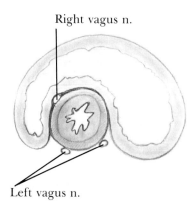

Right vagus n.

Left vagus n.

Fig. 15–8

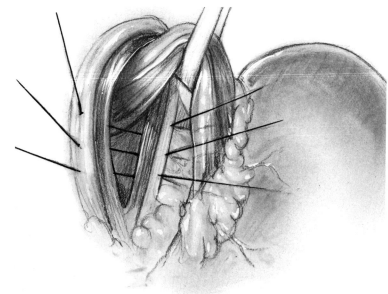

On the greater curvature aspect of the esophagogastric junction there is usually a small fat pad. Excising the fat pad improves adhesion of the gastric wrap to the esophagus.

Fig. 15–9

Repairing the Hiatal Defect

Using 0 Tevdek sutures on a large atraumatic needle, begin at the posterior margin of the hiatal defect and take a bite (1.3–2.0 cm in width) of the crus and its overlying peritoneum on each side of the hiatus. Insert the next suture about 1.0–1.2 cm cephalad and continue this process until the index finger can just be inserted *comfortably* between the esophagus and the margin of the hiatus **(Fig. 15–9)**.

Suturing the Fundoplication

Pass a 40F Maloney dilator into the stomach. Insert the first fundoplication suture by taking a bite of the fundus on the patient's left using 2-0 atraumatic Tevdek. Pass the needle through the seromuscular surface of the gastric lesser curve just distal to the esophagogastric junction; then take a final bite of the fundus on the patient's right. Attach a hemostat to tag this stitch but do not tie it. Each bite should contain 5–6 mm of tissue including submucosa, but it should not penetrate the lumen. Do not pierce any of the vagus nerves with a stitch. To perform a fundoplication without tension, it is necessary to insert the gastric sutures a sufficient distance lateral to the esophagogastric junction. Place additional sutures, as illustrated in **Figure 15–10**, at intervals of about 1 cm. Each suture should contain one bite of fundus, then esophagus, and then the opposite side of the fundus. No more than 2–3 cm of esophagus should be encircled by the fundoplication. Now tie all of these sutures **(Fig. 15–11)**. It should be possible to insert one or two fingers between the

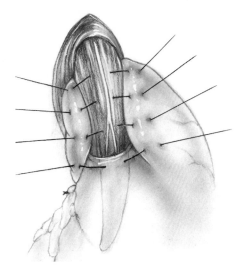

Fig. 15–10

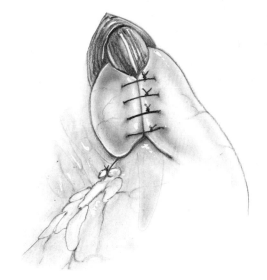

Fig. 15–11

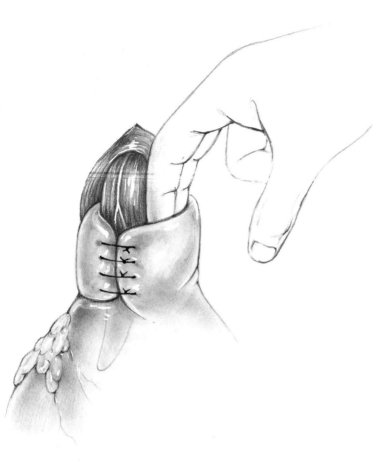

Fig. 15-12

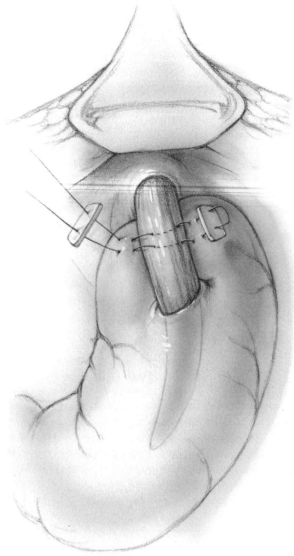

Fig. 15-13

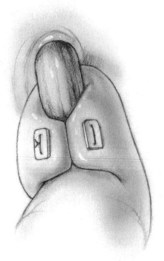

Fig. 15-14

esophagus and the Nissen wrap **(Fig. 15–12)**. If this cannot be done, the wrap is too tight.

A number of surgeons place sutures fixing the upper margin of the Nissen wrap to the esophagus to prevent the entire wrap from sliding downward and constricting the stomach in the shape of an hourglass. DeMeester and Stein, after considerable experience, advocated a Nissen wrap measuring only 1 cm in length, claiming that longer wraps produce postoperative dysphagia in a number of patients. Even with a 60F Maloney bougie in the esophagus, a 1 cm wrap has effectuated excellent control of reflux. They constructed this wrap employing one horizontal mattress suture of 2-0 Prolene buttressed with Teflon pledgets **(Figs. 15–13, 15–14)**.

Optionally, at this point one may invert the layer of fundoplication sutures by inserting a continuous seromuscular layer of 4-0 Prolene Lembert sutures (not illustrated). This layer provides protection against leakage if any of the fundoplication sutures were placed too deep.

Testing Antireflux Valve

Ask the anesthesiologist to inject 300–400 ml saline solution into the nasogastric tube and then withdraw the tube into the esophagus. Now try to expel the saline by compressing the stomach. If the saline cannot be forced into the esophagus by moderate manual compression of the stomach, the fundoplication has indeed created a competent antireflux valve.

Abdominal Closure

Close the abdomen without drainage in routine fashion.

POSTOPERATIVE CARE

Continue nasogastric suction for 1–2 days. Then initiate oral feeding. A barium esophagram is obtained before the patient is discharged. If a satisfactory repair has been accomplished, 3–4 cm of distal esophagus becomes progressively narrower, tapering to a point at the gastroesophageal junction. If this tapering effect is not noted, it suggests that the wrap may be too loose. Successful antireflux procedures, whether by the Nissen, Hill, Belsey, or Collis-Nissen technique, show similar narrowing of the distal esophagus on the postoperative esophagram. A typical postoperative barium esophagram is shown in **Figure 15–15**.

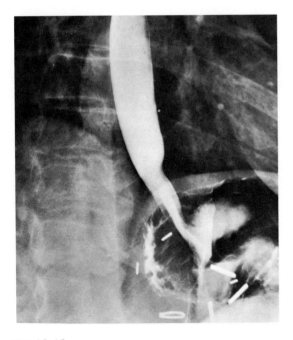

Fig. 15-15

COMPLICATIONS

Dysphagia, usually transient

"Gas bloat" (rare)

Disruption of fundoplication

Slipping downward of fundoplication with obstruction

Postoperative paraesophageal hernia if hiatal defect was not properly closed

Herniation of fundoplication into thorax

Esophageal or gastric perforation by deep necrosing sutures

Persistent gastroesophageal reflux

REFERENCES

Bais JE, Bartelsman JF, Bonjer HJ, et al. Laparoscopic or conventional Nissen fundoplication for gastro-oesophageal reflux disease: randomised clinical trial; the Netherlands Antireflux Surgery Study Group. Lancet 2000;355:170.

DeMeester TR, Stein JH. Minimizing the side effects of antireflux surgery. World J Surg 1992;16:335.

Deschamps C, Trastek VF, Allen MS, et al. Long-term results after reoperation for failed antireflux procedures. J Thorac Cardiovasc Surg 1997;113:545.

Henderson RD, Marryatt G. Total fundoplication gastroplasty; long-term follow-up in 500 patients. J Thorac Cardiovasc Surg 1983;85:81.

Herrington JR Jr. Treatment of combined sliding and paraesophageal hiatal hernia; emphasis on protection of the vagus nerves. Contemp Surg 1983;22:19.

Horgan S, Pohl D, Bogetti D, Eubanks T, Pellegrini C. Failed antireflux surgery: what have we learned from reoperations? Arch Surg 1999;134:809.

Kauer WK, Peters JH, DeMeester TR, et al. A tailored approach to antireflux surgery. J Thorac Cardiovasc Surg 1995;110:141.

Leonardi HK, Crozier RE, Ellis FH. Reoperation for complications of the Nissen fundoplication. J Thorac Cardiovasc Surg 1981;81:50.

Luostarinen ME, Isolauri JO. Randomized trial to study the effect of fundic mobilization on long-term results of Nissen fundoplication. Br J Surg 1999;86:614.

Luostarinen M, Isolauri J, Laitinen J, et al. Fate of Nissen fundoplication after 20 years: a clinical, endoscopic and functional analysis. Gut 1993;34:1015.

Peillon C, Manouvrier JL, Labreche J, et al. Should the vagus nerves be isolated from the fundoplication wrap? A prospective study. Arch Surg 1994;129:814.

Polk HC Jr. Fundoplication for reflux esophagitis: misadventures with the operation of choice. Ann Surg 1976;183:645.

Rieger NA, Jamieson GG, Britten-Jones R, Tew S. Reoperation after failed antireflux surgery. Br J Surg 1994;81:1159.

Rogers DM, Herrington JL, Morton C. Incidental splenectomy associated with Nissen fundoplication. Ann Surg 1980;191:153.

Stirling MC, Orringer MB. Surgical treatment after the failed antireflux operation. J Thorac Cardiovasc Surg 1986;92:667.

Urschel JD. Complications of antireflux surgery. Am J Surg 1993;166:68.

16 Laparoscopic Nissen Fundoplication

INDICATIONS

Symptomatic reflux esophagitis refractory to medical therapy

Barrett's esophagus (consider mucosal ablation)

PREOPERATIVE PREPARATION

Pass a nasogastric tube to decompress the stomach. See Chapter 15.

PITFALLS AND DANGER POINTS

Injury to the esophagus.

Tension pneumothorax due to unrecognized entry into the mediastinal pleura. Even a relatively small tear can allow CO_2 to enter the pleural space and compromise ventilation.

Injury to spleen or stomach.

Failure to create a sufficiently floppy wrap.

OPERATIVE STRATEGY

Several laparoscopic fundoplications have been devised. We prefer the laparoscopic Nissen fundoplication because it is intended to be virtually identical to a well established open procedure when completed. The steps in the dissection are necessarily a bit different from those for the open procedure, and several additional features should be noted.

First, the hiatus is accessed by elevating the left lobe of the liver without dividing its attachments. Second, the esophagus is exposed and mobilized by dissecting the crura with minimal manipulation of the esophagus. The resulting extensive mediastinal dissection that accompanies esophageal mobilization makes approximation of the crura mandatory. Postoperative herniation of the stomach or small intestine may complicate the laparoscopic procedure when this step is omitted. Finally, several short gastric vessels *must* be divided to ensure creating a floppy wrap.

OPERATIVE TECHNIQUE

Room Setup and Trocar Placement

Position the patient with the legs slightly spread and supported on padded stirrups **(Fig. 16–1)**. Position the monitors at the head of the table. We place the primary monitor at the patient's left shoulder, with a secondary monitor at the patient's right, as shown. Some surgeons use a single monitor placed over the head of the operating table. We prefer to stand in

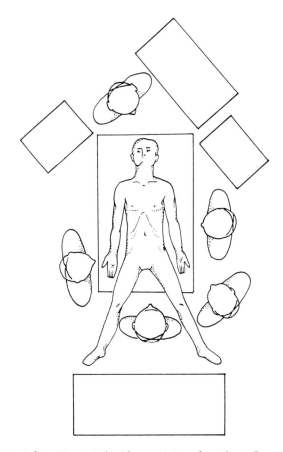

Fig. 16-1 (Reprinted with permission, from Scott-Conner CEH (ed) The SAGES Manual: Fundamentals of Laparoscopy and GI Endoscopy. New York, Springer-Verlag, 1999.)

the usual position, at the patient's side, for the initial puncture and entry into the abdomen. During dissection and suturing, the surgeon should stand between the patient's legs, directly facing the hiatus **(Fig. 16–2)**. When choosing an initial puncture site (to be used for the laparoscope) recall that the hiatus is quite high and deep. The normal umbilical port site may therefore be too low. A trocar pattern must be individualized according to the patient's body habitus. A 30° angled laparoscope is mandatory for easy visualization.

Exposure of the Hiatus

Pass a liver retractor through the right lateral port site. A variety of liver retractors are available, and which one is chosen is largely a matter of the surgeon's preference. We prefer a flexible retractor that becomes rigid and assumes the shape shown in **Figure 16–3** when a screw is turned. The particular retractor shown is composed of many short segments with an internal cable. When the tension on the cable is released, the retractor becomes limp and may be straightened out to pass it through a trocar. Once the retractor is inside the abdomen, the cable is tightened by twisting a knob on the handle. In-

creasing tension on the internal cable forces the articulations to bend into the shape shown. The retractor is bent into shape by tightening the cable in the commodious right subphrenic space and is then passed underneath the liver.

The liver retractor is properly placed when stable exposure is obtained and the diaphragmatic surface is seen behind the left lobe of the liver. It may not be possible to distinguish the actual hiatus at this point. This exposure generally requires that the retractor be "toed in" so the part of the retractor closest to the hiatus has maximal lift applied. The laparoscope and instruments are then insinuated underneath the left lobe of the liver in the working space thus created.

Generally, the stomach and some omentum partially or completely obscure the hiatus even with the liver retracted. Therefore the second part of obtaining exposure entails placing an endoscopic Babcock clamp on the stomach and pulling toward the left lower quadrant **(Fig. 16–4)**.

Dissecting the Hiatus

The esophagus is dissected by clearing the peritoneum off the hiatus and carefully exposing the

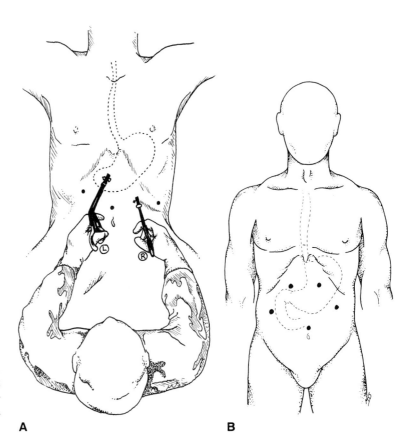

Fig. 16–2 (Reprinted with permission, from Scott-Conner CEH (ed) The SAGES Manual: Fundamentals of Laparoscopy and GI Endoscopy. New York, Springer-Verlag, 1999.)

A   B

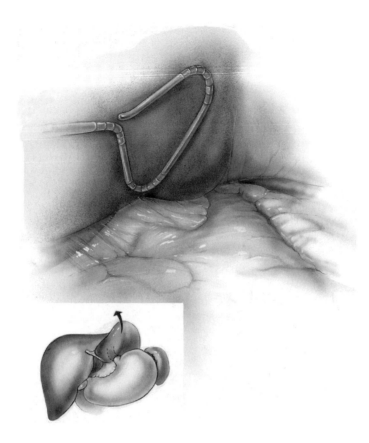

Fig. 16-3

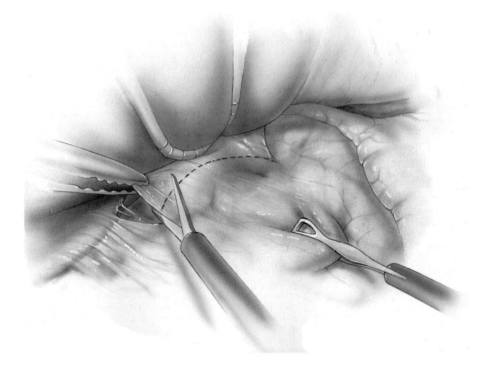

Fig. 16-4

muscular crura. Properly performed, this maneuver automatically exposes the esophagus and creates a posterior window.

Begin the dissection by exposing the right crus. Start by opening the peritoneum just to the right of the probable hiatus. The first step involves dividing the lesser omentum. A grasper is used to elevate the flimsy lesser omentum close to the hiatus, and ultrasonic dissecting scissors are used to divide the omentum (Fig. 16-4).

It is tempting to begin this dissection by opening the transparent part of the omentum farther to the right. If you begin your omental window high, however, near the hiatus, you are less likely to encounter a hepatic artery. This has the additional advantage of keeping the window in the lesser omentum relatively small, which helps anchor the wrap and prevents slipping.

Do not try to identify and dissect the esophagus at this stage. To do so risks perforation. A far safer approach is to dissect and clearly define the muscular hiatus and both crura. First identify the right crus after dividing the peritoneum. Next carry the dissection up over the arch of the crura, concentrating on exposing the muscle fibers of the diaphragm. During this dissection the esophagus becomes obvious by its orientation, longitudinal muscle, and overlying vagus nerve; it may also be gently displaced downward **(Fig. 16–5)** and to the left. The esophagus has a light pink to reddish pink color and characteristic longitudinal striations. If there is uncertainty as to the location of the esophagus, the nasogastric tube may be palpable to light touch with a grasper, or an esophagogastro-duodenoscopy (EGD) scope may be passed and used to elevate and transilluminate the esophagus. These maneuvers are rarely needed.

A closed grasper is used to push the esophagus down. This grasper is introduced parallel to the esophagus through one of the left-sided trocars and is used to probe into the mediastinum by gently pushing the esophagus down.

When the upper part of the hiatus has been cleaned thoroughly, elevate the esophagus gently with a closed grasper and clean the lower part of the *left* crus from the *right* side by working underneath the esophagus **(Fig. 16–6)**. This maneuver produces a window behind the esophagus while minimizing the risk of perforating the esophagus. The esophagus is *never actually grasped*; rather, it is gently displaced to one side or the other using a closed grasper. Frequently the anterior vagus nerve is seen on the right side of the esophagus.

It is fairly common to encounter a sizable vessel next to the esophagus on the right side **(Fig. 16–7)**.

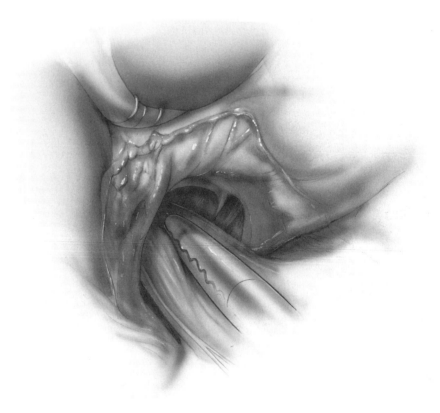

Fig. 16–5

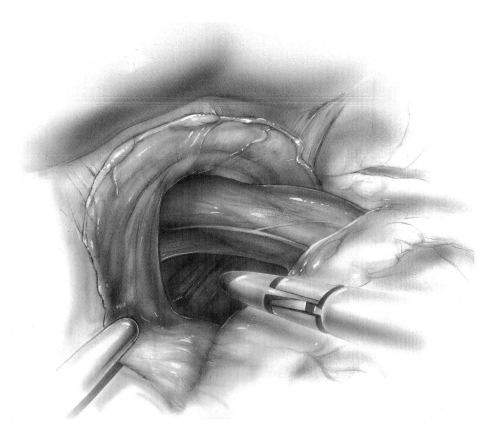

Fig. 16-6

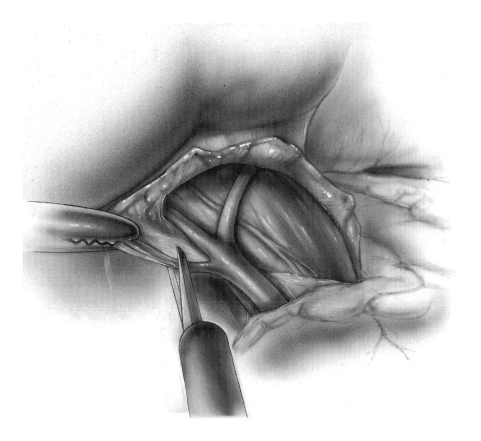

Fig. 16-7

The vessel is smaller than it appears; it looks large because it is closer to the scope than the esophagus. This vessel is usually a branch of the inferior phrenic artery. It must be carefully secured with ultrasonic shears **(Fig. 16–8)**. A replaced hepatic artery, sometimes encountered in this region, is usually larger and is seen to curve away toward the liver rather than pass cephalad toward the diaphragm. If a replaced hepatic artery is encountered, gently displace it to the right (out of the field of surgery) and protect it.

Mobilizing the Esophagus

If the crura have been carefully dissected to create an adequate posterior window, there should be a clear space behind the esophagus and retractors should pass easily. The retractors we prefer are curved and paired. They are designed to be inserted from the left and right sides.

Pass the first retractor from the left side. The design of the retractor shown is similar to that of the liver retractor. It is passed into the abdomen limp, and the cable is tightened to make it assume its working configuration. Once the curve is set, the retractor is rigid and ready for use.

Follow the arc of the circle while passing the retractor. Gently swing it from behind. Do not attempt to create a window with the retractor—the window should already be there. Do not attempt to "hook up" under the esophagus; to do so risks posterior perforation. When the tip of the retractor is seen to emerge from the right side of the space behind the esophagus, lift the esophagus with the retractor **(Fig. 16–9)**.

Pass the second esophageal retractor from the right. Follow the first retractor around, concentrating on the feel of metal on metal as the second retractor "rides" along parallel to the first. Maintain traction on the stomach to help generate a sufficient length of esophagus **(Fig. 16–10)**.

Move the two retractors apart in a spreading movement, parallel to the long axis of the esophagus **(Fig. 16–11)** to enlarge the window behind the esophagus if needed. Generally only one of the retractors is needed for the remainder of the procedure.

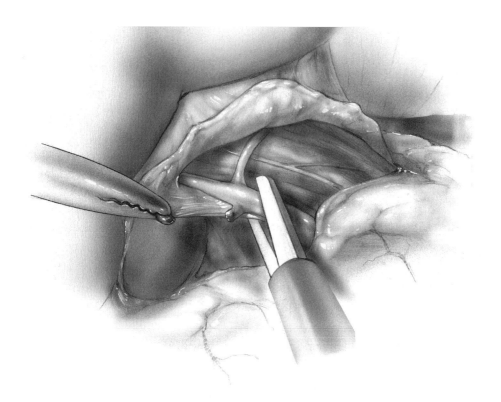

Fig. 16-8

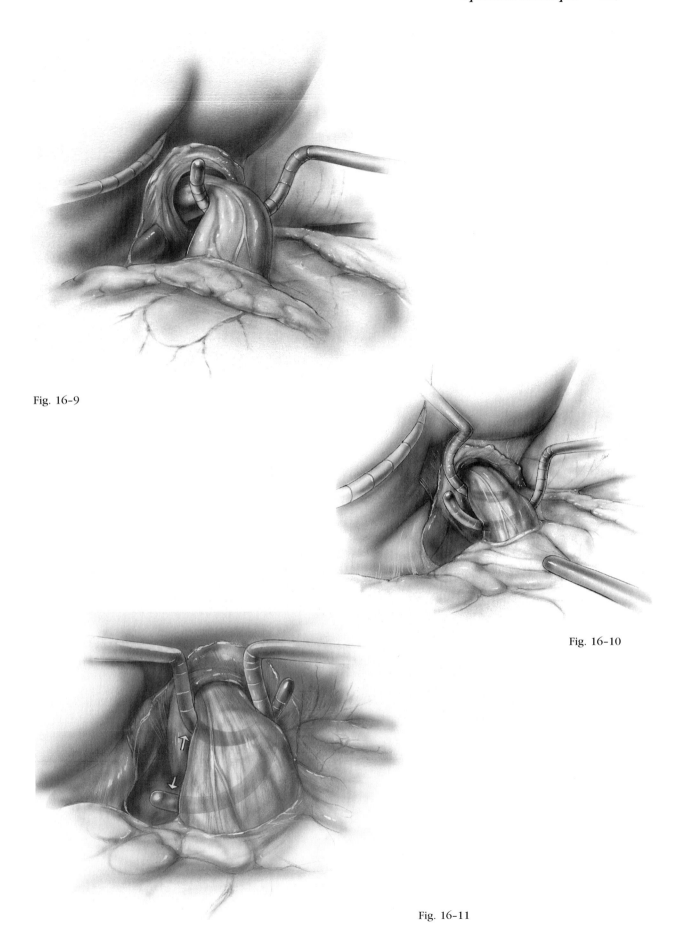

Fig. 16-9

Fig. 16-10

Fig. 16-11

Closing the Hiatus

The hiatus must be closed to avoid herniation of the stomach or small intestine. Place one or two simple sutures of 0 or 2-0 silk and tie them **(Fig. 16–12)**. Leave a gap to avoid overtightening the hiatus, which may cause postoperative dysphagia.

Dividing the Short Gastric Vessels

The short gastric vessels tether the fundus of the stomach to the spleen **(Fig. 16–13a)**. Begin dividing these vessels at a convenient point high on the fundus and work cephalad **(Fig. 16–13b)**. We prefer ultrasonic shears for this division. Test the mo-

Fig. 16-12

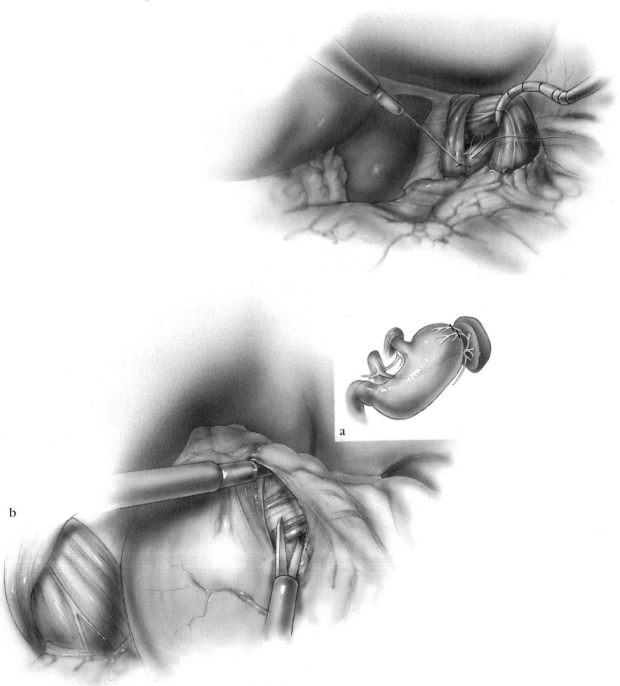

Fig. 16-13a,b

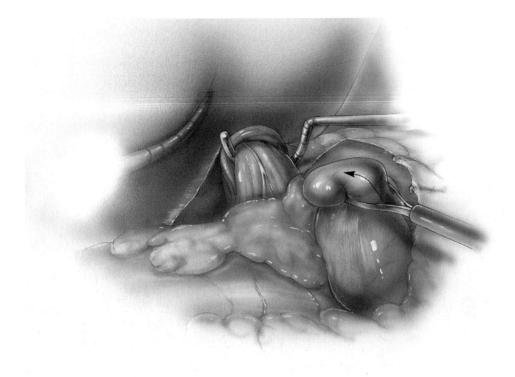

Fig. 16–14a

bility of the fundus by passing it back and forth anterior to the esophagus **(Figs. 16–14a, 16–14b)**.

If at any time there has been concern about injury to the esophagus or stomach, have the anesthesiologist instill methylene blue into the nasogastric tube and look for staining. Repair any areas of concern at this time. Use the wrap to buttress any esophageal repair.

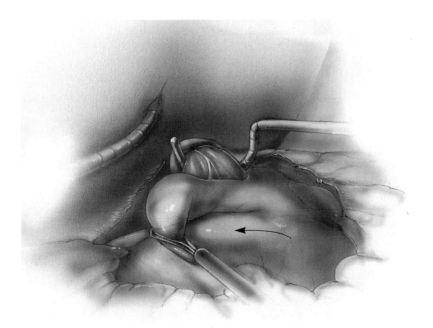

Fig. 16–14b

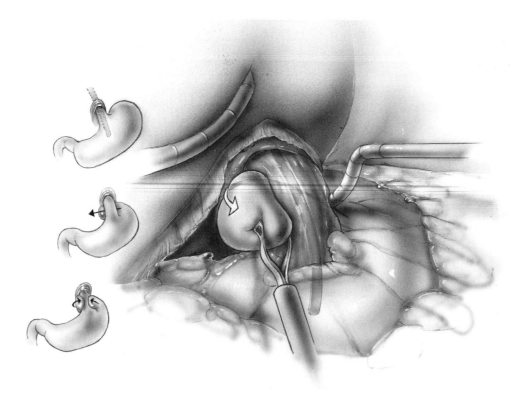

Fig. 16–15a,b,c,d

Creating the Wrap

Remove the esophageal retractors and allow the esophagus to return to its normal anatomic position. Pass Maloney dilators from above. For most adults, sequentially pass dilators until a 56–60F dilator is in place (**Fig. 16–15a**).

Replace the left esophageal retractor and elevate the esophagus. Use an angled grasper to reach behind the esophagus from right to left. Grasp the fun-

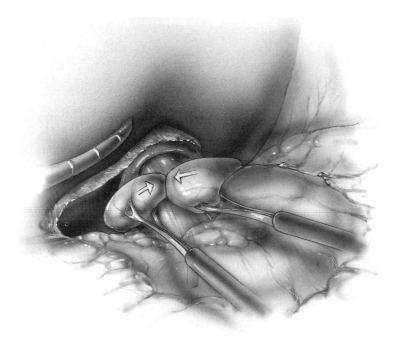

Fig. 16–16

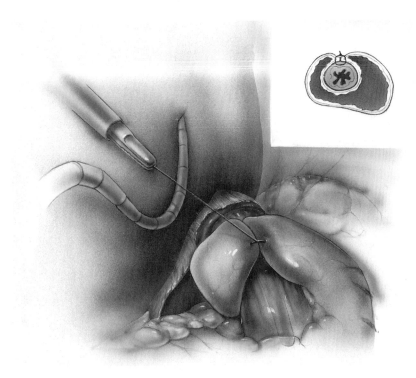

Fig. 16-17

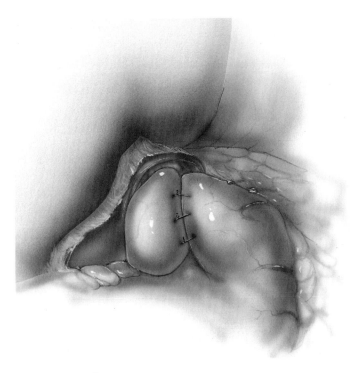

Fig. 16-18

dus and pull it behind the esophagus. It should pass easily **(Fig. 16–15b, 16–15c, 16–15d)**.

Bring additional fundus over from the left side to meet the portion that has been passed behind **(Fig. 16–16)**. The wrap should meet easily and feel "floppy." Avoid the error of creating a twist by pulling the posterior part of the wrap too far to the right. Such a twist may contribute to postoperative dysphagia.

Place three sutures to complete the wrap. Catch a bit of the esophagus with the first suture or two to anchor the wrap well above the stomach **(Fig. 16–17)**. Take care not to take an excessively deep bite and create a perforation. Some surgeons place clips on the knots to mark the location of the wrap. It facilitates postoperative evaluation with barium swallow. The completed wrap should lie easily below the diaphragm **(Fig. 16–18)**.

POSTOPERATIVE CARE

We keep the nasogastric tube in place for the first 24 hours to avoid gastric dilatation. A Hypaque swallow the first postoperative day should demonstrate free passage of Hypaque without extravasation. This is particularly important if there is any question of the integrity of the wrap or esophagus.

COMPLICATIONS

Esophageal perforation

Herniation of viscera through the hiatal opening

Slipped wrap

Dysphagia

REFERENCES

Hunter JG, Trus TL, Branum GD, Waring JP, Wood WC. A physiologic approach to laparoscopic fundoplication for gastroesophageal reflux disease. Ann Surg 1996; 223:673.

Peters JH. Laparoscopic treatment of gastroesophageal reflux and hiatal hernia. In: Scott-Conner CEH (ed) The SAGES Manual: Fundamentals of Laparoscopy and GI Endoscopy. New York, Springer-Verlag, 1999, pp 196–212.

Schauer PR, Meyers WC, Eubanks S, et al. Mechanisms of gastric and esophageal perforations during laparoscopic fundoplication. Ann Surg 1996;223:43.

17 Posterior Gastropexy (Hill Repair)

Surgical Legacy Technique

INDICATIONS

See Chapter 15.

Gastroesophageal reflux.

Successful execution of this operation requires that the esophagus be long enough to suture the esophagogastric junction to the level of the median arcuate ligament without tension (5-7 cm of intraabdominal esophagus).

PREOPERATIVE PREPARATION

See Chapter 15.

PITFALLS AND DANGER POINTS

Hemorrhage from laceration of celiac or inferior phrenic artery

Injury to spleen

Improper calibration of lumen of lower esophageal sphincter

Excessive narrowing of diaphragmatic hiatus

Failure to identify the median arcuate ligament

Injury to left hepatic vein or vena cava when incising triangular ligament to liberate left lobe of liver

OPERATIVE STRATEGY

Dissecting the Median Arcuate Ligament

The median arcuate ligament constitutes the anterior portion of the aortic hiatus, the aperture in the diaphragm through which the aorta passes. The ligament, a condensation of preaortic fascia, arches over the anterior surface of the aorta just cephalad to the origin of the celiac artery and joins the right crus of the diaphragm at its insertion onto the vertebral column. This band of fibrous tissue covers about 3 cm of the aorta above the celiac axis and is in turn covered by crural muscle fibers. It can be identified by exposing the celiac artery and pushing it posteriorly with the finger at the inferior rim of the median arcuate ligament. For Hill's operation, the surgeon dissects the celiac artery and celiac ganglion away from the overlying median arcuate ligament in the midline, avoiding the two inferior phrenic arteries that arise from the aorta just to the right and just to the left of the midline. Nerve fibers from the celiac ganglion must be cut to liberate the median arcuate ligament.

An alternative method for identifying the median arcuate ligament is to visualize the anterior surface of the aorta above the aortic hiatus. A few fibers of preaortic fascia may have to be incised. Then with the left index fingernail pushing the anterior wall of the aorta posteriorly, pass the fingertip in a caudal direction. The fingertip passes behind a strong layer of preaortic fascia and median arcuate ligament. At a point about 2-3 cm caudal to the upper margin of the preaortic fascia, blocking further passage of the fingertip, is the attachment of the inferior border of the median arcuate ligament to the aorta at the origin of the celiac artery. The pulsation of the celiac artery is easily palpated by the fingertip, which is lodged between the aorta and the overlying ligament. Vansant and colleagues believed that the foregoing maneuver constitutes sufficient mobilization of the median arcuate ligament and that the ligament need not be dissected free from the celiac artery and ganglion to perform a posterior gastropexy. We believe that a surgeon who has not had considerable experience liberating the median arcuate ligament from the celiac artery may find Vansant's modification to be safer than Hill's approach. If one succeeds in catching a good bite of the preaortic fascia and median arcuate ligament by Vansant's technique, the end result should be satisfactory.

If the celiac artery or the aorta is lacerated during the course of the Hill operation, do not hesitate to divide the median arcuate ligament and preaortic fascia in the midline. This step may be necessary to expose the full length of the laceration.

Calibrating the Esophagocardiac Orifice

In addition to fixing the esophagocardiac junction to the median arcuate ligament, the Hill operation serves to narrow the entrance of the lower esophagus into the stomach by partially turning in the lesser curvature aspect of the esophagogastric junction. Calibration of this turn-in is important if reflux is to be prevented without at the same time causing chronic obstruction. Hill (1977) used intraoperative manometry to measure the pressure at the esophagocardiac junction before and after completing the gastropexy. He believed that a pressure of 50-55 mm Hg ensures that the calibration is proper. Orringer et al. reported that intraoperative pressures did not correlate at all with pressures obtained at postoperative manometry, perhaps because of the variable influence of preoperative medication and anesthetic agents.

If intraoperative manometry is not used, the adequacy of the repair should be tested by invaginating the anterior wall of the stomach along the indwelling nasogastric tube upward into the esophagogastric junction. Prior to the repair, the index finger can pass freely into the esophagus because of the incompetent lower esophageal sphincter. After the sutures have been placed and drawn together but not tied, the tip of the index finger should be able to palpate the esophageal orifice but should not quite be able to enter the esophagus alongside the 18F nasogastric tube. This method of calibration has been successful in our hands.

Liberating Left Lobe of Liver

As discussed in Chapter 15, liberating the left lobe of the liver is rarely needed.

OPERATIVE TECHNIQUE

Incision and Exposure

With the patient in the supine position, elevate the head of the table about 10°–15° from the horizontal. Make a midline incision from the xiphoid to a point about 4 cm below the umbilicus **(Fig. 17–1)**. Insert a Thompson or Upper Hand retractor to elevate the lower portion of the sternum and draw it forcefully in a cephalad direction. Explore the abdomen for incidental pathology, such as a duodenal ulcer, cholelithiasis, chronic pancreatitis, or colon disease.

Mobilizing the Esophagogastric Junction

Identify the peritoneum overlying the abdominal esophagus by palpating the indwelling nasogastric tube. Divide this peritoneum with Metzenbaum scissors and continue the incision over the right and left branches of the crus **(Fig. 17–2)**. After exposing the crus, elevate this muscle by inserting a peanut sponge dissector between the crus and the esophagus, first on the right and then on the left. Then insert the left index finger to encircle the esophagus by *gentle* dissection. If the esophagus is inflamed owing to inadequately treated esophagitis, it is easy to perforate it by rough finger dissection. Identify and protect both the right and left vagus nerves. Then encircle the esophagus with a latex drain and free it from posterior attachments by dividing the phrenoesophageal ligaments **(Fig. 17–3)**.

Make an incision in the avascular portion of the gastrohepatic ligament. Continue this incision in a cephalad direction toward the right side of the hiatus. When dividing the gastrohepatic ligament it is often necessary to divide an accessory left hepatic

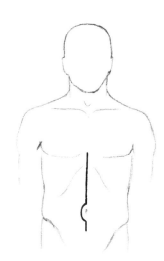

Fig. 17-1

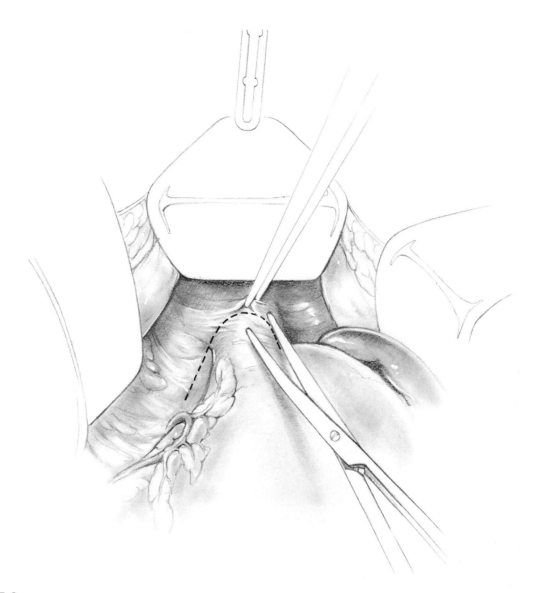

Fig. 17-2

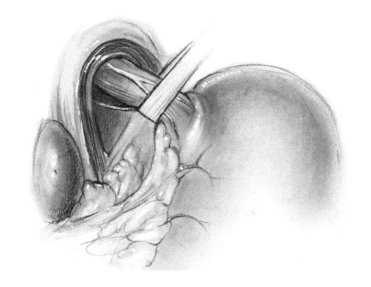

Fig. 17-3

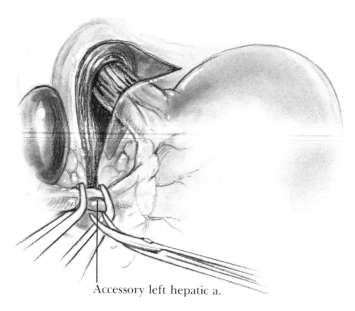

Accessory left hepatic a.

Fig. 17–4

branch of the left gastric artery **(Fig. 17–4)**. At the conclusion of this step, the muscular portion of the crura surrounding the hiatus should be clearly visible throughout the circumference of the hiatus.

The only structure binding the gastric fundus to the posterior abdominal wall now is the gastrophrenic ligament. The best way to divide this ligament is to insert the left hand behind the esophagogastric junction and then bring the left index finger between the esophagogastric junction and the diaphragm. This places the ligament on stretch. Divide this avascular ligament **(Fig. 17–5)** from the esophagogastric junction along the greater curvature down to the first short gastric artery. It is often necessary to divide the first two short gastric vessels to achieve proper mobilization. This may be done by applying a Hemoclip to the splenic side and a 2-0 silk ligature to the gastric side of the short gastric vessel.

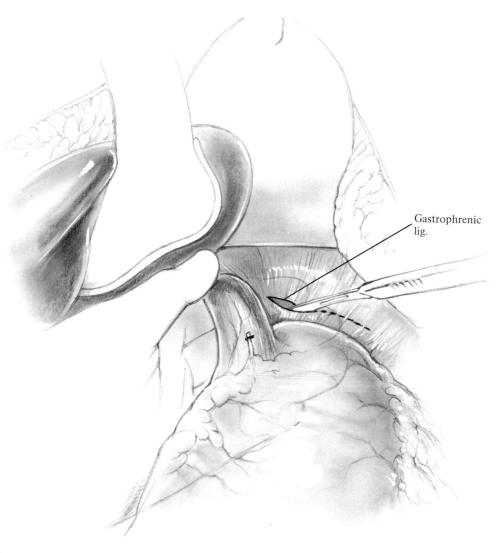

Gastrophrenic lig.

Fig. 17–5

Avoid injuring the spleen by carefully inspecting the anterior surface of this organ prior to dissection in this region. Divide any attachments between the omentum and the splenic capsule, as traction on the omentum would otherwise cause avulsion of the capsule and bleeding.

Inserting the Crural Sutures

Ask the first assistant to retract the esophagus toward the patient's left; then narrow the aperture of the hiatus by approximating the crural bundles behind the esophagus. Use 0 Tevdek atraumatic sutures on a substantial needle. Take a bite of 1.5–2.0 cm of crus on the left and a similar bite on the right. Include the overlying peritoneum together with the crural muscle **(Fig. 17–6)**. Do not tie these sutures at this time but tag each with a small hemostat. It is sometimes helpful to grasp the left side of the crus with a long Babcock or Allis clamp. Do not apply excessive traction with these clamps or sutures, as the crural musculature tends to split along the line of its fibers. Insert three or four sutures of this type as necessary. Then tentatively draw the sutures together and insert the index finger into the remaining hiatal aperture. It should be possible to insert a fingertip into the remaining aperture alongside the esophagus with its indwelling nasogastric tube. Narrowing the hiatal aperture more than this may cause permanent dysphagia and does not help reduce reflux. Do not tie the crural sutures at this point.

Identifying the Median Arcuate Ligament

Hill's Method

After the lower esophagus and proximal stomach have been completely freed, identify the celiac artery and use the left index finger to press it posteriorly into the aorta. If the index finger slides in a cephalad direction, its tip meets the lower border of the median arcuate ligament. Between the aorta and median arcuate ligament are branches of the celiac ganglion as well as the right and left inferior phrenic arteries, which arise from the aorta in this vicinity. It is necessary to divide some of the nerve fibers; but once the inferior margin of the ligament is freed from the aorta in the midline, it is possible to pass an instrument in a cephalad direction without encountering any further resistance. Hill passed a Goodell cervical dilator between the median arcuate ligament and the aorta to protect the aorta while sutures were being inserted into the lower border of the ligament. He stated that if a small diaphragmatic branch of the aorta is disrupted the bleeding often subsides with pressure. However, it is possible for the inexperienced surgeon to induce major hemorrhage by traumatizing the arteries in this vicinity. Caution is indicated.

Vansant's Method

Vansant and colleagues described another technique for identifying and liberating the median arcuate

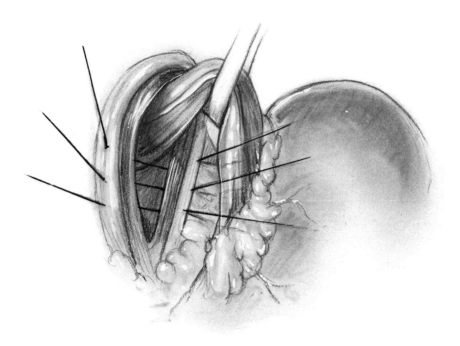

Fig. 17–6

ligament by approaching it from its superior margin: Identify the anterior surface of the aorta in the hiatal aperture between the right and left branches of the crus. Occasionally, it is necessary to dissect away some areolar tissue. With the left index fingernail pressing posteriorly against the aorta about 4 cm cephalad to the diaphragm, slide the index finger in a caudal direction. Deep behind the confluence of the diaphragmatic crura, the tip of the index finger passes behind a dense band of preaortic fascia that crosses over the aorta as the aorta passes through the aortic hiatus in the posterior diaphragm. The width of this band is variable but averages perhaps 3 cm. At the lower margin of this band the fingertip encounters pulsation of the celiac artery, which arises from the anterior wall of the aorta at the inferior margin of the median arcuate ligament. The median arcuate ligament lies between the fingertip and a thin layer of muscle fibers representing the caudal confluence of the diaphragmatic crura. With the index finger in place, Vansant and associates inserted three interrupted atraumatic sutures of no. 1 braided silk into the median arcuate ligament. Each suture is tagged with a hemostat, leaving each needle attached for later use when suturing the posterior gastropexy.

Suturing Posterior Gastropexy

Rotate the esophagogastric junction so the lesser curvature aspect of the stomach faces anteriorly. Then place a large Babcock clamp on the anterior and another clamp on the posterior phrenoesophageal bundle. Between these two bundles the longitudinal muscle fibers of the esophagus can be seen as they join the lesser curvature of the stomach. Where to place the proximal suture is an important consideration. Placing it too high causes excessive narrowing of the esophageal lumen; placing it too low does not increase the intraluminal pressure adequately in the lower esophageal sphincter area. We use 2-0 atraumatic Tevdek and include a few millimeters of adjacent gastric wall together with the phrenoesophageal bundle to ensure that the submucosa has been included in the suture. After placing the upper suture, cross the two ends or insert the first throw of a tie. Then estimate the lumen of the esophagastric junction by invaginating the stomach with the index finger along the indwelling nasogastric tube. If this maneuver is attempted before tying down the suture, the finger passes easily into the lumen of the esophagus in patients who have an incompetent lower esophageal sphincter. After the first suture is tentatively closed, only the tip of the index finger should be able to enter the esophagus. In the absence of intraoperative esophageal manometry, this is the best method for calibrating proper placement of the gastropexy sutures.

If the first suture has been judged to be properly placed, tag it with a hemostat and insert three additional sutures of atraumatic 2-0 Tevdek into the phrenoesophageal bundles, at intervals of about 1 cm, caudal to the first suture. Place a hemostat on each suture as a tag. After all the sutures have been placed, tighten each and again use the index finger to calibrate the lumen of the esophagogastric junction. If it is satisfactory, expose the anterior wall of the aorta in the hiatal aperture behind the esophagus. With the index fingernail closely applied to the anterior wall of the aorta, pass the fingertip in a caudal direction underneath the preaortic fascia and median arcuate ligament down to the point where the fingertip palpates the pulsation of the celiac artery. Then remove the index finger and replace it with a narrow right-angled retractor such as the Army-Navy retractor **(Fig. 17-7)**. Be certain that the retractor is indeed deep to the median arcuate ligament. This retractor serves to protect the aorta while the gastropexy sutures are being inserted through the preaortic fascia.

Identify the proximal suture that has already been placed in the phrenoesophageal bundles and pass the suture through the preaortic fascia. Be sure to take a substantial bite of the tissue anterior to the Army-Navy retractor. Pass the needle deep enough so it makes contact with the metal retractor; otherwise, only some overlying crural muscle fibers may be included in the stitch, which is then not strong enough to ensure a long-term successful result. After the first stitch has been passed through the preaortic fascia, tag it with a hemostat; pass each of the remaining phrenoesophageal sutures through the preaortic fascia by the same technique and tag each with a hemostat (Fig. 17-7).

Another good method to expedite suturing of the median arcuate ligament is to use a large right-angle bronchus clamp. Insert the tip of the clamp behind the median arcuate ligament instead of behind the Army-Navy retractor. Use the clamp to draw the median arcuate ligament vigorously anteriorly. Pass the needle with the suture through the median arcuate ligament just deep to the clamp, which ensures that a large bite of ligament is included in each stitch. Be certain not to injure the underlying aorta with the needle.

At this point check the entire area for hemostasis. Then tie the previously placed crural sutures (Fig. 17-6), narrowing the aperture of the hiatus. After these sutures have been tied, the index finger should pass freely into the hiatal aperture with an indwelling 18F nasogastric tube in the esophagus. If this is not the case, replace the proximal crural suture as necessary. Now tie each of the previously placed *gastropexy* sutures and cut all the ends **(Fig. 17-8)**.

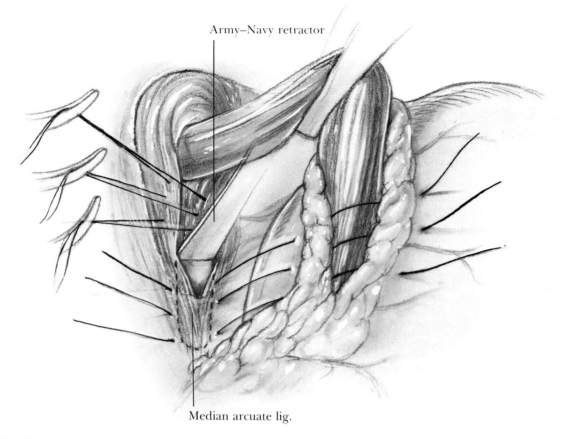

Army–Navy retractor

Median arcuate lig.

Fig. 17-7

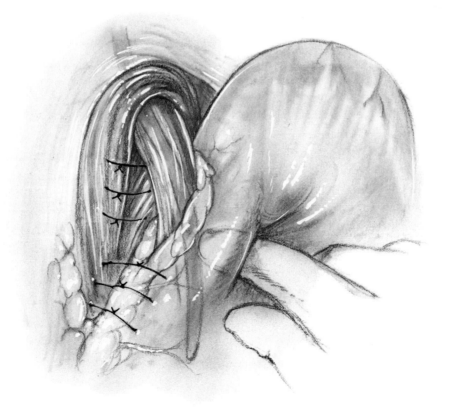

Fig. 17-8

Testing the Antireflux Valve

A simple method for testing the efficacy of the antireflux valve is to have the anesthesiologist inject about 500 ml of saline into the nasogastric tube and then withdraw the tube to a point above the esophagogastric junction. In the presence of a competent antireflux valve, compressing the saline-filled stomach fails to force the saline into the esophagus.

Abdominal Closure

Close the abdomen without drainage in routine fashion.

POSTOPERATIVE CARE

Continue nasogastric suction for 1–2 days.

Obtain a radiograph of the esophagogastric junction after a barium swallow before the patient is discharged from the hospital.

COMPLICATIONS

Dysphagia (usually transient).

Persistence or recurrence of gastroesophageal reflux. This and other complications following the Hill operation, are uncommon.

REFERENCES

Aye RW, Hill LD, Kraemer SJ, Snopkowski P. Early results with the laparoscopic Hill repair. Am J Surg 1994;167:542.

Aye RW, Mazza DE, Hill LD. Laparoscopic Hill repair in patients with abnormal motility. Am J Surg 1997;173:379.

Hill LD. An effective operation for hiatal hernia; an eight year appraisal. Ann Surg 1967;166:681.

Hill LD. Progress in the surgical management of hiatal hernia. World J Surg 1977;1:425.

Orringer MB, Schneider R, Williams GW, Sloan H. Intraoperative esophageal mamometry: is it valid? Ann Thorac Surg 1980;30:13.

Vansant JH, Baker JW, Ross DG. Modification of the Hill technique for repair of hiatal hernia. Surg Gynecol Obstet 1976;143:637.

18 Transthoracic Gastroplasty (Collis) and Nissen Fundoplication

INDICATIONS

Short esophagus due to reflux esophagitis

Recurrent gastroesophageal reflux with stricture after an antireflux procedure

Previous subtotal gastrectomy generally contraindicates a Collis-Nissen procedure

PREOPERATIVE PREPARATION

Dilate the esophageal stricture up to 40F. It can generally be done with Maloney dilators.

Insert a nasogastric tube down to the stricture.

Assessment for colon interposition is prudent in difficult cases (see Chapter 14). Bowel preparation allows colon to be used as a conduit if needed.

When esophagoscopy reveals severe acute ulcerative esophagitis with inflammation and bleeding, a 2- to 3-week period of preoperative intensive medical treatment with cimetidine, omeprazole, or both reduces inflammation and lessens the risk of intraoperative perforation of the esophagus.

PITFALLS AND DANGER POINTS

Esophageal perforation

Hemorrhage resulting from traumatizing or avulsing the accessory left hepatic artery, inferior phrenic artery, ascending branch of the left gastric artery, short gastric vessel, or inferior pulmonary vein

Laceration of spleen

Inadvertent vagotomy

Inadequate suturing, permitting the fundoplication to slip postoperatively

OPERATIVE STRATEGY

Performing an Adequate Gastroplasty

The object of performing a gastroplasty is to lengthen a shortened esophagus for an extent sufficient to prevent tension from being exerted on the antireflux operation and hernia repair. This newly constructed esophagus ("neoesophagus") consists of a tube made from the lesser curvature of the stomach. A 56F Maloney dilator is passed into the stomach, and the tube is constructed by applying an 80 mm linear cutting stapler precisely at the esophagogastric junction parallel to and snugly alongside the Maloney dilator. When the stapler is fired, the esophageal tube is lengthened by as much as 7 cm. If the stapler has been placed snugly against the esophagogastric junction, there are no irregularities or outpouchings at this point.

Mobilizing the Esophagus and Stomach

Not only is it important to mobilize the distal esophagus completely, at least as far up as the inferior pulmonary vein, but the proximal stomach must be entirely free of attachments, just as when a Nissen fundoplication is being performed through an abdominal approach. This operation can be accomplished without tension only with full mobilization. It requires dividing the phrenoesophageal and gastrophrenic ligaments, freeing the hiatus throughout its complete circumference from any attachments to the stomach or lower esophagus, and dividing an accessory left hepatic artery, which courses from the left gastric artery across the proximal gastrohepatic ligament to help supply the left lobe of the liver. After mobilization has been accomplished, the remaining maneuvers in the Collis-Nissen operation are not difficult.

If the esophagus is inadvertently perforated during the dissection, exercise careful judgment when deciding whether it is safe to suture the esophageal laceration or a resection and colon or jejunum interposition is necessary. If it is elected to suture the laceration, try to cover the suture line with a flap of parietal pleura (see Figs. 23-1 to 23-3).

Avoiding Hemorrhage

Avoiding unnecessary bleeding during any operation requires a careful dissection and a knowledge of vascular anatomy. This is especially important when mobilizing the stomach through a thoracic approach because losing control of the accessory left hepatic, short gastric, or inferior phrenic artery causes the proximal bleeding arterial stump to retract deep into the abdomen. Controlling these retracted vessels is difficult and may require laparotomy or at least a peripheral incision in the diaphragm. Preventing this complication is not difficult if the dissection is orderly and the surgeon is aware of the anatomic location of these vessels. Similarly, careful dissection and avoidance of traction along the greater curvature of the stomach helps prevent damaging the spleen.

Avoiding Esophageal Perforation

When the distal esophagus is baked into a fibrotic mediastinum, sharp scalpel dissection is safer than blunt dissection if injury to the esophagus and the vagus nerves is to be avoided. Sometimes the fibrosis terminates 8-9 cm above the diaphragm. If so, the esophagus and the vagus nerves can easily be encircled at this point, which provides a plane for subsequent dissection of the distal esophagus.

OPERATIVE TECHNIQUE

Incision

With the patient under one-lung anesthesia in the lateral position, left side up, make a skin incision in the sixth intercostal space from the costal margin to the tip of the scapula **(Fig. 18–1)**. Then identify the latissimus dorsi muscle and insert the index finger underneath it. Transect this muscle with electrocautery; then divide the underlying anterior serratus muscle in similar fashion **(Fig. 18–2)**. In both cases

it is preferable to divide these muscles somewhat caudal to the skin incision, as it helps preserve muscle function. Then use electrocautery to divide the intercostal muscles along the upper border of the seventh rib **(Fig. 18–3)** and open the pleura. Complete this opening from the costal margin to the region of the lateral spinal muscles. Separate the periosteum and surrounding tissues from a 1 cm segment of the posterior portion of the seventh rib lateral to the spinal muscles. Excise a 1 cm segment of this rib **(Fig. 18–4)**. Then divide the intercostal neurovascular bundle that runs along the inferior border of this rib **(Fig. 18–5)**.

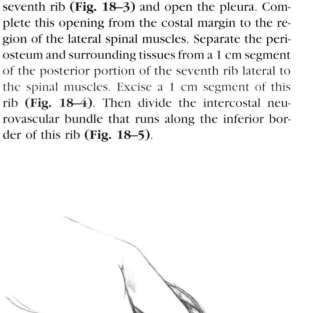

Ant. serratus m.

Intercostal m.

Latissimus dorsi m.

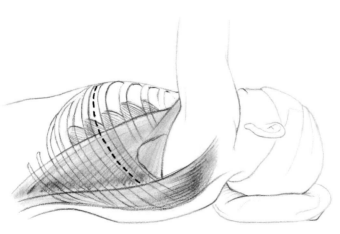

Fig. 18-1

Fig. 18-2

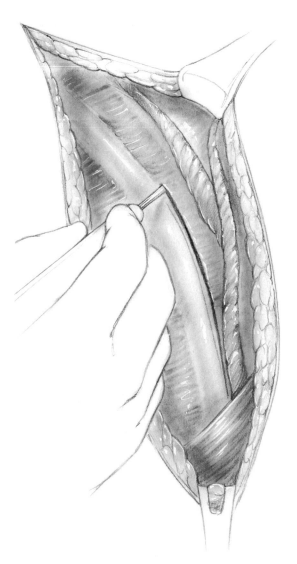

Fig. 18-3

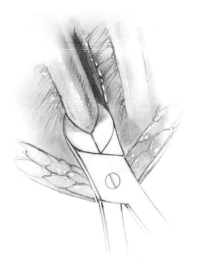

Fig. 18-4

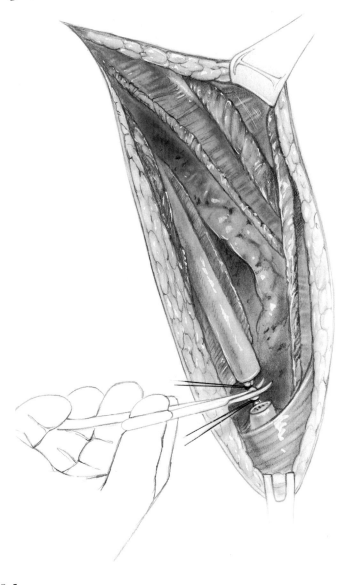

Fig. 18-5

Insert a Finochietto retractor into the incision and gradually increase the distance between the blades of the retractor over a 10-minute period to avoid causing rib fractures. In patients who have undergone previous surgery of the distal esophagus or proximal stomach, do not hesitate to continue this incision across the costal margin, converting it into a thoracoabdominal incision to facilitate dissection on the abdominal aspect of the diaphragmatic hiatus (see Figs. 12-6, 12-7).

Liberating the Esophagus

Incise the inferior pulmonary ligament with electrocautery and then compress the lung and retract it in anterior and cephalad directions using moist gauze pads and Harrington retractors. Incise the mediastinal pleura just medial to the aorta (**Figs. 18–6, 18–7**). Encircle the esophagus with the index finger using the indwelling nasogastric tube as a guide. If this cannot be done easily, it may be necessary to initiate sharp dissection at a somewhat higher level, where the fibrosis may be less advanced. Encircle the esophagus and the vagus nerves with a latex

drain. Continue the dissection of the esophagus from the inferior pulmonary vein down to the diaphragmatic hiatus. After the mediastinal pleura has been incised down to the hiatus, continue the incision anteriorly and divide the pleura of the pericardiophrenic sulcus (Fig. 18-6); otherwise, the medial aspect of the hiatal ring is not visible. If the right pleural cavity has been inadvertently entered, simply place a moist gauze pad over the rent in the pleura to prevent excessive seepage of blood into the right chest and continue the dissection.

Excising the Hernial Sac

Identify the point at which the left branch of the crus of the diaphragm meets the hernial sac. Any attenuated fibers of the phrenoesophageal ligament and preperitoneal fat are made apparent by applying traction to the diaphragm. Incise these tissues and the underlying peritoneum (**Fig. 18-8**). Continue the incision in the peritoneum in a circumferential fashion, opening the lateral and anterior aspects of the hernial sac; expose the greater curvature of the stomach. Insert the left index finger into the sac and continue the

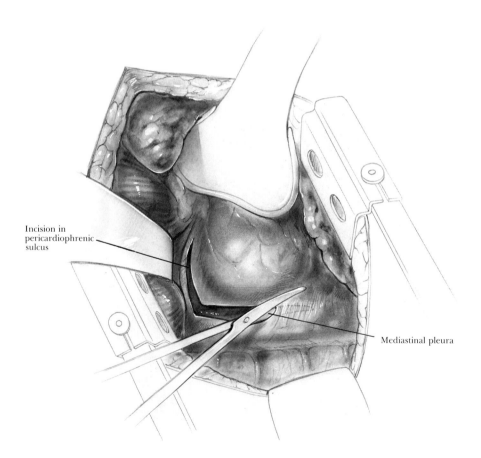

Incision in pericardiophrenic sulcus

Mediastinal pleura

Fig. 18-6

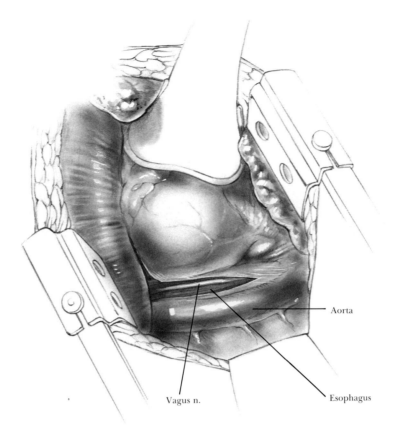

Fig. 18-7

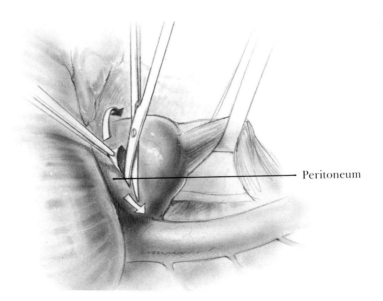

Fig. 18-8

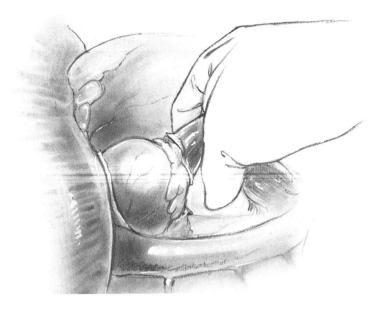

Fig. 18–9

incision along the medial (deep) margin of the hiatus using the finger as a guide **(Fig. 18–9)**. A branch of the inferior phrenic artery may be noted posterolaterally near the left vagus nerve; it is divided and ligated with 2-0 silk. While attempting to circumnavigate the proximal stomach, the index finger in the hernial sac encounters an obstruction on the lesser curvature side of the esophagogastric junction. It represents the proximal margin of the gastrohepatic ligament, which often contains a 2- to 4-mm accessory left hepatic artery coming off the ascending left gastric artery. By hugging the lesser curvature side of the cardia with the index finger, this finger can be passed between the stomach and the gastrohepatic ligament, delivering the ligament into the chest, deep to the stomach.

Identify the artery and ligate it proximally and distally with 2-0 silk. Divide it between the two ligatures **(Fig. 18–10)**. After this step, it should be possible to pass the index finger around the entire circumference of the proximal stomach and encounter no attachments between the stomach and the hiatus. Throughout these maneuvers, repeatedly check on the location of the vagus nerves and preserve them. Excise the peritoneum that constituted the hernial sac.

Dilating an Esophageal Stricture

Ascertain that the esophagus is lying in a straight line in the mediastinum. Ask the anesthesiologist or a surgical assistant to pass Maloney dilators into the esoph-

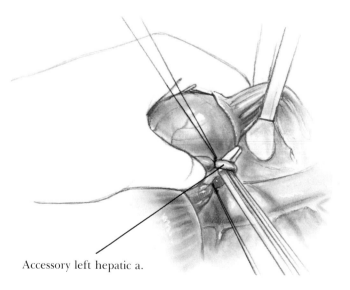

Accessory left hepatic a.

Fig. 18–10

agus through the mouth after removing the indwelling nasogastric tube. As the dilator is passed down the esophagus, guide it manually into the lumen of the stricture. Successively larger bougies are passed, up to size 50–60F, which can be successfully accomplished in probably 95% of cases. Occasionally, forceful dilatation of this type causes the lower esophagus to burst in the presence of unyielding transmural fibrosis. In this case, resect the damaged esophagus and perform a colonic or jejunal interposition between the healthy esophagus and the stomach (see Chapter 14).

Dividing the Short Gastric Vessels

Continue the dissection along the greater curvature of the stomach in an inferior direction until the first short gastric vessel is encountered. Use a long right-angled Mixter clamp to encircle this vessel with two 2-0 silk ligatures. Tie each ligature, leaving at least 1 cm between them. Divide between ligatures. Continue this process until about five proximal short gastric vessels have been divided and about 12-15 cm of greater curvature has been mobilized.

Gastroplasty

Verify that the esophagogastric junction has indeed been completely mobilized. Identify the point at which the greater curvature of the stomach meets the esophagus. Overlying this area is a thin fat pad perhaps 3 cm in diameter. Carefully dissect this fat pad away from the serosa of the stomach and the longitudinal muscle of the esophagus **(Fig. 18–11)**. Avoid damaging the anterior vagus nerve.

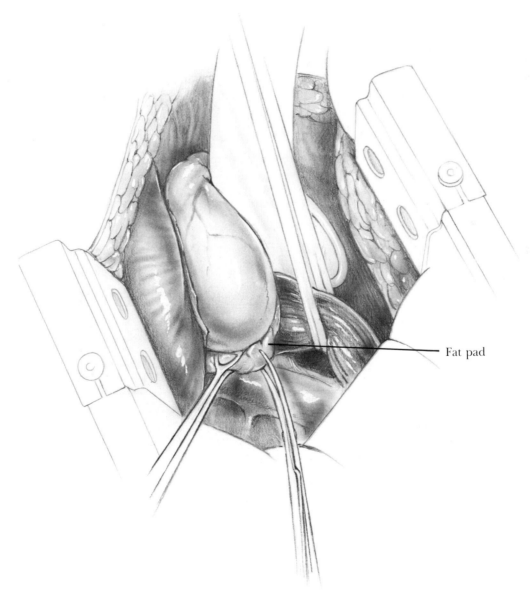

Fat pad

Fig. 18–11

Pass a 56-60F Maloney dilator into the stomach and position it along the lesser curvature. Then apply an 80 mm linear cutting stapler parallel and closely adjacent to the Maloney dilator; a Babcock clamp retracts the greater curvature of the stomach in a lateral direction **(Fig. 18–12)**. Fire the stapler and remove it. Verify that the staples have been shaped into an adequate B and that there are no leaks. Lightly electrocoagulate the everted mucosa. This maneuver will have lengthened the esophagus by approximately 6-7 cm **(Fig. 18–13)**. In most cases no additional length of neoesophagus is necessary because of the greater lengths now available in these stapling devices. Although this step is not shown here, it is wise as a precautionary measure to oversew the staple lines with two continuous Lembert sutures of 4-0 Prolene or PDS: one continuous suture to invert the staple line along the neoesophagus and a second continuous suture to invert the staple line along the gastric fundus. A continuous suture of the Lembert type is suitable, taking care not to turn in an excessive amount of tissue, as it would narrow the neoesophagus unnecessarily.

Performing a Modified Nissen Fundoplication

Because the neoesophagus has utilized a portion of the gastric fundus, there may not be sufficient remaining stomach to perform the Nissen fundoplication in the classic manner. Instead, as seen in **Figure 18–14**, the apex of the gastric fundus is wrapped around the neoesophagus in a counterclockwise fashion.

Before inserting any sutures, remove the indwelling large Maloney dilator and replace it with one of 50F. Place a large hemostatic clip at the site of the new esophagogastric junction (i.e., the junction of the neoesophagus with the stomach) as a radiographic marker. The fundoplication should encircle the neoesophagus in a loose wrap for a distance of 3 cm **(Fig. 18–15)**.

Figure 18-15 illustrates insertion of the first Nissen fundoplication stitch including a 5- to 6-mm bite of gastric wall, then a bite of the neoesophagus, and finally a bite of the opposite wall of the gastric fundus. These bites should be deep to the submucosa

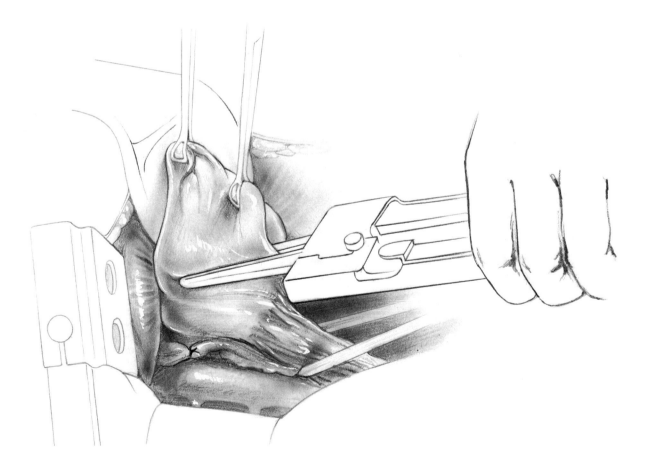

Fig. 18-12

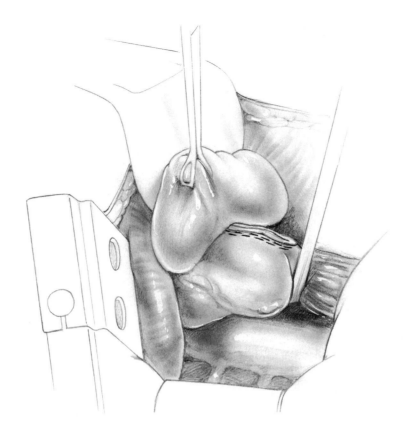

Fig. 18-13

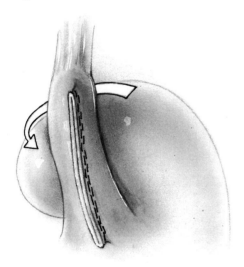

Fig. 18-14

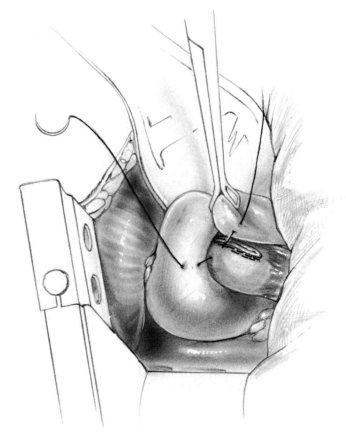

Fig. 18-15

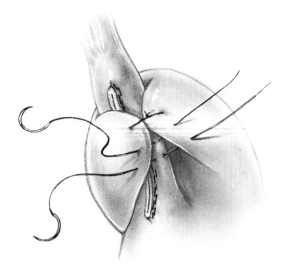

Fig. 18-16

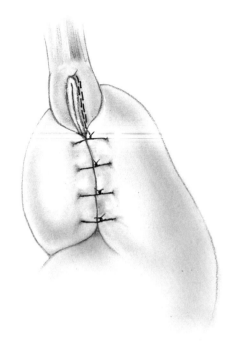

Fig. 18-17

but not into the lumen of the stomach. We prefer 2-0 Tevdek for these sutures. A total of three or four fundoplication sutures are used at 1 cm intervals (**Figs. 18–16, 18–17**). Now remove the Maloney dilator from the esophagus and replace it with a nasogastric tube. **Figure 18–18** illustrates that the fundoplication wrap around the neoesophagus is loose enough to admit the fingertip. Optionally, invert the layer of fundoplication sutures by oversewing it with a continuous Lembert seromuscular suture of 4-0 Prolene (not illustrated).

Closing the Hiatal Defect

Close the defect in the posterior portion of the hiatus by inserting 0 Tevdek interrupted sutures through the right and left margins of the hiatus. Take a bite 1.5-2.0 cm in width and include overlying parietal pleura. After checking for hemostasis, reduce the fundoplication into the abdomen. It should slide down with ease. Then tie each of the sutures, leaving space for the surgeon's fingertip alongside the esophagus or neoesophagus with a nasogastric tube in place (**Figs. 18–19, 18–20**). Place a hemostatic clip at the edge of the hiatus as a marker. It is not necessary to resuture the incision in the mediastinal pleura.

Irrigate the mediastinum and thoracic cavity with warm saline and check for complete hemostasis. Insert a 36F chest tube through a puncture wound below the level of the incision and bring the tube up the posterior gutter above the hilus of the lung. Insert three to five interrupted no. 2 PDS pericostal sutures and tie them to approximate the ribs. Close

the overlying serratus and latissimus muscles in two layers with 2-0 PG continuous sutures. Close the skin with continuous or interrupted fine nylon sutures.

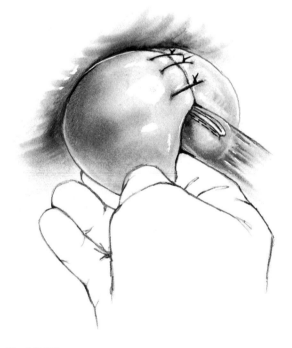

Fig. 18-18

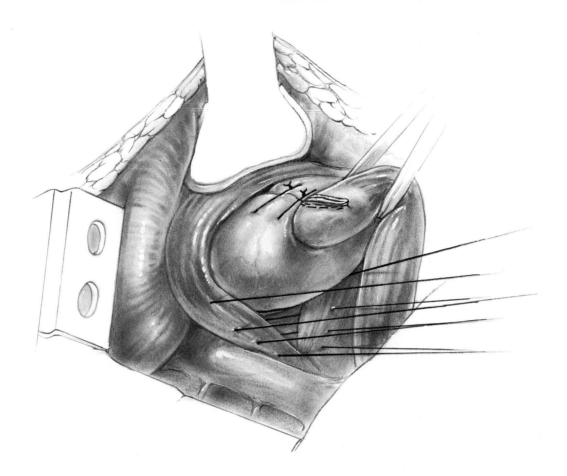

Fig. 18-19

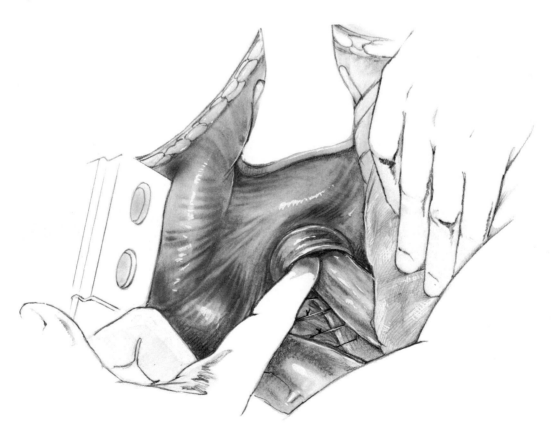

Fig. 18-20

POSTOPERATIVE CARE

Continue nasogastric suction for 1–3 days.

Continue perioperative antibiotics for 24 hours.

Obtain an esophagram (first water-soluble then thin barium) on postoperative day 7.

Remove the chest drainage tube on day 3 unless drainage is excessive.

COMPLICATIONS

Obstruction. Occasionally there is a partial obstruction at the area of the fundoplication due to edema during the first 2 weeks following surgery. If the wrap is too tight, this obstruction may persist.

Recurrent gastroesophageal reflux. This is uncommon after the Collis-Nissen procedure unless the fundoplication suture line disrupts.

Leakage from the gastroplasty or fundoplication sutures. This complication is rare. If the fundoplication sutures are inserted into the lumen of the stomach and the suture is tied with strangulating force, a leak is possible. The risk of this occurring may be reduced by oversewing the fundoplication suture line with a continuous Lembert seromuscular suture.

Necrosis of the gastroplasty tube. This complication was reported by Orringer and Orringer during an operation for recurrent hiatus hernia. They warned that traumatizing the lesser curve of the stomach may doom a gastroplasty tube.

REFERENCES

Gastal OL, Hagan JA, Peters JH, et al. Short esophagus: analysis of predictors and clinical implications. Arch Surg 1999;134:633.

Jobe BA, Horvath KD, Swanstrom LL. Postoperative function following laparoscopic Collis gastroplasty for shortened esophagus. Arch Surg 1998;133:867.

Orringer MB, Orringer JS. The combined Collis-Nissen operation: early assessment of reflux control. Ann Thorac Surg 1982;33:534.

Stirling MC, Orringer MB. Continued assessment of the combined Collis-Nissen operation. Ann Thorac Surg 1989;47:224.

Urschel HC, Razzuk MA, Wood RE, et al. An improved surgical technique for the complicated hiatal hernia with gastroesophageal reflux. Ann Thorac Surg 1973;15:443.

19 Bile Diverting Operations for Management of Esophageal Disease

INDICATIONS

Disabling bile reflux symptoms after esophageal surgery

PREOPERATIVE PREPARATION

Confirm bile reflux by visual inspection at endoscopy, radionuclide scan, or 24-hour pH monitoring.

Insert a nasogastric tube.

PITFALLS AND DANGER POINTS

Injury to liver, pancreas, or stomach
Damaging blood supply to residual gastric pouch

OPERATIVE STRATEGY

Bile Diversion after Failed Antireflux Procedures

Bile diversion is considered only after multiple failed antireflux procedures. Generally vagotomy and antrectomy with bile diversion via a Roux-en-Y reconstruction **(Figs. 19–1, 19–2)** is the procedure of choice. If transabdominal vagotomy does not appear feasible because of excessive scar tissue around the abdominal esophagus, transthoracic or thoracoscopic vagotomy is an alternative.

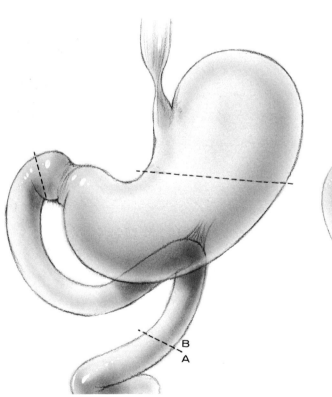

Fig. 19-1

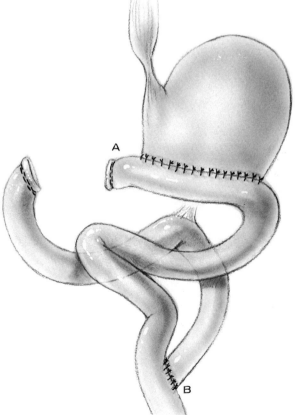

Fig. 19-2

Bile Diversion after Esophagogastrectomy

Bile diversion after esophagogastrectomy is used when bile reflux complicates otherwise successful esophageal resection with esophagogastrectomy. Perform the dissection with extreme care to avoid traumatizing the blood supply to the residual stomach. Generally, the gastric remnant is supplied only by the right gastric and right gastroepiploic vessels. A variation of this procedure, the duodenal switch procedure, is also illustrated.

OPERATIVE TECHNIQUE

Vagotomy and Antrectomy with Bile Diversion

Incision and Exposure

Ordinarily a long midline incision from the xiphoid to a point about 5 cm below the umbilicus is adequate for this operation. Divide the many adhesions and expose the stomach. Evaluate the difficulty of performing a hemigastrectomy, rather than other available operations. Insert an Upper Hand or Thompson retractor and determine if a transabdominal vagotomy is feasible.

Vagotomy

If it is feasible to perform a truncal vagotomy, follow the procedure described in Chapter 25. If dissecting the area of the esophagogastric junction appears too formidable a task, thoracoscopic or transthoracic vagotomy is an option.

Hemigastrectomy

Follow the procedure described in Chapter 30 for performance of a Billroth II gastric resection. Close the duodenal stump by stapling (see Fig. 29-43) or suturing (see Figs. 29-20 to 29-22).

Roux-en-Y Gastrojejunostomy

Create a Roux-en-Y limb of jejunum by the technique described in Figure 34-4. Then perform an end-to-side gastrojejunostomy using sutures (see Figs. 29-34 to 29-40) or staples (see Figs. 29-42 to 29-47). Position this anastomosis so it sits about 1 cm proximal to the stapled closed end of the jejunum (see Fig. 29-49). Complete construction of the Roux-en-Y segment by anastomosing the proximal cut end of the jejunum near the ligament of Treitz to the side of the descending segment of jejunum at a point 60 cm distal to the gastrojejunos-

tomy, as shown in Figures 34-26 to 34-30. Close the defect in the jejunal mesentery with interrupted sutures.

Closure

Close the abdominal wall without drainage in the usual fashion.

Bile Diversion Following Esophagogastrectomy

Incision and Exposure

Make a midline incision from the xiphoid to a point somewhat below the umbilicus. Divide the various adhesions subsequent to prior surgery and expose the pyloroduodenal region. Because of the previous surgery (esophagogastrectomy) **(Fig. 19–3)** this area is now located 5-8 cm from the diaphragmatic hiatus.

Dividing the Duodenum, Duodenojejunostomy, Roux-en-Y Reconstruction

Divide the duodenum at a point 2-3 cm beyond the pylorus. Be careful not to injure the right gastric or right gastroepiploic vessels, as they constitute the entire blood supply of the residual gastric pouch. To di-

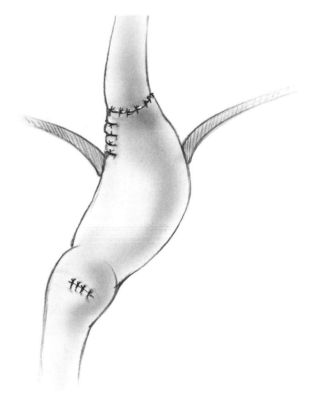

Fig. 19-3

vide the duodenum, first free the posterior wall of the duodenum from the pancreas for a short distance. If possible, pass one jaw of a 55/3.5 mm linear stapler behind the duodenum, close the device, and fire the stapler. Then divide the duodenum flush with the sta-

pling device. Lightly cauterize the everted mucosa and remove the stapler, which leaves the proximal duodenum open. Leave 1 cm of the posterior wall of the duodenum free (**Fig. 19–4**, point A) to construct an anastomosis with the jejunum.

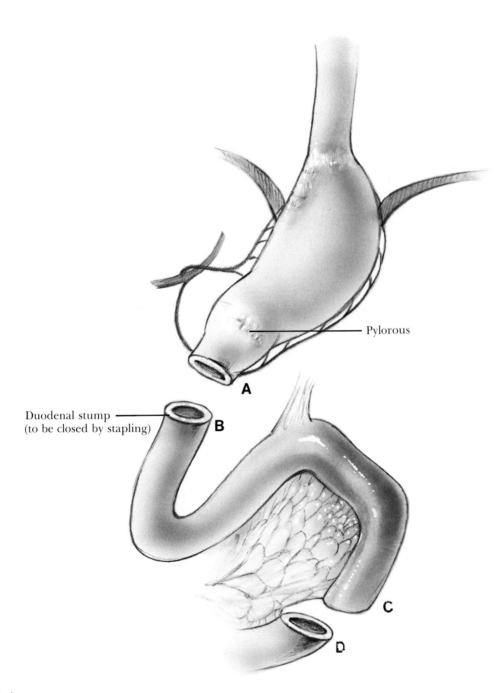

Fig. 19-4

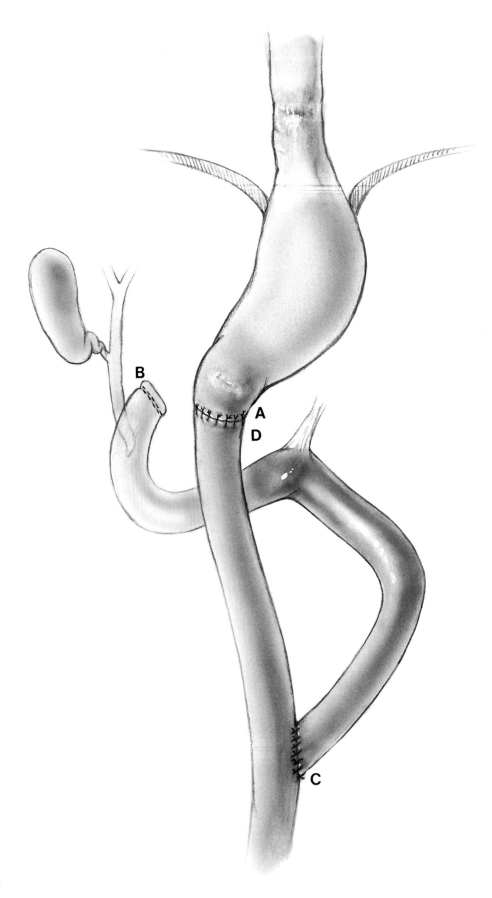

Fig. 19-5

Develop a Roux-en-Y limb of jejunum by the technique described in Figure 34-4. Bring the open distal end of the divided jejunum (Fig. 19-4, point D) to the level of the duodenum. Generally it most comfortably assumes an antecolic position, but occasionally it is feasible to bring it through an incision in the mesocolon (retrocolic).

Establish an end-to-end duodenojejunostomy (**Fig. 19–5**, point A to point D) utilizing one layer of interrupted 4-0 silk for the seromuscular layer and continuous or interrupted sutures of atraumatic 5-0 PG for the mucosal layers (see Figs. 37-2 to 37-10).

Complete the construction of the Roux-en-Y segment by creating an end-to-side jejunojejunostomy at a point 60 cm distal to the duodenojejunostomy using the technique shown in Figures 34-26 to 34-30. Close the defect in the jejunal mesentery with interrupted sutures.

Bile Diversion by Duodenojejunostomy Roux-en-Y Switch Operation

Incision and Exposure

Make a midline incision from the xiphoid to a point about 3-4 cm below the umbilicus.

Duodenojejunostomy

Perform a thorough Kocher maneuver, freeing the head of the pancreas and duodenum anteriorly and posteriorly. Place a marking suture on the anterior wall of the duodenum precisely 3 cm distal to the pylorus. This represents the probable point at which the duodenum will be transected. Now approach the point at which the duodenum and pancreas meet. Divide and carefully ligate the numerous small vessels emerging from the area of the pancreas and entering the duodenum on both anterior and posterior surfaces until a 2 cm area of the posterior wall of duodenum has been cleared. Do not dissect the proximal 2–3 cm of duodenum from its attachment to the pancreas. Dissecting the next 2 cm of duodenum free of the pancreas provides enough length to allow stapled closure of the duodenal stump and a duodenojejunal end-to-end anastomosis. Be careful not to injure the pancreatic segment of the distal common bile duct or the duct of Santorini, which enters the duodenum at a point about 2 cm proximal to the papilla of Vater.

Fig. 19–6

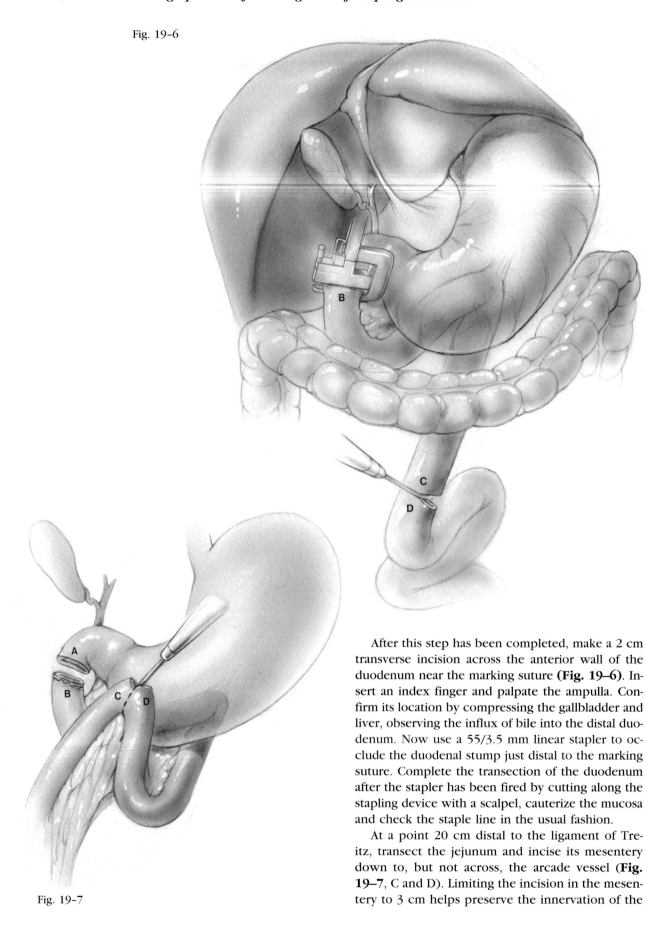

Fig. 19-7

After this step has been completed, make a 2 cm transverse incision across the anterior wall of the duodenum near the marking suture **(Fig. 19–6)**. Insert an index finger and palpate the ampulla. Confirm its location by compressing the gallbladder and liver, observing the influx of bile into the distal duodenum. Now use a 55/3.5 mm linear stapler to occlude the duodenal stump just distal to the marking suture. Complete the transection of the duodenum after the stapler has been fired by cutting along the stapling device with a scalpel, cauterize the mucosa and check the staple line in the usual fashion.

At a point 20 cm distal to the ligament of Treitz, transect the jejunum and incise its mesentery down to, but not across, the arcade vessel **(Fig. 19–7**, C and D). Limiting the incision in the mesentery to 3 cm helps preserve the innervation of the intestinal pacemaker in the upper jejunal mesentery. Bring the distal transected end of the jejunum through a small incision in the mesocolon and make an end-to-end anastomosis between the proximal transected duodenum to the jejunum using 4-0 interrupted silk sutures for the seromuscular layer and 5-0 Vicryl sutures for the mucosa (**Fig. 19–8**, A and C). Then perform an end-to-side jejunojejunostomy to the descending limb of jejunum (Fig. 19-8) at a point 60 cm distal to the duodenojejunostomy by the technique described in Figures 34–26 to 34–30. Eliminate any defect in the mesocolon or the jejunal mesentery by suturing. Irrigate the abdominal cavity and abdominal wound and close the abdomen in the usual fashion without drainage.

COMPLICATIONS

Intestinal obstruction

Anastomotic leak

REFERENCES

Appleton BN, Beynon J, Harikrishnan AB, Manson JM. Investigation of oesophageal reflux symptoms after gastric surgery with combined pH and bilirubin monitoring. Br J Surg 1999;86:1099.

Critchlow JF, Shapiro ME, Silen W. Duodenojejunostomy for the pancreaticobiliary complications of duodenal diverticulum. Ann Surg 1985;202:56.

DeLangen ZL, Slooff MJ, Jansen W. The surgical treatment of postgastrectomy reflux gastritis. Surg Gynecol Obstet 1984;158:322.

DeMeester TR, Fuchs KH, Ball CS, et al. Experimental and clinical results with proximal end-to-end duodenojejunostomy for pathological duodenogastric reflux. Ann Surg 1987;206:414.

Mason RJ, DeMeester TR. Importance of duodenogastric reflux in the surgical outpatient practice. Hepatogastroenterology 1999;46:48.

Oberg S, Peters JH, DeMeester TR, et al. Determinants of intestinal metaplasia within the columnar-lined esophagus. Arch Surg 2000;135:651.

Oberg S, Ritter MP, Crookes PF, et al. Gastroesophageal reflux disease and mucosal injury with emphasis on short-segment Barrett's esophagus and duodenogastroesophageal reflux. J Gastrointest Surg 1998;2:547.

Smith J, Payne WS. Surgical technique for management of reflux esophagitis after esophagogastrectomy for malignancy: further application of Roux-en-Y principle. Mayo Clin Proc 1975;50:588.

Stein HJ, Barlow AP, DeMeester TR, et al. Complications of gastroesophageal reflux disease: role of the lower esophageal sphincter, esophageal acid and acid/alkaline exposure, and duodenogastric reflux. Ann Surg 1992;216:35.

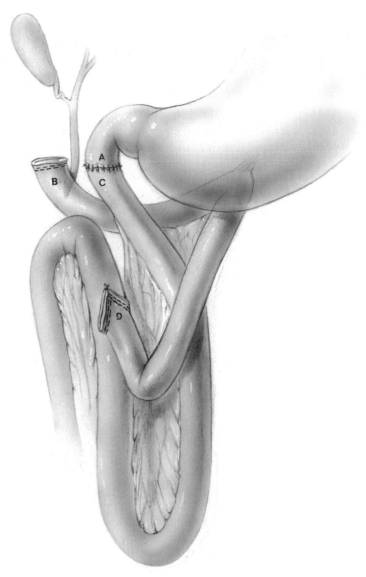

Fig. 19–8

20 Cricopharyngeal Myotomy and Operation for Pharyngoesophageal (Zenker's) Diverticulum

INDICATIONS

Symptomatic Zenker's diverticulum

PREOPERATIVE PREPARATION

Perioperative antibiotics

OPERATIVE STRATEGY

Adequate Myotomy

Performing a cricopharyngeal myotomy is similar to performing a cardiomyotomy. The physiologic upper esophageal sphincter is considerably wider than the anatomic cricopharyngeus muscle. The transverse muscle fibers are only about 2.0–2.5 cm wide, whereas the high pressure zone corresponding to the cricopharyngeus area can be 4 cm wide. Consequently, a proper cricopharyngeal myotomy should not only transect all of the transverse fibers of the cricopharyngeus muscle but also 1–2 cm of the proximal esophagus so the myotomy is at least 4 cm long. The incision in the muscle is carried down to the mucosa of the esophagus, which should bulge out through the myotomy after all the muscle fibers have been divided. Additionally, the mucosa is freed from the overlying muscle over the posterior half of the esophagus.

Is Diverticulectomy Necessary?

If the pharyngoesophageal diverticulum is a small diffuse bulge measuring no more than 2–3 cm in diameter, we perform only a myotomy and make no attempt to excise any part of the diverticulum because after the myotomy there is only a gentle bulge of mucosa and no true diverticulum. On the other hand, longer, finger-like projections of mucosa should be amputated because there have been a few case reports of recurrent symptoms due to the persistence of diverticula left behind in patients in whom an otherwise adequate myotomy had been done. Belsey advocated

suturing the most dependent point of the diverticulum to the prevertebral fascia in the upper cervical region. This procedure effectively up-ends the diverticulum so it can drain freely into the esophageal lumen by gravity. We prefer to amputate diverticula larger than 3 cm rather than perform a diverticulopexy. With application of a stapling device, amputation of the diverticulum takes only about 1 minute of additional operating time, and the results have been excellent.

OPERATIVE TECHNIQUE

Incision and Exposure

With the patient's head turned somewhat toward his or her right, make an incision along the anterior border of the left sternomastoid muscle beginning at a point 2–3 cm above the clavicle **(Fig. 20–1)**. Divide the platysma muscle. Electrocoagulate the bleeding points. Free the anterior border of the sternomastoid muscle and retract it laterally, exposing the omohyoid muscle crossing the field from medial to lateral. Transect this muscle **(Fig. 20–2)**. The diver-

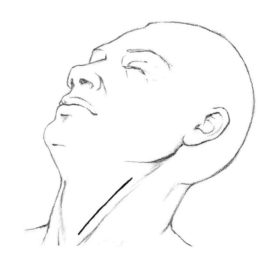

Fig. 20–1

200

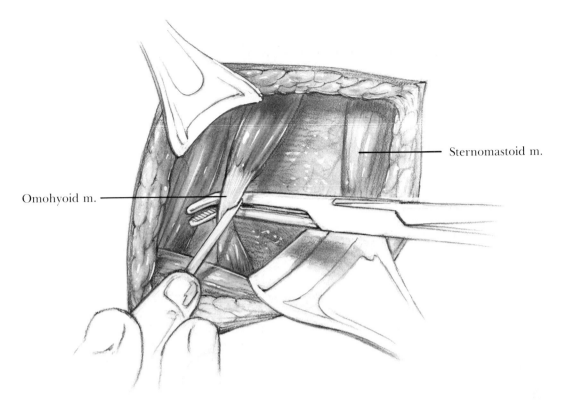

Omohyoid m.

Sternomastoid m.

Fig. 20-2

ticulum is located deep to the omohyoid muscle. Identify the carotid sheath and the descending hypoglossal nerve and retract these structures laterally. The thyroid gland is seen in the medial portion of the operative field underneath the strap muscles. Retract the thyroid gland and the larynx in a medial direction, revealing in most cases a prominent middle thyroid vein **(Fig. 20–3)**. Ligate and divide this vein.

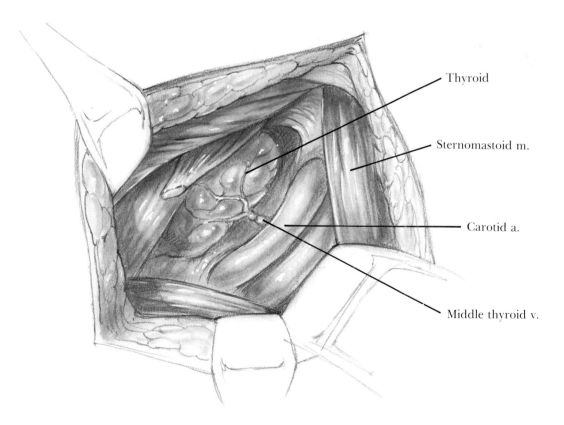

Thyroid

Sternomastoid m.

Carotid a.

Middle thyroid v.

Fig. 20-3

Divide the areolar tissue anterior to the carotid artery and identify the inferior thyroid artery and the recurrent laryngeal nerve. In some patients there appears to be no true left inferior thyroid artery arising from the thyrocervical trunk, in which case the lower thyroid is supplied by branches of the superior thyroid artery. In most patients with the inferior thyroid artery emerging from underneath the carotid artery and crossing the esophagus to supply the lower thyroid (see Figs. 107-10, 107-11), divide and ligate this vessel after identifying the recurrent laryngeal nerve. After this step has been completed, retracting the larynx in an anteromedial direction and the carotid artery laterally exposes the lateral and posterior aspects of the cervical esophagus and the pharyngoesophageal junction. Often it is not necessary to divide the inferior thyroid artery or its branches to develop adequate exposure for diverticulectomy.

Dissecting the Pharyngoesophageal Diverticulum

The pharyngoesophageal diverticulum emerges posteriorly between the pharyngeal constrictor and the cricopharyngeus muscles. Its neck is at the level of the cricoid cartilage, and the dependent portion of the diverticulum descends between the posterior wall of the esophagus and the prevertebral fascia overlying the bodies of the cervical vertebrae. Blunt dissection with the index finger or a peanut sponge generally identifies the most dependent portion of the diverticulum. Grasp it with a Babcock clamp and elevate the diverticulum in a cephalad direction. Mobilize the diverticulum by sharp and blunt dissection down to its neck. If there is any confusion about the anatomy, especially in patients who have undergone previous operations in this area, ask the anesthesiologist to pass a 40F Maloney bougie through the

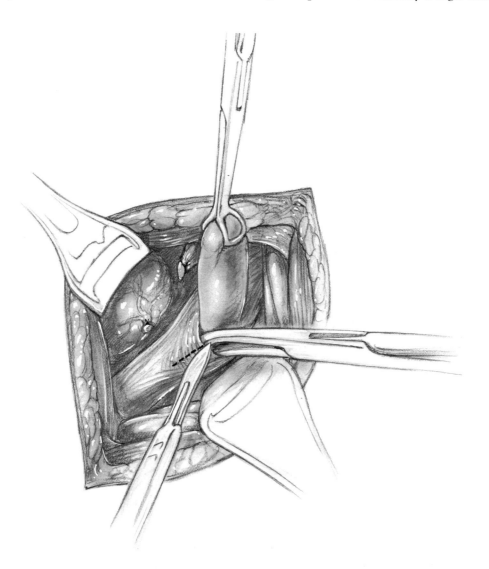

Fig. 20-4

mouth into the cervical esophagus. Guide the tip of the bougie past the neck of the diverticulum so it enters the esophagus. The exact location of the junction between the esophagus and the diverticulum can then be identified. There is generally some fibrous tissue overlying the mucosa of the diverticulum. Lightly incise it with a scalpel near the neck of the sac down to the submucosa. At this point the transverse fibers of the cricopharyngeus muscle are easily identified.

Cricopharyngeal and Esophageal Myotomy

Insert a blunt-tipped right-angled hemostat between the mucosa and the transverse fibers of the cricopharyngeus muscle just distal to the neck of the diverticulum **(Fig. 20–4)**. Elevate the hemostat in the posterior midline and incise the fibers of the cricopharyngeus muscle with a scalpel. Continue this dissection down the posterior wall of the esophagus for a total distance of about 5–6 cm. Now elevate the incised muscles of the cricopharyngeus and the upper esophagus from the underlying mucosal layer over the posterior half of the esophageal circumference by blunt dissection.

After the mucosa has been permitted to bulge out through the myotomy, determine whether the diverticulum is large enough to warrant resection. If so, apply a 30- or 55-mm linear stapler with 3.5 mm staples across the neck of the diverticulum **(Fig. 20–5)**. Close the stapler. Fire the staples and amputate the diverticulum flush with the stapling device. The 40F Maloney dilator in the lumen of the esophagus protects against excising too much mucosa and narrowing the lumen. After removing the stapling

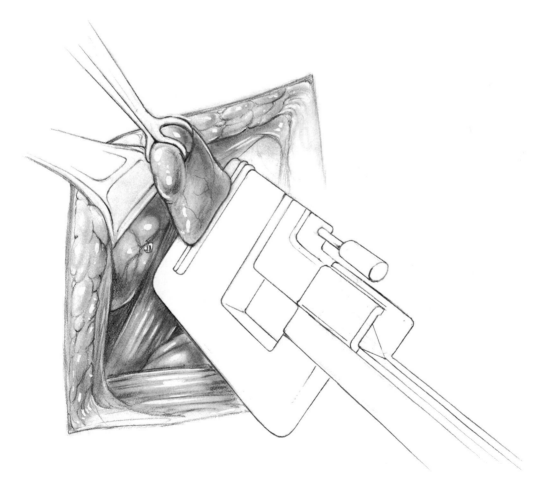

Fig. 20–5

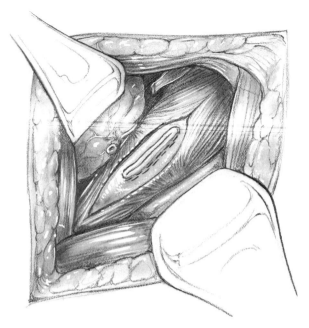

Fig. 20-6

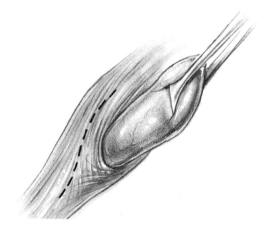

Fig. 20-7

device, carefully inspect the staple line and the staples for proper closure. Check for complete hemostasis **(Fig. 20–6)**.

An alternative method for performing the myotomy is illustrated in **Figure 20–7**, where the incision is initiated 1.0-1.5 cm cephalad to the cricopharyngeus muscle, in the pharyngeal constrictor muscle. It is then continued downward for 4-5 cm. Remove the diverticulum in the usual fashion.

Drainage and Closure

After carefully inspecting the area and ensuring complete hemostasis, insert a medium-size latex drain into the prevertebral space just below the area of the diverticulectomy. Bring the drain out through the lower pole of the incision.

Close the incision in layers with interrupted 4-0 PG sutures to the muscle fascia and platysma. Close the skin with continuous subcuticular sutures of 4-0 PG, interrupted nylon sutures, or skin staples.

POSTOPERATIVE CARE

Remove the drain by postoperative day 4. Initiate a liquid diet on the first postoperative day and progress to a full diet over the next 2-3 days. Continue perioperative antibiotics for a second dose.

COMPLICATIONS

Esophageal fistula. When the fistula is small and drains primarily saliva, it generally closes after a week of intravenous feeding if the patient's operative site has been drained as described above.

Recurrent laryngeal nerve palsy. It is generally temporary, secondary to excessive traction on the thyroid cartilage or to direct trauma to the nerve

Persistent dysphagia. This is due to inadequate myotomy

REFERENCES

Belsey R. Functional disease of the esophagus. J Thorac Cardiovasc Surg 1966;52:164.

Bremner CG. Zenker diverticulum. Arch Surg 1988;133: 1131.

Crescenzo DG, Trastek VF, Allen MS, Deschamps C, Pairolero PC. Zenker's diverticulum in the elderly: is operation justified? Ann Thorac Surg 1998;66:347.

Ellis FH Jr, Crozier RE. Cervical esophageal dysphagia; indications for and results of cricopharyngeal myotomy. Ann Surg 1981;194:279.

Henderson RD, Hanna WM, Henderson RF, Maryatt G. Myotomy for reflux-induced cricopharyngeal dysphagia. J Thorac Cardiovasc Surg 1989;98:428.

Huang B, Payne WS, Cameron AJ. Surgical management for recurrent pharyngoesophageal (Zenker's) diverticulum. Ann Thorac Surg 1984;37:189.

Rocco G, Deschamps C, Martel E, et al. Results of reoperation on the upper esophageal sphincter. J Thorac Cardiovasc Surg 1999;117:28.

Worman LW. Pharyngoesophageal diverticulum—excision or incision? Surgery 1980;87:236.

21 Esophagomyotomy for Achalasia and Diffuse Esophageal Spasm

INDICATIONS

Achalasia

Extended myotomy sometimes performed for diffuse esophageal spasm

PREOPERATIVE PREPARATION

Obtain a barium swallow esophagram.

Perform esophagoscopy with biopsy and brushings of the narrowed portion of distal esophagus if any mucosal abnormalities are noted.

Perform esophageal manometry.

For advanced cases, lavage the dilated esophagus with a Levine tube and warm saline for 1–2 days prior to operation to evacuate retained food particles. Combine this with a liquid diet.

Pass a nasogastric tube into the esophagus the morning of operation.

Administer perioperative antibiotics.

PITFALLS AND DANGER POINTS

Extending the myotomy too far on the stomach

Perforating the esophageal mucosa

Performing an inadequate circumferential liberation of the mucosa

Creating a hiatus hernia

OPERATIVE STRATEGY

Length of Myotomy for Achalasia

Ellis et al. (1980) attributed their low incidence of postoperative gastroesophageal regurgitation (3%) to the fact that the myotomy terminates only a few millimeters beyond the esophagogastric junction. At the esophagogastric junction, several veins run in a transverse direction just superficial to the esophageal mucosa. One does not encounter any other transverse vein of this size during myotomy of the more proximal esophagus. Once these veins are encountered, terminate the myotomy. In no case should more than 1 cm of gastric musculature be divided. Continue the myotomy in a cephalad direction for 1–2 cm beyond the point at which the esophagus begins to dilate. For early cases, where no significant esophageal dilatation is evident, the length of the myotomy should be 5–8 cm.

Choice of Operative Approach

Laparoscopic myotomy is an excellent alternative for patients with achalasia in whom the narrow segment is limited to the distal esophagus (see Chapter 22). Open esophagomyotomy may be performed through a thoracotomy incision (as shown here) or transabdominally. The thoracic approach allows excellent exposure without disrupting the phrenoesophageal ligaments, potentially contributing to postoperative gastroesophageal reflux. It facilitates a long myotomy in cases of diffuse esophageal spasm.

Mucosal Perforation

Mucosal perforation is easily repaired if recognized. It is advisable for the surgeon to test the integrity of the mucosal layer following myotomy by having the anesthesiologist insert 100–200 ml of a methylene blue solution through the nasogastric tube. When a mucosal perforation is identified during the operation, careful suturing of the mucosa generally avoids further difficulty. Some surgeons close the muscle over the perforation and then rotate the esophagus so the myotomy can be performed at a different point on the esophageal circumference. Closing the mediastinal pleura over the esophagus, as we do routinely, helps buttress a sutured perforation of the mucosa (see Figs. 23-1 to 23-3).

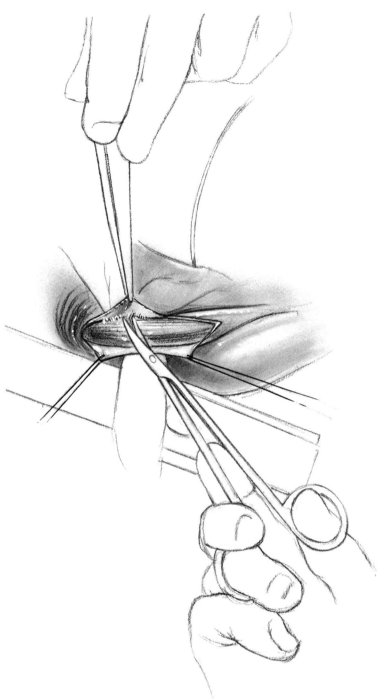

OPERATIVE TECHNIQUE

Incision and Exposure

Place the patient in the full left thoracotomy position. Make a skin incision along the course of the seventh intercostal space. Incise the serratus and latissimus muscles with electrocautery; then make an incision along the upper border of the eighth rib through the intercostal musculature (see Figs. 18-1 to 18-3). Open the pleura for the length of the eighth rib. Insert a Finochietto retractor and gradually increase the space between the seventh and eighth ribs. Divide the inferior pulmonary ligament and retract the left lung in a cephalad and anterior direction using large moist gauze pads and Harrington retractors. Make an incision in the mediastinal pleura overlying the distal esophagus **(Fig. 21–1)**. Then gently encircle the esophagus with the index finger, which is facilitated by the indwelling nasogastric tube. Encircle the esophagus with a latex drain. Be careful to identify and preserve the vagus nerves. Free the esophagus from surrounding structures to the level of the diaphragm but no lower **(Fig. 21–2)**.

Esophagomyotomy for Achalasia

Place the left index finger underneath the distal esophagus. Make a longitudinal incision through both the longitudinal and circular muscle layers of the esophagus until the muscosal surface is exposed **(Fig. 21–3)**. Continue this incision in a cephalad direction for a distance of about 2 cm above the point where the esophagus begins to dilate, or at least 5-7 cm.

Continue the myotomy in a caudal direction as far

Fig. 21-1

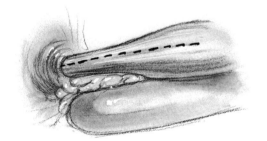

Fig. 21-2

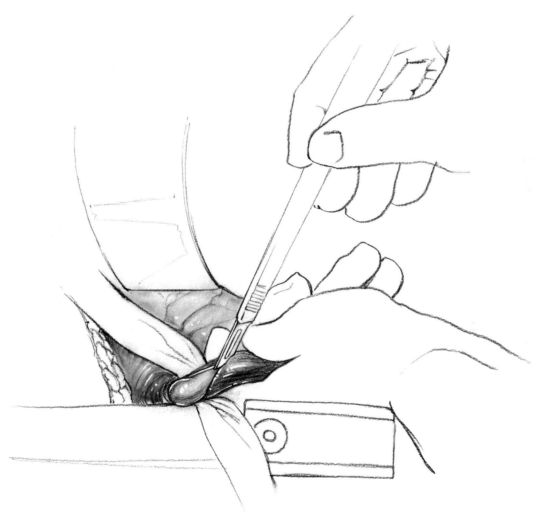

Fig. 21-3

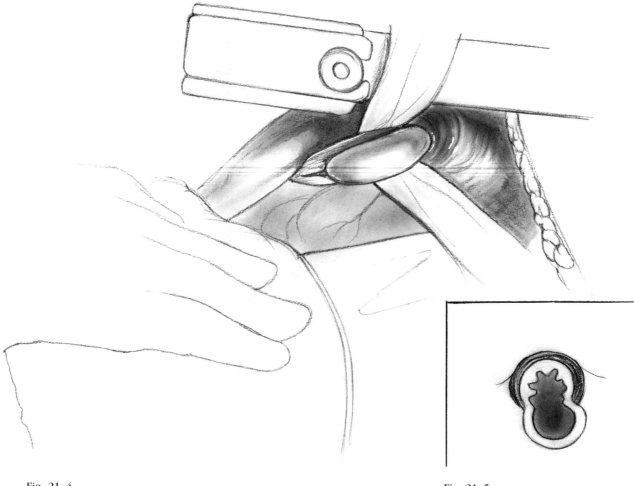

Fig. 21-4

Fig. 21-5

as the esophagogastric junction **(Fig. 21–4)**. This junction can be identified by noting one or two veins crossing transversely over the mucosa deep to the musculature. Do not continue the incision more than 1 cm into the gastric musculature. Another way to confirm the location of the esophagogastric junction is that the gastric musculature differs from that of the esophagus.

To prevent the muscle fibers from reuniting it is important to free at least 50% of the circumference of the mucosa from its muscular coat. This may be accomplished using Metzenbaum scissors to elevate the circular muscle from the underlying mucosa, proceeding medially and then laterally to the initial longitudinal myotomy until the mucosa bulges out, as seen in cross section in **Figure 21–5**. Achieve complete hemostasis by cautious electrocoagulation and fine suture-ligatures, especially in the incised esophageal muscle.

If the mucosa has been inadvertently incised, carefully repair the laceration with one or more 5-0 nonabsorbable sutures. At this point, ask the anesthesiologist to inject a solution of methylene blue into the esophagus to prove that there is no mucosal perforation.

Esophagomyotomy for Diffuse Esophageal Spasm

The technique for performing a myotomy to alleviate diffuse spasm differs from that described for achalasia only in the length of the myotomy. If the lower esophageal sphincter can relax normally when swallowing occurs, do not extend the myotomy to the terminal esophagus. The preoperative manometric assessment of the patient's esophageal contractions determines how far the esophagomyotomy should be extended.

Closure and Drainage

Bring a 30F chest tube out through a stab wound in the ninth intercostal space in the anterior axillary line. Approximate the ribs with two or three pericostal sutures of no. 2 PDS. Close the remainder of the wound in layers, as illustrated in Figures 12-42 to 12-44.

POSTOPERATIVE CARE

Remove the nasogastric tube the day following surgery.

Initiate oral intake of liquids on the first or second postoperative day, if tolerated.

Remove the chest tube as soon as the drainage becomes minimal, about the third or fourth postoperative day.

COMPLICATIONS

Persistent dysphagia. In some cases an inadequate myotomy for achalasia fails to relieve the patient's dysphagia. About 2 weeks following operation in such cases, esophageal dilatation with Maloney dilators may help. If reoperation is needed, consider laparoscopic myotomy, as the problem is generally at the distal end of the myotomy.

Recurrent dysphagia following initial relief of symptoms. It is possible that in these cases the muscular tissues have reunited. A trial of bougienage with Maloney bougies up to 50F may prove successful. Because esophageal carcinoma occasionally complicates long-standing achalasia, patients with recurrent dysphagia following a symptom-free interval after esophagomyotomy should have complete evaluation by radiography, esophagoscopy, and biopsy.

Reflux esophagitis. Although most patients with symptoms of reflux can be handled conservatively, an antireflux operation is required in severe cases.

Diaphragmatic hernia.

Empyema.

REFERENCES

Csendes A, Braghetto I, Mascaro J, Henriquez A. Late subjective and objective evaluation of the results of esophagomyotomy in 100 patients with achalasia of the esophagus. Surgery 1988;104:469.

Donohue PE, Schlesinger PK, Sluss KF, et al. Esophagocardiomyotomy—floppy Nissen fundoplication effectively treats achalasia without causing esophageal obstruction. Surgery 1994;116:719.

Ellis FH. Esophagectomy for achalasia: who, when, and how much? Ann Thorac Surg 1989;47:334.

Ellis FH Jr. Oesophagomyotomy for achalasia: a 22 year experience. Br J Surg 1993;80:882.

Ellis FH Jr, Gibb SP, Crozier RE. Esophagomyotomy for achalasia of the esophagus. Ann Surg 1980;192:157.

Henderson RD, Ryder DE. Reflux control following myotomy in diffuse esophageal spasm. Ann Thorac Surg 1982;34:230.

Hunter JG, Richardson WS. Surgical management of achalasia. Surg Clin North Am 1997;77:993.

Murray GF, Battaglini JW, Keagy BA, et al. Selective application of fundoplication in achalasia. Ann Thorac Surg 1984;37:185.

Orringer MB, Stirling MC. Esophageal resection for achalasia: indications and results. Ann Thorac Surg 1989;47:340.

Pellegrini C, Wetter LA, Patti M, et al. Thoracoscopic esophagomyotomy: initial experience with a new approach for the treatment of achalasia. Ann Surg 1992;216:296.

Skinner DB. Myotomy and achalasia. Ann Thorac Surg 1984;37:183.

22 Laparoscopic Esophagomyotomy

INDICATIONS

Achalasia in which the high-pressure zone is localized to the distal esophagus

PREOPERATIVE PREPARATION

See Chapters 16 and 21.

PITFALLS AND DANGER POINTS

Inadequate myotomy. Careful review of preoperative studies (esophagoscopy, manometry, contrast esophagraphy) helps determine whether the high-pressure zone is limited to the distal esophagus and hence is accessible from the abdominal approach. Intraoperative endoscopy assists in ensuring that an adequate myotomy has been performed.

Esophageal perforation.

Creation of severe gastroesophageal reflux. Overzealous myotomy, extension of the myotomy too far down on the cardia, poor patient selection, and excessive mobilization of the esophagus contribute to postoperative reflux. Selective use of partial fundoplications (Dor and Toupet) is advocated by some surgeons. We believe this is not necessary routinely.

OPERATIVE STRATEGY

The first laparoscopic esophagomyotomies were done through the left chest using a thoracoscope in a manner analogous to the open Heller myotomy (see Chapter 21). As experience with laparoscopic Nissen fundoplication grew, it became obvious that access to the distal esophagus was better through the laparoscopic approach than through the thoracoscopic approach. For the typical patient with achalasia limited to the distal esophagus, laparoscopic approach is easiest. References at the end of the chapter describe the thoracoscopic approach, which is needed when a long myotomy is required for diffuse esophageal spasm. Most surgeons who

perform this procedure are already facile in laparoscopic Nissen fundoplication (see Chapter 16).

Patient Position, Room Setup, Trocar Placement

Use the same patient position and room setup shown for the Nissen fundoplication (see Figs. 16-1, 16-2). Allow room at the head of the table for an esophagogastroduodenoscopy (EGD) scope, which is used at the end of the procedure to judge the adequacy of the myotomy. Typical trocar placement is shown in **Figure 22–1**. Generally five ports are required, and the general considerations discussed in Chapter 16 apply to trocar site placement for this procedure.

Initial Exposure and Esophageal Mobilization

Place a liver retractor and obtain access to the hiatus in the usual fashion (see Figs. 16-3 through 16-5). Concentrate on the anterior dissection. It is not strictly

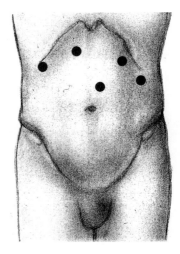

Fig. 22-1 Trocar placement. The supraumbilical trocar and the right subcostal trocar are placed 15 cm from the xiphoid, the left subcostal trocar about 10 cm from the xiphoid. The epigastric trocar is placed as high as the liver edge allows and as lateral as the falciform ligament allows. The left flank port is about 7 cm lateral to the left subcostal trocar.

necessary to mobilize the esophagus fully both anteriorly and posteriorly if the *narrowed segment and the dilated segment above it* are easily visualized once the hiatus has been cleared. Many surgeons believe that preserving the posterior attachments of the esophagus at the hiatus may decrease the incidence of postoperative reflux. Additional length may be gained, if necessary, by minimal additional dissection, sufficient to pass an articulating curved grasper behind the esophagus **(Fig. 22–2a)** and encircling the esophagus with a 6 inch segment of a 0.25-inch Penrose drain **(Fig. 22–2b)**. Grasp the drain and pull down toward the left lower quadrant to lengthen the segment of intraabdominal esophagus.

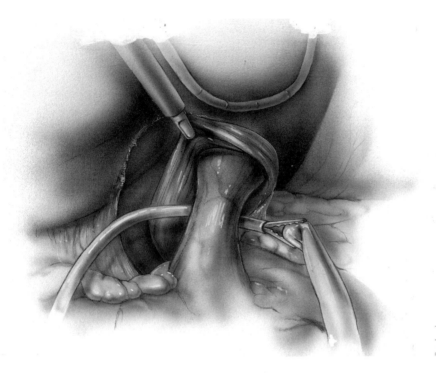

Fig. 22–2a

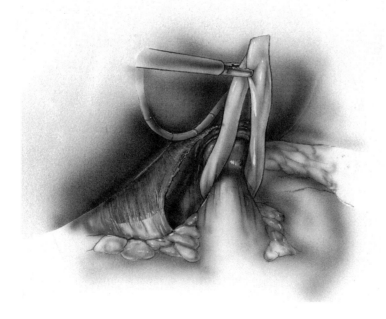

Fig. 22–2b

Myotomy

Begin the myotomy at a convenient location on the midportion of the thickened distal esophagus **(Fig. 22–3a)**. Curved scissors attached to electrocautery are useful for splitting, elevating, lightly cauterizing, and cutting parallel to the longitudinal muscle fibers. Use atraumatic graspers to elevate and pull down on the longitudinal muscle to improve exposure **(Fig. 22–3b)**. The underlying hypertrophied circular muscle fibers then come into view. Release the tension on the Penrose drain (if one was placed) to avoid pushing the walls of the esophagus together, which would increase the probability of injury to the epithelial tube.

Sequentially elevate the circular muscle fibers on the blade of the scissors, lightly cauterize, and cut. As the esophageal wall starts to open, place atraumatic graspers on the left and right cut edges of the muscular tube and pull gently apart and toward the patient's feet.

The epithelial tube is readily identified by its whitish color, smooth texture, and the small blood vessels that cross it. It may appear to balloon out into the field and is easily injured **(Fig. 22–4)**. Elevating the muscle edges helps minimize this tendency.

Extend the myotomy cephalad with the scissors until the circular muscle layer becomes thinner and the esophagus is dilated by sequentially lifting the circular muscle away from the epithelial tube with the blade of the scissors and cutting it **(Figs. 22–5a, 22–5b)**.

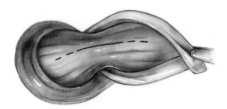

Fig. 22-3a

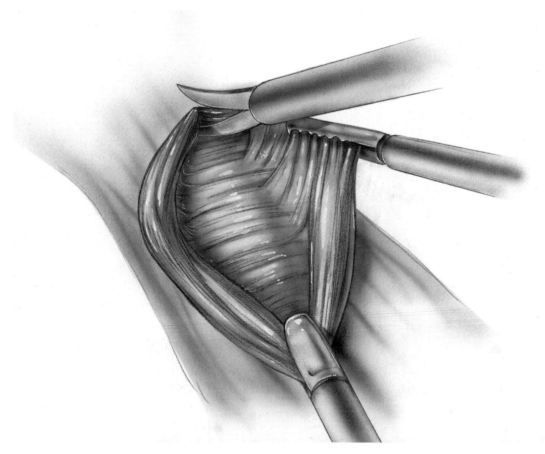

Fig. 22-3b

Fig. 22-4

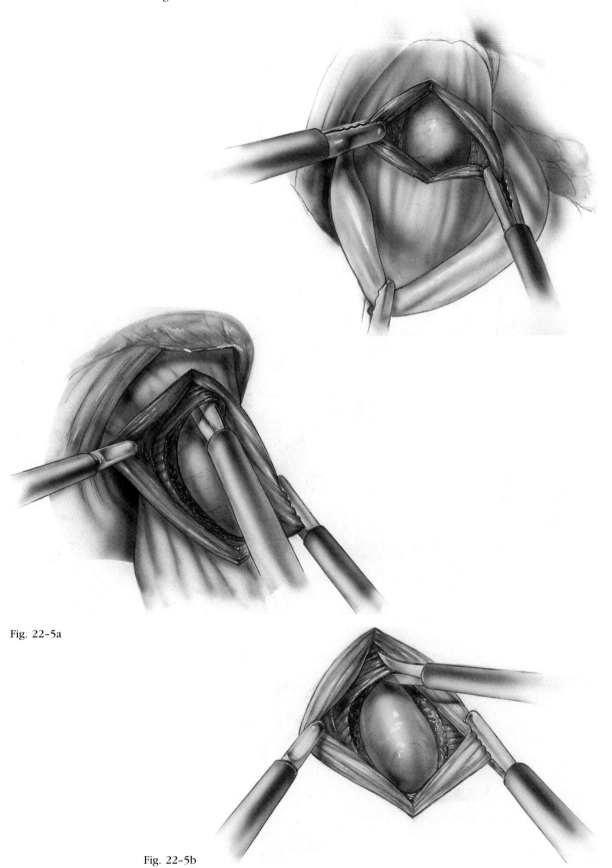

Fig. 22-5a

Fig. 22-5b

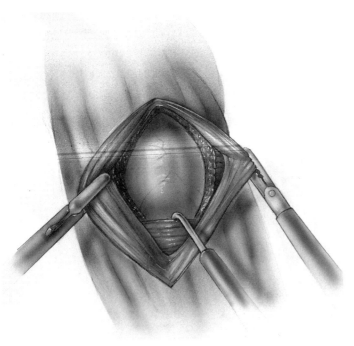

Fig. 22-6

Complete the myotomy distally with hook cautery. Engage the hook under the circular muscle fibers; lift it up to avoid burning the underlying epithelial tube, and pull it down to cauterize and divide the muscle **(Fig. 22–6)**. Some surgeons pass a right-angle clamp under the circular muscle and use it to displace the epithelial tube deep, out of harm's way.

Generally, a complete myotomy must extend about 1 cm onto the stomach **(Fig. 22–7)**. Release all instruments from the esophagus. Pass an EGD scope into the distal esophagus and visualize the gastro-esophageal junction, identifiable by the Z-line where the color changes between whitish esophageal epithelium and pink gastric mucosa. The opening should be patulous if an adequate myotomy was performed.

Irrigate the abdomen with saline and fill the left upper quadrant. Insufflate with the EGD scope and watch for bubbles. The completed myotomy is shown in Figure 22-7.

Fundoplication

Some surgeons perform a partial fundoplication at the conclusion of the procedure. An anterior (Dor) fundoplication is a simple way to buttress a small (repaired) perforation. A posterior partial (Toupet) fundoplication is said to help keep their edges of the myotomy separate. We use a partial fundoplication selectively.

COMPLICATIONS

Inadequate myotomy

Gastroesophageal reflux

Esophageal perforation

REFERENCES

Alves A, Perniceni T, Godeberge P, et al. Laparoscopic Heller's cardiomyotomy in achalasia: is intraoperative endoscopy useful and why? Surg Endosc 1999;13:600.

Dempsey DT, Kalan MM, Gerson RS, Parkman HP, Maier WP. Comparison of outcomes following open and laparoscopic esophagomyotomy for achalasia. Surg Endosc 1999;13:747.

Maher JW. Thoracoscopic esophagomyotomy for achalasia: maximum gain, minimal pain. Surgery 1997;122:836.

Oddsdottir M. Laparoscopic cardiomyotomy. In: Scott-Conner CEH (ed) The SAGES Manual: Fundamentals of Laparoscopy and GI Endoscopy. New York, Springer-Verlag, 1999, pp 213-220.

Patti MG, Pellegrini CA. Minimally invasive approaches to achalasia. Semin Gastrointest Dis 1994;5:108.

Stewart KC, Finley RJ, Clifton JC, et al. Thoracoscopic versus laparoscopic modified Heller myotomy for achalasia: efficacy and safety in 87 patients. J Am Coll Surg 1999;189:169.

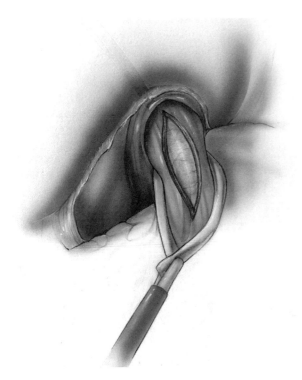

Fig. 22-7

23 Operations for Esophageal Perforation and Anastomotic Leaks

INDICATIONS

Instrumental or emetogenic esophageal perforation

Postoperative leak

PREOPERATIVE PREPARATION

Confirm perforation with diagnostic studies such as chest radiography; for suspected cervical perforations, lateral neck films in hyperextension; computed tomography (CT) scan or esophageal contrast radiographs.

Administer nasoesophageal suction proximal to perforation of the thoracic esophagus.

Insert a thoracostomy tube for pneumothorax.

Maintain fluid resuscitation.

Administer appropriate systemic antibiotics.

Insert appropriate central venous or pulmonary artery pressure monitors.

Control the airway with endotracheal intubation.

PITFALLS AND DANGER POINTS

Delayed diagnosis of the perforation

Inadequate attention to pulmonary function

Inadequate surgery to control continuing contamination

Inadequate drainage

Depending on sutured closure of inflamed esophagus

Suturing a perforated esophagus proximal to an obstruction

Inadequate pleural toilet and lung decortication

OPERATIVE STRATEGY

Visualize and thoroughly explore the region of the perforation. What appears to be a 1 cm perforation may prove to be three to four times that length after it is mobilized from the mediastinal pleura. Débride necrotic material around the perforation if suturing is anticipated. When the defect appears too large or the tissues too inflamed for suturing, it may be possible to apply a roof patch consisting of a flap of muscle pedicle, pleura, or pericardium that is sutured over the perforation. Otherwise, a diversion-exclusion operation or thoracic esophagectomy is necessary.

OPERATIVE TECHNIQUE

Pleural Flap Repair of Thoracic Esophageal Perforation

Incision

Make an incision in the left or right thoracic cavity depending on which side the perforation appears to present on the contrast esophageal radiograph. Generally, the lower half of the esophagus is approached through a left sixth or seventh intercostal space thoracotomy. The uncommon perforations of the upper esophagus are better approached through the right chest.

Exposure; Locating the Perforation

Incise the mediastinal pleura above and below the area of suspected perforation. Free to the mediastinal pleura from the esophagus so the esophagus can be elevated from its bed for thorough exploration. Sometimes the perforation is obscured by a layer of necrotic tissue. If the perforation is not immediately apparent, ask the anesthesiologist to instill air or a solution of methylene blue into the nasoesophageal tube and look for bubbling or the area of blue staining on the esophageal wall. Most patients have a pleural and a significant mediastinal infection with necrosis. Complete débridement of the mediastinum and decortication of the lung with removal of both parietal and visceral peels are used to control infection and ensure maximal lung function. Complete expansion of the lung is the best secondary defense against breakdown of an esophageal repair and helps control any fistula that develops.

Repair

When operation is performed soon (8 hours) after perforation, it may be possible to débride the tissues around the esophagus if marked edema and inflammation have not yet occurred; a viable tissue buttress should always be added to the repair. For suture closure, close the mucosal layer with interrupted sutures of 4-0 or 5-0 nonabsorbable synthetic suture and approximate the muscular layer with interrupted Lembert sutures of 4-0 silk or Prolene. In selected cases, a stapled closure may work. There must be sufficient good tissue to achieve an everted stapled closure without narrowing the lumen. Mobilize the edges of the effect and use Allis clamps to bring the full thickness of the esophageal wall within the jaws of a linear thick tissue stapler. Cover the suture line with a pleural flap. If the perforation is located in the lateral aspect of the esophagus, a simple rectangular flap of pleura is elevated and brought over the suture line. Use many interrupted 4-0 nonabsorbable sutures to fix the pleural flap around the sutured perforation.

When the perforation is not suitable for a sutured closure due to marked edema and inflammation, employ a pleural flap, an intercostal muscle flap, or some other viable buttress as a roof patch over the open defect in the esophagus. First débride the obvious necrotic tissue around the perforation. When the esophagus is too inflamed to hold sutures, it is advisable to exclude the upper esophagus from the gastrointestinal tract by one of the methods described below to supplement the pleural roof patch. With an extensive defect in the esophagus or one located on the posterior surface, outline a large rectangular flap of pleura as illustrated in **Figure 23–1**. In the presence of mediastinitis, the pleura is thickened and easy to mobilize from the posterior thoracic wall. Leave the base of the pedicle attached to the adjacent aorta. Slide the pedicle flap underneath the esophagus **(Fig. 23–2)** so it surrounds the entire organ. Insert multiple 4-0 interrupted nonabsorbable sutures deep enough to catch the submucosa of the esophagus around the entire circumference of the perforation as well as the entire circumference of the esophagus above and below the perforation, as illustrated in **Figure 23–3**.

Drainage

Place the tip of a 36F chest tube near the site of the esophageal perforation. Suture it to the mediastinal tissues with a catgut stitch. Bring this tube out through a small incision through the ninth or tenth interspace in the anterior axillary line. Place a smaller chest tube in the posterior portion of the apex of the chest and bring it out through a second stab wound. Attach both to underwater suction drainage.

Intercostal Muscle Flap Repair of Esophageal Perforation

Another method for bringing viable tissue to the site of an esophageal perforation is to create a vascularized flap of the appropriate intercostal muscle with which to wrap the perforation of the esophagus. If the patient undergoes surgery within the first 8 hours after a perforation, minor débridement and primary suturing generally remedy the situation. However, for perforations that have been leaking for a longer interval before surgery is undertaken, débridement of necrotic tissue and primary suturing may not be adequate; in these situations wrapping with a viable muscle flap may help achieve primary healing. In cases where the perforation is too large for suture closure, a roof patch consisting of viable intercostal muscle sutured to the intact esophagus around the perforation may be effective. Richardson et al. have reported remarkable success with this technique for esophageal defects due to penetrating trauma.

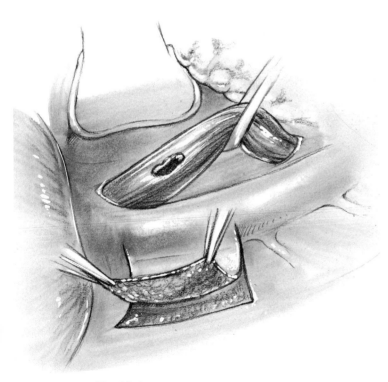

Fig. 23-1

To achieve a viable muscle flap, care must be taken to preserve the intercostal vessels. These vessels must be left attached to the muscle as it is being dis-

sected away from the upper and lower rib borders. **Figure 23-4** illustrates dissection of the full thickness of the intercostal muscle from its attachments

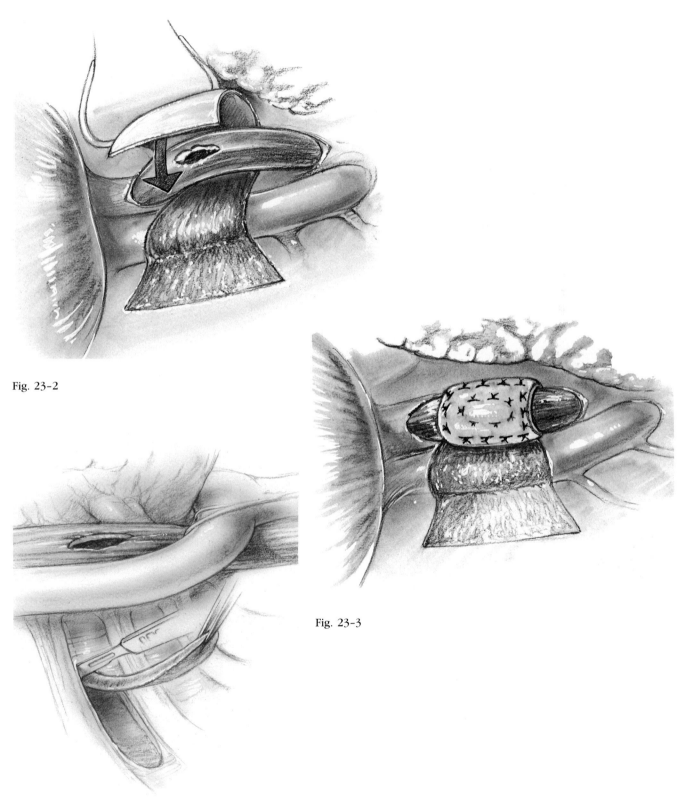

Fig. 23-2

Fig. 23-3

Fig. 23-4

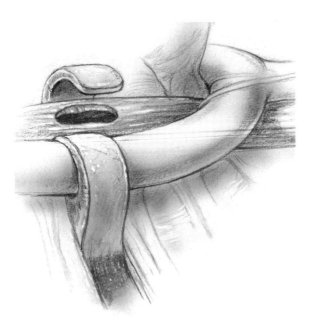

Fig. 23-5

to the adjacent ribs. **Figures 23–5, 23–6**, and **23–7** illustrate application of the intercostal muscle flap as a roof patch over a perforation that was not suitable for sutured closure. Large perforations (longer than the width of the muscle flap) may be difficult to repair by this technique. Drain the mediastinum and chest as described above. If the repair proves to be of poor quality, do not hesitate to resect the esophagus or to apply a temporary occlusion technique to the esophagus, as described below.

Esophageal Occlusion Methods Without Cervical Esophagostomy

When cervical esophagostomy is used for diversion in the neck, it is sometimes difficult to reconstruct the esophagus after the perforation heals. An alternative but less secure method is staple occlusion of the proximal esophagus. Avoid capturing the vagus nerves when stapling the lower esophagus. It is possible to occlude the esophagus above a thoracic perforation through the exploratory chest incision if the thoracic esophagus above the perforation is healthy. A sump-type nasoesophageal suction catheter is placed above the staple line.

Esophageal Diversion by Cervical Esophagostomy

Incision and Exposure

With the patient's head turned toward the right, make an incision along the anterior border of the sternomastoid muscle beginning 2-3 cm below the level of the mandibular angle and continuing down to the clavicle (see Fig. 11-27). Liberate the anterior border of the sternomastoid muscle. Divide the omohyoid muscle if it crosses the operative field. Retract the sternomastoid muscle and carotid sheath laterally and retract the prethyroid muscles medially, exposing the thyroid gland (see Fig. 11-29). Carefully divide the areolar tissue between the thyroid gland and the carotid sheath to expose the inferior thyroid artery and the recurrent laryngeal nerve. In some cases it is necessary to divide the inferior thyroid artery. Preserve the recurrent nerve. Identify the tracheoesophageal groove. Begin the dissection on the

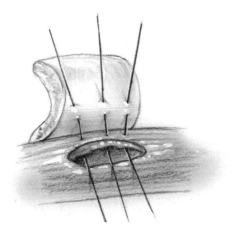

Fig. 23-6

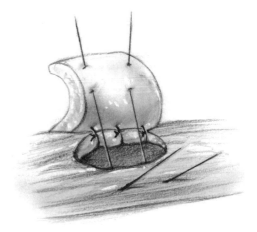

Fig. 23-7

prevertebral fascia and free the esophagus posteriorly. Then encircle the esophagus with the index finger or a right angle clamp, but keep the plane of dissection close to the esophagus; otherwise, it is possible to traumatize the *opposite* recurrent laryngeal nerve or injure the membranous posterior wall of the trachea. After the esophagus has been encircled, pass a latex drain around the esophagus for purposes of traction. Mobilize the esophagus from the level of the hypopharynx down to the upper mediastinum.

Suturing the Esophagostomy

After mobilization is satisfactory, suture the sternomastoid muscle back in place by means of several interrupted 4-0 synthetic absorbable stitches. Close the platysma muscle with interrupted sutures of the same material, leaving sufficient space to suture the esophagostomy to the skin. Then insert interrupted 4-0 PG subcuticular sutures to close the skin, leaving a 3- to 4-cm gap in the closure for the esophagostomy.

Now make a transverse incision across the anterior half of the circumference of the esophagus. Suture the full thickness of the esophagus to the subcuticular layer of skin with interrupted 4-0 absorbable synthetic sutures **(Fig. 23–8)**.

In one case we found that, despite thorough mobilization of the esophagus, the incised esophagus could not be sutured to the skin without tension. A subtotal thyroid lobectomy was carried out. The incised esophagus was then sutured to the platysma muscle with interrupted sutures, leaving the skin in this area open. These steps produced a satisfactory result. As an alternative, mobilize the proximal thoracic esophagus and staple it closed with the linear stapler. Then either return it to its bed and decompress the closed esophageal remnant with a nasoesophageal tube or a lateral pharyngostomy tube or explant it to a subcutaneous position and create a stoma as described below.

Anterior Thoracic Esophagostomy

When a thoracic esophagectomy (Orringer and Stirling 1990) is carried out in these patients, an incision is made in the neck along the anterior border of the sternomastoid muscle. After the esophagus has been delivered through this incision, excise the segment that is nonviable and preserve all the viable esophagus. Make a subcutaneous tunnel from the incision in the neck over the anterior thorax. This tunnel should equal the length of the preserved esophagus. Make the esophagostomy on the anterior wall of the chest by making an incision in the skin and suturing the full

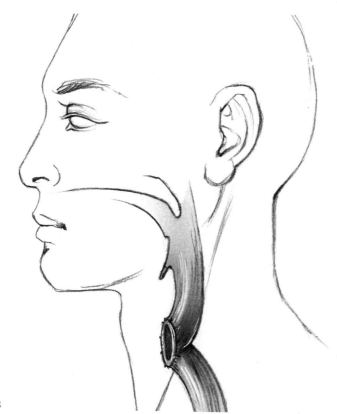

Fig. 23–8

thickness of the esophagus to the subcuticular layer of skin with interrupted 5-0 Vicryl sutures. It is much easier to apply stoma collection bags to the anterior chest than to a cervical esophageal stoma.

Excluding the Esophagus from the Gastrointestinal Tract

Perform a thoracotomy as described for the pleural flap operation. Incise the mediastinal pleura and liberate the esophagus from its bed **(Fig. 23–9)**. The perforation may be sutured or covered with a pleural flap (Fig. 23-3).

Then free the esophagus around its entire circumference distal to the perforation. Urschel et al. occluded the esophagus by surrounding it with a strip of Teflon that was sutured to itself to form a circumferential constricting band. Do not make this band so tight it strangulates the tissue. An umbilical tape may be passed around the Teflon band and tied to ensure the proper degree of constriction. Try to avoid including the vagus nerves in the constricting

band. An alternative method of occluding the lower esophagus is to ligate it with a Silastic tube, such as the Jackson-Pratt catheter **(Figs. 23–10, 23–11)**. This material appears to be less irritating to the tissues than Teflon or umbilical tape. Another alternative is to use the TA-55 stapling device *with 4.8 mm staples* to occlude the esophagus. When applying the staples, separate the vagus nerves from the esophagus so they are not trapped in the staple line. Use staples only if the esophagus is not markedly thickened or inflamed. Otherwise, the thickened tissues may be strangulated by the staples. After a period of 3–4 weeks a gap often appears in this staple line. This gap can usually be dilated by gentle passage of Maloney dilators. If the gap is small, the interventional radiologist can pass a guidewire over which dilating devices may be passed.

Another reported method for occluding the esophagus is passage of no. 2 chromic catgut or PG twice around the esophagus, which is then tied in a snug but not strangulating knot. The esophagus should respond easily to dilatation by the end of 2–4 weeks. It

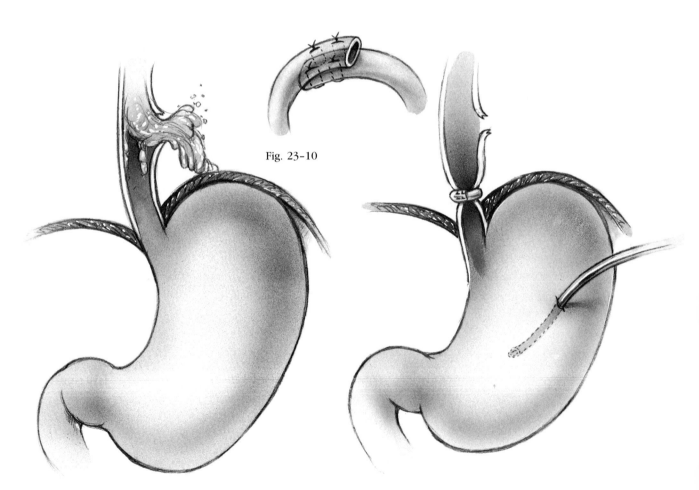

Fig. 23-10

Fig. 23-9   Fig. 23-11

has been reported that even with delayed operations in patients who suffer large lacerations of the thoracic esophagus spontaneous healing occasionally occurs over a period of weeks, so esophageal replacement with either colon or stomach is not necessary.

This technique should be used if the patient has significant reflux. In other circumstances, we eliminate this step altogether because it is a distal obstruction and can prevent healing of a fistula.

To decompress the stomach and prevent pressure against the esophageal closure, a Stamm gastrostomy should be performed. In contrast to the usual location shown in Figure 23–11, it is wise to place this gastrostomy near the lesser curvature of the stomach if possible. In this way, if a gastric pull-up operation is to be performed to replace the esophagus, the gastrostomy defect can be included in the segment of the lesser curvature that is customarily excised when preparing the stomach for advancement into the neck. It does not interfere with the blood supply to the greater curvature.

Finally, place proper drainage tubes to the area of perforation and close the thoracic incision. All of these patients require a tube gastrostomy to decompress the stomach; after the esophageal perforation has healed, the gastrostomy tube is used for purposes of feeding.

POSTOPERATIVE CARE

Most of these patients require *ventilatory support* for several days. Careful *cardiopulmonary monitoring* is a necessity.

Paste a small *drainage* bag or ileostomy bag over the esophagostomy to collect saliva. In patients without an esophagostomy, maintain nasoesophageal sump suction postoperatively.

These patients require intensive *antibiotic* treatment, depending on bacterial cultures of the mediastinum.

Do not remove the thoracotomy drainage tubes until drainage has ceased.

Total parenteral nutrition is necessary until the gastrostomy tube can be used for feeding.

Obtain frequent *chest radiographs* or *CT scans* in a search for loculated collections of pus.

COMPLICATIONS

Esophagocutaneous fistula

Uncontrolled sepsis including empyema or mediastinal abscess

Subphrenic abscess

Limited expansion of lung, requiring surgical decortication after active infection has subsided

REFERENCES

Alexander PV, Hollands M, O'Roaurke IC, Tait N. Intercostal pedicle flap for thoracic esophageal perforations. Aust NZ J Surg 1997;67:133.

Altorjay A, Kiss J, Voros A, Sziranyi E. The role of esophagectomy in the management of esophageal perforations. Ann Thorac Surg 1998;65:1433.

Bardini R, Bonavina L, Pavanello M. Temporary double exclusion of the perforated esophagus using absorbable staples. Ann Thorac Surg 1992;54:1165.

Goldstein LA, Thompson WR. Esophageal perforations: a 15 year experience. Am J Surg 1983;143:495.

Gouge TH, Depan HJ, Spencer F. Experience with the Grillo pleural wrap procedure in 18 patients with perforation of the thoracic esophagus. Ann Surg 1989;209:612.

Iannettoni MD, Vlessis AA, Whyte RI, Orringer MB. Functional outcome after surgical treatment of esophageal perforation. Ann Thorac Surg 1997;64:1609.

Mansour KA, Wenger RK. T-Tube management of late esophageal perforations. Surg Gynecol Obstet 1992;175:571.

Maroney TP, Ring EJ, Gordon RL, et al. Role of interventional radiology in the management of major esophageal leaks. Radiology 1989;170:1055.

Michel L, Grillo HC, Malt RA. Operative and nonoperative management of esophageal perforations. Ann Surg 1981;194:57.

Orringer MB, Stirling MC. Esophagectomy for esophageal disruption. Ann Thorac Surg 1990;49:35.

Paramesh V, Rumisek JD, Chang FC. Spontaneous recanalization of the esophagus after exclusion using nonabsorbable staples. Ann Thorac Surg 1995;59:1214.

Pate JW, Walker WA, Cole FH Jr, et al. Spontaneous rupture of the esophagus: a 30-year experience. Ann Thorac Surg 1989;47:689.

Richardson JD, Tobin GR. Closure of esophageal defects with muscle flaps. Arch Surg 1994;129:541.

Richardson JD, Martin LF, Borzotta AP, Polk HC Jr. Unifying concepts in treatment of esophageal leaks. Am J Surg 1985;149:157.

Sarr MG, Pemberton JH, Payne WS. Management of instrumental perforations of the esophagus. J Thorac Cardiovasc Surg 1982;84:211.

Skinner DB, Little AG, DeMeester TR. Management of esophageal perforation. Am J Surg 1980;139:760.

Thai AP, Hatafuku T. Improved operation for esophageal rupture. JAMA 1964;188:826.

Triggiani E, Belsey R. Oesophageal trauma: incidence, diagnosis, and management. Thorax 1977;32:241.

Urbani M, Mathisen DJ. Repair of esophageal perforation after treatment for achalasia. Ann Thorac Surg 2000;69:1609.

Urschel HC Jr, Razzuk MA, Wood RE, et al. Improved management of esophageal perforation: exclusion and diversion in continuity. Ann Surg 1974;179:587.

Whyte RI, Iannettoni MD, Orringer MB. Intrathoracic esophageal perforation: the merit of primary repair. J Thorac Cardiovasc Surg 1995;109:140.

Wilson SE, Stone R, Scully M, et al. Modern management of anastomotic leak after esophagogastrectomy. Am J Surg 1982;144:94.

Wright CD, Mathisen DJ, Wain JC, et al. Reinforced primary repair of thoracic esophageal perforation. Ann Thorac Surg 1995;60:245.

Part III
Stomach and Duodenum

24 Concepts in Surgery of the Stomach and Duodenum

Michael W. Grabowski
Daniel T. Dempsey

The major indications for gastric surgery are ulcer disease, cancer, and access for feeding (gastrostomy placement). This chapter begins with considerations relevant to those three indications. A brief discussion of alternative choices for a drainage procedure after gastric resection for benign disease or malignancy follows. The chapter concludes with a section on complications. This final section details recognition and management of various postgastrectomy and postvagotomy syndromes.

SURGERY FOR PEPTIC ULCER

The last quarter century has seen dramatic changes in how peptic ulcer disease is evaluated and treated. Although older paradigms such as "no acid no ulcer" remain valid, they have largely been replaced with models relating peptic ulcer to *Helicobacter* infection or nonsteroidal antiinflammatory drug (NSAID) ingestion [1]. Three key advances are responsible for this change: the discovery and evolution of antiacid secretory medications, elucidation of the critical role of *Helicobacter pylori* in the pathogenesis of peptic ulcer, and the evolution of advanced endoscopic/laparoscopic techniques to diagnose and intervene in the natural history of the disease. As a direct result, the indications for surgery and the selection of procedures for peptic ulcer disease are currently being reevaluated. Controversy exists regarding the "best" surgical procedure. In the past extensive operations were utilized because they had the lowest ulcer recurrence rate, although they led to the most morbidity and mortality. The ability to eradicate *H. pylori* and the use of proton pump inhibitors may mitigate the concern about ulcer recurrence [2]. As we have seen in many other areas of surgery, less may become more as we treat peptic ulcer disease during the twenty-first century.

Surgical interventions for the management of peptic ulcer disease fall into two broad categories. Elective operations have been relegated to relative obscurity, and urgent or emergent procedures for the complications of peptic ulcer disease (PUD), most commonly bleeding, perforation, and obstruction, have come to the forefront. Surgeons today must be knowledgeable about the indications for operation and facile in the performance of surgical procedures that are now more commonly accomplished in a nonelective situation. In this section, we review the current concepts related to operative management of PUD.

Gastric Ulcer

Gastric ulceration has traditionally been divided into four types based on location and acid secretory status. Type I gastric ulcers are located in the body of the stomach and are not necessarily associated with high acid output. Type II and III gastric ulcers have some duodenal or prepyloric component and thus are surgically treated more like duodenal ulcers [3]. Their management is discussed below. Lastly, type IV gastric ulcer is relatively uncommon and occurs high on the lesser curvature close to the gastroesophageal (GE) junction.

Elective surgery for intractability of type I gastric ulcer should be preceded by an appropriate biopsy to rule out occult carcinoma. In an emergent operation for gastric ulcer, biopsy must be done because the result may alter the choice of operation. Classically, the procedure of choice for intractable type I benign gastric ulcer has been distal gastrectomy to include the ulcer with reconstruction in a Billroth I (preferred) or Billroth II fashion. The mortality rate for this elective operation is not substantially higher than that for vagotomy and drainage (around 2%), and the operation is definitely more effective in preventing ulcer recurrence, which is about 4% following partial gastrectomy with Billroth I versus up to 20% following vagotomy and drainage. An alternative approach to type I benign gastric ulcer is highly selective vagotomy with excision of the ulcer. In experienced hands this method yields lower morbidity and mortality but an increased chance of ulcer recurrence, in the range of 4–15% [4]. Proponents of the latter approach claim that the patients have fewer postoperative side effects and the procedure may be approached in a minimally invasive fashion. Unfortunately, excision of a lesser curve ulcer can be challenging and may denervate the antrum and pylorus, thwarting the "highly selective" vagotomy. Type IV gastric ulceration poses a challenge because of its relation to the GE junction. Ideally, the ulcer is resected in continuity with a distal gastrectomy and reconstruction with gastroduodenostomy (Pauchet operation). Other options include vagotomy and drainage with biopsy or excision of the ulcer, biopsy of the ulcer followed by distal gastric resection, or Roux-en-Y esophagogastrojejunostomy (Csendes operation). Total gastrectomy for benign gastric ulcer should be avoided.

Emergent surgery for gastric ulceration is most often indicated for perforation or hemorrhage. The procedure to be undertaken is often influenced by the preoperative status of the patient. After controlling hemorrhage or spillage and assessing the possibility of occult carcinoma, the surgeon has several options depending on stability and premorbid risk factors of the patient. Distal gastrectomy addresses the inciting problem and has the lowest recurrence rate but is associated with significant morbidity and mortality in this class of patients [5]. Alternatively, in higher risk or more unstable patients, excision, omental patch, or oversewing of the ulcer with or without vagotomy and pyloroplasty are viable alternatives.

Duodenal Ulcer

Elective surgery for intractable duodenal ulcer is now rare. The surgical options include highly selective vagotomy, truncal vagotomy with drainage procedure, or vagotomy and antrectomy. Any elective surgery for an intractable duodenal ulcer must have extremely low morbidity. Highly selective vagotomy (HSV) has the lowest postoperative morbidity rate while providing an acceptably low recurrence rate [6]. Moreover, HSV can be completed laparoscopically with good results in experienced hands. Thus HSV is considered the primary surgical choice for intractable duodenal ulcer. Truncal vagotomy (TV) with a drainage procedure or TV with antral resection are associated with higher postoperative complication rates and are probably best reserved for failure of HSV in this setting.

Gastric outlet obstruction (GOO) secondary to peptic ulcer disease most often presents a semi-

elective indication for operation. Attempt a trial of medical/endoscopic treatment before undertaking surgery. Fluid resuscitation, nasogastric decompression, acid suppression, and therapy for *H. pylori* are the mainstays of the preoperative regimen. An attempt at endoscopic balloon dilation may yield initial success, but recurrent obstruction is common. The operative choices for GOO include HSV with dilation, HSV and drainage (we prefer gastrojejunostomy to pyloroplasty), truncal vagotomy and drainage, and truncal vagotomy and antrectomy. Our procedure of choice in most patients nowadays is HSV and gastrojejunostomy. Although the ulcer recurrence rate is somewhat higher, the morbidity is clearly lower than vagotomy and antrectomy.

Perforated duodenal ulcer, on rare instances treated in a nonoperative fashion, most often requires urgent surgical intervention. The choice of operation depends on whether a definitive ulcer operation as undertaken. This decision can be clouded today, as most of the published data on this topic predate elucidation of the critical role of *H. pylori* in this disease. Patients with major premorbid medical illness, shock, or delayed diagnosis of perforation are probably best served with omental patch closure (Graham patch) alone. Alternatively, good operative candidates, especially those with a history of peptic ulcer disease, may be better served with closure of the perforation and HSV. The latter approach not only fixes the acute process it provides long-term protection from recurrence with minimal side effects. In some cases, where there is extensive scarring of the pyloric region, truncal vagotomy with drainage may be indicated. Lastly, there is considerable enthusiasm for the laparoscopic management of duodenal ulcer perforation, especially in good risk patients with early diagnosis. Laparoscopic management of this problem most often involves omental patch closure and requires the surgeon to be facile in the techniques of intracorporeal suturing [7].

Although advanced endoscopic techniques may have improved the nonoperative management of bleeding duodenal ulcer, it remains a not infrequent indication for urgent or emergent surgical intervention. The first concern should be management of the bleeding ulcer site. This is most often accomplished via a longitudinal duodenotomy, which may have to be extended through the pylorus. Once the bleeding duodenal ulcer is controlled with sutures of nonabsorbable material, the surgeon is faced with several options. If the pylorus has not been encompassed in the duodenotomy, HSV may be undertaken. If the incision crossed the pylorus (the more common scenario), we prefer truncal vagotomy with closure of the duodenotomy in a pyloroplasty. Although one might consider truncal vagotomy with antrectomy, it carries a higher perioperative risk and probably is not warranted in the current era.

Gastrostomy

Use of the stomach as a portal for feeding or decompression seems to be increasing as more medically complex and terminal patients are encountered. Additionally, the last quarter century has seen the advent of less invasive methods for gaining access to perform gastrostomy [8,9]. Gastrostomy tubes may be placed endoscopically (percutaneous endoscopic gastrostomy, or PEG), laparoscopically, or in a conventional (open) fashion. Each method has its unique advantages and limitations. PEG is a relatively simple method that can be performed outside the operating room and does not require general anesthesia. The limitation of this method lies in the blind nature of the tube insertion and the lack of fixation of the stomach to the inner abdominal wall. Laparoscopic gastrostomy provides direct visualization as well as a method of stomach fixation but is more invasive. Open gastrostomy is the most invasive but may be the only option in certain patients with prior abdominal surgery. The Stamm gastrostomy method is the more commonly used open method today since the introduction of better feeding tubes. The Janeway gastrostomy creates a permanent mucosa-lined gastrocutaneous fistula, obviating the need for continual tube placement. It is less frequently employed. The best gastrostomy tube placement method is that which is individualized to the patient's medical condition and long-term needs and the surgeon's personal experience.

CHOICE OF OPERATION FOR GASTRIC CANCER

Adenocarcinoma of the stomach often extends submucosally much farther than is appreciated on gross examination. Early metastasis is usually to regional lymph nodes, but the lymphatic drainage of the stomach is extensive and often unpredictable. These facts support a generous gastric resection for treatment of this disease, with the ideal being 6 cm of normal tissue proximal and distal to the tumor. For the past two decades the standard operation performed for gastric adenocarcinoma of the body or antrum has been "radical subtotal gastrectomy," which includes (1) a 70–90% distal gastrectomy; (2) ligation of the right gastric, right gastroepiploic, and left gastric arteries at their origin with removal of associated lymphoid tissue; and (3) removal of the lesser and greater omentum. Cancers of the cardia

or fundus are treated with total gastrectomy or proximal subtotal gastrectomy with high ligation of the left gastric artery and removal of the gastrosplenic ligament and lesser omentum together with the crural lymphatic tissue. For lesions close to the GE junction, distal esophagus is usually removed. Despite increasing interest in more extensive surgical procedures for the treatment of gastric adenocarcinoma, none has definitively improved the cure rate of this dreaded disease [10].

Subtotal Versus Total Gastrectomy

Despite the argument for wider resection, routine total gastrectomy for gastric adenocarcinoma should be avoided. When compared to subtotal resection, the operative mortality is higher, the nutritional side effects more devastating, and the cure rate no better after total gastrectomy [11]. Most tumors of the distal stomach are adequately resected with distal subtotal gastrectomy described above. If at least 30% of the proximal stomach remains, continuity is reestablished with the Billroth II gastrojejunostomy. A Billroth I reconstruction should be avoided in cases of gastric malignancy because of the risk of recurrence at the duodenal margin (usually the margin with the least tumor clearance). If 20% or less of the proximal stomach remains, reconstruction should be with a Roux limb or a Billroth II with Braun enteroenterostomy.

Total gastrectomy should be considered for extensive cancers and for proximal gastric cancer [12]. A less attractive alternative for the latter lesion is proximal subtotal gastrectomy. However, in this instance esophagogastrostomy should be assiduously avoided because of the risk of bile esophagitis, which inevitably occurs if pyloroplasty is added. Occasionally we have used a proximal gastrectomy with esophagogastrostomy without pyloroplasty in patients with a poor prognosis. In this instance we always add a feeding jejunostomy. A better option for reconstruction following proximal gastric resection may be isoperistaltic jejunal interposition (Henley loop).

If total gastrectomy is performed (and the surgeon should not hesitate if this operation is necessary to do an adequate curative resection), some sort of jejunal reservoir should be constructed. In our experience, the most satisfactory option is a Roux-en-Y esophagojejunostomy with a J-pouch.

R1 Versus R2 Lymphadenectomy

In general, an R1 resection means complete removal of all perigastric lymph nodes appropriate for the tumor (distal, middle, or proximal gastric tumor)

Table 24-1. Lymphadenectomy for Gastric Cancer (Lymph Node Groups Resected)

Lymph Node Groups Resected	
R1 Resection	R2 Resection
Lower third tumors	
3 Lesser curve	1 Right cardiac
4 Greater curve	7 Left gastric artery
5 Suprapyloric	8 Hepatic artery
6 Infrapyloric	9 Celiac artery
Middle third tumors	
1 Right cardiac	2 Left cardiac
3 Lesser curve	7 Left gastric artery
4 Greater curve	8 Hepatic artery
5 Suprapyloric	9 Celiac artery
6 Infrapyloric	10 Splenic hilar
	11 Splenic artery
Upper third tumors	
1 Right cardiac	5 Suprapyloric
2 Left cardiac	6 Infrapyloric
3 Lesser curve	7 Left gastric artery
4 Greater curve and	8 Hepatic artery
short gastric	9 Celiac artery
	10 Splenic hilar
	11 Splenic artery
	110 Low paraesophageal

(Table 24–1). An R2 resection means an R1 resection plus removal of all lymph nodes along the named arteries to the stomach, again appropriate for the tumor [13]. The R2 dissection requires significant retroperitoneal dissection, and for most gastric tumors includes the anterior leaf of the transverse mesocolon and the anterior capsule of the pancreas. Splenectomy and distal pancreatectomy are not routinely performed, as this extensive surgery has been shown to increase perioperative morbidity without improving the cure rate. The extent of gastric resection is generally the same for R1 and R2 resections for distal gastric tumors (70% distal gastrectomy) and for proximal gastric tumors (total gastrectomy). Most surgeons doing an R2 resection for mid-gastric tumors perform total gastrectomy, whereas those doing an R1 resection may leave a small proximal gastric pouch (10–20%).

The Japanese experience with extended gastrectomy and lymphadenectomy has been favorable. However, prospective evaluations in Western countries have shown higher operative morbidity and mortality rates without any improvement in cure rates [14,15].

Splenectomy

Splenectomy should be performed if the tumor is adherent to the spleen. It should also be considered for tumors of the greater curvature that involve the gastrosplenic ligament. Otherwise, splenectomy should not be part of the routine surgical treatment for gastric adenocarcinoma [16].

Laparoscopy

Should staging laparoscopy be a routine part of the preoperative evaluation of gastric carcinoma? The answer to this question depends somewhat on the surgeon's attitude toward the surgical palliation of incurable gastric cancer. Despite improvements in preoperative staging with dynamic computed tomography (CT) and endoscopic ultrasonography, unexpected liver or peritoneal metastases are found in 10–20% of patients with gastric cancer. In the absence of significant bleeding or impending obstruction from the primary tumor, many surgeons (the authors included) believe that gastrectomy is contraindicated if liver or peritoneal disease is extensive. Laparoscopy helps avoid a major unnecessary operation in this small group of patients.

CHOICE OF DRAINAGE PROCEDURE FOR GASTRIC SURGERY

Pyloroplasty Versus Gastrojejunostomy

If the tissue proximal and distal to the pylorus is relatively normal, pyloroplasty is an attractive option after truncal vagotomy. Although gastrojejunostomy is an equally effective drainage procedure with a comparable incidence of dumping, several problems can occur with this operation [17], including marginal ulceration, internal hernia (under the jejunal loop or through the mesocolon if a retrocolic anastomosis is done), afferent loop obstruction, and bilious vomiting from "circus movement." It may be more difficult to perform a subsequent gastric resection in a patient with a previous pyloroplasty than with a gastrojejunostomy.

Billroth I Versus Billroth II

Gastroduodenostomy (Billroth I) is a useful option for establishing gastrointestinal continuity following distal gastric resection (<50%) for benign disease. Although there are no clinically significant physiologic advantages of Billroth I over Billroth II, the former does avoid the aforementioned problems associated with loop gastrojejunostomy. It also avoids a duodenal stump. Billroth II is the preferred reconstruction after gastrectomy for malignancy.

Billroth II Versus Roux-en-Y

The Roux gastrojejunostomy prevents bile from entering the gastric remnant. This is important if a small gastric remnant (<20%) exists, as performance of Billroth II in this situation often results in intolerable bile reflux esophagitis. Furthermore, a leak at a Roux-en-Y anastomosis does not contain bile or pancreatic enzymes and may be less virulent than a leak following a Billroth II gastrojejunostomy. The disadvantages of the Roux gastrojejunostomy include the need for an additional anastomosis (the enteroenterostomy). In addition, this reconstruction is relatively ulcerogenic, as bile, pancreatic juice, and duodenal secretions do not bathe the gastric anastomosis. Finally, some patients develop significantly delayed gastric emptying following Roux gastrojejunostomy, especially if a generous gastric remnant remains. For these two latter reasons, the Roux-en-Y gastrojejunostomy should not be performed in patients unless a generous gastrectomy (>80%) has been performed.

Roux-en-Y Versus Braun Enteroenterostomy or Henley Loop

Because of problems with delayed gastric emptying following the Roux gastrojejunostomy, some surgeons prefer a loop gastrojejunostomy with a Braun enteroenterostomy to divert most of the bile away from the small gastric remnant [18]. A more complex operation that can be used to minimize bile reflux into a small gastric remnant without bypassing the duodenum is the Henley loop. Here an isoperistaltic loop of jejunum (40 cm) is interposed between the gastric remnant and the duodenum [19]. These options clearly should be considered in patients requiring reoperation because of complications following the Roux gastrojejunostomy.

POSTOPERATIVE COMPLICATIONS

Pulmonary Problems

Atelectasis is probably the most common complication after gastric operation. Adequate analgesia, incentive spirometry, and early ambulation help minimize this problem. Pneumonia is a less common but feared complication. Predisposing factors are atelectasis, vomiting, and preexisting lung disease. Pulmonary embolism is unusual with current prophylactic practices but should be considered in any postoperative patient with acute shortness of breath or chest pain.

Leak

Following a gastric or duodenal operation, any suture line may leak and create a potentially fatal situation. These problems usually are obvious by the fifth or sixth postoperative day and are associated with increasing abdominal pain, fever, distension, and leukocytosis. These findings should prompt an aggressive diagnostic evaluation including obstruction series, contrast CT scan, or Gastrografin upper gastrointestinal (GI) series. Although small leaks can sometimes be managed nonoperatively with a strategically placed drain, most patients benefit from reoperation. Irrigation and drainage of the peritoneal cavity, decompression of the leaking segment (e.g., duodenostomy or gastrostomy), closure or intubation of the leak (or both), and feeding jejunostomy are important aspects of management.

Pancreatitis

Pancreatitis following gastroduodenal operation is generally caused by trauma ("blunt or penetrating") to the gland itself or to the major or minor papilla. Treatment is usually nonoperative except in cases of necrotizing pancreatitis or persistent pancreatic fistula. Either of the papillae can be injured during aggressive dissection of the postbulbar duodenum. More commonly the more proximal minor papilla is occluded or transected. This is usually a self-limited problem unless the patient has pancreas divisum. Occasionally, a duodenal stump leak is misdiagnosed as pancreatitis.

Wound Problems

Wound infection, dehiscence, and herniation occur after major gastric operations. The problems are interrelated in that infection predisposes to the other two complications, and all three share risk factors. Wound infection is related to intraoperative contamination, which is more significant in the setting of acid suppression, gastric cancer, and obstruction. Pulmonary disease, abdominal distension, obesity, infection, malnutrition, and steroid therapy have all been shown to increase the incidence of wound failure.

Delayed Gastric Emptying

In the occasional patient recovering from gastric surgery, the nasogastric tube "cannot be removed" because of persistent nausea and vomiting. Frequently the gastric outlet is anatomically patent. Alternative methods of gastric intubation and alimentation are often preferable to a major reoperation during the first 6 weeks postoperatively when the inflammatory response in the surgical field may be intense. Reoperation during this early postoperative period is often difficult, hazardous, and usually unnecessary. If adequate gastric remnant remains, a gastrostomy may be placed laparoscopically or endoscopically and a tube fed into the jejunum. Alimentation can be given enterally or via total parenteral nutrition. Alternatively, in patients with a small gastric remnant where a Stamm gastrostomy technique is impossible, a decompressing gastric tube can be passed retrograde through the jejunal efferent limb (using a Witzel technique), and another (distal) tube may be placed antegrade as a Witzel feeding jejunostomy. If these patients can be nursed through the first 3 months postoperatively, reoperation is often unnecessary and GI function is satisfactory. Reoperation should thus usually be delayed for 3–6 months after the first operation unless a high-grade or complete mechanical obstruction has been demonstrated in the small intestine. This may represent a process that predisposes to small bowel strangulation (e.g., herniation through the transverse mesocolon or proximal adhesive small bowel obstruction) and should be operated on promptly.

POSTGASTRECTOMY SYNDROMES

A variety of abnormalities affect a small number of patients after gastric surgery [20]. Most result from disturbance of the normal anatomic and physiologic mechanisms that control gastric motor function or from an alteration in the food stream.

Dumping Syndrome

Clinically significant dumping occurs in 5–10% of patients after pyloroplasty, pyloromyotomy, or distal gastrectomy. The symptoms are thought to be a result of the abrupt delivery of a hyperosmolar load into the small bowel. It is usually due to ablation of the pylorus, but decreased gastric compliance with accelerated emptying of liquids (e.g., after HSV) is another accepted mechanism.

"Early" dumping occurs about 15–30 minutes after a meal. The patient becomes diaphoretic, weak, lightheaded, and tachycardic. These symptoms may be ameliorated by recumbence or saline infusion. Diarrhea often follows. A variety of aberrations in GI hormones have been observed.

"Late" dumping usually occurs 2–3 hours after a meal. It represents a form of postprandial hypoglycemia associated with hyperinsulation and is relieved by administration of sugar.

Medical therapy for the dumping syndrome consists of dietary management and a somatostatin analog (octreotide). There is some evidence that adding dietary fiber at mealtime may alleviate the syndrome. It is the rare patient with dumping symptoms who requires an operation. Most patients improve with time (months and even years), dietary management, and medication.

The results of remedial operation for dumping are variable and unpredictable. There are a variety of surgical approaches, none of which works consistently well. There is not a great deal of experience reported in the literature with any of these methods, and long-term follow-up is rare. Operations to be considered for disabling dumping include pyloric reconstruction, takedown of the gastrojejunostomy, and Roux reconstruction [21]. Although the latter has been applied successfully to patients with disabling dumping following distal gastrectomy, it may also prove useful as a Roux-en-Y duodenojejunostomy (i.e., duodenal switch procedure) in the rare patient with disabling dumping following pyloroplasty (we are skeptical of pyloric reconstruction). Long-term acid suppression is advisable.

Diarrhea

Truncal vagotomy is associated with clinically significant diarrhea in 5–10% of patients. It occurs soon after operation and is usually not associated with other symptoms, a fact that helps distinguish it from dumping (see above). The diarrhea may be a daily occurrence, or it may be more sporadic and unpredictable. Possible mechanisms include intestinal dysmotility and accelerated transit, bile acid malabsorption, rapid gastric emptying, and bacterial overgrowth. Some patients with postvagotomy diarrhea respond to cholestyramine, and in others codeine or loperamide are useful.

In the rare patient who is debilitated by postvagotomy diarrhea that is unresponsive to medical management, one surgical option is a 10 cm reversed jejunal interposition placed in continuity 100 cm distal to the ligament of Treitz. Another option is the onlay antiperistaltic distal ileal graft. Both operations can cause obstructive symptoms or bacterial overgrowth (or both).

Gastric Stasis

Gastric stasis following operation on the stomach may be due to gastric motor dysfunction or mechanical obstruction. The gastric motility abnormality may have been preexistent and unrecognized by the operating surgeon. Alternatively, it may be secondary to deliberate or unintentional vagotomy or resection of the dominant gastric pacemaker. An obstruction may be mechanical (e.g., anastomotic stricture, efferent limb kink from adhesions or constricting mesocolon, or a proximal small bowel obstruction) or functional (e.g., retrograde peristalsis in a Roux limb). Gastric stasis presents with vomiting (often of undigested food), bloating, epigastric pain, and weight loss.

Evaluation of a patient with suspected postoperative gastric stasis includes esophagogastroduodenoscopy (EGD), upper gastrointestinal series, gastric emptying scan, and gastric motor testing. Once mechanical obstruction has been ruled out, medical treatment is successful in most cases of motor dysfunction that follows previous gastric surgery. It consists of dietary modification and promotility agents. Intermittent oral antibiotic therapy may be helpful for treating bacterial overgrowth with its attendant symptoms of bloating, flatulence, and diarrhea.

Gastroparesis following vagotomy and drainage may be treated with subtotal (75%) gastrectomy. Billroth II anastomosis with Braun enteroenterostomy may be preferable to Roux-en-Y reconstruction. This latter option may be associated with persistent emptying problems, which subsequently require near-total or total gastrectomy, a nutritionally unattractive option. Delayed gastric emptying following ulcer operation may represent an anastomotic stricture (often due to recurrent ulcer), or proximal small bowel obstruction. The latter should be dealt with at re-operation. Recurrent ulcer usually responds to medical therapy. Endoscopic dilation is occasionally helpful. Gastroparesis following subtotal gastric resection is best treated with near-total (95%) or total gastric resection and Roux-en-Y reconstruction. If total gastrectomy is performed, a jejunal reservoir should be fashioned. Gastric pacing is promising, but it has not achieved widespread clinical usefulness in the treatment of gastric atony.

Bile Reflux Gastritis

Following ablation or resection of the pylorus, most patients have bile in the stomach on endoscopic examination along with some degree of gross or microscopic gastric inflammation [22,23]. Attributing postoperative symptoms to bile reflux is therefore problematic, as most asymptomatic patients also have bile reflux. It is generally accepted that a small subset of patients have bile reflux gastritis; they present with nausea, bilious vomiting, epigastric pain, and quantitative evidence of excess enterogastric reflux. Curiously, symptoms often develop months or years after the initial operation. The differential diagnosis includes afferent or efferent loop obstruction, gastric stasis, and small bowel obstruction. Plain abdominal radiography, upper endoscopy, upper GI series, ab-

dominal CT scans, and gastric emptying scans are helpful for evaluating these possibilities. Bile reflux may be quantitated with gastric analysis or more commonly scintigraphy (bile reflux scan).

Remedial operation eliminates the bile from the vomitus and may improve the epigastric pain, but it is quite unusual to render these patients completely asymptomatic, especially if they are narcotic-dependent. Bile reflux gastritis after distal gastric resection may be treated by Roux-en-Y gastrojejunostomy, Henley loop, or Billroth II gastrojejunostomy with Braun enteroenterostomy. To eliminate bile reflux the Roux limb or Henley loop should be at least 45 cm long, and a Braun enteroenterostomy should be placed a similar distance from the stomach. Excessively long limbs may be associated with obstruction or malabsorption. All operations can result in marginal ulceration on the jejunal side of the gastrojejunostomy and thus are combined with a generous distal gastrectomy. If this has already been done at a previous operation, the Roux or Braun operations may be attractively simple. The benefits of decreased acid secretion following total gastric vagotomy may be outweighed by vagotomy-associated dysmotility in the gastric remnant, especially during the current era when excellent and safe acid suppression is available. The Roux operation may be associated with an increased risk of emptying problems compared to the other two options, but controlled data are lacking. Patients with debilitating bile reflux after gastrojejunostomy can be considered for simple takedown of this anastomosis.

Primary bile reflux gastritis (i.e., no previous operation) is rare and may be treated with duodenal switch operation, essentially an end-to-end Roux-en-Y to the proximal duodenum. The Achilles' heel of this operation is, not surprisingly, marginal ulceration. Thus it should be combined with parietal cell vagotomy and perhaps H_2 blockers.

Roux Syndrome

A subset of patients who have had distal gastrectomy and Roux-en-Y gastrojejunostomy have great difficulty with gastric emptying in the absence of mechanical obstruction. These patients present with vomiting, epigastric pain, and weight loss. This clinical scenario has been labeled the Roux syndrome. Endoscopy may show bezoar formation, dilation of the gastric remnant, or dilation of the Roux limb. An upper GI series confirms these findings and may show delayed gastric emptying. This is better quantitated by a gastric emptying scan, which always shows delayed solid emptying and may show delayed liquid emptying as well.

Gastrointestinal motility testing shows abnormal motility in the Roux limb, with propulsive activity toward rather than away from the stomach. Gastric motility may also be abnormal. Presumably the disordered motility in the Roux limb occurs in all patients with this operation. Why only a subset of patients develop the Roux syndrome is unclear. Perhaps those with disordered gastric motility are at most risk. The disorder seems to be more common in patients with a generous gastric treatment. Truncal vagotomy has also been implicated.

Medical treatment consists of promotility agents. Surgical treatment consists of paring down the gastric remnant. If gastric motility is severely disordered, a 95% gastrectomy should be done. The Roux limb should be resected if it is dilated and flaccid; doing so does not put the patient at risk for short bowel problems. Gastrointestinal continuity may be reestablished with another Roux, a Billroth II with Braun enteroenterostomy, or a Henley loop. Truncal vagotomy should probably not be done. Long-term acid suppression may be necessary.

Gallstones

Gallstone formation following gastric operation is generally thought to result from vagal denervation of the gallbladder with attendant gallbladder dysmotility. Stasis of gallbladder bile leads to sludge and stone formation. Other possible but incompletely investigated possibilities include postoperative ampullary dysfunction and changes in bile composition. It is unclear whether simply dividing the hepatic branches of the anterior vagal trunk (as is frequently done during antireflux and bariatric operations as well as subtotal gastric resection) increases gallstone formation. Although prophylactic cholecystectomy is not justified with most gastric surgery, it should be considered if the gallbladder appears abnormal, especially if subsequent cholecystectomy is likely to be difficult. Similarly, if preoperative evaluation reveals sludge or gallstones or if intraoperative evaluation reveals stones, cholecystectomy should be done if it appears straightforward and the gastric operation has gone well.

Metabolic Problems

Weight loss. Weight loss is common in patients who have undergone vagotomy or gastric resection (or both). The degree of weight loss tends to parallel the magnitude of the operation. It may be insignificant in the large person or devastating in the asthenic female patient. The surgeon should always reconsider before performing a gastric resection for benign disease in a thin girl or woman. The causes of weight loss after gastric surgery generally fall into one of two categories: altered dietary intake or malabsorption. If a stain for fecal fat is negative, it is likely that decreased caloric intake is the problem. This is the most common cause of weight loss after gastric surgery and may be due to small stomach syndrome, postoperative gastroparesis, or self-imposed dietary modification because of dumping or diarrhea. Specific problems may be treated as outlined above. Consultation with an experienced dietitian may prove invaluable.

Anemia. Iron absorption takes place primarily in the proximal gastrointestinal tract and is facilitated by an acidic environment. Intrinsic factor, essential for the enteric absorption of vitamin B_{12}, is produced by the parietal cells of the stomach. Vitamin B_{12} bioavailability is also facilitated by an acidic environment.

With this as background, it is easy to understand why patients who have had a gastric operation are at risk for anemia. Anemia is the most common metabolic side effect in patients who have undergone gastric bypass for morbid obesity. It also occurs in up to one-third of patients who have had a vagotomy or gastric resection (or both). Iron deficiency is the most common cause, but vitamin B_{12} or folate deficiency also occurs, even in patients who have not had total gastrectomy. Of course, patients who have had a total gastrectomy all develop vitamin B_{12} deficiency without parenteral vitamin B_{12}. Gastric bypass patients should be given oral iron supplements and be monitored for iron, vitamin B_{12}, and folate deficiency. Patients who have undergone vagotomy or gastrectomy should be similarly monitored with periodic determination of hematocrit, red blood cell indices, iron and transferrin levels, and vitamin B_{12} and folate levels. Marginal nutritional status should be corrected with oral or parenteral supplementation (or both).

Bone disease. Gastric surgery frequently disturbs calcium and vitamin D metabolism. Calcium absorption occurs primarily in the duodenum, which is bypassed with a gastrojejunostomy. Fat malabsorption may occur because of blind loop syndrome and bacterial overgrowth or because of inefficient mixing of food and digestive enzymes. This can significantly affect absorption of vitamin D, a fat-soluble vitamin. Abnormalities of calcium and vitamin D metabolism can contribute to metabolic bone disease in patients following gastric surgery. The problems usually manifest as pain or fractures years after the gastric operation. Musculoskeletal symptoms should prompt a study of bone density. Dietary supplementation of calcium and vitamin D may be useful for preventing these complications. Routine skeletal monitoring of patients at high risk (e.g., elderly men and women; postmenopausal women) may prove useful for identifying skeletal deterioration that with appropriate treatment can be arrested.

REFERENCES

1. Freston JW. Management of peptic ulcers: emerging issues. World J Surg 2000;24:250.

2. Hopkins RJ, Girardi LS, Turney EA. Relationship between Helicobacter pylori eradication and reduced duodenal and gastric ulcer recurrence: a review. Gastroenterology 1996;110:1244.

3. Johnson HD. Gastric ulcer: classification, blood group characteristics, secretion patterns, and pathogenesis. Ann Surg 1965;162:996.

4. Jamieson GG. Surgery for peptic ulcer disease in the era of H_2 receptor blockers. Dig Dis 1989;7:76.

5. Dempsey DT, Ritchie WP. Gastric ulcer. In: Ritchie WP (ed) Shackelford's Surgery of the Alimentary ract, vol II, 4th ed. Philadelphia, Saunders 1996.

6. Millat B, Fingerhut A, Borie F. Surgical treatment of complicated duodenal ulcers: controlled trials. World J Surg 2000;24:299.

7. Tung WSP, Strasberg SM. Peptic ulcer disease. In: Laparoscopic Surgery Principles and Practice, 1st ed. St. Louis, Quality, 1997.

8. Gauderer MWL, Ponsky JL, Izant RJ. Gastrostomy without laparotomy: a percutaneous endoscopic technique. J Pediatr Surg 1980;15:872.

9. Murayama KM, Schneider PD, Thompson JS. Laparoscopic gastrostomy: a safe method for obtaining enteral access. J Surg Res 1995;58:1.

10. Hartgrink HH, Bonenkramp HJ, van de Velde CJH. Influence of surgery on outcomes in gastric cancer. Surg Oncol Clin North Am 2000;9:97.

11. Bozzetti F, Marubini E, Bonafanti G, et al. Subtotal versus total gastrectomy for gastric cancer: five-year survival rates in a multicenter randomized Italian trial: Italian Gastrointestinal Tumor Study Group. Ann Surg 1999;230:170.

12. Harrison LE, Karpeh MS, Brennan MF. Proximal gastric cancers resected via a transabdominal only approach: results and comparisons to distal adenocarcinoma of the stomach. Ann Surg 1997;225:678.

13. Meyer HJ, Jahne J. Lymph node dissection for gastric cancer. Semin Surg Oncol 1999;17:117.

14. Cuschieri A, Fayers P, Fielding J, et al. Postoperative morbidity and mortality after D1 and D2 resections for gastric cancer: preliminary results of the MRC randomized controlled surgical trial. Lancet 1996;347:995.

15. Bonenkamp JJ, Hermans J, Sasako M, van de Velde CJH. Extended lymph node dissection for gastric cancer. N Engl J Med 1999;340:908.

16. Kitamura K, Nishida S, Ichikawa D, et al. No survival benefit from combined pancreaticosplenectomy and total gastrectomy for gastric cancer. Br J Surg 1999;86:119.

17. Kennedy T, Johnston GW, Love AHG, et al. Pyloroplasty versus gastrojejunostomy: results of a double-blind, randomized controlled trial. Br J Surg 1973;60:949.

18. Vogel SB, Drane WE, Woodward ER. Clinical and radionuclide evaluation of bile diversion by Braun enteroenterostomy: prevention and treatment of alkaline reflux gastritis: an alternative to Roux-en-Y diversion. Ann Surg 1994;219:458.

19. Aronow JS, Matthews JB, Garcia-Aguilar J, et al. Isoperistaltic jejunal interposition for intractable postgastrectomy alkaline reflux gastritis. J Am Coll Surg 1995;180:648.

20. Delcore R, Cheung LY. Surgical options in postgastrectomy syndromes. Surg Clin North Am 1991;71:57.

21. Miedema BW, Kelly KA. The Roux operation for postgastrectomy syndromes. Am J Surg 1991;161:256.

22. Malagelada JR, Phillips SF, Shorter RG, et al. Postoperative reflux gastritis: pathophysiology and long-term outcome after Roux-en-Y diversion. Ann Intern Med 1985;103:178.

23. Ritchie WP Jr. Alkaline reflux gastritis: an objective assessment of its diagnosis and treatment. Ann Surg 1980;192:288.

25 Truncal Vagotomy

SURGICAL LEGACY TECHNIQUE

INDICATIONS

Truncal vagotomy is rarely indicated as an adjunct to management of refractory duodenal ulcer disease or during performance of other procedures (see Chapter 24).

PREOPERATIVE PREPARATION

See Chapter 24.

PITFALLS AND DANGER POINTS

Esophageal trauma

Splenic trauma

Inadequate vagotomy

Disruption of esophageal hiatus with postoperative hiatal hernia; gastroesophageal reflux

OPERATIVE STRATEGY

Avoiding Esophageal Trauma

The best way to avoid trauma to the esophagus is by performing most of the esophageal dissection under *direct vision*. Forceful, blind finger dissection can be dangerous. After the peritoneum overlying the abdominal esophagus is incised **(Figs. 25–1, 25–2, 25–3)**, the crural musculature should be clearly exposed. The next vital step in this sequence is to develop a groove between the esophagus and the adjoining crux on each side. This should be done under direct vision using a peanut dissector **(Fig. 25–4)**. Only after the anterior two-thirds of the esophagus has been exposed is it permissible to insert an index finger and encircle the esophagus.

Avoiding Splenic Trauma

Splenic trauma can be prevented by avoiding any traction that draws the stomach toward the patient's right. Such traction may avulse the splenic capsule because of attachments between the omentum and the surface of the spleen. Consequently, all traction on the stomach should be applied on the lesser curvature side and directed toward the patient's feet. Avulsion of a portion of the splenic capsule, in the absence of gross disruption of the splenic pulp, does not require splenectomy. Application of topical hemostatic agents and pressure may control bleeding satisfactorily.

Preventing Incomplete Vagotomy

In most cases of recurrent marginal ulcer, it turns out that the posterior vagal trunk has not been divided. This trunk is generally the largest trunk encountered. The surgeon's failure to locate the pos-

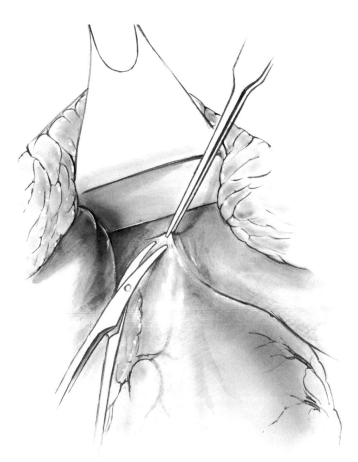

Fig. 25-1

234

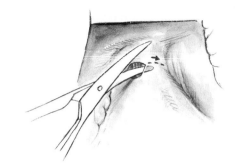

Fig. 25-2

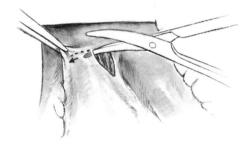

Fig. 25-3

terior vagus suggests inadequate knowledge of the anatomy of the posterior vagus. The right (posterior) vagal trunk is frequently 2 cm or more distant from the right lateral wall of the esophagus. It is often not delivered into the field by the usual maneuver of encircling the esophagus with the index finger. If the technique described below is carefully followed, this trunk is rarely overlooked.

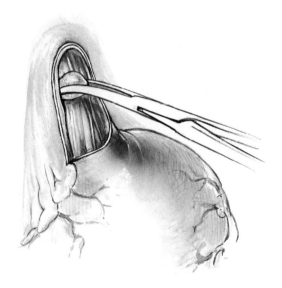

Fig. 25-4

To improve tissue recognition skills the surgeon should place each nerve specimen removed from the vicinity of the esophagus into a separate bottle for histologic examination. Each bottle should have a label indicating the anatomic area from which the nerve was removed. The pathology report that arrives several days after the operation can serve as a test of the surgeon's ability to identify nerves visually. The surgeon may be surprised to find that four or five specimens of nerve have been removed during a complete truncal vagotomy. Frozen section examination is helpful but not conclusive because it cannot prove that all the vagal nerve branches have been removed. The surgeon must gain sufficient skill at identifying nerve trunks to be certain no significant nerve fiber remains.

Hiatus Hernia

Significant hiatal hernia following vagotomy occurs in no more than 1–2% of cases. This percentage can probably be reduced if the surgeon repairs any large defects seen in the hiatus after the dissection has been completed.

OPERATIVE TECHNIQUE

Incision and Exposure

Make a midline incision from the xiphoid to a point about 5 cm below the umbilicus. The incision can be extended into the xiphocostal junction if necessary. Elevate the sternum 8–10 cm by means of an Upper Hand or Thompson retractor. Elevate the upper half of the operating table about 10°. Retract the left lobe of the liver in a cephalad direction utilizing Harrington or Weinberg retractors. In rare instances the triangular ligament must be incised and the left lobe of the liver retracted to the patient's right for exposure (see Chapter 15).

Using long DeBakey forceps and long Metzenbaum scissors incise the peritoneum overlying the abdominal esophagus (Figs. 25-1, 25-2, 25-3). Next identify the muscles of the right and left branches of the crux. Use a peanut dissector to develop a groove between the esophagus and the adjacent crux, exposing the anterior two-thirds of the esophagus (Fig. 25-4). At this point insert the right index finger gently behind the esophagus and encircle it.

Left (Anterior) Vagal Trunks

In our experience, whereas the posterior trunk often exists as a single structure in the abdomen, the anterior vagus divides into two *or more* trunks in more than 50% of cases. The main left trunk generally runs along the anterior wall of the lower esophagus, and the other branches may be closely applied to the longitudinal muscle of the anterior esophagus. The major nerve branches may be accentuated by caudal traction on the stomach, which makes the anterior nerves prominent against the esophagus. After applying hemostatic clips, remove segments from each of the anterior branches **(Fig. 25–5)**. Any suspicious fibers should be removed with forceps and sent to the pathology laboratory for analysis.

Identification of the Right (Posterior) Vagus

The posterior vagal trunk often is situated 2–3 cm lateral and posterior to the right wall of the esoph-

agus. Consequently, its identification requires that when the surgeon's right index finger encircles the lowermost esophagus, proceeding from the patient's left to right, the fingernail should pass over the anterior aorta. The finger should then go a considerable distance toward the patient's right before the finger is flexed. The fingernail then rolls against the *deep* aspect of the right branch of the crural muscle. When this maneuver is completed, the right trunk, a structure measuring 2–3 mm in diameter, is contained in the encircled finger to the right of the esophagus **(Fig. 25–6)**. Its identification may be confirmed in two ways. First, look for a major branch going toward the celiac ganglion. Second, insert a finger above the left gastric artery

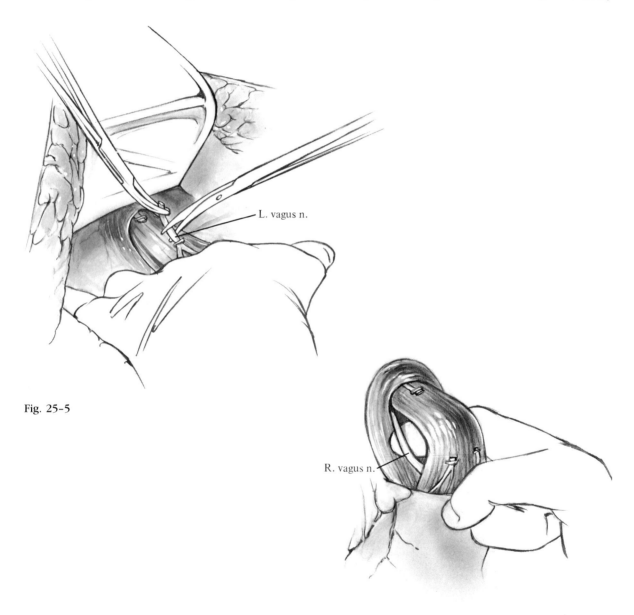

Fig. 25-5

L. vagus n.

R. vagus n.

Fig. 25-6

near the lesser curvature of the stomach and draw the left gastric vessel in a caudal direction. This applied traction to the posterior vagus, which then stands out as a stout cord. The right trunk rarely divides in the abdomen above the level of the esophagogastric junction.

Apply a long Mixter clamp to the nerve; place hemostatic clips above and below the clamp; and remove a 2- to 3-cm segment of nerve and submit it for histologic study. Rotate the esophagus and inspect the posterior wall. All the conclusion of this step the lower 5 cm of esophagus should be cleared of all nerve fibers. One should see only longitudinal muscle throughout its circumference **(Fig. 25–7)**.

Suture of Crural Musculature

If the hiatus admits two or more fingers alongside the esophagus, one or two sutures of 0 Tevdek should be placed to approximate the muscle bundles behind the esophagus, taking care to leave a gap of one fingerbreadth between the esophagus and the newly constructed hiatus. No attempt at fundoplication or any other antireflux procedure need be undertaken unless the patient had symptoms or other evidence of gastroesophageal reflux and esophagitis before the operation. Check hemostasis before going on to the gastric resection or drainage procedure.

POSTOPERATIVE CARE

See Chapter 27.

COMPLICATIONS

Operative perforation of the esophagus. This injury must be carefully repaired with two layers of interrupted sutures. If additional exposure is needed, do not hesitate to extend the abdominal incision into

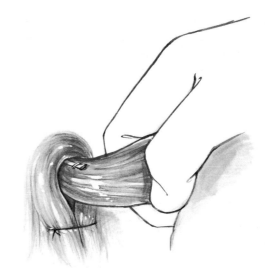

Fig. 25-7

the left sixth or seventh intercostal space. For additional security when repairing a low esophageal tear, cover the suture line with gastric wall by performing a Nissen fundoplication.

Postoperative gastric stasis. Because this complication is unpredictable and difficult to manage, a drainage procedure such as pyloroplasty or gastrojejunostomy is generally done with truncal vagotomy.

REFERENCES

Cuschieri A. Laparoscopic vagotomy. Gimmick or reality? Surg Clin North Am 1992;72:357.

McDermott EW, Murphy JJ. Laparoscopic truncal vagotomy without drainage. Br J Surg 1993;80:236.

Poon R, Chow L, Lim B, Gertsch P. Thoroscopic vagotomy for recurrent ulcer after previous gastric operation. Aust NZ J Surg 1997;67:177.

Roberts JP. Debas HT. A simplified technique for rapid truncal vagotomy. Surg Gynecol Obstet 1989;168:539.

26 Proximal Gastric Vagotomy

SURGICAL LEGACY TECHNIQUE

INDICATIONS

Peptic ulcer disease refractory to medical management

See Chapter 24

PREOPERATIVE PREPARATION

Esophagogastroduodenoscopy to confirm the diagnosis

PITFALLS AND DANGER POINTS

Hematoma of gastrohepatic ligament

Incomplete vagotomy

Damage to innervation of pyloric antrum

Injury to spleen

Necrosis or perforation of lesser curvature of stomach

OPERATIVE STRATEGY

Exposure

The visibility of the area around the lower esophagus is greatly enhanced if the Thompson or the Upper Hand retractor is attached so the blade underlying the lower border of the sternum elevates the sternum and draws it in a cephalad direction.

Prevention of Hematoma and Injury to Gastric Lesser Curve

Hematomas in the region of the gastrohepatic ligament along the lesser curve of the stomach increase the difficulty of identifying the terminal branches of the nerve of Latarjet. Furthermore, rough dissection and hematomas in this area may damage the deserosalized muscle along the lesser curve to such an extent that necrosis may occur. This rare complication is preventable if dissection is performed gently. Resuturing the peritoneum produces inversion of the deserosalized portion of the lesser curve and helps prevent perforation.

Preserving Innervation of the Antrum

The anterior and posterior nerves of Latarjet terminate in a configuration resembling the foot of a crow. This crow's-foot portion maintains innervation of the antrum and pylorus and ensures adequate emptying of the stomach.

Adequacy of Proximal Vagotomy

Hallenbeck et al. demonstrated that the incidence of recurrent postoperative ulcer dropped markedly when they extended the dissection so the lower esophagus was completely freed of any vagal innervation. This required meticulous removal of all nerve branches reaching the lower 5-7 cm of the esophagus and the proximal stomach. Grassi noted that one reason the proximal vagotomy technique fails is that surgeons sometimes overlook a branch leading from the posterior vagus nerve to the posterior wall of the upper stomach. He named it the "criminal nerve." If all the vagal nerve branches that enter the distal esophagus or proximal stomach are divided, interruption of the criminal nerve is included in the dissection.

Postoperative Gastroesophageal Reflux

Extensive dissection in the region of the esophagogastric junction may produce or exacerbate gastroesophageal reflux. Patients with preoperative gastroesophageal reflux should undergo an antireflux procedure at completion of the proximal gastric vagotomy. A posterior gastropexy (see Chapter 17) or a Nissen fundoplication (see Chapter 15) may be done. The choice of procedure depends on the experience of the surgeon and the operative findings.

OPERATIVE TECHNIQUE

Incision and Exposure

With the patient supine, elevate the head of the operating table 10°-15°. Make a midline incision from the xiphoid to a point 5 cm below the umbilicus. Insert an Upper Hand or Thompson retractor to elevate the lower sternum about 8-10 cm. Insert a self-retaining retractor of the Balfour type without excessive tension to separate the margins of the incision. Depending on the patient's body habitus, use a Weinberg or a Harrington retractor to elevate the left lobe of the liver above the esophageal hiatus. On rare occasions this exposure is not adequate, and the triangular ligament of the left lobe of the liver may have to be divided, with the left lobe retracted to the patient's right.

Identification of Right and Left Vagal Trunks

Expose the peritoneum overlying the abdominal esophagus and transect it transversely using long Metzenbaum scissors and DeBakey forceps. Extend the peritoneal incision to uncover the muscular fibers of the crura surrounding the esophageal hiatus (see Figs. 25-1 to 25-3). Separate the anterior two-thirds of the circumference of the esophagus from the adjacent right and left crux of the diaphragm using scissors and peanut-sponge dissection under direct vision (see Fig. 25-4). Then encircle the esophagus with the right index finger.

The right (posterior) vagus nerve is frequently 2 cm or more away from the esophagus. To avoid leaving the posterior vagus behind, pass the finger into the hiatus at the groove between the left branch of the crux and the left margin of the esophagus. Pass the fingernail along the anterior wall of the aorta and curve it anteriorly along the posterior aspect of the right side of the diaphragmatic crux, entering the operative field adjacent to the right crux. As a result of this maneuver, the index finger almost invariably contains both vagal trunks in addition to the esophagus. The right vagus generally is considerably larger than the left and is almost always a single trunk. The left (anterior) vagus can be identified generally at the right anterior surface of the *lower* esophagus. Separate each vagal trunk gently from the esophageal wall, pulling the vagal trunk toward the right and the esophagus to the left. Encircle each vagal trunk with a Silastic loop, brought out to the right of the esophagus.

Identification of Crow's Foot

Pass the left index and middle fingers through an avascular area of the gastrohepatic omentum and enter the lesser sac. This enables the nerves and blood vessels along the lesser curvature of the stomach to be elevated and put on stretch. The anterior nerve of Latarjet, which is the termination of the left vagus trunk as it innervates the anterior gastric wall, can be seen through the transparent peritoneum adjacent to the lesser curvature of the stomach. It intermingles with terminal branches of the left gastric artery, which also go to the lesser curvature. As the nerve of Latarjet reaches its termination, it divides into four or five branches in a configuration that resembles a crow's foot. These terminal branches innervate the distal 6-7 cm of the antrum and pylorus and should be preserved **(Figs. 26-1, 26-2a)**.

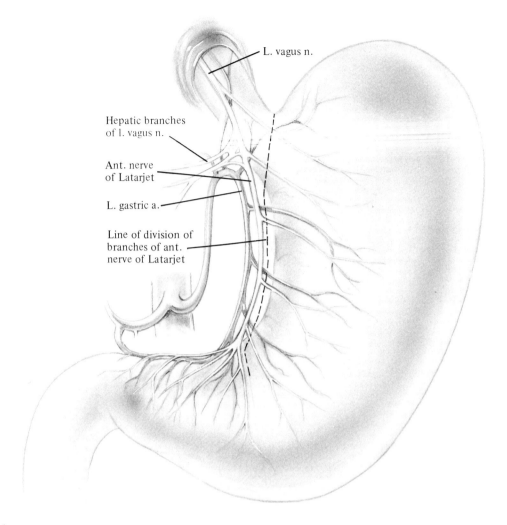

L. vagus n.

Hepatic branches
of l. vagus n.

Ant. nerve
of Latarjet

L. gastric a.

Line of division of
branches of ant.
nerve of Latarjet

Fig. 26-1

Dissection of the Anterior Nerve of Latarjet

After identifying the crow's foot, insert a Mixter right-angle clamp underneath the next cephalad branch of the nerve and the accompanying blood vessels **(Fig. 26–2b)**. This branch is 6–7 cm cephalad to the pyloric muscle. After the clamp has broken through the peritoneum on both sides of these structures, divide them between Adson hemostats and carefully ligate with 4-0 silk **(Fig. 26–2c)**. Alternatively, each branch may be double-ligated before being divided. Repeat the same maneuver many times, ascending the lesser curvature of the stomach and taking care not to include more than one branch in each hemostat. To preserve the innervation of the antrum, the hemostats must be applied close to the

gastric wall so as not to injure the main trunk of the nerve of Latarjet. Take great care not to tear any of these small blood vessels, as they tend to retract and form hematomas in the gastrohepatic ligament obscuring the field of dissection. This is a particular hazard in obese patients. Avoid trauma to the musculature of the gastric wall, as this area of the lesser curvature is not protected by a layer of serosa.

Continue dissection of the anterior layer of the gastrohepatic ligament until the main trunk of the left vagus nerve is reached. Retract this trunk toward the patient's right by means of the umbilical tape. At the conclusion of the dissection, the left vagus nerve should be completely separated from the wall of the esophagus for a distance of 6–7 cm above the esophagogastric junction. Any small nerve branching from the vagus nerve to this portion of the esophagus

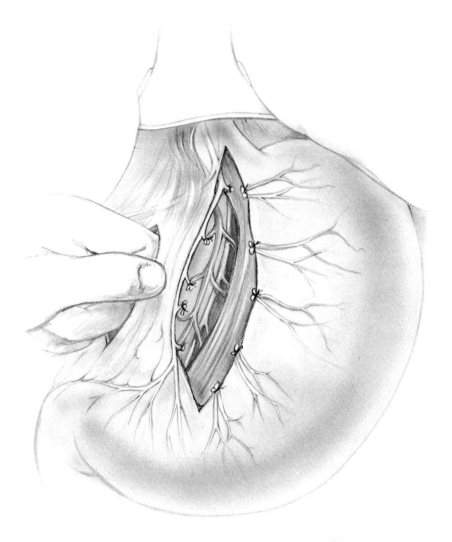

Fig. 26-2a

should be divided. In this fashion all the branches from the left vagus to the stomach are interrupted, with the exception of those innervating the distal antrum and pylorus. Preserve the hepatic branch of the vagus trunk also because it leaves the left vagus and goes to the patient's right on its way to the liver.

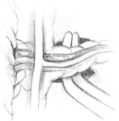

Fig. 26-2b

Dissection of Posterior Nerve of Latarjet

Delineate the posterior leaflet of the gastrohepatic omentum as it attaches to the posterior aspect of the lesser curvature of the stomach. Again, the crow's foot should be identified and preserved. Each branch of the left gastric artery and vein, together with each terminal branch of the *posterior* nerve of Latarjet, should be individually isolated, double-clamped,

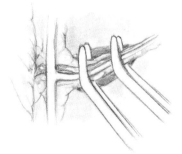

Fig. 26-2c

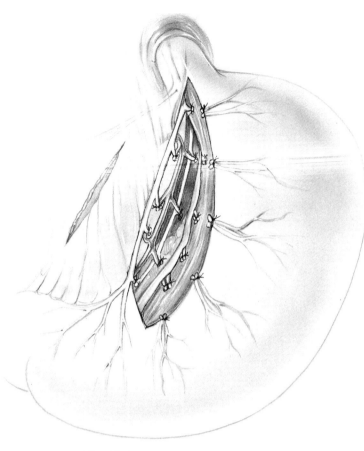

Fig. 26-3

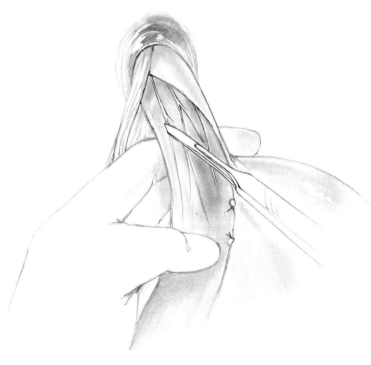

Fig. 26-4

divided, and ligated **(Fig. 26–3)**. Take care to make this division close to the gastric wall to preserve the main nerve of Latarjet. Continue this dissection in a cephalad direction until the previously identified right vagal trunk can be seen alongside the distal esophagus. When this dissection has been properly completed, it becomes evident that the right vagus nerve and the gastrohepatic ligament are situated far to the right of the completely bare lesser curvature. Now dissect away the posterior aspect of the esophagus from the posterior vagus nerve for a distance of 7 cm above the esophagogastric junction so no branches from this trunk can reach the stomach by way of the distal esophagus.

Pay special attention to the criminal nerve of Grassi, which is a branch of the posterior vagal trunk passing behind the esophagus to the posterior wall of the gastric cardia. If the surgeon's left hand can be passed between the freed vagal trunks and the distal esophagus as well as the gastric fundus, it helps ensure that the extent of the dissection has been adequate. In addition, carefully inspect the longitudinal muscle fibers of the distal esophagus. Any tiny fibers resembling nerve tissue should be divided or avulsed from the musculature throughout the circumference of the lower 7 cm of esophagus **(Fig. 26–4)**.

Repair of the Lesser Curvature

Use interrupted 4-0 silk Lembert sutures to approximate the peritoneum over the gastric musculature, thereby reperitonealizing the lesser curvature **(Fig. 26–5)**. Close the abdominal incision in the usual fashion, without drainage.

POSTOPERATIVE CARE

Continue nasogastric suction and intravenous fluids for 48 hours. At the end of this time the patient generally is able to be advanced to a normal diet. Usually the postoperative course is uneventful, and undesirable postoperative gastric sequelae, such as dumping, are distinctly uncommon.

COMPLICATIONS

Recurrent ulceration. Inadequate vagotomy results in recurrent ulceration.

Necrosis. Unique to proximal gastric vagotomy is necrosis of the lesser curvature. Although rare (0.3% of all proximal gastric vagotomy operations), it is often fatal. It probably results from trauma or hematoma of the gastric wall in an area that lacks serosa. Prevention requires accurate dissection as-

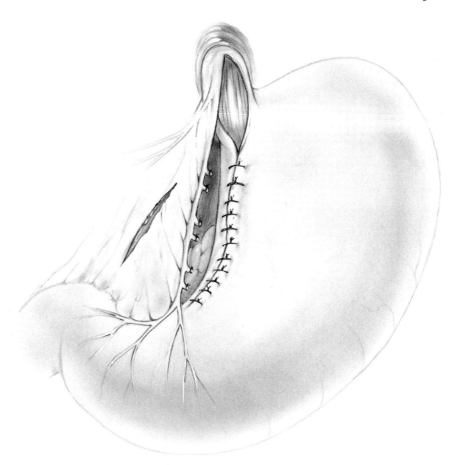

Fig. 26-5

sisted by reperitonealization of the lesser curvature by suturing (Fig. 26-5). Treatment requires early diagnosis and resection.

REFERENCES

Casas AT, Gadacz TR. Laparoscopic management of peptic ulcer disease. Surg Clin North Am 1996;76:515.

Dallemagne B, Weerts JM, Jehaes C, Markiewicz S, Lombard R. Laparoscopic highly selective vagotomy. Br J Surg 1994;81:554.

Donohue PE. Ulcer surgery and highly selective vagotomy—T2K. Arch Surg 1999;134:1373.

Grassi G. Special comment: Anatomy of the "criminal branch" of the vagus and its surgical implications. In: Nyhus LM, Wastell C (eds). Surgery of the Stomach and Duodenum. Boston, Little, Brown, 1977, 61.

Hallenbeck GA, Gleysteen JJ, Aldrete JS. Proximal gastric vagotomy: effects of two operative techniques on clinical and gastric secretory results. Ann Surg 1976;184:435.

Jordan PH Jr. Indications for parietal cell vagotomy without drainage in gastrointestinal surgery. Ann Surg 1989;210:29.

Jordan PH Jr, Thornby J. Parietal cell vagotomy performed with fundoplication for esophageal reflux. Am J Surg 1997;173:264.

Temple MB, McFarland J. Gastroesophageal reflux complicating highly selective vagotomy. Br J Surg 1975;2:168.

Valen B, Halvorsen JF. Reperitonealization of the lesser curve in proximal gastric vagotomy for duodenal ulcer. Surg Gynecol Obstet 1991;173:6.

Wilkinson JM, Hosie KB, Johnson AG. Long-term results of highly selective vagotomy: a prospective study with implications for future laparoscopic surgery. Br J Surg 1994;81:1469.

27 Pyloroplasty (Heineke-Mikulicz and Finney) Operation for Bleeding Duodenal Ulcer

SURGICAL LEGACY TECHNIQUE

INDICATIONS

Pyloroplasty is now primarily used in poor-risk patients undergoing emergency surgery for massive hemorrhage from duodenal ulcer. A vagotomy is generally added (see Chapters 25 and 26).

PREOPERATIVE PREPARATION

Nasogastric suction

Esophagogastroduodenoscopy (endoscopic control of hemorrhage is frequently possible, obviating the need for operation)

Perioperative antibiotics

PITFALLS AND DANGER POINTS

Suture line leak

Inadequate lumen

OPERATIVE STRATEGY

Control of Bleeding

The ulcer is exposed through a generous gastroduodenotomy. The incision begins on the distal antrum, crosses the pylorus, and continues several centimeters down onto the duodenum. The bleeding site must be positively identified. Do not hesitate to extend the incision proximally, or distally if necessary. The arterial anatomy of the stomach is shown in **Figure 27–1**. The most common situation

is a posterior duodenal ulcer eroding into the gastroduodenal artery. Occasionally, a gastric ulcer erodes into the left or right gastric artery, the gastroepiploic arcade, or (rarely) posteriorly into the splenic artery.

Choice of Pyloroplasty

Even if fibrosis and inflammation of the duodenum are present, as they may be with severe ulcer disease, in most cases a Heineke-Mikulicz pyloroplasty is feasible. When the duodenum appears too inflexible to allow performance of this procedure, the Finney pyloroplasty or gastrojejunostomy should be elected. The latter two operations, although slightly more complicated than the Heineke-Mikulicz, ensure production of an adequate lumen for gastric drainage. Because the gastroduodenal incision is optimally positioned slightly differently for the two types of pyloroplasty, it is well to decide which type is to be performed before the incision is made.

OPERATIVE TECHNIQUE

Kocher Maneuver

In most cases pyloroplasty requires a Kocher maneuver (see Figs. 11–14 to 11–16) to provide maneuverability of the tissues: Grasp the peritoneum lateral to the duodenum with forceps and make an incision in this peritoneal layer. Alternatively, in many patients the surgeon's index finger may be insinuated behind the common bile duct and portal vein, pointing toward the ampulla of Vater. The finger then slides toward the patient's right. Overlying the fingertip is

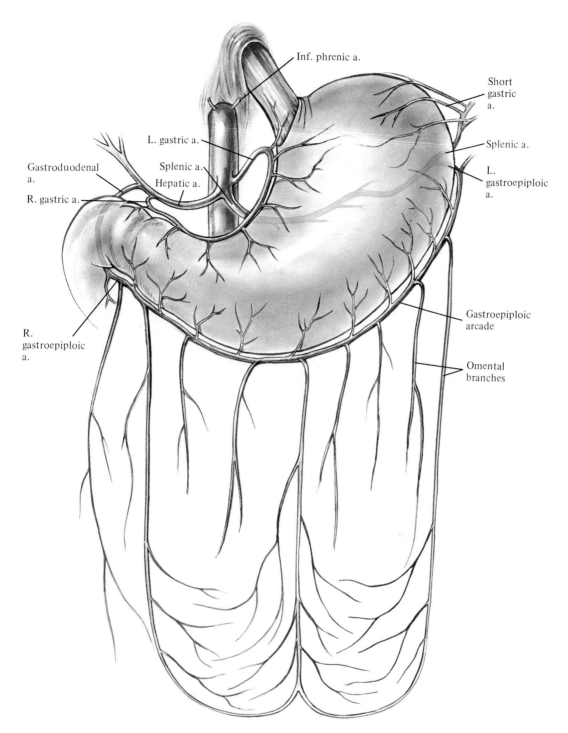

Inf. phrenic a.

Short gastric a.

L. gastric a.

Splenic a.

Gastroduodenal a.

Splenic a.

L. gastroepiploic a.

Hepatic a.

R. gastric a.

Gastroepiploic arcade

R. gastroepiploic a.

Omental branches

Fig. 27-1

not only a thin layer of peritoneum but also an avascular lateral duodenal ligament that attaches the duodenum to the underlying retroperitoneal structures.

Incise the peritoneal layer with scissors or electrocautery and then stretch the lateral duodenal ligament with the fingertip and divide it similarly.

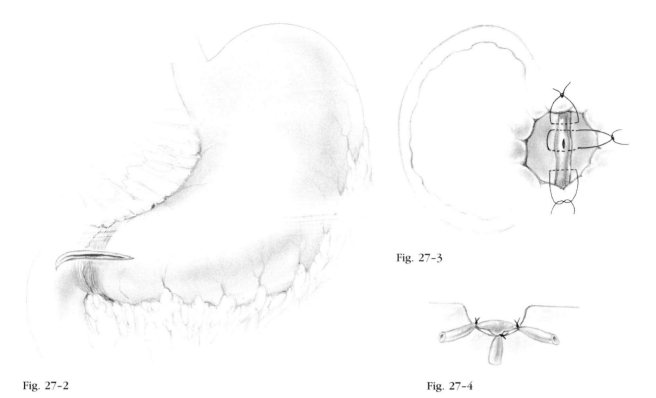

Fig. 27-3

Fig. 27-2   Fig. 27-4

Pyloroduodenal Incision for Heineke-Mikulicz Pyloroplasty

Make a 5 cm incision across the lower antrum, pyloric sphincter, and proximal duodenum, with the incision centered on the pyloric muscle **(Fig. 27–2)**. Apply Babcock clamps to the cephalad and caudad cut ends of the pyloric sphincter and draw them apart to open the incision. Transfix any bleeding points with 4-0 PG or PDS suture-ligatures or with careful electrocoagulation. Close the incision transversely, providing a patulous lumen for gastric drainage.

Emergency Procedure for Bleeding Ulcer

The longitudinal incision across the pylorus and into the proximal 3 cm of the duodenum described above generally provides good visualization of a posterior ulcer that is penetrating the gastroduodenal artery (Fig. 27-2). Do not hesitate to extend this incision proximally or distally as far as necessary to identify the bleeder.

The most common source of duodenal ulcer bleeding is posterior erosion into the gastroduodenal artery (Fig. 27-1). Transfix this artery with 2-0 silk sutures proximal and distal to the bleeding point. Place a third suture on the pancreatic side and deep to the bleeding point **(Figs. 27–3, 27–4)** to occlude a hidden posterior branch of the gastroduodenal

artery. This branch, generally the transverse pancreatic artery, may produce retrograde bleeding following apparently successful proximal and distal ligation of the gastroduodenal artery. Pluck the thrombus from the lumen of the ulcerated artery to determine if hemorrhage control is complete.

The incision in the stomach and duodenum is then closed as a pyloroplasty. If the incision is relatively short, as shown in Figure 27-2, a Heineke-Mikulicz closure is appropriate. A longer incision, or a fibrotic duodenum, may require closure by a Finney pyloroplasty. Both are described in the sections that follow. A Kocher maneuver (see Figs. 11-14 to 11-16) greatly facilitates closure.

Heineke-Mikulicz Pyloroplasty:

Sutures

Use one layer of sutures to prevent excessive tissue inversion. Most techniques call for a through-and-through suture. As the gastric wall is much thicker than the duodenal wall, it is difficult with this technique to prevent eversion of mucosa between the sutures. Consequently, we prefer deep "seromucosal" sutures (see Fig. 4-13) or interrupted Lembert sutures of 4-0 silk. Insert the first suture at the midpoint of the suture line **(Fig. 27–5)**. Proceed with the closure from one corner to the midpoint and then from the other corner to the midpoint, inverting just enough of the seromuscular coat to pre-

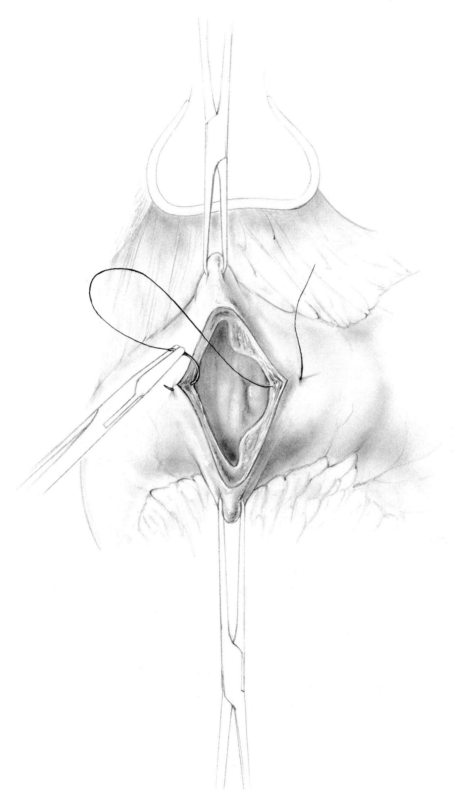

Fig. 27-5

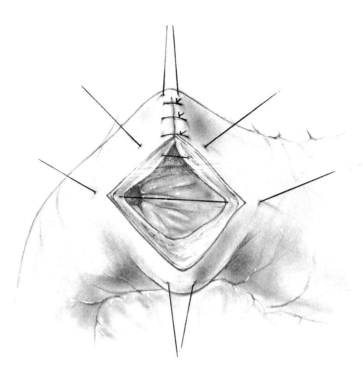

Fig. 27–6

vent outpouching of mucosa between the sutures **(Figs. 27–6, 27–7).**

Then suture omentum loosely over the pyloroplasty. This prevents leakage from the one-layer suture line and adhesions between the suture line and the undersurface of the liver, which may cause angulation and partial obstruction.

Stapling

Instead of suturing the pyloroplasty incision as described above, apply Allis clamps to the incision, approximating the tissues in eversion, mucosa to mucosa. Then apply a 55/4.8 mm linear stapling device to the everted tissues just deep to the line of Allis clamps **(Fig. 27–8)** and fire it. Excise redundant tissue with a scalpel, lightly electrocoagulate the everted mucosa, and remove the stapler. Carefully inspect the staple line to be sure satisfactory B formation has been carried out **(Fig. 27–9).** Control bleeding points by conservative electrocoagulation or 4-0 PG sutures. Place omentum over this stapled closure.

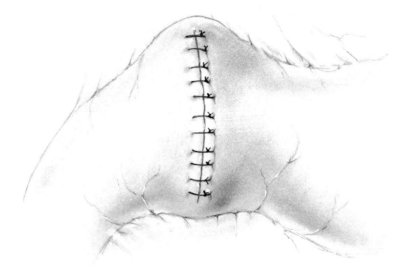

Fig. 27–7

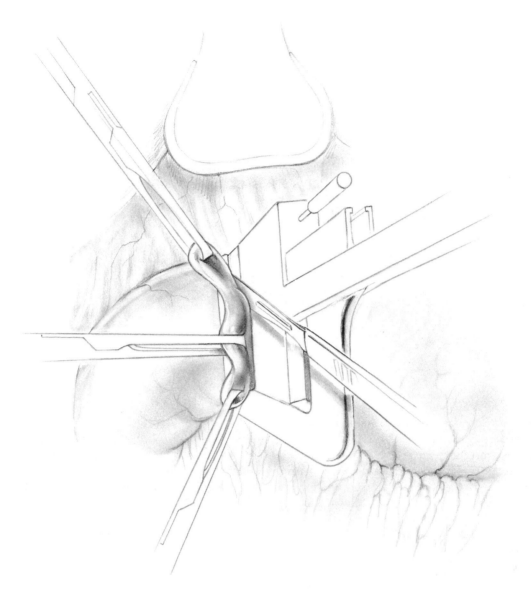

Fig. 27-8

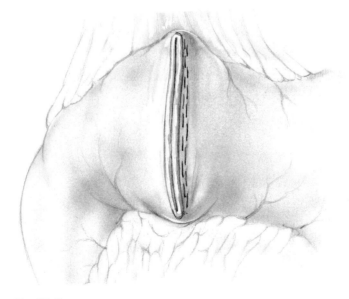

Fig. 27-9

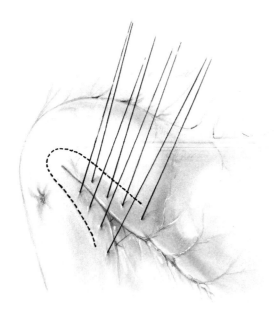

Fig. 27-10

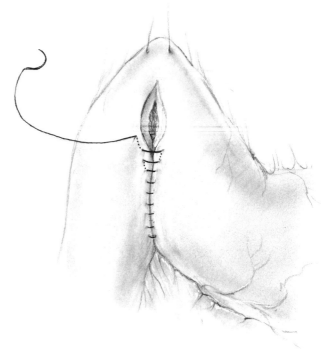

Fig. 27-12

Finney Pyloroplasty

Unlike the anterior midline gastroduodenotomy incision previously described, for the Finney pyloroplasty the gastroduodenal incision is kept close to the greater curvature side of the stomach and the pancreatic side of the proximal duodenum **(Fig. 27–10)** to avoid excessive tension on the anterior suture line. Ideally, the first row of sutures is placed before the incision is made.

Insert a layer of interrupted 4-0 silk Lembert sutures to approximate the greater curvature of the stomach to the superior portion of the proximal duodenum. Place these sutures fairly close to the greater curvature of the stomach and to the junction of the duodenum and pancreas. Continue this suture line for a distance of 5-6 cm from the pylorus (Fig. 27-10).

When the sutures have been tied, make an inverted U-shaped incision along a line 5-6 mm superficial to the suture line (Fig. 27-10). Carry this incision through

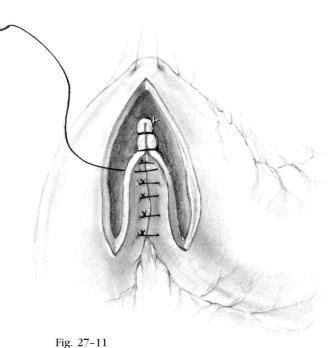

Fig. 27-11

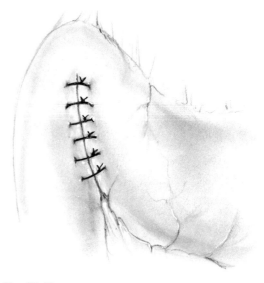

Fig. 27-13

the full thickness of the pyloric sphincter. After the incision has been made, the mucosal surface of both the gastric antrum and duodenum can easily be seen.

Begin the mucosal suture at the inferior surface of the divided pyloric sphincter. Pass a needle armed with 3-0 atraumatic PG through the full thickness of stomach and duodenum at the pyloric sphincter and tie it **(Fig. 27–11)**. Continue the suture in a caudal direction as a continuous locked stitch until the lowermost portion of the incision is reached. Then pass the needle from inside out on the stomach side. Approximate the anterior mucosal layer by means of a continuous Connell or Cushing suture **(Fig. 27–12)**, which should be terminated when the cephalad end of the incision is reached. Close the anterior seromuscular layer by means of interrupted 4-0 silk Lembert sutures **(Fig. 27–13)**. At the conclusion the lumen should admit two fingers.

POSTOPERATIVE CARE

Administer nasogastric suction for 1–3 days.

COMPLICATIONS

Complications following this operation are rare, although delayed gastric emptying occurs occasionally, as does suture-line leakage. Dumping symptoms may occur.

Reversal of Pyloroplasty or Gastrojejunostomy

About 1–2% of patients who have undergone truncal vagotomy and pyloroplasty or gastrojejunostomy develop severe symptoms of dumping, diarrhea, or bilious vomiting of such severity that surgical correction may be indicated. Reconstruction of the pylorus is required in rare circumstances. Martin and Kennedy described reconstruction of the pylorus in nine patients who underwent a Heineke-Mikulicz pyloroplasty and three with a Finney pyloroplasty. There was marked improvement in three-fourths of the patients whose complaints were dumping and diarrhea.

One can surgically reverse a pyloroplasty by reopening the transverse incision, identifying both cut ends of the pyloric sphincter, reapproximating the sphincter by interrupted sutures, and closing the incision in a longitudinal direction, thereby restoring normal anatomy.

REFERENCES

Berne CJ, Rosoff L. Peptic ulcer perforation of the gastroduodenal artery complex. Ann Surg 1969;169:141.

Branicki FJ, Coleman SY, Pritchett CJ, et al. Emergency surgical treatment for nonvariceal bleeding of the upper part of the gastrointestinal tract. Surg Gynecol Obstet 1991;172:113.

Martin CJ, Kennedy T. Reconstruction of the pylorus. World J Surg 1982;6:221.

Robles R, Parrilla P, Lujan JA, et al. Long-term follow-up of bilateral truncal vagotomy and pyloroplasty for perforated duodenal ulcer. Br J Surg 1995;82:665.

Wang BW, Mok KT, Chang HT, et al. APACHE II score: a useful tool for risk assessment and an aid to decision-making in emergency operation for bleeding gastric ulcer. J Am Coll Surg 1998;187:287.

28 Gastrojejunostomy

INDICATIONS

Gastrojejunostomy is performed for duodenal or gastric outlet obstruction when other procedures are not possible.

PREOPERATIVE PREPARATION

See Chapter 24.

PITFALLS AND DANGER POINTS

Postoperative gastric bleeding

Anastomotic obstruction

OPERATIVE STRATEGY

Traditionally, gastrojejunal anastomoses have been placed on the posterior wall of the antrum to improve drainage. However, posterior drainage is dependent drainage only when the patient is lying in bed flat on his or her back, and it is questionable whether the average patient spends enough hours in this position to warrant the additional difficulty of placing the gastrojejunostomy in a posterior location. We prefer to perform an anterior gastrojejunostomy along the greater curvature of the antrum, situated no more than 5–7 cm from the pylorus.

OPERATIVE TECHNIQUE

Incision

Make a midline incision from the xiphoid to the umbilicus.

Freeing the Greater Curvature

Beginning at a point about 5 cm proximal to the pylorus, double-clamp, divide, and individually ligate the branches of the gastroepiploic vessels on the greater curvature of the stomach, separating the greater omentum from the greater curvature of the stomach for a distance of 6–8 cm.

Gastrojejunal Anastomosis: Suture Technique

Identify the ligament of Treitz and pass the jejunum in an antecolic fashion, so that the bowel runs from the patient's left to right. Make a 5 cm longitudinal scratch mark with the back of a scalpel blade on the antimesenteric border of the jejunum, beginning at a point no more than 12–15 cm from the ligament of Treitz. This point marks the eventual incision into the jejunum for the anastomosis.

Because of the large size of the anastomosis, a continuous suture technique is satisfactory. After freeing a 6 cm segment of the greater curvature from the omentum, initiate (close to the greater curve) a continuous Lembert suture of atraumatic 3-0 PG on the left side of the anastomosis and approximate the seromuscular coats of the stomach and jejunum for a distance of about 5 cm (**Fig. 28–1**). Lock the last posterior Lembert suture. Then make incisions, 5 cm long, on the antimesenteric border of the jejunum and along the greater curvature of the stomach. Begin approximating the posterior mucosal layer at the midpoint of the incision using a double-armed suture of 3-0 PG. Insert and tie the first suture. Continue the suture toward the patient's left as a continuous locked suture, penetrating both mucosal and seromuscular coats. Terminate it at the left lateral margin of the incision. At this time, with the second needle initiate a similar type stitch from the midpoint to the right lateral margin of the incision (**Fig. 28–2a**). Approximate the anterior mucosal layer by means of a continuous Connell or continuous Cushing-type stitch. The two sutures should meet anteriorly

252

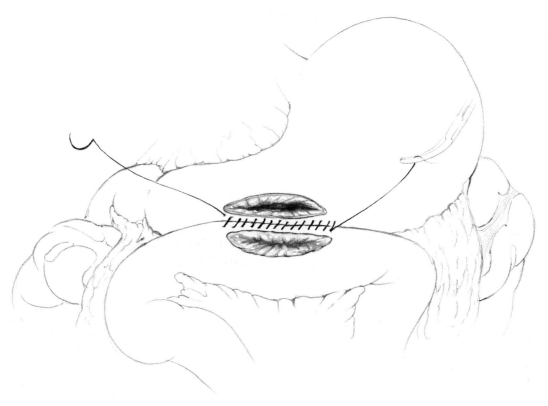

Fig. 28-1

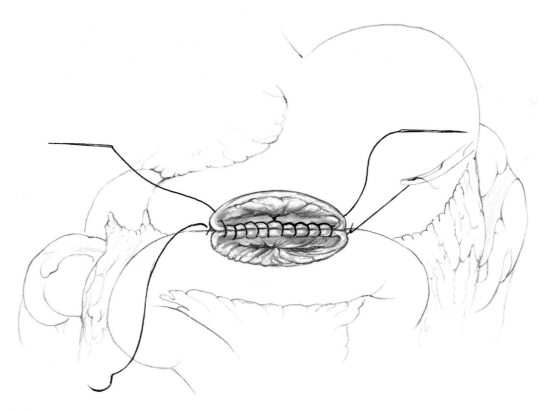

Fig. 28-2a

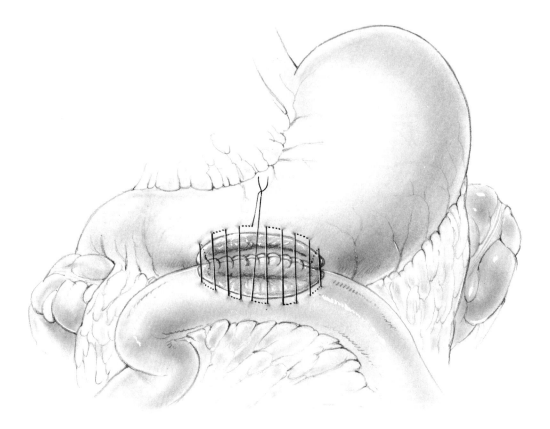

Fig. 28–2b

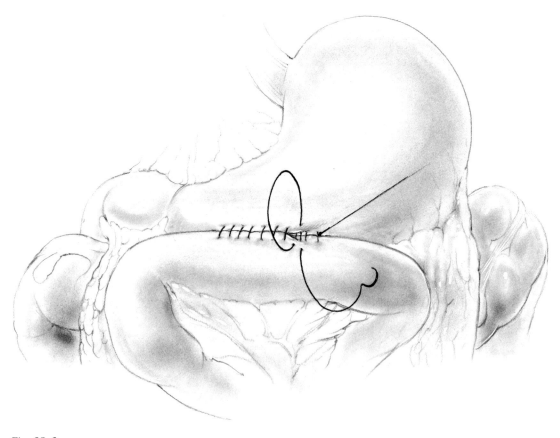

Fig. 28–3

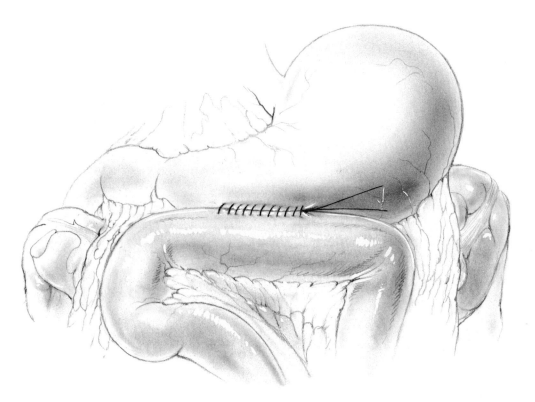

Fig. 28-4

near the midline and be tied to each other **(Fig. 28–2b)**.

Close the anterior seromuscular layer with the same curved needle utilized for the posterior layer. It should progress as a continuous Lembert suture **(Fig. 28–3)** from the right lateral margin of the anastomosis toward the left lateral margin. Terminate the suture by tying it to itself **(Fig. 28–4)**. The anastomosis should admit two fingers.

Stapling Technique

Identify the proximal jejunum and bring it to an antecolonic position as described above. With

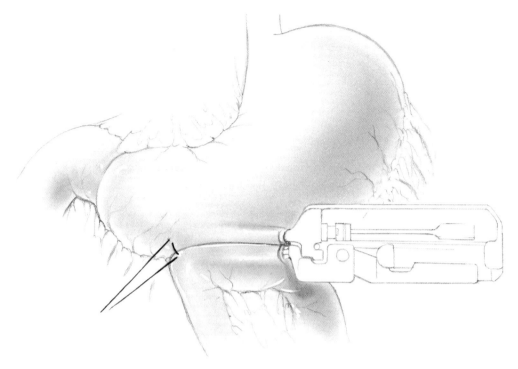

Fig. 28-5

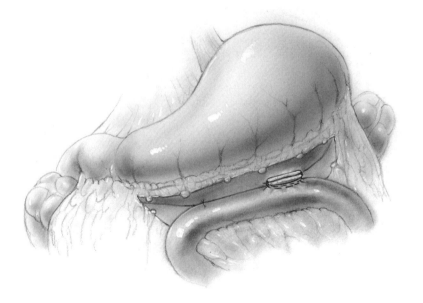

Fig. 28-6

electrocautery make a stab wound on the antime-senteric side of jejunum at a point 12-15 cm from the ligament of Treitz. Make a second stab wound along the greater curvature of the stomach at a point about 10 cm from the pylorus. Insert one fork of the cutting linear stapling device into the jejunum and one fork into the stomach **(Fig. 28–5)**. Align the je-junum so its antimesenteric border is parallel to the fork of the stapler and lock the device. Check the proposed gastrojejunal staple line to ensure that the forks of the stapler include no tissue other than stomach and jejunum. Fire the stapler and remove it.

Apply Allis clamps to the anterior and posterior terminations of the staple line. Inspect the staple line carefully for bleeding and control any bleeding point by cautious electrocoagulation or insertion of 4-0 PG atraumatic suture-ligatures.

Closure of Stab Wound

Approximate the remaining defect in the anastomosis in an everting fashion by applying several Allis clamps. Apply a 55 mm linear stapler deep to the Allis clamps. If the gastric wall is of average thickness use 3.5 mm staples; otherwise a larger size is necessary. Fire the stapler and excise the redundant tissue with Mayo scissors. Lightly electrocoagulate the everted mucosa and remove the stapling device. The lumen should admit two fingers without difficulty. Place a 4-0 seromuscular Lembert suture to fix the stomach to the jejunum on the right lateral margin of the newly stapled anastomosis **(Fig. 28–6)**.

POSTOPERATIVE CARE

Administer nasogastric suction for 1–3 days.

COMPLICATIONS

Gastric bleeding is a rare complication, occurring in 1–2% of cases. *Anastomotic leakage and obstruction* are even less common than gastric bleeding. At times an apparently satisfactory gastrojejunostomy is anatomically patent but *fails to empty* well.

REFERENCES

Csendes A, Maluenda F, Braghetto I, et al. Prospective randomized study comparing three surgical techniques for the treatment of gastric outlet obstruction secondary to duodenal ulcer. Am J Surg 1993;166:45.

Salky B. Laparoscopic gastric drainage procedures. Semin Laparosc Surg 1999;6:224.

Soetikno RM, Carr-Locke DL. Expandable metal stents for gastric-outlet, duodenal, and small intestinal obstruction. Gastrointest Endosc Clin North Am 1999;9:447.

29 Gastrectomy (Antrectomy) for Peptic Ulcer

SURGICAL LEGACY TECHNIQUE

INDICATIONS

See Chapter 24.

PREOPERATIVE PREPARATION

See Chapter 24.

PITFALLS AND DANGER POINTS

Inadequate duodenal stump closure

Trauma to pancreas resulting in postoperative acute pancreatitis

Incomplete removal of distal antrum

Splenic trauma

Injury to common bile duct or ampulla of Vater during ulcer dissection

Inadequate lumen in gastroduodenal anastomosis (Billroth I) with postoperative obstruction

Inadvertent gastroileostomy (Billroth II)

Excessive length of afferent limb (Billroth II)

OPERATIVE STRATEGY

Choice of Billroth I or Billroth II Reconstruction

Although each reconstruction has its proponents, it has been difficult to demonstrate convincing evidence of the superiority of one method over the other. Successful completion of a Billroth I recon-

struction requires pliable duodenum that can be brought to the gastric remnant without tension. The Billroth II reconstruction avoids tension by creating a duodenal stump and an end-to-side gastrojejunostomy.

Billroth II: Duodenal Stump

Most of the serious postoperative complications of gastric surgery involve failure of the duodenal stump closure. This leads to disruption and duodenal fistula or trauma to the pancreas, which results in acute pancreatitis. Because these complications result from persistent efforts to dissect the duodenum away from the pancreas when there is advanced fibrosis surrounding a penetrating duodenal ulcer, the simplest means to prevent trouble is for the surgeon to become aware early in the operation that the duodenal dissection is fraught with danger. It is not necessary to excise the ulcer if there is pliable duodenum proximal to the ulcerated area.

When a difficult duodenum is identified early during the operation, perform either vagotomy with a drainage procedure or proximal gastric vagotomy instead of attempting resection. If as a result of poor judgment the surgeon gets into difficulty after having broken into a posterior penetrating duodenal ulcer, the Nissen technique, the Cooper modification of it, or catheter duodenostomy may prove lifesaving. A successful Nissen maneuver requires that the anterolateral wall of the duodenum be pliable and of fairly normal thickness. If this wall is shrunken and contracted with fibrosis or is acutely inflamed, it may not be suitable for inversion into the pancreas by the Nissen-Cooper method.

Catheter Duodenostomy

If there is any doubt about the security of the duodenal stump suture line, insert a catheter into the duodenum for postoperative decompression. It provides a valuable safety valve and prevents disruption of the duodenal suture line in most instances.

Marginal Ulcer Following Billroth II

Among the causes of postoperative marginal ulcer is erroneous transection of the antrum proximal to the pylorus, leaving antral mucosa in contact with the alkaline bilious secretions. Although an error of this type is not committed in the presence of normal anatomy, this mistake is indeed possible when the area is obscured by inflammation and fibrosis. When the landmarks of the pyloric sphincter are obscured, use frozen section biopsy to confirm the absence of antral mucosa and the presence of Brunner's glands at the cut end of the duodenal stump.

Splenic Trauma

Traction on the greater curvature of the stomach is the most common cause of splenic injury, which results in avulsion of a portion of the splenic capsule adherent to the greater omentum. If downward traction on the stomach is needed, apply it to the lesser curvature. These minor capsular avulsion injuries can generally be managed by direct pressure over a sheet of topical hemostatic agent.

Ligating the Bleeding Point in Duodenal Ulcers

The most common source of bleeding in patients who undergo emergency surgery for massive hemorrhage is a posterior duodenal ulcer eroding into the gastroduodenal artery (see Fig. 27–1). See Chapter 27 for details on proper management of this problem.

Avoiding Postoperative Wound Infection

Patients who undergo gastric resection for an ulcer in the presence of chronic obstruction or massive hemorrhage are more prone to develop postoperative wound infection than are patients who undergo elective surgery for a duodenal ulcer. Perioperative antibiotics help decrease the incidence of this complication.

OPERATIVE TECHNIQUES: BILLROTH I AND II

Incision

The incision should be midline, from the xiphoid to a point 5 cm below the umbilicus. Use an Upper Hand or Thompson retractor to elevate the lower margin of the sternum and a Harrington retractor to elevate the lower surface of the liver. Perform a vagotomy when indicated (see Chapter 25).

Evaluation of Duodenal Pathology

It is not easy to evaluate the potential difficulty of dissecting the posterior wall of the duodenum off the pancreas by simple inspection. Just how difficult the procedure may be is not known until the posterior dissection is initiated. Pay attention to the quality and flexibility of the anterior wall of the duodenum. If the wall is soft and maneuverable, it can be useful should a Nissen-type stump closure become necessary. A markedly fibrotic, rigid, or edematous anterior wall indicates that closing the stump will be difficult. Marked edema or scarring in the region of the pylorus, pancreas, and hepatoduodenal ligaments is a relative contraindication to gastrectomy.

When the surgeon is uncertain of the nature of the pathology, a short incision may be made in the proximal duodenum to visualize ulcer pathology. This enables the surgeon to make a more accurate estimate of the technical expertise required to perform the resection. When in doubt, it is better to perform a vagotomy and drainage procedure or a proximal gastric vagotomy than a heroic duodenal dissection, as fatal duodenal leakage or acute pancreatitis may follow the dissection.

Dissection of Greater Curvature

Incise the avascular portion of the gastrohepatic ligament to the right of the lesser curvature and pass the left hand behind the lesser curvature and antrum of the stomach, emerging deep to the gastroepiploic arcade along the greater curvature of the stomach

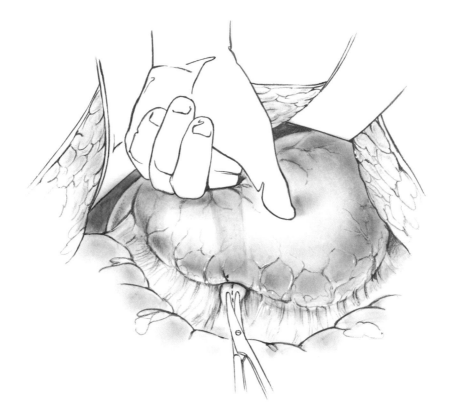

Fig. 29-1

(Fig. 29–1). This maneuver elevates the greater omentum from the underlying mesocolon, which contains the middle colic artery. Isolate the branches going from the gastroepiploic arcade to the greater curvature of the stomach, then double-clamp and divide each. Continue this process up along the greater curve of the stomach until the halfway point be-

tween the pylorus and the diaphragm is reached **(Fig. 29–2)**.

Next dissect the distal segment of the gastroepiploic arcade from the antrum. Perform the distal 4 cm of this dissection with care, as a number of fragile veins in the vicinity of the origin of the right gastroepiploic vessels are easily torn. As this dissection progresses, divide the congenital avascular attachments between the back wall of the antrum and the pancreas. Completion of this dissection frees the entire distal half of the gastric greater curvature.

Division of Left Gastric Vessels

Select a point on the lesser curvature about halfway between the esophagogastric junction and the pylorus. This point serves as a reasonably good approximation of the upper margin of the antral mucosa. Insert a large hemostat between the lesser curvature and the adjacent vascular bundle, which are divided between additional hemostats. Place two ligatures, consisting of 0 silk or a double strand of 2-0 silk, on the proximal side and another on the specimen side **(Fig. 29–3a, 29–3b)**. Preferably there is at least a 1 cm stump of left gastric artery beyond these ties. Inspect the pedicle carefully for hemostasis, as occasionally the bulky ligature permits a

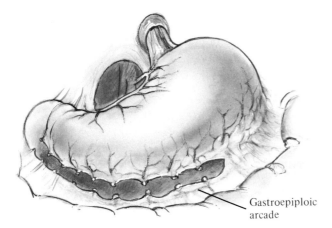

Gastroepiploic arcade

Fig. 29-2

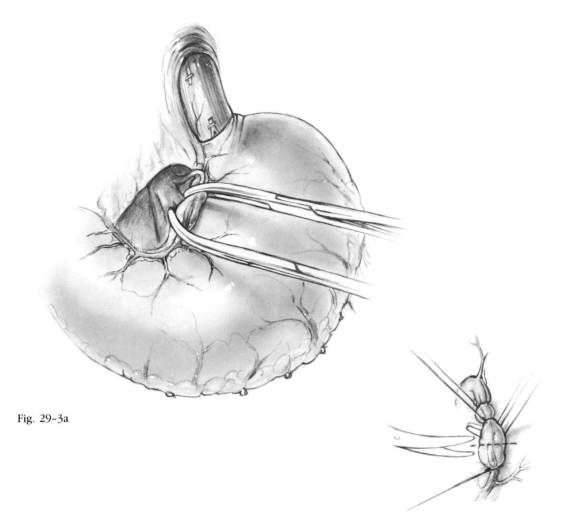

Fig. 29-3a

Fig. 29-3b

trickle of blood to continue through the lumen of the artery. Several additional small venous branches to the lesser curvature may require individual ties, as they are easily torn during insertion of these mass ligatures.

Division of Stomach

If vagotomy is adequate, no more than 50% of the stomach need be removed **(Fig. 29–4)**. This is accomplished by applying Allen clamps for a distance of 3–4 cm at an angle of 90° to the greater curvature of the stomach. The amount of stomach in the Allen clamp should equal the width of the gastrojejunal or gastroduodenal anastomosis to be performed in a subsequent step.

After the gastric wall has been incised midway between these two clamps, apply a 90/4.8 mm linear stapler at a somewhat cephalad angle to close the lesser curvature portion of the residual gastric pouch

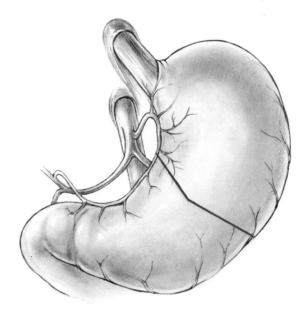

Fig. 29-4

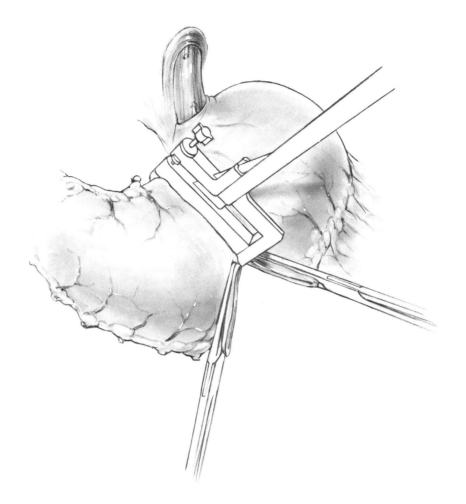

Fig. 29-5

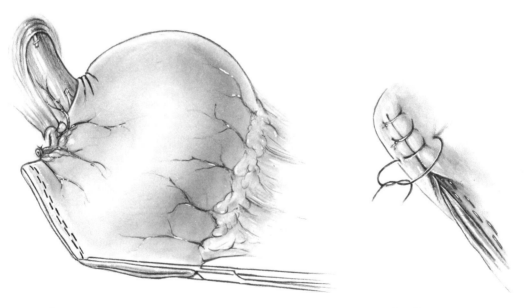

Fig. 29-6a

Fig. 29-6b

(**Fig. 29–5**). Fire the stapler. Place another Allen clamp opposite the stapler and divide the gastric tissue flush with the stapler. Lightly electrocauterize the gastric mucosa before removing the stapling device (**Fig. 29–6a**). Invert the stapled portion of the gastric pouch using a layer of interrupted 4-0 silk Lembert sutures (**Fig. 29–6b**). Apply a gauze pad over the exposed mucosa on the specimen side and fix it in place with umbilical-tape ligatures, leaving the Allen clamps in position.

When a stapling device is not used, the lesser curvature should be divided between Allen clamps (**Fig. 29–7**) and then closed in several layers. For the first layer use 3-0 PG on a straight intestinal needle. Initiate this suture on the lesser curvature of the gastric pouch just underneath the Allen clamp. Then pass the

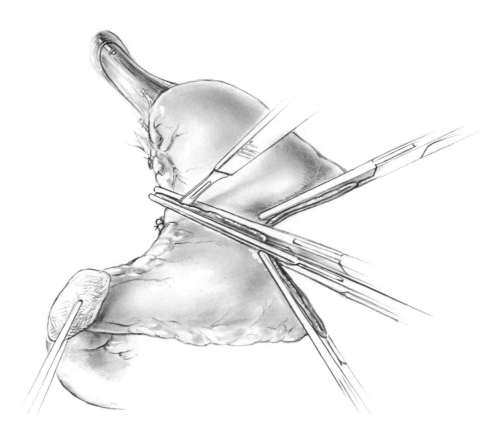

Fig. 29-7

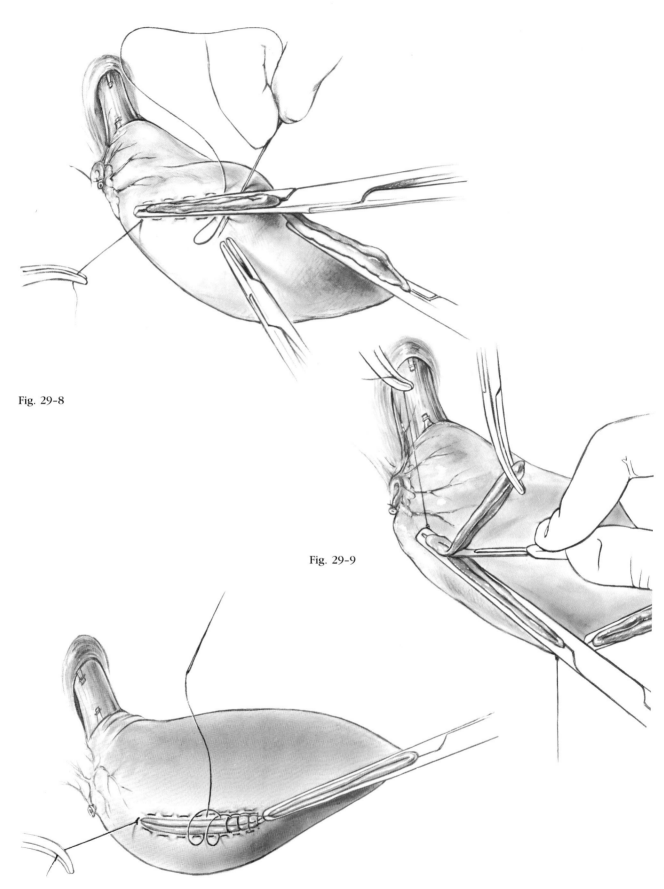

Fig. 29-8

Fig. 29-9

Fig. 29-10

straight needle back and forth underneath the Allen clamp to make a basting stitch, terminating it at the base of the Allen clamp **(Fig. 29–8)**. After trimming excess gastric tissue **(Fig. 29–9)** remove the Allen clamp, return the same suture to its point of origin as a continuous locked suture **(Fig. 29–10)**, and tie it to its point of origin. This completes hemostasis of this suture line. Then invert the mucosa using one layer of interrupted 4-0 silk Lembert sutures **(Fig. 29–11)**.

Duodenal Dissection in the Absence of Advanced Pathology

Identify, ligate, and divide the right gastric artery **(Fig. 29–12)**. Apply traction to the specimen in an anterior direction to expose the posterior wall of the duodenum and the anterior surface of the pancreas. Five or six small blood vessels can usually be identified proceeding from the pancreas to the back wall of the duodenum. Divide each between Crile hemostats and ligate each with 3-0 or 4-0 silk. If there has been some scarring in this area, the stump of a small artery may retract into the substance of the pancreas. In this case,

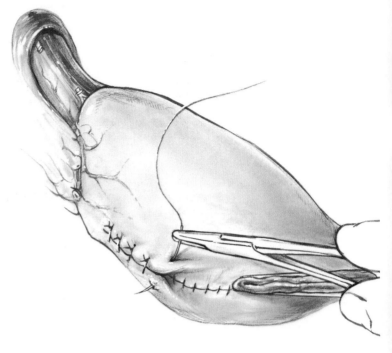

Fig. 29-11

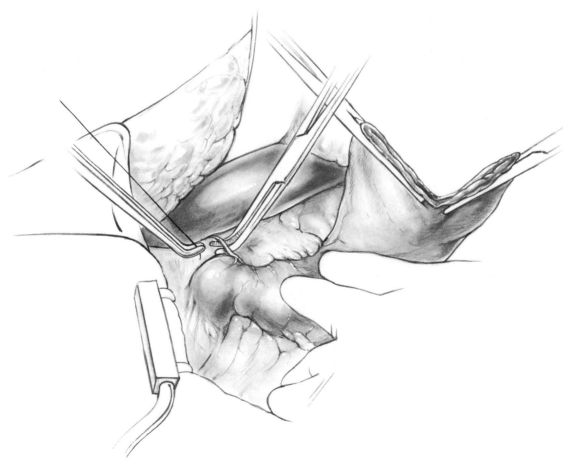

Fig. 29-12

control the bleeding with a mattress suture of 4-0 silk. No more than 1.5 cm of the posterior duodenal wall should be freed from the underlying pancreas, as this amount is adequate for turning in the duodenal stump or for gastroduodenal end-to-end anastomosis. Keep the dissection in a plane close to the posterior wall of the duodenum.

Division of Duodenum

Apply an Allen clamp immediately distal to the pylorus and transect the duodenum flush with the clamp, which should be left on the specimen **(Fig. 29–13)**. Before discarding the specimen, remove the clamp and inspect the distal end of the specimen to ascertain that a rim of duodenal mucosa has been removed. This ensures that there is no remaining antral mucosa left behind in the duodenal stump. If there is still a question, the presence or absence of the antrum should be confirmed by frozen section examination of the distal end of the specimen.

Insert an index finger into the duodenal stump to check the location of the ampulla of Vater. The ampulla is situated on the posteromedial aspect of the descending duodenum at a point approximately 7 cm behind the pylorus. Occasionally the orifice of the duct of Santorini can be palpated along the back wall of the duodenum. If the duodenal dissection has not continued beyond the gastroduodenal artery, there need be no concern about damage to the duct of Santorini or the main pancreatic duct. When the dissection continues beyond this point, special attention must be paid to these structures. If the duct of Santorini is divided, close the open duct with a

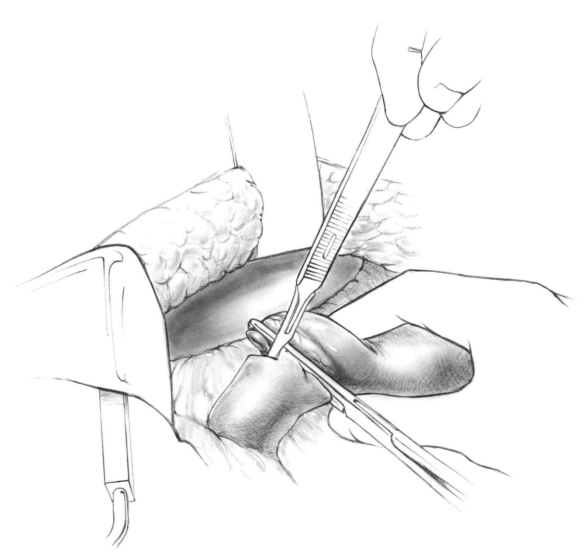

Fig. 29–13

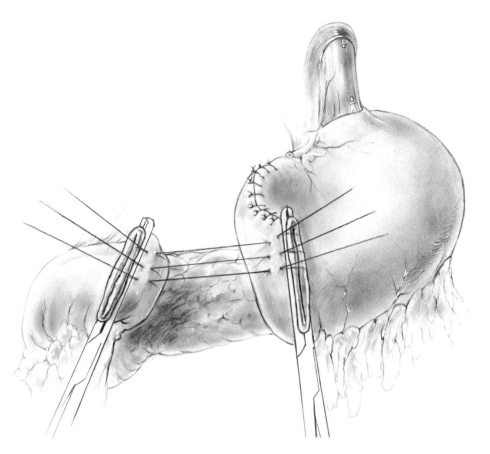

Fig. 29-14

fine nonabsorbable suture-ligature. If the ampulla
has been divided inadvertently and is separated from
the duodenum, replant it into the duodenal stump
or into a Roux-en-Y segment of the jejunum.

Billroth I Gastroduodenal Anastomosis

When at least 1 cm of healthy posterior duodenal
wall is available, a routine gastroduodenal anastomosis is constructed. The Allen clamp previously applied to the unsutured portion of the gastric pouch
should contain a width of stomach approximately
equal to the diameter of the duodenal stump. Insert
the corner sutures by the Cushing technique. Complete the remainder of the posterior layer with interrupted 4-0 silk seromuscular Lembert sutures
(Fig. 29–14). To prevent postoperative obstruction,
take care not to invert an excessive amount of tissue.

Remove the Allen clamp and approximate the mucosal layer using a double-armed 4-0 PG suture, initiating it at the midpoint of the posterior layer where
the knot is tied **(Fig. 29–15)**. Take small bites as a

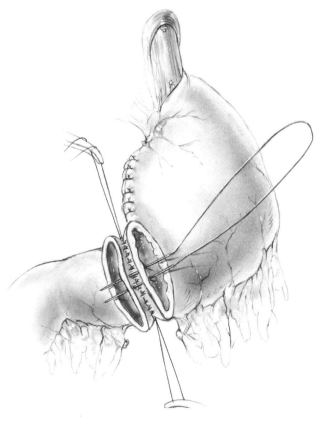

Fig. 29-15

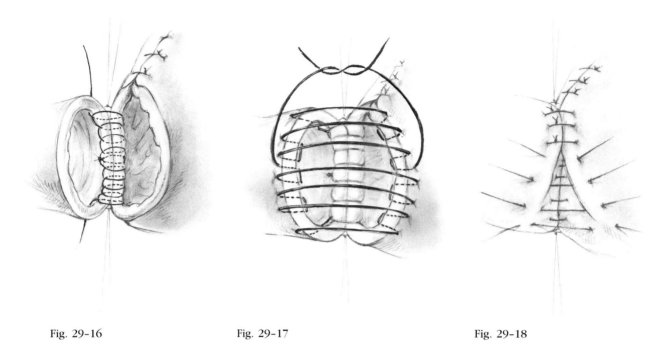

Fig. 29-16   Fig. 29-17   Fig. 29-18

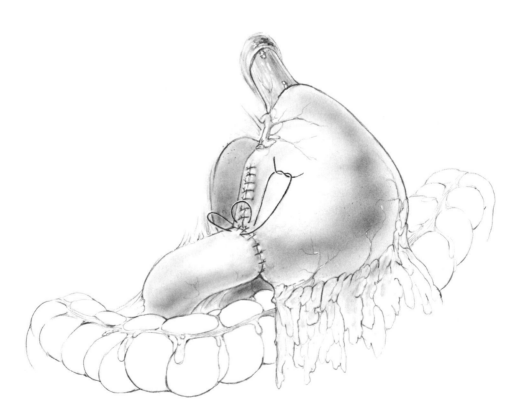

Fig. 29-19

continuous locked suture is inserted **(Fig. 29–16)**. Control any bleeding points by absorbable suture-ligature or electrocautery. Approximate the anterior mucosal layer with a continuous Connell or Cushing suture, which should be terminated at the midpoint of the anterior layer **(Fig. 29–17)**. Reinforce this suture line by a seromuscular layer of interrupted 4-0 silk Lembert sutures **(Fig. 29–18)**. At the "angle of sorrow," where the Hofmeister shelf of the gastric pouch meets the duodenal suture line at its lateral margin, insert a crown stitch by taking seromuscular bites of the anterior wall of the gastric pouch and then of the posterior wall of the gastric pouch, returning to catch the wall on the duodenal side **(Fig. 29–19)**. If the sutures have been properly inserted, the lumen should admit the tip of the surgeon's thumb. Loosely suture omentum over the anastomosis.

Billroth II: Closure of Duodenal Stump

Close the healthy duodenal stump with an inverting Connell suture of 4-0 PG supplemented by a layer of interrupted 4-0 silk Lembert sutures. Initiate the Connell suture by placing a half purse-string stitch at the right lateral margin of the duodenum. Continue this strand to the middle and initiate a second strand of 4-0 PG at the left margin of the duodenal stump. Continue this also to the middle of the stump and terminate it by tying it to the first strand **(Fig. 29–20)**.

Though it is simple to insert a layer of interrupted Lembert seromuscular sutures as a second layer when the tissues are not thickened **(Figs.**

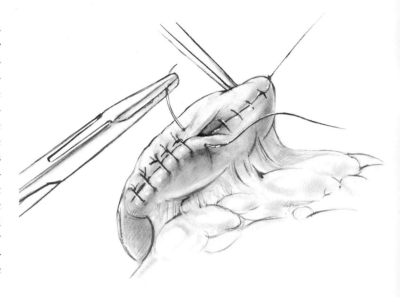

Fig. 29-21

29–21, 29–22), suturing the fibrotic duodenum requires judgment and skill. If the stitch is placed deep through the mucosa and then tied with strangulating force, a fistula may result. Once a small leak occurs, the powerful duodenal digestive juices may erode the adjacent tissue with *disastrous* results.

After the Connell suture has been completed, use forceps to test the flexibility of the tissue by pushing down tentatively on the suture line. Manipulating the tissue in this manner increases the accuracy of one's judgment about the best place for the Lembert sutures. A common error is to insert the seromuscular Lembert stitch too close to the Connell suture line. If this is done with a pliable duodenum of normal thickness, no harm results. However, sewing thick, fibrotic tissue into apposition without first sufficiently inverting the Connell suture line creates a

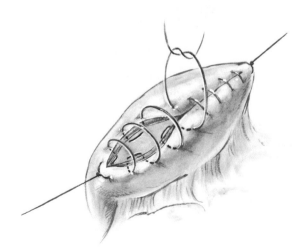

Fig. 29-20

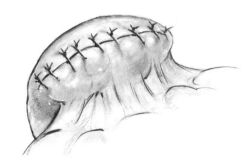

Fig. 29-22

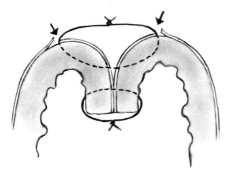

Fig. 29-23a

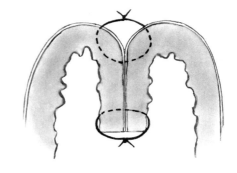

Fig. 29-23b

lateral shearing force that causes a small tear when the suture is tied **(Fig. 29–23a)**. If the suture also penetrates the mucosa of the duodenum, this mishap, combined with excessive shearing force, may produce a duodenal fistula. The fistula can be prevented if the surgeon inverts the Connell suture line for a distance of 2–3 mm before placing the Lembert suture **(Fig. 29–23b)**. If the duodenal serosa has a small tear after the Lembert suture is tied, the above error (Fig. 29-23a) was committed or the suture was tied too tightly.

Billroth II: Dissection of Difficult Duodenum

If the posterior duodenal wall and adjacent pancreas are replaced by fibrosis, a scalpel dissection, rather than scissors dissection, should be used **(Fig. 29–24)**. It is not necessary to apply hemostats when incising dense scar tissue, but it is important to keep the plane of dissection close to the posterior wall of the duodenum, thereby avoiding trauma to the pancreas. When the dissection enters the posterior duo-

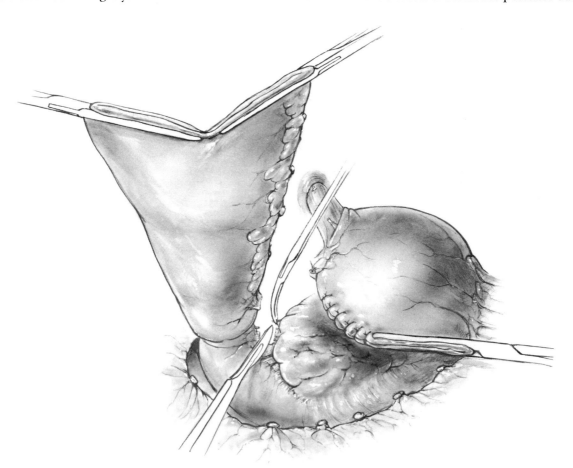

Fig. 29-24

denum at the site of the penetrating ulcer, this "window" in the duodenum should be enlarged by an incision extending proximally from the ulcer toward the pylorus. The incision permits the surgeon's index finger to be inserted into the duodenal lumen. With the finger as a guide, dissection around the borders of the ulcer may be resumed.

It is obviously not necessary to remove the *base of the ulcer* during this dissection. The base of the ulcer is really the anterior surface of the pancreas, which should not be disturbed. When the duodenum is dissected from the pancreas beyond the dense scar tissue, small hemostats may again be applied to the vessels on the pancreatic side. The vessels are then divided; and any bleeding from the duodenum, which is generally minimal in the presence of fibrosis, can be ignored. If the dissection is successful, the caudal lip of the ulcer is dissected away from the duodenum; and after a few more millimeters of dissection the posterior duodenal wall may assume a fairly normal appearance. Liberate 1.5 cm of posterior duodenal wall. If at any point it appears that liberating the caudal lip of the ulcer is becoming dangerous, terminate the dissection and close the stump using the Nissen-Cooper technique (see below).

Another contraindication to further dissection of the caudal lip of the ulcer is proximity to the ampulla of Vater. Check this possibility by frequently palpating with the index finger in the duodenal lumen. After an adequate segment of posterior duodenum has been liberated, closure may be performed as described above (Figs. 29-20 through 29-22).

When a posterior duodenal or pyloroduodenal penetrating ulcer involves the hepatoduodenal ligament, it may be necessary to identify the course of the common bile duct. Make an incision in the proximal common bile duct and pass a 16F catheter or no. 4 Bakes dilator through the ampulla. Palpate this guide to confirm the position of the duct and avoid damaging it.

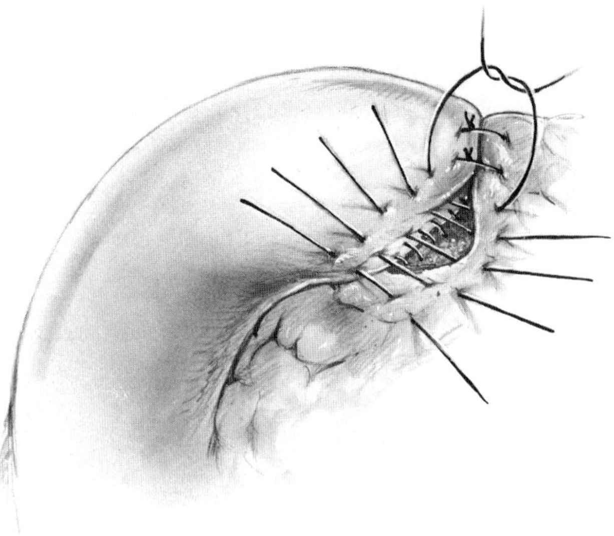

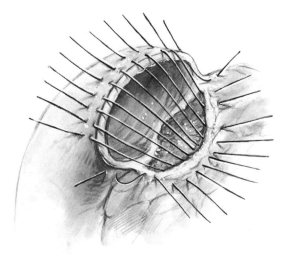

Fig. 29-26

Closure of Difficult Stump by Nissen-Cooper Technique

When it is deemed hazardous to free the posterior duodenum beyond a callous ulcer, perform a Kocher maneuver to gain additional mobility of the duodenum. Then accomplish closure by inserting interrupted 4-0 silk Lembert sutures to attach the free anterior and anterolateral walls of the duodenum to the distal lip of the ulcer **(Fig. 29–25)**. Use a second layer of Lembert sutures to invert the first suture line by suturing the pliable anterior wall to the proximal lip of the ulcer and to the adjacent pancreatic capsule **(Fig. 29–26)**. Devised by Nissen and Cooper, this technique was used extensively by Harrower. A variation of it **(Fig. 29–27)** involves inserting the first layer of sutures to attach the free

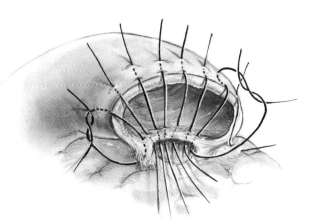

Fig. 29-25

Fig. 29-27

anterior wall of the duodenum to the proximal lip of a large ulcer crater. This may be reinforced by a layer of Lembert sutures between the duodenum and adjacent pancreatic capsule. It is *essential* that the anterior wall of the duodenum be soft, pliable, and long enough for use in the Nissen-Cooper maneuver without causing tension on the suture line. A Kocher maneuver must be performed to liberate the duodenum for this type of closure.

Closure of Difficult Duodenal Stump

Duodenal Stenosis

Occasionally, chronic duodenal ulcer disease produces an annular stenosis at some point in the proximal 3–4 cm of the duodenum. If there is no active bleeding, it is safe to close a healthy duodenum proximal to an ulcer. On the other hand, it is unwise to attempt inversion of the duodenal stump proximal to an area of marked stenosis. There simply is not enough room to invert the normal diameter of proximal duodenum into a stenotic segment. In such cases the duodenum should be dissected down to the point of stenosis and perhaps 1 cm beyond (**Fig. 29–28**). It is then a simple matter to turn in the stenosed area. Usually only three or four interrupted Lembert sutures of 4-0 silk are required for each of the two layers because of their narrow diameter (**Fig. 29–29**).

Catheter Duodenostomy

Catheter duodenostomy is designed to protect the integrity of a difficult duodenal stump closure. Properly performed this technique, which prevents buildup of intraluminal pressure against the newly sutured stump, has been surprisingly safe. If there is doubt about the integrity of the duodenal stump suture line, place a 14F whistle-tip or Foley catheter through a tiny incision in the lateral wall of the descending duodenum. This maneuver is easier to per-

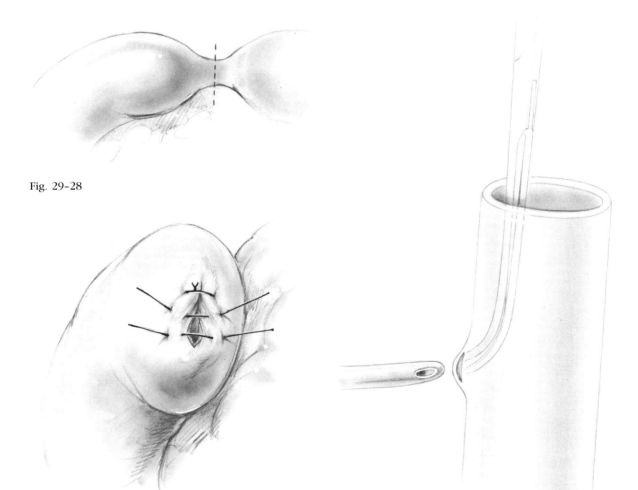

Fig. 29–28

Fig. 29–29

Fig. 29–30

form before the duodenal stump is closed. Pass a right-angled (Mixter) clamp into the open duodenum, press the tip of the clamp laterally against the duodenal wall, and make a 3 mm stab wound to allow the tip of the clamp to pass through the duodenal wall. Use the Mixter clamp to grasp the tip of the catheter and draw it into the duodenal lumen **(Fig. 29–30)**. Close the incision around the catheter with a 4-0 silk purse-string suture. Wrap the catheter with omentum and bring it out through a stab wound in the abdominal wall, *leaving some slack* to allow for postoperative abdominal distension. Suture the catheter to the skin with heavy silk. In addition, bring a latex Penrose drain from the area of the duodenotomy out through a separate stab wound in the lateral abdominal wall **(Fig. 29–31)**.

There may be some occasions when the surgeon finds it impossible to invert the duodenal stump, even with the techniques described earlier. This happens rarely, but if it does occur the catheter may be placed directly in the stump of duodenum, which should be closed as well as possible around the catheter. The lateral duodenostomy is much preferred, however.

Following the operation, place the catheter on low suction until the patient passes flatus; then connect the catheter to a plastic bag for gravity drainage. Irrigate the catheter twice each day with 5 ml sterile saline. If the patient does well, remove the drain by the eighth postoperative day. Three days later partly withdraw the duodenostomy catheter so its tip lies just outside the duodenum. Apply low suction. If the volume of drainage does not exceed 100 ml per day, gradually withdraw the catheter over the next day or two.

Duodenal Closure with Surgical Staples

If the duodenal wall is not thickened markedly with fibrosis or edema, and if an 8- to 10-mm width of duodenum is available, the stump may be closed safely using a 55 mm linear stapling device. Apply the stapler to the duodenal stump before dividing the specimen. After the stapler has been fired, apply an Allen clamp on the specimen side and, with a scalpel, transect the stump flush with the stapling device **(Fig. 29–32)**. Lightly electrocauterize the everted mucosa of the duodenal stump before removing the stapling device. There is no need to invert this closure with a layer of sutures. Experimental and clinical evidence shows that despite the eversion of duodenal mucosa seem with this closure, healing is essentially equal to that seen with the sutured duodenal stump. Generally, we cover the stapled stump with omentum or the pancreatic capsule with a few sutures, but we do not invert the mucosa.

When the duodenal wall is at all thickened, use large (4.8 mm) staples to reduce the degree of compression applied to the tissues by the stapling device. There should be blood circulation to the narrow rim of tissue that lies distal to the staple line, which generally manifests as slight oozing from the tissues despite the staples. It must again be emphasized that if the duodenal wall is so diseased it

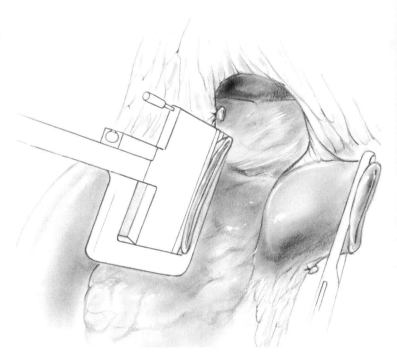

Fig. 29-31   Fig. 29-32

probably would not heal if closed by sutures, stapling will fail as well.

Closure of Difficult Duodenal Stump by Billroth I Gastroduodenostomy

In the hands of an expert such as Nyhus, "If one can close the duodenum, one can anastomose to it." Although it is not always necessary to liberate the distal tip of the ulcer crater, the duodenum should be dissected away from the pancreas at least to this point. The usual technique of gastroduodenal anastomosis, as described in Figures 29-14 through 29-19, must be modified. In the region of the ulcer crater only one posterior layer of interrupted 4-0 silk sutures should be inserted, taking a bite of stomach, underlying fibrosed pancreas, and the distal lip of the ulcer crater and duodenum, with the knot tied inside the lumen **(Fig. 29–33)**. If the ulcer crater is so deep the posterior anastomotic suture line cannot be buttressed by the underlying pancreatic bed of the ulcer, use of this technique may be hazardous. Because surgery for duodenal ulcer declined during the 1990s, fewer surgeons have had the opportunity to develop experience and judgment in managing the difficult duodenum. It is not wise for the inexperienced surgeon to perform a Billroth I anastomosis unless the above precautions are followed.

Billroth II Gastrojejunal Anastomosis

Although there are many variations of the technique for constructing Billroth II anastomoses, we have preferred a short-loop antecolic anastomosis of the Schoemaker-Hofmeister type. It does not seem to matter whether the afferent segment of the jejunum is attached to the greater curvature of the gastric pouch or to the lesser curvature. The distance from the ligament of Treitz to the gastric pouch should be no more than 12-15 cm. The major portions of the transverse colon and omentum should be brought to the patient's right for the antecolic anastomosis.

Score the antimesenteric aspect of the jejunum with the back of a scalpel blade. Place the first posterior suture line posterior to but parallel with this scratch line. This maneuver ensures that the stoma is placed accurately and may help prevent postoperative obstruction of the gastric outlet. Attach the jejunum to the gastric pouch with interrupted 4-0 silk seromuscular Lembert sutures placed about 5 mm apart **(Fig. 29–34)**. Leave the first and last stitches long and tag them with a hemostat. Cut all the remaining silk tails.

If any gastric wall protrudes from the Allen clamp, remove the excess with a scalpel incision flush with the clamp **(Fig. 29–35)**. Then use electrocautery to

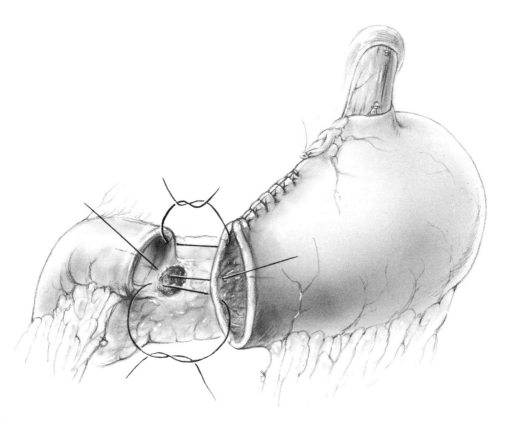

Fig. 29-33

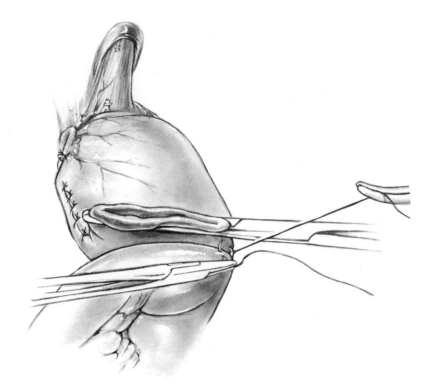

Fig. 29-34

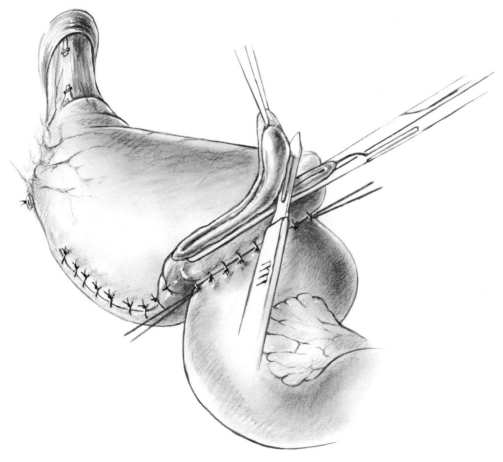

Fig. 29-35

make an incision along the antimesenteric scratch line in the jejunum. Open the mucosa of the jejunum (**Fig. 29–36**). Control bleeding points with electrocautery. The incision in the jejunum should be a few millimeters shorter than the diameter of the opening in the gastric pouch.

Remove the Allen clamp and open the gastric pouch. Carefully control any bleeding points on the anterior aspect of the gastric pouch by means of 4-0 PG suture-ligatures. The posterior wall is controlled by the mucosal locked suture. Initiate this suture at the midpoint of the posterior layer with a double-armed 3-0 PG suture, which should be inserted through the full thickness of the gastric and jejunal walls and tied (**Figs. 29–37a, 29–37b, 29–37c**). Start a continuous locked suture from the midpoint and go first to the right and then to the left. Complete the anterior mucosal layer with a continuous Connell or Cushing suture. Initiate the suture line first at the right-hand margin of the anastomosis (**Fig. 29–38a**) and then on the left (**Fig. 29–38b**), working both needles toward the midpoint, where the two strands should be tied to each other (**Fig. 29–38c**). Complete the anterior layer with a row of interrupted 4-0 silk seromuscular Lem-

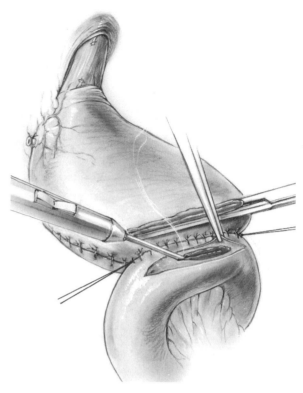

Fig. 29-36

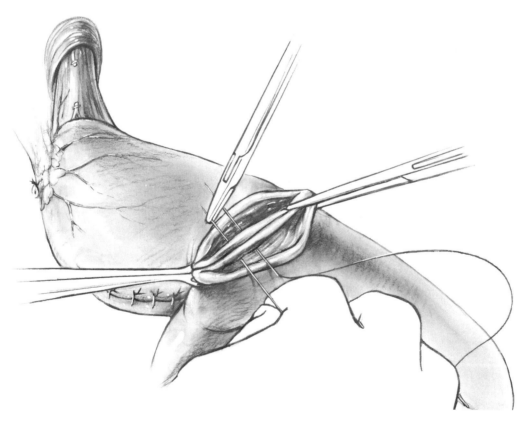

Fig. 29-37a

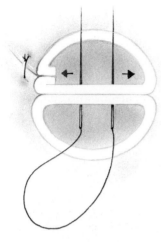

Fig. 29-37b

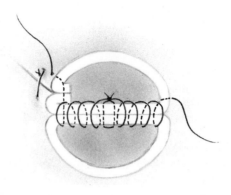

Fig. 29-37c

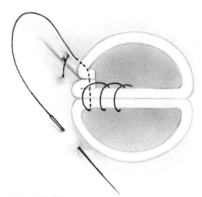

Fig. 29-38a

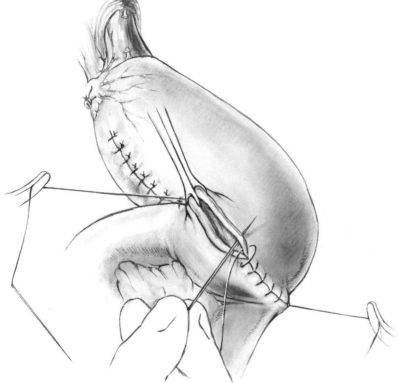

Fig. 29-38b

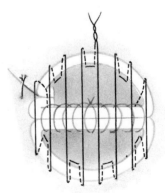

Fig. 29-38c

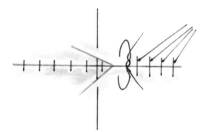

Fig. 29-38d

bert sutures **(Fig. 29–38d, 29–39)** on curved needles. At the medial margin of the anastomosis (the "angle of sorrow") insert a crown stitch **(Fig. 29–40)**. Occasionally, two crown sutures are inserted for added security.

For the poor-risk patient, minimize anesthesia time by inserting the seromuscular suture layer in over-and-over continuous Lembert fashion using 3-0 PG instead of interrupted silk. The mucosal layer may be closed using the same technique as described above. When this anastomosis is performed with care, there seems to be no disadvantage to using continuous PG seromuscular suture.

Billroth II Gastrojejunal Anastomosis by Stapling Technique

Isolate the vasa brevia along the greater curvature individually by passing a Kelly hemostat behind the vessels. Tie them or secure them with a clipping and dividing instrument that divides the vessels and applies stainless steel clips to both cut ends simultaneously **(Fig. 29–41)**. When stapling is used, it is not necessary to close the lesser curvature as a separate step. Instead, apply a 90/4.8 mm linear stapler across the entire stomach, tighten it, and fire **(Fig. 29–42)**. Apply a large Payr clamp to the specimen side of the stomach and divide the stomach flush with the stapling device by a scalpel. Lightly electrocauterize the everted mucosa and remove the stapler. Close the duodenal stump with the 55 mm linear stapler as previously described and remove the specimen **(Fig. 29–43)**.

It is imperative that the nasogastric tube not be permitted to lie anywhere in the vicinity of the staple line during this step. If the nasogastric tube becomes trapped in the gastric staple line, it cannot be removed without another laparotomy.

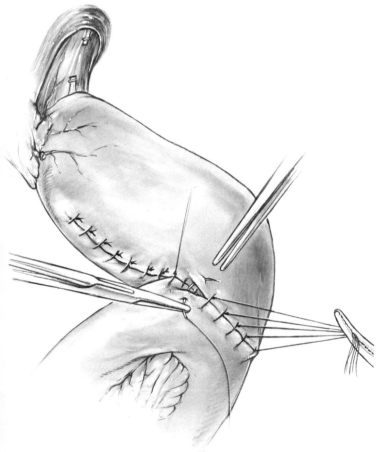

Fig. 29-39

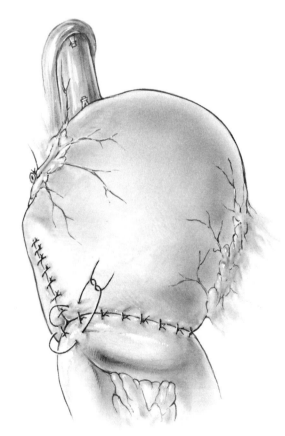

Fig. 29-40

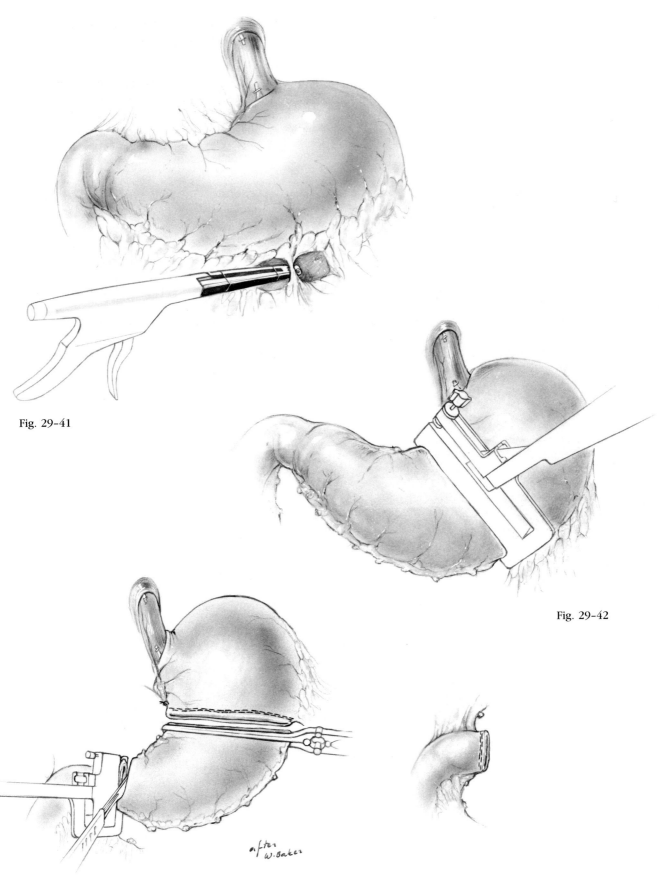

Fig. 29-41

Fig. 29-42

Fig. 29-43

after
W. Baker

Next identify the ligament of Treitz and bring a segment of proximal jejunum in antecolic fashion to the greater curvature side of the gastric pouch. Approximate the antimesenteric border of the jejunum with a 4-0 silk suture to a point on the greater curvature of the stomach about 2 cm proximal to the staple line. Make small stab wounds in the gastric pouch and jejunum adjacent to this suture and just deep to it. Then insert the cutting linear stapling device so one fork enters the gastric pouch parallel to the staple line and the other fork enters the jejunum and is placed exactly along the antimesenteric border **(Fig. 29–44)**. Take care not to allow any other organ or tissue to intrude between the stomach and jejunum being grasped by the stapling device. When this stapler has been inserted to the 4- or 5-cm mark, close and lock it (Fig. 29-44). Then reinspect the area. There should be a 2 cm width of posterior gastric wall between the staple line and the proposed anastomotic staple line. Also, the gastric and jejunal tissues should be exactly apposed to each other in the hub of the stapling device. At this point fire and remove the stapler.

Apply Allis clamps to the anterior and posterior terminations of the staple line and carefully inspect the mucosal surface of the stapled anastomosis for bleeding. Arterial spurting from the gastric wall oc-

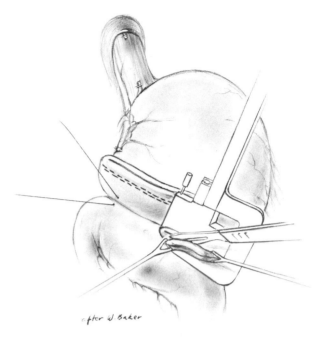

after W. Baker

Fig. 29-45

curs occasionally. When it does, transfix the vessel with a fine PG suture-ligature.

Control lesser bleeding by cautious electrocoagulation. Multiple bleeding points are seen on rare occasions. The entire mucosal suture line should then be oversewn with a locked continuous suture of 4-0 PG. The needle must be inserted deep to the staples when performing this maneuver. It should be necessary in no more than 1–2% of all cases.

After hemostasis is ensured, approximate the gastric and jejunal layers of the open stab wounds in an everting fashion with several Allis or Babcock clamps. Close the defect with one application of a 55 mm linear stapler deep to the line of Allis clamps **(Fig. 29–45)**. *This staple line must include the anterior and posterior terminations of the anastomotic staple line,* guaranteeing that there is no defect between the two lines of staples. Excise the redundant tissue, lightly electrocoagulate the everted mucosa, and remove the stapler. Alternatively, close the stab wound defect in an inverting fashion by various suturing techniques. Then place a single 4-0 silk seromuscular suture at the right termination of the stapled anastomosis **(Fig. 29–46)**. The gastrojejunal stoma should admit two fingers. A three-dimensional representation of the anastomosis is shown in **Figure 29–47**.

Drainage and Closure

Whenever the surgeon thinks the duodenal closure is less than perfect after a Billroth II operation, a

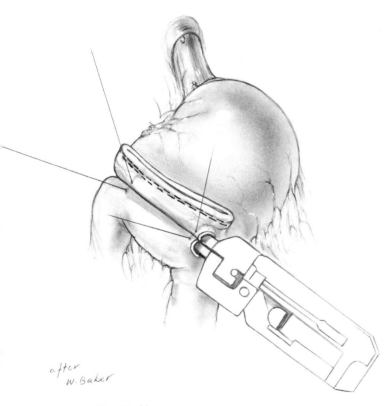

after W. Baker

Fig. 29-44

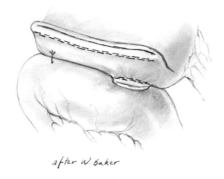

after W. Baker

Fig. 29-46

closed-suction drain should be brought out from the vicinity of the duodenal stump through a stab wound in the right upper quadrant. The drain should be separated from the duodenal suture line by a layer of omentum. Accomplished this way, drainage does no harm to the patient. Close the abdominal wall in the usual fashion after taking pains to ensure that the efferent limb of the jejunum descends freely and without kinks.

POSTOPERATIVE CARE

Nasogastric suction should be continued for several days. Oral intake can be resumed when there is evidence of bowel function. For the first 4-6 weeks following gastric resection the diet should be low in carbohydrates and fluids and high in protein and fat to reduce the osmolarity of the meals. Liquids should largely be eliminated from meals and be consumed

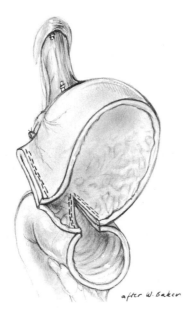

after W. Baker

Fig. 29-47

beginning 1 hour after meals. Sweet drinks should be avoided. If this course is followed, the transitory dumping symptoms, which many patients experience during the early postgastrectomy period, are avoided. Generally, after 4-6 weeks patients can enjoy an unlimited diet.

COMPLICATIONS

Duodenal fistula. In the presence of an adequate drain, the appearance of duodenal content in the drainage fluid with no other symptoms may not require vigorous therapy. On the other hand, if there are signs of spreading peritoneal irritation, prompt relaparotomy is indicated. If no drain was placed during the initial operation, immediate relaparotomy is undertaken whenever there is reason to suspect duodenal leakage. On rare occasions relaparotomy can be performed before there is intense inflammatory reaction of the duodenal tissues, and the defect may be closed by suture. This is seldom possible, however. If suturing the virgin duodenum at the first operation was not successful, an attempt at secondary suturing fails unless considerable additional duodenum can be freed from the pancreas for a more adequate closure. In most cases the operation is done to provide excellent drainage. A small sump-suction drain should be inserted into the fistula and additional latex and sumps placed in the area. If a controlled duodenocutaneous fistula can be achieved, it generally closes after a few weeks of total parenteral nutrition. Prescribing a somatostatin analog to reduce duodenal and pancreatic secretion is also helpful.

Leaks from Billroth I gastroduodenal anastomoses, though rare, are even more serious than from duodenal stump (Billroth II) procedures. Generally they are treated by the Graham technique of closing a perforated duodenal ulcer with a segment of viable omentum (see Figs. 27-3, 27-4). Multiple sump drains should also be inserted.

Acute pancreatitis. Acute pancreatitis is a serious complication that is best avoided by preventing trauma to the pancreas during the initial operation. Therapy is identical to that for acute pancreatitis in the patient who has not undergone an operation.

Gastric outlet obstruction. Obstruction in the gastroduodenal anastomosis is generally due to inversion of too much tissue, which produces a mechanical block. If this condition does not respond after a period of conservative treatment, reoperation to convert to a Billroth II anastomosis is probably necessary.

Be aware that the Billroth II gastrojejunal anastomosis occasionally develops an outlet obstruction

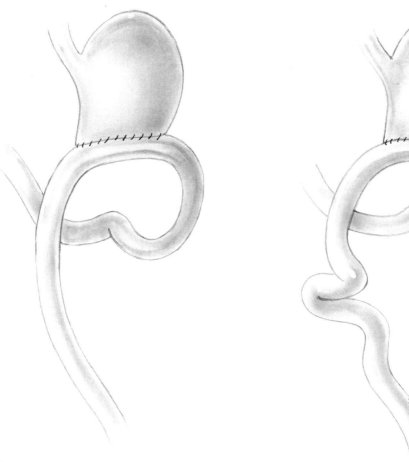

Fig. 29–48

Fig. 29–49

that appears due to malfunction of the efferent loop of the jejunum. This diagnosis can be confirmed by inserting a gastroscope well into the efferent and afferent limbs of the jejunum, which demonstrates the absence of any mechanical stomal obstruction. Relaparotomy in these cases is of no value. Generally, several weeks of conservative treatment with nutritional support is successful. Passage of a small feeding tube into the efferent limb allows direct enteral support until function recovers.

Alkaline reflux gastritis. Alkaline reflux gastritis may require conversion of the Billroth II to a Roux-en-Y reconstruction **(Fig. 29–48, 29–49)**. Transect the afferent limb of jejunum at its point of entry into the gastric pouch. Use a TA-55 stapler to close the gastric side of the jejunum; then anastomose the open end of the afferent segment to the side of the efferent segment of the jejunum. This anastomosis should take place at a point 60 cm distal to the gastrojejunostomy. It converts the efferent limb of the jejunum to a Roux-en-Y configuration. Vagotomy is necessary to prevent marginal ulceration following this type of Roux-en-Y anastomosis. Although some

surgeons routinely use a Roux-en-Y reconstruction for all gastric surgery, severe hypomotility (Roux stasis syndrome) occasionally follows this procedure and can be difficult to manage. Miedema and Kelly described an alternative reconstruction using an uncut Roux limb as a prophylactic measure.

Afferent loop obstruction, afferent loop syndrome. Acute mechanical blockage of the afferent stoma, often accompanied by jejunogastric intussusception or internal hernia, causes an acute closed-loop obstruction that manifests as excruciating upper abdominal pain and retching. Gastrointestinal radiography reveals complete block at the afferent stoma, which can be confirmed by endoscopy. This situation is a surgical emergency because if the distended afferent loop bursts lethal peritonitis results. Obviously, emergency surgery for correction of the obstruction is essential.

Intermittent afferent limb obstruction causes postprandial pain that is relieved by bilious vomiting. Because the efferent limb is patent, the vomitus may not contain food. Exploration and jejunojejunostomy allow drainage of the afferent limb into the efferent limb.

Most afferent loop symptomatology can be prevented by ensuring that the distance between the ligament of Treitz and the gastric pouch is never more than 12–15 cm. These problems do not occur after a Billroth I reconstruction.

Dumping syndrome. The "dumping syndrome" may occur in any patient whose pylorus has been rendered nonfunctional. It is more common in patients of asthenic habitus who have never achieved normal body weight, even before surgery. Dietary alteration generally controls dumping. Slow introduction of concentrated carbohydrate loads, particularly in liquid form (e.g., apple juice), may help avoid the problem.

Marginal ulcer. One cause of recurrent ulcer is the surgeon's having left behind gastrin-secreting antral mucosa on the duodenal stump following a Billroth II gastrectomy. Unrecognized Zollinger-Ellison syndrome also can cause recurrent ulcer after what would otherwise be an adequate ulcer operation.

Malabsorption. Anemia may be due to inadequate iron absorption. Folic acid and vitamin B_{12} deficiencies develop on rare occasions following gastrectomy. Another late complication is osteomalacia or osteoporosis caused by poor calcium or vitamin D absorption. Steatorrhea and diarrhea develop in some cases and may contribute to malnutrition. These patients should be studied for the presence of gluten enteropathy, which may be unmasked by the gastrectomy. Although almost all the early complications are manageable, malabsorption and malnutrition many years after a gastrectomy are difficult to treat. These complications seem rare, however, following a 40–50% gastrectomy.

REFERENCES

Aranow JS, Matthews JB, Garcia-Aguilar J, Novak G, Silen W. Isoperistaltic jejunal interposition for intractable postgastrectomy alkaline reflux gastritis. J Am College Surg 1995;180:648.

Austen WG, Baue AE. Catheter duodenostomy for the difficult duodenum. Ann Surg 1964;160:781.

Burch JM, Cox CL, Feliciano DV, Richardson RJ, Martin RR. Management of the difficult duodenal stump. Am J Surg 1991;162:522.

Burden WR, Hodges RP, Hsu M, O'Leary JP. Alkaline reflux gastritis. Surg Clin North Am 1991;71:33.

Eagon JC, Miedema BW, Kelly KA. Postgastrectomy syndromes. Surg Clin North Am 1992;72:445.

Goh P, Tekant Y, Isaac J, Kum CK, Ngoi SS. The technique of laparoscopic Billroth II gastrectomy. Surg Laparosc Endosc 1992;2:258.

Gowen GF. Delayed gastric emptying after Roux-en-Y due to four types of partial obstruction. Ann Surg 1992;215:363.

Harrower HW. Closure of the duodenal stump after gastrectomy for posterior ulcer. Am J Surg 1966;111:488.

Herrington JL Jr. Vagotomy-antrectomy: how I do it. Acta Chir Scand Suppl 1992;72:335.

Jones RC, McClelland RN, Zedlitz WH, Shires GT. Difficult closures of the duodenal stump. Arch Surg 1967;94:696.

Karlstrom L, Kelly KA. Roux-Y gastrectomy for chronic gastric atony. Am J Surg 1989;157:44.

Miedema BW, Kelly KA. The Roux stasis syndrome: treatment by pacing and prevention by use of an "uncut" Roux limb. Arch Surg 1992;127:295.

Nyhus LM, Wastell C. Surgery of the Stomach and Duodenum. Boston, Little, Brown, 1977, p 368.

Sawyers JL. Management of postgastrectomy syndromes. Am J Surg 1990;159:8.

30 Perforated Peptic Ulcer

INDICATIONS

Perforated gastric ulcer. Not all free perforations of gastric ulcers are susceptible to simple plication techniques. Often the ulcer is large and surrounded by edema. When the perforation occurs on the posterior surface of the antrum, adequate repair by plication techniques is generally not possible. Gastric ulcers have a high rate of recurrence. For these reasons, in a good-risk patient in whom the diagnosis of perforation has been made reasonably early, gastric resection is *preferred* to simple plication. If for technical reasons a sound plication cannot be constructed, gastric resection is *mandatory*, regardless of the risk, as a recurrent gastric leak into the peritoneal cavity is almost always fatal.

Perforated duodenal ulcer. If a perforated duodenal ulcer is treated with a simple closure, about one-third of patients remain nonsymptomatic without further treatment. Effective medical therapy has diminished the role for vagotomy in this setting. Laparoscopic plication (see Chapter 31) is an option in properly selected patients.

PREOPERATIVE PREPARATION

Fluid and electrolyte resuscitation, primarily with a balanced salt solution

Nasogastric suction

Systemic antibiotics

Monitoring of hourly urine output, central venous pressure, or pulmonary artery wedge pressure, as indicated

PITFALLS AND DANGER POINTS

Inadequate fluid and electrolyte resuscitation

Inadequate closure of perforation

OPERATIVE STRATEGY

The most important initial step of the operative strategy is to determine, on the basis of the principles discussed above, whether the patient should be treated by plication or resection. On technical grounds alone, large defects in the stomach or duodenum are better handled by resection than by attempted plication. If it appears that plication of a duodenal ulcer would produce obstruction, resection is safer. An alternative is excising the perforation as part of a pyloroplasty incision (see Chapter 27).

For most perforated duodenal ulcers an attempt to close the defect by sutures alone often results in the stitch tearing through the edematous tissue. It is preferable to place a plug of viable omentum over the defect and use through-and-through sutures to hold the omentum in contact with the wall of the duodenum. This practice avoids tension on the sutures. It is important to irrigate the abdominal cavity thoroughly with large quantities of saline to remove the contamination.

OPERATIVE TECHNIQUE OF PLICATION

Incision

A midline incision from the xiphoid to the umbilicus provides good exposure and can be made rapidly.

Identification of Perforation

By following the lesser curvature aspect of the stomach down to the pylorus, the perforation along the anterior wall of the duodenum generally becomes quickly evident (**Fig. 30–1**). In some cases it is sealed off by omentum or the undersurface of the liver. If this area is not the site of the perforation, search the entire stomach carefully, up to the esophagus and including the entire posterior surface of the stomach in the lesser sac. Rarely, a perforation is found somewhere in the small intestine or colon (e.g., secondary to a sharp fishbone).

Plication of Perforation

Generally, insert 3-0 silk (or PG) on an atraumatic intestinal needle beginning at a point about 5 mm above the perforation. Bring the stitch out at a point 5 mm distal to the perforation and leave it untied.

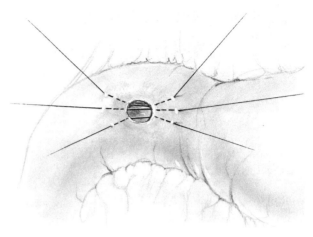

Fig. 30-2

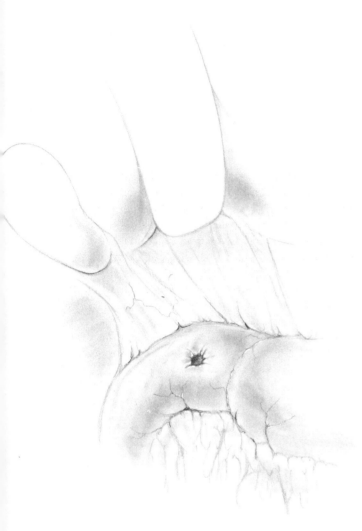

Fig. 30-1

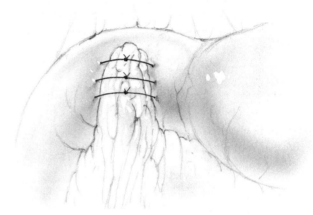

Fig. 30-3

Two additional sutures of the same types are needed for the average perforation. Next, isolate a viable segment of omentum and place it over the perforation. Tie the three sutures over the plug of omentum to fasten it in place **(Figs. 30–2, 30–3)**. It is *not* necessary to approximate the margins of the hole in the duodenum but only to cap it with viable omental tissue.

Peritoneal Lavage

Using large volumes of warm saline, thoroughly lavage the peritoneal cavity with multiple aliquots until the gastric contents and fibrin are removed from the surfaces of the bowel and peritoneum.

Abdominal Closure

Consider needle catheter jejunostomy if the patient is malnourished. Close the midline incision without drainage using the modified Smead-Jones technique as described in Chapter 3. Unless the patient has ad-

vanced peritonitis, the skin may be closed in routine fashion.

POSTOPERATIVE CARE

Nasogastric suction

Acid-reducing therapy

Test for *Helicobacter pylori* and treat if positive

Intravenous fluids

Systemic antibiotics, guided to aerobic and anaerobic cultures obtained at surgery

Enteral feeding by needle catheter jejunostomy for malnourished patients

COMPLICATIONS

Subphrenic and subhepatic abscesses occur mainly in patients whose operations have been delayed more than 8-12 hours after the perforation.

Duodenal obstruction, caused by the plication, should be suspected if gastric emptying has not returned to normal by the eighth or ninth postoperative day. It may be confirmed by a gastrointestinal contrast study.

Reperforation of the duodenal ulcer occurs in rare cases, and the surgeon must be alert to detect this complication. When it does occur, gastric resection is mandatory if there is to be any hope of stopping the duodenal leak.

REFERENCES

Donovan AJ, Berne TV, Donovan JA. Perforated duodenal ulcer: an alternative therapeutic plan. Arch Surg 1998;133:1166.

Jordan GL Jr, Angel RT, DeBakey ME. Acute gastroduodenal perforation: comparative study of treatment with simple closure, subtotal gastrectomy and hemigastrectomy and vagotomy. Arch Surg 1966;92:449.

Ng EK, Lam YH, Sung JJ, et al. Eradication of Helicobacter pylori prevents recurrence of ulcer after simple closure of duodenal ulcer perforation: randomized controlled trial. Annal Surg 2000;231:153.

Sharma R, Organ CH Jr, Hirvela ER, Henderson VJ. Clinical observation of the temporal association between crack cocaine and duodenal ulcer perforation. Am J Surg 1997;174:632.

Stabile BE. Redefining the role of surgery for perforated duodenal ulcer in the Helicobacter pylori era. Ann Surg 2000;231:159.

Svanes C, Lie RT, Svanes K, Lie SA, Soriede O. Adverse effects of delayed treatment for perforated peptic ulcer. Ann Surg 1994;220:168.

31 Laparoscopic Plication of Perforated Ulcer

INDICATIONS

Simple anterior perforated duodenal ulcer

PREOPERATIVE PREPARATION

Nasogastric suction

Intravenous hydration

Antibiotics

PITFALLS AND DANGER POINTS

Incomplete closure

Duodenal obstruction

Incorrect diagnosis

OPERATIVE STRATEGY

Laparoscopic plication is appropriate when a simple anterior perforated duodenal ulcer is diagnosed. The operation may be conceptualized in four steps: confirming the diagnosis and peritoneal toilet, exposing the perforation, selecting the omental patch, and securing the patch in place.

This procedure is not suitable for large perforations or perforations for which the extent cannot be easily determined (e.g., large duodenal ulcers that appear to wrap around toward the posterior duodenal wall). Gastric perforations may be better handled by resection.

OPERATIVE TECHNIQUE

Position the patient supine. The room setup and trocar placement are similar to those for laparoscopic cholecystectomy (see Figs. 8-1, 67-4). An angled laparoscope may facilitate looking down onto the duodenal surface.

Thoroughly examine the peritoneal cavity, suctioning away any fluid or debris. Generally, the liver is adherent to the duodenum, partially or completely closing the perforation. Irrigate and aspirate the subphrenic spaces and all four quadrants of the abdomen.

Pass a closed grasper through one of the right sub-

costal ports and use it to tease the liver gently away from the duodenum by blunt dissection. If the perforation is relatively fresh, the gelatinous fibrin adhesions are easy to sweep away **(Fig. 31–1)**.

Pass the grasper laterally to open the subhepatic space and elevate the liver. Pass a suction irrigator through the epigastric port and irrigate **(Fig. 31–2)**.

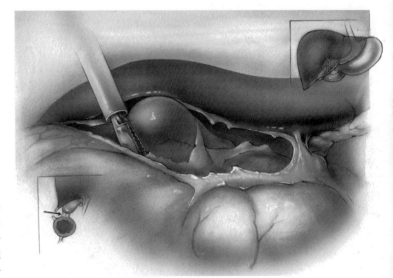

Fig. 31-1

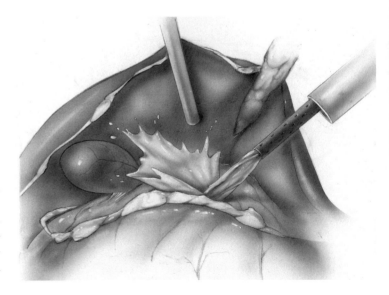

Fig. 31-2

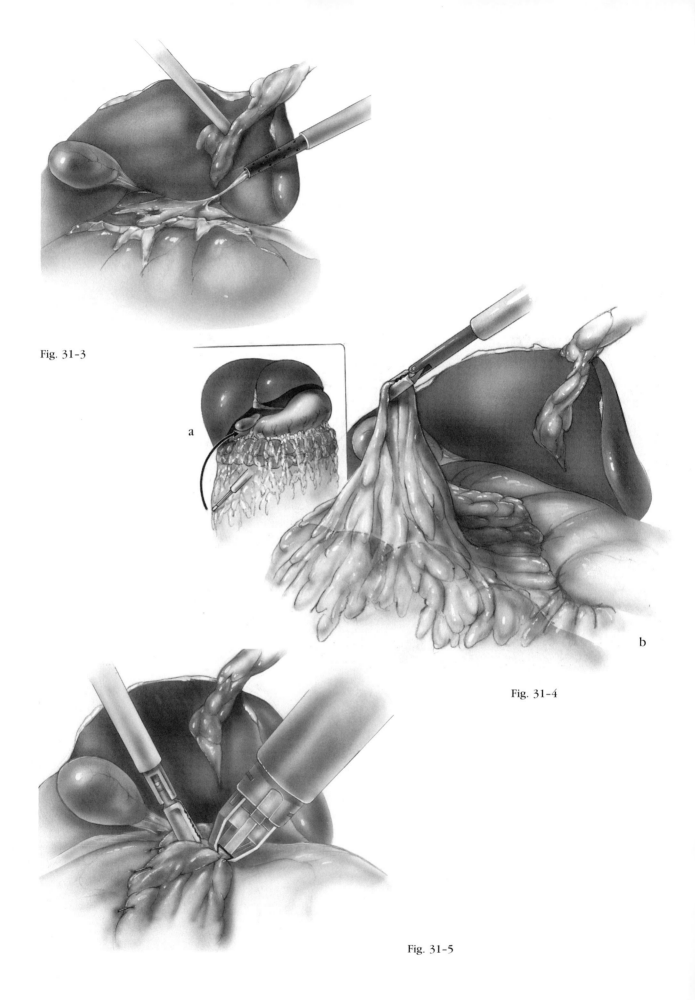

Fig. 31-3

a

b

Fig. 31-4

Fig. 31-5

With sufficient irrigation and possibly some gentle rubbing with the tip of the suction-irrigator, the fibrin peels away revealing the perforation **(Fig. 31–3)**. Confirm that the perforation is amenable to omental plication (a small, anterior duodenal perforation that is easily visualized).

Choose a soft, supple piece of omentum for the patch. This may require pulling a piece up from the lower abdomen, as the omentum near the perforation may be thickened and edematous **(Fig. 31–4a)**. Confirm that the section of omentum chosen reaches the site of perforation easily and without tension **(Fig. 31–4b)**.

There are two methods for securing the patch: stapling and suturing. Both are described here.

Securing the Patch with a Hernia Stapler

When the stapler is used to secure the patch, a series of staples are placed on both sides of the patch in such a fashion that one limb of each staple goes through the omentum and the other goes directly into the duodenum. There is danger that the staple does not adequately secure a purchase in the duodenum if both limbs go through the omentum first. Close the stapler slowly. As it begins to engage the tissue, pull back slightly to prevent inadvertent injury to the back wall of the duodenum **(Fig. 31–5)**. Place a series of staples on each side of the patch.

Suturing the Patch

Suturing the patch is relatively straightforward. Three or four sutures are placed across the perforation and tied over the omentum **(Fig. 31–6)**. It is generally easier to take a seromuscular bite of each side of the duodenum than to attempt to place a through-and-through suture (as shown for the open procedure). It is usually easier to tie these sutures as they are placed (rather than at the end of the procedure). Begin at the apex and proceed toward the laparoscope.

Testing the Patch

Confirm the security of the patch closure by injecting air into the nasogastric tube and watching for air bubbles under saline. Place a drain in the subphrenic space if desired **(Fig. 31–7)**.

Esophagogastroduodenoscopy

An esophagogastroduodenoscopy (EGD) scope is used by some as an adjunct. The endoscope is passed into the duodenum and the perforation visualized. A grasping forceps is passed through the perforation

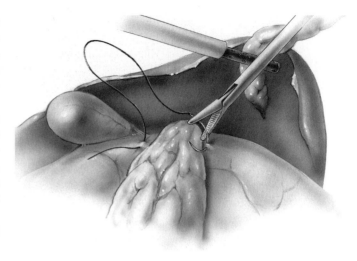

Fig. 31–6

and used to stabilize the omentum during suturing. Visualizing the duodenum with the scope at the end ensures that staples or sutures have not been placed too deeply. Insufflation with the scope replaces injection of the air through the nasogastric tube when the patch is tested. We have not found it necessary to use an EGD scope in these cases.

POSTOPERATIVE CARE

Postoperative care is the same as that required for the open procedure. Generally a day or two of nasogastric suction is required until the gastric ileus subsides, and it allows additional time for the patch closure to become secure. Antibiotic treatment is the same as that used for an open procedure. The first postoperative week is dominated by the physiologic

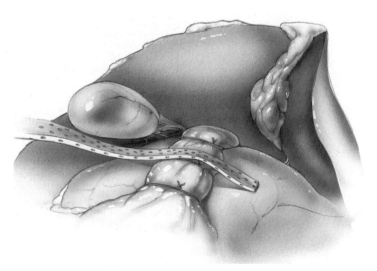

Fig. 31–7

response to the perforation and associated peritonitis. The advantages of the laparoscopic approach generally do not become obvious until the second or third week after surgery.

COMPLICATIONS

Failure to recognize a malignant perforation

Inadequate patch closure resulting in continuing sepsis

Subphrenic or subhepatic abscess

REFERENCES

Darzi A, Cheshire NH, Somers SS, et al. Laparoscopic omental patch repair of perforated duodenal ulcer with an automated stapler. Br J Surg 1993;80:1552.

Lau W-Y, Leung K-L, Kwong K-H, et al. A randomized study comparing laparoscopic versus open repair of perforated peptic ulcer using suture or sutureless technique. Ann Surg 1996;224:131.

Nathanson LK, Easter DW, Cuschieri A. Laparoscopic repair/peritoneal toilet of perforated duodenal ulcer. Surg Endosc 1990;4:232.

32 Gastrostomy

INDICATIONS

Gastric decompression without the need for a tube traversing the esophagogastric junction or the nasopharynx. A tube across the esophagogastric junction renders the distal esophageal sphincter ineffective. Gastroesophageal reflux with pneumonia or esophageal stricture may result.

Gastric tube feeding.

PITFALLS AND DANGER POINTS

Gastric leak into the peritoneal cavity

OPERATIVE STRATEGY

The Stamm gastrostomy is fast and relatively safe. When the gastrostomy is no longer needed, removal of the tube usually results in prompt closure of the tract.

For patients who require long-term gastric tube feeding, the Janeway gastrostomy is more convenient than the usual Stamm gastrostomy, as the Janeway construction does not require an indwelling tube. Percutaneous endoscopic gastrostomy is an alternative for many patients. The Stamm and Janeway gastrostomies can also be performed laparoscopically.

When constructing a tube gastrostomy, the gastrostomy opening must be carefully sutured to the anterior abdominal wall around the stab wound made for the exit of the tube. Otherwise, gastric contents may leak out around the tube and escape into the abdominal cavity.

OPERATIVE TECHNIQUE

Stamm Gastrostomy

When performed as part of another abdominal procedure, the abdominal incision has already been made. If necessary, it can be extended upward into the epigastrium to expose the stomach. When gastrostomy is performed as a single procedure, a short upper midline incision generally suffices.

Chose a location in the midportion of the stomach, closer to the greater curvature than to the lesser curvature **(Fig. 32–1)**. Using 2-0 atraumatic PG or silk, insert a circular purse-string suture with a 1.5 cm diameter.

Grasp the left side of the incised linea alba with a Kocher clamp and elevate it. Then make a stab wound through the middle third of the left rectus muscle at the level of the purse-string suture. Pass a Kelly hemostat through the stab wound from the peritoneum outward and use it to grasp the tip of

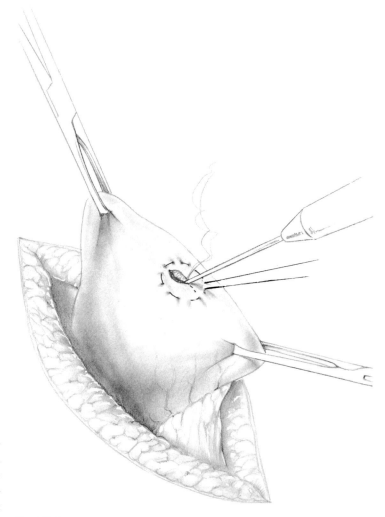

Fig. 32-1

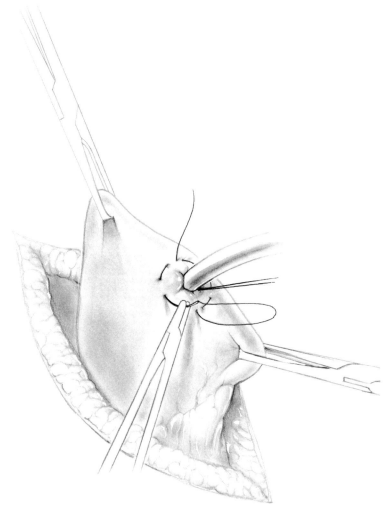

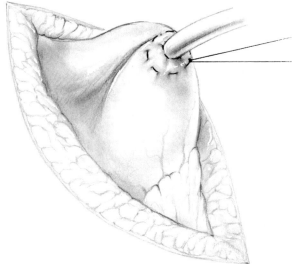

Fig. 32-2

Fig. 32-3

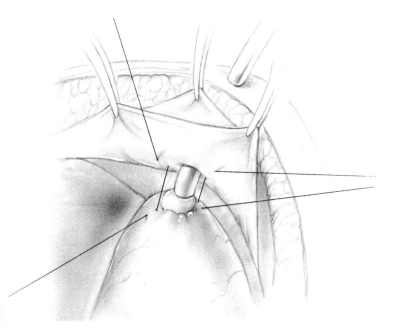

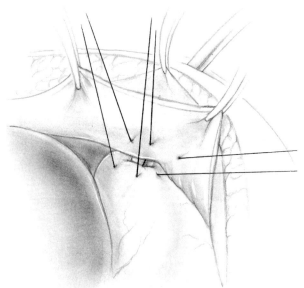

Fig. 32-4

Fig. 32-5

an 18F Foley, Malecot, or mushroom catheter. Draw the catheter into the abdominal cavity with the hemostat. With electrocautery make a stab wound in the anterior gastric wall in the middle of the previously placed purse-string suture (Fig. 32–1). Insert the catheter into the stomach, tighten the purse-string suture, and tie it to invert the gastric serosa **(Fig. 32–2)**. Invert this purse-string suture, in turn, with a second concentric 2-0 PG or silk purse-string suture **(Fig. 32–3)**. If a Foley catheter was used, inflate the balloon, and draw the stomach toward the anterior abdominal wall. Insert Lembert sutures of PG or silk in four quadrants around the catheter to sew the stomach to the anterior abdominal wall around the stab wound **(Fig. 32–4)**. When these four Lembert sutures are tied, the anterior gastric wall is firmly anchored to the abdominal wall **(Fig. 32–5)**.

Janeway Gastrostomy, Stapled

Make a 10- to 12-cm midline incision in the mid-epigastrium. Local anesthesia may be used in the poor-risk patient. Apply Babcock clamps to the anterior gastric wall near the lesser curvature; then apply a cutting linear stapling device **(Fig. 32–6)**. Fire the device, laying down four rows of staples, and incise for a distance of about 4 cm between the staples **(Fig. 32–7)**. This maneuver provides a tunnel of gastric mucosa about 4 cm in length, which is sufficient to pass through the abdominal wall. Reinforce the line of staples with a layer of continuous or interrupted 3-0 atraumatic PG seromuscular Lembert sutures to invert the staples **(Fig. 32–8)**.

Make a vertical incision about 1.5 cm long in the skin overlying the middle third of the left rectus muscle. Deepen the incision through the rectus muscle with the aid of electrocautery and then dilate it by inserting the index finger.

Grasp the gastric nipple and draw it to the outside by passing a Babcock clamp into the incision in the rectus muscle. This brings the gastric wall into contact with the anterior abdominal wall, to which it should be fixed with two Lembert sutures of 3-0 PG. Then transect the tip of the gastric nipple with Mayo scissors, leaving enough gastric tissue to reach the skin level. Insert an 18F catheter into the stomach to test the channel. Mature the gastrostomy with interrupted 3-0 PG sutures, which should pass through the entire thickness of the gastric nipple and catch the subcuticular layer of the skin.

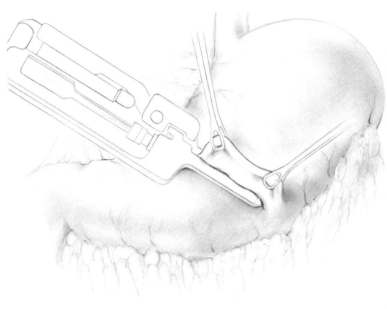

Fig. 32-6

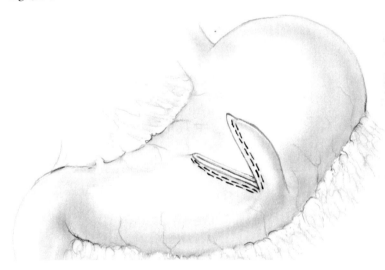

Fig. 32-7

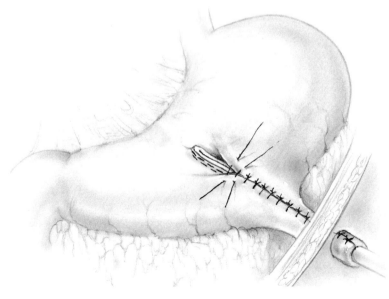

Fig. 32-8

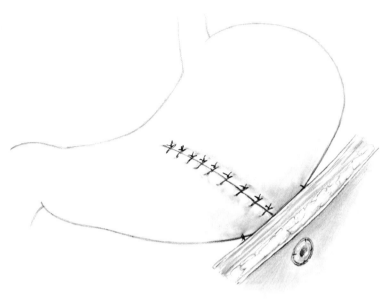

Fig. 32-9

Close the abdominal incision in the usual fashion and apply a sterile dressing **(Fig. 32–9)**. Leave the catheter in place until the wound heals.

After healing has taken place, gastric feeding can be started by inserting a catheter into the stomach while the nutrients are being administered. The catheter is removed between meals.

REFERENCES

Bergstrom LR, Larson DE, Zinsmeister AR, Sarr MG, Silverstein MD. Utilization and outcomes of surgical gastrostomies and jejunostomies in an era of percutaneous endoscopic gastrostomy: a population-based study. Mayo Clin Proc 1995;70:829.

Cosentini EP, Sautner T, Gnant M, et al. Outcomes of surgical, percutaneous endoscopic, and percutaneous radiologic gastrostomies. Arch Surg 1998;133:1076.

Duh QY, Senokozlieff-Englehart AL, Choe YS, et al. Laparoscopic gastrostomy and jejunostomy: safety and cost with local vs general anesthesia. Arch Surg 1999; 134:151.

Gadacz TR. Laparoscopic gastrostomy. In Scott-Conner CEH (ed) The SAGES Manual: Fundamentals of Laparoscopy and GI Endoscopy. New York, Springer-Verlag, 1999, pp 221-226.

Gauderer MW. Gastrostomy techniques and devices. Surg Clin North Am 1992;72:1285.

Molloy M, Ose KJ, Bower RH. Laparoscopic Janeway gastrostomy: an alternative to celiotomy for the management of a dislodged percutaneous gastrostomy. J Am Coll Surg 1997;185:187.

Murayama KM, Johnson TJ, Thompson JS. Laparoscopic gastrostomy and jejunostomy are safe and effective for obtaining enteral access. Am J Surg 1996;172:594.

33 Radical Subtotal Gastrectomy

INDICATIONS

Adenocarcinoma of the distal stomach

PREOPERATIVE PREPARATION

Endoscopic biopsy and ultrasonography.

Computed tomography and other imaging studies as appropriate to stage.

Nutritional rehabilitation by tube feeding when feasible or by total parenteral nutrition when indicated.

Mechanical and antibiotic bowel preparation. This is important for two reasons: (1) the stomach and necrotic tumor may be colonized by virulent bacteria; and (2) concomitant colon resection may be needed if the middle colic artery is involved with tumor.

Perioperative systemic antibiotics.

PITFALLS AND DANGER POINTS

Inadequate resection

Injury to pancreas, spleen

Ischemia of gastric pouch if splenectomy is performed

See Chapter 29

OPERATIVE STRATEGY

Extent of Resection

Radical subtotal gastrectomy is an en bloc resection designed to accomplish three things: (1) remove the distal stomach with adequate clean proximal and distal margins; (2) remove regional lymph nodes in continuity for staging and tumor control; and (3) in appropriate cases remove segments of adjacent organs

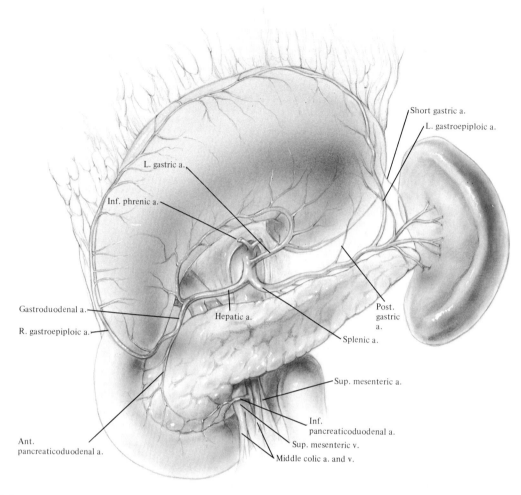

L. gastric a.

Inf. phrenic a.

Short gastric a.

L. gastroepiploic a.

Gastroduodenal a.

R. gastroepiploic a.

Hepatic a.

Post.
gastric
a.

Splenic a.

Sup. mesenteric a.

Inf.
pancreaticoduodenal a.

Sup. mesenteric v.

Ant.
pancreaticoduodenal a.

Middle colic a. and v.

Fig. 33-1

involved by direct extension. **Figure 33–1** shows the stomach lifted up to display the vascular anatomy, and **Figure 33–2** shows the regional anatomy to demonstrate the close proximity of the stomach to the pancreas, liver, and transverse mesocolon.

Frozen sections are helpful for evaluating *proximal and distal margins*. As with many gastrointestinal malignancies, gastric cancer may extend submucosally for several centimeters beyond the obvious tumor mass.

A common classification system for *gastric lymphadenectomy* uses the term R1 lymph node dissection for resection of lymph nodes in the immediate vicinity of the stomach (perigastric nodes). For distal cancers it would include nodes along vascular arcades that parallel the lesser curvature, greater curvature, and suprapyloric and infrapyloric areas. The more extensive R2 lymphadenectomy includes all of those nodes as well as the right cardiac, left gastric artery, celiac, and hepatic artery nodes. En bloc resection of the superior leaf of the transverse mesocolon and the pancreatic capsule is generally included.

For carcinomas located more proximally but still able to be encompassed by a subtotal gastrectomy, the R1 lymphadenectomy consists of right cardiac nodes as well as the previously mentioned lesser curvature, greater curvature, suprapyloric, and infrapyloric nodes removed during R1 dissection for more distal lesions. The R2 lymph node dissection for more proximal lesions adds the left cardiac, left gastric artery, hepatic artery, celiac, splenic hilar (optional), and splenic artery nodes to those previously listed (R1 for proximal lesions).

The technique described in this chapter removes the R1 and some of the R2 nodes, a common strategy employed in the United States. References at the end of the chapter give information about even more radical lymphadenectomies utilized by surgeons in other parts of the world where gastric cancer is more common.

Gastric cancer can involve any contiguous organ by *direct extension*. Generally such extension is obvious on the preoperative imaging studies, but the surgeon must be prepared to excise in continuity.

Posteriorly, the tumor can invade the body or tail of the pancreas, the middle colic artery, or the transverse colon, all of which can be included in the specimen. Invasion of the aorta contraindicates resection. Extension into the left lobe of the liver is amenable to resection, as is extension into the crura of the diaphragm. Generally survival is poor when extensive tumor dictates excision of adjacent organs.

For large carcinomas of the distal stomach, the left gastric artery may be ligated at its origin and included in the specimen, together with the nodes along the lesser curvature of the stomach and the lesser omentum. Hepatic artery node dissection down to the pylorus is included, together with any visible subpyloric and right gastric nodes and the lymph glands around the origin of the right gastroepiploic artery and the upper border of the pancreas. The spleen is not removed because the short gastric vessels provide the blood supply to the gastric pouch. Adjacent organs are included when there is evidence of direct invasion. Total gastrectomy is done if most of the lesser curve of the stomach is invaded.

Splenectomy or No Splenectomy

Splenectomy allows the most complete removal of splenic hilar lymph nodes and has been advocated to allow radical lymphadenectomy. It is distinctly unusual, however, for a resectable antral lesion to involve splenic and pancreatic lymph nodes. Consequently, it appears unnecessary to perform routine splenectomy for lesions of the distal stomach. A major drawback of including the spleen in a resection that also involves ligation of the left gastric artery *at its origin* is that ischemia or gangrene of the residual gastric pouch may develop. After left gastric ligation and division of the left gastroepiploic artery, the blood supply of the residual gastric pouch is limited. There is often a posterior gastric branch that arises from the splenic artery proximal to the origin of the left gastroepiploic artery. It is possible to preserve this artery if care is taken during the operation, but it is a small vessel and is easily traumatized. In addition, there are collateral branches from the inferior phrenic vessels and intramural circulation from the esophagus. Finally, concomitant splenectomy is associated with an increased risk of subphrenic abscess and other septic complications. Studies in the United States have shown no benefit and considerable associated morbidity from concomitant splenectomy.

Blood Supply to Residual Gastric Pouch

As mentioned above, whenever the left gastric artery is divided at its origin and splenectomy is performed, the blood supply to the gastric pouch may be inad-

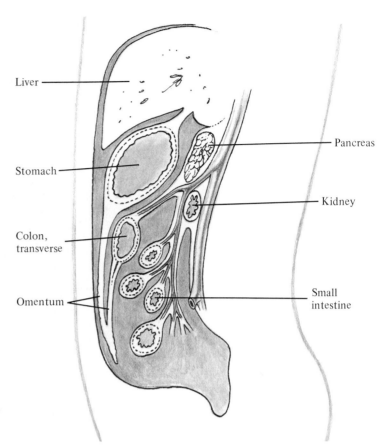

Fig. 33-2

equate. Thus one should avoid splenectomy in these cases unless so little gastric pouch is left behind that it may receive adequate nourishment through the intramural channels from the esophagus if the posterior gastric and inferior phrenic collaterals prove inadequate. If there is any doubt about the adequacy of the blood supply, perform a total gastrectomy.

Duct of Santorini

When carcinoma approaches the pyloric region, microscopic spread into the proximal 4-5 cm of the duodenum is possible. When as much as 5 cm of the duodenum is mobilized, the dissection has progressed beyond the gastroduodenal artery. In this area there is a risk that the duct of Santorini will be transected. Because the duodenal wall is free of inflammation in cases of this type, this structure may well be identifiable, in which case it should be divided and ligated. If the duct of Santorini communicates with the duct of Wirsung, the pancreatic juice then drains freely into the larger duct, and there should be no postoperative difficulty. In some cases the duct of Santorini does not communicate with the main duct, in which event, despite the ligature, a pancreatic fistula may

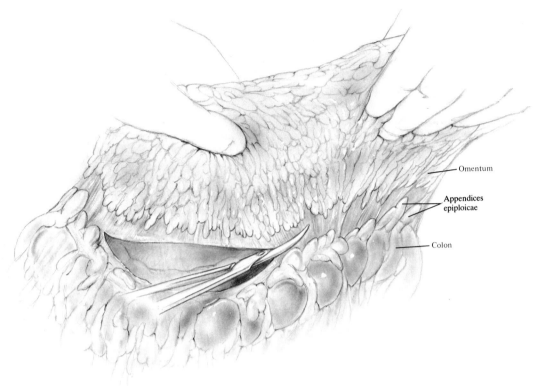

Fig. 33-3

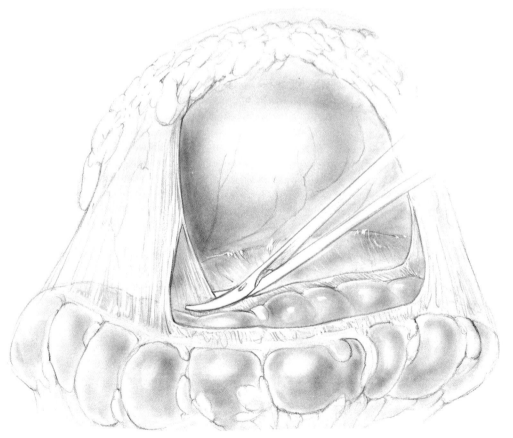

Fig. 33-4

well develop. This situation probably requires a secondary operation to anastomose a Roux-en-Y segment of the jejunum to the transected duct for internal drainage. Fortunately, in most cases the two ducts do communicate.

OPERATIVE TECHNIQUE

Incision and Exposure

An upper midline incision extending from the xiphoid to several centimeters below the umbilicus gives good exposure for this procedure. Place an Upper Hand or Thompson retractor to elevate the lower sternum.

Resection

Radical subtotal gastrectomy differs from gastrectomy for peptic ulcer disease in terms of the dissection and the extent of resection. The reconstruction is essentially the same and is not repeated here.

Begin with a thorough exploration of the abdomen. Metastatic disease not detected on preoperative imaging studies does not preclude resection for palliation in selected patients. Evaluate the location and mobility of the tumor; determine whether adjacent structures must be resected or if a total gastrectomy (see Chapter 34) is more appropriate.

Omentectomy

Separate the entire gastrocolic omentum from the transverse colon by scalpel and scissors dissection through the avascular embryonic fusion plane, as seen in the coronal section of the abdomen in Figure 33-2. Be alert to the difference in texture and color of the fat in the epiploic appendices of the colon and that of the omentum. Considerable bleeding can be avoided by keeping the plane of dissection between the appendices and the omentum **(Fig. 33–3)**. Next elevate the omentum from the transverse mesocolon **(Fig. 33–4)**. Take care to avoid damage to the mesocolon and middle colic artery. Expose the anterior surfaces of the pancreas and duodenum, along with the origin of the right gastroepiploic vessels. Ligate the latter at their origin with 2-0 silk and divide them, sweeping all adjacent lymph nodes toward the specimen **(Fig. 33–5)**.

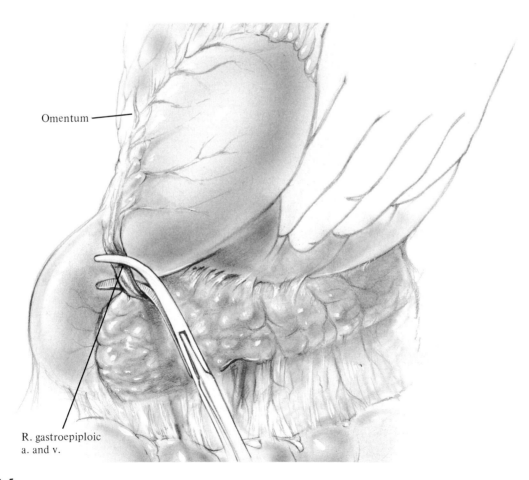

Omentum

R. gastroepiploic
a. and v.

Fig. 33-5

Celiac Axis Dissection and Division of Left Gastric Vessels

With the greater curvature of the stomach elevated and retracted toward the patient's right, it is a simple matter to palpate the left gastric artery as it travels from the region of the aorta, anteriorly, to meet the lesser curvature of the stomach. When there is tumor in this area, the splenic or hepatic artery may be followed in a proximal direction. It leads to the celiac axis and to the origin of the left gastric artery. By dissecting the areolar and lymphatic tissue away, the artery may be skeletonized **(Fig. 33–6)**. A blunt-tipped Mixter right-angle clamp is helpful for delineating the circumference of the artery. Use the clamp to pass 2-0 silk ligatures around the vessel. After it has

been double-ligated, divide it. The coronary vein, which is situated just caudal to the artery, often is identified first during the course of the dissection. It too should be divided and ligated and the lymphatic tissue swept toward the specimen. At the conclusion of this step, the superior border of the adjacent pancreas and the anterior surface of the celiac axis and the aorta should be free of lymphatic tissue.

Hepatic Artery Node Dissection

Make an incision in the peritoneum overlying the common hepatic artery as it leaves the celiac axis. Carry this incision down to the origin of the gastroduodenal artery. Lymph nodes overlie the hepatic artery; dissect them toward the lesser curve of the

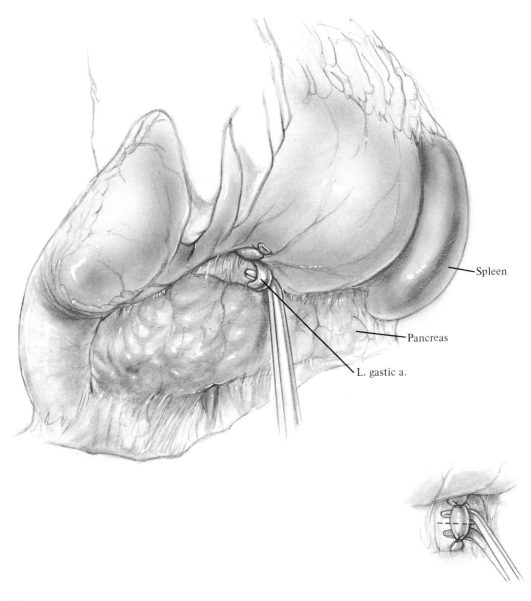

Spleen

Pancreas

L. gastic a.

Fig. 33-6

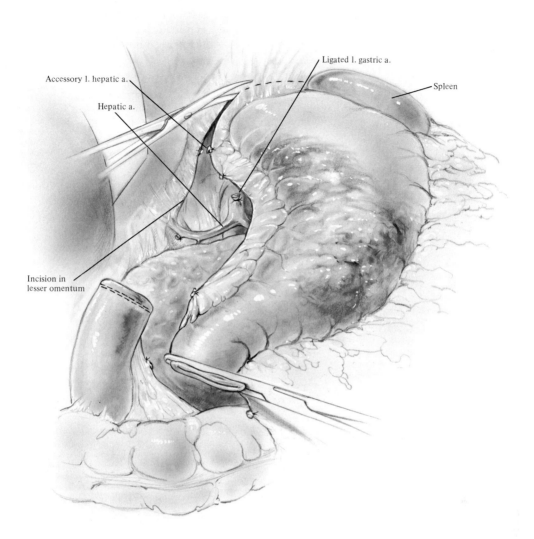

Accessory l. hepatic a.

Hepatic a.

Ligated l. gastric a.

Spleen

Incision in lesser omentum

Fig. 33-7

gastric specimen, leaving the artery skeletonized (**Fig. 33–7**). If desirable, the lymph node dissection may be pursued to the hilus of the liver by skeletonizing the hepatic artery, portal vein, and common bile duct. Adequate data are not yet available to indicate how extensive the lymph node dissection should be.

Suspicious nodes in the subpyloric region and the superior margin of the pancreas are excised and the splenic artery skeletonized up to the distal end of the pancreas.

Division of Duodenum

Divide and ligate the right gastric artery. Perform a Kocher maneuver and dissect the duodenum from the anterior surface of the pancreas for a distance of 5 cm. If a stapled closure of the duodenum is elected,

apply the 55/4.8 mm linear stapler to the duodenal stump. Fire the stapler and apply an Allen clamp to the specimen side of the duodenum. Divide the duodenum flush with the stapling device, as in Figure 29-43. Ligate the distal end of the specimen with umbilical tape behind the Allen clamp and remove the clamp. Cover the distal end of the specimen with a sterile rubber glove, which is fixed in place with an additional umbilical tape ligature. When it is elected to suture the duodenal stump, follow the technique illustrated in Figures 29-20 through 29-22.

With the additional mobility thus attained, reassess the extent of the tumor and plan a line of resection along the greater and lesser curvatures. The usual radical subtotal gastrectomy encompasses approximately 80% of the stomach, leaving a small gastric remnant. An 8- to 10-cm margin beyond the tumor is advisable.

In some cases it requires hand-tailoring the Hofmeister shelf rather than using the standard stapling technique described in Chapter 30. If it does not appear possible to preserve a small gastric remnant and still obtain a good proximal margin, proceed with total gastrectomy (see Chapter 34).

Reconstruction is generally by antecolic Billroth II anastomosis, as shown in Figures 29–34 through 29–36. No drains are placed.

POSTOPERATIVE CARE

Postoperative care is identical to that following gastrectomy for peptic ulcer (see Chapter 29). Enteral or total parenteral nutrition is added to the regimen when indicated.

COMPLICATIONS

Complications are similar to those following gastrectomy for peptic ulcer (see Chapter 29), but subphrenic and subhepatic sepsis is more common because of the increased bacterial contamination associated with carcinoma.

REFERENCES

Bonenkamp JJ, Hermans J, Sasako M, van de Velde CJ. Extended lymph-node dissection for gastric cancer: Dutch Gastric Cancer Group. N Engl J Med 1999;340:908.

Bozzetti F, Marubini E, Bonfanti G, et al. Subtotal versus total gastrectomy for gastric cancer: five year survival rates in a multicenter randomized Italian trial: Italian Gastrointestinal Tumor Study Group. Ann Surg 1999; 230:170.

Harrison LE, Karpeh MS, Brennan MF. Total gastrectomy is not necessary for proximal gastric cancer. Surgery 1998;123:127.

Kasukura Y, Fujii M, Mochizuki F, Kochi M, Kaiga T. Is there a benefit of pancreaticosplenectomy with gastrectomy for advanced gastric cancer? Am J Surg 2000; 179:237.

Maehara Y, Hasuda S, Koga T, et al. Postoperative outcome and sites of recurrence in patients following curative resection of gastric cancer. Br J Surg 2000;87:353.

Roukos DH, Lorenz M, Encke A. Evidence of survival benefit of extended (D2) lymphadenectomy in Western patients with gastric cancer based on a new concept: a prospective long-term follow-up study. Surgery 1998; 123:573.

Siewert JR, Bottcher K, Stein HJ, Roder JD. Relevant prognostic factors in gastric cancer: ten-year results of the German Gastric Cancer Study. Ann Surg 1998;228:449.

Smith JW, Brennan MF. Surgical treatment of gastric cancer: proximal, mid, and distal stomach. Surg Clin North Am 1992;72:381.

Wanebo HJ, Kennedy BJ, Winchester DP, Stewart AK, Fremgen AM. Role of splenectomy in gastric cancer surgery: adverse effect of elective splenectomy on long term survival. J Am Coll Surg 1997;185:177.

Yoo CH, Noh SH, Shin DW, Choi SH, Min JS. Recurrence following curative resection for gastric carcinoma. Br J Surg 2000;87:236.

34 Total Gastrectomy

INDICATIONS

Zollinger-Ellison syndrome

Adenocarcinoma of the stomach

Gastric leiomyosarcoma or other malignancy

Life-threatening hemorrhage from extensive erosive gastritis (rarely)

PREOPERATIVE PREPARATION

See Chapter 33.

PITFALLS AND DANGER POINTS

Improper reconstruction of alimentary tract, which can lead to postoperative reflux alkaline esophagitis.

Erroneous diagnosis of malignancy. Patients have undergone total gastrectomy when surgeons have misdiagnosed a large posterior penetrating ulcer as a malignant tumor. Because benign gastric ulcer can be cured by relatively simple surgery, this error may have serious consequences for the patient. If preoperative gastroscopic biopsy has been negative, perform a gastrotomy and with a scalpel or a biopsy punch obtain a direct biopsy of the edge of ulcer in four quadrants.

Inadequate anastomotic technique, resulting in leak or stricture.

Sepsis in wound or subhepatic and subphrenic spaces due to contamination by gastric contents.

Failure to identify submucosal infiltration of carcinoma in the esophagus or duodenum beyond the line of resection.

OPERATIVE STRATEGY

Exposure

If the primary lesion is a malignancy of the body of the stomach that does not invade the lower esophagus, a midline incision from the xiphocostal junction to a point 6–8 cm below the umbilicus may prove adequate for total gastrectomy if the Upper Hand or Thompson retractor is used to elevate the lower sternum. If the tumor is approaching the esophagogastric junction, it may be necessary to include 6–10 cm of lower esophagus in the specimen to circumvent submucosal infiltration by the tumor. In this case a left thoracoabdominal incision is indicated, as described in Chapter 12. Never attempt to construct an esophageal anastomosis without excellent exposure.

Esophageal Anastomosis

We prefer an end-to-side esophagojejunal anastomosis because it permits invagination of the esophagus into the jejunum, which in turn results in a lower incidence of leakage. With end-to-end esophagojejunostomy, invagination would result in constriction of the lumen.

The lumen of the anastomosis can be further increased if the anterior wall of the esophagus is left 1 cm longer than the posterior wall. This converts the anastomosis from a circular shape to an elliptical one, adding to its circumference.

Prevention of Reflux Alkaline Esophagitis

An anastomosis between the end of the esophagus and the side of the jejunum combined with a side-to-side

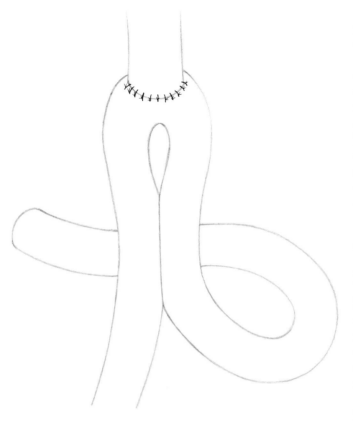

Fig. 34-1

jejunojejunostomy **(Fig. 34–1)** results in a high incidence of *disabling* postoperative alkaline esophagitis. *This must be prevented by utilizing the Roux-en-Y principle in all cases.* The distance between the esophagojejunal anastomosis and the jejunojejunal anastomosis must be 60 cm or more to prevent reflux of the duodenal contents into the esophagus. This is a far more important consideration than is construction of a jejunal pouch for a reservoir, and we no longer create such a pouch in these cases.

Extent of the Operation

See Chapter 33.

Microscopic submucosal infiltration may occur in the esophagus as far as 10 cm proximal to a grossly visible tumor and occasionally well down into the duodenum. Frozen section microscopic examination of both the esophageal and duodenal ends of the specimen should be obtained to avoid leaving behind residual submucosal carcinoma.

The lymph nodes along the celiac axis should be swept up with the specimen when the left gastric artery is divided at its origin. The lymphatics along the hepatic artery also should be removed, along with those at the origin of the right gastroepiploic artery. Whether it is beneficial to skeletonize the he-

patic artery and portal vein all the way to the hilus of the liver is not clear.

Routine resection of the body and tail of the pancreas may increase the mortality rate from this operation because pancreatic complications can occur; at the same time it has not been proved that this additional step improves a patient's long-term survival. However, if the tail of the pancreas shows evidence of tumor invasion, this portion of the pancreas should certainly be included in resection. The anatomy of the structures involved in this operation can be seen in Figure 33-1.

OPERATIVE TECHNIQUE

Incision and Exposure

In many cases adequate exposure is obtained by a midline incision from the xiphocostal junction to a point 6 cm below the umbilicus, along with the use of an Upper Hand or Thompson retractor. When the carcinoma involves the lower esophagus, a left thoracoabdominal approach should be used.

Exploration and Determination of Operability

Tumors are considered nonresectable when there is posterior invasion of the aorta, vena cava, or celiac axis. Invasion of the body or tail of the pancreas is not a contraindication to operation; nor is invasion of the left lobe of the liver, as these structures can be included in the specimen if necessary.

When there is only a moderate degree of distant metastasis in the presence of an extensive tumor, a palliative resection is indicated *if it can be done safely.*

Invasion of the root of the mesocolon, including the middle colic artery, does not contraindicate resection if leaving these structures attached to the specimen removes the tumor. This often requires concomitant resection of a segment of the transverse colon. It is surprising that in some patients removing a short segment of the main middle colic artery does not impair the viability of the transverse colon so long as there is good collateral circulation.

Omentectomy, Lymph Node Dissection, and Division of Duodenum

The initial steps are performed as described in Chapter 33. The dissection begins with a complete omentectomy, ligation of the right gastroepiploic vessels at their origin, and division of the duodenum. The lesser omentum is followed up to the left gastric

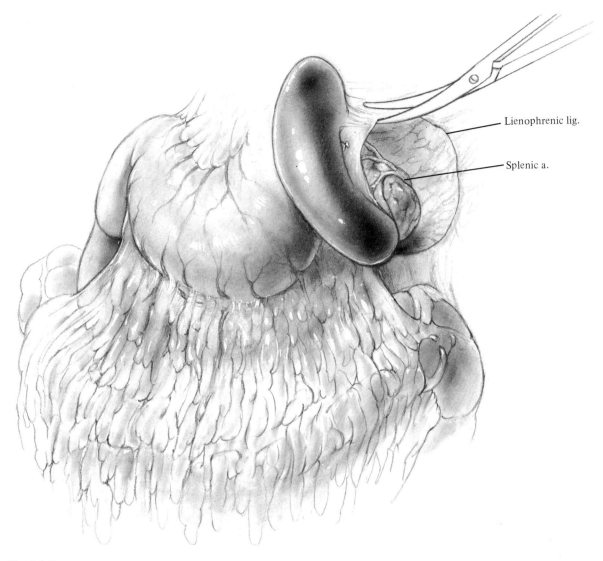

Lienophrenic lig.

Splenic a.

Fig. 34–2

artery, which is ligated at its origin. Nodal tissue is removed with the lesser omentum. If splenectomy is planned, it is frequently done as the first step.

Splenectomy

Splenectomy is performed only when tumor encroaches on the spleen or splenic hilum. With a scalpel or Metzenbaum scissors incise the avascular lienophrenic ligament that attaches the lateral aspect of the spleen to the undersurface of the diaphragm (Fig. 34–2). As this incision reaches the inferior pole of the spleen, divide the lienocolic ligament; the posterior surface of the pancreatic tail can then be seen. The tail can be elevated gently from the retroperitoneal space. Palpate the splenic artery near the distal end of the pancreas, encircle it with 2-0 silk, and ligate it and the splenic vein. Divide these vessels

between ligatures, releasing the tip of the pancreas from the hilus of the spleen. Incise a fold of posterior parietal peritoneum along the upper border of the body of the pancreas to separate the pancreas from the specimen. The spleen may be left attached to the greater curvature of the stomach, or it may be more convenient to divide and ligate the short gastric vessels and remove the spleen as a separate specimen. For the retroperitoneal dissection, expose the fascia of Gerota and the left adrenal gland. If there is evidence of tumor invasion, include these structures in the specimen.

Dissection of the Esophagocardiac Junction: Vagotomy

After the triangular ligament has been divided, retract the left lobe of the liver to the patient's right and incise the peritoneum overlying the abdominal esophagus. Using a peanut dissector, dissect the esophagus away from the right and left branches of the diaphragmatic crux. Then encircle the esophagus with the index finger and perform a bilateral truncal vagotomy, as described in Chapter 25. Incise the peritoneum overlying the right crux (see Fig. 33-7). Identify the cephalad edge of the gastrohepatic ligament, which contains an accessory left hepatic branch of the left gastric artery. Divide this structure between clamps at a point close to the liver, completing division of the gastrohepatic ligament.

Pass the left hand behind the esophagocardiac junction, a maneuver that delineates the avascular gastrophrenic and any remaining esophagophrenic

ligaments, all of which should be divided **(Fig. 34–3)**, freeing the posterior wall of the stomach. To minimize further spill of neoplastic cells into the esophageal lumen, occlude the esophagogastric junction with umbilical tape or staples applied with the 55 mm linear stapler.

Preparation of Roux-en-Y Jejunal Segment

After identifying the ligament of Treitz, elevate the proximal jejunum from the abdominal cavity and inspect the mesentery to determine how it can reach the apex of the abdominal cavity for the esophagojejunal anastomosis. In some patients who have lost considerable weight before the operation, the je-

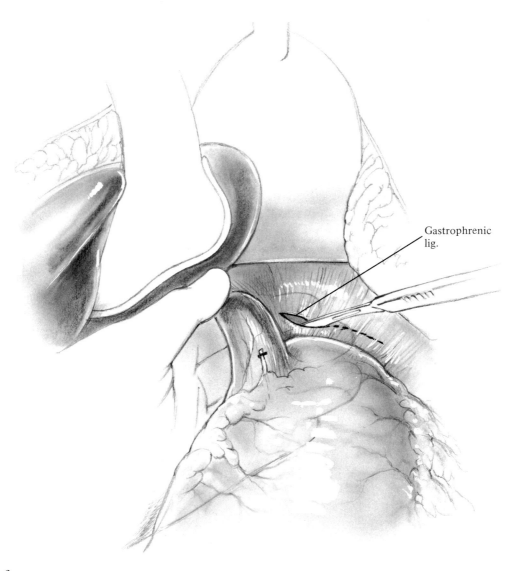

Gastrophrenic lig.

Fig. 34-3

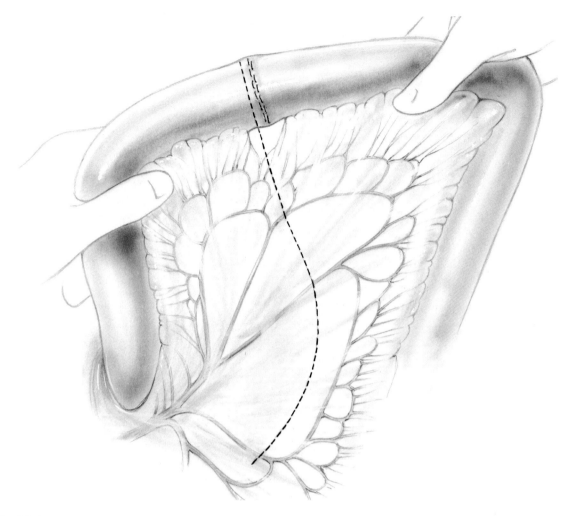

Fig. 34-4

junum reaches the esophagus without the need to divide anything but the marginal artery. In patients whose jejunal mesentery is short, it may be necessary to divide several arcade vessels. Transillumination is a valuable aid for dissecting the mesentery without undue trauma.

Generally, the point of division of the jejunum is about 15 cm distal to the ligament of Treitz, between the second and third arcade vessels. Make an incision in the mesentery across the marginal vessels and divide and ligate them with 3-0 silk. Divide and ligate one to three additional arcade vessels to provide an adequate length of the jejunum to reach the esophagus without tension **(Fig. 34-4)**.

Apply a 55/3.5 mm linear stapler to the point on the jejunum previously selected for division. Fire the stapler. Apply an Allen clamp just proximal to the stapler and divide the jejunum flush with the stapler.

Lightly electrocauterize the everted edge and remove the stapler.

Next make a 3- to 4-cm incision in the avascular portion of the transverse mesocolon to the left of the middle colic artery. Deliver the stapled end of the jejunum through the incision in the mesocolon to the region of the esophagus. After the jejunal segment is properly positioned, suture the defect in the mesocolon to the wall of the jejunum to prevent herniation later.

End-to-Side Sutured Esophagojejunostomy

The anticipated site of the esophageal transection is 6–10 cm above the proximal margin of the visible tumor. If the diaphragmatic hiatus is excessively large, narrow it with one or two 2-0 silk sutures **(Fig.**

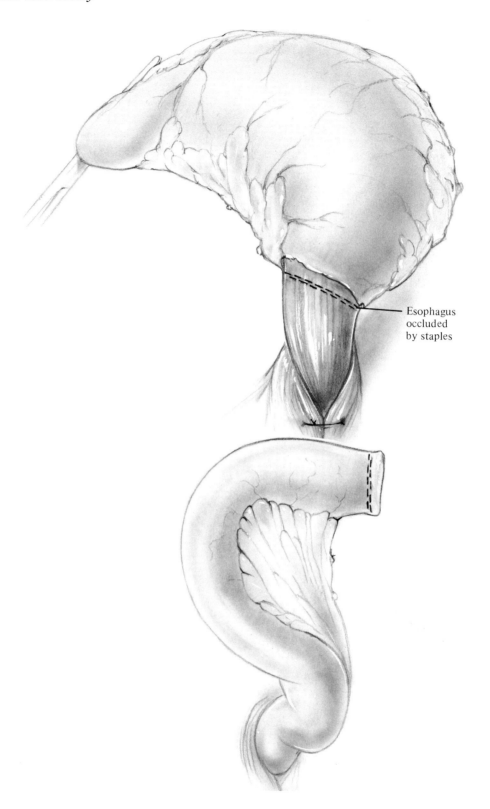

Esophagus
occluded
by staples

Fig. 34-5

34–5). Then insert several interrupted 3-0 silk sutures between the undersurface of the diaphragm and the posterior wall of the jejunum to prevent tension on the anastomosis caused by gravity. The sutures should be placed in the jejunum sufficiently posterior to preserve the antimesenteric border for anastomosis.

Before beginning to construct the anastomosis, mark the exact site of the anticipated jejunal incision by making a scratch with a scalpel along the antimesenteric border of the jejunum. This serves as a guide for inserting the first layer of esophagojejunal sutures. Then place the specimen on the patient's chest, which exposes the posterior wall of the esophagus for the first layer of anastomotic sutures. Place a 4-0 atraumatic silk Cushing suture beginning at the right lateral portion of the esophagus. With the same needle take a bite at the right lateral margin of the jejunal scratch mark. Place a similar suture at the left lateral margins of the esophagus and jejunum. Apply

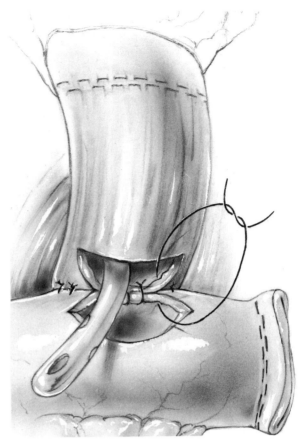

Fig. 34-7

hemostats to each suture, as none is tied until the suture line has been completed **(Fig. 34–6).** Note that the anticipated incision in the jejunum is slightly longer than the diameter of the esophagus.

With three or four additional Cushing sutures of 4-0 silk, complete the posterior seromuscular layer of the anastomosis by successive bisection (see Figs. 4-19, 4-20). After inserting the sutures but before tying them, it is helpful to divide the posterior wall of the esophagus. Do this in a transverse manner, using a scalpel, until the mucosa has been transacted. Complete the incision with Metzenbaum scissors, leaving the anterior wall of the esophagus intact. Now tie and cut the sutures but leave the right and left lateralmost sutures long, with the identifying hemostats attached.

Make an incision in the antimesenteric border of the jejunum, as previously marked. Excise redundant mucosa if necessary. Control excessive bleeding with 4-0 PG suture-ligatures or careful electrocoagulation. Now approximate the posterior mucosal layers by interrupted sutures of atraumatic 5-0 Vicryl, with the knots tied inside the lumen **(Fig. 34–7).** Instruct the anesthesiologist to pass the nasogastric tube farther down the esophagus. When the tube appears in the esophageal orifice, guide it down the jejunum.

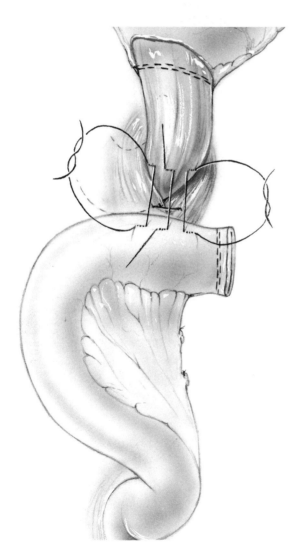

Fig. 34-6

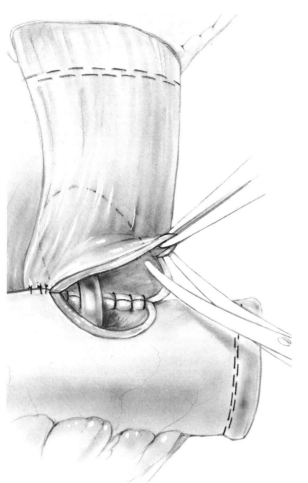

Fig. 34-8

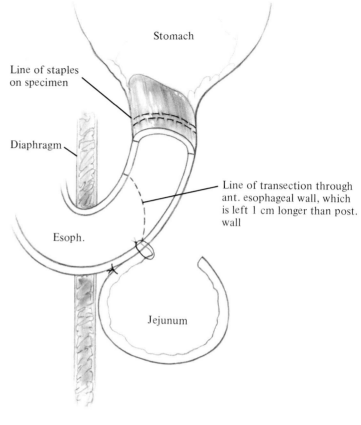

Stomach

Line of staples
on specimen

Diaphragm

Esoph.

Jejunum

Line of transection through
ant. esophageal wall, which
is left 1 cm longer than post.
wall

Fig. 34-9

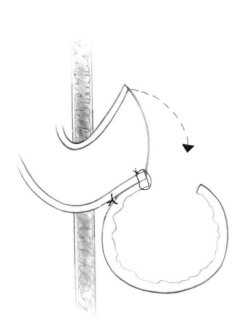

Fig. 34-10

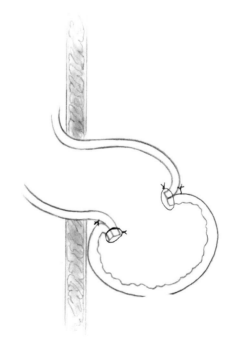

Fig. 34-11

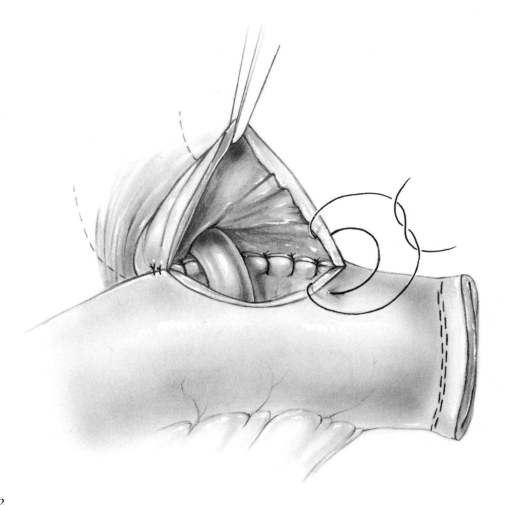

Fig. 34-12

Divide the remaining esophagus so the anterior wall is 1 cm longer than the already anastomosed posterior wall **(Figs. 34–8, 34–9, 34–10, 34–11)**. Remove the specimen and ask the pathologist to perform a frozen section examination of both the proximal and distal margins. If the frozen section examination is positive for malignancy, further excision is indicated.

Approximate and invert the anterior mucosal layer by 5-0 Vicryl sutures, interrupted, with the knots tied inside the lumen **(Fig. 34–12)**. If it is difficult to invert the mucosa by this technique, the procedure may be accomplished with interrupted "seromucosal" sutures of 5-0 Vicryl, 4–5 mm wide, inserted to include the cut end of the esophageal muscularis and mucosa (Fig. 4-13).

Complete the final anastomotic layer by inserting interrupted 4-0 silk Cushing sutures to approximate the outer layers of the esophagus and jejunum **(Fig. 34–13)**. Each suture should encompass a bite of about 5 mm of esophagus and jejunum. The peritoneum overlying the diaphragmatic hiatus can now be brought down over the anastomosis. Attach it to the

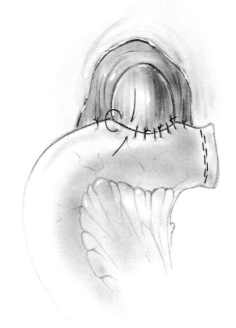

Fig. 34-13

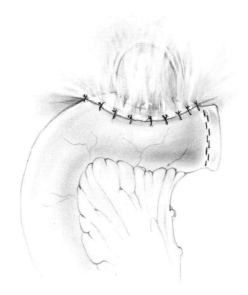

Fig. 34-14

anterior wall of the jejunum by several interrupted 4-0 silk stitches **(Fig. 34–14)**. A sagittal section of the completed anastomosis is seen in **Figure 34–15**.

On occasion the esophagus appears to be unusually narrow secondary to spasm or atrophy. In this case *gentle* digital dilatation by the surgeon before constructing the anastomosis may accomplish a somewhat larger anastomotic lumen than would otherwise be the case. If desired, it is possible to perform the anastomosis over a 40F Hurst or Maloney esophageal bougie instead of the nasogastric tube.

End-to-Side Stapled Esophagojejunostomy

An end-to-side esophagojejunostomy performed with a circular stapler requires easy access to 4–5 cm of relaxed esophagus with good exposure to en-

able the surgeon to inspect the anastomosis carefully at its conclusion. After the esophagus has been transected and the specimen removed, insert a guy suture of 3-0 silk in each of the four quadrants of the esophagus, going through all layers. Attach a hemostat to each suture. Then insert a purse-string suture of 2-0 Prolene no more than 3–4 mm proximal to the cut edge of the esophagus. Attach a hemostat to the completed purse-string suture. Now check the diameter of the esophagus by first gently dilating it with the middle finger or thumb. Then gently insert the smallest lubricated sizer. Vigorous attempts to dilate the esophagus would result in a tear along the mucosa. It may require resecting considerably more esophagus than is convenient. It is not wise to try to repair a tear of this type and use the damaged tissue for an anastomosis. For this reason, be gentle during dilatation. If the sizer does not enter the esophagus readily, convert to a sutured anastomosis as described above. We prefer to use a 28- or 31-mm cartridge when possible. In a patient who has suffered from chronic esophagogastric obstruction, the esophagus may well admit the larger cartridge.

Bring the previously prepared Roux-en-Y segment of jejunum and pass it through an incision in the avascular part of the transverse mesocolon. The jejunum should easily reach the esophagus with 6–7 cm to spare. Gently dilate the lumen of the jejunum and in-

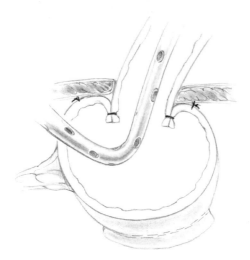

Fig. 34-15

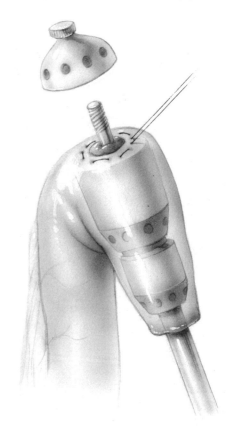

Fig. 34-16

sert the lubricated cartridge of the circular stapler into the open end of the jejunum, as in **Figure 34–16**. Remove the anvil from the cartridge before inserting it into the jejunum. Make a small incision over the rod of the stapler through the elbow of the jejunum so the rod can penetrate the antimesenteric border of the jejunum. Then insert a 2-0 Prolene purse-string suture around this rod and tie the suture.

Have the assistants grasp the four guy sutures and gently stretch the opening of the esophagus by applying mild traction. This loosens the purse-string suture. Gently insert the well lubricated anvil into the lumen of the esophagus and tie the purse-string suture as illustrated in **Figure 34–17**. With most stapling devices this is most easily done before reattaching the anvil to the stapler. Reattach the anvil to the device and be certain the screw is tight. Now turn the screw at the base of the stapler so the anvil is approximated to the cartridge. When this has been completed, fire the device by pulling the trigger. Then turn the wing nut the appropriate number of turns counterclockwise, rotate the device, and ma-

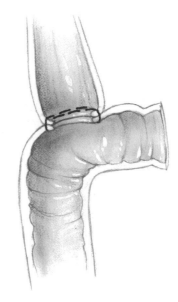

Fig. 34-18

nipulate the anvil in such fashion as to withdraw the stapler from the anastomosis. At this point it is important to insert the index finger into the open end of the jejunum **(Fig. 34–18)**. The index finger should go easily through the anastomosis into the esophagus and in a caudal direction into the distal jejunum. If this finger exploration is satisfactory, apply a 55/3.5 mm linear stapler to the jejunum, as seen in **Figure 34–19**. Apply the stapler at a point

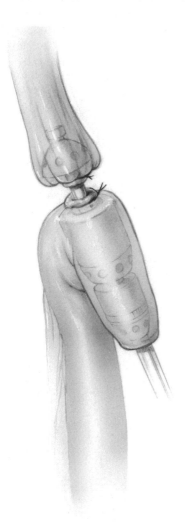

Fig. 34-17

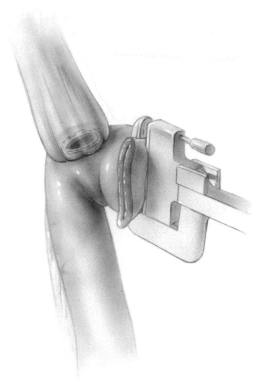

Fig. 34-19

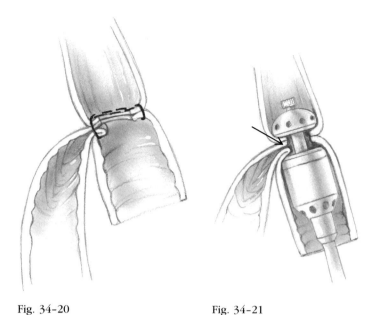

Fig. 34-20   Fig. 34-21

about 1–2 cm away from the anastomosis. Close the jaws of the linear stapler and fire it. Then amputate the redundant jejunum and lightly electrocauterize the exposed mucosa. It is important to amputate the jejunum close to the anastomosis so no blind loop develops.

If the finger exploration was not satisfactory, and the index finger goes from the open end of the jejunum directly into the esophagus but cannot enter the distal jejunum, as shown in **Figure 34–20**, the surgeon has committed the error of permitting the shoulder of the cartridge to carry the left wall of the jejunum **(Fig. 34–21)** along with it so it is enclosed within the anastomosis, thus totally occluding the entrance into the efferent limb of the jejunum. This serious error can be prevented if the surgeon closely observes the passage of the cartridge, as shown in Figure 34-16, to be certain it slides past the side wall of the jejunum to abut the antimesenteric border completely. If such an error was made, the anastomosis must be repeated.

Roux-en-Y Jejunojejunostomy

Sutured Version

Attention should now be directed to restoring the continuity of the small intestine by doing an end-to-side anastomosis between the cut end of the proximal jejunum and the side of the Roux-en-Y limb. This anastomosis should be made 60 cm from the esophagojejunal anastomosis to prevent bile reflux. After the proper site on the antimesenteric border of jejunum has been selected, make a longitudinal scratch mark with a scalpel. Use interrupted 4-0 silk Lembert sutures for the posterior seromuscular layer of the end-to-side anastomosis **(Fig. 34–22)**. When all these sutures have been placed, make an incision along the previously marked area of the jejunum and remove the Allen clamp from the proximal segment of the jejunum. Approximate the mucosal layers using 4-0 chromic catgut or PG double-armed with straight needles **(Fig. 34–23)**. Take the first stitch in the middle of the posterior layer and tie it. Close the remainder of the posterior mucosal layer with a continuous locked suture **(Fig. 34–24)**. Approxi-

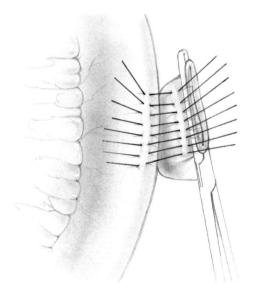

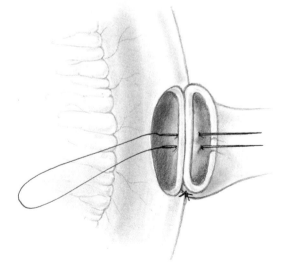

Fig. 34-22   Fig. 34-23

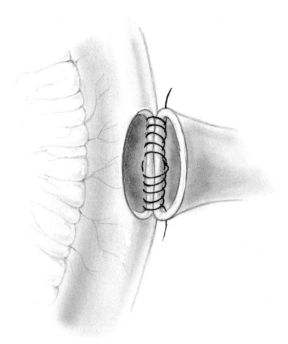

Fig. 34-24

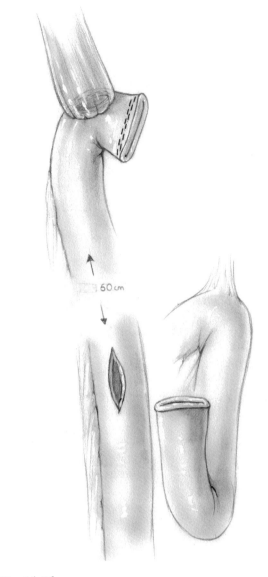

mate the anterior mucosal layer with a continuous suture of either the Connell or Cushing type. Then close the final anterior seromuscular layer with interrupted 4-0 silk Lembert sutures **(Fig. 34–25)**. Test the lumen by invaginating the jejunum with the index finger.

Stapled Version

In most cases, we prefer to perform the Roux-en-Y jejunojejunostomy with a stapling technique. To ac-

Fig. 34-26

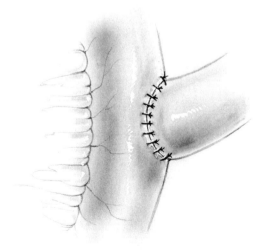

complish this, the proximal segment of the jejunum is approximated to the Roux-en-Y limb. With electrocautery make a 1.5 cm longitudinal incision on the antimesenteric border. Insert a linear cutting stapling device: one fork in the descending segment of the jejunum and the other fork in the open end of the proximal segment of the jejunum **(Fig. 34–26)**. Be certain the *open end of the proximal segment of jejunum is placed so the opening faces in a cephalad direction.* If the limbs of the jejunum are not joined in this manner, there is increased risk of narrowing the lumen of the jejunum. When the sta-

Fig. 34-25

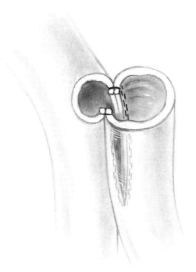

Fig. 34-27

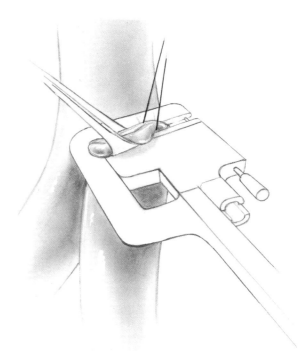

Fig. 34-29

pler is in place, lock it and fire; it can be seen that the first layer of the anastomosis has been completed in a side-to-side fashion between the antimesenteric borders of the two segments of the jejunum (**Fig. 34–27**).

To close the remaining defect in the anastomosis, apply Allis clamps to the right- and left-hand terminations of the staple line. Insert a guy suture into the midpoint of the remaining defect on the proximal segment of the jejunum and pass it through the midpoint of the defect on the distal segment of the jejunum (**Fig. 34–28**). When the guy suture approximates these two points, apply Allis clamps to

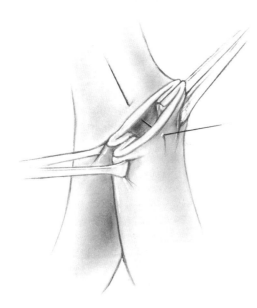

Fig. 34-28

the right side of the defect to approximate the two segments of the jejunum in an everting fashion. Complete this part of the anastomosis by applying and firing the TA-55 stapling device deep to the Allis clamps and the guy suture (**Fig. 34–29**). Excise the redundant mucosa flush with the stapling device but preserve the guy suture. Lightly electrocoagulate the everted mucosa.

Use Allis clamps again to close the remaining defect and apply the 55/3.5 mm linear stapler once more deep to the Allis clamps and the guy suture. When the stapler is fired and the redundant mucosa excised, the anastomosis is complete. It can be seen that the lumen is quite large (**Fig. 34–30**). Close the remaining potential defects between the mesentery of the proximal and distal jejunum with interrupted sutures of 4-0 silk to prevent herniation.

Modifications of Operative Technique for Patients with Zollinger-Ellison Syndrome or Benign Disease

When total gastrectomy is being performed for the Zollinger-Ellison syndrome or benign disease, several modifications are indicated. First, it is not necessary to excise considerable lengths of the esophagus or duodenum. These structures are divided close to the margins of the stomach. Second, it is

we do not insert drains in the abdominal cavity. Otherwise, a 6 mm Silastic Jackson-Pratt catheter may be brought out from the vicinity of the anastomosis through a puncture wound in the abdominal wall and attached to closed-suction drainage.

POSTOPERATIVE CARE

Administer nasogastric suction for 3–4 days.

Administer perioperative antibiotics.

Administer enteral feedings by way of the needle catheter jejunostomy (if placed) after the patient recovers from anesthesia.

As with other esophageal anastomoses, nothing should be permitted by mouth until the seventh postoperative day, at which time an esophagram should be obtained in the radiography department. If no leakage is identified, a liquid diet is initiated that may be increased rapidly according to the patient's tolerance.

Long-term postoperative management requires all patients to be on a dietary regimen that counteracts dumping. The diet should be high in protein and fat but low in carbohydrate and liquids. Frequent small feedings are indicated. Liquids should not be consumed during or 1–2 hours after meals to prevent hyperosmolarity in the lumen of the proximal jejunum. Some patients require several months of repeated encouragement to establish adequate caloric intake following total gastrectomy. Others seem to do well with no dietary restrictions.

Dietary supplements of vitamins, iron, and calcium as well as continued parenteral injections of vitamin B_{12} are necessary for long-term management of patients following total gastrectomy.

COMPLICATIONS

Sepsis of the abdominal wound or the subphrenic space is one complication that follows surgery for an ulcerated gastric malignancy. Early diagnosis and management are necessary.

Leakage from the esophagojejunal anastomosis is the most serious postoperative complication but occurs rarely if proper technique has been used. A minor degree of leakage may be managed by prompt institution of adequate drainage in the region, supplemented every 8 hours by injecting 15 ml of saline with suitable antibiotics through the drainage catheter. A nasogastric tube of the sump type should be passed to a point just proximal to

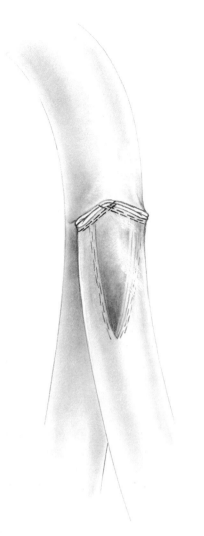

Fig. 34-30

not necessary to remove the spleen or omentum, and the greater curvature dissection can be carried out by dividing each of the vasa brevia between the greater curvature of the stomach and the greater omentum, leaving the omentum behind. Third, dissection of the lymph nodes in the region of the celiac axis, hepatic artery, and pancreas is not indicated. Except for the foregoing modifications, the technique is essentially the same as for cancer operations; however, the incidence of postoperative complications is far lower in patients with Zollinger-Ellison syndrome.

Wound Closure

Irrigate the abdominal cavity with saline. Consider placing a needle-catheter jejunostomy in malnourished patients. If hemostasis is excellent and the anastomoses have been performed with accuracy,

the esophagojejunal anastomosis for continuous suction. Nutritional support is essential, as are systemic antibiotics. In more serious cases, a diverting cervical esophagostomy may be required. Fortunately, a properly performed Roux-en-Y anastomosis diverts duodenal and pancreatic enzymes from the leak. If the Roux-en-Y technique has not been used, exteriorization of the jejunal segment, temporary occlusion of the distal esophagus, and cervical esophagostomy become necessary to control the septic process.

REFERENCES

Hayes N, Ng EK, Raimes SA, et al. Total gastrectomy with extended lymphadenectomy for "curable" stomach cancer: experience in a non-Japanese Asian center. J Am Coll Surg 1999;188:27.

Maeta M, Yamashiro H, Saito H, et al. A prospective pilot study of extended (D3) and superextended para-aortic lymphadenectomy (D4) in patients with T3 or T4 gastric cancer managed by total gastrectomy. Surgery 1999;125:325.

35 Exposure of the Third and Fourth Portions of the Duodenum

INDICATIONS

Tumor

Bleeding

Trauma

PREOPERATIVE PREPARATION

Nasogastric tube

Endoscopy and biopsy possibly for tumors of the third and fourth portions of the duodenum

Computed tomography (CT) of the abdomen

PITFALLS AND DANGER POINTS

Trauma to superior mesenteric artery or vein

Trauma to pancreas

OPERATIVE STRATEGY

Because the third portion of the duodenum is located behind the superior mesenteric vessels and transverse mesocolon, approaching it directly would be hazardous. Liberating the right colon and small bowel mesentery from their attachments to the posterior abdominal wall permits the surgeon to elevate the right colon and entire small bowel to a position over the patient's thorax. This changes the course of the superior mesenteric and middle colic vessels so they travel directly cephalad, leaving the transverse portion of the duodenum completely exposed.

After liberating the right colon by incising the peritoneum of the right paracolic gutter, the renocolic attachments are divided. Continuing in this plane, the surgeon can then free the entire mesentery of the small intestine in an entirely avascular dissection. It is important to devote special attention

to the superior mesenteric vein as it emerges from the pancreas; rough traction in the area may avulse one of its branches, producing troublesome bleeding.

When planning a resection of the third and fourth portions of the duodenum, it must be noted that to the right of the superior mesenteric vessels the blood supply of the third portion of the duodenum arises from many small branches of the inferior pancreaticoduodenal arcade. These vessels must be dissected, divided, and ligated delicately, one by one, to avoid pancreatic trauma and postoperative acute pancreatitis. The distal duodenum is not attached to the body of the pancreas to the left of the superior mesenteric vessels: Its blood supply arises from branches of the superior mesenteric artery, as does that of the proximal jejunum. These branches are easily identified and controlled.

If the pancreas has not been invaded, it is possible to resect the third and fourth portions of the duodenum for tumor and then construct an anastomosis between the descending duodenum and the jejunum, so long as the ampulla is not involved. When working in this area, it is essential that the ampulla of Vater be identified early during the dissection.

OPERATIVE TECHNIQUE

Incision

A long midline incision from the mid-epigastrium to the pubis gives excellent exposure for this operation.

Liberation of Right Colon

Open the peritoneum of the right paracolic gutter with Metzenbaum scissors. Insert an index finger to separate the peritoneum from underlying fat and areolar tissue, which provides an avascular plane. When the hepatic flexure is encountered, electrocautery can help control bleeding as the peritoneum is cut. It is not necessary to dissect the greater omentum off the transverse colon during this operation. It is important, however, to continue the division of the paracolic peritoneum around the inferior portion of the cecum and to move on medially to liberate the terminal ileum, all in the same plane **(Fig. 35–1)**. Identify the renocolic ligament at the medial margin of Gerota's fascia. Division of this thin, ligamentous structure completely frees the right mesocolon.

Liberation of Small Bowel Mesentery

Insert the left index finger underneath the remaining avascular attachments between the mesentery of the small bowel and the posterior wall of the abdomen; incise these attachments until the entire small intestine up to the ligament of Treitz is free and can be positioned over the patient's thorax. This configuration resembles the anatomy of patients who have a congenital failure of rotation or malrotation of the bowel **(Fig. 35–2)**.

Resection of Duodenum

There is no structure lying over the third and fourth portions of the duodenum or proximal jejunum at this time. If a tumor of the duodenum is to be resected, it is important to determine now if it is safe to do so. If some portion of the pancreas has been invaded, a decision must be made whether a partial or total pancreatectomy is indicated for the patient's pathology. If the duodenum is free, dissection is best begun by identifying the blood supply of the distal duodenum, dividing each vessel between clamps, and ligating. As the pancreatic head is approached, perform this dissection with delicacy. It is possible to identify and divide each of the small vessels arising from the pancreas. This frees the duodenum and permits resection and anastomosis.

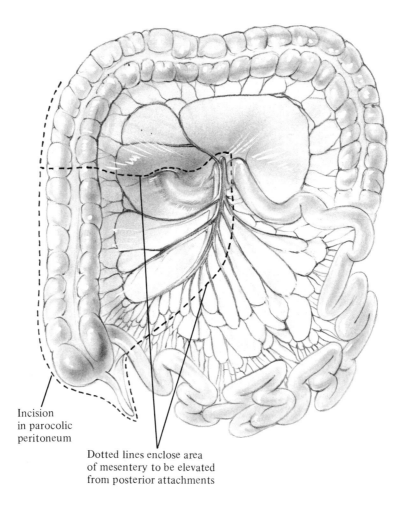

Incision
in parocolic
peritoneum

Dotted lines enclose area
of mesentery to be elevated
from posterior attachments

Fig. 35–1

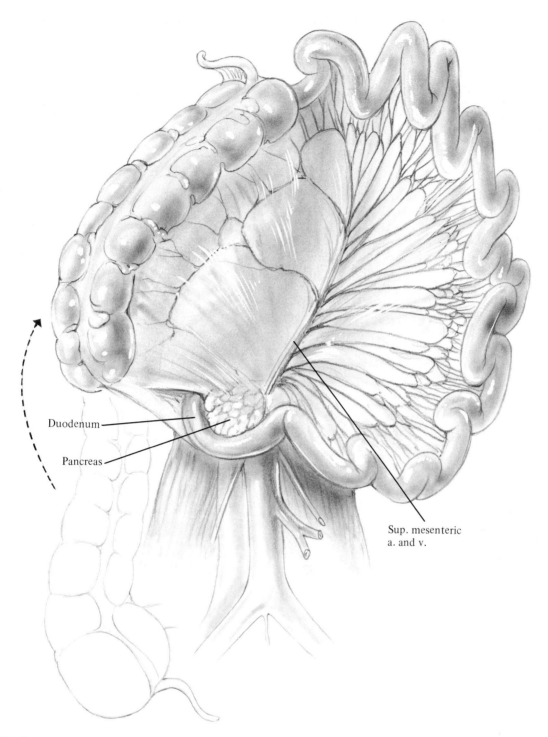

Duodenum

Pancreas

Sup. mesenteric
a. and v.

Fig. 35–2

About 1 cm of the duodenum should be freed from the pancreas proximal to the point of transection. This permits an end-to-end anastomosis between the proximal duodenum and a segment of the jejunum that is brought over for this purpose. Mere closure of the distal duodenum plus a gastrojejunostomy is not a satisfactory operation, as the proximal duodenum would eventually dilate to huge proportions and form a blind loop. If for some reason the end of the duodenum is suitable for closure but not for anastomosis, a side-to-side anastomosis between the second portion of the duodenum and proximal jejunum is a good alternative.

Closure

After the anastomosis has been performed, return the right colon and small bowel to the abdomen. Make no attempt to reestablish the posterior attachments of the mesentery. Close the abdomen in routine fashion.

POSTOPERATIVE CARE

Aside from applying nasogastric suction until bowel function has resumed with the passage of flatus, postoperative care is routine. Acute pancreatitis is a possible complication of any dissection in the region of the pancreas. So long as the serum amylase level remains elevated and the patient shows any signs of acute pancreatitis, nasogastric suction should be continued until no danger exists.

COMPLICATIONS

Pancreatitis

Anastomotic leaks

REFERENCES

Androulakis J, Colborn GL, Skandalakis PN, Skandalakis LJ, Skandalakis JE. Embryologic and anatomic basis of duodenal surgery. Surg Clin North Am 2000;80:171.

Asensio JA, Demetriades D, Berne JD, et al. A unified approach to the surgical exposure of pancreatic and duodenal injuries. Am J Surg 1997;174:54.

Cattell RB, Braasch JW. A technique for the exposure of the third and fourth portions of the duodenum. Surg Gynecol Obstet 1960;111:379.

Nauta RJ. Duodenojejunostomy as an alternative to anastomosis of the small intestine at the ligament of Treitz. Surg Gynecol Obstet 1990;170:172.

Part IV
Small Intestine and Appendix

36 Concepts in Surgery of the Small Intestine and Appendix

Samir S. Awad
Michael W. Mulholland

In general surgery multiple surgical diseases involve the small intestine or appendix and require knowledge relating to operations on the small bowel. This chapter introduces the concepts necessary to operate on the small bowel and appendix safely.

The small bowel begins with the jejunum at the ligament of Treitz and ends with the terminal ileum as it joins the cecum. Procedures commonly performed on the small bowel include small bowel resection and anastomosis, enterolysis for small bowel obstruction, stricturoplasty for treatment of strictures secondary to inflammatory bowel disease, Meckel's diverticulectomy, and open and laparoscopic appendectomy.

SMALL BOWEL RESECTION WITH ANASTOMOSIS

Common indications for small bowel resection and anastomosis include resection of tumor, injury secondary to blunt or penetrating trauma, and inflammatory conditions such as Crohn's disease and ischemic enteritis. Small bowel tumors are rare and can be difficult to diagnose because symptoms are usually insidious in onset and vague in presentation. To diagnose a small intestinal neoplasm at an early stage, the surgeon must include that possibility in the differential diagnosis. Benign tumors include adenomas, leiomyomas, lipomas, and hemangiomas. Patients may present with bright red blood per rectum or melena with resultant anemia. These tumors can also be a lead point for intussusception and cause obstructive symptoms [1].

Primary malignant tumors include adenocarcinoma, carcinoid, lymphoma, and sarcoma. Patients present with symptoms that include bleeding, ob-

struction, and perforation; and they may have carcinomatosis at exploration. The poor prognosis associated with malignant tumors of the small bowel is a result of the long delay between the onset of symptoms and diagnosis of the lesion. Less commonly, malignant tumors present as acute obstruction or perforation [1].

Traumatic injuries to the small bowel can occur as a result of penetrating or blunt trauma, with 85% of injuries secondary to penetrating trauma. Injuries to the small bowel secondary to blunt trauma are often difficult to diagnose and must be included in the differential diagnosis when the mechanism of blunt injury involves sudden deceleration and compression. Injuries range from simple perforation to areas of devitalized small bowel with compromised blood supply. Initial management of these injuries follows the basic principles of trauma resuscitation. Once an injury is confirmed, the patient is taken to the operating room; after a thorough exploration, an intraoperative decision is made regarding primary repair versus segmental resection, as described below [2].

About 60% of patients with Crohn's disease have involvement in the small bowel (10% jejunum, 50% ileum). Patients may present with high-grade obstruction and sepsis, but operation is more commonly indicated for failure of medical therapy. The operative procedure of choice depends on whether the patient has had prior small bowel resection and on the location of the diseased segment. For example, patients who present with symptomatic Crohn's enteritis affecting the terminal ileum that does not resolve with medical management can be treated with small bowel resection. Patients who have had prior resections and are symptomatic due to chronic strictures may be treated with stricturoplasty (see below).

In the elective setting, once a mass in the small bowel is localized or a resection is planned for a segment of bowel involved with Crohn's disease, the patient undergoes mechanical bowel preparation with magnesium sulfate. One dose of prophylactic preoperative intravenous antibiotic is administered that covers skin and intestinal flora [3]. A standard midline incision is made, and systematic exploration of the abdomen is undertaken. Examination begins with palpation of the liver, gallbladder, pancreas, and retroperitoneum, with biopsy of any suspicious lesions. The small bowel is then eviscerated with meticulous visual inspection and palpation of the mesenteric and antimesenteric borders of the small bowel and mesentery from the ligament of Treitz to the terminal ileum. All the peritoneal surfaces are then inspected followed by careful palpation of the large bowel down to the rectum. Following this step the segment of small bowel of interest is identified, and the remainder of the small bowel is carefully packed away out of the operative field. For tumors of the small bowel, a safe margin is then measured, typically about 5 cm on either side of the lesion; and that segment of bowel is resected with its associated mesentery. Malignant tumors are treated with a wide excision that includes local mesenteric lymph nodes. For patients with Crohn's disease, an isolated obstructed segment of small bowel is treated by resection. Bowel conservation is currently the goal, with resection proceeding to grossly negative margins.

For the emergency patient who presents with perforation and spillage of intestinal contents due to a malignancy, intestinal ischemia, or iatrogenic or traumatic injury, attention must be paid to rapid diagnosis and resuscitation followed by immediate exploration. The abdomen is explored systematically, and any area of hemorrhage from the blood supply to the small bowel is identified and controlled. Next, any area of perforation is identified, and spillage is controlled. The cause of the perforation or compromise to the small bowel blood supply is identified, and an intraoperative decision is made regarding primary repair versus resection of small bowel. For small perforations secondary to penetrating trauma, primary repair in the transverse direction can be performed if the perforation involves less than 50% of the diameter of the small bowel. For larger perforations and for areas of small bowel with a compromised blood supply, a resection with primary anastomosis may be performed following the principles outlined below. The only major contraindications to small bowel resection with anastomosis are a questionable blood supply or a patient whose condition on the operating room table is pre-

carious. In these situations, both ends of the divided bowel are exteriorized as enterostomies and the anastomosis is completed at a later time.

Prior to dividing the segment of intestine, an adequate length of small bowel must be freed proximal and distal to the area to be resected to ensure a tension-free anastomosis. A good blood supply is required for optimal healing. This criterion is determined by noting pulsatile flow in the region where the bowel is transected. When dividing the mesentery, hematomas should be avoided, as they may impair circulation. Care must be taken to avoid excessive spillage of enteric contents after transecting the bowel and while performing the anastomosis. Control may be accomplished using nontraumatic bowel clamps that are carefully applied to the small bowel while avoiding clamping the mesentery. Once the bowel is divided, accurate apposition of the seromuscular coats is essential because optimal healing of an anastomosis requires serosa-to-serosa approximation. Care must be taken when handling the bowel wall with forceps, as improper use may cause trauma to the bowel wall. Once the sutures are placed, excessive force should not be applied when tying; otherwise, strangulation of the bowel wall can occur. Finally, when the sutures are placed, care must be taken to ensure that the bowel walls are not collapsed lest the back wall is caught by the suture, causing an obstruction. A variety of techniques exist for performing the anastomosis, ranging from hand-sewn to stapled anastomoses. Each technique is covered in detail in Chapter 37.

ENTEROLYSIS FOR SMALL BOWEL OBSTRUCTION

Acute small bowel obstruction is a significant surgical problem that is often challenging diagnostically and therapeutically to the general surgeon. Intestinal obstruction is defined as the failure of progression of intestinal contents distally secondary to blockage of the intestinal lumen from an intrinsic or extrinsic lesion [4,5]. The small bowel may become obstructed for a variety of reasons, including adhesions from prior laparotomy (60%), benign and malignant tumors (20%), strangulated hernia (10%), inflammatory processes with narrowing of the lumen (5%), volvulus or intussusception (3%), and other miscellaneous conditions (2%) such as gallstone ileus [5].

Patients who present with an acute small bowel obstruction often complain of colicky pain followed by vomiting, constipation progressing to obstipation, or loose diarrhea secondary to passage of stool distal to the obstruction. Physical examination reveals a distended, tympanitic abdomen with hyperactive (early) or absent (late) bowel sounds. Abdominal radiographs reveal dilated loops of bowel, air-fluid levels, and a paucity of colonic air. Selective use of radiologic techniques, including water-soluble contrast and computed tomography (CT) studies, are helpful for characterizing the nature of the obstruction.

Despite the clinical and radiologic presentation, patients suffering from this condition are often difficult to assess and require careful evaluation and management [6]. In one study, senior surgeons were not able to determine preoperatively whether strangulation had taken place more than 50% of the time [7]. For patients who present with a partial intestinal obstruction, as suggested by a significant amount of air in the colon and the intermittent passage of flatus with no signs of fever, leukocytosis, systemic symptoms, or signs of peritonitis, a trial of conservative management with nasogastric suction, intravenous hydration, and close observation with serial examinations is warranted. Patients suffering from an acute complete obstruction, confirmed by the clinical and radiographic picture, should be operated on as soon as rehydration and correction of electrolytes has taken place, usually within 12–24 hours from the onset of symptoms [8]. When strangulation is suspected, rapid resuscitation is initiated and continued in the operating room.

The initial management of small bowel obstruction begins with replacement of fluid losses, correction of electrolyte abnormalities, and decompression of the bowel through nasogastric suctioning. Patients with suspected complete obstructions and those with partial obstructions that do not resolve are taken to the operating room. After administration of a dose of preoperative antibiotic that covers skin and intestinal flora, an attempt is made to enter the abdominal cavity through a scar-free area. Once the abdominal cavity is entered, the extent of adhesions in the vicinity of the incision can be determined. Through the use of gentle traction and countertraction, adhesions between loops of bowel and the abdominal wall are identified and transected with Metzenbaum scissors, freeing the small bowel from the abdominal wall on both sides. Because of dilated loops of bowel proximal to the obstruction, it is often necessary to decompress the bowel to improve exposure, preserve viability, and permit abdominal closure.

Decompression is accomplished by milking the intestinal contents proximally to a nasogastric tube placed in the stomach. It is not advisable to create a gastrotomy or an enterotomy to place a long tube for the purpose of intraoperative decompression. Care must be taken when handling dilated loops of

bowel, as injury to the bowel or tearing of the mesentery can occur. It is important to have patience and proceed from easy, thin adhesions to denser adhesions. Once a segment of small bowel is freed, it is traced to the nearest loop of bowel with adhesions. This process is continued until the adhesions causing the obstruction are relieved.

Once adhesiolysis is complete, the small bowel must be reinspected along its entire length to determine if there are any serosal tears or inadvertent enterotomies and to determine viability. Small serosal tears with intact submucosa can be left unrepaired. If the mucosa is bulging, approximating the serosa on either side by interrupted Lembert stitches in a transverse direction repairs the area. Determining the viability of a segment of small bowel that has been freed can be difficult. Clues such as improved color and visible, palpable mesenteric pulsations are not reliable. Any area in question should be wrapped in warm packs and reevaluated in 15 minutes. If the question of viability continues fluorescein staining and Doppler evaluation should be performed. If there are extensive areas of small bowel in question, a second-look operation should be planned in 24-hours to preserve as much bowel as possible.

A vexing problem for the general surgeon is the patient who presents with recurrent bouts of obstruction secondary to adhesions. Recurrent obstructions occur in 10–15% of cases. Several techniques have been used in an attempt to prevent this complication. The strategy employed has been to fix the intestinal loops into a streamline configuration such that when adhesions do form obstruction does not occur. Historically, stitch plication of the small bowel consisted of suturing parallel loops of bowel together, incorporating both bowel wall and mesentery [9]. This procedure requires significantly long operating times and is associated with substantial morbidity. It has not been shown to prevent recurrent obstruction. Because of failure, long intraluminal (Baker) tube stents were introduced. These tubes are placed through the nose or through a gastrotomy and left in place for 2 weeks. Even though there are single-institution successful reports of these techniques, no prospective studies have been performed to demonstrate conclusively that long intestinal tubes prevent recurrent obstruction [10,11].

SMALL INTESTINAL STRICTUROPLASTY

Multiple intestinal strictures are common sequelae of chronic inflammation in patients with Crohn's disease. Up to 30% of patients who have undergone resection for Crohn's disease require another operation. Because of this high recurrence rate, radial resections for repeated bouts of intestinal obstruction secondary to strictures are inadvisable. Stricturoplasty has emerged as a useful technique for treating these narrowed segments of small bowel and serves as a valuable adjunct in the treatment of Crohn's disease [12-14]. Stricturoplasty should be considered for patients with short, fibrotic strictures (15-35% of Crohn's patients), a previous resection of more than 100 cm of small bowel, rapid symptomatic recurrence within 1 year of the previous resection, or evidence of short-bowel syndrome. Stricturoplasty is contraindicated in patients with peritonitis secondary to intestinal perforation, enteroenteric fistulas at the site of stricture, multiple strictures in a short segment, malnutrition, or hemorrhagic strictures [5,13,14].

There are two types of stricturoplasty: the Heineke-Mikulicz and Finney varieties **(Figs. 36–1, 36–2)**. The Heineke-Mikulicz stricturoplasty is useful for short segments of narrowing (less than 8 cm in length), whereas the Finney stricturoplasty is useful for longer narrowed segments (more than 10 cm). The Heineke-Mikulicz stricturoplasty involves dividing the stricture longitudinally along its short course including 1–2 cm of normal bowel proximally and distally. The enterotomy is then closed transversely, as shown. When a longer segment of narrowing is found, the Finney stricturoplasty can be performed, as in Figure 36-2. If intraluminal ulceration is seen, the bowel is biopsied to exclude malignancy. Results of stricturoplasty are favorable and reveal that it is a safe, effective procedure in selected patients with Crohn's disease. Stric-

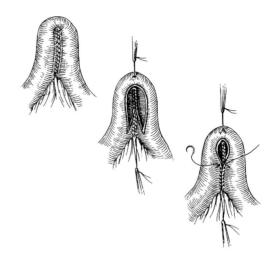

Fig. 36-2. (Reproduced, with permission, from Bell RH Jr., Rikkers LF, Mulholland MW (eds) Digestive Tract Surgery: A Text and Atlas. Philadelphia: Lippincott Williams Wilkins, 1996.)

turoplasty is associated with a 28% reoperation rate, comparable to resection while preserving the length and function of small bowel [5].

MECKEL'S DIVERTICULUM

Meckel's diverticulum is the most common developmental anomaly of the small bowel, occurring in 2% of the population. The diverticulum is a remnant of the attachment of the small bowel to the embryologic yolk sac. Meckel's diverticula arise from the antimesenteric border of the distal 100 cm of the small bowel. Ectopic tissue is found in approximately 50% of diverticula and consists of gastric tissue in 60-85% of cases and pancreatic tissue in 5-16%. Bleeding may occur as a result of ulceration in the presence of acid-secreting mucosa.

Diagnosing Meckel's diverticulum is often difficult and should be considered in patients with unexplained abdominal pain, nausea and vomiting, or intestinal bleeding. The clinical picture can mimic acute appendicitis, intestinal obstruction, Crohn's disease, and peptic ulcer disease. The most useful diagnostic method is a technetium-99m pertechnetate scan, which is dependent on uptake of the isotope in heterotopic gastric tissue.

Meckel's diverticulum is encountered incidentally during elective abdominal surgery, during exploration for acute abdomen, during exploration for acute gastrointestinal bleeding, or after preoperative localization. Options for treatment include diverticulectomy, segmental small bowel resection, or simple observation. For symptomatic diverticula that are bleeding or acutely inflamed, a segmental resection

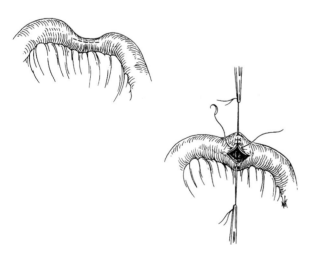

Fig. 36-1. (Reproduced, with permission, from Bell RH Jr., Rikkers LF, Mulholland MW (eds) Digestive Tract Surgery: A Text and Atlas. Philadelphia: Lippincott Williams Wilkins, 1996.)

with primary anastomosis is recommended that includes surrounding small bowel. For the incidental, asymptomatic diverticulum, a simple diverticulectomy with standard suture or stapled techniques can be performed. A diverticulectomy may also be done laparoscopically if the diverticulum is localized preoperatively or found to be the cause of symptoms during exploratory laparoscopy. If the condition is noted incidentally in association with other intraabdominal pathology, observation may be appropriate and safe. An appendectomy is often performed in the same setting to avoid future diagnostic confusion.

APPENDECTOMY

The evaluation and treatment of acute appendicitis has remained essentially unchanged for most individuals who present with this disease. Although advancements have been made in laboratory analysis and imaging via ultrasonography and helical CT, nothing can replace careful evaluation by an experienced surgeon. Appendicitis remains a diagnosis based primarily on history and physical examination, with further studies being useful adjuncts in atypical cases. Confusion is more likely to occur in the very young or the very old [15,16]. The treatment of acute appendicitis continues to be early surgical intervention.

Patients typically present with periumbilical visceral pain that over time migrates and localizes to the right lower quadrant. This pain can be associated with nausea with or without vomiting, low grade fever, anorexia, and diarrhea. Laboratory evaluation reveals leukocytosis with a left shift. With atypical presentations, for women of childbearing age, and for obese patients, ultrasonography in experienced hands and helical CT offer the highest yield in terms of specificity, sensitivity, and predictive value when used as adjuncts to the physical examination. Despite these tests, the diagnosis is often difficult.

When the presentation is classic, the diagnosis is made on clinical grounds. The patient is taken to the operating room, and an appendectomy is performed. (Refer to Chapters 40 and 41 for details of the technique.)

Laparoscopic appendectomy has emerged as a possible alternative to the open technique. Although laparoscopic appendectomy offers advantages to women of childbearing age and obese individuals, its routine use is not indicated based on current reports in the literature. A meta-analysis of 16 randomized controlled trials in adults revealed that laparoscopic appendectomy had consistently longer operating times and minimally reduced hospital stay, but there was a decrease in postoperative pain and an earlier return to normal activity. Wound infections were found more often in the open surgery groups, but a trend toward increased intraabdominal abscesses occurred in the laparoscopy group. The overall comparison suggests that there is little advantage to laparoscopic appendectomy over the open technique [17-19].

Occasionally when operating for presumed acute appendicitis the general surgeon identifies other pathology as the etiology of the patient's right lower quadrant pain. Common findings include inflammatory bowel disease or an appendiceal mass such as a carcinoid or mucocele. For patients found to have Crohn's disease at operation, an appendectomy can be performed safely so long as the base is not involved. Carcinoid tumors of the appendix are typically small, firm, circumscribed yellow tumors. When encountered, simple appendectomy with resection of the mesoappendix is adequate treatment for carcinoids less than 1 cm. For carcinoids more than 2 cm or smaller tumors with involved nodes, right hemicolectomy should be performed. Mucoceles of the appendix can be benign or malignant. An appendectomy is adequate treatment for benign tumors, but care must be taken to avoid rupture, as pseudomyxoma peritonei has been reported. Right hemicolectomy should be performed for mucous papillary adenocarcinoma.

In summary, multiple concepts must be adhered to for one to be successful when operating on the small bowel and appendix. Operating on the small bowel is usually safe unless the blood supply is impaired or active acute inflammation, edematous or dilated bowel, or advanced peritoneal sepsis is present. In most situations small bowel resection with primary anastomosis for benign, malignant, or traumatic disease, an enterolysis for small bowel obstruction, a stricturoplasty for a stricture secondary to Crohn's disease, Meckel's diverticulectomy, and appendectomy can be safely performed when the above principles are followed.

REFERENCES

1. Schwartz SI, Ellis H. Maingot's Abdominal Operations. Norwalk, CT, Appleton & Lange, 1990.
2. Feliciano DV, Moore EE, Mattox KL. Trauma 3rd ed. Norwalk, CT, Appleton & Lange, 1996.
3. Nichols RL. Surgical antibiotic prophylaxis. Med Clin North Am 1995;79:509.
4. Bell RH, Rikkers LF, Mulholland MW. Digestive Tract

Surgery. A Text and Atlas. Philadelphia, Lippencott-Raven, 1996.

5. Cameron JL. Current Surgical Therapy, 6th ed. St. Louis, Mosby, 1998.

6. Wilson MS, Ellis H, Menzies D, et al. A review of the management of small bowel obstruction: members of the Surgical and Clinical Adhesions Research Study (SCAR). Ann R Coll Surg Engl 1999;81:320.

7. Sarr MG, Bulkley GB, Zuidema GD. Preoperative recognition of intestinal strangulation obstruction: prospective evaluation of diagnostic capability. Am J Surg 1983;145:176.

8. Bass KN, Jones B, Bulkley GB. Current management of small-bowel obstruction. Adv Surg 1997;31:1.

9. Childs WA, Phillips RB. Experience with intestinal plication and a proposed modification. Ann Surg 1960; 152:258.

10. Weigelt JA, Snyder WH, Normal JL. Complications and results of 160 Baker tube plications. Am J Surg 1980; 140:810.

11. Ramsey SG, Shuk A. Nasogastrointestinal intraluminal tube stenting in the prevention of recurrent small bowel obstruction. Aust NZ J Surg 1983;53:7.

12. Becker JM. Surgical therapy for ulcerative colitis and Crohn's disease. Gastroenterol Clin North Am 1999; 28:371.

13. Fazio VW, Galandiuk S, Jagelman DG, et al. Stricturoplasty in Crohn's disease. Ann Surgery 1989;210:621.

14. Fazio VW, Tjandra JJ. Stricturoplasty for Crohn's disease with multiple long strictures. Dis Colon Rectum 1993;36:71.

15. Wilcox RT, Traverso LW. Have the evaluation and treatment of acute appendicitis changed with new technology? Surg Clin North Am 1997;77:1355.

16. Birnbaum BA, Wilson SR. Appendicitis at the millennium. Radiology 2000;215:337.

17. Fingerhut A, Millat B, Borrie F. Laparoscopic versus open appendectomy: time to decide. World J Surg 1999;23:835.

18. Slim K, Pezet D, Chipponi J. Laparoscopic or open appendectomy? Critical review of randomized, controlled trials. Dis Colon Rectum 1998;41:398.

19. Golub R, Siddiqui F, Pohl D. Laparoscopic versus open appendectomy: a metaanalysis. J Am Coll Surg 1998; 186:545.

37 Small Bowel Resection and Anastomosis

INDICATIONS

Tumor

Trauma

Strangulation

Perforation

Crohn's enteritis with complications

Ischemic enteritis

PREOPERATIVE PREPARATION

Nasogastric intubation in selected cases (obstruction, perforation)

Perioperative antibiotics

PITFALLS AND DANGER POINTS

Small bowel anastomosis is generally safe unless the blood supply is impaired or advanced peritoneal sepsis is present. When a small bowel anastomosis fails because of technical errors, the leak almost invariably occurs at the mesenteric border, where the serosa has not been adequately cleared of blood vessels and fat.

OPERATIVE STRATEGY

Successful Bowel Anastomosis Requirements

1. *Good blood supply*. Determine this by noting pulsatile flow after dividing a terminal arterial branch in the region where the bowel is to be transected. There should be no hematoma near the anastomosis, as it could impair circulation.
2. *Accurate apposition of the seromuscular coats*. There should be no fat or other tissue between the two bowel walls being sutured. The seromuscular suture must catch the submucosa, where most of the tensile strength of the intestine is situated. Optimal healing of an anastomosis requires serosa-to-serosa approximation. De-

vote special attention to the mesenteric border of any anastomosis. This is the point at which several terminal blood vessels and accompanying fat are dissected from the bowel wall to provide visibility for accurate seromuscular suture placement. Clear fat and blood vessels from a 1 cm wide area of serosa around the circumference of an anastomosis. This allows increased accuracy for suture placement without causing ischemia.
3. *Sufficient mobility of the two ends of bowel*. A sufficient length of bowel must be freed proximal and distal to each anastomosis to ensure there is no tension on the healing suture line. Remember to allow for some degree of foreshortening if postoperative distension occurs.
4. *No excessive force*. Force must not be excessive when tying the anastomotic sutures, as it would result in strangulation of tissue. If the suture should inadvertently have been placed through the full thickness of the bowel and into the lumen, the strangulated tissue will cause a leak. Tie sutures with no more tension than is needed to approximate both intestinal walls.
5. *No excessive force applied to the forceps*. When manipulating the ends of the bowel to be anastomosed there must be no excessive force. If the imprint of forceps teeth is visible on the serosa after the forceps have been removed, the surgeon obviously compressed the tissue with too much force. Pass the curved needle through the tissue with a rotatory motion to minimize trauma. As discussed in Chapter 4, it does not matter whether an intestinal anastomosis is sutured or stapled so long as proper technique is employed.
6. *Learn the pitfalls*. One must learn the pitfalls (technical and conceptual) before constructing stapled intestinal anastomoses. Study the strategy of avoiding the complications of surgical stapling (see Chapter 5).
7. *Avoid common errors*. One must avoid the common errors seen among neophytes learning the art of anastomotic suturing:

Do not insert the outer layer of seromuscular sutures with the collapsed bowel resting on a flat surface. An even worse error consists in putting the left index finger underneath the back of the anastomosis while inserting the anterior seromuscular sutures. Both errors make it possible to pass the seromuscular suture through the bowel lumen and catch a portion of the posterior wall. When the sutures are tied, an obstruction is created. Although some of these sutures may later tear out of the back wall in response to peristalsis, others remain permanently in place and produce a stenosis. To prevent this complication, simply have the assistant *grasp the tails of the anastomotic sutures that have already been tied*. Skyward traction on these sutures keeps the lumen of the anastomosis open while the surgeon inserts additional sutures.

Another error consists in inserting anastomotic sutures while the bowel is under linear tension. This practice stretches the bowel wall so it becomes relatively thin, making it difficult to enclose a substantial bite of tissue in the suture. *A sufficient length of intestine, proximal and distal, should be loosely placed in the operative field*. After the first seromuscular bite has been taken, the needle is ready to be reinserted into the wall of the opposite segment of intestine. At this time it is often helpful to use forceps to elevate the distal bowel at a point 3–4 cm distal to the anastomosis. Elevation relaxes this segment of the bowel and permits the suture to catch a substantial bite of tissue, including the submucosa. Each bite should encompass about 4–5 mm of tissue. These stitches should be placed about 4–5 mm from each other.

Contraindications to Anastomosis

Because of the excellent blood supply and substantial submucosal strength of the small bowel, anastomoses are often successful even in the presence of such adverse circumstances as intestinal obstruction and gross contamination of the abdominal cavity. Consequently, the only major contraindications to a primary small bowel anastomosis are peritoneal sepsis, a questionable blood supply, or a patient whose condition on the operating table is precarious. In these cases both ends of the divided small bowel may be brought to the skin as temporary enterostomies or simply stapled closed and returned to the abdomen for a planned second look.

OPERATIVE TECHNIQUE

Small Bowel Anastomosis by Suturing

Incision

Use a midline vertical incision for the best exposure of the small bowel.

Division of Mesentery

Expose the segment of intestine to be resected by laying it flat on a moist gauze pad on the abdominal wall. With a scalpel make a V-type incision in the mesentery to be removed, carrying it through the superficial peritoneal layer only, to expose the underlying blood vessels **(Fig. 37–1)**. Apply medium-size hemostats in pairs to the intervening tissue. Divide the tissue between hemostats and ligate each with 2-0 PG. After the wedge of mesentery has been completely freed, apply Allen clamps to the bowel on the specimen sides. Apply noncrushing intestinal clamps proximally and distally to prevent spillage of intestinal contents. Remove the diseased segment of intestine by scalpel division.

Open Two-Layer Anastomosis

Considerable manipulative trauma to the bowel wall can be avoided if the anterior seromuscular layer of sutures is the first layer to be inserted. This should be done by successive bisection (see Chapter 4). First, use 4-0 silk on an atraumatic needle and insert a seromuscular suture on the antimesenteric border followed by a second suture on the mesenteric bor-

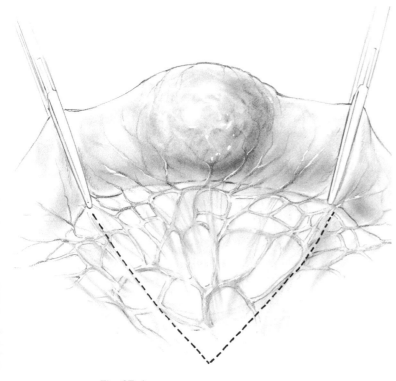

Fig. 37-1

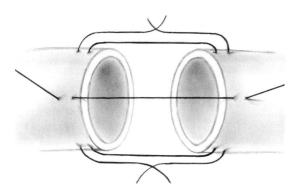

Fig. 37-2

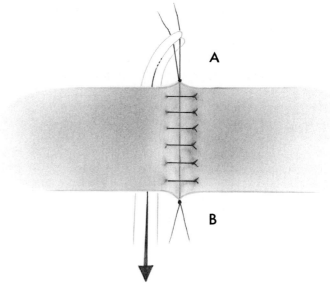

Fig. 37-3b

der **(Fig. 37–2)**. Tie both sutures. Next, bisect the distance between these two sutures and insert and tie the third Lembert suture at this point. Follow this sequence until the anterior seromuscular layer has been completed **(Fig. 37–3a)**. Retain the two end sutures as guys, but cut the tails of all the remaining sutures. *Rotate the bowel by passing guy suture A behind the anastomosis* **(Fig. 37–3b)** so the posterior layer is on top **(Fig. 37–3c)**.

Close the mucosal layer with a running 5-0 double-armed PG suture. Insert the two needles at the midpoint of the deep layer **(Fig. 37–4)**. Tie the suture and close the posterior layer, which should

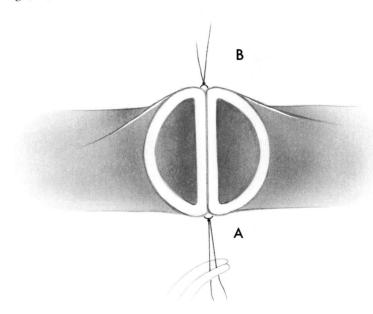

Fig. 37-3c

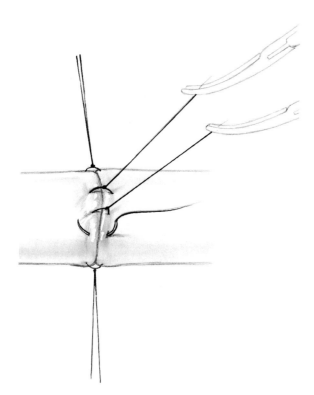

Fig. 37-3a

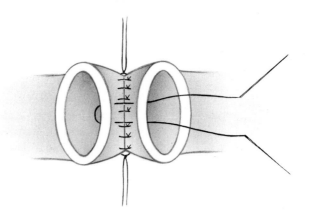

Fig. 37-4

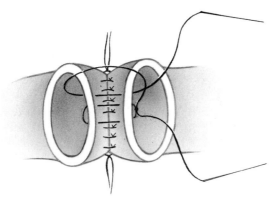

Fig. 37-5

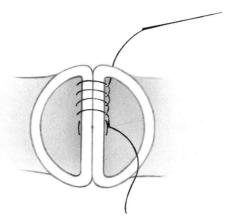

Fig. 37-6

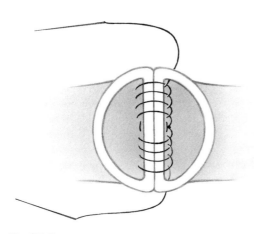

Fig. 37-7

insert the final seromuscular layer of interrupted 4-0 silk Lembert sutures **(Fig. 37–10)**. The technique of successive bisection is not necessary in the final layer because the two segments of bowel are already in accurate apposition.

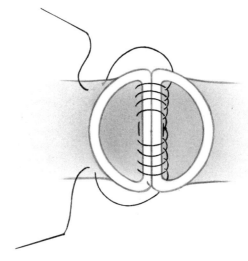

Fig. 37-8

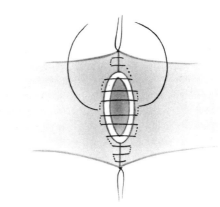

Fig. 37-9

include mucosa and a bit of seromuscular tissue, with a continuous locked suture **(Figs. 37–5, 37–6, 37–7)**. Turning in the corners with this technique is simple. Bring the needle from inside out through the outer wall of the intestine **(Fig. 37–8)**. Then complete the final mucosal layer using the Connell technique or a continuous Cushing suture **(Fig. 37–9)**. After this mucosal layer has been completed,

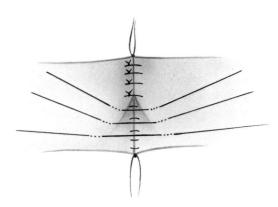

Fig. 37-10

After all the suture tails have been cut, carefully inspect for imperfections in the suture line, especially at the mesenteric margin. Test the patency of the lumen by invaginating one wall of the intestine through the anastomosis with the tip of the index finger.

Open One-Layer Anastomosis

The first step in constructing an end-to-end anastomosis in one layer is identical to the steps in Figures 37-2 and 37-3a. Insert interrupted 4-0 silk Lembert sutures on the anterior seromuscular layer. Cut the tails of all the sutures except the two at the end and rotate the bowel to expose the opposite, unsutured bowel (Figs. 37-3b, 37-3c). Approximate this too with interrupted 4-0 silk *seromuscular* Lembert sutures, paying special attention to the mesenteric border, where fat and blood vessels may hide the seromuscular tissue from view if the dissection has not been thorough.

After the anastomosis is completed, check it closely for defects. Test the size of the lumen by invaginating the wall with a fingertip.

Alternatively, instead of Lembert sutures "seromucosal" stitches may be inserted (**Fig. 37–11**). This suture enters the seromuscular layer and, like the Lembert sutures, penetrates the submucosa; but instead of emerging from the serosa, the needle emerges just beyond the junction of the cut edge of the serosa and underlying mucosa. This stitch has the advantage of inverting a smaller cuff of tissue than does the Lembert or Cushing technique and may therefore be useful when the small bowel lumen is exceedingly small. When inserted properly the seromucosal suture inverts the mucosa but not to the extent seen with the Lembert stitch.

Closure of Mesentery

Close the defect in the mesentery by a continuous suture of 2-0 PG on a large, intestinal-type needle. Take care not to pierce the blood vessels.

Small Bowel Anastomosis Using Stapling Technique

In our experience, the most efficient method for stapling the small bowel is a two-step functional end-to-end technique. It requires the two open-ended segments of the small bowel to be positioned so their antimesenteric borders are in apposition. Insert a cutting linear stapling device, one fork in the proximal and the other fork in the distal segment of

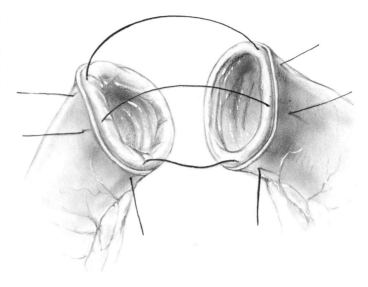

Fig. 37-11

the intestine (**Fig. 37–12**). Fire the stapling instrument, which forms one layer of the anastomosis in an inverting fashion (**Fig. 37–13**). Apply Allis clamps to the anterior and posterior terminations of the

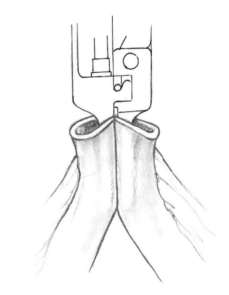

Fig. 37-12

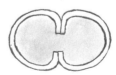

Fig. 37-13

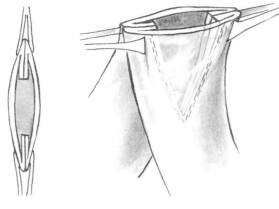

Fig. 37-14   Fig. 37-15

staple line. Then draw the two Allis clamps apart **(Figs. 37–14, 37–15)**. Close the remaining defect in the anastomosis in an everting fashion after applying four or five Allis clamps to maintain apposition of the walls of the proximal and distal segments of bowel **(Fig. 37–16)**.

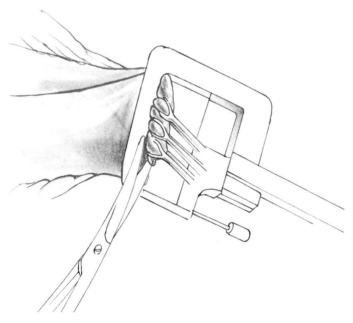

Fig. 37-16

After all the Allis clamps have been aligned, staple the bowel in eversion by applying a 90/3.5 mm linear stapling device just deep to the Allis clamps (Fig. 37-16). If the bowel wall is thick, use 4.8 mm staples. It is essential that the line of staples cross both the anterior and posterior terminations of the anastomotic staple line to avoid gaps in the staple line. Fire the stapler and excise the redundant bowel flush with the stapling device using Mayo scissors. Lightly electrocoagulate the everted mucosa.

Carefully inspect the staple line to be sure each staple has formed a proper B. Bleeding may be controlled by conservative electrocautery or by using interrupted 4-0 atraumatic PG sutures.

Close the defect in the mesentery with a continuous 2-0 atraumatic PG suture. If feasible, cover the everted mucosa by the mesenteric suture line to minimize the possibility of it becoming a nidus of adhesion formation. Cover the anastomosis with a layer of omentum, whenever possible, to prevent adhesions.

POSTOPERATIVE CARE

Administer nasogastric suction until bowel function resumes.

COMPLICATIONS

Although it is uncommon for the patient to develop complications following a small bowel anastomosis, postoperative obstruction does occasionally occur. Anastomotic leaks accompanied by intraperitoneal sepsis or enterocutaneous fistula are rare except after resection in the face of sepsis or when mesenteric circulation is impaired.

REFERENCES

Carty NJ, Keating J, Campbell J, et al. Prospective audit of an extramucosal technique for intestinal anastomosis. Br J Surg 1991;78:1439.

Chassin JL, Rifkind KM, Sussman B, et al. The stapled gastrointestinal tract anastomosis: incidence of postoperative complications compared with the sutured anastomosis. Ann Surg 1978;188:689.

38 Enterolysis for Intestinal Obstruction

INDICATIONS

Enterolysis is indicated for acute cases of complete small bowel obstruction. It is frequently performed as an incidental procedure when the previously operated abdomen must be reentered.

PREOPERATIVE PREPARATION

Institute nasogastric suction promptly.

Initiate fluid and electrolyte resuscitation.

Administer perioperative antibiotics.

PITFALLS AND DANGER POINTS

Inadvertent laceration and spillage of the contents of the intestine is a hazard of this procedure. Failure to identify and relieve all points of obstruction can occur unless the entire small bowel is dissected free.

OPERATIVE STRATEGY

Dissect carefully and patiently to avoid spillage of intestinal contents. Bacterial overgrowth occurs rapidly when the contents stagnate. Massive distension with thinning of the bowel make it much more likely to occur and more serious if it happens.

Enter the abdomen through a scar-free area and carefully dissect the bowel from the underside of the abdominal wall. Adhesions are commonly dense in the region of the old scar.

Separate loops of bowel, working from regions of easy dissection toward those where it is difficult. The additional exposure gained by doing the easy dissection first facilitates work in the more difficult parts. Work on the collapsed region (distal to the obstruction) first, if possible, and keep the dilated proximal bowel in the abdomen as long as possible.

After all adhesions have been freed, repair any injured segments and evaluate intestinal viability. Determine whether operative decompression is needed prior to closure.

OPERATIVE TECHNIQUE

Incision and Bowel Mobilization

A long midline incision is preferable. In the case of a previous midline incision, start the new incision 3–5 cm cephalad to the upper margin of the scar so the abdomen can be entered through virgin territory. If the old scar extends from xiphoid to pubis, enter through the cephalad part of the incision, where it is likely that only the stomach or the left lobe of the liver (rather than distended loops of bowel) will be encountered.

Carry the skin incision through the old scar and down to the linea alba. After opening the upper portion of the incision, identify the peritoneal cavity and then carefully incise the remainder of the scar. If entry into the peritoneum is difficult, lift up on the skin and subcutaneous tissues on both sides of the incision to create locally negative intraabdominal pressure and gently continue to incise with a scalpel. As soon as the peritoneum is entered, air flows into the peritoneal cavity and creates a safe zone for continued

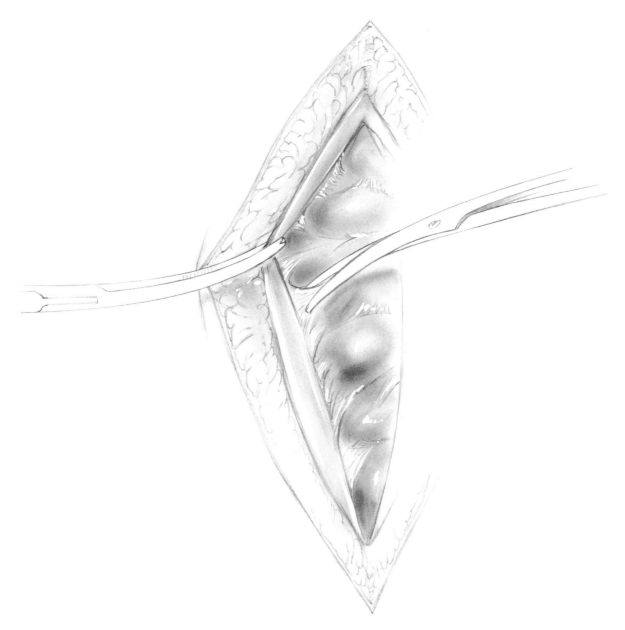

Fig. 38–1

dissection. At the same time dissect away any ad-herent segments of underlying intestine **(Fig. 38–1)**.

Approach to Densely Adherent Abdomen

Whereas the content of the normal small intestine is sterile, with intestinal obstruction the stagnation of bowel content results in overgrowth of virulent bacteria with production of toxins. When these sub-stances spill into the peritoneal cavity, the likelihood of postoperative mortality and infection increases significantly. To avoid this mishap, dissection should be done carefully and patiently.

The basic dissection strategy consists in entering the abdominal cavity through a scar-free area. Even though an old midline scar is frequently used to reen-ter an abdomen to relieve an obstruction, it is ad-vantageous to make some part of the incision through an area of the abdomen above or below the old scar. Access to the peritoneal cavity through an unscarred area often gives the surgeon an opportunity to assess the location of adhesions in the vicinity of the antic-ipated incision. After the free abdominal cavity is en-tered and any adherent segments of intestine are freed, the remainder of the incision is carefully done.

Attach Allis clamps to the peritoneum and linea alba on one side of the incision and have the assistant lift up on the clamps. Metzenbaum scissors can generally then be insinuated behind the various layers of avascular adhesions to incise them (Fig. 38-1). If the left index finger can be passed underneath a loop of bowel adherent to the abdominal wall, it helps guide the dissection. The aim is to free all the intestine from the anterior and lateral abdominal wall, first on one side of the incision and then on the other, so the anterior and lateral layers of parietal peritoneum are completely free of intestinal attachments **(Fig. 38–2)**.

Once the intestine has been freed, trace a normal-looking segment to the nearest adhesion. If possible insert an index finger into the leaves of the mesentery, separating the two adherent limbs of the intestine. By gently bringing the index finger up between the leaves of the mesentery the adherent layer can often be stretched into a fine, filmy membrane, which is then easily divided with scissors **(Fig. 38–3)**. In general, the strategy is to insinuate either

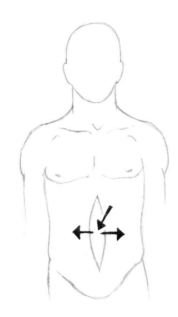

Fig. 38-2

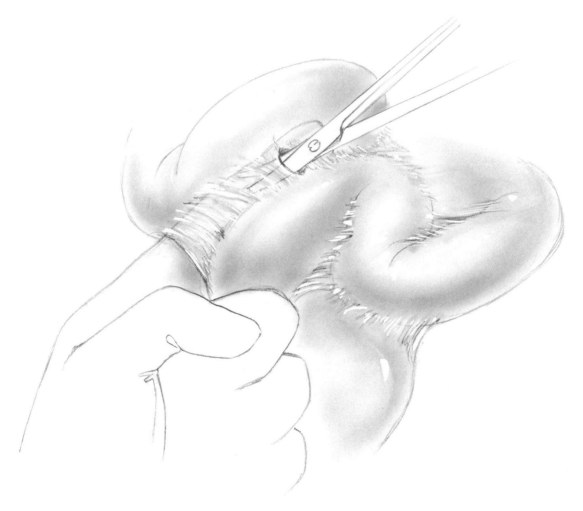

Fig. 38-3

the left index finger or closed blunt-tipped curved Metzenbaum scissors underneath an adhesion to delineate the plane and then withdraw the closed scissors and cut the fibrous layer. A guiding principle is *to perform the easy dissection first*. If this principle is always followed, the difficult portion of a dissection becomes easy. Avoid tackling a dense adherent mass directly; if the loops of intestine going to and coming from the adherent mass are dissected on their way in and on their way out of the mass of adhesions, a sometimes confusing collection of intestine can be easily untangled.

In the case of an acute small bowel obstruction, frequently there are only one or two adhesions and a markedly distended proximal bowel. When this occurs, be careful not to permit the distended bowel to leap out of a small portion of the incision, as it may be torn inadvertently in the process. If possible, first deliver the collapsed bowel (distal to the point of obstruction) and then trace it retrograde up to the point of obstruction. The adhesion can then be divided under direct vision and the entire bowel freed.

Free the remainder of the bowel of adhesions, from the ligament of Treitz to the ileocecal valve. Accomplish this task by delicate dissection with Metzenbaum scissors, alternately sliding the scissors underneath a layer of fibrous tissue to visualize its extent and then cutting the adhesion. This can be done more efficiently if the left index finger can be insinuated in such a way as to circumscribe the adherent area, or if the index finger can be brought between the leaves of mesentery separating the adherent bowel, thereby placing the adhesion on stretch and making it visible (Fig. 38-3). In some cases there are adhesions of a cartilaginous nature, especially in patients whose obstruction is due to multiple malignant implants. Bold scalpel incisions should be made to divide adhesions of this type. Again, by doing the easy dissection first, the difficult parts become easier.

Relaparotomy for Early Postoperative Obstruction

We most often reenter the same incision, usually in the midline, to reexplore the postoperative abdomen. Because most relaparotomy operations are done after the eighth to tenth postoperative day, some sharp dissection may be necessary to enter the abdomen.

To divide adhesions in these cases, many of the loops of bowel can be separated by inserting the index finger between the leaves of adjoining mesentery. By elevating the finger, the adhesion can be stretched between the bowel segments. Often the adhesion can be disrupted by pinching it *gently* between the thumb and index finger without damaging the serosa of the bowel.

Operative Intestinal Decompression

If the diameter of the small bowel appears to be so distended that closing the incision would be difficult, operative decompression of the bowel makes the abdominal closure simpler and may improve the patient's postoperative course. Decompression may also lessen the risk of inadvertent laceration of the tensely distended intestine.

We prefer to use the Baker intestinal tube, which is a 270 cm long tube with a 5 ml balloon at its tip, for this procedure. It may be passed through the patient's nose by the anesthesiologist or introduced by the surgeon through a Stamm gastrostomy. It is then passed through the pylorus with the balloon deflated. The balloon is partially inflated and the tube milked around the duodenum to the ligament of Treitz and then down the small intestine. Meanwhile, intermittent suction is applied to aspirate gas and intestinal contents. Caution should be exercised when milking the tube through the intestine, as the distended bowel has impaired tensile strength and can easily be torn. In patients who have relatively few adhesions, the Baker tube may be removed at the conclusion of the decompression and a nasogastric tube substituted for postoperative suction. In the rare case where the bowel has sustained extensive serosal damage, the Baker tube may be left in place for 2-3 weeks to perform a "stitchless plication" (see Chapter 39).

Repair of Damage to Bowel Wall

Small areas of intestine from which the serosa has been avulsed by dissection require no sutures for repair if the submucosa has remained intact. This is evident in areas where some muscle fiber remnants remain. Otherwise, when only thin mucosa bulges out and the mucosa is so transparent that bubbles of fluid can be seen through it, the damage is extensive enough to require inversion of the area with interrupted or continuous seromuscular 4-0 PG Lembert sutures. Large areas of damage should be repaired transversely by one or two layers of Lembert sutures in a transverse manner. Extensive damage requires bowel resection with anastomosis by sutures or stapling.

If a segment of bowel is of questionable viability, replace it in the abdomen and cover the incision with warm, moist packs. Reevaluation in 10–15 minutes often reveals that the bowel has regained some color, tone, and peristalsis indicative of recovering perfusion.

Closure

After decompressing the bowel, replace it in the abdominal cavity. If there has been any spillage, thoroughly irrigate the abdominal cavity with large volumes of warm saline solution. Close the abdominal wall in the usual fashion with a modified Smead Jones technique (see Chapter 3).

POSTOPERATIVE CARE

Nasogastric or long intestinal tube suction (or both) are required postoperatively until evidence of bowel function returns. This is manifested by active bowel sounds or the passage of flatus or stool per rectum.

When a Baker tube must remain in place postoperatively because of extensive serosal damage or some other indication for a "stitches plication" (see Chapter 39), it is generally necessary to insert a nasogastric tube in the other nostril to decompress the upper gastrointestinal tract. Our policy is to avoid filling both nostrils with intestinal tubes. It is far preferable in these cases to insert the long Baker tube through a newly constructed Stamm gastrostomy, thereby leaving one nostril free.

Antibiotics are given perioperatively.

COMPLICATIONS

Recurrent intestinal obstruction

Intestinal fistula or peritonitis

39 Baker Tube Stitchless Plication

Surgical Legacy Technique

INDICATIONS

Operations for intestinal obstruction due to extensive adhesions, when the patient has already undergone numerous similar operations

Extensive serosal damage following division of many adhesions

PREOPERATIVE PREPARATION

See Chapter 38.

Nasogastric suction should be initiated before the operation.

PITFALLS AND DANGER POINTS

Trauma to the bowel while passing the Baker tube

Reverse intususception when the tube is removed

OPERATIVE STRATEGY

Adhesions tend to form again after enterolysis. Plication attempts to prevent multiple recurrent adhesions by holding the bowel in a prearranged orderly fashion (**Fig. 39–1**) during the period of adhesion formation. In this manner, any adhesions that develop presumably form between loops of intestine that are held in gentle curves, minimizing the chances of recurrent adhesive obstruction.

The Baker tube may be passed through a Stamm gastrostomy (preferred), a jejunostomy, or under rare circumstances retrograde through a cecostomy. It is not advisable to pass the tube via the nasogastric route, as the tube must remain in place for at least 10 days. A nasogastric tube may be required to decompress the stomach postoperatively.

OPERATIVE TECHNIQUE

Enterolysis of the entire small bowel should be performed as the first step of this operation. Create a Stamm gastrostomy (see Figs. 32-1 through 32-5). The Baker tube is an 18F 270 cm long intestinal tube with a balloon at the end and a dual lumen. The primary lumen may be placed for suctioning the bowel to decompress it during tube passage

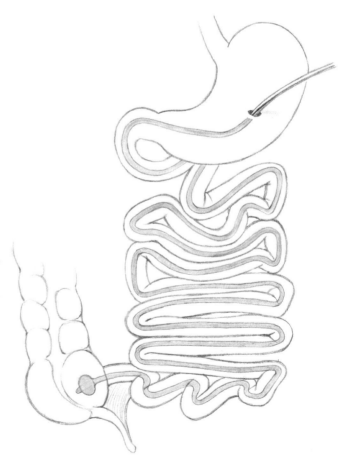

Fig. 39-1

and during the early postoperative period. The second lumen controls inflation and deflation of the balloon.

Pass the sterile Baker tube into the gastrostomy and then through the pylorus; partially inflate the balloon. By milking the balloon along the intestinal tract the tube may be drawn through the entire length of the intestine. Supply intermittent suction to the tube to evacuate gas and intestinal contents. Pass the balloon through the ileocecal valve and inflate it to 5 ml.

Distribute the length of the intestine evenly over the length of the tube. Then arrange the intestine in the shape of multiple Ss. Irrigate the peritoneal cavity and close the abdomen in the usual fashion. If there has been any spillage of bowel contents during the dissection, if gangrenous bowel has been resected, or if an enterotomy has been performed for intestinal decompression, do not close the skin incision, as the incidence of wound infection is extremely high.

When local factors contraindicate a gastrostomy, pass the Baker tube through a stab wound near McBurney's point and construct a cecostomy by the Stamm technique. Insert a purse-string suture using 3-0 PG in a portion of the cecum near the stab wound. Make a puncture wound in the center of the purse-string suture, insert the Baker tube, and hold the purse-string suture taut. To pass the Baker tube through the ileocecal valve, make a 3- to 4-mm puncture wound in the distal ileum. Then insert a Kelly hemostat into the wound and pass the hemostat into the cecum. Grasp the Baker tube with the hemostat and draw the tube into the ileum. Close the puncture wound with sutures.

Inflate the balloon of the Baker tube and milk the balloon in a cephalad direction until the tip of the Baker tube has reached a location proximal to the point of obstruction and to any area of bowel that has suffered serosal damage. Suction all the bowel contents through the Baker tube and deflate the balloon.

Insert a second 3-0 PG purse-string suture, inverting the first purse-string suture. Then suture the cecostomy to the abdominal wall with one 3-0 PG suture in each quadrant surrounding the abdominal stab wound.

POSTOPERATIVE CARE

Connect the Baker tube to low wall suction. Deflate the balloon at the end of the Baker tube on the second postoperative day. We cut off the port after balloon deflation to ensure that the balloon is not inadvertently reinflated. The tube itself must stay in place for 14–21 days if a stitchless plication is to be achieved. An additional nasogastric tube may be required for several days. Prolonged ileus due to preoperative obstruction or the manipulation of bowel required to pass the tube is common.

When bowel function returns, remove the Baker tube from the suction and allow the patient to eat. Simply clamp the tube and leave it in place as a stent. When it is time to remove the Baker tube, do so gradually, with the balloon deflated to avoid creating (reverse) intusussception.

Antibiotics are given postoperatively to patients who have had an intraoperative spill of intestinal contents.

POSTOPERATIVE COMPLICATIONS

Wound infection

REFERENCES

Baker JW. Stitchless plication for recurring obstruction of the small bowel. Am J Surg 1968;116:316.

Childs WA, Phillips RB. Experience with intestinal plication and a proposed modification. Ann Surg 1960; 152:258.

Noble TB. Plication of small intestine as prophylaxis against adhesions. Am J Surg 1937;35:41.

40 Appendectomy

INDICATIONS

Acute appendicitis

Interval appendectomy following conservative treatment of appendiceal abscess

Mucocele of appendix

Adenocarcinoma and carcinoid of appendix may require right colon resection in addition to appendectomy, especially if there is suspicion of metastases in lymph nodes

PREOPERATIVE PREPARATION

Diagnostic studies: ultrasonography and computed tomography (CT) of the appendix (if necessary)

Intravenous fluids

Perioperative antibiotics

Nasogastric tube if ileus is present

PITFALLS AND DANGER POINTS

Inadvertent laceration of inflamed cecum during blunt dissection

Inadequate control of blood vessels in edematous mesoappendix

OPERATIVE STRATEGY

Incision

When the diagnosis is clear, use a McBurney incision, which splits the muscles along the lines of their fibers, each in a somewhat different direction. The healed scar with this incision is usually quite strong, and the cosmetic result is good. For most cases the incision proves to be centered over the base of the appendix. If the exposure is inadequate, the incision may be carried in a medial direction by dividing the rectus sheath. If necessary, the right rectus muscle itself may be transected to expose the pelvic organs. If it is obvious that the exposure is inadequate, even

with an extension (e.g., if a perforated ulcer is found), make a new vertical incision suitable to the pathology and close the McBurney incision. If the diagnosis is uncertain, the laparoscopic approach (see Chapter 41) or even a midline laparotomy incision may be preferable.

Management of Appendiceal Stump

In most cases acute appendicitis is the result of a closed-loop obstruction due to an appendiceal fecalith. The base of the appendix, which is proximal to the obstructing fecalith, usually is fairly healthy even in the presence of advanced inflammation or even if the remainder of the organ is gangrenous. This makes ligature or inversion of the appendiceal stump a safe procedure.

After the appendix has been removed, the stump may be managed by simple ligation or by inversion with a purse-string suture around its base. There does not appear to be proof of the superiority of either method, although a purse-string inversion may produce fewer adhesions than a simple ligation, which permits eversion of some of the mucosa. Inversion is preferable in simple cases; but if the area is edematous, making inversion difficult, simple ligation is preferable.

Indication for Drainage

The presence of inflammation or even generalized peritonitis due to a perforated appendix is not an indication for external drainage. Close the abdominal wall without drainage after thoroughly irrigating the abdominal cavity and pelvis. If an abscess with rigid walls is encountered, drain the cavity with a closed-suction drain. Leave the skin wound open in cases of perforated appendix to avoid wound sepsis.

OPERATIVE TECHNIQUE

Incision

Draw an imaginary line from the right anterior superior iliac spine to the umbilicus. At a point 3–4

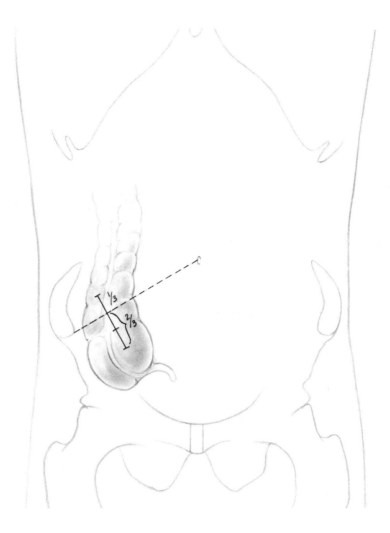

Fig. 40-1

cm medial to the anterior spine, draw a line perpendicular to this line **(Fig. 40–1)**. This is the general direction of the McBurney skin incision. About one-third of the incision should be above the imaginary line between the iliac spine and umbilicus and two-thirds below this line. The average length of this incision is 6 cm.

Deepen this incision through the external oblique aponeurosis, along the line of its fibers **(Fig. 40–2)**. Start the incision with a scalpel and extend it with Metzenbaum scissors. Then elevate the medial and lateral leaves of the external oblique aponeurosis

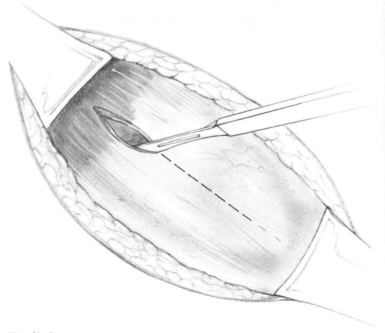

Fig. 40-2

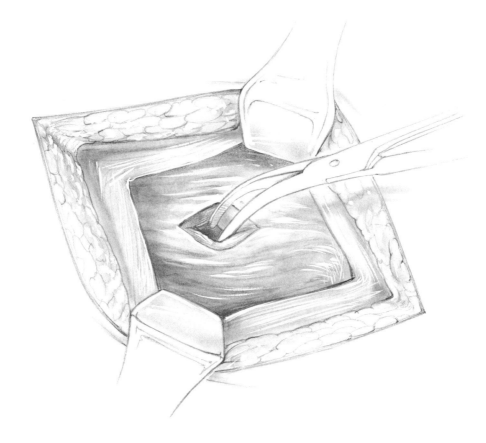

Fig. 40-3

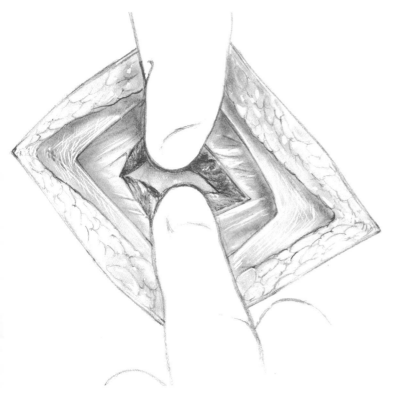

Fig. 40-4

from the underlying muscle and separate them between retractors **(Fig. 40–3)**.

Note that the internal oblique muscle, which is fairly thick, and the transversus muscle, which is deep to the internal oblique, run in a transverse direction. Make an incision just below the level of the anterosuperior iliac spine into the thin fascia of the internal oblique muscle. Then insert a Kelly hemostat to separate the muscle fibers of the internal oblique and underlying transversus muscle (Fig. 40-3). Using either two Kelly hemostats or both index fingers, enlarge this incision sufficiently to insert small Richardson retractors **(Fig. 40–4)**.

Obtain adequate hemostasis of one or two vessels in the internal oblique muscle with electrocautery; then note the layer of fat that adjoins the peritoneum. Tease this fat off the peritoneum lateral to the rectus muscle to identify a clear area. Elevate it between two hemostats and make an incision into the peritoneal cavity **(Fig. 40–5)**. Enlarge the incision sufficiently to insert Richardson retractors and explore the region.

For additional exposure in a medial direction when, for example, it is necessary to identify a woman's pelvic organs, a medial extension of about 2 cm can be made across the anterior rectus sheath, after which a similar division of the posterior sheath can be carried out and the rectus muscle retracted medially. The inferior epigastric vessels may be encountered and generally can also be retracted medially.

When the lateral extremity of the McBurney incision must be extended, the surgeon has two choices: (1) Close the McBurney incision and make a separate vertical incision of adequate length for exposure. (2) If additional exposure of only a few centimeters is needed, the oblique and transverse muscles may be deliberately divided with electrocautery in a cephalad direction along the lateral portion of the abdominal wall. Be aware that if this vertical extension along the lateral abdominal wall is continued for *more than* 4–5 cm, two or more intercostal nerves are likely to be divided, resulting in muscular weakness of the lower abdomen. If a 4- to 5-cm extension of the incision is closed carefully, generally no serious problems of weakness or herniation develop.

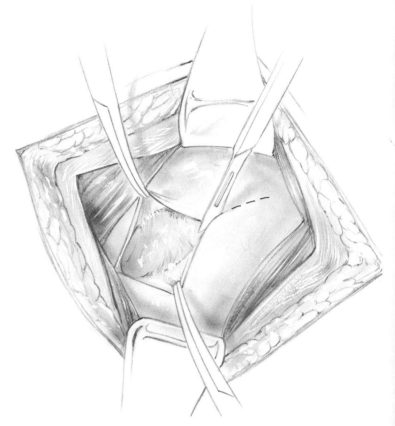

Fig. 40–5

Delivery of Appendix

Insert small Richardson retractors into the peritoneal cavity and grasp the anterior wall of the cecum with a moist gauze pad **(Fig. 40–6)**. With the cecum partially exteriorized, identify the appendix. If the appendix cannot be seen, exploration with the index finger may reveal an inflammatory mass consisting of inflamed appendix and mesoappendix. It can usually be delivered into the incision by gentle digital manipulation around the borders of the mass.

If this palpatory maneuver is not successful in locating the appendix, follow the taenia on the anterior wall of the cecum in a caudal direction. This leads to the base of the appendix, which can then be grasped in a Babcock clamp. Apply a second Babcock clamp to the tip of the appendix and deliver it into the incision.

Division of Mesoappendix

If the base of the mesoappendix is not thick, it may be encompassed by a single ligature of 2-0 PG. Otherwise, divide the mesoappendix between serially applied hemostats and ligate each with 2-0 or 3-0 PG

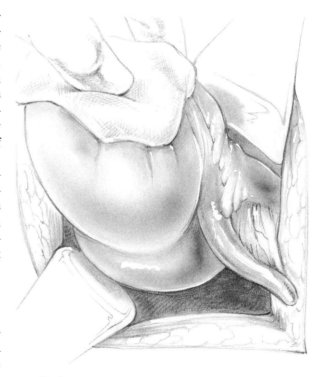

Fig. 40–6

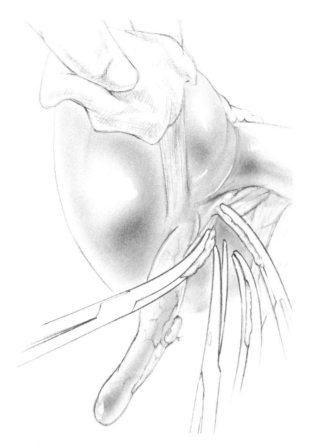

Fig. 40-7

until the base of the appendix has been dissected free **(Fig. 40–7)**.

Ligation of Appendiceal Stump

Hold the tip of the appendix in a Babcock clamp and double-ligate the base with 2-0 PG or chromic catgut at a point 4-6 mm from the cecum. Apply a straight hemostat to the appendix 1 cm distal to the ligature; then transect the appendix with a scalpel 5-6 mm distal to the ligature **(Fig. 40–8)** and remove the specimen. The appendiceal stump may be lightly sterilized by applying electrocautery to the exposed mucosa, or it may simply be returned to the abdominal cavity **(Fig. 40–9)**.

Inversion of Appendiceal Stump

To invert the stump, insert a purse-string suture around the base of the appendix using 3-0 PG or silk on an atraumatic needle. The radius of this suture should exceed the anticipated length of the appendiceal stump **(Fig. 40–10)**. Apply a small straight hemostat to the base of the appendix at a point 5-6 mm from the cecum. Apply a second hemostat 1 cm distal to the first. Using a scalpel, transect the appendix just distal to the first hemostat **(Fig. 40–11)**, which should now be used to invert the stump into the previously placed purse-string suture **(Fig. 40–12)**. As the first knot is being tied, gradually withdraw the hemostat, completing the purse-string tie. The single suture should be sufficient; if there is some doubt of its adequacy, it may be reinforced with a figure-of-eight suture of the same material. Many surgeons ligate the base of the appendix before inverting it.

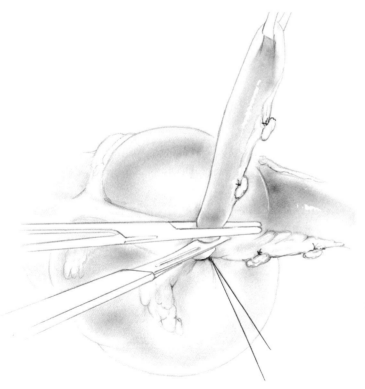

Fig. 40-8

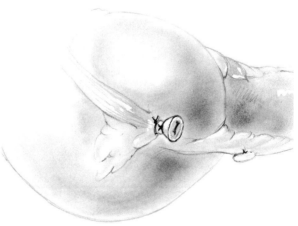

Fig. 40-9

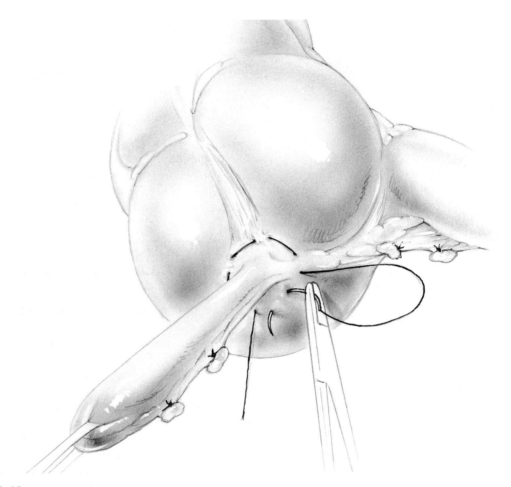

Fig. 40-10

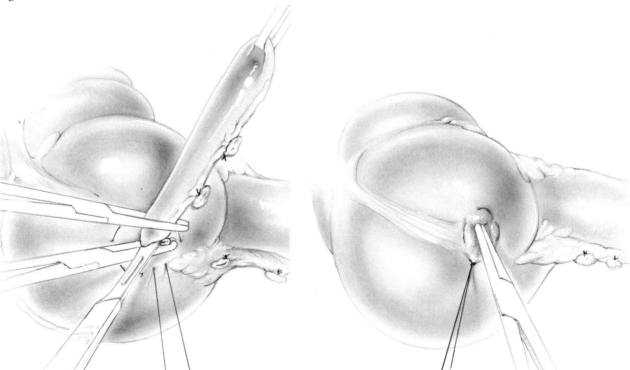

Fig. 40-11

Fig. 40-12

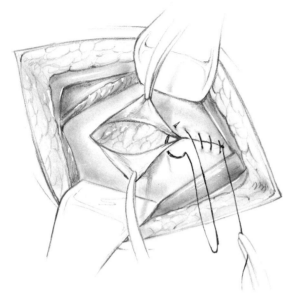

Fig. 40-13

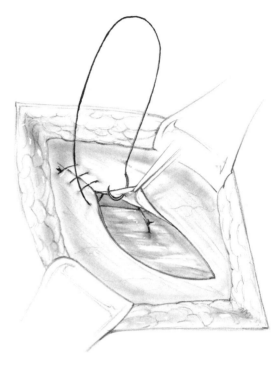

Fig. 40-15

Closure of Incision

Irrigate the right lower quadrant and pelvis with a dilute antibiotic solution; then apply four hemostats to the cut ends of the peritoneum. Close the peritoneum with continuous 3-0 atraumatic PG sutures **(Fig. 40–13)**. Close the internal oblique and transversus muscles as a single layer with interrupted sutures of 2-0 PG tied loosely **(Fig. 40–14)**. Close the external oblique aponeurosis with continuous or interrupted sutures of 2-0 PG **(Fig. 40–15)**.

If intraperitoneal pus or a gangrenous appendix is present, do not close the skin incision. Rather, place a few vertical mattress sutures of 4-0 nylon but do not tie them. Insert just enough gauze into the incision to keep the skin edges separated.

POSTOPERATIVE CARE

In the absence of pus or perforation, postoperative antibiotics need not be administered beyond the operative period. Otherwise, appropriate systemic antibiotics are indicated. Most patients recover rapidly following an appendectomy and rarely require intravenous fluid for more than 1 day. If the skin wound has been packed open, change the packing daily. If the area is clean, tie the previously placed skin sutures on the fourth postoperative day or perform a delayed closure with skin tapes.

COMPLICATIONS

Postoperative *sepsis*, in the form of peritonitis or a pelvic abscess, is the most serious postoperative complication of an appendectomy. If the patient is febrile after the fourth or fifth postoperative day, perform a daily rectal or pelvic examination to try to detect a pelvic abscess. Often it can be discovered when the tip of the examining finger feels a fluctuant, tender mass pressing on the anterior wall of the rectum or cul-de-sac. If the abscess has progressed on antibiotic

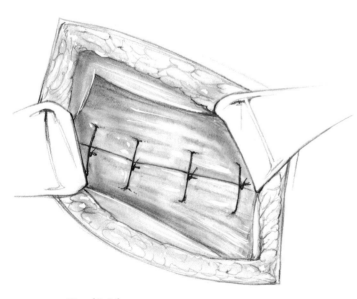

Fig. 40-14

therapy, incision and drainage may be performed with general anesthesia. To do so, dilate the anus and then pass a needle into the palpable mass. Aspiration should reveal pus just deep to the rectal wall. If pus is found, insert a hemostat along the needle tract to make 1- to 2-cm opening for drainage. CT scans or sonography are useful for identifying abdominal and pelvic abscesses, which often can be drained percutaneously by the interventional radiologist.

Wound infection following an appendectomy for a perforated appendicitis is another cause of fever. It can be prevented by delaying closure of the skin. When a wound abscess is detected, open the overlying skin for drainage.

Intestinal *obstruction* due to adhesions occasionally occurs during the postoperative period, especially when there is some degree of peritonitis. Early relaparotomy is indicated for a complete obstruction.

41 Laparoscopic Appendectomy

INDICATIONS

Acute appendicitis

Right lower quadrant pain of unknown etiology, especially in women of reproductive age

Interval appendectomy

PREOPERATIVE PREPARATION

See Chapter 40.

Place an indwelling bladder catheter for any laparoscopic procedure that involves the pelvis or lower abdomen.

PITFALLS AND DANGER POINTS

Injury to bladder from trocars or instruments

Injury to cecum from traction or dissection

Incomplete appendectomy, resulting in a retained stump

See Chapter 40

OPERATIVE STRATEGY

The laparoscopic approach allows the surgeon to make a thorough visual inspection of the abdominal cavity and hence is especially useful in cases in which the diagnosis is questionable. The procedure differs from open appendectomy in that the base of the appendix usually presents first and is divided first followed by the mesentery. A pretied ligature or staples are used to secure the base. The stump is generally not inverted. The choice of approach (open versus laparoscopic) should not influence the decision to drain or not to drain (see Chapter 40) or the duration of antibiotic therapy. These decisions should be based on the extent of the purulent and inflammatory process found at laparoscopic exploration. Other causes of lower abdominal pain, such as an inflamed Meckel's diverticulum or torsion of an ovarian cyst, may also be treated laparoscopically.

The laparoscopic approach is not advisable if an appendiceal mucocele is found, as spillage of mucocele contents may seed the peritoneal cavity with malignant cells.

OPERATIVE TECHNIQUE

Position the patient supine on the operating table. Tuck both arms at the sides; if the arms remain on armboards, they limit the ability of the camera-holder and the first assistant to move cephalad as needed. Position the monitors at the foot of the bed. If only one monitor is being used, place it along an imaginary line of sight from the umbilicus through McBurney's point. Decompress the bladder with a Foley catheter. A typical room layout is shown in **Figure 41–1**.

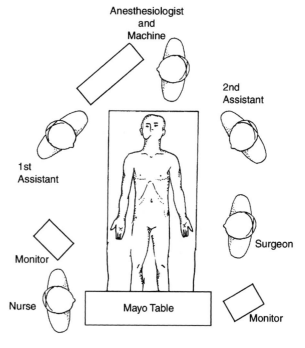

Fig. 41-1

352

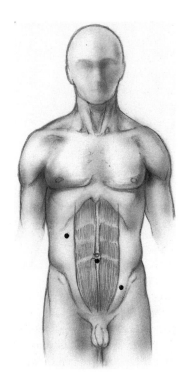

Fig. 41-2

It is important to have sufficient working distance from the right lower quadrant. Consider the location of the umbilicus relative to McBurney's point. For most patients a supraumbilical location is best for the first trocar. Place secondary trocars in the right mid-clavicular or anterior axillary line and left lower quadrant (lateral to the rectus muscle to avoid the inferior epigastric vessels) **(Fig. 41–2)**.

Thoroughly explore the abdomen and confirm the diagnosis. Examination of the female adnexae is facilitated by gently sweeping up one tube and ovary to displace the uterus to one side and then the other. Use a closed grasper or Babcock clamp to push and elevate gently, rather than grasp, the adnexae **(Fig. 41–3)**.

Exposure is enhanced by placing the patient in Trendelenburg position with the right side up. Gently sweep the omentum and small intestine medially to expose the cecum, which may be recognized by its size and white color and the presence of taeniae **(Fig. 41–4a)**. In the most common situation, the appendix lies underneath the terminal ileum and is tethered posteriorly by its mesentery **(Fig. 41–4b)**. Pulling the cecum cephalad causes at least part of the appendix, most commonly the base, to come into view **(Fig. 41–4c)**. The maneuver commonly used during open surgery (pulling the cecum cephalad, toward the patient's left shoulder) may obscure the view by pulling the cecum closer to the umbilically placed laparoscope. A straight cephalad pull, toward the patient's right shoulder, avoids this problem.

Pass an endoscopic Babcock clamp through the left lower quadrant trocar and gently pull the cecum toward the patient's left shoulder in such a way as to roll the lateral aspect of the cecum toward you. The base of the appendix should come into view. Grasp the appendix near its base with a Babcock or an atraumatic grasper. Pull straight up toward the anterior abdominal wall. Identify the base and confirm its location by the convergence of taeniae on the cecum.

There are two major ways to secure the base of the appendix: with an endoscopic stapler or a pretied suture ligature. Both methods are described here.

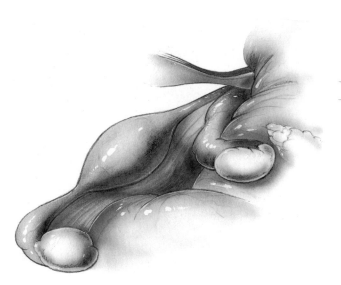

Fig. 41-3

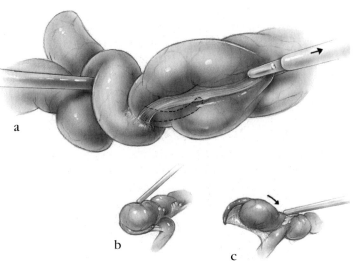

Fig. 41-4a,b,c

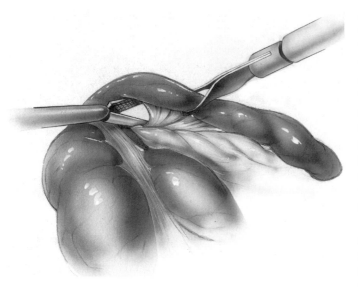

Fig. 41-5

Stapled Closure

Withdraw the Babcock clamp and replace it with a Maryland dissector or right-angle clamp. Insert the point of this dissection instrument into the groove between the fatty mesentery of the appendix and the appendix, immediately adjacent to the base **(Fig. 41–5)**. Sometimes the appendiceal mesentery is thin

or transparent at this point. Take care not to injure the cecum with the tip of the clamp. If necessary, begin creating the window just above the termination of the appendix to ensure that the tips of the clamp do not inadvertently injure the cecum behind the mesentery, where it cannot be seen. Gently open and spread, withdraw, close, and reinsert the instrument until the tip passes completely through the mesentery at this point. Enlarge this window until it is at least 1 cm in diameter. We prefer the endoscopic right-angle clamp for the task of enlarging the window once it has been established. Reconfirm that the window is exactly at the base of the appendix.

Withdraw the dissecting instrument and insert an endoscopic stapler through the 12 mm left lower quadrant port. The hinge of the stapler must be completely outside the trocar for the stapler to open properly. It may be necessary to pass the stapler behind and beyond the appendix, along the right gutter toward the right subphrenic space to have sufficient distance to open the stapler fully. Open the stapler. Withdraw the stapler (and trocar if necessary) and maneuver the narrower jaw (anvil) through the window in the mesentery. Visualize the tip of the anvil emerging on the far side of the appendix. Rotate the stapler as needed to optimize visualization of the appendix, mesentery, stapler, and cecum. Pull up on the appendix and push down on the stapler as you close the jaws of the sta-

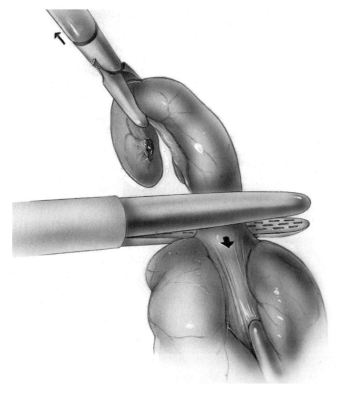

Fig. 41-6

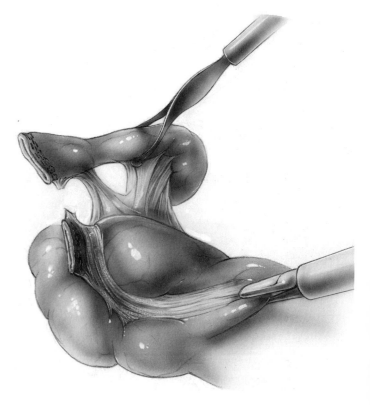

Fig. 41-7

pler **(Fig. 41–6)**; this move maximizes the chances of positioning the stapler properly (across the base so no appendiceal remnant is left). Close, but do not fire, the stapler. Rotate the stapler back and forth to visualize the proposed site of transection fully. Fire the stapler.

Open the stapler and release any adherent tissue. It may be necessary to divide a small amount of tissue with scissors. If this must be done, visually confirm that the staple line extends to the full length of the appendiceal base **(Fig. 41–7)**. Move the stapler to a safe location; close and remove it.

If necessary, reposition the appendix, now tethered only by its mesentery, so the mesentery is clearly seen. Frequently the mesentery is widest at its attachment to the appendix and then narrows as the branches of the appendicular artery converge on the trunk vessel. By identifying a narrower portion of the mesentery, it may be possible to secure it with a single application of the stapler. Reload the stapler and pass and fire it as previously described. Alternatively, use endoscopic clips to secure individual vessels **(Fig. 41–8)**. Carefully inspect the staple lines for completeness and hemostasis. Control any bleeding by endoscopic clips or suture.

Ultrasonic dissection forceps may be used instead of the stapler to divide and control the mesentery.

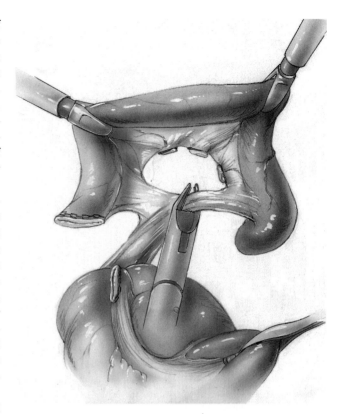

Fig. 41-8

Pretied Ligature

Alternatively, the mesentery may be divided first by clips or an ultrasonic dissecting forceps. A pretied ligature is then used to secure the base.

Identify individual branches of the appendicular artery and make windows in the mesentery between these vessels using a Maryland dissector or a right-angle clamp. Place clips on the vessels and divide them, as shown in Figure 41-8. Do not attempt to skeletonize the vessels, as they are likely to tear. Sequentially divide the mesentery along a line from the free edge toward the appendiceal base.

After completely dividing the mesentery, pass a pretied ligature into the field through the left lower quadrant trocar. Shorten the loop slightly. Avoid letting the ligature come in contact with viscera, as the loop is easier to manipulate while still dry and relatively stiff (rather than damp and limp).

Drop the appendix. Pass a Babcock clamp or atraumatic grasper through the loop of the ligature and grasp the appendix at its midportion. Pull the appendix through the loop while maneuvering and shortening the loop. Use the knot-pusher as a finger to position the knot at the base and slowly tighten the ligature **(Fig. 41–9)**.

We prefer to place two ligatures side by side on the base and a clip or a third ligature on the specimen

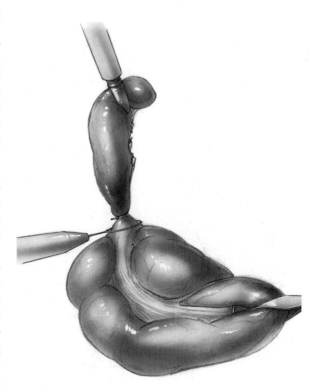

Fig. 41-9

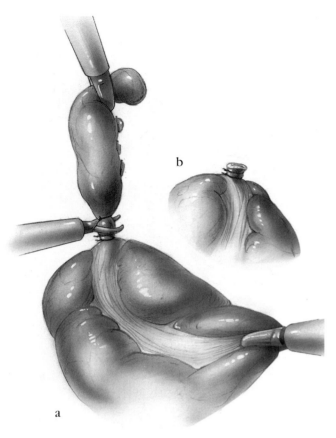

Fig. 41-10a,b

side. Divide the appendix **(Fig. 41–10a)**. Inspect the stump to verify the ligatures are in a good position **(Fig. 41–10b)**. Cauterize the exposed mucosa lightly.

Removal of the Appendix

A small, minimally inflamed appendix may be drawn completely into the left lower quadrant trocar; the

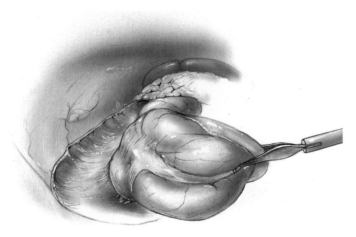

Fig. 41-12

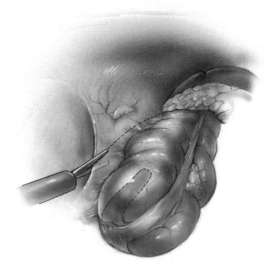

Fig. 41-11

trocar (containing the specimen) can then be completely removed and replaced. A specimen bag is used for larger, more inflamed, gangrenous or perforated appendices.

Management of the Retrocecal Appendix

The appendix is occasionally completely retrocecal and cannot be visualized without mobilizing the cecum and right colon. Incise the line of Toldt from the cecum up to the vicinity of the hepatic flexure **(Fig. 41–11)** with hook cautery, scissors (with cautery attachment), or ultrasonic shears. Grasp the cut edge of peritoneum adherent to the right colon and pull the right colon medially while lysing any residual adhesions by sharp and blunt dissection **(Fig. 41–12)**.

The appendix is then found on the back wall of the cecum, generally adherent to the cecum with fibrous bands. It may be so encased in fibrous tissue it is difficult to identify at first. Tactile perception from the Babcock clamp may help identify the appendix, which feels like a small, firm cylinder compared with the softer cecum.

Grasp the appendix near its base and sequentially lyse the fibrous adhesions that tether the appendix to the cecum **(Fig. 41–13)**. Sharp dissection with scissors or ultrasonic shears is best. Remove the appendix in the usual fashion.

Closure of Trocar Sites and Postoperative Care

If purulent material is encountered, close the fascia as usual but leave the skin open. Necrotizing fasci-

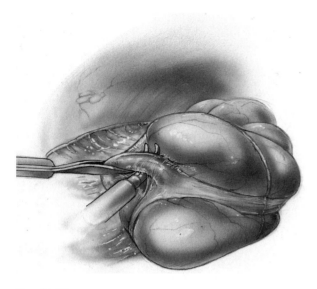

Fig. 41–13

itis has been reported as a rare complication and is more likely in obese patients.

The patient may have an ileus for several days, especially if the appendix was gangrenous or perforated. Because the events of the first postoperative week are determined by the extent of the pathology, the immediate advantage of the laparoscopic approach may not be obvious.

Continue antibiotics as you would as if the oper-

ation had been performed as an open procedure. In other words, if you would have given antibiotics for 1 week following open appendectomy for perforated appendicitis with local peritonitis, follow this regimen after laparoscopic appendectomy for the same pathology.

COMPLICATIONS

Abdominal wall infection (discussed above)

Pelvic or abdominal abscess

Retained appendiceal stump (causing recurrent appendicitis)

REFERENCES

Apelgren KN. Laparoscopic appendectomy. In Scott-Conner CEH (ed) The SAGES Manual: Fundamentals of Laparoscopy and GI Endoscopy. New York, Springer-Verlag, 1999, pp 275–280.

Apelgren KN, Cowan BD, Metcalf AM, Scott-Conner CEH. Laparoscopic appendectomy and the management of gynecologic pathologic conditions found at laparoscopy for presumed appendicitis. Surg Clin North Am 1996;76:469.

Macarulla E, Vallet J, Abad JM, et al. Laparoscopic versus open appendectomy: a prospective randomized trial. Surg Laparosc Endosc 1997;7:335.

Part V
Large Intestine

42 Concepts in Surgery of the Large Intestine

Danny M. Takanishi
Fabrizio Michelassi

This chapter provides a comprehensive overview of essential concepts relating to the operative approach and strategy for colon and rectal surgery. Additional information is contained in the technical chapters that follow and the references at the end of the chapter.

BENIGN CONDITIONS

Diverticular Disease

Diverticulosis is defined by the presence of diverticula. Bleeding and septic complications are the major surgical concerns. Surgical management depends on the site of colonic involvement, the frequency of "attacks," elective or emergent basis, and the presence of synchronous lesions. Only 1% of patients with diverticulosis require surgery. The sigmoid and descending colon are most commonly involved, although generalized colonic involvement (pandiverticulosis) may occur.

Diverticulitis, the most common condition complicating diverticulosis, occurs in approximately 10–25% of patients [1,2]. Symptoms include pain and tenderness in the left lower quadrant, altered bowel habits, nausea, fever, and if the involved segment of colon is in contact with the bladder, urinary symptoms (frequency, dysuria, pneumaturia, fecaluria). A palpable mass may be noted in the lower abdomen or pelvis. Leukocytosis with a left shift is common. Computed tomography (CT) is the best confirmatory test. It provides additional information concerning transmural extension and abscess formation as well as the presence or absence of adjacent organ involvement [3]. Image-guided percutaneous drainage may obviate the need for emergent surgery if an abscess is detected. After resolution of the acute attack, endoscopic evaluation is valuable for assessing the extent of disease and ruling out synchronous pathology.

Initial therapy depends on clinical findings. Patients with mild tenderness and low grade fever may be cared for on an outpatient basis with oral antibiotics and a clear liquid diet. Patients with symptoms and signs severe enough to require hospitalization require intravenous broad-spectrum antibiotics, hydration, and bowel rest (and possibly nasogastric decompression). Most patients improve within 48-72 hours. Surgery is generally not indicated for the first such attack unless the course is complicated by perforation and free peritonitis or abscess formation. About 30-45% of patients have recurrent attacks and require surgical intervention [1,4].

The optimal treatment is resection of the primary disease with primary anastomosis. This can certainly be carried out after successful antibiotic treatment and gentle mechanical bowel preparation. Patients who fail antibiotic therapy should undergo a two-stage operation with segmental resection of the diseased segment of bowel, primary anastomosis, and a proximal loop ileostomy or colostomy. If an abscess has been encountered in the pelvis, an omental flap can be developed to fill the abscess cavity and separate it from the colorectal anastomosis. If the planned anastomosis seems to lie within the evacuated abscess cavity, it is wiser to perform a segmental resection with an end-colostomy and a Hartmann's rectal closure or mucous fistula. The gastrointestinal continuity can be reestablished at a later time. This approach is also preferred for cases of free perforation with generalized peritonitis.

There is little role for colonic diversion without resection. This temporizing approach is reserved primarily for the rare, high-risk individual with extensive co-morbidities, abscess formation, or localized peritonitis, who would not tolerate a major operative procedure. In this case a proximal diverting loop colostomy or loop ileostomy must be complemented by abscess drainage (operatively or percutaneously with radiographic guidance) to control sepsis. Staged resection and closure of the diverting stoma is performed at a later date.

Diverticulitis may occasionally present with signs of complete *obstruction*. In otherwise asymptomatic patients (absence of pain, tenderness, systemic signs of infection), resection of the affected segment with end-colostomy and Hartmann's closure of the rectosigmoid is generally performed. Another option is on-table colonic lavage with resection, primary anastomosis, and possibly a proximal loop diverting stoma. In the poorest-risk patient a diverting transverse loop colostomy is still an option as an initial step to a staged resection.

Patients with two or more documented episodes of diverticulitis or with a history of complications from diverticular disease (bleeding, high grade partial obstruction due to cicatricial narrowing, fistulas) are candidates for elective resection. Elective resection should be considered after the first episode of diverticulitis in young patients (less than 40 years old) and those who are immunosuppressed [1,2,4,5]. Although resection can be performed 1–3 weeks following the attack of acute diverticulitis, if all the signs of local inflammation have receded rapidly many surgeons prefer to delay the operation for 2–3 months, allowing complete patient recovery and resolution of the inflammatory reaction. Delaying definitive therapy beyond 3 months puts the patient at increased risk of recurrence with no additional technical advantage.

After standard mechanical and antibiotic bowel preparation resection is based on the gross extent of disease and should include all indurated and hypertrophied bowel. Generally the sigmoid colon is primarily involved, and resection can be limited to this region. The rectum does not need to be elevated from the presacral space. Unless the mesentery is so inflamed and edematous it becomes easier to divide it close to its base, it may be resected close to the bowel wall, a concept that holds true for all benign diseases with an inflammatory component. The anastomosis is done using bowel that is soft, pliable, and free of diverticula. The splenic flexure often requires mobilization to ensure a tension-free anastomosis.

Diverticulosis is one of the most common causes of massive *lower gastrointestinal bleeding*, especially in the elderly. In most patients the bleeding stops. If episodes recur or if there is any hemodynamic instability during the first episode, surgical intervention is mandatory. If the site can be localized, by endoscopic means or arteriography, segmental resection can be done. In an emergency situation with an unstable patient, a two-stage procedure is best, with primary resection and colostomy as the first step. If the bleeding site cannot be localized, an abdominal colectomy may be necessary after preoperative proctosigmoidoscopy has ruled out the presence of a bleeding site in the rectum and rectosigmoid. Whether a primary anastomosis is per-

formed in the emergency setting or delayed for an elective procedure depends in part on the patient's hemodynamic and overall condition. If bleeding stops and the bleeding site had been identified, elective one-stage resection is carried out after bowel preparation.

Colovesical fistulas are the most common of all diverticular fistulas. Most are suspected on clinical presentation, with CT scanning probably the most sensitive test for confirming the clinical diagnosis. After appropriate bowel preparation, it is usually possible to perform one-stage, primary resection of the diseased sigmoid, with immediate anastomosis. The area of involvement in the bladder is generally small, and it may be excised and repaired by primary closure. If available, an omental interposition flap may be utilized. A Foley catheter is left in place for 7–10 days postoperatively to maintain bladder decompression.

Colonoscopy is the examination of choice for patients with chronic, occult blood loss and may also be useful for moderately severe lower gastrointestinal bleeding in the hemodynamically stable patient. If hemorrhage can be temporarily controlled, bowel preparation may be instituted and one-stage, segmental resection with primary anastomosis may be feasible.

For patients who are exsanguinating rapidly, volume resuscitation is paramount. Angiography is the test of choice and localizes the bleeding site in 75% of cases [6]. Selective infusion of vasopressin to stop or decrease the rate of hemorrhage followed by limited, segmental resection of the colon may be feasible. If brisk hemorrhage continues and angiography does not localize the source, subtotal colectomy should be performed after preoperative proctosigmoidoscopy has ruled out the rectum as the site of bleeding. Whether a primary anastomosis is performed in the emergency setting or delayed to an elective situation depends in part on the patient's hemodynamic and overall condition.

Volvulus

Volvulus of the colon results from twisting of the mesentery, most commonly in the cecum and sigmoid. It is believed that the underlying predisposing factors include an elongated mesentery or a narrow base [7]. The resulting clinical presentation is one of bowel obstruction, which may progress rapidly to strangulation, gangrene, and perforation. The sigmoid is the site most frequently involved. Plain radiographs of the abdomen may demonstrate the dilated loop of colon in the right upper quadrant ("omega loop"), and barium enema demonstrates a "bird's beak" appearance of the barium terminating at the level of the torsion. If no peritoneal signs are present, perform rigid proctosigmoidoscopy to reduce and decompress the bowel. If the mucosa appears viable, a large red rubber tube can then be inserted through the rigid proctosigmoidoscope to stent the rectosigmoid junction and decompress the proximal colon. Subsequently, mechanical preparation can be instituted and elective one-stage sigmoid resection done, given the high recurrence rate if this approach is not taken [7]. If the volvulus cannot be reduced or if any evidence of impending gangrene is detected, emergent laparotomy is indicated. After operative reduction, the involved segment is resected as part of a planned two-stage procedure with an end-colostomy and mucous fistula or Hartmann's pouch. Alternatively in low-risk patients, intraoperative intestinal lavage can be performed and a primary colorectal anastomosis fashioned.

Cecal volvulus is the next most common colonic volvulus. It presents as small bowel obstruction. Plain radiographs of the abdomen may demonstrate features of a small bowel obstruction in association with a dilated cecum in the left upper quadrant. Emergency laparotomy is required. First reduce the volvulus and assess the viability of the bowel. If the bowel is viable, cecopexy is performed. A tube cecostomy can be added to increase the chances of a successful cecopexy. Simple reduction is inadequate and attended by a significant recurrence rate. Evidence of impending gangrene requires resection. Options include an end-ileostomy with mucous fistula. Primary anastomosis is safe in patients who are hemodynamically stable and in whom perforation or contamination has not occurred.

Ischemic Colitis

Ischemic colitis is heterogeneous in terms of etiology, anatomic site of involvement, presentation, and degree of severity [8]. Although all areas of the colon can be involved, the splenic flexure and rectosigmoid (watershed areas) seem to be at particular risk [8,9]. Significant morbidity and mortality are in large part due to underlying conditions. A high index of suspicion is necessary for diagnosis. Many patients experience left flank and left lower quadrant pain, diarrhea, and blood per rectum. Colonoscopy is the diagnostic tool of choice. Plain radiographs of the abdomen and CT scans are useful primarily to exclude other causes of abdominal pain or the complications of perforation, pneumatosis, and portal vein air. Barium enema no longer has a role in the diagnosis and workup of this disease.

Initial treatment is supportive and consists of fluid resuscitation, bowel rest (possibly with nasogastric decompression), correction of anemia, and broad-spectrum antibiotics. Most attacks (80–90%) are self-limiting and heal with this approach. All require colonoscopy 6–8 weeks after the event. A small percentage (2%) of patients develop strictures [8,9]. Surgical resection is required if obstructive symptoms develop, or if cancer cannot be definitively excluded. After appropriate bowel preparation, an elective one-stage procedure is done, resecting the diseased segment of colon and performing the anastomosis in noninvolved, normal, viable bowel.

In a small group of cases ischemia progresses to necrosis and frank gangrene. These patients are quite toxic and ill, with evidence of sepsis, hemodynamic instability, and eventual shock. This mandates emergent laparotomy. The goals of surgery are (1) to assess the extent of ischemia by evaluating mesenteric flow (palpation, Doppler, intravenous fluorescein dye combined with a Wood's lamp) and by endoscopic evaluation of mucosal viability; and (2) to resect all nonviable, compromised bowel. Normal mucosa must be present at the margins of the resection. In general, an end-colostomy and a Hartmann's pouch or mucous fistula should be created (the latter has the unique advantage of allowing direct evaluation of the mucosa for evidence of ongoing ischemia); in the rare hemodynamically stable, low-risk patient, intraoperative cleansing of the proximal large bowel can be followed by a primary anastomosis. Another option is extension of the resection to include a subtotal colectomy with an ileorectal anastomosis. If the involvement is confined to the right colon, a primary anastomosis is feasible, provided there has been no major contamination and the patient is hemodynamically stable. If a primary anastomosis has been fashioned but there are doubts about intestinal viability, a planned second-look laparotomy is scheduled within 24 hours.

Rectal Prolapse

Complete rectal prolapse (procidentia) presents with intussusception of the rectum into the anal canal [10], with the descent of all layers of the rectum through the anus. All patients should therefore undergo endoscopic evaluation to rule out a tumor etiology serving as the lead point and to assess for ulceration or other complications.

Surgical options all aim to correct the abnormal anatomy. Broadly categorized, techniques for repair are based on either an abdominal or a perineal approach. Factors considered during selection of a particular procedure include age, overall performance status, and the advantages or disadvantages of each technique [10,11].

Abdominal approaches include rectopexy alone, segmental resection alone, or a combination of the two. Rectopexy (e.g., the Ripstein procedure) (see Chapter 56) involves complete rectal mobilization to the pelvic floor with division of the lateral stalks. Suture rectopexy utilizes simple suturing of the rectum to the sacral fascia (posterior rectopexy) or the peritoneum, pelvic brim, or uterus (anterior rectopexy). Variations of this procedure diverge with the manner in which the rectum is suspended; nonreabsorbable sutures, Ivalon sponge (Wells' procedure), or Teflon/Marlex mesh (Ripstein procedure) have been well described [10,11]. Recurrence rates range from 2% to 16%, and complications include obstruction secondary to mesh wraps or sepsis related to the foreign body (e.g., full-thickness decubitus and pelvic abscesses). Segmental resection alone has also been successful, with recurrence rates comparable to those seen with the pexy procedures [11]. Associated complications are few, consisting primarily of anastomotic dehiscence. The lowest recurrence rates have been noted with the combination suture rectopexy and sigmoid resection.

Perineal approaches include simple encirclement of the anus and rectosigmoidectomy. The Thiersch procedure (see Chapter 63) has evolved over time but is rarely used owing to the high rates of recurrence and septic complications. Perineal rectosigmoidectomy involves resecting the prolapsed bowel starting 1–2 cm proximal to the dentate line. A primary anastomosis and a levatorplasty are then performed concomitantly. Recurrence rates vary significantly, from approximately 3% up to 60% in some series [12]. Theoretically, the reduction in rectal reservoir function could potentially result in urgency or incontinence.

It is generally accepted that transabdominal approaches are associated with lower rates of recurrence than the perineal approaches, which have higher recurrence rates but are safer options in high-risk or elderly patients [10,11]. What is still debatable and controversial is which procedures result in better functional outcomes. Unfortunately, too few randomized trials have compared the functional outcomes of the various techniques. Hence this important issue has not been addressed adequately.

Familial Polyposis and Hereditary Colon Cancer Syndromes

Familial adenomatous polyposis (FAP) is the phenotypic result of a germline mutation of the adenomatous polyposis coli (*APC*) gene on chromosome 5q21 [13]. The disease is characterized by multiple adenomatous polyps in the large bowel that can be complicated by bleeding, obstruction (uncommon), a protein-losing enteropathy, and of considerable significance the development of adenocarcinomas. Extraintestinal manifestations are also common. The penetrance of this gene is high; this fact and the associated risk for carcinoma have provided the rationale to pursue a surgical approach as early as the late teenage years.

Current appropriate treatment requires total removal of the colorectal mucosa to avoid the later development of carcinoma, a complication that generally afflicts these patients by the age of 40, if not sooner. Although proctocolectomy with ileostomy removes the risk of colorectal cancer, it is obviously attended by loss of transanal defecation. This option, nowadays, is usually reserved for patients with advanced cancer of the rectum or anal incontinence. To avoid a permanent stoma, surgeons once performed subtotal colectomy with ileorectal anastomosis combined with electrocautery destruction of the remaining rectal polyps. Obviously, the remnant mucosa required close surveillance for the development of carcinoma. Review of the literature demonstrated a 30% incidence of rectal cancers after 20 years, so this procedure was indicated in only a small number of selected patients.

Today complete removal of colorectal cancer risk and maintenance of transanal defecation is achieved with a restorative proctocolectomy with ileal pouch/anal anastomosis [14]. The technique is described in Chapter 48. An alternative technique utilizing a stapled anastomosis (ileal pouch/distal rectal anastomosis) may yield slightly better functional results at the expense of risking recurrent polyposis in the retained mucosa, which presumably would render patients at higher risk for the development of dysplasia and adenocarcinoma. Currently, it is not possible to quantify the risk for the individual patient. Mutational analysis to pinpoint the specific locus of the gene mutation in the *FAP* gene in an individual patient may prove to be a method of selecting who can safely undergo an ileorectal anastomosis and who requires an ileal pouch/anal procedure or proctocolectomy because of a high risk for rectal cancer development in the retained rectum.

Hereditary nonpolyposis colorectal cancer (HNPCC) syndrome is the most common inherited disease predisposing to the development of colorectal cancer after FAP. This autosomal dominant syndrome is characterized by right-sided colon cancer usually by age 40–45 years, and increased incidence of synchronous and metachronous colorectal cancer, and an excess of extracolonic cancers, such as endometrial, ovarian, and upper gastrointestinal lesions. The predisposition to cancer in patients with HNPCC syndrome arises from germline mutations in mismatch repair (*MMR*) genes. A total abdominal colectomy is recommended as an alternative to lifetime endoscopic surveillance for selected *MMR* gene mutation carriers with colon adenomas. Prophylactic colectomy should be considered for patients whose colons are difficult to scope or for those in whom endoscopic polypectomy may be technically difficult.

Inflammatory Bowel Disease

Crohn's Colitis

Surgery is indicated for intractability (including individuals dependent on high doses of immunosuppressive agents and steroids), septic complications, chronic bleeding and anemia, stricture formation, fulminant colitis or toxic megacolon, and the development of dysplasia or adenocarcinoma [15]. Surgical treatment must be tailored to the anatomic extent of the macroscopic disease. If the colitis is limited to the right colon, a right hemicolectomy can suffice; if it extends past the splenic flexure, and the rectosigmoid is devoid of disease, an abdominal colectomy with ileosigmoid anastomosis is necessary. In the presence of pancolitis, a proctocolectomy with terminal ileostomy is the procedure of choice. A restorative proctocolectomy with ileal pouch/anal anastomosis is contraindicated in Crohn's disease because of the high risk of perineal and pelvic septic complications and the high Crohn's disease recurrence rate in the ileal pouch.

In case of fulminant colitis or toxic megacolon, many patients undergo total colectomy and end-ileostomy, with further surgery after a recovery period of 2–3 months. Completion proctectomy or an ileorectal anastomosis may be appropriate if the rectal stump is not diseased and there is good anal sphincter function without significant perineal disease [16]. In this acute emergency setting the colon is exquisitely friable. Exercise great care during operative manipulation to prevent rupture and peritoneal contamination. Do not attempt to separate the omentum from the transverse colon, as it may lead to inadvertent colonic perforation or may violate walled-off microabscesses.

Patients with extensive perineal disease complicated by acute and chronic sepsis should be treated by a staged approach with total colectomy and a short rectal pouch about 5 cm or less in length. Concomitant with this Hartmann coloproctectomy, fistulous tracts are opened and perirectal abscesses are drained. With subsequent resolution of perineal sepsis, intersphincteric resection of the rectal stump by a perineal approach can then be undertaken. This approach has significantly diminished the risk of perineal wound complications.

Although segmental colon resection is associated with a higher recurrence rate than proctocolectomy with ileostomy, it may avoid or delay a permanent stoma and facilitates retaining as much colon mucosa as possible. This is especially desirable in patients who have already suffered a sizable loss of small intestine. Thus sigmoid or left-sided colon disease is usually treated with a sigmoid or left colectomy; isolated rectal disease can be treated with abdominoperineal proctectomy with end-colostomy [17,18].

Anorectal complications of Crohn's disease must be approached based on their severity and extension and on the status of the rectal mucosa. If the rectum is not diseased, perianal abscesses can be drained, anorectal stenosis dilated, fistula in ano surgically treated, and rectovaginal fistula repaired with good expectation of complete healing. If the perineal disease is severe or the rectal mucosa is diseased (or both), a rectal ablative procedure is the only surgical procedure that can avoid the complications and return the patient to a satisfactory quality of life.

A genetically engineered monoclonal antibody, Infliximab, has been found to be efficacious in a randomized trial for treating fistulas in Crohn's disease patients. Long-term follow-up is necessary; but if these data are validated, this agent may prove to offer another option to the challenging and often complex management of perineal Crohn's fistulas.

Ulcerative Colitis

Unlike Crohn's disease, which can affect any portion of the gastrointestinal tract, ulcerative colitis is limited to the colon and rectum. The surgical indications are similar for both diseases, however, and include medical intractability, fulminant colitis and toxic megacolon, stricture formation, hemorrhage, and the presence of dysplasia and carcinoma [15,19]. In the pediatric population, delayed growth and maturation may also be an indication, though less so than for Crohn's disease.

Proctocolectomy/end-ileostomy has the advantage of removing the entire target end-organ and curing the patient, usually with one surgical procedure. Although a major disadvantage is that the procedure results in a permanent stoma, it represents the best option for individuals with poor anal sphincter function, an advanced rectal carcinoma, and advanced age [15]. A variation on this theme is construction of a continent, or Kock, ileostomy. The benefit of this approach is that it allows patients an opportunity to maintain control over evacuation, but the technique is not without complications.

The ileal pouch/anal procedure is probably the most popular option in terms of patient preference. With experience in major centers accruing since the 1980s along with concomitant long-term patient follow-up, this operation has an excellent success rate and good functional results [20–26]. In the absence of dysplastic or malignant degeneration a complete mucosectomy is not mandatory, and the ileoanal anastomosis can be performed with a circular stapler 0.5–2.0 cm proximal to the dentate line. This modification makes the procedure easier, increases the chance of avoiding a temporary ileostomy (one-step restorative proctocolectomy with ileoanal pouch anastomosis), allows the procedure to be performed in obese patients, and maintains the lower rectal mucosa with its proprioceptive sensation indispensable for distinguishing flatus from liquid and solid stool.

Total abdominal colectomy and ileorectal anastomosis has been used in the past. Because of the retained rectum, ongoing surveillance for the early detection of dysplasia or carcinoma is mandatory [27–31]. This approach therefore is limited to patients with rectal sparing (which is unusual given that the disease has a tendency to manifest in the rectum first), elderly patients, and patients whose ulcerative colitis is complicated by a stage IV colon cancer.

Subtotal colectomy/end-ileostomy is the favored approach in patients with fulminant colitis intractable to medical therapy, toxic megacolon, or acute bleeding. In most cases, the subjects are severely ill individuals, many of whom are debilitated, on high-dose steroids, or highly catabolic with systemic manifestations of hemodynamic instability or sepsis. This procedure removes the diseased colon, allowing resolution of the systemic manifestations and quiescence of the associated rectal involvement. After a period of recovery, patients remain candidates for a completion proctectomy with the creation of an ileal pouch/anal procedure. From an operative standpoint this staged approach has the added advantage of allowing associated pelvic inflammation to subside. Pelvic dissection in the acute setting causes potentially more blood loss and greater risk of injury to the pelvic autonomic nerves or rectum during dissection, further compounding the risk of pelvic septic complications [32].

Indeterminate Colitis

In approximately 5–10% of patients with inflammatory colitis the diagnosis of Crohn's or ulcerative colitis is still equivocal even after a thorough endoscopic and histopathologic evaluation. In patients with medically intractable disease requiring surgery, in both the emergent setting and the elective setting, the preferred approach is generally subtotal colectomy with end-ileostomy and closure of the rectal stump [33]. This approach allows for the possibility of a completion restorative proctectomy and ileal pouch/anal procedure if the histologic evaluation of the specimen demonstrates ulcerative colitis, while avoiding the unfortunate situation of performing an ileal pouch/anal procedure in an individual later diagnosed as having Crohn's disease [34].

Polyps

The *hyperplastic polyp* is the most common type of polyp. It tends to be diminutive, is often multiple, harbors no malignant potential, and is easily removed endoscopically by simple biopsy in most cases. *Adenomatous polyps* and *villous adenomas* are premalignant lesions, based on observations of their natural history and an improved understanding of the molecular events in the adenoma–carcinoma sequence of colorectal cancer [35]. The risk of invasive cancer increases with polyp size, morphology (sessile), and histology (degree of villous component) [35–37]. Most polyps are initially excised endoscopically. Lesions less than 2 cm are amenable to endoscopic polypectomy; larger lesions may require partial snare excision or multiple piecemeal excisions. If histopathologic examination of the specimen excludes the presence of carcinoma, endoscopic removal is all that is needed. If the polyp cannot be removed endoscopically or is extremely large (and malignancy cannot be excluded), the patient must undergo operative polypectomy or segmental colon resection [35]. In these cases it is useful to inject the site with India ink at endoscopy to facilitate intraoperative identification.

Subsequent management is guided by the presence of invasive cancer and the likelihood of lymph node metastasis. Haggit et al. developed a prognostic schema that may be used to identify patients adequately treated by endoscopic excision alone [37,38]. Endoscopic removal of a polyp found to have malignant degeneration is considered sufficient if the following conditions have been met.

1. Endoscopic removal has provided an adequate margin of resection.
2. The lesion is well to moderately differentiated.
3. There is no lymphovascular invasion.
4. There is no evidence of invasion of the submucosa of the colonic wall.

All patients treated in this fashion require follow-up colonoscopy in 3-6 months to assess for local recurrence. If the polyp shows malignant degeneration, the margins of excision are less than 2 mm, and there is invasion of the submucosa, a poor histologic grade, or lymphatic/vascular invasion, the patient stands at increased risk for lymph node involvement or local recurrence by the carcinoma. In these instances, segmental colectomy is generally selected.

Cyclooxygenase-2 (COX-2) inhibitors may modify the management of colonic polyps in the future. Accumulating data suggest that this class may diminish the risk of developing adenomas and carcinomas [39]. Investigations are currently underway to elucidate the role these compounds play in colorectal carcinogenesis. This holds the promise of a potentially effective strategy in the nonoperative management of premalignant tumors of the colon and rectum.

MALIGNANT CONDITIONS

Colorectal Cancer

Extent of Resection

The surgical management of colorectal carcinoma is based on two principles: rendering patients disease-free when feasible and palliating any symptoms attributable to the malignancy. The concept of the "extent of resection" for curative intent has undergone considerable evolution as better understanding of the magnitude of lymphadenectomy and proximal, distal, and radial margins has accrued. In the case of colon cancers, resection is generally based on the vascular anatomy to ensure removal of the entire lymph node drainage basin [39]. This complete mesenteric excision frequently is associated with proximal and distal margins longer than 5-6 cm, which are more than adequate to minimize anastomotic and locoregional recurrences. The radial margin, not a frequent issue in colon cancers, becomes a consideration when the tumor invades adjacent organs. In this case, en bloc resection of the involved adjacent organs or viscera is required, provided distant disease is not present to preclude curative resection.

In the case of rectal cancer, including distal and radial margins is equally important to prevent locoregional recurrences, but it is rendered more challenging by the desire to save the anal sphincter complex and by the anatomic constraints of the pelvis. Optimal initial treatment is important, as local recurrences are often not salvageable for cure, and up to 25% of patients dying from rectal cancers have

disease limited strictly to the pelvis. In addition, pelvic recurrences are quite symptomatic, with bleeding, tenesmus, anal sphincter dysfunction and incontinence, pelvic sepsis, bowel and urinary obstruction, and severe perineal pain secondary to bone and nerve plexus involvement [39]. Neoadjuvant or adjuvant radiation therapy (with or without chemotherapy) forms a major part of the multimodality approach to treating rectal carcinomas to enhance locoregional control.

Contemporary studies have not demonstrated any survival benefit of "high" lymphovascular ligation of a major vessel compared to a "low" ligation closer to the cancer [39]. Extended pelvic lymphadenectomy or high ligation of the inferior mesenteric artery for surgical management of rectal cancer has conferred no survival benefit, and current practice emphasizes ligation of the inferior mesenteric artery distal to the origin of the left colic artery [39]. The role of the sentinel node biopsy is being evaluated.

The surgical approach to a rectal cancer also depends on its distance from the anal verge. For cancers proximal to 5-7 cm from the anal verge, adequate oncologic clearance and gastrointestinal continuity restoration may be achieved with a low anterior resection using modern anastomotic techniques [40]. For coloanal anastomosis at the level of the dentate line, a colonic J-pouch reservoir may be added (see Intestinal Pouch Reservoirs, below).

Colorectal Cancer with Synchronous Pathology

Synchronous lesions are relatively common in colorectal carcinoma; hence there is a need to study the entire colon preoperatively or intraoperatively, generally by total colonoscopy. In a series of 228 patients with colorectal cancer evaluated at the University of Chicago, 45.6% had synchronous lesions and 11.0% required a surgical resection more extensive than what would have been dictated by the primary tumor [41]. Eleven patients (4.9%) had synchronous adenocarcinoma, in agreement with already reported data.

Synchronous Benign or Premalignant Conditions

In the case of coexisting *diverticular disease*, oncologic considerations and the location of significantly diseased bowel guide the extent of resection. The anastomosis must be constructed in a region of healthy tissue without diverticula or muscular hypertrophy.

Synchronous polyps outside the planned resection field should be addressed. If the colon cancer and the synchronous polyp(s) are present within the same segment of colon, a standard resection is performed. If the involved areas are noncontiguous, attempt preoperative endoscopic resection. If the polyp is confirmed to be benign but too large for endoscopic resection, colostomy with operative polypectomy combined with segmental colon resection may be a feasible option. If the polyp is located on the mesenteric side or is too large for surgical resection through a colostomy or if it harbors a malignancy, an extended colon resection is often necessary to remove both the polyp and the cancer and to avoid two anastomotic suture lines.

In the setting of *ulcerative colitis*, the principles of resection are based on the need to remove the target organ and the primary tumor concomitantly. With ulcerative colitis this often requires a restorative proctocolectomy with construction of an end-ileostomy or ileal pouch/anal procedure. A proctocolectomy will ileostomy may be necessary for rectal cancers. A subtotal colectomy with ileorectal anastomosis may be an alternative in the presence of a metastatic colon cancer.

The goals of management for *familial polyposis* are analogous to that for ulcerative colitis. Optimal management generally involves a restorative proctocolectomy to remove all involved diseased large bowel at risk for the development of metachronous carcinomas and avoid a permanent stoma. Proctocolectomy with ileostomy may be necessary in the presence of a rectal cancer.

A total abdominal colectomy is recommended for *MMR gene mutation carriers* with a colon carcinoma. Postmenopausal women should be advised to consider a prophylactic hysterectomy and bilateral salpingo-oophorectomy.

Synchronous Cancer

The reported incidence of synchronous cancers varies between 1.5% and 10.7% [41]. The approach is to treat each cancer conceptually as a separate lesion. If the two are within a contiguous portion of colon, a standard primary resection is done; if they involve two noncontiguous regions, an extended resection is done so only one anastomosis must be created. It may necessitate subtotal colectomy.

Preoperative Evaluation

Total colonoscopy with appropriate biopsy is the "gold standard" for diagnosis and confirmation of the presence of malignancies and synchronous pathology. Careful histologic evaluation is important for both cancer and benign conditions. Barium enema examination and the newer virtual reality imaging

(still investigational) have limited roles because tissue sampling is not possible [39]. These studies are used primarily when total colonoscopy is not feasible.

Precise measurement of location for carcinoma of the rectum is generally done by digital rectal examination and rigid proctosigmoidoscopy. Each assesses the distance between the anal verge and the lower border of the tumor. Digital examination also allows assessment of the distance between the anorectal ring and the distal edge of the tumor. It is this distance that determines, in part, the surgical options available to an individual patient, most importantly the feasibility of sphincter preservation. Digital evaluation also provides an initial determination of tumor size, depth, location, and mobility. Finally, it assists in identifying those tumors potentially amenable to local excision techniques.

Precise preoperative staging assists in proper surgical planning and has become increasingly important as multimodality (including neoadjuvant) treatment gains widespread popularity. Standard staging studies include chest radiography or thoracic CT and CT of the abdomen and pelvis to determine if measurable pulmonary, hepatic, or peritoneal metastases are present and if adjacent organ involvement exists. Ultrasonography, in experienced hands, is equivalent to the CT scan as an imaging modality to detect liver metastases. Both have supplanted the use of liver chemistries for this goal [39]. Magnetic resonance imaging is not thought to offer additional advantage. Other staging studies (CT scans of the head or bone scans) are used only in symptomatic patients [39].

Digital examination and endorectal ultrasonography are more accurate than CT scans for determining the *local extent of rectal cancer* [39,42]. Endorectal ultrasonography is particularly useful for measuring the precise depth of invasion and the status of the perirectal lymph nodes.

Determination of the *carcinoembryonic antigen (CEA) level* has no value for preoperative staging of a colon or rectal carcinoma. It may be helpful as a baseline, however, for postoperative follow-up.

Finally, *patient age and overall performance status* (including co-morbid medical illnesses, nutritional status) are important issues when determining the timing and selection of the surgical procedure(s). Assessment of the general status is important when choosing the operative approach. High-risk, elderly patients with multiple co-morbidities are better served by less extensive resections, with attendant decreased anesthesia time, more rapid recovery, and less morbidity and mortality. Advanced age alone is not considered a contraindication to operative intervention in the emergent or the elective setting. Patients who are debilitated, cachectic, or otherwise infirm may require nutritional support and restitution of metabolic and intravascular volume deficits before any planned procedure (if delay does not further compromise the patient's condition).

Obesity may preclude restoration of gastrointestinal continuity and maintenance of transanal defecation because of technical constraints. Patients must be informed of this possibility during preoperative treatment planning discussions. Stoma site selection also poses a significant challenge in this group of patients (see Intestinal Stomas, below).

Neoadjuvant Therapy for Rectal Adenocarcinoma

Trials of preoperative (neoadjuvant) or postoperative radiation therapy for rectal adenocarcinoma have shown decreased local recurrence in the treated cohorts [43–53]. Perceived advantages of preoperative versus postoperative radiotherapy include optimal radiosensitivity of well oxygenated neoplastic cells still undisturbed by the surgical dissection and the possibility of decreasing the size of the perirectal infiltration allowing for a negative radial margin. In addition, preoperative radiotherapy avoids irradiation of the freshly fashioned anastomosis. The preoperative dose delivered and the duration of that delivery continue to be sources of considerable debate. A randomized trial from Lyon demonstrated that a longer interval to surgery (6–8 weeks compared to 2 weeks) resulted in significantly better tumor regression and downstaging with no differences appreciated in terms of local control, survival, or complication rate at a median follow-up of approximately 3 years [54]. Although most reports indicate that better local control is achievable with pre- or postoperative adjuvant therapy of advanced rectal cancers, most reports fail to demonstrate that neoadjuvant therapy translates into improved control and overall survival when compared to postoperative treatment [47,51,52].

Squamous Carcinoma of the Anus

The *Nigro protocol* is used for squamous cell carcinoma of the anal region. This combined regimen of external beam radiation, 5-fluorouracil, and mitomycin C allows preservation of sphincter function and yields improved 5-year survival compared to that of historical controls who underwent abdominoperineal resection. Overall 5-year survival rates with modern modifications of this protocol exceed 80% [55,56]. For those with persistent or recurrent disease, salvage abdominoperineal resection may result in more than 50% long-term survival [56].

Surgical Approach and Strategy

Preoperative Preparation

Although *mechanical bowel preparations* have been used for decades, currently no clinical trial data support this practice. A meta-analysis based on three clinical trials showed that patients who underwent mechanical bowel preparation had a higher rate of wound infections and anastomotic leaks. The prevailing concern regarding the potential risk of intraoperative peritoneal contamination and the facilitation of intraoperative colonic manipulation continues to favor use of mechanical bowel preparations. Polyethylene glycol (colonic lavage) solutions are most commonly used. A clear liquid diet for 1–2 days prior to the operative procedure is another component of the traditional bowel preparation.

The concept of *antimicrobial prophylaxis* has been studied extensively for years. Debate centers on the optimum route of administration, what constitutes the best antibiotic, and the value of combination regimens of oral and parenteral agents. The most common regimens include preoperative oral neomycin and erythromycin only, parenterally administered second-generation cephalosporins only, and a combination of the two. Oral antibiotics should be given within 24 hours of the procedure. The timing of parenteral agents is guided by the goal of adequate tissue levels at operation. This generally means dosing one-half hour before the skin incision.

The extent or need for *postoperative parenteral antibiotic administration* is also unknown. From the standpoint of prophylaxis there appears to be no benefit beyond two or three doses postoperatively or for a period beyond 24 hours.

Patients who have been on *steroids* as part of their medical regimen for inflammatory bowel disease or collagen-vascular disorders require preoperative pharmacologic doses in preparation for the metabolic stress of general anesthesia and a major operative procedure. Supplementation is done to prevent precipitation of adrenal insufficiency during the perioperative period. A "rapid taper" schedule is followed over the subsequent days until the patient is at the preoperative oral dose equivalent. A sample regimen is hydrocortisone intravenously 100 mg q8h on the day of surgery, followed by 75 mg q8h for the next 24 hours, then 50 mg q8h for 24 hours, then 50 mg q12h by postoperative day 3.

Laparotomy Versus Laparoscopy

Open laparotomy is the traditional approach and is emphasized in the chapters that follow. The procedure begins with thorough evaluation of the extent of disease and assessment for associated diseases before planned resection. This includes evaluation of adjacent organ involvement and regional lymph node involvement and determination of the presence or absence of distant (usually hepatic) disease. All four quadrants of the abdomen are examined, including the entire small bowel, along with careful exploration of the pelvis and gynecologic organs and all peritoneal surfaces.

Innovations in *minimally invasive surgery* have been extended to colorectal surgery, and many "open" procedures have been adapted to this approach [57–68]. Comparative studies continue to accrue, substantiating earlier hypotheses of safety and feasibility. Accurate comparative assessments of diminished postoperative pain and ileus, shorter hospital stay, shortened postoperative convalescence compared to that after open procedures, and cost differences continue to be areas of some controversy. Preliminary analyses of data demonstrate that an equivalent resection may be accomplished [39,57,58,61,62,64,65]. Laparoscopy is also useful for staging and abdominal exploration prior to laparotomy for recurrent or metastatic disease. By detecting peritoneal implants, laparoscopy may spare patients the morbidity of an unnecessary laparotomy in this setting [39]. Port-site metastases in patients who have undergone the procedure with a "curative" resection remain a concern. Trials are currently in progress to determine the exact incidence of this phenomenon and to elucidate its etiology.

Alternatives to Formal Resection of Rectal Cancer

Simple transanal excision is the most common local approach to rectal polyps and cancers. With the patient in lithotomy or jack-knife position, an anal retractor is placed for exposure and a headlight utilized to visualize the anorectal canal. The tumor is excised with electrocautery obtaining a full-thickness biopsy (deep margin is perirectal fat) with a 1 cm margin around the tumor. The defect may be left open or closed with absorbable sutures. Complications are rare, and there is no postoperative pain. This approach is used [36,39] in tumors that are

Well to moderately differentiated

Small (<3 cm)

Nonulcerated

Involve less than one-fourth the circumference of the rectum

Exophytic

Mobile

Tis or T1 lesions (as determined by endorectal ultrasonography)

Demonstrating no evidence of lymphovascular invasion

Without palpable perirectal lymphadenopathy

Within 10 cm of anal verge.

Positive margins or unfavorable histopathologic characteristics require surgical resection. Data from clinical trials show that *adjuvant radiation* reduces recurrence rates significantly after transanal excision in well selected patients, in contrast to surgery alone [39]. These data must be interpreted with caution because many of these studies are small with short follow-up; and so far there has been no evidence that this combination of treatment has any effect on overall survival. Along this line of thought, T2 lesions have been subjected to chemoradiation as adjuvant treatment, particularly because of the higher likelihood of regional node involvement with increasing depth of invasion [39]. This modality has been associated with low morbidity (less than 10%) and no operative mortality. Yet with the maturation of some clinical studies, the recurrence rates for locally resected T2 lesions approximate 15–25% even after postoperative chemotherapy, suggesting that formal resection is still the treatment of choice for these tumors.

Transanal endoscopic microsurgery offers a transanal approach to lesions located in the proximal rectum and rectosigmoid. Essentially, a large-bore proctoscope allows resection of the tumor with specially constructed graspers, scissors, needle-holders, and cautery while viewing the procedure on a video screen. Full-thickness excision with primary closure is achieved. This approach is utilized primarily for adenomas and Tis and T1 cancers. Local recurrence rates appear comparable to those seen with open surgical approaches, with less morbidity and shorter hospitalization [69–73].

Electrocoagulation and *laser fulguration* represent other transanal ablative techniques. These techniques are limited in that full-thickness resections and wide margins usually cannot be obtained [74]. Hence they should be restricted to patients whose medical condition and general status precludes major surgery and those who already have identifiable distant metastasis.

The *posterior approach* may be useful for resecting benign rectal polyps that would otherwise be difficult to reach through the anal route because of size, location, or distance from the anal verge. This approach is ideal for polyps located 7–13 cm from the anal verge, especially if located on the anterior or lateral rectal wall.

Endocavitary irradiation (papillon technique) is based on use of a low-voltage generator to irradiate a rectal carcinoma through a proctoscope. This has the benefit of a more limited extent of radiation injury compared to external beam irradiation, and adjacent organs are therefore spared injury. This factor is exploited using large doses (up to 15,000 cGy) directed to the tumor bed, often combined with an iridium 192 implant [75,76]. It is done as an outpatient procedure for cure or palliation. The morbidity is minimal, except that many patients require local anesthesia or sedation owing to the large proctoscope utilized, and some develop varying degrees of incontinence due to sphincter injury. Again, a major disadvantage of this procedure and similar "ablation" techniques is the absence of an intact specimen to allow comprehensive histologic examination, which may influence the decision for additional therapy. For this reason, when a local approach is chosen the choice is usually between a transanal approach (with or without endoscopic microsurgery) or a posterior approach.

Specific Interoperative Considerations During Operations for Colorectal Cancer

Many techniques, such as the Turnbull "no touch" technique were previously advocated in an attempt to minimize locoregional and distant failure [77]. As our understanding of cancer biology has improved based on observational, natural history studies and the advent of molecular biology and cancer genetics, it has become increasingly clear that to a great extent it is the biology of the specific tumor that governs disease-free survival. However, analysis of data involving patterns of recurrence has allowed formulation of a few principles that may affect the disease-free interval and ultimately survival.

The most significant surgeon-controlled factor that diminishes the risk of local recurrence is an operative conduct aimed at obtaining *negative proximal, distal, and radial resection margins*. This may necessitate the use of intraoperative frozen section control and en bloc resection if there is adjacent organ involvement. Suture line recurrence constitutes a form of local failure, and strategies to prevent this occurrence are similar to those expounded to prevent local recurrences in general.

Minimize manipulation of the tumor and, in particular, avoid breaching the colonic wall with significant spillage of tumor cells into the peritoneal cavity. It is not clear exactly what tumor inoculum size is necessary for implantation and propagation to occur, as host factors play an important role. If the involved

segment of large bowel is adherent to an adjacent organ or structure, perform an en bloc resection rather than attempting to dissect the tumor free in patients where the resection has curative intent.

The surgical principles governing control of locoregional recurrence pertain to prevention of distant failure as well. There is a growing body of literature that substantiates the theory that inadequate local control, by virtue of persistent disease, increases the propensity for distant disease [39].

Strategies for Complex Situations

Patients who are *septic* because of abscess or perforation require fluid resuscitation and broad-spectrum parenteral antibiotics. Initial antibiotic coverage should include agents effective against Enterobacteriaceae and obligate anaerobes such as *Bacteroides* species and *Clostridium*. Bowel rest is also an important component of management, as many patients have an associated ileus depending on the degree of the septic insult.

In instances of *colonic perforation*, whether due to benign or malignant disease, an emergent resection to control the septic process is imperative. Constructing an anastomosis in the presence of peritoneal contamination, especially if generalized, is attended by a significant risk of anastomotic leakage. Consequently, the most common and safest option is represented by a segmental colon resection with a proximal end-stoma and closure of the distal colon or construction of a mucous fistula. Alternatively, if the perforation is localized and walled off, resection with primary anastomosis and proximal diverting loop ileostomy is often possible. This approach has the advantage of not requiring a formal laparotomy to reconstitute gastrointestinal continuity at a later time. If a good-risk, healthy patient is found to have a localized cecal perforation, an ileocolonic anastomosis following right colectomy may be done, provided the two intestinal segments to be anastomosed are free of inflammation. The anastomosis should be placed in the upper abdomen, away from the abscess cavity. Omentum may be used to wrap the anastomosis as an added precaution. If contamination and inflammation are not well localized or if the patient has significant co-morbidity, hemodynamic instability, or pulmonary insufficiency, primary anastomosis is hazardous and should not be attempted. For more extensive colonic involvement, as may be the case with fulminant colitis with perforation, or in the setting with a cecal perforation resulting from a distal left colonic carcinoma obstruction, a subtotal colectomy with end-ileostomy and mucous fistula or Hartmann's pouch may be the best option.

The approach to management of *abscesses* is analogous to that for a localized perforation, with a few additional principles. First, any undrained inflammatory exudate and pus must be evacuated. Second, depending on the degree of necrosis and the age of the abscess, débridement may be required to remove all devitalized tissue. Drain placement may be necessary for the perioperative period, depending on the degree of residual contamination. Finally, an omental flap may be useful to fill the drained abscess cavity and separate it from the abdominal cavity.

Fistulas can usually be managed by one-stage, primary resection of the diseased segment of colon, with primary anastomosis after bowel preparation. If there is an associated abscess with substantial contamination and sepsis, the procedure may require staging. The abscess cavity may have to be drained, débrided, and filled with an omental flap. Reconstruction of the gastrointestinal continuity may have to be delayed in favor of a proximal stoma and distal Hartmann pouch/mucous fistula. Alternatively, a primary anastomosis with proximal diverting loop ileostomy may be undertaken.

In patients with *large bowel obstruction* the standard approach has been a stage resection with creation of an ostomy and later reconstruction of the gastrointestinal tract. This is due, in large part, to an inability to prepare the obstructed colon adequately combined with concern of fashioning an anastomosis using dilated, edematous bowel. Three techniques warrant discussion, as they are useful adjuncts in the management of this condition. For the first two techniques, intestinal decompression and lavage, data attest to the safety, efficacy, cost-effectiveness, and improved quality of life that has resulted from their implementation [78-84]. For the third technique, use of metallic stents, data are sparse but nevertheless promising.

Intestinal decompression involves creating a colotomy proximal to the site of obstruction and within the confines of the intestinal segment to be resected to decompress the proximal bowel with a large-bore catheter or suction device [79-81]. This generally takes 10-15 minutes. A theoretic benefit is decreased colonic distension, which facilitates abdominal closure and improves colonic perfusion and tone. The technique appears to be safe and efficacious.

On-table intestinal lavage (intraoperative antegrade irrigation) has gained favor as a method to cleanse the colon mechanically at surgery and to facilitate one-stage colonic resection and primary anastomosis. Key elements to the successful outcome of this approach are the absence of significant peritoneal

contamination, no intraoperative hemodynamic instability, and a patient with an otherwise excellent performance status with minimal co-morbid disease [82-84]. The most common method involves mobilizing the obstructed colon and distal intestinal transection; draining the proximal intestinal end into a large bucket via a plastic conduit (the authors prefer an ultrasonographic/endoscopic plastic sleeve); placing a large Foley catheter into the cecum (often via the stump of the removed appendix) and securing it in place with a purse-string suture; and lavaging the colon with saline until the effluent is clear [79,82]. This technique is more cumbersome than intestinal decompression and requires a longer time to complete (approximately 30-45 minutes). Currently, no prospective randomized trial has compared the outcome of intestinal decompression alone to decompression plus on-table colonic lavage prior to primary colon anastomosis. One retrospective analysis demonstrated no additional benefit with the addition of lavage [82].

Metallic stents or endoprostheses have been used for benign strictures and malignant obstruction [85-89]. Data from small, single-institution series show excellent results, probably attributable in part to careful patient selection. The procedures have been easily adapted to endoscopic or fluoroscopic deployment, are well tolerated, can be performed on an outpatient basis with minimal sedation, and provide palliation (to avoid colostomy in a terminally ill patient) or allow mechanical bowel preparation in anticipation of a single-stage resection and anastomosis.

Primary Anastomosis versus Staged Procedures

Patients presenting with *malignant large bowel obstruction* generally undergo a staged resection and creation of a temporary ostomy with later takedown of the ostomy to restore gut continuity. Although options for on-table decompression and cleansing exist, as previously described, many of these patients are elderly and have associated medical illnesses that preclude prolonged anesthesia.

An attempt to construct an anastomosis in the presence of *generalized peritoneal contamination* is associated with a significant risk of anastomotic leakage. Hemodynamic instability, pulmonary and renal insufficiency, and even frank shock argue for a short but definitive operation that does not further compromise the tenuous physiologic status of these patients. Therefore the prevailing standard of care dictates that in the presence of generalized peritonitis or septic shock (or both) a primary anastomosis is contraindicated. Occasionally, in the presence of walled-off perforations or localized abscesses a primary anastomosis can be fashioned as detailed above.

Hemodynamic instability predisposes a patient to systemic perioperative morbidity and mortality as a result of impaired end-organ perfusion and oxygen delivery (e.g., risk of cardiac ischemic events or cerebrovascular accident) and to local complications related to anastomotic integrity and dehiscence. Additionally, the clinical manifestation of hemodynamic instability itself is a harbinger of an underlying disease process that generally defines an already poor-risk patient population. Thus if colonic resection is required, a staged approach is often a better option than fashioning a primary anastomosis.

Patients who are *severely malnourished* lack physiologic reserves for wound healing and the immune response to potential infectious agents. A staged approach (rather than primary anastomosis) allows an adequate interval for restitution of the patient to an anabolic phase and positive nitrogen balance.

Patients with medically intractable *indeterminate colitis* should undergo subtotal colectomy with end-ileostomy and closure of the rectal stump. This approach spares patients a permanent ileostomy and allows the possibility of a restorative proctectomy and ileal pouch/anal procedure if histopathologic examination of the specimen demonstrates ulcerative colitis, while avoiding performing an ileal pouch/anal procedure in an individual later diagnosed as having Crohn's disease.

Technical Factors for Safe Anastomosis

A properly constructed anastomosis is attended by a dehiscence rate of less than 2%. Reported data reveal that the radiographic leak rate is actually much higher than the appreciated clinically detected rate, particularly for rectal cancer, though the clinical significance of this finding is not clear. To obtain these excellent results, proper patient selection (as described above) and attention to the following technical details is of utmost importance.

The cut edge of the mesentery of each intestinal segment should have *demonstrable pulsatile arterial blood flow*. The bowel wall should be pink, soft, and pliable; and the transected edge should demonstrate bleeding or mild oozing of bright red blood, confirming an intact blood supply. Intramural hematomas at the site of the anastomosis or a hematoma in the adjacent mesentery may impair blood flow and should be avoided by handling and manipulating the bowel and mesentery gently during mobilization, resection, and construction of the anastomosis.

Accurate seromuscular apposition must be achieved. Submucosa must be included in each suture, as this layer contributes to anastomotic strength, a function of its connective tissue component. Great care should be exercised to be certain there are no blood clots or pericolonic fat (mesentery or appendices epiploicae) interposed between the two ends of the bowel at the anastomosis. This often requires that a 1 cm cuff of bowel be completely cleared of fat, mesentery, and epiploic appendices. Most anastomotic leaks appear to occur on the mesenteric side of the bowel, presumably related to inadequate clearing of supporting, investing fatty tissue of the mesentery. If a hand-sewn technique is elected, good inversion of all layers of the bowel should be achieved without compromising luminal patency. Sutures should be tied to obtain tissue approximation, avoiding excessive force and strangulation necrosis of the bowel wall, which would result in anastomotic dehiscence.

The *mesenteric defect* should be closed with absorbable or nonabsorbable, interrupted or continuous suture technique to prevent an internal hernia. The exception to this rule is represented by the mesenteric defect obtained after a distal rectosigmoid or low anterior resection. The risk of internal herniation after these resections and anastomoses is sufficiently low that attempts to close these mesenteric defect are usually not pursued.

The anastomosis must be constructed *without tension*. Adequate mobilization may require division of peritoneal attachments and ligaments, such as those that suspend the splenic flexure.

Avoid contamination during intestinal mobilization and resection or at the time of the construction of the anastomosis. This requires proper technique during the mobilization phase, use of noncrushing bowel clamps on both ends of the bowel during bowel resection and anastomotic construction, and simultaneous liberal use of laparotomy pads to partition off the anastomotic site from the rest of the peritoneal cavity. Irrigation of the peritoneal cavity prior to abdominal closure also dilutes bacterial counts and limits the degree of any contamination.

Accumulation of blood (or serum) in the vicinity of an anastomosis not only may compromise the blood supply to the anastomosis but may provide a nidus for infection. Subsequent localized sepsis may predispose to abscess formation and anastomotic dehiscence. Treatment begins with prevention. Principles of meticulous hemostasis and asepsis require ardent adherence. Transient, early postoperative closed suction drainage of the presacral space may be a useful adjunct for resections carried distal to the peritoneal reflection to prevent accumulation of blood and tissue fluid.

Closure of the pelvic peritoneum may result in considerable *perianastomotic deadspace*. This may result in the collection of tissue exudate, which invites infection. The pelvic peritoneum is thus best left open to allow the small bowel to descend into the pelvis and fill the deadspace. Other options include creating an omental pedicle flap or a rectus muscle flap and bringing it down into the pelvis, effectively obliterating any deadspace [90].

Distal obstruction causes anastomotic failure. All efforts are made to ensure that there is no coexisting distal obstruction prior to construction of any bowel anastomosis. Preoperative radiographic contrast studies and pre- or intraoperative endoscopic studies provide useful information in this regard.

Other Factors Affecting Anastomotic Healing

Preoperative radiation therapy was believed by many to be the Achilles heel of the neoadjuvant approach to treatment of rectal cancers. Although irradiation impairs healing, in the setting of rectal cancer the anastomotic complication rates of preoperative irradiation have compared favorably to those seen with adjuvant approaches.

Prolonged administration of *high-dose steroids* impairs wound healing. This class of drugs results in muscle- and protein-wasting, a condition that predisposes to negative nitrogen balance and a catabolic state. After prolonged steroid administration there is weakening of the cellular desmosomic plaques and inhibition of fibroblast activity, which account for the slower anastomotic healing noted in humans (confirmed in animal models by measuring bursting pressures of colonic anastomoses as the endpoint) [91–95]. To complicate matters, immune function, a necessary component of wound healing and important for minimizing infectious complications, is suppressed.

Carcinoma at the anastomotic margin contributes to anastomotic leakage and "suture-line" recurrence. This situation is rarely encountered today, as the principles of negative proximal and distal margins are well appreciated, and the use of intraoperative frozen section control of resection margins (if close or in doubt) is standard practice.

Technical Considerations and Adjuncts

After constructing an ileal pouch/anal anastomosis without a diverting ileostomy, it is advisable to *drain the pouch* for 5–7 days by way of a transanal

catheter. This allows drainage of secretions, blood and fecal material, avoids overdistension of the pouch, and minimizes suture-line dehiscences. The same concept can be used after closing a rectal stump during an emergency colectomy, especially if the closure has been challenging and the rectum appears tense with blood and secretions.

Biodegradable intraluminal tubes have proved feasible adjuncts for construction of anastomoses in the setting of septic processes and colonic obstruction in both animal models and humans [96,97]. Many materials have been used for this purpose, with the most popular being latex condoms. Results in small prospective series have demonstrated that the use of these devices is safe and technically uncomplicated. The risk of dehiscence and other complications in the setting of unprepared colon and even in instances of prior radiotherapy have been minimal. The technique generally involves using a sterile ring of a latex condom, which is sutured to the mucosa and submucosa of the proximal end of the bowel used for the anastomosis, followed by creation of the bowel anastomosis itself. The "tube" essentially intraluminally bridges or "bypasses" the anastomosis, which presumably allows better healing to occur by minimizing contact with stool.

The use of an *omental flap* can be desirable as it has many advantages in selected circumstances. Indeed, the omentum appears to be a major source of leukocytes and macrophages during intraabdominal septic processes, has angiogenic properties, has the ability to fill deadspaces and abscess cavities, and partitions off inflamed organs or an anastomosis to prevent generalized peritonitis or dehiscences. Furthermore, it can be used to exclude the small bowel from the pelvis when adjuvant therapy is likely during postoperative treatment of a rectal cancer [90].

There are differing opinions regarding the efficacy of *wrapping colorectal anastomoses with omentum*. Many surgeons traditionally have wrapped omentum (if enough is available to make it feasible) around colorectal anastomoses with the intent of reducing the risk or consequence of anastomotic leaks. A prospective, randomized French trial reported in 1999 demonstrated absolutely no benefit to this approach for colon or rectal anastomoses [90]. Omental wrapping of colorectal anastomoses does not appear to provide any additional benefit over the use of meticulous principles of surgical technique for anastomotic construction.

If *disparity exists between two ends of bowel*, there are a number of options that may be employed to construct an anastomosis. One maneuver is called the Cheatle slit, described in Figure 43-10, which involves creating a longitudinal incision along the antimesenteric border of the smaller limb of bowel to be anastomosed. Subtotal colectomy and low anterior resection are attended by a significant discrepancy between the two limbs of bowel. Use of a Cheatle slit in these circumstances to create an end-to-end-anastomosis is often difficult owing to the large disparity of the size of the two intestinal lumens and the location of the anastomosis deep in the pelvis. A side-to-end anastomosis (ileoproctostomy or coloproctostomy) is usually an easier alternative. Furthermore, the end of the rectum can be invaginated into the side of the ileum or colon for additional protection against leakage without risking stenosis due to the relatively large anastomosis that can be achieved by this method. Alternatively, a side-to-side functional end-stapled anastomosis can be fashioned by initially stapling the two intestinal ends side by side with a linear stapler; the common lumen can then be closed by firing a second linear stapler across.

INTESTINAL POUCH RESERVOIRS

Creation of intestinal pouch reservoirs is an integral component of restorative proctocolectomy for ulcerative colitis and familial polyposis. The pouches are of varied configurations, each with its own proponents, but the purpose served is identical, all with demonstrated excellent functional outcomes [98].

The *J-pouch* is a double-loop reservoir that has become the most common pouch because it is simple and easy to construct. It may be the best option for a narrow pelvis in an obese individual because it is less bulky than other configurations. It also may be the best option when performing a stapled anastomosis because of the ease at passage of the stapling device. The J-pouch offers minimal difficulty with evacuation and emptying; and in general, the functional results are good when the pouch is at least 15 cm in length. A brief comment regarding *colonic* J-pouches is in order. Similar to small bowel J-pouches, a 6- to 8-cm colonic pouch appears to improve the functional results after a proctectomy with coloanal anastomoses for treatment of rectal cancer. Stool frequency and urgency appear to be reduced compared to straight coloanal anastomoses [99–101]. This advantage is most apparent during the first 1–2 years of construction, after which equivalent functional outcomes tend to occur. Some studies advocating this approach have demonstrated a tendency toward a reduced incidence of anastomotic complications with the colonic J-pouch procedure, an observation that needs to be substantiated by larger studies.

H-pouch (also called the lateral H-pouch) is a double-loop reservoir designed to enhance the efficiency of pouch evacuation by placing the two segments of ileum in an isoperistaltic configuration [98]. The functional results are good if strict attention is paid to creating a short spout and a pouch length less than 12 cm. Two loops, placed in a slightly staggered alignment with respect to each other, may be an alternative to a J-pouch for patients with a short mesentery, rendering it difficult for the reservoir to reach the anus. As with the S-pouch, this configuration may pose difficulty with passage of stapling devices to create a stapled anastomosis. Additionally, like the S- and W-pouches, this type has the disadvantage of being more difficult to construct.

The *S-pouch* has a distal spout. This triple-loop configuration is helpful if there is technical difficulty with the pouch reaching the anus. It is more time-consuming to construct, as would be expected, and patients may experience difficulty with pouch evacuation, particularly if the outlet is longer than 2 cm [98].

The *W-pouch* is a quadruple-loop pouch with some important advantages over other pouches. In patients with partial loss of the terminal ileum this construction allows maintenance of pouch reservoir capacity (largest capacity of all types) [98]. Patients who fail other configurations in terms of functional results of high stool frequency and nocturnal incontinence may benefit from conversion to a large-capacity W-pouch, which results in decreased stool frequency. A disadvantage of this pouch is that its construction is difficult and time-consuming.

INTESTINAL STOMAS

Intestinal stomas can be broadly categorized as temporary or permanent. The goal governing construction of a stoma is to allow the patient to return to an active life style. This is facilitated by appropriate stoma placement and protrusion to avoid local complications, especially those related to skin breakdown and appliance malfunction. The appropriate stoma site must be selected preoperatively for all elective procedures and for most emergent ones. Adequate mesenteric mobilization is necessary for stoma protrusion. End-ileostomies should protrude more than end-colostomies (1.0–1.5 cm vs. 0.5–1.0 cm) in view of the more liquid effluent. Protrusion helps bowel contents from seeping between the wafer of the appliance and the peristomal skin; it also prevents peristomal skin irritation and breakdown. Additional precautions include placement of sutures in the dermis during stomal maturation to prevent potential hypertropic scarring and intestinal cell implantation in the epidermis, which may render proper adherence of appliances difficult [102, 103]. A snug fascial opening prevents postoperative herniation.

Preoperative site selection is important, as improper siting may result in poor fit of the appliance, with leakage and skin breakdown. Ideally, the site is chosen and marked preoperatively by the surgeon in consultation with an enterostomal therapist [104]. The location should be flat and away from skin creases and the costal or iliac margins; it should be in an area of normal, healthy-appearing skin that is visible to the patient. Have the patient sit, stand, and bend to select the best site. In general, the optimal location is approximately one-third the distance from the umbilicus to the anterior superior iliac spine. Place the stoma higher in obese individuals so they can see it.

One of the issues with temporary stomas is the *timing of closure* with restoration of gastrointestinal continuity. The underlying problem necessitating creation of the stoma should have been addressed and rectified. There should obviously be no distal obstruction. Anal sphincter mechanisms must be intact and function normally to ensure continence. Traditional teaching dictated that the surgeon wait 60–90 days before attempting closure. The purpose was to allow adequate time for overall recovery of the general physiologic status and adequate anastomotic healing if the temporary ostomy was created for the purpose of "protecting" an anastomosis. This time interval is more empiric than scientific, and no randomized, controlled trials have been conducted that have specifically identified the optimal timing for stomal closure. Certainly there are retrospective data that support ostomy closure prior to this interval without prohibitive complications [102,105,106].

Loop ileostomies are temporary stomas often created in the setting of sphincter-preservation procedures for rectal cancer, ulcerative colitis, and familial polyposis. These stomas require careful attention to detail during construction because the relatively high-volume effluent is highly irritating to the skin. In general, a site in the ileum is selected as distal as possible to maintain maximal absorptive surface area of the terminal ileum (the bowel distal to this site becomes effectively defunctionalized). If the loop ileostomy is performed in conjunction with a colorectal or coloanal anastomosis, the loop ileostomy should be placed 8–10 cm proximal to the ileocecal valve to facilitate subsequent closure. The mesentery is not fixed to the parietal peritoneum, thereby

facilitating ease of takedown at a later time. A variation of this technique involves complete transection of the intestinal lumen with closure of the distal segment without division of the mesentery; both ends are brought out through the same abdominal wall site.

Cecostomy, used frequently in the past, is rarely performed today. Situations in which the procedure should be considered include the following: (1) patients with cecal volvulus at high risk of recurrence in whom resection of the colon is not necessary; and (2) patients with "pseudoobstruction" of the colon (Ogilvie syndrome) in whom an exploratory laparotomy was performed for presumptive mechanical obstruction and none was found or in whom repeated colonoscopies failed to decompress the distended colon and the patient develops signs and findings of impending cecal perforation. The procedure may be indicated during performance of an appendectomy when the wall of the cecum is indurated and friable and resection of the cecum is not otherwise desirable. Finally, it may be useful in the presence of an impending perforation of the cecum secondary to a mechanical obstruction of the colon. When the cecal diameter is more than 10 cm (measured on abdominal radiographs), there is appropriate concern about cecal perforation. If tenderness accompanies this finding, cecal exploration is mandatory to rule out ischemic necrosis of the cecal wall secondary to increased intraluminal pressure. Attempting a decompressing transverse colostomy without cecal evaluation risks a catastrophic perforation in areas of serosal tears and ischemic necrosis.

A cecostomy can be fashioned as a *tube* or a *skin-sutured cecostomy*. A tube cecostomy is more easily and expeditiously performed; and after it is no longer needed, the resulting fistula usually closes spontaneously soon after withdrawing the tube. Conversely, it requires significant nursing care and frequent irrigation and often becomes obstructed by semisolid fecal material. A skin-sutured cecotomy is a better decompressing and cleansing stoma, requiring much less nursing care, although it requires formal surgical closure when it is no longer needed.

Loop colostomies are rarely used nowadays. Preference is usually given to the loop ileostomy because of its ease of construction and subsequent closure. The only remaining indication to use of the loop colostomy is probably the bed-ridden patient with an unresectable, obstructing left colon cancer.

The *Kock continent ileostomy* involves complementary construction of a pouch and a continent "nipple valve." This modification obviates the requirement for patients to wear an appliance to collect and contain ileal excretions. Evacuation involves intubation of the pouch by the patient a few times daily. This operation is attended by many complications that require reoperation (in the range of 15-20% and up to 30% in some large series). As a result, the Kock ileostomy cannot be recommended for general use. This procedure may be considered in patients who are severely opposed to wearing a stomal appliance because of personal preference or peristomal complications and those who have previously undergone total proctocolectomy with a failed ileal pouch/anal procedure. This procedure is contraindicated in those with Crohn's disease and relatively contraindicated if a significant small bowel resection has previously been done, in those over 60 years of age, in obese patients, and in the presence of significant associated psychiatric illness. Furthermore, patients must be highly motivated and well informed about the procedure, its attendant complications, and the significant possibility of additional surgery to rectify complications.

POSTOPERATIVE CARE

Nasogastric intubation, long a mainstay of the postoperative management of patients who undergo large bowel operations, was done on the premise that it served the purpose of gut decompression until bowel function returned. Disadvantages of routine nasogastric intubation include impairment of lower esophageal sphincter function predisposing to gastroesophageal reflux with consequent esophagitis, an increase in nasopharyngeal secretions and risk of developing paranasal sinusitis, and impairment of coughing and pulmonary toilet, which increases the risk of perioperative pulmonary morbidity. Numerous randomized trials have shown no benefit for nasogastric decompression, and this modality is therefore probably best limited to patients who require extensive intraoperative dissection because of adhesions, those who experience nausea, emesis, and abdominal distension during the perioperative period, and the cohort operated on because of intestinal obstruction or sepsis. In the elective setting, postoperative nasogastric decompression is not routinely necessary.

Similarly, the initiation of *postoperative feeding* has changed over the past two decades. Early practice was based, to an extent, on animal studies that illustrated that before the seventh postoperative day the intrinsic tensile strength of a wound was inadequate to withstand a disruptive force. Extrapolating to humans, many believed that it made sense to "rest" an anastomosis of the colon for 5-7 days following an operation. It was believed that any minor imperfection in the anastomosis had an opportunity to heal without resulting in leakage. Current standard practice calls for institution of oral feedings as soon as evidence of bowel function is present (usually normoactive bowel sounds in a nondistended patient who has or has not yet passed flatus or stool). Chronologically, this occurs between the third and fifth postoperative day. Surgical tradition has resulted in institution of clear liquids first, advancing to a general diet based on the patient's ability to "tolerate" the intake (absence of nausea, emesis, or cramping, with passing of flatus and stool). No randomized studies exist to substantiate the efficacy of commencing with a clear liquid diet and advancing it rather than instituting a general diet at the outset of the return of bowel function. Randomized trials have shown that early oral feeding (starting on the first postoperative day) after elective colorectal surgery is safe and generally well tolerated [107,108].

Colorectal surgery generally requires a *postoperative hospital stay* of 5-10 days. Patients were and still are traditionally discharged from the hospital when they are clinically stable and afebrile, able to tolerate an adequate oral intake to maintain hydration and nutritional repletion, have bowel function, and their pain is controlled through oral medications. Many factors hinder discharge: nausea, emesis, ileus, pain, fatigue, and the inability to care for drains, tubes, and ostomies competently. Laparoscopy has failed to reveal a consistent benefit for early discharge. A combination multimodality rehabilitation regimen with early oral nutrition, mobilization, and effective pain relief has reduced hospital stays for colorectal procedures to 2 days [109]. The success of this technique requires a motivated patient and an anesthesia team carefully integrated into the process at all steps. It requires use of epidural anesthesia with limited oral and parenteral narcotics (which contribute to bowel dysmotility) and limitation of crystalloid use intraoperatively to diminish bowel edema, and thus speed the return of function. In our experience this is a safe, efficacious regimen and has far-reaching consequences in cost-containment without sacrificing or compromising patient care.

Management of Altered Sphincter Function

During convalescence, after restorative procto-colectomies for ulcerative colitis or familial polyposis and after sphincter-saving procedures for rectal cancers, attention is directed at careful evaluation of stool frequency, volume and consistency, urgency, degree of incontinence if present, constipation or difficulty with evacuation, development of anal stenosis, and occurrence of pouchitis. If incontinence occurs, it must be quantitated by recording the number of nocturnal and diurnal episodes, the need to wear a protective pad, and incontinence to flatus, liquid, or solid stools.

Changes in diet and administration of drugs to alter intestinal motility may ameliorate the frequency and consistency of bowel movements over time. Incontinence and stool frequency tend to disappear with time. Ileoanal or coloanal stenoses may have to be mechanically dilated under anesthesia to ease difficulty of evacuation. In the absence of a coloanal stenosis, suppositories or Fleet's enemas may be necessary to initiate a bowel movement.

Urogenital Function

Low pelvic dissections for benign or malignant disease may be associated with complications such as urinary retention, dyspareunia, impotence (secondary to parasympathetic nerve damage), retrograde ejaculation (resulting from sympathetic nerve injury), and the development of rectourethral or rectovaginal fistulas. Preoperatively, a surgeon is well advised to pay careful attention to signs and symptoms of urogenital functional abnormalities.

Meticulous attention to detail during pelvic dissections, particularly for benign diseases that do not require extensive mesorectal resections, prevents the occurrence of some but not all of these complications. Some, such as urinary retention, though relatively frequent, are self-limiting; and resolution occurs with time. Others are more disabling and may severely affect the quality of life. Patients who are candidates for procedures attended by these risks require in-depth counseling to ensure an informed decision.

CANCER SURVEILLANCE

Most colorectal cancer recurrences (80–85%) occur within the first 2 years of surgical resection for "curative intent" [39]. Up to two-thirds of patients whose lesions were resected for cure develop recurrent disease. Some of these patients may still be cured, particularly those with disease limited to the pelvis and those with isolated hepatic or pulmonary metastases. These patterns of failure have led surgeons to monitor patients closely during the first 2 years. If at 5 years patients are disease-free, the likelihood of recurrence decreases to 5% or less [39]. Many centers advocate patient evaluation every 3–4 months for the first 2–3 years, every 6 months for the remainder of the 5 years, then annually. Complete history and physical examination, stool for Hemoccult testing, hemoglobin and hematocrit levels assessing for anemia, liver function testing, carcinoembryonic antigen (CEA) assay, chest radiography, CT of the abdomen and pelvis, yearly endoscopy, transrectal ultrasonography (rectal cancer), radiolabeled-anti-CEA antibody imaging, and fluorodeoxyglucose positron emission tomography (if the plasma CEA level is rising) have been utilized. The most effective strategy for follow-up remains controversial. Many studies fail to demonstrate a statistically significant increase in survival based on early detection of recurrences, prior to the development of symptomatic disease [39].

POUCH SURVEILLANCE

Pouchitis is the most common long-term morbidity associated with ileal pouch/anal anastomoses [110–113]. For unknown reasons, this condition occurs more frequently in patients who have had ulcerative colitis than in those with familial polyposis; and the incidence is even higher if pancolitis or extraintestinal manifestations were present. Among the many theories to explain this phenomenon are pouch outflow obstruction, stasis and bacterial overgrowth, abnormal mucus secretion, reduced levels of free fatty acids in the pouch, oxygen free radical injury secondary to ischemia, presence of antineutrophil cytoplasmic antibodies, and pouches that are created "too" large [110]. Clinically, patients present with low grade fever, fatigue and malaise, and frequent loose stools or frank diarrhea occasionally with passage of blood or associated with pelvic pain, cramps, and urgency, often with soiling and incontinence. The mucosa becomes inflamed with progression to ulceration in severe cases. In more than 50% of patients the first episode occurs within the first year of surgery, with the initial risk highest during the first 6 months after surgery [111,112].

Therapy often comprises a course of metronidazole or fluoroquinolone antibiotics. Daily dosing may be necessary for chronic pouchitis. If it fails, antiinflammatory agents are used (e.g., steroids or 5-aminosalicylic acid enemas). Approximately 10% of patients with pouchitis become intractable to medical therapy (chronic pouchitis). Follow-up in this cohort should include both endoscopic and histologic evaluation for the development of high-grade dysplasia. If this ensues, pouch removal is necessary because of the high risk of malignancy (particularly if villous atrophy is also noted). Conversion to an end-ileostomy with pouch removal may also be necessary because of the poor functional results associated with chronic pouchitis [114]. New biologic response-modifying modalities are currently under investigation and may prove to be promising alternatives for nonoperative management of this entity [115].

REFERENCES

1. Roberts PL, Veidenheimer MC. Current management of diverticulitis. Adv Surg 1994;27:189.

2. Ferzoco LB, Raptopoulos V, Silen W. Acute diverticulitis. N Engl J Med 1998;338:1521.

3. Smith TR, Cho KC, Morehouse HT, et al. Comparison of computed tomography and contrast enema evaluation of diverticulitis. Dis Colon Rectum 1990; 33:1.

4. Schecter S, Mulvey J, Eisenstat TE. Management of uncomplicated acute diverticulitis: results of a survey. Dis Colon Rectum 1999;42:470.

5. Eusebio EB, Eisenberg MM. Natural history of diverticular disease of the colon in young patients. Am J Surg 1973;125:308.

6. Parker BM, Obeid FN, Sorensen VJ, et al. The management of massive lower gastrointestinal bleeding. Am Surg 1993;9:676.

7. Ballantyne GH, Brandner MD, Beart RW Jr, et al. Volvulus of the colon: incidence and mortality. Ann Surg 1985;202:83.

8. Bower TC, Ischemic colitis. Surg Clin North Am 1993;73:1037.

9. Gandhi SK, Hanson MM, Vernava AM, et al. Ischemic colitis. Dis Colon Rectum 1996;39:88.

10. Kim DS, Tsang CBS, Wong WD, et al. Complete rectal prolapse: evolution of management and results. Dis Colon Rectum 1999;42:460.

11. Madoff RD, Mellgren A. One hundred years of rectal prolapse surgery. Dis Colon Rectum 1999;42:441.

12. Altemeier WA, Culbertson WR, Schowengerdt C, et al. Nineteen years experience with the one-stage perineal repair of rectal prolapse. Ann Surg 1971;173: 993.

13. Kinzler KW, Nilbert MC, Su L-K, et al. Identification of FAP locus genes from chromosome 5q21. Science 1991;253:661.

14. Kartheuser AN, Parc R, Penna CP, et al. Ileal pouch-anal anastomosis as the first choice operation in patients with familial adenomatous polyposis: a ten-year experience. Surgery 1996;119:615.

15. Michelassi F. Indications for surgical treatment in ulcerative colitis and Crohn's disease. In Michelassi F, Milsom JW (eds) Operative Strategies in Inflammatory Bowel Disease. New York, Springer-Verlag, 1999, pp 150–153.

16. Heppell J, Farkouh E, Dube S, et al. Toxic megacolon: an analysis of 70 cases. Dis Colon Rectum 1986;29: 789.

17. McLeod RS. Resection margins and recurrent Crohn's disease. Hepatogastroenterology 1990;37:63.

18. Heimann TM, Greenstein AJ, Lewis B, et al. Prediction of early symptomatic recurrence after intestinal resection in Crohn's disease. Ann Surg 1993;218:294.

19. Farouk R, Pemberton JH. Surgical options in ulcerative colitis. Surg Clin North Am 1997;77:85.

20. Milsom JW. Restorative proctocolectomy with ileoanal anastomosis. In Michelassi F, Milsom JW (eds) Operative Strategies in Inflammatory Bowel Disease. New York, Springer-Verlag, 1999, pp 173–183.

21. Gemlo BT, Wong WD, Rothenberger DA, et al. Ileal pouch-anal anastomosis: patterns of failure. Arch Surg 1992;127:784.

22. Fazio VW, Ziv Y, Church JM, et al. Ileal pouch-anal anastomoses complications and function in 1005 patients. Ann Surg 1995;222:120.

23. Miller R, Bartolo DC, Orrom WJ, et al. Improvement of anal sensation with preservation of the anal transition zone after ileoanal anastomosis for ulcerative colitis. Dis Colon Rectum 1990;33:414.

24. McIntyre PB, Pemberton JH, Beart RW, et al. Double-stapled vs. hand-sewn ileal pouch-anal anastomosis in patients with chronic ulcerative colitis. Dis Colon Rectum 1994;37:430.

25. Luukkonen P, Jarvinen HJ. Stapled vs. hand-sutured ileoanal anastomosis in restorative proctocolectomy: a prospective, randomized study. Arch Surg 1993; 128:437.

26. Gozzetti G, Poggioli G, Marchetti F, et al. Functional outcome in hand-sewn vs. stapled ileal pouch-anal anastomosis. Am J Surg 1994;168:325.

27. Khubchandani IT, Kontostolis SB. Outcome of ileorectal anastomosis in an inflammatory bowel disease surgery experience of three decades. Arch Surg 1994;129:866.

28. Longo WE, Oakley JR, Laverly IC, et al. Outcome of ileorectal anastomosis for Crohn's colitis. Dis Colon Rectum 1992;35:1066.

29. Ekbom A, Helmick C, Zack M, et al. Ulcerative colitis and colorectal cancer: a population-based study. N Engl J Med 1990;323:1228.

30. Pinczowski D, Ekbom A, Baron J, et al. Risk factors for colorectal cancer in patients with ulcerative colitis: a case-control study. Gastroenterology 1994;107: 117.

31. Taylor BA, Pemberton JH, Carpenter HA, et al. Dysplasia in chronic ulcerative colitis: implications for colonoscopic surveillance. Dis Colon Rectum 1992; 35:950.

32. Ziv Y, Fazio VW, Church JM, et al. Safety of urgent restorative proctocolectomy with ileal pouch-anal anastomosis for fulminant colitis. Dis Colon Rectum 1995;38:345.

33. Price AB. Overlap in the spectrum of nonspecific inflammatory bowel disease—"colitis indeterminate." J Clin Pathol 1978;31:567.

34. McIntyre PB, Pemberton JH, Wolff BG, et al. Indeterminate colitis: long-term outcome in patients after ileal pouch-anal anastomosis. Dis Colon Rectum 1995;38:51.

35. Stein BL, Coller JA. Management of malignant colorectal polyps. Surg Clin North Am 1993;73:47.

36. Cooper HS, Deppisch LM, Gourly WK, et al. Endoscopically removed malignant colorectal polyps: clinicopathologic correlations. Gastroenterology 1995; 108:1657.

37. Haggitt RC, Glotzbach RE, Soffer EE, et al. Prognostic factors in colorectal carcinomas arising in adenomas: implications for lesions removed by endoscopic polypectomy. Gastroenterology 1985;89:328.

38. Nivatvongs S, Rojanasakul A, Reiman HM, et al. The risk of lymph node metastases in colorectal polyps with invasive adenocarcinoma. Dis Colon Rectum 1991;34:323.

39. Laverly IC, Lopez-Kostner F, Pelley RJ, et al. Treatment of colon and rectal cancer. Surg Clin North Am 2000;80:535.

40. Hautefeuille P, Valleur P, Perniceni T. Functional and oncologic results after coloanal anastomosis for low rectal carcinoma. Ann Surg 1988;207:61.

41. Bat L, Neumann G, Shemesh E. The association of synchronous neoplasm with occluding colorectal cancer. Dis Colon Rectum 1985;28:149.

42. Kahn H, Alexander A, Rakinic J, et al. Preoperative staging of irradiated rectal cancers using digital rectal examination, computed tomography, endorectal ultrasound, and magnetic resonance imaging does not accurately predict T0,N0 pathology. Dis Colon Rectum 1997;40:140.

43. Fisher B, Wolmark N, Rockette H, et al. Postoperative adjuvant chemotherapy or radiation therapy for rectal cancer: results from the NSABP protocol R-01. J Natl Cancer Inst 1988;90:21.

44. Jessup JM, Bothe A, Stone MD, et al. Preservation of sphincter function in rectal carcinoma by a multimodality treatment approach. Surg Oncol Clin North Am 1992;1:137.

45. Papillon J, Gerard JP. Role of radiotherapy in anal preservation for cancer of the lower third of the rectum. Int J Radiat Oncol Biol Phys 1990;19:1219.

46. Minsky BD, Cohen AM, Enker WE, et al. Combined modality therapy of rectal cancer: decreased acute toxicity with the preoperative approach. J Clin Oncol 1992;10:1218.

47. Hyams DM, Mamounas EP, Petrelli N, et al. A clinical trial to evaluate the worth of preoperative multimodality therapy in patients with operable carcinoma of the rectum: a progress report of the national surgical breast and bowel project protocol r-03. Dis Colon Rectum 1997;40:131.

48. Bernini A, Deen KI, Madoff RD, et al. Preoperative adjuvant radiation with chemotherapy for rectal cancer: its impact on stage of disease and the role of endorectal ultrasound. Ann Surg Oncol 1996;3:131.

49. Shumate CR, Rich TA, Skibber JM, et al. Preoperative chemotherapy and radiation therapy for locally advanced primary and recurrent rectal carcinoma. A report of surgical morbidity. Cancer 1993;71:3690.

50. Minsky BD. Sphincter preservation in rectal cancer. Preoperative radiation therapy followed by low anterior resection with coloanal anastomosis. Semin Radiat Oncol 1998;8:30.

51. Mendenhall WM, Bland KI, Copeland EM III, et al. Does preoperative radiation therapy enhance the probability of local control and survival in high-risk distal rectal cancer? Ann Surg 1992;215:696.

52. Vauthey JN, Marsh RW, Zlotecki RA, et al. Recent advances in the treatment and outcome of locally advanced rectal cancer. Ann Surg 1999;229:745.

53. Wagman R, Minsky BD, Cohen AM, et al. Sphincter preservation in rectal cancer with preoperative radiation therapy and coloanal anastomosis: long term follow-up. Int J Radiat Oncol Biol Phys 1998;42:51.

54. Francois Y, Nemoz CJ, Baulieux J, et al. Influence of the interval between preoperative radiation therapy and surgery on downstaging and on the rate of sphincter-sparing surgery for rectal cancer: the Lyon R90-01 randomized trial. J Clin Oncol 1999;17:2396.

55. Cho CC, Taylor CW III, Padmanabhan A, et al. Squamous cell carcinoma of the anal canal: management with combined chemoradiation therapy. Dis Colon Rectum 1991;34:675.

56. Nigro ND. The force of change in the management of squamous-cell cancer of the anal canal. Dis Colon Rectum 1991;34:482.

57. Franklin M, Rosenthal D, Abrego-Medina D, et al. Prospective comparison of open vs. laparoscopic colon surgery for carcinoma. Dis Colon Rectum 1996;39(suppl):35.

58. Milsom J, Bohm B, Hammermofer K, et al. A prospective, randomized trial comparing laparoscopic versus conventional techniques in colorectal cancer surgery: a preliminary report. J Am Coll Surg 1998; 187:46.

59. Philips EH, Franklin M, Caroll BJ, et al. Laparoscopic colectomy. Ann Surg 1992;216:703.

60. Puente I, Sosa JL, Sleeman D, et al. Laparoscopic-assisted colorectal surgery. J Laparoendosc Surg 1994;4:1.

61. Stage J, Schulze S, Moller P, et al. Prospective randomized study of laparoscopic versus open colonic resection for adenocarcinoma. Br J Surg 1997;84:391.

62. Talac R, Nelson H. Laparoscopic colon and rectal surgery. Surg Clin North Am 2000;9:1.

63. Eijsbouts QAJ, Heuff G, Sietses C, et al. Laparoscopic surgery in the treatment of colonic polyps. Br J Surg 1999;86:505.

64. Larach SW, Patankar SK, Ferrara A, et al. Complications of laparoscopic colorectal surgery: analysis and comparison of early vs. latter experience. Dis Colon Rectum 1997;40:592.

65. Kockerling F, Schneider C, Reymond MA, et al. Early results of a prospective multicenter study on 500 consecutive cases of laparoscopic colorectal surgery: laparoscopic colorectal surgery study group. Surg Endosc 1998;12:37.

66. Franklin ME Jr, Dorman JP, Jacobs M, et al. Is laparoscopic surgery applicable to complicated colonic diverticular disease? Surg Endosc 1997;11:1021.

67. Muckleroy SK, Ratzer ER, Fenoglio ME. Laparoscopic colon surgery for benign disease: a comparison to open surgery. J Soc Laparoendosc Surg 1999;3:33.

68. Sardinha TC, Wexner SD. Laparoscopy for inflammatory bowel disease: pros and cons. World J Surg 1998;22:370.

69. Heintz A, Morschel M, Jumginger T. Comparison of results after transanal endoscopic microsurgery and radical resection for T1 carcinoma of the rectum. Surg Endosc 1998;12:1145.

70. Saclarides TJ. Transanal endoscopic microsurgery: a single surgeon's experience. Arch Surg 1998;133:595.

71. Winde G, Nottberg H, Keller R, et al. Surgical cure for early rectal carcinomas (T1): transanal endoscopic microsurgery vs. anterior resection. Dis Colon Rectum 1996;39:969.

72. Kreis ME, Jehle EC, Haug V, et al. Functional results after transanal endoscopic microsurgery. Dis Colon Rectum 1996;39:1116.

73. Smith LE, Ko ST, Saclarides T, et al. Transanal endoscopic microsurgery: initial registry results. Dis Colon Rectum 1996;39(suppl):79.

74. Salvati EP, Rubin RJ, Eisenstat TE, et al. Electrocoagulation of selected carcinoma of the rectum. Surg Gynecol Obstet 1988;166:393.

75. Papillon J. Intracavitary irradiation of early rectal cancer for cure: a series of 186 cases. Dis Colon Rectum 1994;37:88.

76. Papillon J. Surgical adjuvant therapy for rectal cancer: present options. Dis Colon Rectum 1994;37:144.

77. Turnbull RB, et al. Cancer of the colon: the influence of the no-touch isolation technique on survival rates. Ann Surg 1967;166:420.

78. Lau PW, Lo CY, Law WL. The role of one stage surgery in acute left-sided colonic obstruction. Am J Surg 1995;169:406.

79. MacKenzie S, Thomson SR, Baker LW. Management options in malignant obstruction of the left colon. Surg Gynecol Obstet 1992;174:337.

80. Naraynsingh V, Rampayl R, Maharaj D, et al. Prospective study of primary anastomosis without colonic lavage for patients with an obstructed left colon. Br J Surg 1999;86:1341.

81. Nyam DCNK, Seow Choen F, Leong AFPK, et al. Colonic decompression without on-table irrigation for obstructing left-sided colorectal tumours. Br J Surg 1996;83:786.

82. Forloni B, Reduzzi R, Paludetti A, et al. Intraoperative colonic lavage in emergency surgical treatment of left-sided colonic obstruction. Dis Colon Rectum 1998;41:23.

83. Kressner U, Autonsson J, Ejerblad S, et al. Intraoperative colonic lavage and primary anastomosis and alternative to Hartmann procedure in emergency surgery of the left colon. Eur J Surg 1994;160:287.

84. Murray JJ, Schoetz DJ, Coller JA, et al. Intraoperative colonic lavage and primary anastomosis in nonelective colon resection. Dis Colon Rectum 1991;34:527.

85. Rey JF, Romanczyk MG. Metal stents for palliation of rectal carcinoma: a preliminary report on 12 patients. Endoscopy 1995;27:501.

86. Saida Y, Sumiyama Y, Nagao J, et al. Stent endoprosthesis for obstructing colorectal cancers. Dis Colon Rectum 1996;39:552.

87. Mainar A, DeGregorio Ariza MA, Tejero E, et al. Acute colorectal obstruction: treatment with self-expandable metallic stent scheduled surgery: results of a multicenter study. Radiology 1999;210:65.

88. Binkert CA, Ledermann H, Jost R, et al. Acute colonic obstruction: clinical aspects and cost-effectiveness of preoperative palliative treatment with self-expanding metallic stents: a preliminary report. Radiology 1998;206:199.

89. Akle CA. Endoprostheses for colonic strictures. Br J Surg 1998;85:310.

90. O'Leary DP. Use of the greater omentum in colorectal surgery. Dis Colon Rectum 1999;42:533.

91. Del Rio JV, Beck DE, Opelka FG. Chronic perioperative steroids and colonic anastomosis healing in rats. J Surg Res 1996;66:138.

92. Eubanks TR, Greenberg JJ, Dobrin PB, et al. The effects of different corticosteroids on the healing colonic anastomosis and cecum in a rat model. Am Surg 1997;63:266.

93. Furst MB, Stromber BV, Blatchford GJ, et al. Colonic anastomoses: bursting strength after corticosteroid treatment. Dis Colon Rectum 1994;37:12.

94. Ziv Y, Church JM, Fazio VW, et al. Effect of systemic steroids on ileal pouch-anal anastomosis in patients with ulcerative colitis. Dis Colon Rectum 1996;39:504.

95. Cali RL, Ssmyrk TC, Blatchford GJ, et al. Effect of prostaglandin E_1 and steroid on healing colonic anastomoses. Dis Colon Rectum 1993;36:1148.

96. Ruiz PL, Facciuto EM, Facciuto ME, et al. New intraluminal bypass tube for management of acutely obstructed left colon. Dis Colon Rectum 1995;38:1108.

97. Yoon WH, Song IS, Chang ES. Intraluminal bypass technique using a condom for protection of coloanal anastomosis. Dis Colon Rectum 1994;37:1046.

98. Michelassi F, Takanishi D, McLeod RS, et al. Ileal reservoirs. In Michelassi F, Milsom JW (eds) Operative Strategies in Inflammatory Bowel Disease. New York, Springer-Verlag, 1999, pp 186–214.

99. Joo JS, Latulippe JF, Alabaz O, et al. Long-term functional evaluation of straight coloanal anastomosis and

colonic J-pouch: is the functional superiority of colonic J-pouch sustained? Dis Colon Rectum 1998; 41:740.

100. Dehni N, Tiret E, Singland JD, et al. Long-term functional outcome after low anterior resection: comparison of low colorectal anastomosis and colonic J-pouch-anal anastomosis. Dis Colon Rectum 1998;41: 817.

101. Read TE, Kodner IJ. Protectomy and coloanal anastomosis for rectal cancer. Arch Surg 1999;134:670.

102. Shellito PC. Complications of abdominal stoma surgery. Dis Colon Rectum 1998;41:1562.

103. Feinberg SM, McLeod RS, Cohen Z. Complications of loop ileostomy. Am J Surg 1987;153:102.

104. Bass EM, Del Pino A, Tan A, et al. Does preoperative stoma marking and education by the enterostomal therapist affect outcome? Dis Colon Rectum 1997; 40:440.

105. Parks SE, Hastings PR. Complications of colostomy closure. Am J Surg 1985;149:672.

106. Hull TL, Kobe I, Fazio VW. Comparison of handsewn with stapled loop ileostomy closures. Dis Colon Rectum 1996;39:1086.

107. Reissman P, Teoh TA, Cohen SM, et al. Is early oral feeding safe after elective colorectal surgery? A prospective randomized trial. Ann Surg 1995;222:73.

108. Nessim A, Wexner SD, Agachan F, et al. Is bowel confinement necessary after anorectal reconstructive surgery? A prospective randomized, surgeon-blinded trial. Dis Colon Rectum 1999;42:16.

109. Kehlet H, Mogensen T. Hospital stay of 2 days after open sigmoidectomy with a multimodal rehabilitation programme. Br J Surg 1999;86:227.

110. Mignon M, Stettler C, Phillips SF. Pouchitis—a poorly understood entity. Dis Colon Rectum 1995;38:100.

111. Stahlberg D, Gullberg K, Liljeqvist L, et al. Pouchitis following pelvic pouch operation for ulcerative colitis: incidence, cumulative risk, and risk factors. Dis Colon Rectum 1996;39:1012.

112. Hurst RD, Molinari M, Chung TP, et al. Prospective study of the incidence, timing, and treatment of pouchitis in 104 consecutive patients after restorative proctocolectomy. Arch Surg 1996;131:497.

113. Nicholls RJ, Banerjee AK. Pouchitis: risk factors, etiology, and treatment. World J Surg 1998;22:347.

114. Keranen U, Luukkonen P, Jarvinen H. Functional results after restorative proctocolectomy complicated by pouchitis. Dis Colon Rectum 1997;40:764.

115. Sandborn WJ, McLeod R, Jewell DP. Medical therapy for induction and maintenance of remission in pouchitis: a systematic review. Inflamm Bowel Dis 1999; 5:33.

43 Right Colectomy for Cancer

INDICATIONS

Malignancy of the ileocecal region, ascending colon, and transverse colon

PREOPERATIVE PREPARATION

Colonoscopy to confirm the diagnosis and exclude other pathology
Computed tomography (CT) of abdomen
Mechanical and antibiotic bowel preparation
Perioperative antibiotics

PITFALLS AND DANGER POINTS

Injury or inadvertent ligature of superior mesenteric vessels

Laceration of retroperitoneal duodenum

Trauma to right ureter

Avulsion of branch between inferior pancreaticoduodenal and middle colic veins

Failure of anastomosis

OPERATIVE STRATEGY

The extent of the resection depends on the location of the tumor. For tumors of the cecum, the main trunk of the middle colic artery may be preserved **(Fig. 43–1)**. For tumors of the hepatic flexure or

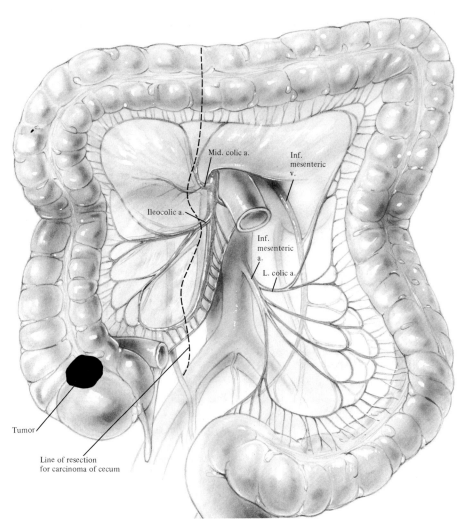

Mid. colic a.

Inf. mesenteric v.

Ileocolic a.

Inf. mesenteric a.

L. colic a.

Tumor

Line of resection for carcinoma of cecum

Fig. 43-1

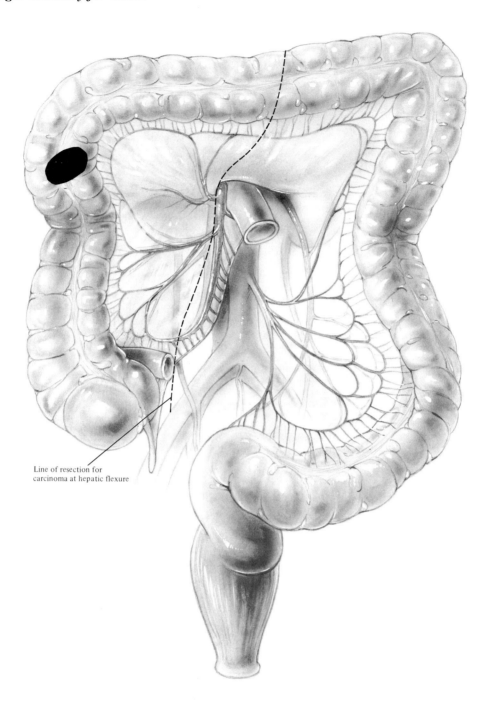

Line of resection for
carcinoma at hepatic flexure

Fig. 43-2

right transverse colon, it is necessary to ligate this vessel and resect additional colon **(Figs. 43–2, 43–3)**.

There are several anatomic advantages to the "no touch technique" described here, although the oncologic advantages are still debated. First, a dissection initiated at the origins of the middle colic and ileocolic vessels makes it possible to perform a more complete lymph node dissection in these two critical areas. Second, by devoting full attention to the lymphovascular pedicles early during the operation, before the anatomy has been distorted by traction

or bleeding, the surgeon gains thorough knowledge of the anatomic variations that may occur in the vasculature of the colon. Finally, the surgeon becomes adept at performing the most dangerous step of this procedure—high ligation of the ileocolic vessels—without traumatizing the superior mesenteric artery and vein.

In most cases when the vascular pedicles are ligated close to their points of origin, it can be seen that the right colon is supplied by two vessels: the ileocolic trunk and the middle colic artery. The mid-

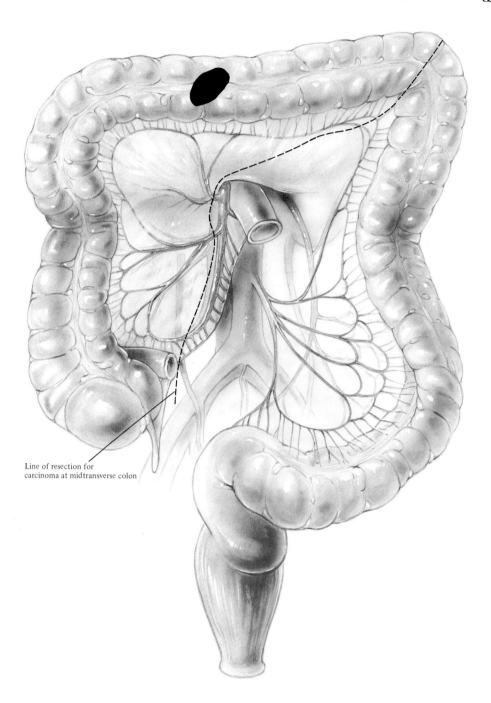

Line of resection for
carcinoma at midtransverse colon

Fig. 43-3

dle colic artery generally divides early in its course into right and left branches. The left branch forms a well developed marginal artery that connects with the left colic artery at the splenic flexure. When the proximal half of the transverse colon is removed, the left colic connection of this marginal artery supplies the remaining transverse colon. *Rarely*, a patient does not have good arterial flow from the divided marginal artery. In such a case the splenic flexure and sometimes the descending and sigmoid colon may have to be resected.

After the two major lymphovascular pedicles have been divided and ligated, the remainder of the mesentery to the right colon and the mesentery to the distal segment of the ileum should be divided. If occluding clamps are applied to the anticipated points of transection of the transverse colon and the ileum at this time, the entire specimen can be seen to be isolated from any vascular connection with the patient. This is all done before there is any manipulation of the tumor—hence the "no touch" technique. The specimen may now be removed by the traditional method of incising the peritoneum in the right paracolic gutter and elevating the right colon.

OPERATIVE TECHNIQUE (Right and Transverse Colectomy)

Incision

Make a midline incision from the mid-epigastrium to a point about 8 cm below the umbilicus. Explore the abdomen for hepatic, pelvic, peritoneal, and nodal metastases. A solitary hepatic metastasis may well be resected at the same time the colectomy is performed. A moderate degree of hepatic metastasis is not a contraindication to removing a locally resectable colon carcinoma. Inspect the primary tumor but avoid manipulating it at this stage.

Ligature of Colon Proximal and Distal to Tumor

Insert a blunt Mixter right-angle clamp through an avascular portion of the mesentery close to the colon, distal to the tumor, and draw a 3 mm umbilical tape through this puncture in the mesentery. Tie the umbilical tape firmly to occlude the lumen of the colon completely. Carry out an identical maneuver at a point on the terminal ileum, thereby completely occluding the lumen proximal and distal to the tumor.

Omental Dissection

For a carcinoma located in the hepatic flexure, divide the adjacent omentum between serially applied

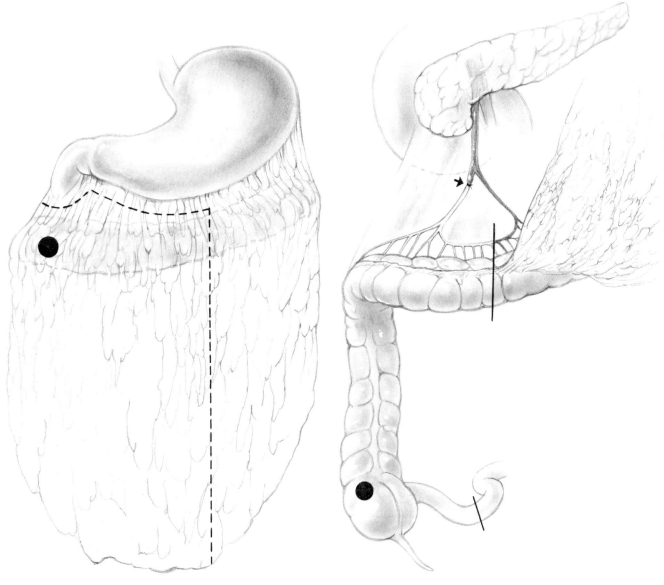

Fig. 43–4   Fig. 43–5

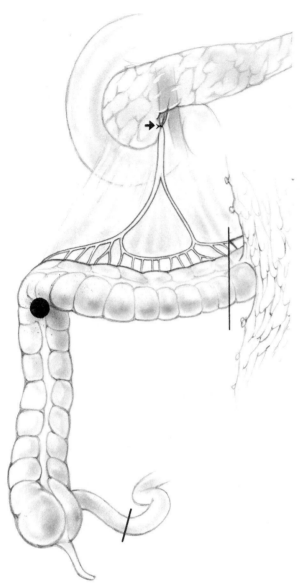

Fig. 43-6

not necessary to divide the middle colic vessels before they branch (Fig. 43–1). The left branch of the middle colic vessel may be preserved and the right branch divided and ligated just beyond the bifurcation **(Fig. 43–5)**.

During operations for tumors near the hepatic flexure of the transverse colon, dissect the middle colic vessels up to the lower border of the pancreas (Figs. 43-2, 43-3, 43-6). Be careful not to avulse a fairly large collateral branch that connects the inferior pancreaticoduodenal vein with the middle colic vein **(Fig. 43–7)**. If this is torn, considerable bleeding follows, as the proximal end of the pancreaticoduodenal vein retracts and is difficult to locate. Gentle dissection is necessary, as these structures are fragile. Place a Mixter clamp deep to the middle colic vessels at the appropriate point; then draw a 2-0 silk ligature around the vessels and ligate them. Sweep any surrounding lymph nodes down toward the specimen and place a second ligature 1.5 cm distal to the first. Divide the vessels 1 cm beyond the proximal ligature. Divide the mesocolon toward the point on the transverse colon already selected

Kelly hemostats just distal to the gastroepiploic arcade of the stomach **(Fig. 43–4)**. If the neoplasm is located in the cecum, there appears to be no merit in resecting the omentum. The omentum may be dissected (with scalpel and Metzenbaum scissors) off the right half of the transverse colon through the avascular plane, resecting only portions adhering to the cecal tumor. After this has been accomplished, with the transverse colon drawn in a caudal direction the middle colic vessels can be seen as they emerge from the lower border of the pancreas to cross over the retroperitoneal duodenum.

Division of Middle Colic Vessels

During operations for carcinoma of the cecum and the proximal 5-7 cm of the ascending colon, it is

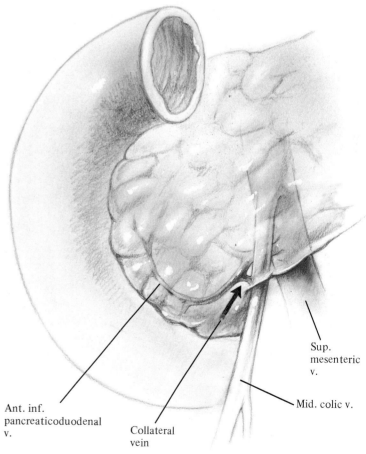

Ant. inf.
pancreaticoduodenal
v.

Collateral
vein

Sup.
mesenteric
v.

Mid. colic v.

Fig. 43-7

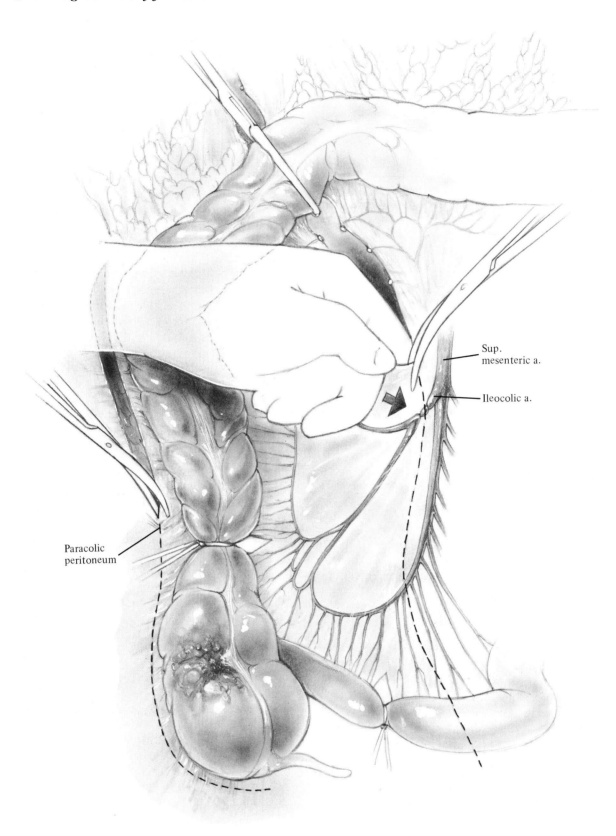

Sup.
mesenteric a.

Ileocolic a.

Paracolic
peritoneum

Fig. 43-8

for division. Divide and ligate the marginal artery and clear the transverse colon of fat and areolar tissue in preparation for an anastomosis. Now apply an Allen clamp to the transverse colon, but to minimize bacterial contamination of the abdominal cavity do not transect the colon at this time.

Division of Ileocolic Vessels

Retract the transverse colon in a cephalad direction. Pass the left index finger deep to the right mesocolon **(Fig. 43–8)**, inserting the finger through the incision already made in the transverse mesocolon. Gentle finger dissection should disclose, in front of the fingertip, a fairly large artery with vigorous pulsation; it is the ileocolic arterial trunk (Fig. 43–8). As the surgeon's index finger moves toward the patient's left, it palpates the adjacent superior mesenteric artery. After identifying these two major vessels, it is a simple matter to incise the peritoneum overlying the ileocolic artery with Metzenbaum scissors. By gentle dissection, remove areolar and lymphatic tissue from the circumference of the ileocolic artery and vein. After rechecking the location of the superior mesenteric vessels, pass a blunt Mixter right-angle clamp underneath the ileocolic artery and vein. Ligate the vessels individually with 2-0 silk ligatures and divide them at a point about 1.5 cm distal to their junctions with the superior mesenteric vessels.

Division of Ileal Mesentery

Pass the left index finger behind the remaining right mesocolon into an avascular area of 3–4 cm. This can be divided and leads to the mesentery of the terminal ileum. For neoplasms close to the ileocecal junction, include 10–15 cm of ileum in the specimen.

For tumors near the hepatic flexure, no more than 8–10 cm of ileum need be resected. In any case, divide the ileal mesentery between Crile hemostats applied serially until the wall of the ileum has been encountered. After ligating each of the hemostats with 3-0 or 2-0 PG, clear the areolar tissue from the circumference of the ileum in preparation for an anastomosis and apply an Allen clamp to this area. At this point the specimen has been isolated from any vascular connection with the host.

Division of Right Paracolic Peritoneum

Retract the right colon in a medical direction and make an incision in the peritoneum of the paracolic gutter (Fig. 43–8). The left index finger may be inserted deep to this layer of peritoneum, which should then be transected over the index finger with Metzenbaum scissors or electrocautery. Continue this dissection until the hepatic flexure is free of lateral attachments. Rough dissection around the retroperitoneal duodenum may lacerate it inadvertently, so be aware of its location. Next, identify the right renocolic ligament and divide it by Metzenbaum dissection. When this is accomplished, the fascia of Gerota and the perirenal fat may be gently swept from the posterior aspect of the right mesocolon. Continue this dissection caudally, eventually unroofing the ureter and gonadal vessel.

Identification of Ureter

If the location of the ureter is not immediately evident, identify the right common iliac artery. The undisturbed ureter generally crosses the common iliac artery where it bifurcates into its internal and external branches. If the ureter is not in this location, elevate the lateral leaflet of the peritoneum, as the ureter may be adhering to the undersurface of this peritoneal flap. The ureter is often displaced by retraction of the peritoneal flap to which it adheres. If the ureter is not present on the lateral leaflet of peritoneum, similarly elevate and seek it on the medial leaflet of the peritoneum. Typical ureteral peristalsis should occur when the ureter is compressed with forceps.

The right colon remains attached to the peritoneum now only at the inferior and medial aspects of the cecum and ileum. There should be no difficulty dividing it.

Division of Ileum and Colon

Protect the abdomen with large gauze pads and remove the specimen and the Allen clamps that had been applied to the ileum and transverse colon. If necessary, linen-shod Doyen noncrushing intestinal clamps may be applied to occlude the ileum and transverse colon at a point at least 10 cm from their

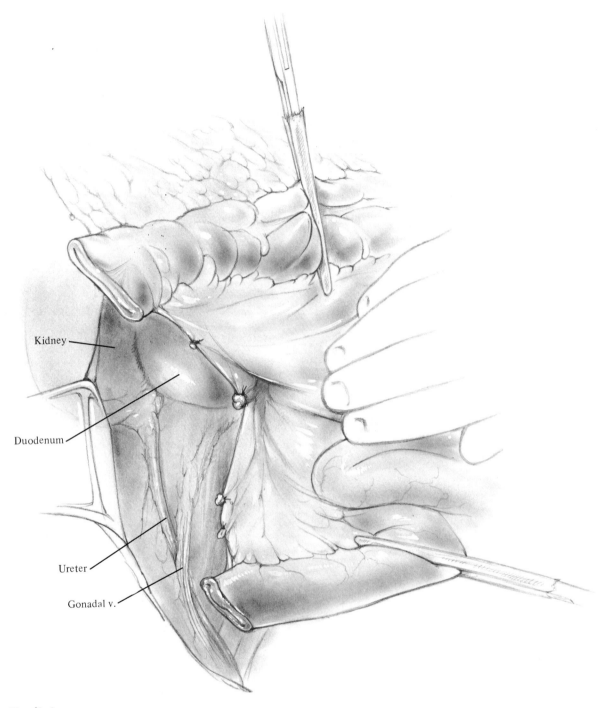

Kidney

Duodenum

Ureter

Gonadal v.

Fig. 43-9

cut edges in preparation for an open, two-layer end-to-end anastomosis **(Fig. 43–9)**.

Before the anastomosis is begun, the blood supply must be carefully evaluated. Generally there is no problem with the terminal ileum if no hematoma has been induced. Test the adequacy of the blood supply to the cut end of the colon by palpating the pulse in the marginal artery. For additional data about the blood supply, divide a small arterial branch near the cut end of the colon and observe the pulsatile arterial flow. If there is any question about the vigor of the blood supply, resect additional transverse colon.

Ileocolic Two-Layer Sutured End-to-End Anastomosis

Align the cut ends of the ileum and transverse colon to face each other so their mesenteries are not twisted. Because the diameter of ileum is narrower than that of the colon, make a Cheatle slit with Metzenbaum scissors on the antimesenteric border of the ileum for a distance of 1–2 cm to help equalize these two diameters **(Fig. 43–10)**. Do not round off the corners of the slit.

Insert the first seromuscular layer of interrupted sutures using 4-0 silk on atraumatic needles. Initiate this layer by inserting the first Lembert suture at the antimesenteric border and the second at the mesenteric border to serve as guy sutures. Attach hemostats to each of these sutures. Drawing the two hemostats apart makes insertion of additional sutures by successive bisection more efficient **(Fig. 43–11)**. Now complete the anterior seromuscular layer of the anastomosis by inserting interrupted

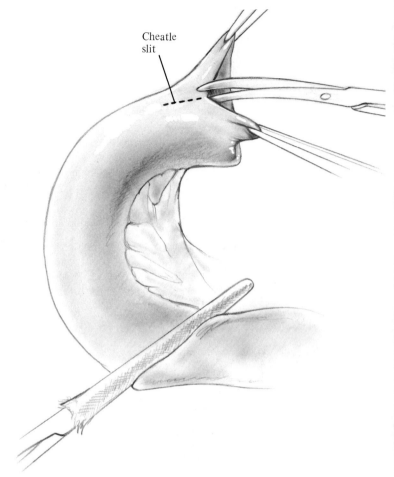

Fig. 43–10

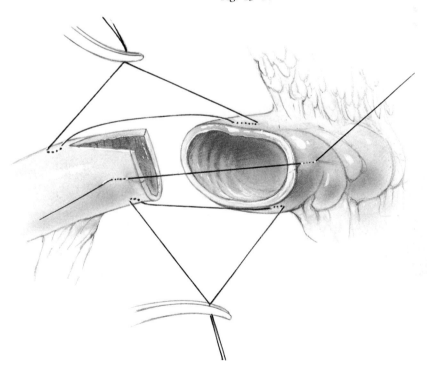

Fig. 43–11

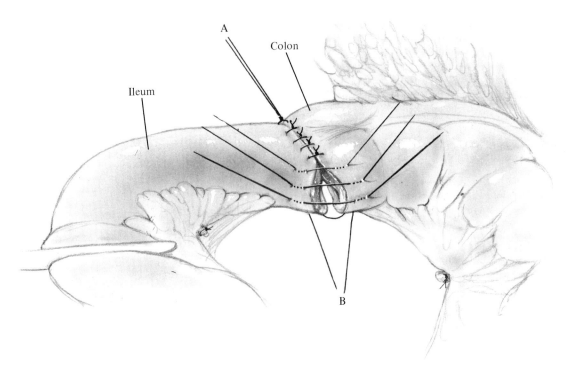

Fig. 43-12

Lembert seromuscular sutures **(Fig. 43–12)**. After the entire anterior layer has been inserted and tied, cut the tails of all the sutures except the two guy sutures.

To provide exposure for the mucosal layer, invert the anterior aspect of the anastomosis by passing the hemostat containing the antimesenteric guy suture **(Fig. 43–13**, A) through the rent in the mesentery deep to the ileocolonic anastomosis. Then draw the mesenteric guy suture (Fig. 43-13, B) in the opposite direction and expose the mucosa for application of the first layer of mucosal sutures **(Fig. 43–14)**. Use 5-0 PG, double-armed, and begin the first suture at the midpoint **(Fig. 43–15a)**. Then pass the suture

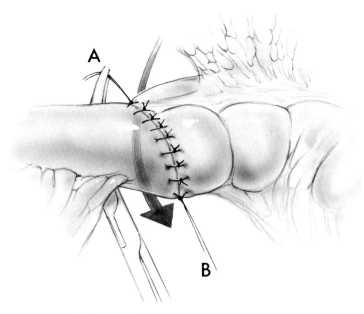

Fig. 43-13

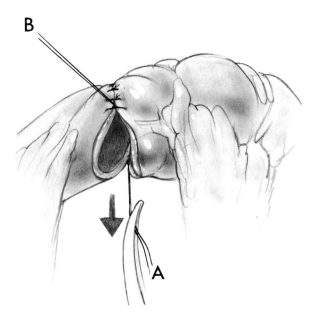

Fig. 43-14

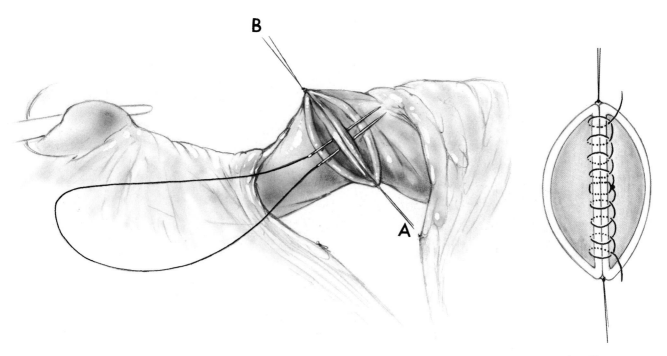

Fig. 43-15a

Fig. 43-15b

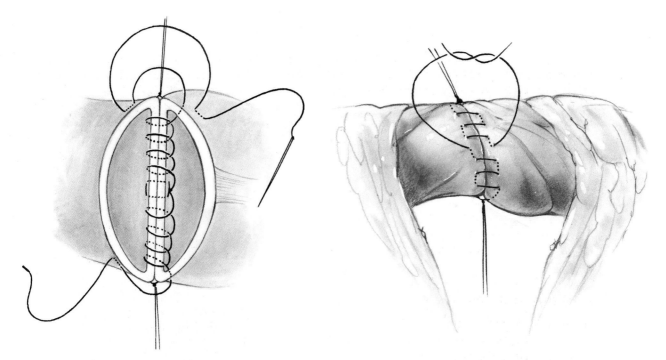

Fig. 43-15c

Fig. 43-16

in a continuous fashion toward the patient's right to lock each stitch. Take relatively small bites (4 mm). When the right margin of the suture line is reached, tag the needle with a hemostat; with the second needle initiate the remainder of the mucosal approximation, going from the midpoint of the anastomosis toward the patient's left in a continuous locked fash-

ion **(Fig. 43–15b)**. When this layer has been completed **(Fig. 43–15c)**, close the superficial mucosal layer of the anastomosis with continuous Connell or Cushing sutures beginning at each end of the anastomosis. Terminate the mucosal suture line in the midpoint of the superficial layer by tying the suture to its mate **(Fig. 43–16)**.

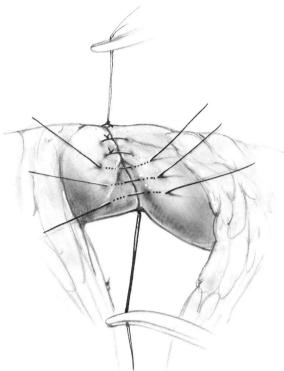

Fig. 43-17

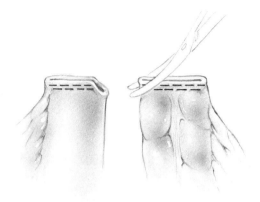

Fig. 43-18

Accomplish the final seromuscular layer by inserting interrupted 4-0 silk Lembert sutures **(Fig. 43–17)**. Devote special attention to ensuring a secure closure at the mesenteric border. Then cut all the sutures and test the lumen with thumb and forefinger to gauge the width of the anastomotic stoma. It should admit the tip of the thumb.

Close the defect in the mesentery by continuous 2-0 PG sutures. Take care to avoid occluding important vessels running in the mesentery during the course of the continuous suture. If desired, a one-layer anastomosis can be constructed by the technique described above, simply by omitting the mucosal suture. If it is accomplished without error, the result is as successful as after the two-layer method.

Anastomosis by Stapling, Functional End-to-End

To perform a stapled anastomosis, clear an area of mesentery and apply the 55/3.5 mm linear stapler transversely across the colon. Transect the colon flush with the stapler using a scalpel. Carry out the identical procedure at the selected site on the ileum. Alternatively, the bowel may be stapled and divided with the linear cutting stapler. Some oozing of blood should be evident despite the double row of staples. Control excessive bleeding by carefully applying electrocoagulation or chromic sutures. Align the ileum and colon side by side and with heavy scissors excise a triangular 8 mm wedge from the an-

timesenteric margins of both ileum and colon **(Fig. 43–18)**.

Insert one of the two forks of the cutting linear stapling instrument into the lumen of the ileum and the other into the colon, *hugging the antimesenteric border* of each **(Fig. 43–19)**. Neither segment of intestine should be stretched, as it may result in excessive thinning of the bowel, leaving inadequate substance for the staples to grasp. After ascertaining that both segments of the bowel are near the hub of the stapler, fire the device; this should result in a side-to-side anastomosis 4–5 cm long. Unlock and remove the device and inspect the staple line for bleeding and possible technical failure when closing the staples.

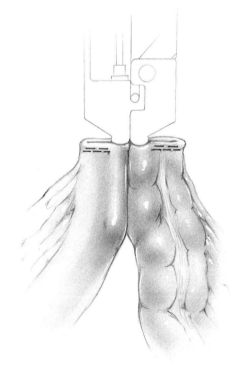

Fig. 43-19

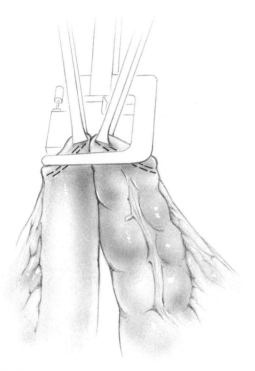

Fig. 43-20

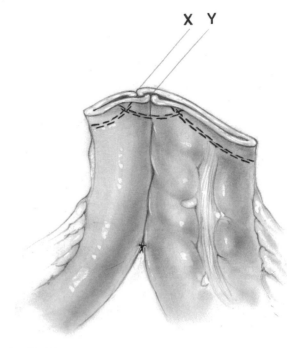

Fig. 43-22

Now apply Allis clamps to the remaining defect in the anastomosis and close it by a final application of the 55/3.5 mm linear stapling instrument **(Fig. 43-20)**. Take care to include a portion of *each of the previously applied staples lines* in the final application of the stapler. However, when applying the Allis clamps, do not align points X and Y **(Fig. 43-21)** exactly opposite each other, as it would result in six staple lines meeting at one point. The alignment of these two points, as shown in **Figure 43-22**, produces the best results. Check the patency of the anastomosis by invaginating the colon through the anastomosis, which should admit the tips of two fingers. Then lightly touch the everted mucosa with the electrocautery instrument. During closure of the mesentery, cover the everted staple lines with adjoining mesentery or omentum if convenient.

We have modified Steichen's method of anastomosing ileum to colon, making it simpler by eliminating two applications of the stapler. With our technique the first step is to insert the cutting linear stapling device, one fork into the open end of ileum and the other fork into the open colon. Then fire the stapler, establishing a partial anastomosis between the antimesenteric borders of ileum and colon, as seen in Figure 43-21. Apply four or five Allis clamps to approximate the lips of the ileum and colon (in eversion) taking care that points X and Y are not in apposition. Then apply a 90/3.5 mm linear stapler underneath the Allis clamps and fire the staples. The end result is illustrated in **Figure 43-23**. In our experience this is the most efficient and reliable method for constructing an ileocolonic anastomosis.

Wound Closure

The surgical team now changes gloves and discards all instruments used up to this point. Irrigate the op-

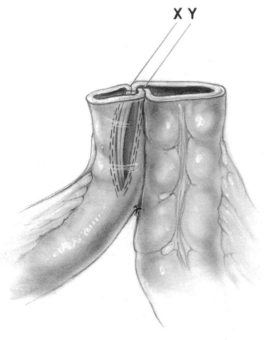

Fig. 43-21

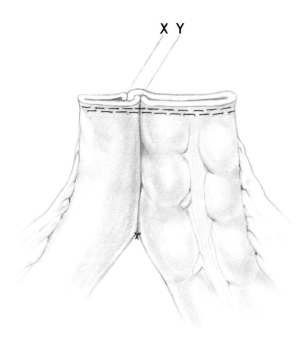

Fig. 43–23

erative field with saline. Cover the anastomosis with omentum if possible. Close the abdomen in routine fashion without drainage.

POSTOPERATIVE CARE

Continue nasogastric suction for 1–3 days.

Delay oral intake of liquid and food until the fifth or sixth postoperative day.

If ileus persists, delay oral intake further and perform CT of the abdomen to exclude abscess, obstruction, or leak.

In the absence of preoperative intraabdominal sepsis, discontinue antibiotics after the operation.

COMPLICATIONS

Leakage from an ileocolonic or colocolonic anastomosis may manifest as peritonitis, colocutaneous fistula, or localized intraperitoneal abscess. Localized or spreading peritonitis should be managed by prompt relaparotomy and exteriorization of both ends of the anastomosis.

Sepsis in the subhepatic, subphrenic, or pelvic areas is an occasional complication of anastomoses of the colon, even in the absence of leakage. CT of the abdomen generally provides the diagnosis, and percutaneous drainage is usually successful.

Wound infection requires prompt removal of all overlying skin sutures to permit wide drainage of the entire infected area.

REFERENCES

Furstenberg S, Goldman S, Machado M, Jarhult J. Mini-laparotomy approach to tumors of the right colon. Dis Colon Rectum 1998;41:997.

Heili MJ, Flowers SA, Fowler DL. Laparoscopic-assisted colectomy: a comparison of dissection techniques. J Soc Laparoendosc Surg 1999;3:27.

Leung KL, Meng WC, Lee JP, et al. Laparoscopic-assisted resection of right-sided colonic carcinoma: a case-control study. J Surg Oncol 1999;71:97.

Metcalf AM. Laparoscopic colectomy. Surg Clin North Am 2000;80:1321.

Schirmer BD. Laparoscopic colon resection. Surg Clin North Am 1996;76:571.

Young-Fadok TM, Nelson H. Laparoscopic right colectomy: five-step procedure. Dis Colon Rectum 2000; 43:267.

Young-Fadok TM, Radice E, Nelson H, Harmsen WS. Benefits of laparoscopic-assisted colectomy for colon polyps: a case-matched series. Mayo Clinic Proc 2000; 75:344.

44 Left Colectomy for Cancer

INDICATIONS

Whereas malignancies of the proximal three-fourths of the transverse colon require excision of the right and transverse colon, cancers of the distal transverse colon, splenic flexure, descending colon, and sigmoid are treated by left hemicolectomy **(Figs. 44–1, 44–2)**.

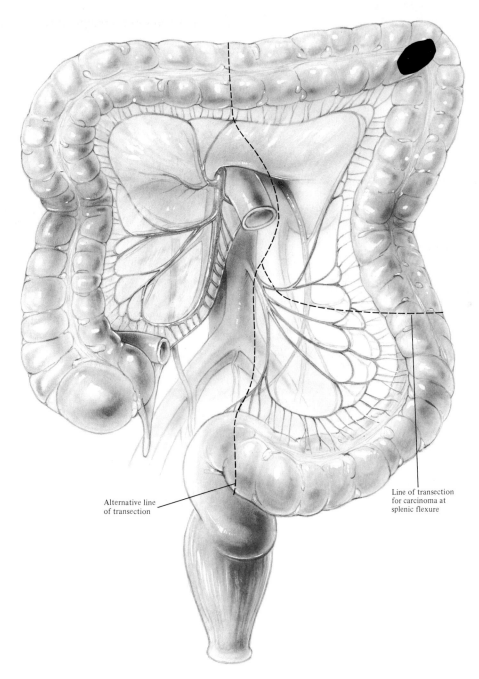

Alternative line of transection

Line of transection for carcinoma at splenic flexure

Fig. 44-1

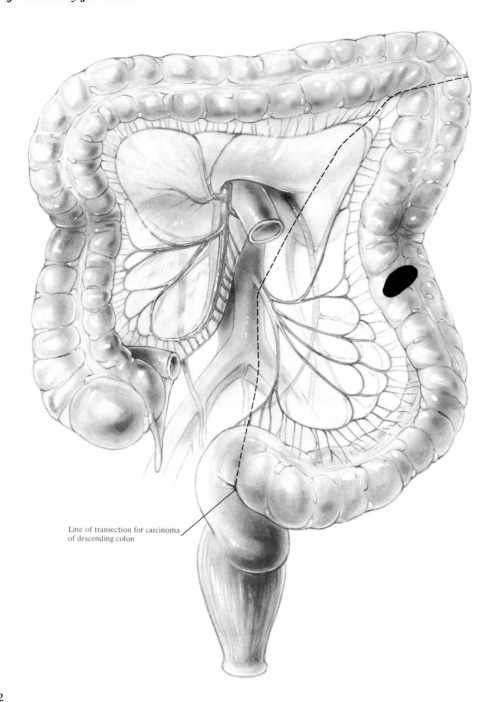

Line of transection for carcinoma of descending colon

Fig. 44-2

PREOPERATIVE PREPARATION

See Chapter 43.

PITFALLS AND DANGER POINTS

Injury to spleen

Injury to ureter

Failure of anastomosis

OPERATIVE STRATEGY

Extent of Dissection

Lymph draining from malignancies of the left colon flows along the left colic or sigmoidal veins to the inferior mesenteric vessels. In the usual case, the inferior mesenteric artery should be divided at the aorta and the inferior mesenteric vein at the lower border of the pancreas.

Except for treating lesions situated in the distal sigmoid, the lower point of division of the colon is through the upper rectum, 2-3 cm above the promontory of the sacrum (Figs. 44-1, 44-2). Presacral elevation of the rectal stump need not be carried out, and the anastomosis should be intraperitoneal. The blood supply of a rectal stump of this length, arising from the inferior and middle hemorrhoidal arteries, is almost invariably of excellent quality. The blood supply of the proximal colonic segment, arising from the middle colic artery, generally is also excellent, provided care is exercised not to damage the marginal vessel at any point in its course.

Liberation of Splenic Flexure

The splenic flexure of the colon may be completely liberated without dividing a single blood vessel if the surgeon can recognize anatomic planes accurately. The only blood vessels going to the colon are those arising from its mesentery. Bleeding during the course of this dissection arises from three sources.

1. Frequently, *downward traction on the colon and its attached omentum* avulses a patch of splenic capsule to which the omentum adheres. It is worthwhile to inspect the lower pole of the spleen at the *onset* of this dissection and to divide such areas of adhesion with Metzenbaum scissors under direct vision before applying traction.
2. Bleeding arises when the *surgeon does not recognize the plane* between the omentum and appendices epiploica attached to the distal transverse colon. The appendices may extend 1-3 cm cephalad to the transverse colon. When they are divided inadvertently, bleeding follows. Note that the character of the fat in the omentum is considerably different from that of the appendices. The former has the appearance of multiple small lobulations, each 4-6 mm in diameter, whereas the appendices epiploica contain fat that appears to have a completely smooth surface. If the proper plane between the omentum and appendices can be identified, the dissection is bloodless.
3. Bleeding can arise from the *use of blunt dissection* to divide the renocolic ligament. This ruptures a number of veins along the surface of Gerota's capsule, which overlies the kidney. Bleeding can be prevented by accurately identifying the renocolic ligament, delineating it carefully, and then dividing it with Metzenbaum scissors along the medial margin of the renal capsule.

Although the classic anatomy books do not generally describe a "renocolic ligament," it can be identified as a thin structure (see Figs. 44-4, 44-5) extending from the anterior surface of the renal capsule to the posterior surface of the mesocolon.

There are three essential steps to safe liberation of the splenic flexure. First, the obvious one is to incise the parietal peritoneum in the left paracolic gutter going cephalad to the splenic flexure. Second, dissect the left margin of the omentum from the distal transverse colon as well as from the left parietal peritoneum near the lower pole of the spleen (in patients who have this attachment). The third, least well understood step, is to identify and divide the renocolic ligament between the renal capsule and the posterior mesocolon. Then pass the index finger deep to this ligament in the region of the splenic flexure (see Fig. 44-5); this plane leads to the lienocolic ligament, which is also avascular and may be divided by Metzenbaum scissors provided this ligament is separated from underlying fatty tissue by finger dissection. The fatty tissue may contain an epiploic appendix with a blood vessel. After the lienocolic ligament has been divided, the index finger should lead to the next avascular "ligament," which extends from the pancreas to the transverse colon. This pancreaticocolic "ligament" comprises the upper portion of the transverse mesocolon. Dividing it frees the distal transverse colon and splenic flexure, except for the mesentery. For all practical purposes the renocolic, lienocolic, and pancreaticocolic "ligaments" comprise one continuous avascular membrane with multiple areas of attachment.

No-Touch Technique

The no-touch technique is more difficult to apply to lesions of the left colon than to those on the right. In many cases it can be accomplished by liberating the sigmoid colon early in the procedure, identifying and ligating the inferior mesenteric vessels, and dividing the mesocolon—all before manipulating the tumor. Care must be taken to identify and protect the ureter.

In some cases the tumor's location or the obesity of the mesocolon make this approach more cumbersome for the surgeon, unlike the situation on the right side where the anatomy lends itself to adoption of the no-touch method as a routine procedure. Most surgeons content themselves with minimal manipulation of the tumor while they use the opera-

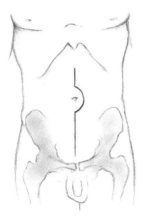

Fig. 44-3a

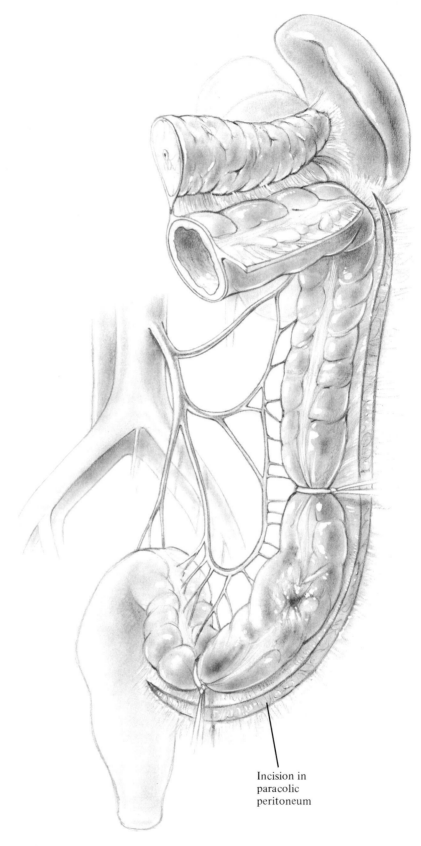

Incision in
paracolic
peritoneum

Fig. 44-3b

tive sequence of first liberating the left colon and then ligating the lymphovascular attachments.

Technique of Anastomosis

Because the anastomosis is generally intraperitoneal and the rectal stump is largely covered by peritoneum, the leak rate in elective cases is less than 2%. Anastomosis may be done by the end-to-end technique or the Baker side-to-end method based on the preference of the surgeon.

If a stapling technique is desired, we prefer the functional end-to-end anastomosis (see Figs. 44-35 through 44-38). A circular stapling device (see Figs. 45-25 through 45-31) may also be used, but the internal diameter of the anastomosis resulting from this technique may be slightly narrow.

OPERATIVE TECHNIQUE

Incision and Exposure

Make a midline incision from a point about 4 cm below the xiphoid to the pubis **(Fig. 44–3a)** and open and explore the abdomen. Insert a Thompson retractor to elevate the left costal margin; it improves the exposure for the splenic flexure dissection. Exteriorize the small intestine and retract it to the patient's right. Apply umbilical tape ligatures to occlude the colon proximal and distal to the tumor.

Liberation of Descending Colon and Sigmoid

Standing at the patient's left, make a long incision in the peritoneum of the left paracolic gutter between the descending colon and the white line of Toldt **(Fig. 44–3b)**. Use the left index finger to elevate this peritoneal layer and continue the incision upward with Metzenbaum scissors until the right-angle curve of the splenic flexure is reached. At this point the peritoneal incision must be moved close to the colon; otherwise the incision in the parietal peritoneum tends to continue upward and laterally toward the spleen. Similarly, with the index finger leading the way, use Metzenbaum scissors to complete the incision in a caudal direction, liberating the sigmoid colon from its lateral attachments down to the rectosigmoid region.

Division of Renocolic Ligament

With the descending colon retracted toward the patient's right, a filmy attachment can be visualized covering the renal capsule and extending medially to attach to the posterior surface of the mesocolon **(Fig. 44–4)**. Most surgeons bluntly disrupt this renocolic attachment, which resembles a ligament, using a gauze pad in a sponge-holder; but this maneuver often tears small veins on the surface of the renal capsule and causes unnecessary bleeding. In-

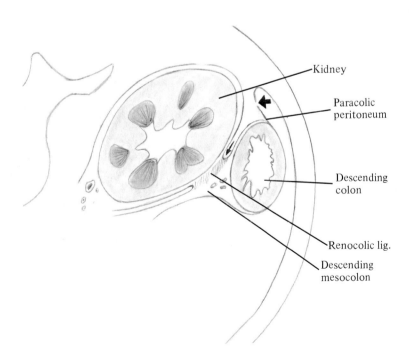

Fig. 44-4

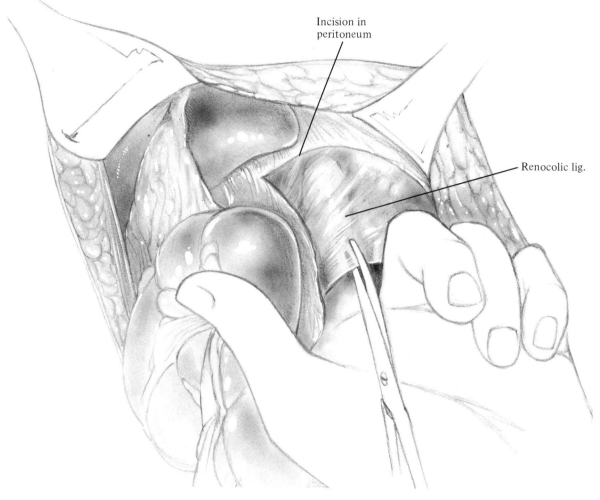

Fig. 44-5

stead, divide this structure with Metzenbaum scissors near the junction of the medial margin of the renal capsule and the adjacent mesocolon. Once the incision is initiated, delineate this fibrous structure by elevating it over an index finger **(Fig. 44–5)**. After the renocolic ligament has been divided, the upper ureter and gonadal vein lie exposed. Trace the ureter down to its entrance into the pelvis and encircle it with a Silastic loop tag for future identification.

Splenic Flexure Dissection

The lower pole of the spleen can now be seen. Sharply divide any adhesions between the omentum and the capsule of the spleen to avoid inadvertent avulsion of the splenic capsule (due to traction on the omentum). If bleeding occurs because the

splenic capsule has been torn, it can usually be controlled by applying a piece of topical hemostatic agent. Occasionally sutures on a fine atraumatic needle are helpful.

At this stage identify and divide the attachments between the omentum and the lateral aspect of the transverse colon. Remember to differentiate carefully between the fat of the appendices epiploica and the more lobulated fat of the omentum (see Operative Strategy, above). Free the omentum from the distal 10-12 cm of transverse colon **(Fig. 44–6)**. If the tumor is located in the distal transverse colon, leave the omentum attached to the tumor and divide the omentum just outside the gastroepiploic arcade.

Return now to the upper portion of the divided renocolic ligament. Insert the *right* index finger underneath the upper portion of this ligament and pinch it between the index finger and thumb; this

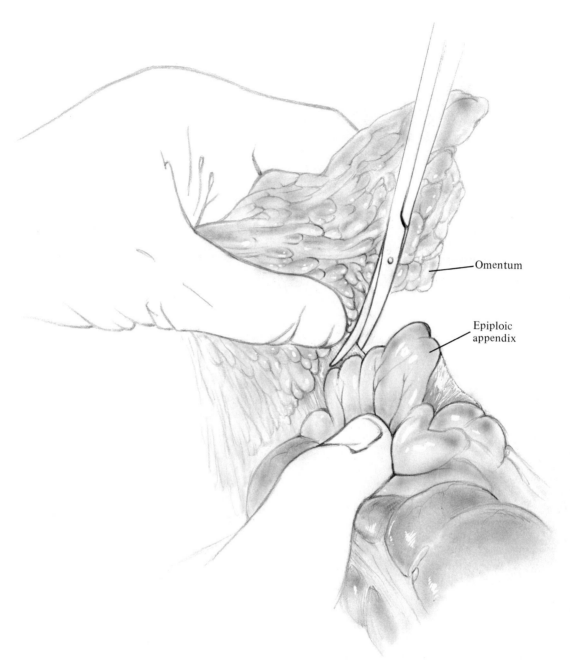

Fig. 44-6

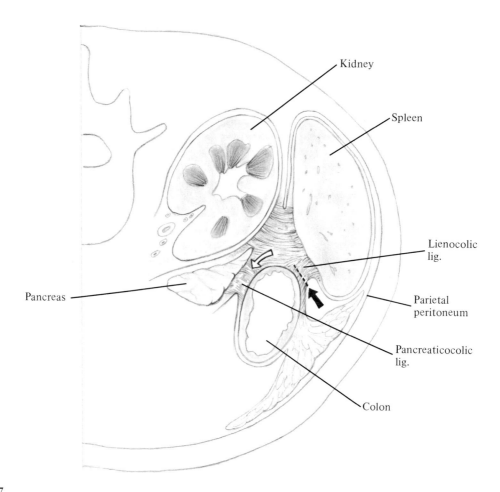

Kidney

Spleen

Lienocolic
lig.

Parietal
peritoneum

Pancreaticocolic
lig.

Pancreas

Colon

Fig. 44-7

maneuver localizes the lienocolic ligament **(Fig. 44–7)**. The ligament should be divided by the first assistant guided by the surgeon's right index finger. By inserting the index finger 5-6 cm farther medially, an avascular pancreaticocolic "ligament" **(Figs. 44-7, 44–8)** can be identified. It is an upper extension of the transverse mesocolon. After this structure has been divided, the distal transverse colon and splenic flexure become free of all posterior attachments. Control any bleeding in the area by suture-ligature or electrocautery.

Ligation and Division of Inferior Mesenteric Artery

Make an incision on the medial aspect of the meso-colon from the level of the duodenum down to the promontory of the sacrum. The inferior mesenteric artery is easily identified by palpation at its origin from the aorta. Sweep the lymphatic tissue in this vicinity downward, skeletonizing the artery, which should be double-ligated with 2-0 silk at a point about 1.5 cm from the aorta **(Fig. 44–9)** and then divided. Sweep the preaortic areolar tissue and lymph nodes toward the specimen. It is not necessary to skeletonize the anterior wall of the aorta, as it could divide the preaortic sympathetic nerves, which would result in sexual dysfunction in male patients. If the preaortic dissection is carried out by gently sweeping the nodes laterally, the nerves are not divided inadvertently. Now divide the inferior mesenteric vein as it passes behind the duodenoje-junal junction and pancreas.

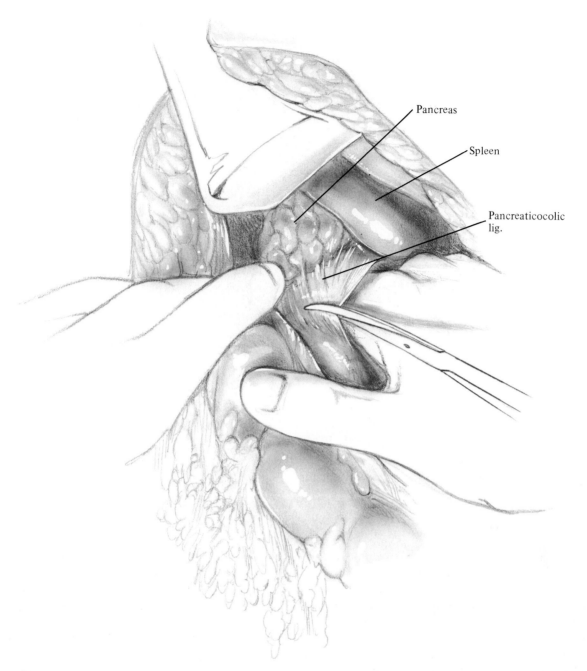

Pancreas

Spleen

Pancreaticocolic
lig.

Fig. 44-8

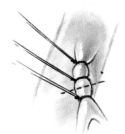

Fig. 44-9

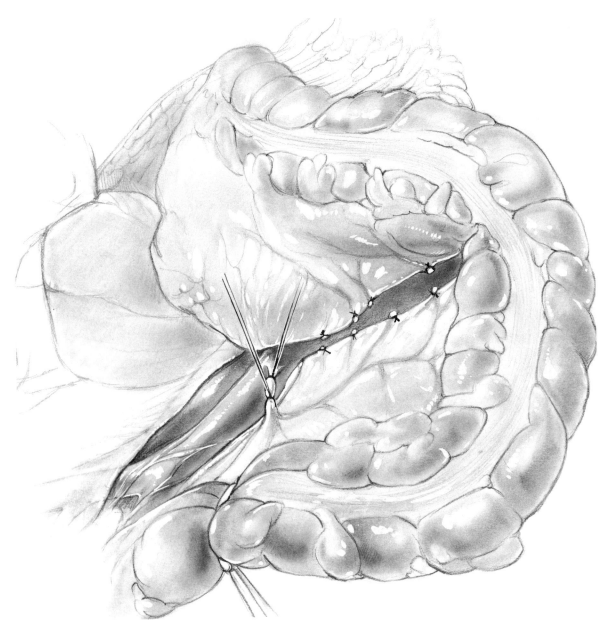

Fig. 44-10

Division of Mesocolon

Depending on the location of the tumor, divide the mesocolon between clamps up to and including the marginal artery **(Fig. 44–10)**.

Ligation and Division of Mesorectum

Separate the distally ligated pedicle of the inferior mesenteric artery and the divided mesocolon from the aorta and iliac vessels down to the promontory of the sacrum. Divide the vascular tissue around the rectum between pairs of hemostats sequentially un-

til the wall of the upper rectum is visible. Then free the rectal stump of surrounding fat and areolar tissue at the point selected for the anastomosis. This point should be 2–3 cm above the promontory of the sacrum, where three-fourths of the rectum is covered anteriorly and laterally by peritoneum.

Insertion of Wound Protector

Insert a Wound Protector ring drape or moist laparotomy pads into the abdominal cavity to protect the subcutaneous panniculus from contamination when the colon is opened.

Division of Colon and Rectum

Expose the point on the proximal colon selected for division. Apply an Allen clamp to the specimen side. Divide the colon after applying a Doyen or other type of nontraumatic clamp to avoid contamination. Completely clear the areolar tissue and fat from the distal centimeter of the proximal colon so the serosa is exposed throughout its circumference. Handle the distal end of the specimen in the same manner by applying an Allen clamp to the specimen side. Now divide the upper rectum and remove the specimen. Suction the rectum free of any contents. Apply no clamp. Use fine PG or PDS sutures to control any bleeding from the rectal wall. Completely clear surrounding fat and areolar tissue from a cuff of rectum 1 cm in width so seromuscular sutures may be inserted accurately.

End-to-End Two-Layer Anastomosis, Rotation Method

There are eight steps to the end-to-end two-layer anastomosis, rotation method.

1. Check the *adequacy of the blood supply* of both ends of the bowel. Confirm that a *cuff of at least 1 cm of serosa* has been cleared to the areolar tissue and blood vessels at both ends of the bowel.
2. *Rotate the proximal colonic segment* so the mesentery enters from the right lateral margin of the anastomosis. Leave the rectal segment undisturbed **(Fig. 44–11)**.
3. If the diameter of the lumen of one of the segments of bowel is significantly narrower than the other, *make a Cheatle slit*, 1-2 cm long, on the antimesenteric border of the narrower segment of bowel (see Figs. 43–10, 43–11).
4. *Insert the first layer of seromuscular sutures*. If the rectal stump is not bound to the sacrum and if it can be rotated easily for 180°, it is more efficient to insert the anterior seromuscular layer as the first step of the anastomosis.
5. Insert interrupted 4-0 silk atraumatic Lembert seromuscular guy sutures, first to the lateral border of the anastomosis and then to the medial border. Using the technique of successive bisection, place the third Lembert suture on the anterior wall halfway between the first two (Fig. 44-11). Each stitch takes about 5 mm of tissue (including the submucosa) from the rectum and then from the descending colon.
6. After all the anterior sutures have been inserted, *tie them and cut all the suture tails* except for those of the two end guy sutures, which should be grasped in hemostats **(Fig. 44–12)**. Pass a he-

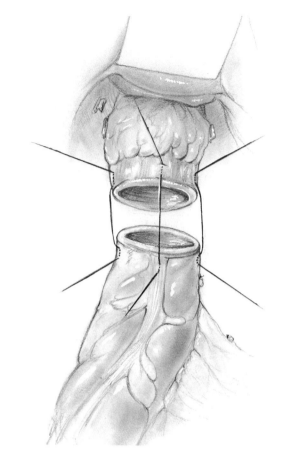

Fig. 44-11

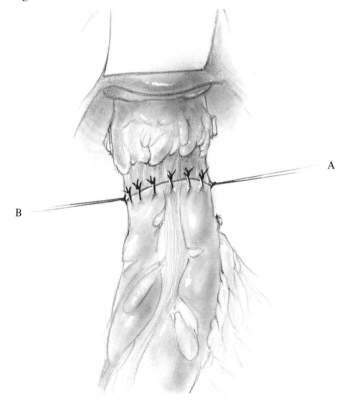

Fig. 44-12

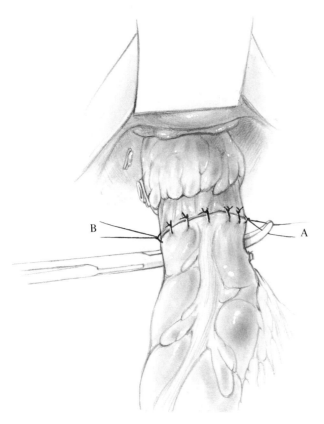

Fig. 44-13

mostat underneath the suture line, grasp the right lateral stitch **(Fig. 44–13,** A), and rotate the anastomosis 180° **(Fig. 44–14)**.

7. Place a double-armed 5-0 Vicryl or PG *suture in the middle of the deep mucosal layer* **(Fig. 44–15a)**. Complete this layer with a continuous locked suture through the full thickness of the bowel **(Fig. 44–15b)**. Then, with the same two needles and using a continuous Connell or Cushing suture, complete the remainder of the mucosal approximation **(Fig. 44–16)**.

8. Approximate the *final seromuscular layer* with interrupted 4-0 atraumatic Lembert silk sutures **(Fig. 44–17)**. After all the suture tails are cut, permit the anastomosis to rotate back 180° to its normal position.

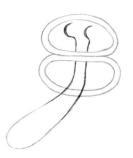

Fig. 44-15a

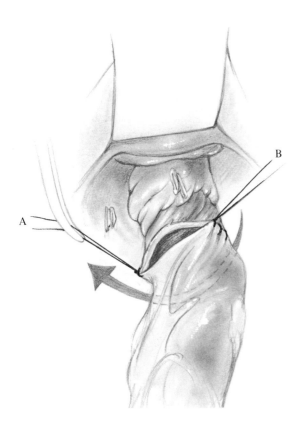

Fig. 44-14

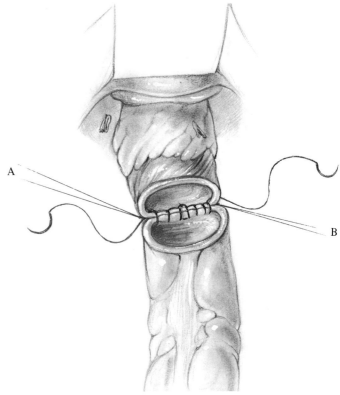

Fig. 44-15b

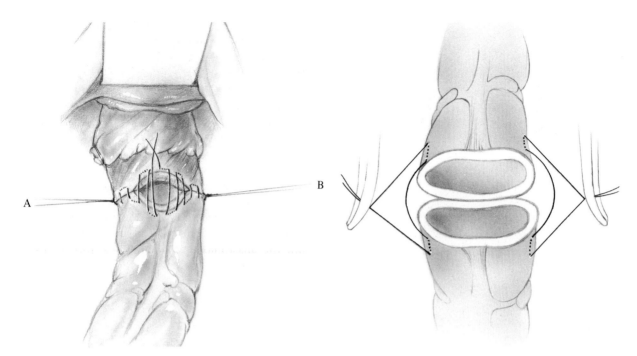

Fig. 44-16

Fig. 44-18

End-to-End Anastomosis, Alternative Technique

When the rectum and colon cannot be rotated 180° as required for the method described above, an alternative technique must be used in which the posterior seromuscular layer is inserted first. To do this, insert a seromuscular suture of 4-0 silk into the left side of the rectum and the proximal colon. Do not tie this suture; grasp it in a hemostat and use it as the left guy suture. Place a second, identical suture on the right lateral aspects of the rectum and proximal colon and similarly hold it in a hemostat **(Fig. 44–18)**.

Insert interrupted 4-0 silk seromuscular Lembert sutures **(Fig. 44–19)** to complete the posterior layer

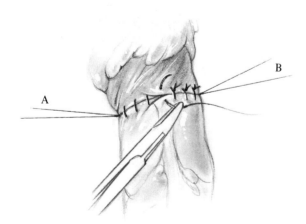

Fig. 44-17

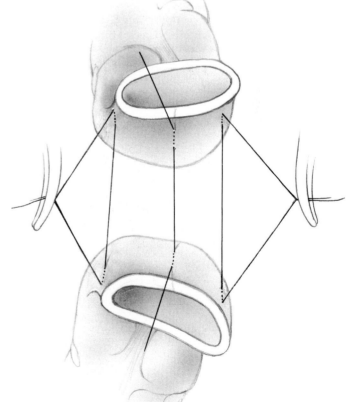

Fig. 44-19

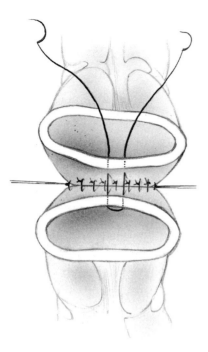

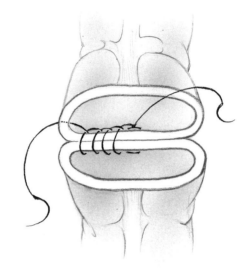

Fig. 44-22

Fig. 44-20

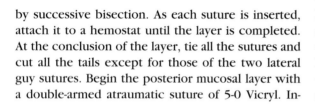

by successive bisection. As each suture is inserted, attach it to a hemostat until the layer is completed. At the conclusion of the layer, tie all the sutures and cut all the tails except for those of the two lateral guy sutures. Begin the posterior mucosal layer with a double-armed atraumatic suture of 5-0 Vicryl. In-

sert the suture in mattress fashion in the midpoint of the posterior layer of mucosa and tie it **(Fig. 44–20)**. Use one needle to initiate a continuous locked suture, taking bites averaging 5 mm in diameter and going through all coats of bowel **(Fig. 44–21)**. Continue this in a locked fashion until the left lateral margin of the anastomosis is reached **(Fig. 44–22)**. At this point pass the needle from the inside to the outside of the rectum and hold it temporarily in a hemostat.

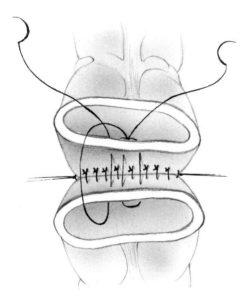

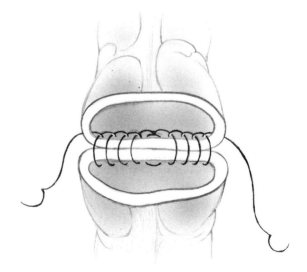

Fig. 44-21

Fig. 44-23

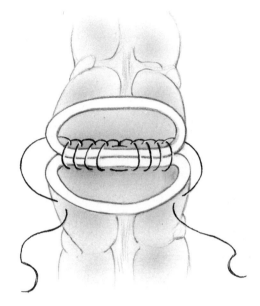

Fig. 44-24

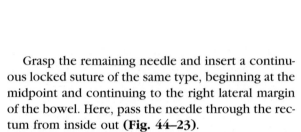

Fig. 44-26

Grasp the remaining needle and insert a continuous locked suture of the same type, beginning at the midpoint and continuing to the right lateral margin of the bowel. Here, pass the needle through the rectum from inside out **(Fig. 44–23)**.

Standing on the left side of the patient, use the needle on the right lateral aspect of the anastomosis to initiate the anterior mucosal layer. Insert continuous sutures of either the Cushing or Connell type

to a point just beyond the middle of the anterior layer. Then grasp the needle emerging from the left lateral margin of the incision and insert a similar continuous Connell or Cushing stitch. Complete the anterior mucosal layer by tying the suture to its mate and cutting the tails of these sutures **(Fig. 44–24, 44–25)**.

Complete the anterior seromuscular layer by inserting interrupted 4-0 silk atraumatic Lembert sutures **(Fig. 44–26)**. Now carefully rotate the anastomosis to inspect the integrity of the posterior layer. Test the diameter of the lumen before closing

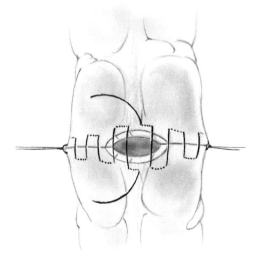

Fig. 44-25

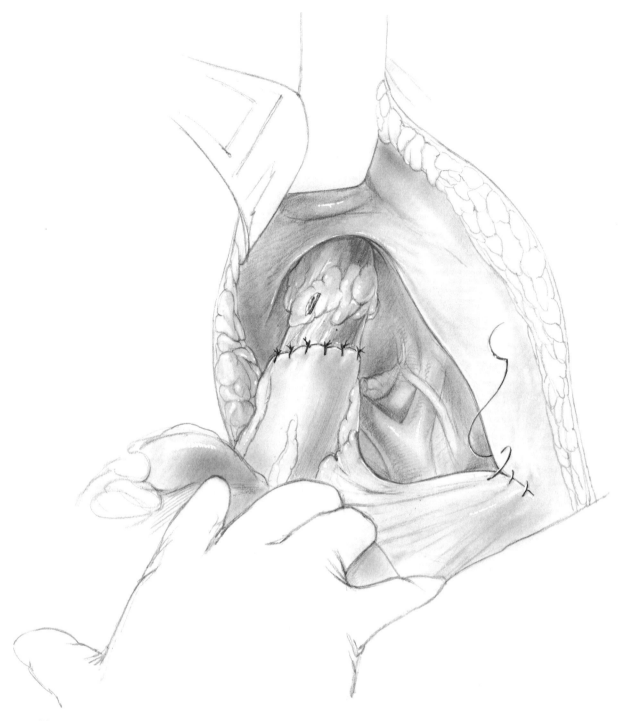

Fig. 44-27

the mesentery by invaginating the colon through the lumen gently with the thumb and forefinger. Then close the mesentery with continuous 2-0 PG sutures **(Fig. 44–27)**. Leave the peritoneal defect in the left paracolic gutter unsutured.

Stapled Colorectal Anastomosis

To construct a stapled colorectal anastomosis, first close the proximal descending colon with a 55/3.5 mm linear stapling device **(Fig. 44–28)**. Apply an

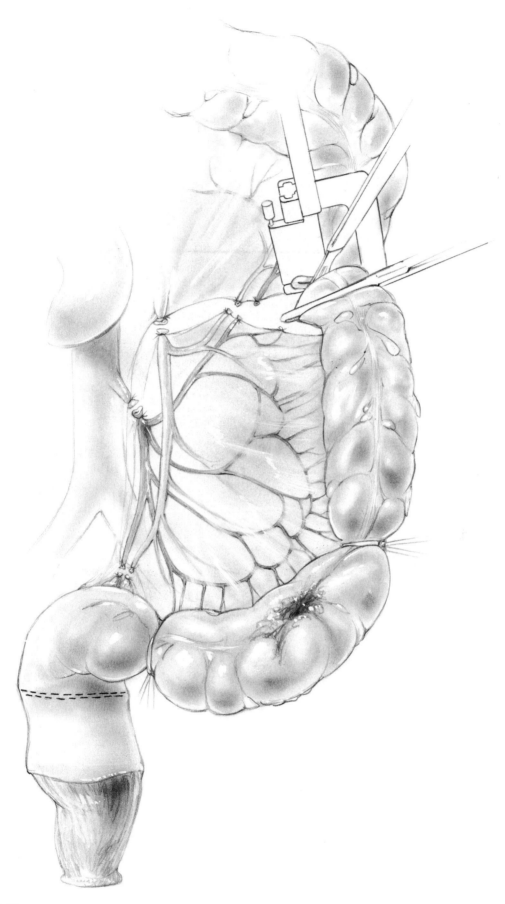

Fig. 44-28

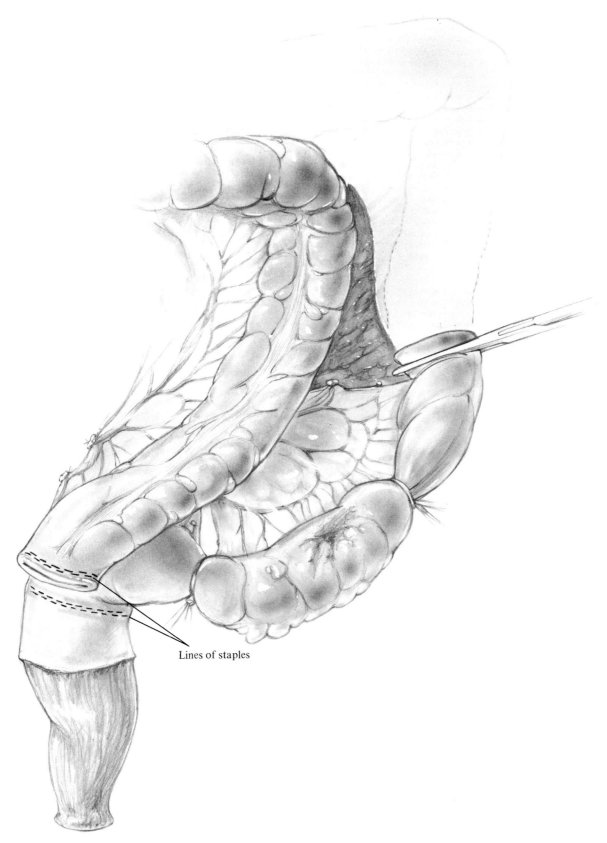

Lines of staples

Fig. 44-29

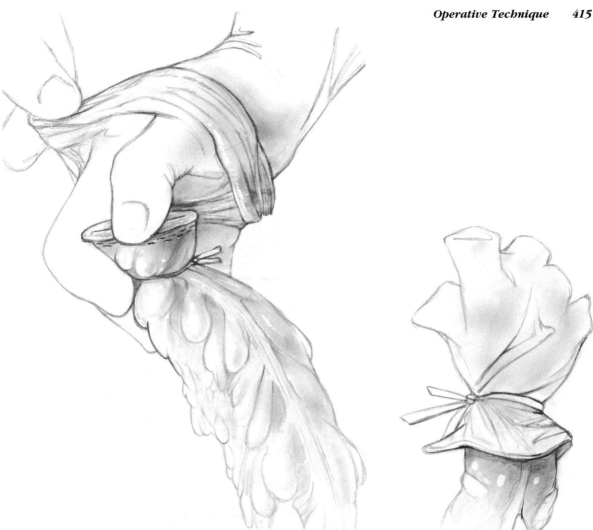

Fig. 44-30

Fig. 44-31

Allen clamp to the specimen side and divide the colon flush with the stapler. Remove the stapler **(Fig. 44–29)** and replace the Allen clamp with an umbilical tape ligature covered with a sterile rubber glove **(Figs. 44–30, 44–31)**. Alternatively, divide the colon with a cutting linear stapler. Then direct attention to the rectum, a segment of which was previously cleared of surrounding fat and vascular tissue. Use the 55/3.5 mm linear stapling device (Fig. 44-28) to apply a layer of staples to this segment of rectum. Do not remove the specimen; retain it so mild upward traction on it can stabilize the rectum during application of the stapling device (Fig. 44-29).

Make a stab wound on the antimesenteric border of the proximal colon at a point 5-6 cm proximal to the staple line. A scalpel blade or electrocautery may be used to make this incision. Make a second stab wound in the anterior wall of the rectal stump at a point 1 cm distal to the staple line already in place **(Fig. 44–32)**. Approximate the two stab

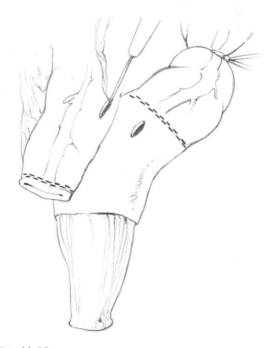

Fig. 44-32

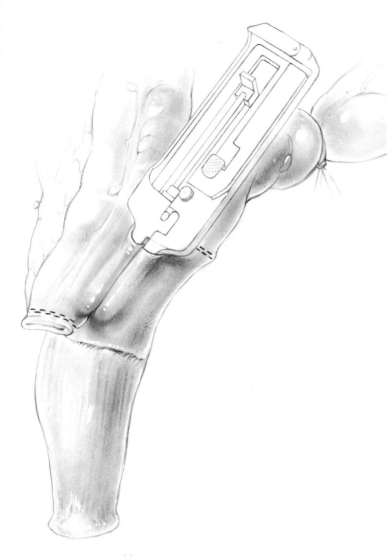

Fig. 44-33

wounds opposite each other, placing the proximal colonic segment anterior to the rectal stump. Insert the linear cutting stapling device, with one fork in the rectal stump and the other in the proximal colonic segment **(Fig. 44–33)**. Allis clamps or guy sutures may be used to approximate the rectum and colon in the crotch of the stapler. Fire and remove the stapler; then carefully inspect the staple line for any defects or bleeding. Close the remaining defect with a continuous inverting 4-0 PG atraumatic su-

ture to the mucosa. Reinforce this closure with a layer of interrupted 4-0 silk atraumatic seromuscular Lembert sutures **(Fig. 44–34)**. Carefully inspect all the staple lines to ascertain that the staples have closed properly into the shape of a B. Bleeding points may require careful electrocoagulation or fine suture ligatures. Transect the rectosigmoid just above the rectal staple line (Fig. 44–34) and remove the specimen.

Stapled Colocolonic Functional End-to-End Anastomosis: Chassin's Method

When the lumen of one segment of bowel to be anastomosed is *much* smaller than the other, as in many ileocolonic anastomoses, the stapling technique illustrated in Figures 43-21 and 43-23 is the simplest method. When a stapled anastomosis is constructed distal to the sacral promontory, the circular stapling technique (see Chapter 45) is preferred. However, for all other intraperitoneal anastomoses of small and large bowel, we have developed a modification of the end-to-end anastomosis. This modification, described in the following steps, avoids the possibility that six rows of staples are superimposed, one on the other, as may happen with the Steichen method.

1. Align the two open ends of bowel to be anastomosed side by side with the antimesenteric borders of each in contact.
2. Insert the linear cutting stapling instrument, placing one fork in each lumen **(Fig. 44–35)**. Draw the mesenteric borders of the bowel in the direction opposite to the location of the stapler. Avoid bunching too much tissue in the crotch of the stapling device. Lock and fire the instrument.
3. After unlocking the stapling instrument, withdraw it from the bowel. Apply Allis clamps to the extremities of the GIA staple line **(Fig. 44–36, point A, shows the first extremity)**.
4. Place the 90 mm linear stapler in the proper position and fire it **(Fig. 44–37)**. Excise the redundant bowel with Mayo scissors and lightly electrocoagulate the everted mucosa.

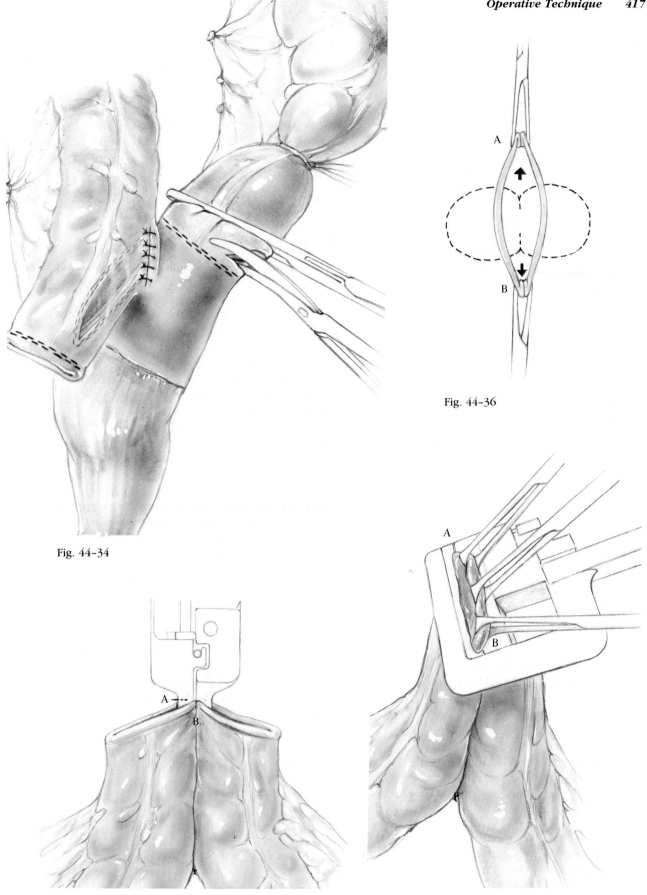

Fig. 44-34

Fig. 44-36

Fig. 44-35

Fig. 44-37

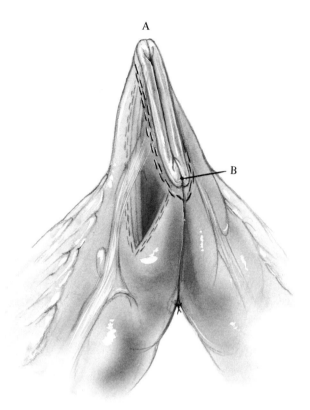

Fig. 44-38

5. Remove the linear stapler **(Fig. 44–38)** and carefully inspect the entire anastomosis for the proper B formation of staples.
6. Finally, insert a single 4-0 atraumatic silk seromuscular Lembert suture at the base of the anastomotic staple line (Fig. 44-38). This prevents any

undue distracting force from being exerted on the stapled anastomosis.

Closure

Discard all contaminated surgical gloves and instruments. Irrigate the abdomen. Most surgeons prefer to close the defect in the mesocolon (Fig. 44-27). A continuous suture of 2-0 PG is suitable for this purpose, although the defect is usually so large that omitting this step does not seem to lead to internal bowel herniation. Close the abdominal incision in routine fashion without placing any drains in the peritoneal cavity.

POSTOPERATIVE CARE

See Chapter 43.

COMPLICATIONS

See Chapter 43.

REFERENCES

Bergamaschi R, Arnaud JP. Intracorporeal colorectal anastomosis following laparoscopic left colon resection. Surg Endosc 1997;11:800.

Weiss EG, Wexner SD. Laparoscopic segmental colectomies, anterior resection, and abdominoperineal resection. In Scott-Conner CEH (ed) The SAGES Manual. Fundamentals of Laparoscopy and GI Endoscopy. New York, Springer-Verlag, 1999, pp 286-299.

45 Low Anterior Resection for Rectal Cancer

INDICATIONS

Low anterior resections are performed to treat malignant tumors of the middle and upper thirds of the rectum, 6-14 cm from the anal verge.

PREOPERATIVE PREPARATION

Mechanical and antibiotic bowel preparation

Computed tomography (CT) of abdomen and pelvis

Endorectal ultrasonography

Other staging studies as indicated

See Chapter 42

PITFALLS AND DANGER POINTS

Anastomotic failure

Presacral hemorrhage

Trauma to rectal stump during presacral dissection

Ureteral damage

OPERATIVE STRATEGY

Prevention of Anastomotic Complications

Anastomotic complications are rare when the resection is high and the anastomosis is intraperitoneal (see Chapter 44). Conversely, a low anterior resection with a colorectal anastomosis below the peritoneal reflection is clinically and radiographically much more prone to leak. The low colorectal anastomosis offers additional difficulty for several reasons.

1. *Anatomic exposure is often difficult.* This is especially true in men, whose pelvis is narrow, and obese patients. Difficulty with exposure often requires the surgeon's hand to be held at an awkward angle, so it is easy to make small tears in the rectum when inserting sutures.

2. *It is easy to mistake mucosa for the muscular layer* owing to the lack of serosal cover over the retroperitoneal rectum. If sutures or staples are erroneously inserted into the mucosal instead of the submucosal and muscular layers, the anastomosis will leak because the mucosa itself has little tensile strength. Identify the longitudinal muscle covering the rectum and be sure to incorporate this layer in the suture line.

3. *The diameter of the rectal ampulla frequently measures in excess of 5-6 cm*, and the lumen of the proximal colon, after proper bowel preparation, is often half this size. The anastomotic technique used must be capable of correcting this disparity.

4. When the surgeon has not achieved perfect hemostasis in the pelvis, *a hematoma forms in the presacral space*. It frequently becomes infected and develops into an abscess, which may erode through the colorectal suture line.

5. If the pelvic peritoneal floor is closed above the colorectal anastomosis, deadspace may surround the anastomosis, which is especially conducive to leakage in the anastomosis. The peritoneal pelvic floor is not resutured after the colorectal anastomosis is completed.

6. Do not leave any empty space in the hollow of the sacrum behind a low anastomosis. For most low anterior resections, we free the attachments of the splenic flexure (see Figs. 44-4 to 44-8) so the descending colon has sufficient redundancy that relaxed colon fills the sacral space behind the anastomosis. If this step cannot be accomplished, fill the empty space in the pelvis by lengthening the omentum sufficiently that it can be delivered to the presacral space.

7. We have virtually eliminated leakage by adopting the side-to-end (Baker) colorectal anastomosis. This permits the diameter of the anastomosis to be exactly equal to that of the lumen of the commodious rectal ampulla. Healthy-sized bites of tissue may be enclosed in the sutures with no dan-

ger of postoperative stenosis. In effect, at the conclusion of the anastomosis, *the rectal ampulla has been invaginated into the side of the proximal colon* (see Fig. 45-23). Placing the anastomosis within 1 cm of the closed end of the proximal colon eliminates the danger of developing a blind-loop syndrome.

8. Following a low anastomosis we routinely insert a closed suction drain into the presacral space, bringing it out through a puncture wound in the left lower quadrant.

9. Although the use of staples for low colorectal anastomoses has been demonstrated to be safe by numerous studies, it is important to observe all the precautions described below to ensure uneventful healing.

Which Colorectal Anastomosis: Sutured, Circular Stapled, or Double Stapled?

Sutured colorectal anastomoses, described below, have been demonstrated to be safe when performed with delicacy of technique by a skilled surgeon on well dissected healthy tissues. Lesions 9–10 cm from the anal verge can generally be removed and a sutured colorectal anastomosis performed. However, when the surgeon resects lesions lower than 10 cm from the anal verge, suturing the colorectal anastomosis can be difficult. Insertion of the circular stapler into the rectum allows construction of a safe colorectal stapled anastomosis with greater ease for the surgeon than is true for the sutured anastomosis.

If the cancer resection has left a rectal stump situated so low in the pelvis that even insertion of the purse-string suture becomes difficult (lesions at 6–8 cm), use the Roticulator 55 mm linear stapler (U.S. Surgical Corp.) to close the proximal edge of the rectal stump rather than a purse-string suture. Passing the circular stapler into the rectum then permits construction of a circular colorectal anastomosis through the linear staple line closing the proximal edge of the rectal stump. This method is especially suitable for the lowest colorectal anastomoses.

Extent of Lymphovascular Dissection

Goligher (1975) advocated routine ligation of the inferior mesenteric artery at the aorta not only for lesions of the descending colon but also for rectal cancer. When this is done, the entire blood supply of the proximal colon must come through the marginal artery all the way from the middle colic artery (**Fig. 45–1**). Although this proves adequate in most patients, there is a danger that the surgeon may not recognize those patients whose blood supply is not sufficient. We believe the risk of this occurring is greater than the benefits that may accrue to the patient by routinely amputating the extra 3 cm of inferior mesenteric artery. It is important that the blood supply to the proximal colon undergoing anastomosis not only be adequate but be optimal before this segment is used in a low colorectal anastomosis. Consequently, in the usual case of rectal cancer we transect the inferior mesenteric artery just distal

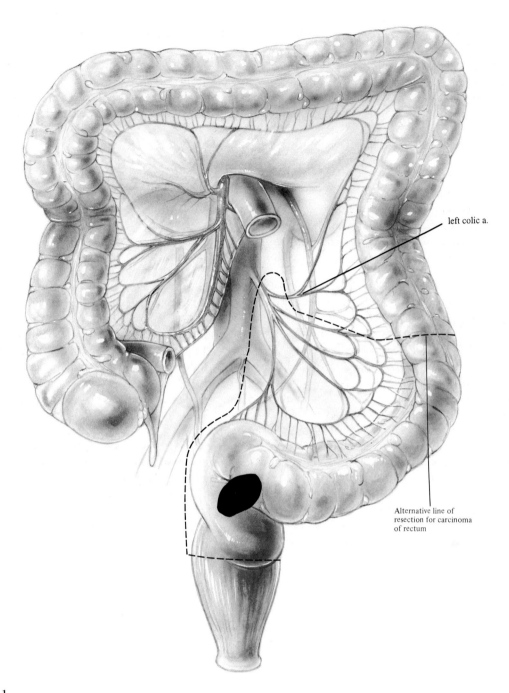

left colic a.

Alternative line of
resection for carcinoma
of rectum

Fig. 45-1

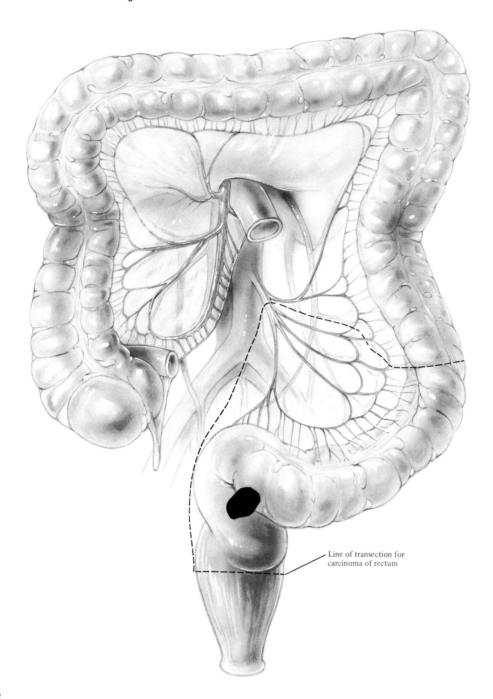

Fig. 45-2

to the origin of the left colic vessel **(Fig. 45–2)**. Even if only the ascending branch of the left colic artery is preserved, there usually is vigorous arterial pulsation in the mesentery of the descending colon. For obese patients, transillumination of the mesentery is helpful for identifying the junction between the inferior mesenteric and left colic arteries.

If the inferior mesenteric artery is ligated proximal to the takeoff of the left colic artery, be sure always to liberate the splenic flexure and resect most of the descending colon unless it can be proven that the circulation through the marginal artery at a lower level is vigorous. This can be accomplished only by demonstrating pulsatile flow from a cut arterial branch at the proposed site of the transection of the colon. *Poor blood flow leads to poor healing*.

In the usual rectal cancer case the sigmoid colon is removed and the descending colon is used for anastomosis. This generally requires liberation of the splenic flexure, which can be accomplished in a few minutes once the surgeon has mastered the technique.

Indications for Complementary Colostomy or Loop Ileostomy

When there is difficulty constructing a low colorectal anastomosis and it is likely the surgeon has created a less-than-perfect anastomosis, a complementary diverting right transverse loop colostomy or loop ileostomy should be constructed. It may be closed as early as 2 weeks after the low anterior resection if a barium enema shows a normal anastomosis.

Presacral Dissection: Prevention of Hemorrhage

Contrary to what apparently is a widely held perception, radical cancer surgery does not require stripping the tissues from the sacrum down to the periosteum. Dissection of the perirectal tissues proximal to the carcinoma is necessary for removal of *tumor emboli* in the lymph nodes and lymphatic channels. If tumor has widely invaded the mesorectum and presacral tissues, it is generally beyond cure by radical surgery.

There is a network of veins lying on the presacral periosteum that drain into the sacral foramina (see Fig. 45-8b). When these veins are torn by blunt dissection, clamping or ligation to control the hemorrhage that results often is impossible, as the torn vessel retracts into the foramen. The massive venous hemorrhage that follows may not be stemmed by ligating the hypogastric arteries. Most intraoperative fatalities during total proctectomy are caused by this type of presacral venous hemorrhage.

Nivatvongs and Fang (1986) described a method for controlling massive hemorrhage from a torn presacral branch of the basivertebral vein. Because the blood pours out of one of the sacral foramina, they proposed occluding the foramen with a titanium thumbtack (Hemorrhage Occluder Pin; Surgin, Placentia, CA, USA), that is left permanently in place. To accomplish this step effectively, first demonstrate that the blood is emerging from a single foramen. If the bleeding is controlled by applying the fingertip to one foramen, applying the thumbtack will be effective. In some cases stuffing some cottonoid Oxycel (oxidized cellulose) into the foramen before inserting the thumbtack may be helpful.

If the surgeon cannot *quickly* control lacerated presacral veins with a stitch, a thumbtack, or bone wax, the bleeding area should be covered with a sheet of Surgicel over which a large gauze pack is placed, filling the sacral hollow. This practice almost always controls the hemorrhage.

Unless the presacral vessels are directly invaded by a bulky tumor of the mid-rectum, massive pre-sacral venous hemorrhage is entirely preventable. Blunt hand dissection of the presacral space is not a desirable technique. The surgeon's hand does not belong in this area until scissors or electrocautery dissection under direct vision has freed all the perirectal tissues from any posterior attachments to the sacrum. This should be done with long Metzenbaum scissors combined with gentle upward traction on the rectum. As the scissors are inserted on each side of the midline, the perirectal tissues can easily be lifted in an anterior direction *without removing the thin layer of endopelvic fascia that covers the presacral veins*. When the presacral dissection stays in the proper plane, the presacral veins are hidden from view by this layer of fascia (see Fig. 45-8a). Occasionally, branches of the middle sacral vessels enter the perirectal tissues from behind and can be divided by electrocautery.

This dissection is easily continued down to the area of the coccyx, where the fascia of Waldeyer becomes somewhat dense as it goes from the anterior surfaces of the coccyx and sacrum to attach to the lower rectum (see Fig. 45-10). Attempts to penetrate this fascia by blunt finger dissection may rupture the rectum rather than the fascia, which is strong. This layer must be incised sharply with scissors or a scalpel, after which one can see the levator diaphragm. When the posterior dissection has for the most part been completed, only *then* should the surgeon's hand enter the presacral space to sweep the dissection toward the lateral pelvic walls. This maneuver helps define the lateral ligaments. The dissection should be bloodless.

Other points of hemorrhage in the pelvic dissection may occur on the lateral walls. They can usually be readily identified and occluded by ligature. Pay close attention also to the left iliac vein, which may be injured during the course of the dissection. As most serious bleeding during pelvic dissections is of venous origin, ligation of the hypogastric arteries is rarely indicated.

Presacral Dissection: Preservation of Hypogastric Nerves

As the rectum is elevated from the presacral space and the anterior surface of the aorta cleared of areolar and lymphovascular tissue, a varying number of preaortic sympathetic nerves of the superior hypogastric plexus can be identified. They are the contribution of the sympathetic nervous system to the bilateral inferior hypogastric (pelvic) plexuses. In male patients their preservation is necessary for normal ejaculation. After they cross the region of the aortic bifurcation and sacral promontory, they coalesce into two major nerve bundles, called the hypogastric nerves. Each nerve, which may have one to three strands, runs toward the posterolateral wall of the pelvis in the vicinity of the hypogastric artery (see Figs. 45-4, 45-6). With most malignancies of the distal rectum these nerves can be preserved without compromising the patient's chances of cure.

After the inferior mesenteric artery and vein are divided and the lymphovascular tissues are elevated from the bifurcation of the aorta by blunt dissection, the sympathetic nerves remain closely attached to the aorta and need not be damaged if the dissection is performed gently. At the promontory of the sacrum, if the rectum is dissected as described above, the right and left hypogastric nerves can be seen posterior to the plane of dissection and can be preserved provided there is sufficient distance separating them from the tumor. There also seems to be diminution in the incidence of bladder dysfunction after nerve preservation.

Ureteral Dissection

To prevent damage to the ureters, these delicate structures must be identified and traced well down into the pelvis. The normal ureter crosses the common iliac artery, at which point this structure bifurcates into its external and internal branches. Because the ureter and a leaf of incised peritoneum are often displaced during the course of dissection, if the ureter is not located in its usual position the undersurfaces of both the lateral and medial leaves of peritoneum should be inspected. The identity of the ureter can be confirmed if pinching or touching the structure with forceps results in typical peristaltic waves. If doubt exists, the anesthesiologist may be instructed to inject indigo carmine dye intravenously, which strains the ureter blue unless the patient is oliguric at the time of injection. The ureter should be traced into the pelvis beyond the point at which the lateral ligaments of the rectum are divided.

OPERATIVE TECHNIQUE

Incision and Position

Patients who have lesions within 14 cm of the anal verge should be placed in the same modified lithotomy position utilizing Lloyd-Davies or Allen leg rests, as described in Chapter 46 for abdominoperineal proctectomy **(Figs. 45–3a, 45–3b)**. The second assistant stands between the patient's abducted thighs for the pelvic portion of the operation, and the surgeon works from the patient's left. In this position the surgeon may judge, after the tumor is mobilized, whether an anterior anastomosis, abdominoperineal proctectomy, or end-to-end anastomosis with the EEA stapling device is suitable. These techniques are best done with the patient in this position. A midline incision, extending from a point about 6 cm below the xiphoid process down to the pubis, is used.

Exploration and Evisceration of Small Bowel

Palpate and inspect the liver. A moderate amount of metastasis is not a contraindication to a conservative version of the anterior resection. Explore the remainder of the abdomen and then eviscerate the small bowel into a plastic intestinal bag or moist gauze pads.

Mobilization of Sigmoid

Expose the left lateral peritoneal gutter. Occlude the lumen of the colon by ligating the distal sigmoid with umbilical tape. Draw the sigmoid colon medially to

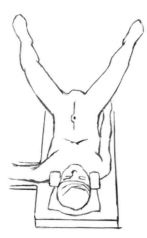

Fig. 45-3a

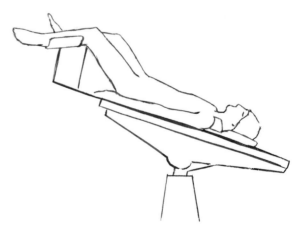

Fig. 45-3b

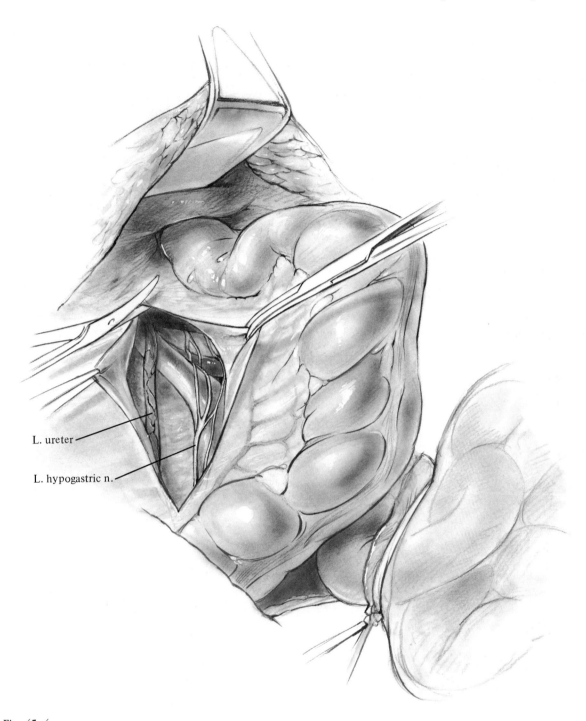

L. ureter

L. hypogastric n.

Fig. 45-4

expose and divide several congenital attachments between the mesocolon and the posterolateral parietal peritoneum with scissors **(Fig. 45–4)**. Extend the incision in the peritoneum cephalad as far as the splenic flexure.

Identify the left ureter and tag it with a Silastic loop for later identification. Use scissors to continue the peritoneal incision along the left side of the rec-

tum down to the rectovesical pouch. Identify the course of the ureter well down into the pelvis. Now retract the sigmoid to the patient's left and make an incision on the right side of the sigmoid mesocolon. The incision should begin at a point overlying the bifurcation of the aorta and should continue in a caudal direction along the line where the mesosigmoid meets the right lateral leaf of peritoneum in the pre-

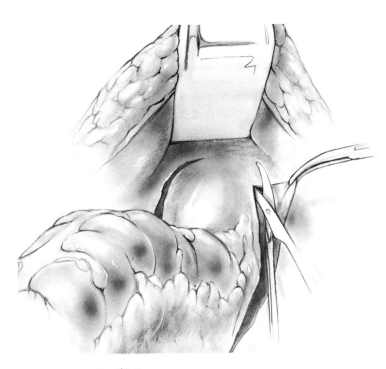

Fig. 45-5

sacral space. After the right ureter has been identified, carry the incision down toward the rectovesical pouch **(Figs. 45–5, 45–6)**.

If the exposure is convenient, incise the peritoneum of the rectovesical pouch, or the rectouterine pouch in female patients (Fig. 45-5). If the exposure is not convenient, delay this step until the presacral dissection has elevated the rectum sufficiently to bring the rectovesical pouch easily to the field of vision.

Lymphovascular Dissection

Apply skyward traction to the colon and gently separate the gonadal vein from the lateral leaf of the mesocolon, allowing it to fall posteriorly. Insert an index finger between the deep margin of the mesosigmoid and the bifurcation of the aorta to feel the pulsation of the inferior mesenteric artery lying superficial to the finger. In markedly obese patients this vessel may be divided and ligated at the level of

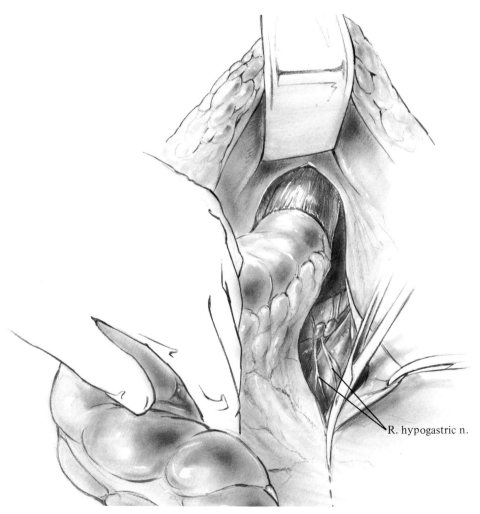

R. hypogastric n.

Fig. 45-6

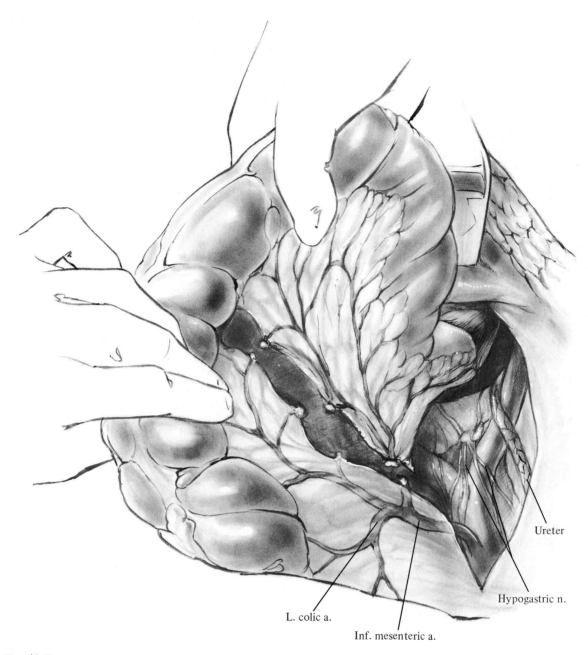

Ureter

Hypogastric n.

L. colic a.

Inf. mesenteric a.

Fig. 45-7

the aortic bifurcation without further dissection. In most patients, however, it is simple to incise the peritoneum overlying the origin of the inferior mesenteric artery and to sweep the areolar and lymphatic tissue downward until one sees the point at which the inferior mesenteric artery gives off the left colic branch **(Fig. 45–7)**. In routine cases divide the inferior mesenteric vessels between 2-0 ligatures just distal to this junction. Then make a superficial scalpel incision along the surface of the mesocolon: Begin at the point where the inferior mesenteric vessels were divided and continue to the descending colon or upper sigmoid. Complete the division of the mesentery along this line by dividing it between serially applied Kelly hemostats and then ligating with 2-0 silk or PG (Fig. 45-7). In nonobese patients it is feasible to incise the peritoneum up to the point where a vessel is visualized and then apply hemostats directly to each vessel as it is encountered. With this technique, the surgeon encounters only one or two vessels on the way to the marginal artery of the colon.

Sweep the mesosigmoid and the lymphovascular bundle distal to the ligated inferior mesenteric ves-

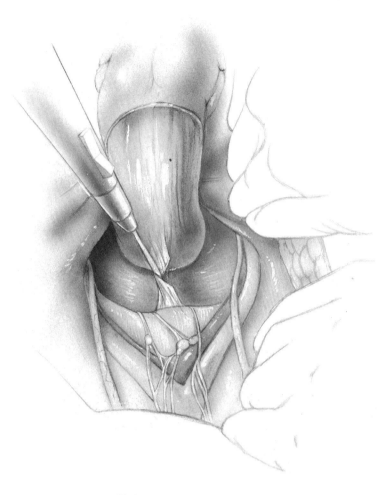

Fig. 45-8a

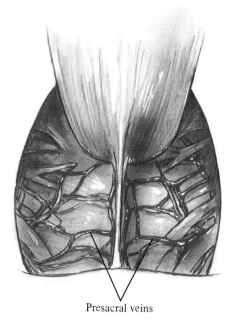

Presacral veins

Fig. 45-8b

sels off the anterior surfaces of the aorta and common iliac vessels by blunt dissection. Leave the preaortic sympathetic nerves intact. To minimize the time during which the patient's abdomen is exposed to possible fecal contamination, do not divide the descending colon at this stage.

Presacral Dissection

With the lower sigmoid on steady upward retraction, it becomes evident that there is a band of tissue extending from the midsacral region to the posterior rectum and mesorectum. On either side of this dense band there is only areolar tissue. Stoutly resist any tendency to insert a hand into the presacral space. Instead, use long, closed Metzenbaum scissors as a blunt dissector **(Fig. 45–8a)**. Insert it first to the right of the midline behind the rectum; by gently elevating the mesorectum the proper presacral plane is then entered. Repeat this maneuver identically on the left side of the midsacral line. Then direct attention to the remaining band of tissue, which contains branches of the middle sacral artery, and divide it with the electrocautery (Fig. 45-8a).

At this time the surgeon sees a thin layer of fibroareolar tissue covering the sacrum. If a shiny layer of sacral periosteum, ligaments, or the naked presacral veins can be seen **(Fig. 45–8b)**, the plane of dissection is *too deep*, presenting a danger of major venous hemorrhage. Elevate the *distal* rectum from the lower sacrum with gauze in a spongeholder. If the dissection has been completed properly, as described, note that the preaortic sympathetic nerves divide into two major trunks in the upper sacral area and then continue laterally to the right and left walls of the pelvis (see Figs. 45-4, 45-6). Gently dissect these nerves from the posterior wall of the specimen unless the nerves have been invaded by tumor.

Now insert a hand into the presacral space, with the objective not of penetrating more deeply toward the coccyx but, rather, of extending the presacral dissection laterally to the right and to the left, so the posterior aspect of the specimen is elevated from the sacrum as far as the lateral ligaments on each side. Place the lateral ligament on the left side on stretch by applying traction to the rectum toward the right. Place a right-angle Mixter clamp underneath the lateral ligament and divide the tissue with electrocautery **(Fig. 45–9)**.

Carry out a similar maneuver to divide the right lateral ligament. Before dividing each lateral ligament, recheck the position of the respective ureter and hypogastric nerve to be certain they lie away from the point of division. Then divide the fascia of

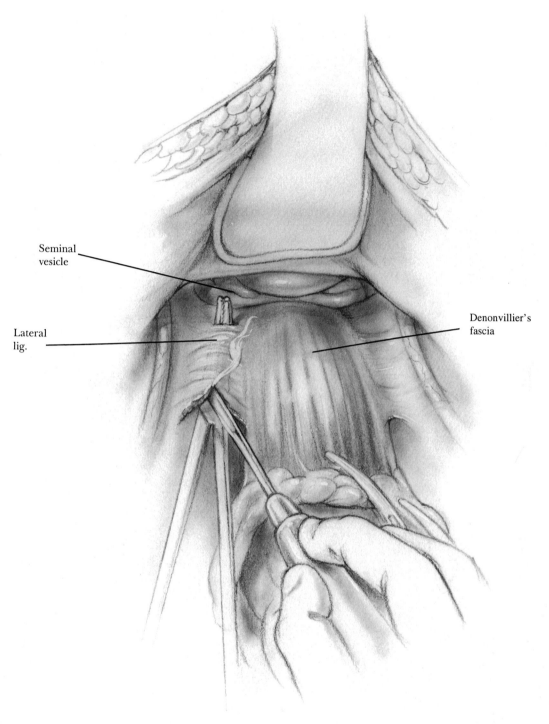

Seminal vesicle

Lateral lig.

Denonvillier's fascia

Fig. 45-9

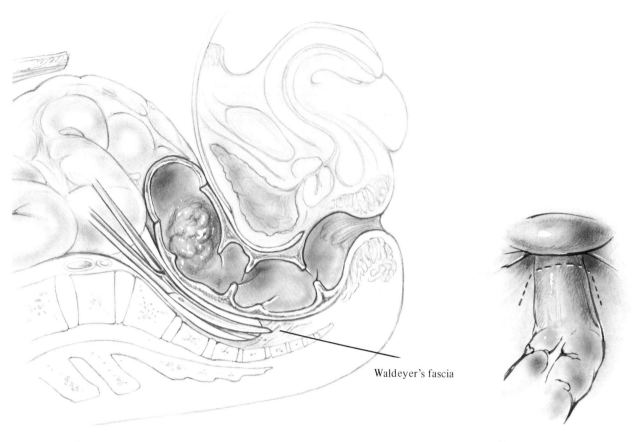

Fig. 45-10

Fig. 45-11a

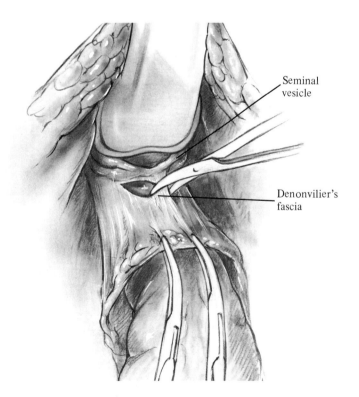

Fig. 45-11b

Seminal vesicle

Denonvilier's fascia

Waldeyer, which extends from the coccyx to the posterior rectal wall **(Fig. 45–10)**.

Now direct attention to the anterior dissection. Use a Lloyd-Davies bladder retractor to pull the bladder (in women, the uterus) in an anterior and caudal direction. If the peritoneum of the rectovesical pouch has not already been incised, perform this maneuver now, thereby connecting the incisions in the pelvic peritoneum previously made on the right and left sides of the rectum **(Fig. 45–11a)**. Apply one or more long hemostats or forceps to the posterior lip of the incised peritoneum of the rectovesical pouch. Place traction on these hemostats to draw the peritoneum and Denonvilliers' fascia in a cephalad and posterior direction, and use Metzenbaum scissors dissection to separate the rectum from the seminal vesicles and prostate **(Fig. 45–11b)**. Use blunt finger dissection to further separate the rectum from the posterior wall of the prostate. Finally, secure hemostasis in this region by cauterizing multiple bleeding points.

In female patients the anterior dissection is somewhat simpler. With a Harrington retractor elevating the uterus, use scalpel dissection to initiate the plane of dissection separating the peritoneum and fascia of Denonvilliers from the posterior lip of the cervix until the proximal vagina has been exposed. Some surgeons routinely perform bilateral salpingo-oophorectomy in women who have rectal and sigmoid cancer because the ovaries are sometimes a site of metastatic deposit. Whether this step is of value has not been ascertained. We do not perform this maneuver in the absence of visible metastasis to the ovaries.

Pelvic Hemostasis

The entire pelvic dissection, if properly performed, entails minimal blood loss. Although hemostatic clips may control clearly identified vessels along the lateral wall of the pelvis, they are not useful in the presacral area. Here the vessels consist of thin-walled veins, which are easily torn by metallic clips at the time of application or during the act of sponging the area later.

Except in the case of a small, clearly defined bleeding point that can be held in a forceps, electrocautery may also be hazardous, as the coagulating tip may act as a scalpel and convert the bleeding point to a major venous laceration. Here a ball-tipped electrode is safer than one with a blade or pointed tip.

See the discussion above, under Operative Strategy, concerning the use of a thumbtack to control massive presacral bleeding localized to a single foramen. Almost invariably, presacral bleeding results from a tear in one or more of the veins that drain into a sacral foramen. When hemorrhage occurs, the area of bleeding should be covered by a sheet of topical hemostatic agent over which pressure is applied with a large gauze pack. Place omentum between the pack and the anastomosis. If the area of bleeding is only 1–2 cm in diameter, removing the gauze pack may be attempted at a later stage in the operation, leaving a small patch of hemostatic agent. Unless this maneuver produces complete hemostasis, replace the gauze pack in the presacral space and leave it there for 24–48 hours. Then remove it by relaparotomy under general anesthesia.

Mobilization of Proximal Colon

If the previously selected point on the descending colon does not easily reach down into the pelvis, mobilize the remainder of the descending colon by incising first the peritoneum in the paracolic gutter and then the "renocolic" ligament. Liberate the en-

tire splenic flexure according to the steps described in Chapter 44. Considerable additional length may be obtained by dividing the transverse branch of the left colic artery (Fig. 45-1). Completely clear the fat and mesentery from a 1 cm width of serosa at the point selected for dividing the descending colon.

Preparation of Rectal Stump

When the rectum is divided at a low level, the mesorectum is no longer a single pedicle traveling along the posterior surface of the rectum. Rather, it fans out into multiple branches. Select a point 4–5 cm distal to the lower border of the tumor and seek the plane between the muscularis of the rectum and the surrounding blood vessels. This plane can sometimes be palpated with the finger; and at other times a large blunt-nosed hemostat can be insinuated into it. In most patients this vascular layer can be divided by electrocoagulation after passing a right-angle clamp between the vasculature and the rectal wall.

Well delineated longitudinal muscle fibers should now be visible all around the lower rectum at the site selected for the anastomosis. At this time place a large right-angle clamp across the entire lumen of the rectum below the tumor.

Irrigation of Rectal Stump

If there is any question as to the adequacy of the bowel preparation, insert a Foley catheter with a 5 ml bag into the rectum. Attach the catheter to plastic tubing to permit the intermittent inflow and drainage of 500 ml of sterile water. This not only removes retained fecal matter but lyses any shed tumor cells. After the irrigation is completed and the rectum is emptied, remove the catheter and apply a large right-angle clamp distal to the tumor to occlude the rectal lumen.

Selection of Anastomotic Technique

Use the side-to-end suture technique for a low colorectal anastomosis at or just below the peritoneal reflection. Alternatively, a circular stapling device may be used. At higher levels, the techniques described in Chapter 44 are also suitable. See also the discussion under Operative Strategy, above.

Side-to-End Low Colorectal Anastomosis (Baker)

Turn to the previously cleared area on the descending colon that is to be used for the anastomosis. Apply a 55/3.5 mm linear stapler across this cleared area and fire the staples **(Fig. 45–12)**. Place an Allen clamp 1 cm distal to the stapler to occlude the specimen side. Divide the colon flush with the stapling device using a scalpel and lightly cauterize the everted mucosa **(Fig. 45–13)**. Ligate the specimen side with umbilical tape. After the Allen clamp is removed, apply a sterile rubber glove over the ligated end and tie the glove in place with another umbilical tape ligature **(Figs. 45–14a, 45–14b)**. Alter-

natively, divide the colon with a linear cutting stapler. Retain this segment of colon containing the specimen temporarily to provide traction on the rectal stump.

Bring the stapled end of the proximal colon down into the pelvis and line it up tentatively with the rectal stump 4–5 cm beyond the tumor. Place a scratch mark along the antimesenteric border of the descending colon beginning at a point 1 cm proximal

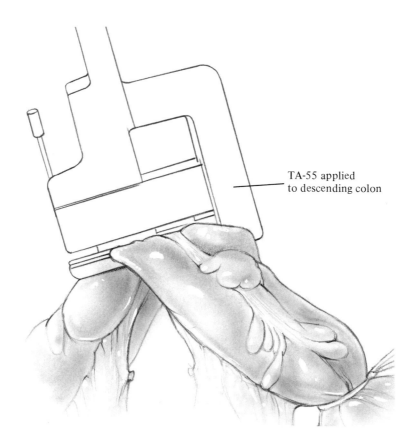

TA-55 applied
to descending colon

Fig. 45-12

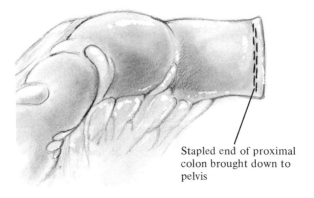

Stapled end of proximal
colon brought down to
pelvis

Fig. 45-13

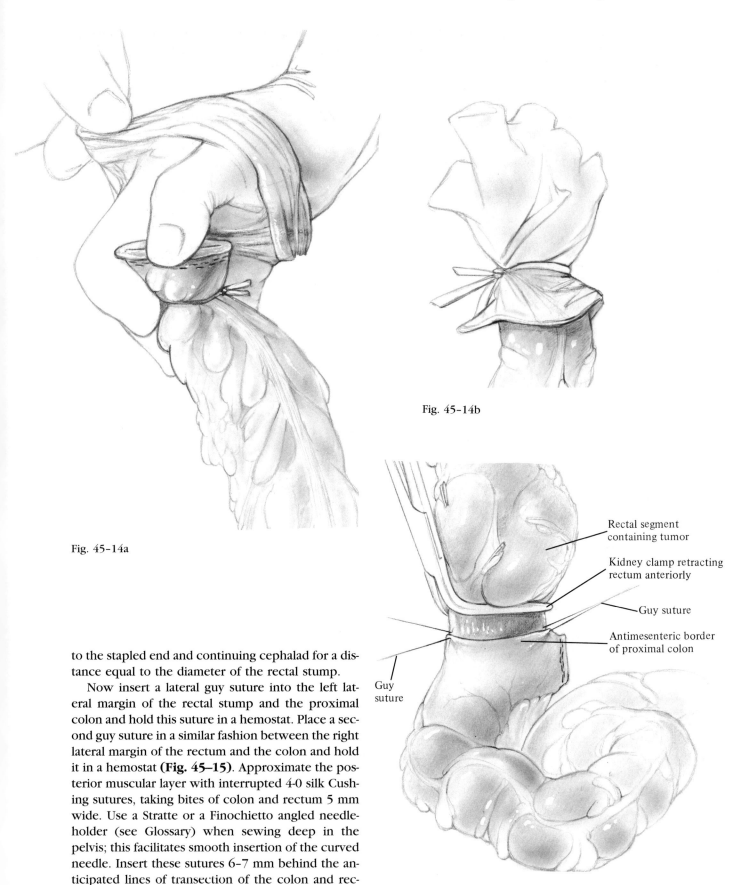

Fig. 45-14b

Fig. 45-14a

Fig. 45-15

Rectal segment
containing tumor

Kidney clamp retracting
rectum anteriorly

Guy suture

Antimesenteric border
of proximal colon

Guy
suture

to the stapled end and continuing cephalad for a distance equal to the diameter of the rectal stump.

Now insert a lateral guy suture into the left lateral margin of the rectal stump and the proximal colon and hold this suture in a hemostat. Place a second guy suture in a similar fashion between the right lateral margin of the rectum and the colon and hold it in a hemostat **(Fig. 45–15)**. Approximate the posterior muscular layer with interrupted 4-0 silk Cushing sutures, taking bites of colon and rectum 5 mm wide. Use a Stratte or a Finochietto angled needleholder (see Glossary) when sewing deep in the pelvis; this facilitates smooth insertion of the curved needle. Insert these sutures 6-7 mm behind the anticipated lines of transection of the colon and rectum. The preferred technique is successive bisection

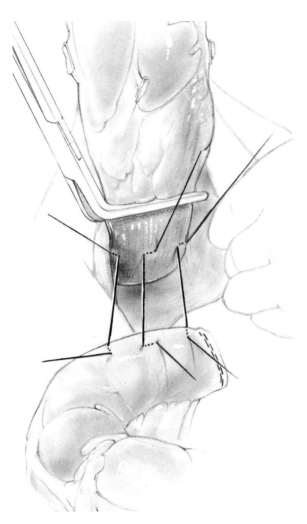

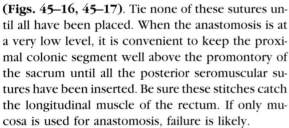

Fig. 45-16

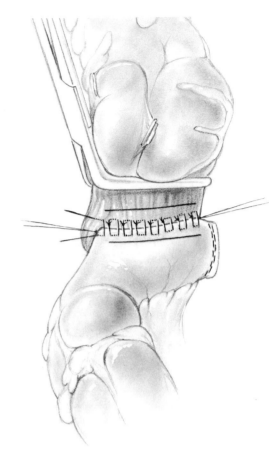

Fig. 45-17

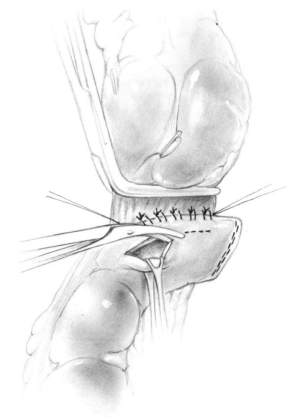

Fig. 45-18

(Figs. 45–16, 45–17). Tie none of these sutures until all have been placed. When the anastomosis is at a very low level, it is convenient to keep the proximal colonic segment well above the promontory of the sacrum until all the posterior seromuscular sutures have been inserted. Be sure these stitches catch the longitudinal muscle of the rectum. If only mucosa is used for anastomosis, failure is likely.

Incise the previous scratch mark in the proximal colonic segment with a scalpel and Metzenbaum scissors **(Fig. 45–18)**. Make a similar incision along a line 6-7 mm proximal to the sutures already placed in the rectum.

If exposure is difficult, it is sometimes helpful to maintain gentle traction on the tails of the Cushing sutures to improve exposure while suturing the mucosa. Then cut the tails of the Cushing sutures successively as the mucosal sutures are inserted. Otherwise, cut all the Cushing sutures at one time,

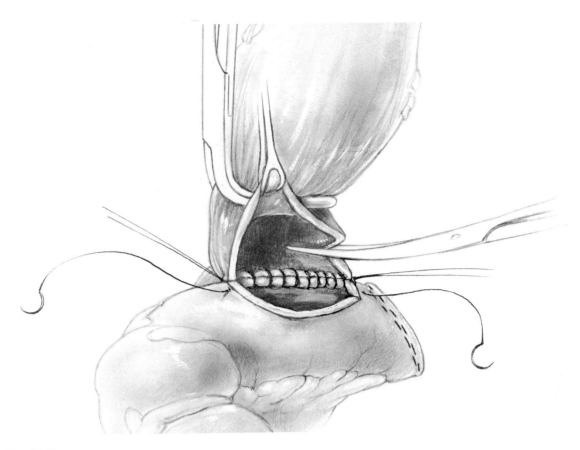

Fig. 45-19

except for the two lateral guy sutures, which should be retained for the moment.

Begin the posterior mucosal closure at the midpoint of the posterior layer using an atraumatic suture of 3-0 PG. Start a continuous locked suture at the midpoint and continue it to the right lateral margin. The second suture of the same material should progress from the midpoint toward the left lateral margin of the suture line **(Fig. 45–19)**.

Divide the anterior wall of the rectum below the large right-angle clamp and remove the specimen. Request an immediate frozen section histologic examination of the distal margin of the specimen to rule out the presence of cancer. If tumor cells are found at the margin, resection of additional rectum is indicated.

Now approximate the anterior mucosal layer by a continuous suture of the Connell or Cushing type **(Fig. 45–20)**. Accomplish this by grasping the needle, which has completed the posterior mucosal layer and is now in the lumen at the right margin of the anastomosis, and passing it from inside out through the rectum. The suture line should progress from the right lateral margin toward the midpoint of

the anterior layer. When this has been reached, grasp the second needle, located at the left lateral margin of the posterior mucosal layer. Use this needle to complete the anterior mucosal layer from the left lat-

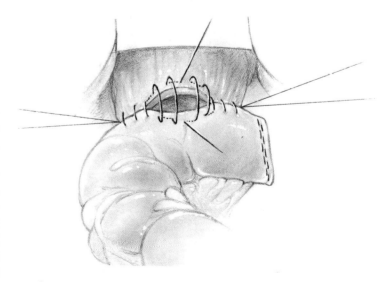

Fig. 45-20

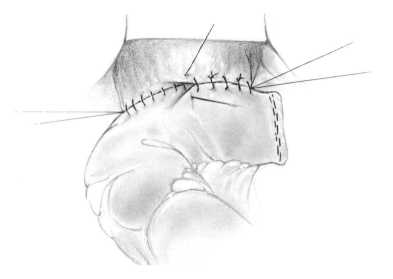

Fig. 45-21

eral margin to the midpoint where the anterior mucosal layer is terminated with the mucosa completely inverted (Fig. 45-20).

Close the anterior muscular layer with interrupted 4-0 atraumatic silk Lembert or Cushing sutures **(Figs. 45–21, 45–22)**. Insert this row of sutures about 6 mm away from the mucosal suture line to accomplish a certain amount of invagination of the rectum into the colon. Because the dimension of the side-to-end lumen is large narrowing does not result. A sagittal section of the anastomosis in **Figure 45–23** illustrates this point. After the anasto-

mosis is completed, carefully inspect the posterior suture line for possible defects, which if present can be corrected by additional sutures.

At this point cut the sutures and thoroughly irrigate the pelvis with a dilute solution of antibiotics. The large defect in the peritoneum need not be closed. This omission has brought no noticeable ill effect, probably because the defect is so large as not to entrap any small intestine permanently.

Make a final check to ensure there is no tension on the colorectal suture line. If there is, additional proximal colon must be liberated. There must be sufficient slack that the colon *fills up the hollow of the sacrum* on its way to the anastomosis, thereby eliminating any deadspace.

Alternative to Colorectal Side-to-End Anastomosis

When the surgeon does not find it practicable to leave the specimen attached to the rectal stump for purposes of traction (the preferred technique described above), an alternative method may be used for the anastomosis. After the first step in the Baker method (Fig. 45-12) has been completed, remove the specimen by a scalpel incision across the rectum distal to the right-angle clamp. This leaves the rectal stump wide open. To prevent the short rectal stump from retracting beyond the prostate, apply long (30 cm) Allis clamps to the right and left corners of the rectal stump. Then insert a Lloyd-Davies bladder retractor deep to the prostate for exposure.

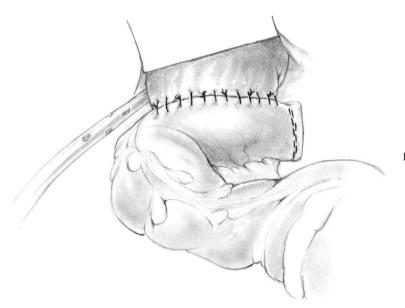

Fig. 45-22

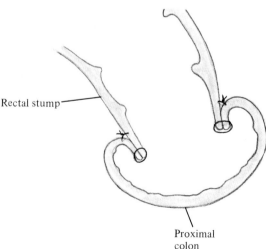

Fig. 45-23

Bring the previously prepared segment of descending colon down to the sacral promontory. The end of this segment of colon should have already been occluded by application of the linear stapling device. Make an incision on the antimesenteric border of the colon beginning 1 cm from the stapled end and continuing proximally for 4–5 cm, which is the approximate diameter of the rectal ampulla.

Insert a guy suture of atraumatic 4-0 silk from the left lateral wall of the rectal stump to the termination of the incision in the colon. Grasp this suture in a hemostat without tying it. Place a similar suture in the right lateral walls of the rectal stump and colon.

Close the remainder of the posterior wall with interrupted horizontal mattress sutures of atraumatic 4-0 silk. Place the first suture at the midpoint of the posterior layer. Using a curved needle, begin the stitch on the mucosal side of the proximal colon and go from inside out through all layers of colon. Then pass the needle from outside in into the rectal stump. It is vitally important that the muscularis of the rectum be included in this bite. Often the muscularis retracts 1 cm or more beyond the protruding rectal mucosa.

Bring the same needle back from inside out on the rectal stump and then from outside in on the proximal colon. Leave this suture untied but grasp it in a hemostat. When it is tied at a later stage in the procedure, the knot lies on the mucosa of the colon.

Place the second horizontal mattress suture halfway between the first suture and the *left* lateral guy suture by the same technique. Place the third suture so it bisects the distance between the midpoint of the posterior layer and the *right* lateral guy suture. Place the remaining stitches by the technique of successive bisection until this layer is complete **(Fig. 45–24)**.

The colon should slide down against the rectal stump while the assistant holds the ends of all the sutures taut. Tie the sutures and leave the tails long, grasping each again in a hemostat. Retaining the long tails of these stitches and applying mild upward traction improves the exposure for insertion of the mucosal sutures. The remainder of the anastomosis is similar to that described above for the Baker technique.

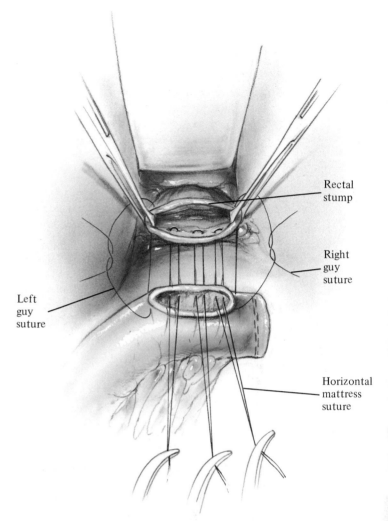

Fig. 45–24

Circular Stapled Low Colorectal Anastomosis

To use the circular stapling technique for low colorectal anastomosis, place the patient in the Lloyd-Davies position, with thighs abducted, anus exposed, and sacrum elevated on a small sandbag. For tumors situated 6–9 cm above the anal verge, it is necessary to dissect the rectum down to the levator diaphragm, which requires complete division of Waldeyer's fascia posteriorly, dissection of the anterior rectum away from the prostate to the level of the urethra, and division of the lateral ligaments down to the levators.

Unless the patient has a narrow pelvis, the entire levator diaphragm then comes into view (**Fig. 45–25**). All of the perirectal lymphatics readily peel off the levator musculature. Then follow the posterior wall of the rectum down to the puborectalis muscle, which marks the cephalad margin of the anal canal. Take care not to continue dissecting beyond the puborectalis, as it is easy to enter the intersphincteric plane and liberate the rectum down to the anal verge. An anastomosis to the skin of the anal canal is technically feasible but would result in excision of the internal sphincter together with the specimen because the intersphincteric space is the natural plane of dissection one enters from above.

Place a large right-angle renal pedicle clamp across the rectum about 1 cm beyond the lower edge of the tumor. Then divide the upper colon between Allen clamps at the site previously selected for this purpose. Ligate the cut distal end of the descending colon with umbilical tape and cover it with a sterile rubber glove (Figs. 45-14a, 45-14b). Bring the proximal colon down into the pelvis. There should be sufficient slack in the colon to fill the hollow of the sacrum on its way to the site of the anastomosis. If not, liberate the transverse colon to achieve sufficient slack.

Next, remove the Allen clamp and gently dilate the colon with appropriate sizers or a Foley catheter balloon. Dilating the colon may prove the most frustrating step of the entire operation. Be careful *not to produce any serosal tears* during this maneuver. It is advisable to use the largest cartridge possible to ensure an ample lumen.

Then insert a 2-0 Prolene continuous over-and-over whip-stitch starting at the left margin of the proximal cut end of the colon (**Fig. 45–26a**). Ascertain that all fat and mesentery have been dissected off the distal 1.5 cm of colon so no fat or blood vessels are interposed between the layers of bowel included in the staple line. If blood vessels are trapped in the staple line, firing the stapler may produce significant bleeding in the rectal lumen,

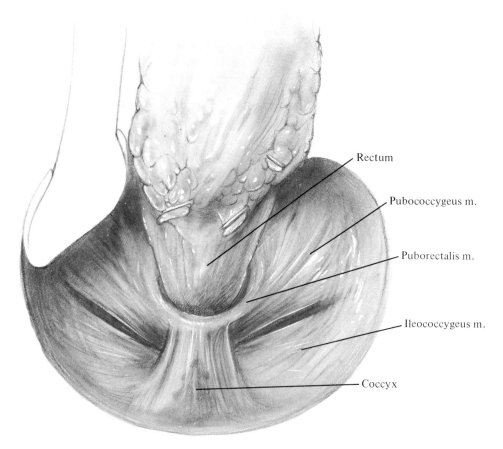

Rectum

Pubococcygeus m.

Puborectalis m.

Ileococcygeus m.

Coccyx

Fig. 45-25

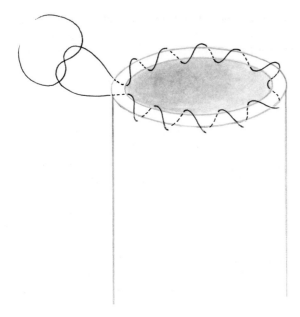

Fig. 45–26a

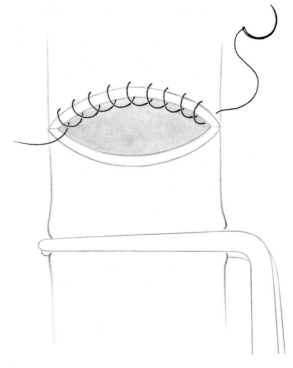

Fig. 45–26c

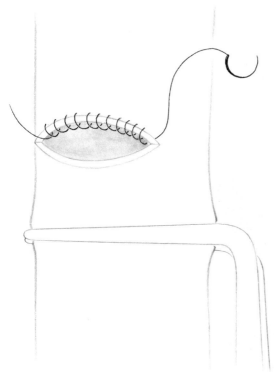

Fig. 45–26b

which is difficult to control. Alternatively, a purse-string instrument (see Fig. G-33) may be used instead of a whip-stitch.

Insert a sterile short proctoscope into the anal canal and aspirate the rectum of its contents. Thoroughly irrigate the rectum with sterile water to wash out any desquamated tumor cells and remove the proctoscope.

Next, insert an over-and-over whip-stitch into the rectal stump. To accomplish this, make an incision through the full thickness of the rectal wall on its left anterolateral aspect, leaving a 4 cm margin beyond the tumor. Place traction on the right-angle clamp to maintain exposure of the lower rectum. Initiate a 2-0 atraumatic Prolene over-and-over whip-stitch at the left lateral corner of the rectal stump **(Fig. 45–26b)**. As this stitch progresses along the anterior wall of the rectum toward the patient's right, divide more and more rectal wall **(Fig. 45–26c)**. Continue the same suture circumferentially along the posterior wall of the rectum until the

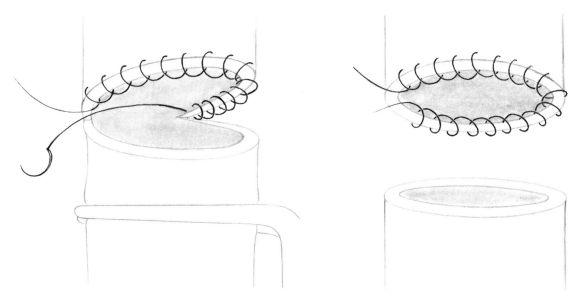

Fig. 45-26d

Fig. 45-26e

point of origin at the left lateral wall is reached and the specimen is completely detached **(Figs. 45–26d, 45-26e)**. Do not attempt to insert the whip-stitch *after* the specimen has been detached because the rectal stump would retract beyond the prostate and suturing from above would be impossible in the case of tumors of the mid-rectum (6-10 cm above the anal verge). Each bite should contain 4 mm of full-

thickness rectal wall, and the stitches should be no more than 6 mm apart to prevent gaps when the suture is tied. A 1.5-2.0 cm width of muscular wall of rectum behind the whip-stitch should be cleared of fat, blood vessels, and areolar tissue. When the staples are fired, there should be no fat or mesentery between the muscular wall of the rectum and the seromuscular wall of the proximal colon. Grasp both

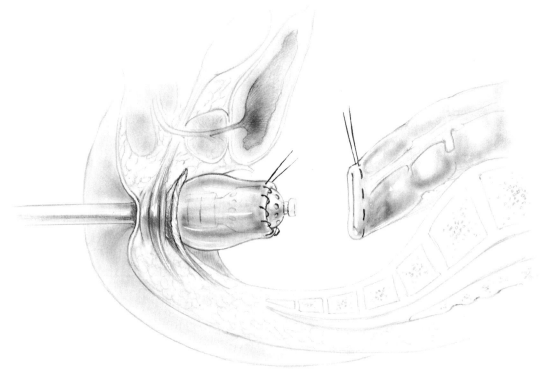

Fig. 45-27

ends of the Prolene purse-string suture in a hemostat. Irrigate the pelvis.

Now move to the perineal portion of the operative field. Check that the stapler is correctly assembled. Because devices from different manufacturers vary, it is crucial to be familiar with the circular stapling device in use. Lubricate the tip of the stapling device with sterile surgical jelly. Insert the device into the anal canal and the rectum with the trigger handles pointing anteriorly **(Fig. 45–27)**. Slowly push the anvil of the stapler through the lower rectal purse-string suture, then rotate the wing nut at the end counterclockwise until the device is wide open. Tie the rectal purse-string suture firmly around the shaft of the stapler **(Fig. 45–28)** and cut the tails 5 mm from the knot.

Apply three Allis clamps in triangular fashion to the cut end of the proximal colon, the lumen of which has been dilated so the colon may be brought over the cap of the circular stapler. When this has been accomplished, tie the colonic purse-string suture and cut its tails 5 mm from the knot **(Fig. 45–29)**. It is vital to observe the integrity of the two purse-string sutures, as any gap in the purse-string closures can cause a defect in the anastomosis.

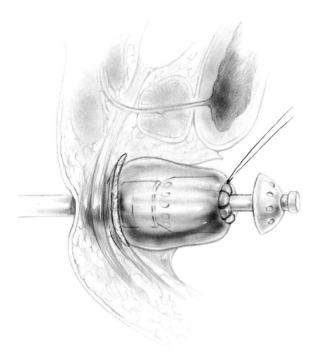

Fig. 45-28

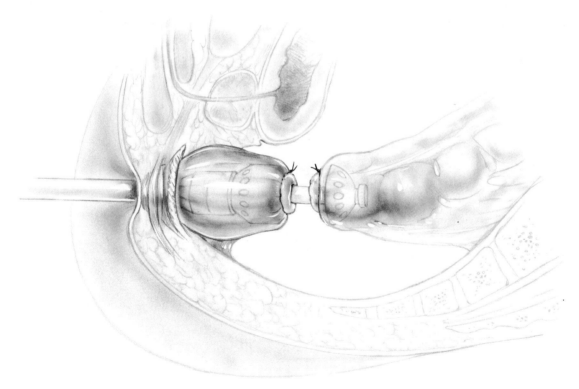

Fig. 45-29

are not grasped between the anvil and the cartridge during this step.

Unlock the trigger handles and then strongly compress them by applying a firm grip **(Fig. 45–31)**. Check the strength of the compression by observing if the black mark on the shaft of the instrument is in the proper location. If this step is done properly, two circular, concentric rows of staples are fired against an anvil, and a circular scalpel blade excises the tissues compressed by the two purse-string sutures in the rectum and colon, resulting in a circular stapled anastomosis.

Now rotate the wing nut counterclockwise the recommended number of turns to open the device and separate the anvil from the cartridge. Rotate the stapler at least 180° to the right and then to the left to free any adherent tissue. Remember that the anvil cap is larger than the inner diameter of the anastomosis. Extract the anvil by depressing the stapling device handle toward the floor, thereby elevating the anterior lip of the anvil. Extract this lip first; then deliver the posterior lip by elevating the handle. It is sometimes helpful if the assistant grasps the anterior rectal stump with a gauze pad or inserts a Lembert suture to stabilize the staple line while the anvil is being extracted **(Figs. 45–32, 45–33)**.

After the instrument has been removed, turn the thumb screw on the cap of the staple cartridge counterclockwise and remove the cap containing the anvil to reveal the segments of rectum and colon that have been amputated. The cartridge should contain two complete circles, each resembling a small

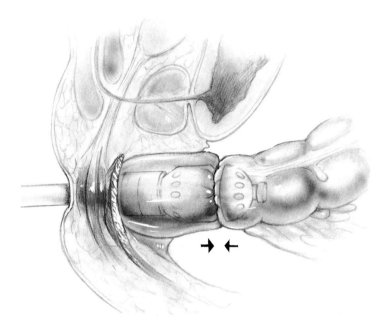

Fig. 45-30

Now *completely* close the circular stapler by rotating the wing nut in a clockwise fashion **(Fig. 45–30)**. Check the vernier marks to confirm complete closure. This approximates the anvil to the staple cartridge. If closure is not complete, the staples are too far from the anvil and do not close to form the B shape. Be sure the vagina, bladder, and ureters

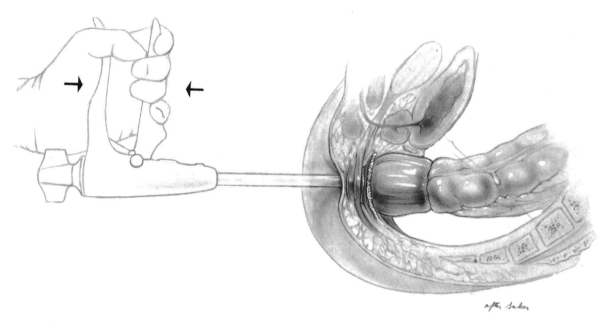

Fig. 45-31

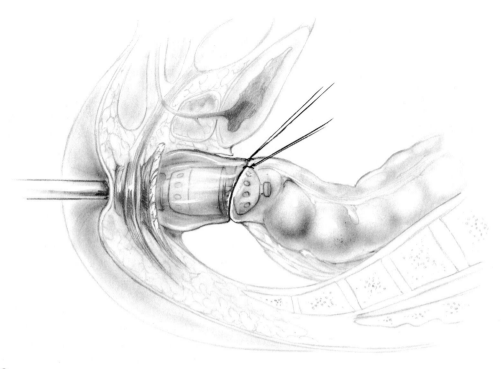

Fig. 45–32

doughnut. One represents the proximal margin of the rectum and the other the distal margin of the proximal colon. Any gap in either of the two circles of bowel indicates a defect in the stapled anastomosis caused by the bowel pulling out of the purse-string suture before being stapled. Locate and repair any such defects. Consider a complementary colostomy or loop ileostomy.

Now check the integrity of the stapled anastomosis by digital examination. An additional test of integrity is to flood the pelvis with sterile saline. Wait until all air bubbles have disappeared and then apply an atraumatic Doyen clamp to the colon above the anastomosis. The assistant then inserts an Asepto-type syringe or a Foley catheter into the anus and pumps air into the rectum while the surgeon palpates the colon. When the colon is inflated with air under only a moderate degree of pressure, observe the pool of saline for air bubbles. The absence of air bubbles is fairly reliable evidence of an intact anastomosis. If air bubbles are detected, attempt to find the source of the leak and repair it with sutures. Create a transverse colostomy if the leak cannot be located or if the suture repair seems unreliable. Another method is to insert a Foley catheter into the rectum and, through it, instill a sterile solution of methylene blue dye. Inspect the anastomosis for leakage of the dye. Use a sterile angled dentist's

mirror to help observe the posterior aspect of the anastomosis.

Double-Stapled Technique for Very Low Colorectal Stapled Anastomosis

There are several situations in which the double-stapled method is advantageous. First, when the rec-

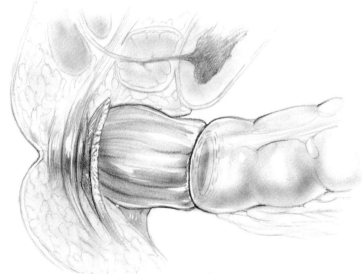

Fig. 45–33

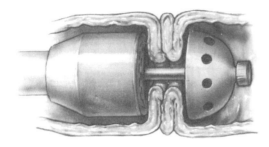

Fig. 45-34

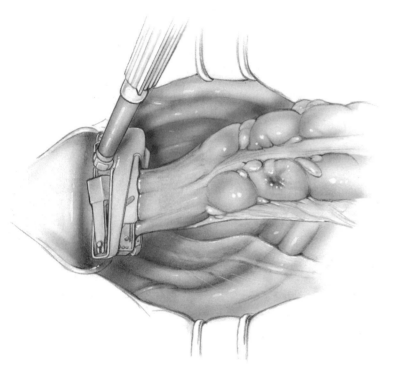

Fig. 45–35

tum is unusually thick or large, even the largest circular stapler cartridge is too small to accommodate the large bulk of tissue. Forcing this large bulk of tissue into the cartridge results in extruding some of the tissue between the colon and rectum being anastomosed (**Fig. 45–34**). Because the tissue is devitalized, it may interfere with healing and cause leakage. When the rectum is bulky, instead of a purse-string suture apply the Roticulator-55 stapler and close the rectum with a line of staples. Then ampu-

tate the specimen. If a circular stapling device is inserted into the rectum, the circular stapled colorectal anastomosis does not encompass a large bulk of rectum, only a relatively thin circle of rectum (Fig. 45–38). Second, it is possible to close the rectal stump at a significantly lower level, as it is much simpler to apply the stapler in this location than to insert a purse-string suture. Third, in patients who have undergone a Hartmann operation, when performing the colorectal anastomosis to the stump of rectum left behind after the Hartmann operation inserting the circular stapling device into the rectal stump makes reversal of the Hartmann operation much simpler than would construction of a sutured colorectal anastomosis.

Anterior resection of the rectum proceeds in the same manner as described above, except that the dissection generally continues farther into the pelvis than the average case, as the Roticulator-55 can be inserted closer to the anal canal than other methods of excising the rectum. After dissection is completed, using the usual retractors on the bladder or uterus, apply the Roticulator-55 to encompass the entire lower rectum and no adjacent pelvic tissues (**Fig. 45–35**). Dissect the rectum down to the longitudinal muscle on all sides. After firing the stapler, apply a long-angled clamp to occlude the proximal rectum and then use the scalpel to divide the rectum flush with the proximal margin of the Roticulator device (**Fig. 45–36**). Locate the upper end of the specimen. Divide the colon and remove the specimen. Insert a 2-0 Prolene purse-string suture close to the cut margin of the colon; then insert the detached anvil into the colon and tie the purse-string suture (**Fig. 45–37**).

Insert the circular stapler cartridge, with the shaft containing the trocar recessed, through the anus into the rectum. Advance the instrument cautiously to the staple line of the closed rectal stump. Rotate the wing nut at the base of the stapler to advance the trocar through the rectal stump. Aim at a spot just anterior to the midpoint of the staple line. When the trocar has emerged through the rectal stump, remove the trocar (Fig. 45-37). Now engage the anvil shaft into the cartridge shaft. Under direct vision, slowly close the wing nut in such fashion that the anvil and the cartridge are properly approximated

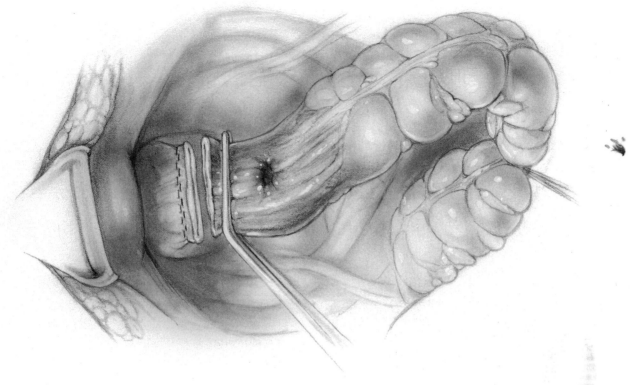

Fig. 45-36

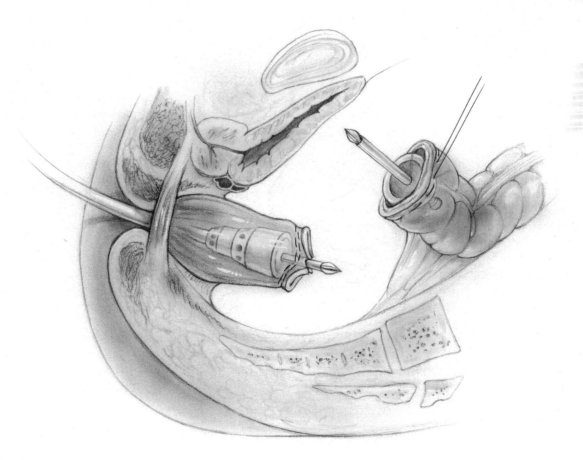

Fig. 45-37

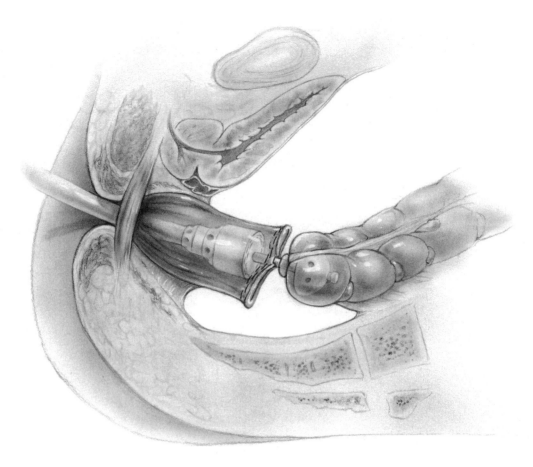

Fig. 45-38

(Fig. 45–38). Then fire the stapler **(Fig. 45–39).** Now open the stapler and remove it as previously described. Carefully check the anastomosis and both "doughnuts" as previously described.

Pitfalls and Danger Points of Circular Stapled Colorectal Anastomosis

Most defects in the staple line are the result of an imperfect purse-string suture. If this suture does not hold the entire cut end of the bowel close to the shaft of the stapling instrument, the staples cannot catch the complete circumference of the colon or rectum, resulting in a defect and postoperative leakage. If complete doughnut-like circles of full-thickness rectum and colon can be identified after the device has been fired, it indicates that the staples have passed through complete circles of bowel and there should be no defect.

Low colorectal circular stapled anastomoses fail also when too much bowel is left beyond the purse-string sutures. When an excessive volume of tissue is admitted into the cartridge, the capacity of the cartridge is exceeded. This results in extrusion of tis-

sue when the cartridge is compressed against the anvil. The devitalized extruded tissue may emerge between the two walls of stapled bowel and interfere with healing. It is also essential to remove fat from the two bowel walls in the area where the staples are to be inserted.

One important exception to use the whip-stitch is where the rectal diameter is large. When a whip-stitch is used to compress a large rectum, it is sometimes impossible to snug the entire diameter up close to the shaft of the stapling device. In this case close the rectum with a linear stapler and use the double-stapled method.

An additional pitfall should be noted. If the trigger handles of the instrument are not compressed fully, the circular scalpel blade fires incompletely. The staples may be driven home, but the redundant colon and rectum within the anvil *are not cut*. Forceful removal of the stapling device under these conditions disrupts the entire anastomosis.

When the anvil cannot be disengaged easily, do not use force. Rather, make a colotomy incision on the antimesenteric border of the upper colon 3–4 cm above the staple line. Then unscrew and remove

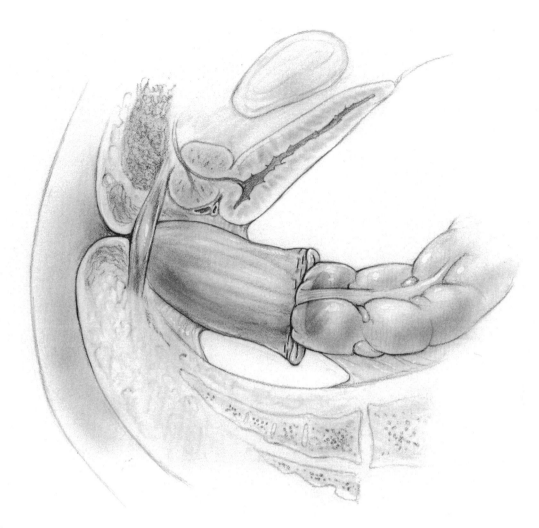

Fig. 45-39

the anvil through the colotomy. Extracting the stapler from the anus is now a simple matter. Inspect
the interior of the anastomosis through the colotomy
opening. If a septum of inverted bowel remains in the
lumen inside the circle of staples, excise the septum
using a Potts angled scissors. Close the colotomy with
a 55 mm linear stapler.

An obvious cause of failure is the erroneous use
of a cartridge or stapler that has been fired already.
In this case the circular blade may function, but
there are no staples; the surgeon is left with two cut
ends of bowel, but no anastomosis. To avoid this error, before attaching the anvil look closely into the
cartridge to be certain it is properly loaded with staples and a circular blade.

Unless the stapler is fully opened, it cannot be removed from the rectum after firing the staples. This
mishap occurs because the anastomosed bowel is
still being grasped between the staple cartridge and
the anvil, and forceful attempts to dislodge the stapler disrupt the anastomosis.

As mentioned above, if the screw that caps the
anvil is not screwed on tightly or if the wing nut
near the handle is not completely closed before
the staples are fired, the space between the staple
cartridge and the anvil is excessive. It prevents
proper closure of the legs of the staples, in which
case the anastomosis may pull apart at the slightest stress. Never use hemostatic clips on any part
of the colon or rectum that may be included in the
stapled anastomosis because these metal clips prevent proper function of the staples and the stapler
blade.

Intraluminal hemorrhage following a stapled
anastomosis occurs if mesenteric blood vessels have
been trapped in the staple line and are transected
by the blade. Bleeding may be controlled by cautious
electrocautery through a proctoscope or by inserting sutures through a proximal colotomy.

When the stapled anastomosis is situated at or
above the cephalad margin of the anal sphincter
muscles (i.e., at or above the puborectalis compo-

nent of the levator muscle), fecal continence is not lost. However, because the proximal colon segment does not function as a reservoir, the patient defecates frequently during the first few months. Each peristaltic contraction results in evacuation of a small, formed stool; but there is no inadvertent loss of stool or liquid. On the other hand, if the anastomosis is at or below the dentate line, the loss of the internal sphincter results in some degree of fecal incontinence for 3-6 months and *sometimes permanently*.

Goligher (1979) described insertion of the purse-string suture into the rectal stump by a transanal approach after dilating the anus and inserting a self-retaining bivalve Parks rectal retractor. Goligher recommended this maneuver in cases where the purse-string suture cannot be inserted from the abdominal approach. Unfortunately, this technique results in excision of the internal sphincter muscle and produces some degree of fecal incontinence if the stapled anastomosis is placed at or below the dentate line. If the transanal approach is used, make every effort to insert the purse-string or whip-stitch into the rectal stump in the upper segment of the anal canal to ensure retention of the internal sphincter muscle. If the rectal stitch cannot be properly applied, one can perform a transanal end-to-end sutured anastomosis by the method of Parks, which makes a point of preserving the internal sphincter muscle. *A coloanal anastomosis may be constructed by a technique similar to that described in Chapter 48 for the ileoanal pouch.*

When the rectal stump is too short to insert a purse-string stitch from above, it is usually possible to use the Roticulator stapler instead (Fig. 45-35). We are enthusiastic about the double-staple technique for colorectal anastomoses that are so low it would be difficult to use sutures. We have resected tumors 6 cm from the anal verge using the stapler with a 2 cm margin of normal tissue, performing a successful stapled anastomosis flush with the upper margin of the anal canal.

Complementary colostomy and presacral drainage should be used following a stapled anastomosis under the same conditions that would lead the surgeon to use these modalities following a sutured colorectal anastomosis. We routinely employ closed-suction presacral drainage for low extraperitoneal anastomoses.

For stapled intraperitoneal anastomoses above the pelvis, we prefer a functional end-to-end anastomosis (see Figs. 44-35 through 44-38) rather than the circular stapled procedure. The latter often takes more time and is prone to more technical complications than the functional end-to-end method.

Wound Closure and Drainage

Remove the wound protector drape. The surgical team should change its gloves and discard all contaminated instruments. Thoroughly irrigate the abdominal cavity and wound with an antibiotic solution. Close the incision in the usual fashion.

POSTOPERATIVE CARE

Nasogastric suction for 3-5 days

No oral intake for the first 4-6 days

Continuation of perioperative antibiotics for 24 hours

Constant bladder drainage via Foley catheter for 6-7 days

Presacral suction catheters attached to closed suction drainage

Drainage catheter removed after 5 days unless there is significant drainage volume

Radiation therapy for selected patients, depending on the stage of disease

COMPLICATIONS

Bladder dysfunction may follow low anterior resection, especially in men with prostatism, but it is much less common than after abdominoperineal proctectomy. Generally, function resumes after 6-7 days of bladder drainage.

Pelvic sepsis secondary to anastomotic leakage is the most common serious complication following low colorectal anastomosis. Any patient with fever, leukocytosis, and ileus following low anterior resection should be assumed to have a leaking anastomosis and a pelvic abscess. Clinical manifestations of this complication commonly occur between the sixth and ninth postoperative days. Cautious digital examination of the rectum by the surgeon may prove to be diagnostic if the finger discloses a defect in the suture line, generally on its posterior aspect. Careful proctoscopic examination may disclose evidence of a defect in the suture line.

The presence of pelvic sepsis can almost always be confirmed by pelvic CT and can often be treated by CT-guided percutaneous catheter drainage. A patient may have sustained a pelvic abscess even in the absence of a definite defect in the suture line. Consequently, a patient who is febrile and toxic should undergo drainage of any septic process if CT-guided percutaneous catheter drainage is not successful. In some cases the patient also requires fecal diversion by transverse colostomy or loop ileostomy.

Patients with mild systemic symptoms who are suspected of having a pelvic infection may be treated by food withdrawal, intravenous antibiotics, and hyperalimentation. Occasionally, a presacral abscess drains into the rectum through the anastomosis without making the patient seriously ill. It must be remembered, however, that anastomotic leakage and pelvis sepsis constitute potentially lethal complications that often require vigorous management.

Sexual dysfunction in men may follow low anterior resection, especially in patients with large tumors and who require extensive dissection of the presacral space, lateral ligaments, and prostatic area.

REFERENCES

Baker JW. Low end to side rectosigmoidal anastomosis. Arch Surg 1950;61:143.

El Pakkastie T, Luukkonen PE, Jarvinen HJ. Anastomotic leakage after anterior resection of the rectum. Eur J Surg 1994;160:293.

Enker WE, Thaler HT, Cranor ML, Polyak T. Total mesorectal excision in the operative treatment of carcinoma of the rectum. J Am Coll Surg 1995;181:335.

Goligher JC. Surgery of the Anus, Rectum, and Colon, 3rd ed. London, Bailliere, 1975, p 662.

Goligher JC. Use of circular stapling gun with peranal insertion of anorectal purse-string suture for construction of very low colorectal or colo-anal anastomoses. Br J Surg 1979;66:501.

Longo WE, Milsom JW, Lavery IC, et al. Pelvic abscess after colon and rectal surgery: what is optimal management? Dis Colon Rectum 1993;36:936.

Nivatvongs S, Fang DT. The use of thumbtacks to stop massive presacral hemorrhage. Dis Colon Rectum 1986; 29:589.

Parks AG, Thomson JPS. Per-anal endorectal operative techniques. In Rob C, Smith R (eds) Operative Surgery, Colon, Rectum, and Anus, 3rd ed. London, Butterworths, 1997, 157.

Stolfi VM, Milson JW, Lavery IC, et al. Newly designed occluder pin for presacral hemorrhage. Dis Colon Rectum 1992;35:166.

Surtees P, Ritchie JK, Phillips RKS. High versus low ligation of the inferior mesenteric artery in rectal cancer. Br J Surg 1990;77:618.

Zu J, Lin J. Control of presacral hemorrhage with electrocautery through a muscle fragment pressed on the bleeding vein. J Am Coll Surg 1994;179:351.

46 Abdominoperineal Resection for Rectal Cancer

INDICATIONS

Malignancy of distal rectum or anus not amenable to sphincter-preserving techniques

PREOPERATIVE PREPARATION

Sigmoidoscopy and biopsy

Barium enema or colonoscopy

Computed tomography (CT) of abdomen and pelvis

Endorectal ultrasonography and other staging studies as indicated

Correction of anemia if necessary

Mechanical and antibiotic bowel preparation

Indwelling Foley catheter in bladder

Nasogastric tube

Perioperative antibiotics

PITFALLS AND DANGER POINTS

Hemorrhage

   Presacral veins

   Left iliac vein

   Middle hemorrhoidal artery

   Hypogastric arterial branches

   Gastrointestinal vessels

Rupture of rectum during dissection

Colostomy ischemia, producing postoperative necrosis

Colostomy under excessive tension, leading to postoperative retraction and peritonitis

Separation of pelvic peritoneal suture line, causing herniation and obstruction of small intestine.

Inadequate mobilization of pelvic peritoneum, resulting in failure of newly constructed pelvic floor to descend completely; resulting empty space encourages sepsis

Genitourinary

   Ureteral trauma, especially during dissection in the vicinity of lateral ligaments of the rectum; inadvertent ureteral ligation; especially during reconstruction of pelvic floor

   Urethral laceration during dissection of perineum in male patients

OPERATIVE STRATEGY

Abdominal Phase

The initial abdominal phase of the dissection is essentially identical to that performed for a low anterior resection. See Chapter 45 for a detailed discussion of the strategy relevant to this phase.

Colostomy

The colostomy may be brought out through the left lower quadrant musculature, the midline abdominal incision, or the belly of the left rectus muscle. If the colostomy is brought out laterally, the 3- to 5-cm gap between the colon and the lateral portion of the abdominal wall should be closed or a retroperitoneal colostomy performed; otherwise the small bowel may become incarcerated in the lateral space. On the other hand, if the colostomy is brought out somewhere near the midline of the abdomen, there is no need to close this space, which becomes so large that movement of small bowel can take place freely without complication.

Goligher (1958) reported a method of bringing the colostomy out through a retroperitoneal tunnel to the opening in the abdominal wall sited in the lateral third of the rectus muscle a few centimeters below the umbilicus. When the peritoneal pelvic floor is suitable for closure by suturing, this technique is another satisfactory method of creating the sigmoid colostomy (see Figs. 46–19 to 46–22).

To prevent necrosis of the colostomy, confirm that there is adequate arterial blood flow to the distal portion of the exteriorized colon, equivalent to that required if an anastomosis were made at this point. Even in the presence of adequate arterial flow, ischemia of the colostomy may occur if an obese mesentery is constricted by a tight colostomy orifice.

Postoperative retraction of the colostomy may result if abdominal distension causes the abdominal wall to move anteriorly. For this reason the limb of colon to be fashioned into a colostomy should protrude without tension for 5 cm beyond the level of the abdominal skin before any suturing takes place.

Pelvic Floor

Because intestinal obstruction due to herniation of the ileum into a defect in the reconstructed pelvic floor is a serious complication, a number of surgeons now omit the step of resuturing the pelvic peritoneum. If no attempt is made to reperitonealize the pelvic floor, the small bowel descends to the level of the sutured levators or subcutaneous layers of the perineum. Intestinal obstruction during the immediate postoperative period does not appear to be common following this technique. However, if intestinal obstruction does occur at a later date, it becomes necessary to mobilize considerable small bowel, which is bound down by dense adhesions in the pelvis. It often results in damage to the intestine, requiring resection and anastomosis to repair it. Thus it appears logical to attempt primary closure of the pelvic peritoneum to prevent this complication, provided enough tissue is available for closure without undue tension. The peritoneal floor should be *sufficiently lax to descend to the level of the reconstructed perineum.* This eliminates the deadspace between the peritoneal floor and the other structures of the perineum. As total proctectomy is done primarily to remove lesions of the lower rectum, there is no need for radical resection of the perirectal peritoneum. One should conserve as much of this layer as possible. If it appears that a proper closure is not possible, it is preferable to leave the floor entirely open. Otherwise the deadspace between the peritoneal diaphragm and the perineal floor often leads to disruption of the peritoneal suture line and to bowel herniation. Creating a vascularized pedicle of omentum is a good way to fill the pelvic cavity with viable tissue and to prevent the descent of small bowel into the pelvis.

Perineal Phase
Position

Turning the patient to a prone position provides the best exposure for the surgeon but imposes a number of disadvantages on the patient. First, circulatory equilibrium may be disturbed by turning the patient who is under anesthesia. Also, changing positions prolongs the operative procedure, as it is not possible to have one member of the surgical team close the abdominal incision while the perineal phase is in process. Similar objections can be raised about the lateral Sims position.

For these reasons we favor the position described here. The patient lies supine, with the sacrum elevated on a folded sheet or sandbag and the lower extremities supported by Lloyd-Davies leg rests, causing the thighs to be widely abducted but flexed only slightly; the legs are supported and moderately flexed. This mild flexion of the thighs does not interfere in any way with the abdominal procedure, and the second assistant can stand comfortably between the patient's legs while retracting the bladder (see Figs. 45-3a, 45-3b).

Whether the abdominal and perineal phases are carried on synchronously by two operating teams or one team does the complete procedure, positioning the patient in this manner gives the surgeon the option of doing some portions of the procedure from below and then switching to the abdominal field in response to the exigencies of a particular step. It facilitates safe lateral dissection of large tumors and complete hemostasis in the pelvis. Some vessels may be easier to control from below, and others should be clamped from above. In addition, after the surgeon has completed suturing the pelvic peritoneum, suction can be applied from below to determine if there is a deadspace between the pelvic floor and the perineal closure. After removing the specimen it is fairly simple to have closure of both the abdomen and perineum proceed simultaneously.

Closure of Perineum

Primary closure of the perineum is now routine, particularly if there has been no fecal spillage in the pelvis during the course of resection, and good hemostasis has been accomplished. Primary healing has been obtained in most of our patients operated on for malignancy when the perineum is closed per primam with insertion of a closed-suction drainage catheter. Suction applied to the catheter draws the reconstructed peritoneal pelvic floor downward to eliminate any empty space.

In patients with major presacral hemorrhage, tamponade the area with a sheet of topical hemostatic agent covered by a large gauze pack, which is brought out through the perineum. Remove the gauze in the operating room on the first or second postoperative day after correcting any coagulopathy and achieving full resuscitation.

In patients who have experienced major pelvic contamination during the operation, the perineum should be closed only partially and drained with both latex and sump drains. In female patients, management of the perineum depends on whether one has elected to remove the posterior vagina. For small anterior malignancies, the adjacent portion of the posterior vagina may be removed with the specimen, leaving sufficient vagina for primary closure with PG. When the entire posterior vaginal wall has been removed along with large anterior lesions, the perineum should be closed with sutures to the levator muscles, subcutaneous fat, and skin. This leaves a defect at the site of the vaginal excision through which loose gauze packing should be inserted. If there is primary healing of the perineal floor, granulation fills this cavity and vaginal epithelium regenerates in 1–3 months. Vaginal resection need not be done for tumors confined to the posterior portion of the rectum.

Dissection of Perineum

The most serious pitfall during perineal dissection is inadvertent transection of the male urethra. This can be avoided if the anterior part of the dissection is delayed until the levator muscles have been divided throughout the remainder of the circumference of the pelvis and the prostate identified. It is important not to divide the rectourethralis muscle at a point more cephalad than the plane of the posterior wall of the prostate (see Fig. 46-11). Alternatively, one should identify the transverse perineal muscles. If the dissection is kept on a plane posterior to these muscles, the urethra is out of harm's way.

Hemostasis

All bleeding during the perineal dissection can be controlled by accurate application of electrocautery. Here, as elsewhere during abdominal surgery, if electrocautery is applied to a vessel that is well isolated from surrounding fat, ligature is not necessary. Whether electrocautery is applied directly to a bleeding point or to forceps or a hemostat depends on the preference of the surgeon. With the cautery device it is possible to obtain complete control of bleeding in this area without undue loss of blood or time.

OPERATIVE TECHNIQUE

Position

Place the patient in the supine position, with the sacrum elevated on several folded sheets or a sandbag and the thighs flexed only slightly but abducted sufficiently to allow adequate exposure of the perineum. The legs should be flexed slightly and the calves padded with foam rubber and supported in Lloyd-Davies leg rests (see Figs. 45-3a, 45-3b). If the thighs are not flexed excessively, there is no interference with performance of the abdominal phase of the operation. The second assistant should stand between the patient's legs during the abdominal phase. Bring the indwelling Foley catheter over the patient's groin and attach it to a plastic tube for gravity drainage into a bag calibrated to facilitate measurement of hourly urine volume. In men, fix the scrotum to the groin with a suture. Close the anal canal with a heavy purse-string suture.

Carry out routine skin preparation of the abdomen, perineum, and buttocks. Drape the entire area with sterile sheets. After these steps have been completed, the operation can be performed with two teams working synchronously or by one team alternating between the abdomen and the perineum.

Incision and Exploration: Operability

Make a midline incision beginning at a point above the umbilicus and continuing to the pubis (see Fig. 45-3a). Separate the pyramidalis muscles as the pubis is approached because getting an extra 1–2 cm closer to the pubis improves the exposure significantly. Open the peritoneum and carry out a general exploration.

In most cases the resectability of a rectal carcinoma cannot generally be determined until a later step in the operation, when the presacral space is open. Accurate preoperative staging has eliminated most of these intraoperative dilemmas. When a tumor invades the sacrum posteriorly or the prostate anteriorly, attempting to core out the rectum by forcing a plane through the tumor is a fruitless and sometimes dangerous endeavor. If much tumor is left behind in the presacral space, the palliation attained is negligible because if it invades the presacral nerves it produces the most distressing of all symptoms in this disease, extreme perineal pain. On the other hand, many tumors are firmly adherent to the sacrum without having invaded it. These lesions should be resected. Cases of borderline resectability may benefit from preoperative neoadjuvant therapy. Local invasion of the ureter does not contraindicate resection, as the divided ureter at this low level can be implanted into the bladder.

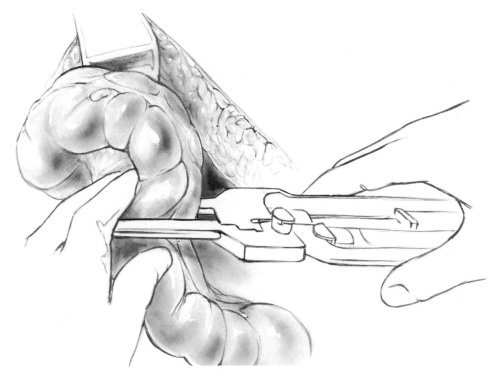

Fig. 46-1a

Mobilization of Sigmoid, Lymphovascular Dissection, and Presacral Dissection

The abdominal phase of this operation proceeds down to the levator diaphragm, as previously outlined (see Figs. 45-4 through 45-11).

The last step in the abdominal portion of the procedure is to divide the sigmoid colon at a point that permits the proximal colon to be brought out of the abdominal incision with at least 5 cm of slack to form an end-colostomy. Use the GIA stapling device, which simultaneously applies staples and divides the colon **(Figs. 46–1a, 46–1b)**. Tie a rubber glove over the end of the distal sigmoid to preserve sterility (see Figs. 45-14a, 45-14b). After this step abandon the abdominal dissection temporarily and initiate the perineal stage.

Pelvic Hemostasis

Obtain pelvic hemostasis as previously described (see Chapter 45). Sometimes bleeding is more easily controlled after the perineal phase is completed. If massive hemorrhage is encountered and cannot be controlled, place gauze packs in the pelvis and remove them in 24-48 hours through the perineum.

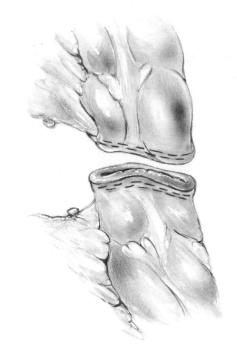

Fig. 46-1b

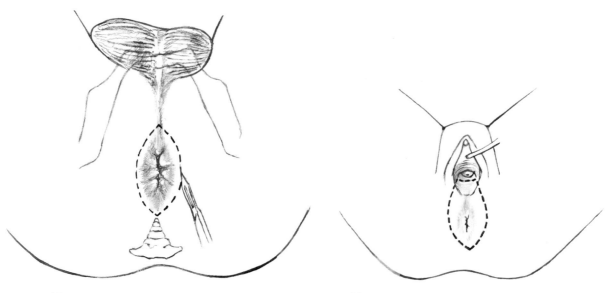

Fig. 46–2   Fig. 46–3

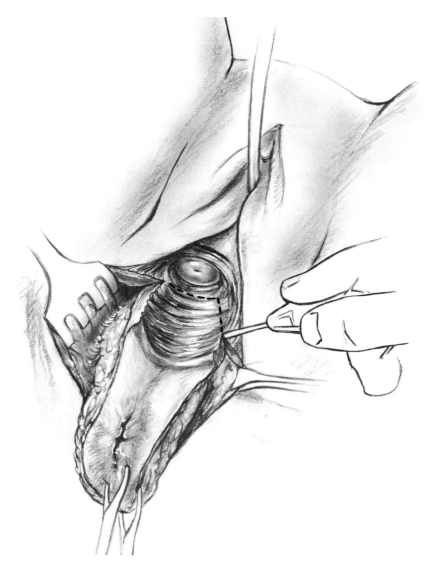

Fig. 46–4

Perineal Dissection

The anus is already closed by a heavy, silk purse-string suture. In male patients make an elliptical incision in the skin beginning at a point 3–4 cm anterior to the anal orifice and terminating at the tip of the coccyx **(Fig. 46–2)**. In female patients with small posterior lesions make the incision from a point just behind the vaginal introitus to the tip of the coccyx. For anterior lesions in women, leave a patch of posterior vagina, including the posterior portion of the vaginal introitus, attached to the rectum in the region of the tumor **(Figs. 46–3, 46–4)**.

In all cases carry the scalpel incision down into the perirectal fat and then grasp the ellipse of skin to be removed in three Allis clamps. While the anus is retracted to the patient's right, have the assistant insert a rake retractor to draw the skin of the perineum to the patient's left. Then incise the perirectal fat down to the levator diaphragm **(Fig. 46–5)**. Generally, two branches of the inferior hemorrhoidal vessels appear in the perirectal fat just superficial to the levators. Each may be secured by electrocautery. Accomplish the identical procedure on the right side of the perineum.

After identifying the anococcygeal ligament at the tip of the coccyx, use electrocautery to divide this ligament transversely from its attachment to the tip of the coccyx **(Figs. 46–6, 46–7)**. Note at this point that if the surgeon's index finger is inserted anterior to the tip of the coccyx it may be unable to enter the presacral space. A dense condensation of fascia (Waldeyer's fascia) attaches the posterior rectum to the presacral and precoccygeal area. If this fascia is torn off the sacrum by blunt technique, the presacral venous plexus may be entered, producing hemorrhage. Therefore Waldeyer's fascia must be incised at the termination of the abdominal portion of the presacral dissection or at the present stage during

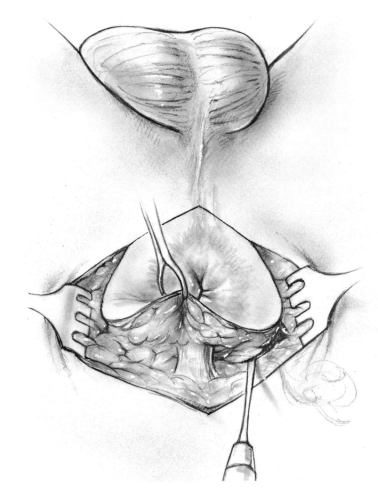

Fig. 46-5

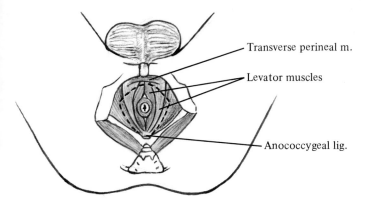

Transverse perineal m.

Levator muscles

Anococcygeal lig.

Fig. 46-6

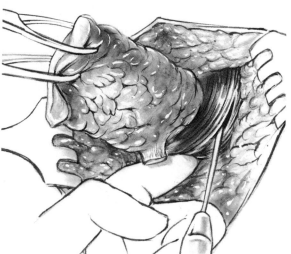

Fig. 46-7

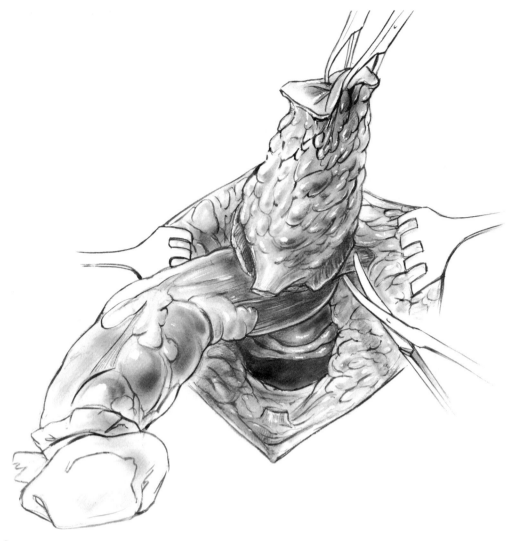

Fig. 46-8

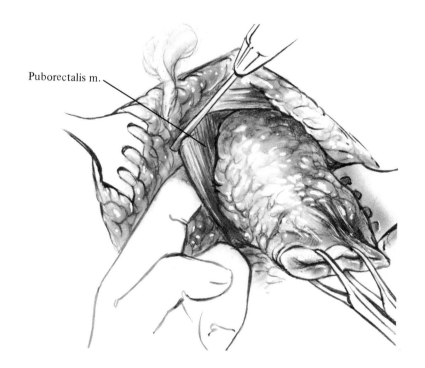

Puborectalis m.

Fig. 46-9

perineal dissection. From the perineal aspect this is a simple maneuver, as it requires only sharp division of the fascia with a scalpel or electrocautery in the plane just deep to the anococcygeal ligament. As soon as this is accomplished it becomes evident that the abdominal and perineal phases of the dissection have joined.

The surgeon should then insert the left index finger underneath the left side of the levator diaphragm and, with the coagulating current, transect the levator muscles upward beginning from below, leaving a portion of the diaphragm attached to the specimen (Fig. 46-7). Continue this incision in the muscular diaphragm up to the region of the puborectalis sling on the anterior aspect of the perineum but not through it.

Use the identical procedure to divide the right-hand portion of the levator diaphragm. Because the greatest danger of the perineal dissection in men is the risk of traumatizing the urethra, delay the anterior portion of the dissection until all the other landmarks in this area have been delineated. To facilitate this delineation, the transected rectosigmoid specimen may be delivered through the opening in the posterior perineum at this time **(Fig. 46–8)**. Insert an index finger underneath the puborectalis muscle and transect it with electrocautery (Figs. 46-8,

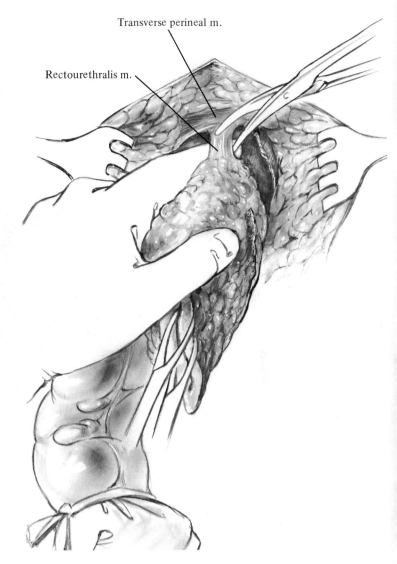

Transverse perineal m.

Rectourethralis m.

Fig. 46-11

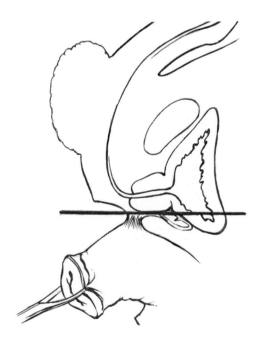

Fig. 46-10

46-9). The prostate was exposed during the abdominal dissection; at this time palpate it and visualize it from below. Make a projection of the plane along the posterior aspect of the prostate gland **(Fig. 46–10)**. Where this plane crosses the rectourethralis muscle, the muscle may be transected safely and the specimen removed **(Fig. 46–11)**. Another landmark, sometimes difficult to identify in obese patients, is the superficial transverse perineal muscles. The anterior plane of dissection should be posterior to these muscles. Finally, divide the remaining attach-

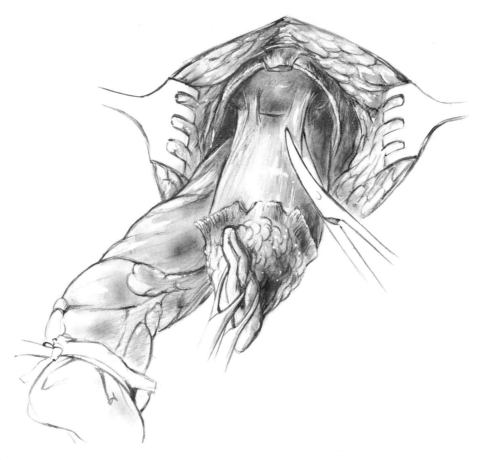

Fig. 46-12

ments to the prostate **(Fig. 46–12)** and remove the specimen.

The above precautions do not apply in women. If the vagina is to be preserved, the anterior dissection should follow a plane just posterior to the vagina. The wall of the vagina should not be traumatized or devascularized during this dissection, as it might well lead to a perineovaginal fistula, which is difficult to manage. It is better to excise the posterior wall of the vagina than to devascularize it partially during the dissection. If the posterior wall of the vagina is to be removed, use electrocautery to continue the perineal skin incision across the vaginal introitus (Fig. 46-4). Complete hemostasis is easily attained when the vagina is incised by electrocautery. Leave a patch of vagina of appropriate dimensions attached to the specimen. Irrigate the presacral space with a dilute antibiotic solution. Hemostasis should be absolute and complete and is easily accomplished using electrocautery and ligatures as one assistant works from above and the surgeon works from below.

Management of Pelvic Floor

In women whose posterior vaginal wall remains intact and in all men, the perineum may be closed per primam if there has been no fecal contamination and if hemostasis is excellent. First, accomplish presacral

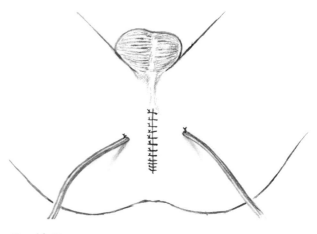

Fig. 46-13

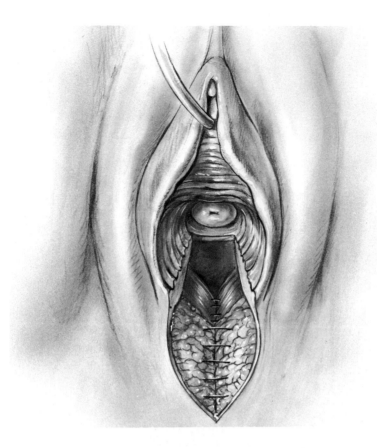

Fig. 46-14

drainage by inserting one or two closed-suction drainage catheters, each 6 mm in diameter. Introduce one catheter through a puncture wound of the skin in the posterior portion of the perineum about 4 cm to the left of the coccyx and a second through a similar point at the right. Suture each catheter to the skin surrounding its exit wound **(Fig. 46–13)**. Place the tips of the catheters in the presacral space. In some cases the posterior levator diaphragm may be partially reconstructed using 2-0 PG sutures. Accomplish the remainder of the perineal closure with one or two layers of interrupted PG to the subcutaneous fat and a subcuticular suture of 4-0 PG to close the skin. As soon as the abdominal surgeon has closed the pelvic peritoneum, apply continuous suction to the two drainage catheters to draw the peritoneum down to the newly reconstructed pelvic floor. The surgeon's aim must be to *eliminate any possible deadspace* between the peritoneal closure and the pelvic floor. These closed suction drains may also be brought out via a stab wound in the lower abdominal wall.

When the posterior vaginal wall and the specimen have been excised, attempt to fabricate a substitute posterior wall with interrupted PG sutures to the perineal fat and to the residual levator muscle

(Fig. 46–14). If this can be accomplished, within a few months after the operation the vaginal mucosa grows over this newly constructed pelvic floor, restoring the vaginal tube. Pack the posterior defect loosely with sterile gauze. Bring the gauze out through the newly reconstructed vaginal introitus after the remainder of the perineal fat and skin have been closed, as described above **(Fig. 46–15)**. If it

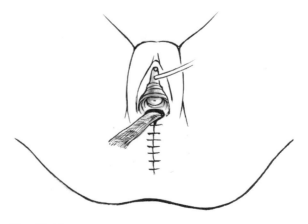

Fig. 46-15

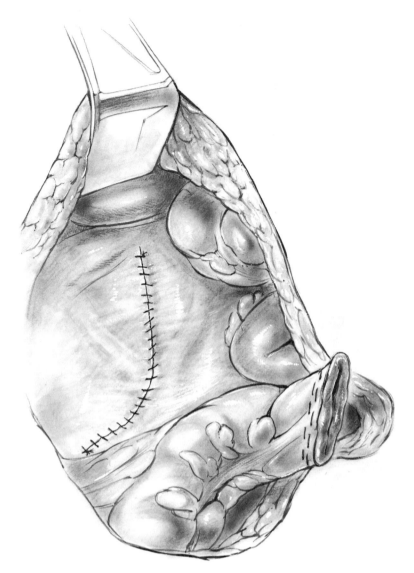

Fig. 46-16

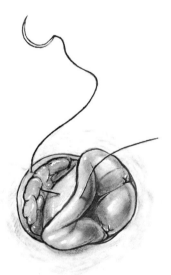

Fig. 46-17

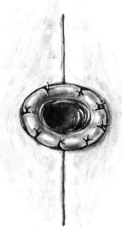

Fig. 46-18

is deemed desirable, a sump catheter can be brought out from the presacral space through the same defect, but it is not done routinely.

While the assistant is closing the perineum, the surgeon should return to the abdominal approach to dissect the pelvic peritoneum free from its surrounding attachments to the lateral pelvic walls and bladder. This enables the peritoneum to be closed without tension **(Fig. 46–16)**. Use a continuous atraumatic suture of 2-0 PG. If there is insufficient peritoneum to permit the peritoneal diaphragm to descend to the level of the newly constructed perineal floor, leave the peritoneum completely unsutured.

Colostomy

The colostomy may be brought out through the upper portion of the midline incision, in which case it is not necessary to close the intraperitoneal gap lateral to the colostomy. Through the midline incision, at a point where 5 cm protrudes from the anterior abdominal skin surface without tension, bring out the segment of colon previously selected to form the colostomy. If this point is near the umbilicus, excise the umbilicus for more postoperative cleanliness. Close the abdominal wall with one layer of monofilament 1-0 PDS; an index finger should fit without tension between the colostomy and the next adjoining suture. Close the skin above and below the colostomy with a continuous subcuticular suture of 4-0 PG. Before closing the skin, irrigate with a dilute antibiotic solution.

After these steps have been completed, excise the line of staples previously used to occlude the colon. Immediately mature the colostomy, using interrupted or continuous sutures of 4-0 PG to attach the full thickness of the colon to the subcuticular plane of the skin **(Figs. 46–17, 46–18)**. No additional sutures are necessary to attach the colon to the fascia or to any other layer of the abdominal wall.

When the peritoneal pelvic floor is suitable for reconstruction by suturing, the retroperitoneal type of colostomy may be performed. Elevate the previously incised peritoneum of the left paracolic gutter from the lateral abdominal wall by finger dissection. Continue until a hand is freely admitted up to the point in the lateral portion of the rectus muscle that has been previously selected for the colostomy **(Figs.**

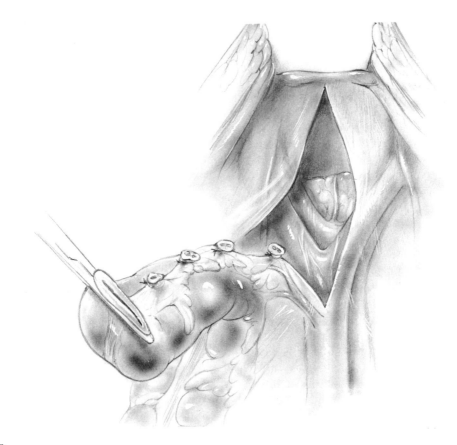

Fig. 46-19

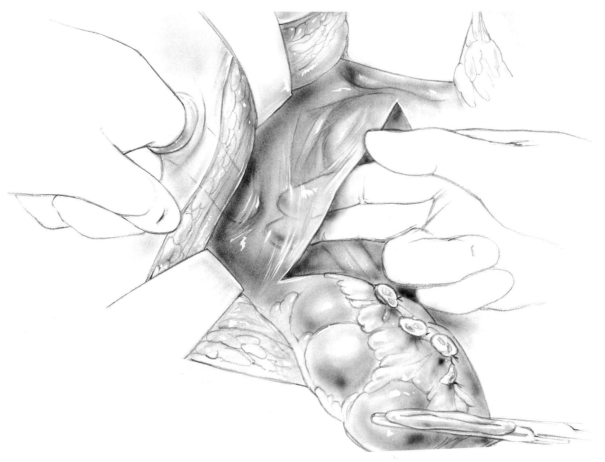

Fig. 46-20

46–19, 46–20), generally about 4 cm below the level of the umbilicus.

Excise a circle of skin about the size of a nickel and expose the fascia of the left rectus muscle. Make cruciate incisions in the anterior rectus fascia, separate the rectus muscle fibers bluntly, and incise the underlying posterior rectus sheath and peritoneum. The aperture in the abdominal wall should be large enough to admit two fingers.

Bring the colon through the retroperitoneal tunnel and out the opening made for the colostomy **(Fig. 46–21)**. Begin the suture line that closes the pelvic peritoneum near the bladder. Continue this suture of 2-0 atraumatic PG in a cephalad direction, closing the entire defect by suturing the free edge of the peritoneum to the anterior seromuscular wall of the sigmoid colon as it enters the retroperitoneal tunnel to become a colostomy **(Fig. 46–22)**. Then close the abdominal incision. Mature the colostomy by a mucocutaneous suture as described above. Attach a temporary colostomy bag to the abdominal wall at the conclusion of the operation.

POSTOPERATIVE CARE

Continue perioperative antibiotic therapy, which had been initiated an hour before the start of operation, for 6 hours postoperatively.

Discontinue nasogastric suction in 24 hours unless the patient develops abdominal distension.

The Foley catheter in the bladder generally remains until the seventh postoperative day.

Perineal Care

Patients who have undergone excision of the posterior vagina have a small amount of gauze packing inserted into the perineum through the residual vaginal defect. This gauze should be removed on the third day, followed by daily saline irrigation of the area. As soon as the patient can sit comfortably, initiate sitz baths daily and discontinue irrigation.

The patients who have had large gauze packs inserted in the presacral region to control hemorrhage should be brought back to the operating room on the first or second postoperative day so the pack can be removed under general anesthesia. The sheet of topical hemostatic agent that had been applied to the sacrum is left undisturbed. The patient should be observed briefly to ascertain that the hemorrhage is under complete control. If the abdominal contents descend to occupy the cavity in the presacral space that had been created by the gauze packing, the perineal floor can be closed tightly around two closed-

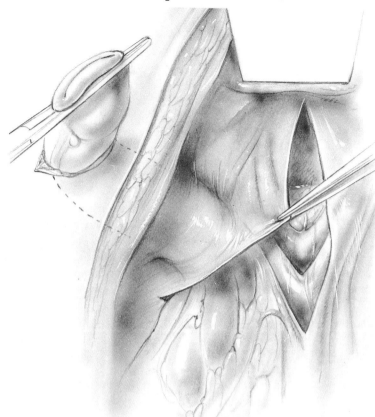

Fig. 46–21

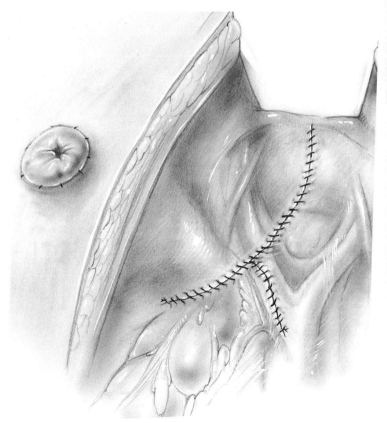

Fig. 46–22

suction drains, as described above. If a large dead-space remains, insert a sump and several latex drains and close the pelvic floor loosely around them.

Most of our patients leave the operating room with the perineum closed per primam. After perineal drainage ceases, generally on the fifth postoperative day, remove the catheters.

Administer sitz baths twice daily to provide symptomatic relief of perineal soreness. Chronic perineal sinus may occur, especially following a proctectomy for colitis. The etiology of this complication, which may persist for years, is not clear, but chronic sepsis and inadequate drainage are the probable causes. Local treatment by curettage, irrigation with a pulsating water jet as noted by Sohn and Weinstein (1977), and perineal hygiene remedy most chronic sinuses. Frequent shaving is necessary to prevent loose hair from entering deep into the sinus and producing a foreign-body granuloma.

Colostomy Care

Observe the colostomy daily through the transparent bag to detect signs of possible necrosis. That the colostomy does not function during the first 6–7 days following the operation need not be a cause for concern if the patient does not develop abdominal distension or cramps. If there is no function beyond this date, abdominal radiography must be performed to rule out an obstruction of the small bowel.

The patient should begin receiving instructions about daily colostomy irrigation during the second week of hospitalization. No patient should leave the hospital before acquiring the skills necessary to perform the irrigation effectively. It is important to understand that the aim of colostomy irrigation is not simply to wash out the distal few inches of colon. Patients sometimes insert a catheter a few inches into the colon, and when the water runs into the colon they permit it promptly to run out alongside the catheter. This is ineffective. Water is instilled into the distal colon for the purpose of dilating the area sufficiently to produce a reflex peristaltic contraction that evacuates the entire distal colon. For many patients this requires injection of more than 1 liter of water before they begin to feel "crampy" discomfort. At this point the catheter should be removed and the patient encouraged to keep the colostomy orifice occluded for a few more minutes, until peristalsis is well underway.

Some patients use a cone-shaped device through which the fluid channel passes, to occlude the lumen. In other cases the patient is able to occlude the lumen by lightly grasping and manually compressing the abdominal wall around the inflow catheter or cone. There are many variations in devices and techniques for colostomy management: When one fails, however, it usually is because the patient has not retained the injected fluid long enough for distension of the distal colon to occur. Without such distension there can be no reflex peristaltic contraction.

All patients must be urged to exercise extreme caution when passing the catheter or any other irrigating device to avoid the possibility of perforating the colon. This complication may occur even in patients who have had 15–20 years of experience irrigating their colostomy. It is generally heralded promptly by the onset of severe abdominal pain during the irrigation. The patient should be urged to report *immediately* for examination if pain occurs at any time during irrigation.

COMPLICATIONS

Acute intestinal obstruction. The small intestine may become obstructed by adhesion to the pelvic suture line or herniation through a defect in the pelvic floor. Adhesions elsewhere in the abdomen, which may occur after any abdominal procedure, can also cause obstruction. If colostomy function has not begun by the sixth or seventh postoperative day, radiographs of the abdomen should be obtained. If small bowel obstruction appears to have occurred and there is no evidence of strangulation, a *brief* trial of a long intestinal tube may be initiated. If this is not promptly successful (3–4 days), secondary laparotomy for relief of the obstruction is indicated.

Hemorrhage. Hemorrhage is rare in properly managed cases. If there is evidence of significant bleeding (by vital signs and laboratory tests or by visible bleeding from the perineal drains), prompt reoperation is preferable to expectant management.

Sepsis. Sepsis that occurs following primary closure of the perineal wound is generally not difficult to detect. It is accompanied by fever, local pain, and purulent drainage through the suction catheters. Under these conditions the perineal incision should be opened sufficiently to insert two fingers, a sump, and several latex or Penrose drains. If this measure does not relieve the infection quickly, the entire wound may be reopened and a gauze pack inserted. The gauze should be changed at least once daily.

Bladder obstruction. Because many men who undergo proctocolectomy for carcinoma are at an age when prostatic hypertrophy is common, this factor combined with the loss of bladder support in the absence of the rectum and some degree of nerve injury leads to a high incidence of urinary tract obstruction. If the obstruction cannot be managed by conservative means, urologic consultation and prostatectomy may be necessary.

Sexual impotence. Some studies have indicated that virtually all operations for radical removal of malignancies in the middle and lower rectum of men have been followed by sexual impotence, although Goligher's (1958) findings were not as bleak. This complication has been rare after operations for benign disease when special precautions are observed (see Chapter 49).

Colostomy complications. Ischemia, retraction, or prolapse of the colostomy may occur if the colostomy is not properly constructed. Parastomal hernia is an occasional late complication.

Chronic perineal sinus. Although a persistent sinus is rare after a properly managed resection for carcinoma, it appears to be common following operations for inflammatory bowel disease. If all the local measures fail and the sinus persists for several years, Silen and Glotzer (1974) recommended a saucerization procedure that consisted of excising the coccyx and the chronically infected wall of the sinus down to its apex. After saucerization, persistent attention to encouraging healing from the bottom has proved successful. Another technique is insertion of a perforated split-thickness skin graft following local débridement and cleansing.

REFERENCES

Anderson R, Turnbull RB Jr. Grafting the unhealed perineal wound after coloproctectomy for Crohn's disease. Arch Surg 1976;111:335.

Goligher JC. Extraperitoneal colostomy or ileostomy. Br J Surg 1958;46:97.

Lechner P, Cesnik H. Abdominopelvic omentopexy: preparatory procedure for radiotherapy in rectal cancer. Dis Colon Rectum 1992;35:1157.

Meade PG, Blatchford GJ, Thorson AG, Christensen MA, Tement CA. Preoperative chemoradiation downstages locally advanced ultrasound-staged rectal cancer. Am J Surg 1995;170:609.

Niles B, Sugarbaker PH. Use of the bladder as an abdominopelvic partition. Am Surg 1989;55:533.

Nivatvongs S, Fang DT. The use of thumbtacks to stop massive presacral hemorrhage. Dis Colon Rectum 1986;29:589.

Silen W, Glotzer DJ. The prevention and treatment of the persistent perineal sinus. Surgery 1974;75:535.

Sohn N, Weinstein MA. Unhealed perineal wound lavage with a pulsating water jet. Am J Surg 1977;134:426.

Weiss EG, Wexner SD. Laparoscopic segmental colectomies, anterior resection, and abdominoperineal resection. In Scott-Conner CEH (ed) The SAGES Manual: Fundamentals of Laparoscopy and GI Endoscopy. New York, Springer-Verlag, 1999, pp 286–299.

47 Subtotal Colectomy with Ileoproctostomy or Ileostomy and Sigmoid Mucous Fistula

INDICATIONS

See Chapter 42 for discussion of issues related to the choice of operative procedure.

Familial polyposis

Chronic ulcerative colitis

Crohn's colitis

PREOPERATIVE PREPARATION

Patients with cachexia may require nutritional support.

Adrenal suppression may be present in patients who have been on steroids for a long time.

For *emergency* colectomy, restitution with blood and electrolytes should be accomplished.

Perioperative antibiotics are prescribed.

PITFALLS AND DANGER POINTS

Operative contamination of the peritoneal cavity with colonic contents, leading to sepsis (with toxic megacolon)

Improper construction of ileostomy

OPERATIVE STRATEGY

When choosing an emergency operative procedure for the patient with complications of inflammatory bowel disease (hemorrhage, perforation, toxic megacolon), consider both the immediate problem and the long-term result. Remember that sphincter-sparing procedures are now available for most of these patients, even when the rectum is involved by disease. Whenever possible retain the rectosigmoid, as it allows restorative proctocolectomy (see Chapter 48) to be performed at a later date.

Sepsis is not uncommon following an emergency colectomy for inflammatory bowel disease and its complications. In Crohn's disease one often finds a fistula to the adjacent bowel or to the skin. In some cases paracolic abscesses are encountered, making gross contamination of the peritoneal cavity inevitable.

When resecting a toxic megacolon, the surgeon should be aware that the colon, especially the distal transverse colon and splenic flexure, may have the consistency of wet tissue paper and can be ruptured by even minimal manipulation. This causes massive, sometimes fatal contamination of the abdominal cavity, and it must be avoided. Make no attempt to dissect the omentum off the transverse colon, as it may unseal a perforation. Elevation of the left costal margin by a Thompson retractor generally provides good exposure of the splenic flexure.

Intraoperative tube decompression may decrease the risk of perforating the colon. Divide the mesentery at a point of convenience nearer to the colon, rather than performing extensive mesenteric excision (as is done for malignancy). Minimize postoperative ileostomy problems by constructing an ileostomy that protrudes permanently from the abdominal wall, like a cervix, for 2 cm. This helps prevent the contents of the small bowel from leaking between the appliance and the peristomal skin. It also greatly simplifies the patient's task of placing the appliance accurately. Finally, close the gap between the cut edge of ileal mesentery and the lateral abdominal wall to avoid internal herniation.

OPERATIVE TECHNIQUE

Placement of Ileostomy

On the day before the operation the surgeon should obtain a face-plate from an ileostomy appliance, or some facsimile, and apply it tentatively to the patient's abdominal wall. Test proper placement with the patient sitting erect. In some patients, if the appliance is not properly placed the rim strikes the costal margin or the anterior spine of the ilium. Generally, the proper location is somewhere near the outer margin of the right rectus muscle, about 5 cm lateral to the midline and 4 cm below the umbilicus. In this position the face-plate generally does not impinge on the midline scar, the umbilicus, the anterior superior spine, or the costal margin no matter what position the patient assumes. If the wafer covers the incision, we prefer a subcuticular skin closure for better skin approximation. The stoma should also be sited so the patient can see it when he or she is erect.

Operative Position

If there is a possibility that the colectomy and total proctectomy will be performed in one stage, position the patient in Lloyd-Davies leg rests (see Figs. 45-3a, 45-3b). Otherwise, the usual supine position is satisfactory.

Incision

We prefer a midline incision because it does not interfere with the ileostomy appliance. It also leaves the entire left lower quadrant free of scar in case ileostomy revision and reimplantation become necessary in the future. On the other hand, many surgeons use a left paramedian incision to permit a wider margin between the ileostomy and the scar. The incision should extend from the upper epigastrium down to the pubis **(Fig. 47–1)**. Because the splenic flexure is foreshortened in many cases of ulcerative colitis and toxic megacolon, exposure for this area is often good, with the Thompson retractor applied to the left costal margin.

Evacuation of Stool

For patients undergoing an operation for acute toxic megacolon, insert a heavy purse-string suture on the anterior surface of the terminal ileum. Make a small enterotomy in the center of the purse-string suture and pass a suction catheter through it, threading the catheter across the ileocecal valve into the cecum. After decompressing the colon, remove the tube and tie the purse-string suture.

Dissection of Right Colon and Omentum

Make an incision in the right paracolic peritoneum lateral to the cecum and insert the left index finger

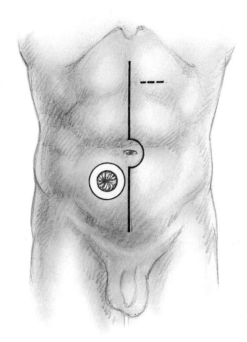

Fig. 47-1

to elevate the avascular peritoneum, which should be divided by scissors in a cephalad direction **(Fig. 47–2)**. If local inflammation has produced increased vascularity in this layer, use electrocautery to carry out the division. Throughout the dissection keep manipulation of the colon to a minimum. Continue the paracolic incision around the hepatic flexure, exposing the anterior wall of the duodenum.

For emergency operations for toxic megacolon, divide the omentum between Kelly hemostats 5 cm above its line of attachment to the transverse colon. If the omentum is fused to the transverse mesocolon, it may be divided simultaneously with the mesocolon in one layer. In most *elective* operations, the omentum can be dissected off the transverse colon through the usual avascular plane **(Fig. 47–3)**.

Dissection of Left Colon

Remain at the patient's right side and make an incision in the peritoneum of the left paracolic gutter in the line of Toldt, beginning at the sigmoid. With the aid of the left hand elevate the avascular peritoneum and divide it in a cephalad direction with Metzenbaum scissors. Carry this incision up to and around the splenic flexure **(Fig. 47–4)**. Mobilize the splenic flexure as described in Chapter 44 (see Figs. 44-5 through 44-8). In patients who suffer from toxic megacolon, perform this dissection with extreme caution so as not to perforate the colon.

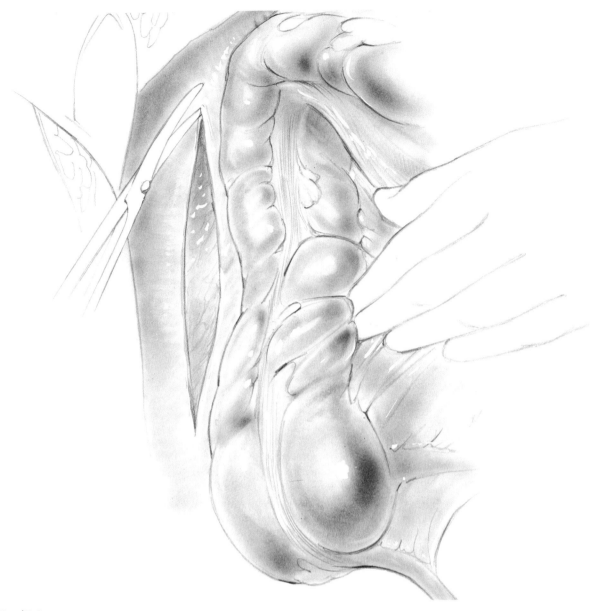

Fig. 47-2

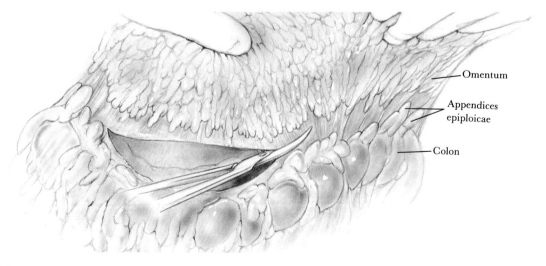

Omentum

Appendices
epiploicae

Colon

Fig. 47-3

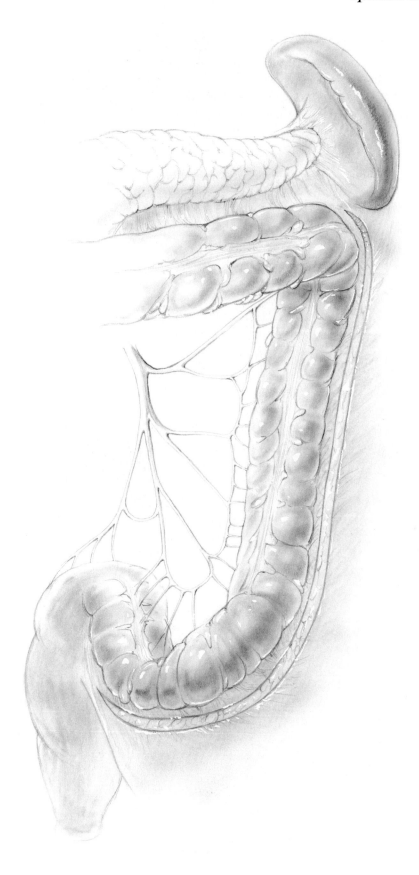

Fig. 47-4

Division of Mesocolon

Turn now to the ileocecal region. If the terminal ileum is not involved in the disease process, preserve its blood supply and select a point of transection close to the ileocecal valve. Divide the mesocolon along a line indicated in **Figure 47–5**. Because most patients who require this operation are thin, each vessel can be visualized, double-clamped, and divided accurately. Ligate each vessel with 2-0 PG or silk ligatures and divide the intervening avascular mesentery with Metzenbaum scissors. In the same way, sequentially divide and ligate the ileocolic branches and the right colic, middle colic, two branches of the left colic, and each of the sigmoidal arteries.

Ileostomy and Sigmoid Mucous Fistula

The technique of fashioning a permanent ileostomy, including suturing the cut edge of the ileal mesen-

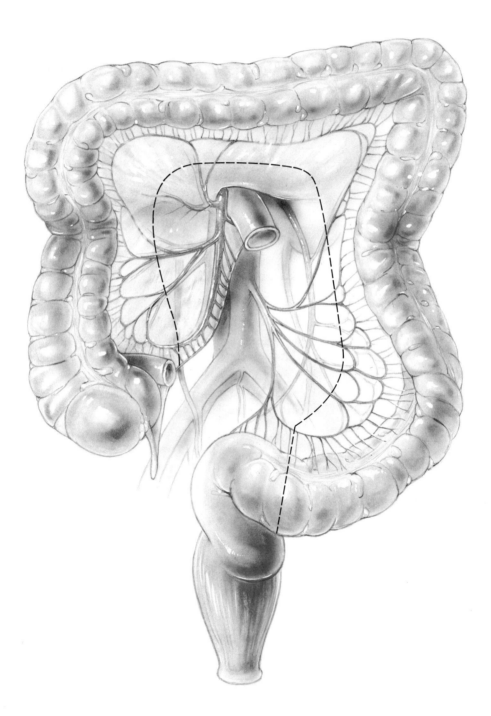

Fig. 47-5

tery to the right abdominal wall, is depicted in Figures 50-1 through 50-9. After the sigmoid mesentery has been divided up to a suitable point on the wall of the distal sigmoid, divide the colon with De-Martel clamps (as shown) or a linear cutting stapler. Bring this closed stump of the rectosigmoid through the lower pole of the incision **(Fig. 47–6)**. Fix the rectosigmoid stump to the lower pole with a few 3-0 PG sutures, approximating the mesocolon and the appendices epiploicae to the anterior rectus fascia. Close the abdominal incision around the mucous fistula.

Ileoproctostomy

When an ileorectal anastomosis is elected, we prefer the side-to-end modified Baker technique (see Figs. 45-12 through 45-23) for the colorectal anastomosis. After the mesentery has been cleared at the point selected for transection of the ileum, apply transversely and fire a 55/3.5 mm linear stapler. Apply an Allen clamp to the specimen side of the ileum and with a scalpel transect the ileum flush with the stapler. Lightly cauterize the everted mucosa and remove the stapling device. Inspect the staple line to ensure that proper B formation of the staples has occurred.

Divide the mesentery of the rectosigmoid up to the point on the upper rectum that has been selected for transection, which is generally opposite the sacral promontory. Apply a right-angle renal pedicle clamp to the colon to exclude colonic contents from the field. Dissect fat and mesentery off the serosa of the rectum at the site to be anastomosed. Make a linear scratch mark on the antimesenteric border of the ileum beginning at a point 1 cm proximal to the staple line and continuing in a cephalad direction for a distance equal to the diameter of the rectum, usually 4-5 cm.

The first layer should consist of interrupted 4-0 silk seromuscular Cushing sutures inserted by the successive bisection technique. After the sutures are tied, cut all the tails except for the two end sutures, to which small hemostats should be attached. Then make incisions on the antimesenteric border of the

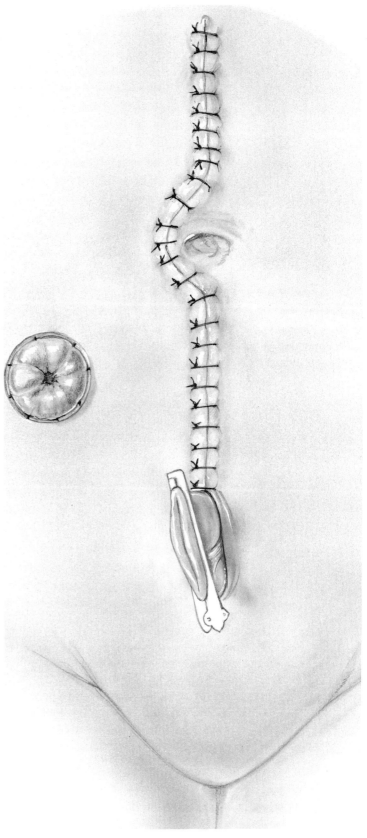

Fig. 47-6

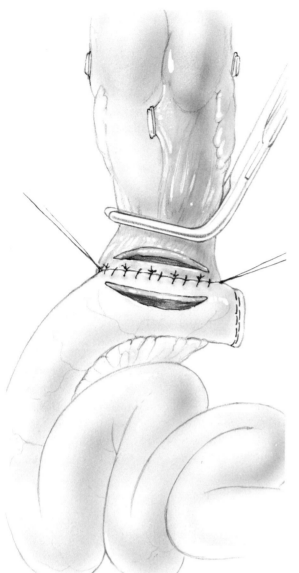

Fig. 47-7

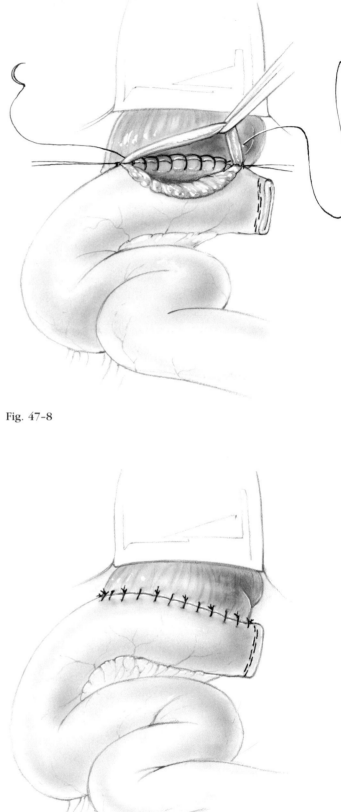

Fig. 47-8

Fig. 47-9

ileum and the back wall of the rectum **(Fig. 47–7)**. Initiate closure of the posterior mucosal layer by inserting a double-armed 5-0 PG suture in the middle point of the posterior layer and tying it. With one needle insert a continuous locked suture to approximate all the coats of the posterior layer, going from the midpoint to the right corner of the anastomosis. Use the other needle to perform the same maneuver going from the midpoint to the left **(Fig. 47–8)**. Amputate the specimen. Then use a continuous Cushing, Connell, or seromucosal suture to approximate the anterior mucosal layer, terminating the suture line at the midpoint of the anterior layer. Close the final anterior seromuscular layer with interrupted 4-0 silk Cushing sutures **(Fig. 47–9)**. If possible, cover the anastomosis with omentum.

Approximate the cut edge of the ileal mesentery to the cut edge of the right lateral paracolic peritoneum with a continuous 2-0 atraumatic PG suture. Do not close the left paracolic gutter. Irrigate the abdominal cavity.

Subtotal Colectomy Combined with Immediate Total Proctectomy

When a proctectomy is performed at the same stage as a subtotal colectomy, occlude the rectosigmoid by a layer of TA-55 staples. Apply an Allen clamp to the specimen side of the colon, which should be transected with removal of the specimen. Construct the ileostomy as depicted in Figures 50–1 through 50–9. Then perform abdominoperineal proctectomy by the technique described in Chapter 49.

Needle-Catheter Jejunostomy

Consider performing needle-catheter jejunostomy in any patient suffering from malnutrition to permit enteral feeding immediately after surgery.

Closure of the Abdominal Incision

Close the abdominal wall in routine fashion without drains (see Chapter 3).

POSTOPERATIVE CARE

Continue nasogastric suction (when indicated) and intravenous fluids until there is good ileostomy function. If there was no operative contamination, discontinue the operative antibiotics within 6 hours. Otherwise, continue antibiotics, modifying as indicated by the operative findings and the postoperative course.

In the operating room apply a Stomahesive disk to the ileostomy after cutting a properly sized opening. Over the disk place a temporary ileostomy bag. Instruct the patient in the details of ileostomy management and encourage him or her to join one of the organizations of ileostomates, where considerable emotional support can be derived by meeting patients who have been successfully rehabilitated.

COMPLICATIONS

Intraabdominal abscess is more common after colon resection for inflammatory bowel disease than for other conditions. When signs of intraabdominal infection appear, prompt laparotomy or percutaneous computed tomography-guided catheter drainage for evacuation of the abscess is indicated.

Intestinal obstruction due to adhesions is not rare following this group of operations because of the extensive dissection. If nonoperative treatment does not bring a prompt response, laparotomy for enterolysis becomes necessary.

Leakage of the anastomosis may follow ileoproctostomy. In case of a major leak, immediate laparotomy for a diverting loop ileostomy (see Chapter 51) followed by pelvic drainage is mandatory. Alternatively, the anastomosis may be taken down and the ileum brought out as a terminal ileostomy.

REFERENCES

Chevalier JM, Jones DJ, Ratelle R, et al. Colectomy and ileorectal anastomosis in patients with Crohn's disease. Br J Surg 1994;81:1379.

Longo WE, Oakley JR, Lavery IC, Church MJ, Fazio VW. Outcome of ileorectal anastomosis for Crohn's colitis. Dis Colon Rectum 1992;35:1066.

48 Ileoanal Anastomosis with Ileal Reservoir Following Total Colectomy and Mucosal Proctectomy

INDICATIONS

Selected patients requiring proctocolectomy for ulcerative colitis, in whom preservation of continence is desired

Familial polyposis

CONTRAINDICATIONS

Cohn's disease

Perianal fistulas

Rectal muscular cuff that is strictured and fibrotic, not soft and compliant

PREOPERATIVE PREPARATION

Treat inflammation and ulcerations of the lower rectum preoperatively. If the patient has had a subtotal colectomy and ileostomy, it may be necessary to treat the rectum with steroid enemas or free fatty acid enemas.

Nutritional rehabilitation is applied when necessary.

Perioperative antibiotics as prescribed.

Nasogastric tube is inserted.

Foley catheter is placed in the bladder.

Endoscopy of ileum via the ileostomy is undertaken when Crohn's disease is suspected after subtotal colectomy.

If one-stage colectomy with reconstruction is anticipated, appropriate mechanical and antibiotic bowel preparation is indicated.

PITFALLS AND DANGER POINTS

Performing an inadequate mucosectomy, which may produce a cuff abscess and possibly lead later to carcinoma

Establishing inadequate pelvic, reservoir, or anastomotic hemostasis, which may result in postoperative hemorrhage or hematoma

Injuring the nervi erigentes or the hypogastric nerves so sexual impotence or retrograde ejaculation results

Failing to diagnose Crohn's disease, resulting in Crohn's ileitis in the reservoir

Using improper technique when closing the temporary loop ileostomy, which leads to postoperative leakage or obstruction

OPERATIVE STRATEGY

Multiple techniques have been described for restorative proctocolectomy. The method described here has served well and accomplishes maximum ablation of the abnormal mucosa. An alternative technique avoids the mucosal proctectomy altogether and creates the anastomosis between the anus and the perineal pouch by means of a double stapling technique. A roticulating linear stapler and circular stapler are used in a manner analogous to that described in Chapter 45. The anastomosis is constructed 1–2 cm above the dentate line, leaving some transitional zone epithelium behind. References at the end of the chapter detail operative results with various techniques and give additional technical details for other methods.

Mucosectomy

The mucosectomy is performed most easily with the patient in the prone jacknife position. The dissection is expedited by injecting a solution of epinephrine (1:200,000) into the submucosal plane. It is performed as the first stage in the procedure; if the rectum is so badly diseased that mucosectomy cannot be reasonably accomplished, the operative plan must be modified. Generally, proctocolectomy is then required.

Good fecal continence can be maintained if the mucosa is dissected away from the rectum up to a point no more than 1–2 cm above the puborectalis, the upper end of the anal canal. This amount of dissection can generally be accomplished transanally with less difficulty in the adult patient than occurs when using the abdominal approach. There must be complete hemostasis in the region of the retained rectum. Generally, careful electrocoagulation can accomplish this end.

Some surgeons advocate the use of a Cavitron ultrasonic aspirator (CUSA) to facilitate the mucosal proctectomy. Frozen-section histologic examination of the excised mucosa may be helpful for ruling out Crohn's disease.

Abdominal Dissection

When performing the colectomy, transect the ileum just proximal to its junction with the ileocecal valve to preserve the reabsorptive functions of the distal ileum. If a previous ileostomy is being taken down, again preserve as much terminal ileum as possible.

Rectal Dissection

When dissecting the rectum away from the sacrum, keep the dissection immediately adjacent to the rectal wall. Divide the mesenteric vessels near the point where they enter the rectum and leave the major portion of the "mesentery" behind. In this way the hypogastric nerves are preserved.

Similarly, when the lateral ligaments are divided, make the point of division as close to the rectum as possible to avoid dividing the parasympathetic nerves essential for normal male sexual function. Anteriorly, the dissection proceeds close to the rectal wall posterior to the seminal vesicles and Denonvilliers' fascia down to the distal end of the prostate.

Division of Waldeyer's Fascia

In the adult patient it is not possible to expose the levator diaphragm unless the fascia of Waldeyer is divided by sharp dissection. This layer of dense fascia is attached to the anterior surface of the sacrum and coccyx and attaches to the posterior wall of the rectum. Unless it is divided just anterior to the tip of the coccyx, it is not possible to expose the lower rectum down to the level of the puborectalis muscle.

Temporary Loop Ileostomy and Ileostomy Closure

The loop ileostomy (see Chapter 51) completely diverts the fecal stream, yet is simple to close. It should be used whenever there is the slightest doubt as to the integrity of the anastomoses in the pelvis.

Ileoanostomy

To facilitate anastomosing the ileum or the ileal reservoir to the anus, it is helpful to flex the thighs on the abdomen to a greater extent than is usually the case when the patient is placed in the lithotomy position for a two-team abdominoperineal operation. Be certain the rectal mucosa has been divided close to the dentate line. Otherwise, it will be necessary to insert sutures high up in the anal canal where transanal manipulation of the needle is extremely difficult. Also, it is important to remove all of the diseased mucosa in this operation to eliminate the possibility of the patient developing a rectal carcinoma at a later date.

One method of achieving exposure with this anastomosis is to insert the bivalve Parks retractor with large blades into the rectum. Then draw the ileum down, between the open blades of the retractor, to the dentate line. Insert two sutures between the ileum and the anterior wall of the anus. Insert two more sutures between the ileum and the posterior portion of the dentate line. Now remove the Parks retractor. Remove the large blades from the retractor and replace them with small blades. Then carefully insert the blades of the Parks retractor into the lumen of the ileum and open the retractor slowly.

With the Parks retractor blades in place, continue to approximate the ileum to the dentate line with 12–15 interrupted sutures of 4-0 Vicryl. This requires that the retractor be loosened and rotated from time to time to provide exposure of the entire circumference of the anastomosis. Be certain to include the underlying internal sphincter muscle together with the epithelial layer of the anal canal when inserting these sutures.

An alternative, more effective method of exposing the anastomosis is to use a Gelpi retractor with one arm inserted into the tissues immediately distal to the dentate line at about 2 o'clock while the second arm of this retractor is placed at 8 o'clock. A second Gelpi retractor is inserted into the anus with one arm at 5 o'clock and the second at 11 o'clock. If the patient is properly relaxed, these two retractors ensure visibility of the whole circumference of the cut end of the anorectal mucosa at the dentate line. Then draw the ileum down into the anal canal and complete the anastomosis.

Constructing the Ileal Reservoir

We prefer a J-loop ileal reservoir that is constructed by making a side-to-side anastomosis in the distal segment of the ileum. We do not include the elbow of the J-loop in the staple line, thereby ensuring that there is no possibility of impairing the blood supply to the ileoanal anastomosis. The terminal end of the ileum is occluded with staples. Although it is possible to establish an ileoanal anastomosis using a circular stapler, we prefer to suture this anastomosis because we like to be sure that no rectal mucosa has been left behind.

OPERATIVE TECHNIQUE

Mucosal Proctectomy Combined with Total Colectomy

When the mucosa of the distal rectum is devoid of visible ulcerations and significant inflammation, mucosal proctectomy may be performed at the same time as total colectomy. In these cases perform the colectomy as described in Chapter 47. Be certain to divide the mesentery of the rectosigmoid close to the bowel wall to avoid damaging the hypogastric and parasympathetic nerves. Also, divide the branches of the ileocolic vessels close to the cecum to preserve the blood supply of the terminal ileum. It is important to transect the ileum within 1-2 cm of the ileocecal valve. Preserving as much ileum as possible salvages some of the important absorptive functions of this organ.

Use a cutting linear stapler to divide the terminal ileum. Lightly cauterize the everted mucosa. Mobilize the entire colon down to the peritoneal reflection, following the procedures illustrated in Figures 44-5, 44-8, and 47-1 to 47-5. Divide the specimen with a cutting linear stapler at the sigmoid level.

Divide the rectosigmoid mesentery close to the bowel wall to avoid interrupting the hypogastric nerves (see Fig. 49-1). Divide the lateral ligaments close to the rectum and divide Denonvilliers' fascia proximal to the upper border of the prostate. Keep the dissection *close to the anterior and lateral rectal walls* in men to minimize the incidence of sexual impotence. After dividing Waldeyer's fascia (see Fig. 45-10) expose the puborectalis portion of the levator diaphragm (see Fig. 45-25).

At this time, transect the anterior surface of the rectal layer of muscularis in a transverse direction down to the mucosa. Make this incision in the rectal wall about 2-4 cm above the puborectalis muscle. Now dissect the muscular layer away from the mucosa. Injecting a solution of 1:200,000 epinephrine between the mucosa and muscularis expedites this dissection. After the muscle has been separated from 1-2 cm of mucosa anteriorly, extend the incision in the muscularis layer circumferentially around the rectum. Use Metzenbaum scissors and a peanut sponge dissector for this step. Achieve complete hemostasis by accurate electrocoagulation. Continue the mucosal dissection until the middle of the anal canal has been reached. Divided the mucosal cylinder at this point, remove the specimen, and leave an empty cuff of muscle about 2-4 cm in length above the puborectalis, which marks the proximal extent of the anal canal. If any mucosa has been left in the anal canal proximal to the dentate line, it can be removed transanally later in the operation.

Alternatively, one may perform the rectal mucosectomy prior to opening the abdomen. This method is described in the next section of this chapter.

Perineal Approach

We agree with the suggestion of Sullivan and Garnjobst (1982) that the rectal mucosal dissection is best performed as the initial step in the operation, regardless of whether the procedure is combined with a simultaneous total colectomy. If it is not possible to dissect the mucosa away from the internal sphincter, perform an ileostomy and abdominoperineal total proctectomy instead of a restorative proctocolectomy.

Performing the mucosal proctectomy with the patient in the prone position affords better exposure than is available in the lithotomy position. After inducing endotracheal anesthesia, turn the patient face down and elevate the hips by flexing the operating table or by placing a pillow under the hips. Also place a small pillow under the feet and spread the buttocks apart by applying adhesive tape to the skin and attaching the tape to the sides of the operating table. Gently dilate the anus until it admits three fingers. Obtain exposure by using a large Hill-Ferguson, a narrow Deaver, or a bivalve Pratt (or Parks) retractor. Inject a solution of 1:200,000 epinephrine in saline in the plane just deep to the mucosa, immediately proximal to the dentate line around the circumference of the anal canal (**Fig. 48–1**). Now make a circumferential incision in the transitional epithelium immediately cephalad to the dentate line. Using Metzenbaum scissors, elevate the mucosa and submucosa for a distance of 1-2 cm circumferen-

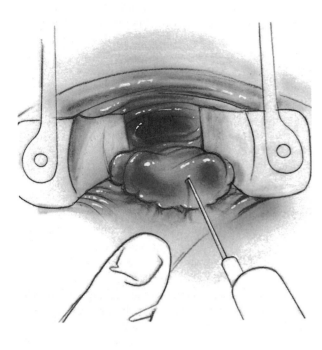

Fig. 48-1

tially from the underlying circular fibers of the internal sphincter muscle **(Fig. 48–2)**. Apply several Allis clamps to the cut end of the mucosa. Maintain hemostasis by accurate electrocoagulation using the needle tip attachment on the electrocautery. It is helpful to roll up two 10 × 20 cm moist gauze

sponges soaked in a 1:200,000 epinephrine solution and insert this roll into the rectum. This step facilitates the dissection between mucosa and muscle.

Continue the dissection to a point 4–6 cm above the dentate line **(Fig. 48–3)**. As the dissection continues cephalad, exposure is obtained by inserting two narrow Deaver retractors the assistant holds in varying positions appropriate to the area being dissected.

After an adequate tube of mucosa 4–6 cm in length has been dissected, insert a purse-string suture near the apex of the dissected mucosal tube and amputate the mucosa distal to the suture. Submit this specimen to the pathologist for frozen-section histologic examination. Insert into the denuded rectum a loose gauze pack that has been moistened with an epinephrine solution. Reposition the patient on his or her back with the lower extremities elevated on Lloyd-Davies stirrups (see Figs. 45-3a, 45-3b).

Abdominal Incision and Exposure

In patients who have undergone a previous subtotal colectomy with a mucous fistula and an ileostomy, reopen the previous long vertical incision, free all of the adhesions between the small bowel and the peritoneum, and liberate the mucous fistula from the abdominal wall. Divide the mesentery between Kelly hemostats along a line close to the posterior wall of the sigmoid and rectosigmoid until the peritoneal reflection is reached. Incise the peritoneal reflection to the right and to the left of the rectum. Continue the dissection downward and free the vascular and areolar tissue from the wall of the rectum. Then elevate the rectum out of the presacral space and in-

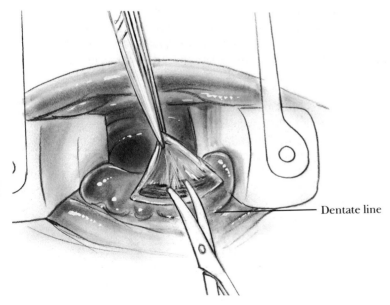

— Dentate line

Fig. 48-2

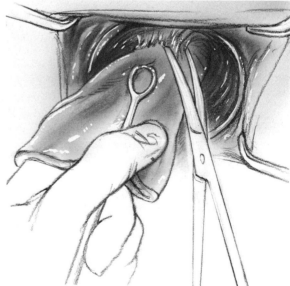

Fig. 48-3

cise the peritoneum of the rectovesical or rectouterine pouch (see Fig. 45-9). Keep the dissection close to the rectal wall, especially in male patients, to avoid the nervi erigentes and the hypogastric nerves. Pay special attention to dividing the lateral ligaments close to the rectum and avoid the parasympathetic plexus between the prostate and the rectum.

With a long-handled scalpel incise Waldeyer's fascia (see Fig. 45-10) between the tip of the coccyx and the posterior wall of the rectum. Enlarge this incision with long Metzenbaum scissors. In male patients incise Denonvilliers' fascia (see Fig. 45-11) on the anterior wall of the rectum proximal to the prostate and the seminal vesicles. Separate the prostate from the rectum. These last two maneuvers permit exposure of the levator diaphragm. Palpating the rectum at this time should enable the surgeon to detect the level at which the purse-string suture was placed in the mucosa during the first phase of this operation. If this purse-string suture is not palpable, ask the assistant to place a finger in the rectum from the perineal approach to help identify the apex of the previous mucosal dissection. Now transect the rectum with electrocautery and remove the specimen. Remove the gauze packing that was previously placed in the rectal stump and inspect the muscular cylinder, which is all that remains of the rectum. This consists of the circular muscle of the internal sphincter surrounded by the longitudinal muscle of the rectum. All of the mucosa has been removed down to the dentate line. Check for complete hemostasis.

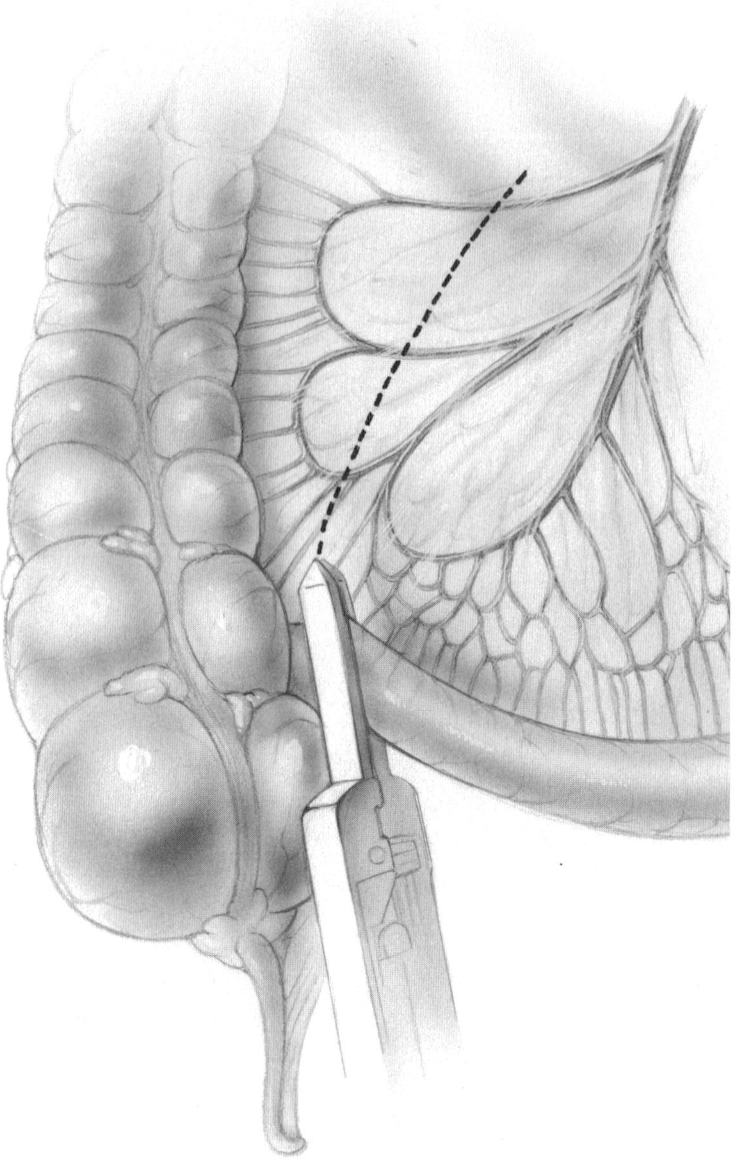

Constructing the Ileal Reservoir

In patients who have had a previous ileostomy, carefully dissect the ileum away from the abdominal wall, preserving as much ileum as possible. Apply a 55/3.5 mm linear stapler across a healthy portion of the terminal ileum. Fire the stapler and amputate the scarred portion of the ileostomy. Lightly cauterize the everted mucosa and remove the stapling device. Now liberate the mesentery of the ileum from its attachment to the abdominal parietes. For patients who have not undergone a previous ileostomy, divide the terminal ileum with a cutting linear stapling device and divide the mesentery along the path indicated in **Figure 48-4**. Freeing the small bowel mesentery from its posterior attachments (see Figs. 35-1, 35-2) and all other adhesions may elongate the mesentery sufficiently that the ileal reservoir reaches the anal canal *without tension*.

Now select a point on the ileum about 20 cm from its distal margin that will serve as the future site of the ileoanal anastomosis. If this point on the ileum can be brought 6 cm beyond the symphysis pubis, one can be assured that there will be no tension on the anastomosis. Otherwise, further lengthen the mesentery by incising the peritoneum on the anterior and posterior surfaces of the ileal mesentery. Burnstein and associates reported that these relaxing incisions each contributed 1 cm to the length of the ileal mesentery. Obtain additional length, if necessary, by applying traction to the anticipated elbow of the J-pouch **(Fig. 48-5)**, transilluminating the mesentery, and selectively dividing branches of the loop formed by the superior mesenteric and ileocolic arteries as shown in **Figure 48-6**.

Be certain that the blood supply to the terminal ileum remains vigorous and that there is no tension

Fig. 48-4

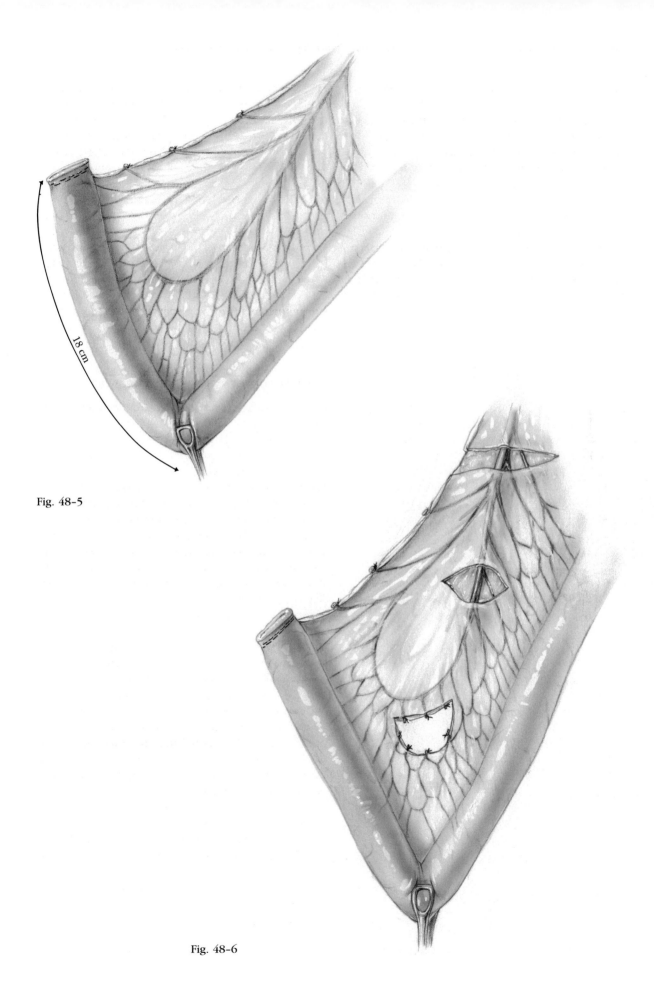

Fig. 48-5

Fig. 48-6

on the ileoanal anastomosis. Take great care to isolate and ligate each vessel in the ileal mesentery individually, especially if the mesentery is thickened from scar tissue or obesity, to avoid postoperative bleeding. If an inadequately ligated vessel retracts into the mesentery, the resulting tense hematoma may produce ileal ischemia.

Now align the distal ileum in the shape of a U, each limb of which measures about 18 cm. Create a side-to-side stapled anastomosis between the antimesenteric aspects of the ascending and descending limbs of this U. Make a transverse stab wound 9 cm proximal to the staple line of the terminal ileum. Make a second transverse stab wound in the descending limb of ileum just opposite the first stab wound **(Fig. 48–7)**. Insert an 80 mm linear cutting stapler in a cephalad direction, one fork in the descending limb and one fork in the ascending limb of jejunum. Remember that this anastomosis is created on the *antimesenteric* borders of both limbs of the jejunum. Fire the stapler, creating an 8 cm side-to-side anastomosis. Withdraw the stapling device and inspect the staple line for bleeding. Electrocauterize bleeding points cautiously. Then reinsert the device into the same two stab wounds but direct the stapler in a caudal direction **(Fig. 48–8)**. Lock the device

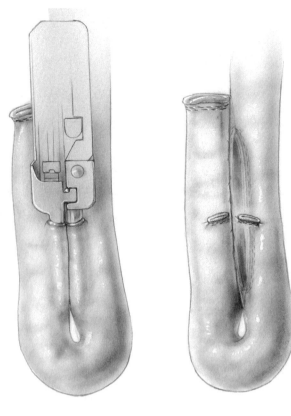

Fig. 48-8   Fig. 48-9

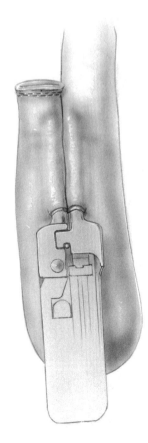

Fig. 48-7

and fire the staples. Remove the stapler and inspect for bleeding. Inspect the staple line via the stab wounds and electrocauterize the bleeding points. The patient should now have a completed side-to-side stapled anastomosis about 16 cm in length. We prefer to leave an intact circular loop of ileum distal to the side-to-side anastomosis to ensure that the bowel to be anastomosed has not been traumatized.

The ileal reservoir is now complete except for the remaining stab wound through which the stapling device was previously inserted. Apply Allis clamps to approximate, in a transverse direction, the walls of the ileum in preparation for transverse application of a 55/3.5 mm linear stapling device, which will accomplish everted closure of the defect. Be certain that the superior and inferior terminations of the previous staple lines are included in the stapler before firing it. Also, avoid the error of trying to fire the linear stapler when the two terminations of the previous staple lines are in exact apposition (see Figs. 43–21 to 43–23). After firing the stapler, lightly electrocauterize the everted mucosa and carefully inspect the staple line to be sure of proper B formation **(Fig. 48–9)**.

Alternatively, *sutures* may be used to construct the side-to-side anastomosis. Make longitudinal incisions along the antimesentric borders of both the ascending and descending limbs of the ileum. Achieve hemostasis with electrocautery. Insert interrupted sutures to approximate the bowel walls at the proximal and distal margins of the anastomosis with 3-0 Vicryl sutures. Insert another suture at the midpoint between these two. Then use a straight atraumatic intestinal needle with 3-0 Vicryl starting at the apex of the posterior portion of the anastomosis and use a continuous locked suture, encompassing all the layers of the bowel. Accomplish closure of the anterior layer of the anastomosis by means of a continuous seromucosal or Lembert suture (see Figs. 4-13, 4-14). Carefully inspect all aspects of the side-to-side anastomosis, both front and back, to be certain there are no defects or technical errors.

Ileoanal Anastomosis

Before passing the elbow of the ileal reservoir down through the anus, recheck the position of the pelvis and buttocks on the operating table. The perineum should project beyond the edge of the table. The simplest method for exposing the dentate line for the anastomosis is to insert two Gelpi retractors, one at right angles to the other. The prongs of the retractors should be inserted fairly close to the dentate line so the transected anorectal junction can be seen. Insert the first Gelpi retractor in the axis between 2 and 8 o'clock and the second between 5 and 11 o'clock. If exposure is not adequate, it may be helpful to readjust the stirrups so the thighs are flexed on the abdomen. This position makes it more convenient to apply retractors to the anus.

After making certain that hemostasis in the pelvis is complete, insert two long Babcock clamps through the anus and grasp the dependent portion of the ileal reservoir. Bring this segment of ileum into the anal canal. Be certain that the bowel has not been twisted during this maneuver and that the mesentery lies flat *without significant tension* on the planned anastomosis. Make a longitudinal incision along the dependent border of the ileal reservoir. Cauterize the bleeding points. Apply traction sutures to the incised ileum, one to each quadrant **(Fig. 48–10)**. Construct a one-layer anastomosis be-

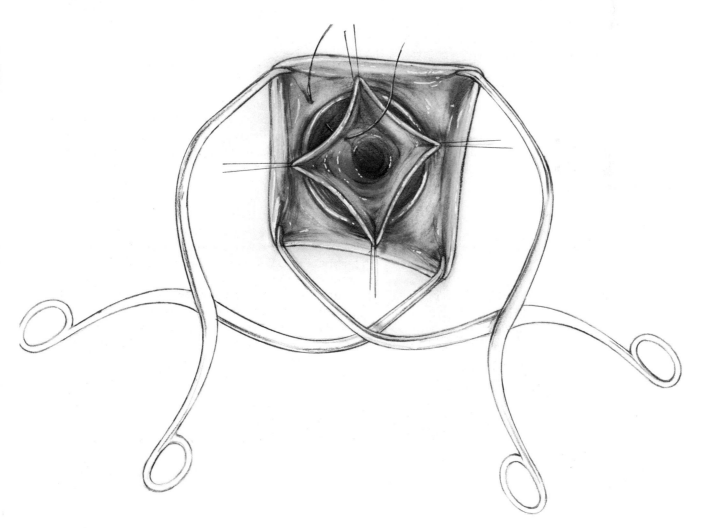

Fig. 48-10

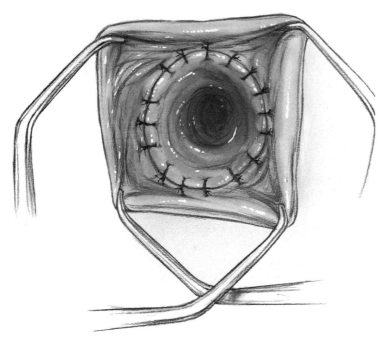

Fig. 48-11

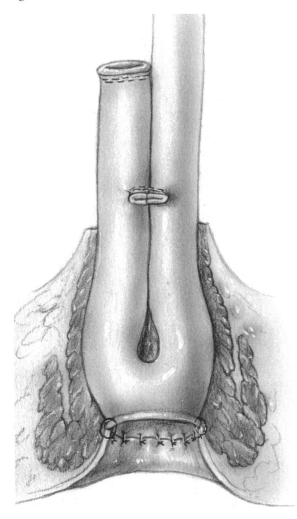

Fig. 48-12

tween the ileum and the dentate line of the anus. Be sure to include in each stitch a 4 mm bite of underlying internal sphincter muscle as well as anal epithelium. Use atraumatic 4-0 PG or PDS sutures **(Fig. 48–11)**. If the anal canal is deep, a double-curved Stratte needle-holder (see Figs. G-17, G-18) is helpful. Insert the first four sutures at 12, 6, 3, and 9 o'clock. Then continue to insert sutures by the method of successive bisection (see Figs. 4-19, 4-20). The resulting ileoanal anastomosis should be widely patent (Fig. 48-11). If desired, the ileal reservoir may now be inflated with a methylene blue solution to check for possible defects in the reservoir staple or suture lines. **Figure 48–12** illustrates the completed anastomosis.

Loop Ileostomy

Until more evidence has accumulated to demonstrate that this step is not necessary, we believe that these patients should have a temporary diverting loop ileostomy (see Chapter 51). If the patient has a defect in the abdominal wall that remains after dismantling a previous ileostomy, it is generally possible to use the same site for the loop ileostomy. Insert a large Babcock clamp through the opening in the abdominal wall and grasp the antimesenteric aspect of a segment of ileum proximal to the ileal reservoir. Select a segment of ileum that does not exert any tension whatever on the ileal reservoir. Construct the loop ileostomy as described later (see Figs. 51-1 through 51-4).

Drainage and Closure

Hematoma or infection in the space between the rectal cuff and the ileal reservoir may produce fibrosis and impair fecal continence. Consequently, at this point in the operation make every effort to achieve complete hemostasis in the rectal cuff and in the pelvis. Insert one or two Jackson Pratt silicone closed-suction drains through puncture wounds in the abdominal wall down to the rectal cuff. Some believe it is important to place a layer of sutures between the proximal cut end of the rectal cuff and the ileal reservoir. Although we do not believe that these sutures can compensate for an inadequate ileoanal anastomosis, they may help prevent tension on the pouch.

Close the abdominal wall with interrupted No. 1 PDS by the modified Smead-Jones technique described in Chapter 3. Close the skin with interrupted fine nylon or skin staples. Then mature the loop ileostomy as described above if this step has not already been done.

POSTOPERATIVE CARE

Continue perioperative antibiotics for 24 hours. Continue nasogastric suction until the ileostomy begins to function. Remove the closed-suction drains from the pelvis between postoperative days 4 and 6, depending on the volume of drainage. (Inject 25 mg kanamycin in 25 ml saline into the drainage catheters every 8 hours.)

Until the loop ileostomy is closed, perform weekly or biweekly digital examinations of the ileoanal anastomosis to prevent the development of a stricture. About 8 weeks following operation, rule out anastomotic defects by direct inspection and palpation. If there has been uneventful healing with no evidence of hematoma or sepsis in the pelvis, perform a barium enema to visualize the ileal reservoir. If both these procedures are negative, close the loop ileostomy. Following closure of the loop ileostomy, regulation of the bowel movements takes time and sometimes requires dietary adjustment and medication to achieve optimum continence.

COMPLICATIONS

An abscess may occur in the rectal cuff or pelvis. This complication has been reported during the early postoperative period and, remarkably, 2 and 6 months after operation in other cases. If the loop ileostomy is still in place, most cuff abscesses can be treated by drainage directly through the anastomosis. Pelvic abscesses may require laparotomy or computed tomography-guided percutaneous catheter insertion for drainage. With proper precautions postoperative sepsis is rare.

Hematoma in pelvis or in reservoir.

Anastomotic dehiscence or stricture.

Wound infection.

Urinary tract infection.

Excessive number of stools.

Fecal incontinence.

Pouchitis (more likely to occur in patients with in-flammatory bowel disease). Treatment with metronidazole may be sufficient.

Pouch surveillance is performed in patients with familial polyposis syndromes. Polyps have been known to form in the ileal reservoir.

Acute intestinal obstruction due to adhesions.

REFERENCES

Burnstein MJ, Schoetz DJ Jr, Collier JA, et al. Technique of mesenteric lengthening in ileal reservoir–anal anastomosis. Dis Colon Rectum 1987;30:863.

Cohen Z, McLeod RS, Stephen W, et al. Continuing evolution of the pelvic pouch procedure. Ann Surg 1992;216:506.

Dehni N, Schlegel RD, Cunningham C, et al. Influence of a defunctioning stoma on leakage rates after low colorectal anastomosis and colonic J pouch-anal anastomosis. Br J Surg 1998;85:1114.

Fazio VW, O'Riordain MG, Lavery IC, et al. Long-term functional outcome and quality of life after stapled restorative proctocolectomy. Ann Surg 1999;230:575.

McCourtney JS, Finlay IG. Totally stapled restorative proctocolectomy. Br J Surg 1997;84:808.

Meagher AP, Farouk R, Dozois RR, Kelly KA, Pemberton H. J-Ileal pouch–anal anastomosis for chronic ulcerative colitis: complications and long-term outcome in 1310 patients. Br J Surg 1998;85:800.

Michelassi F, Hurst R. Restorative proctocolectomy with J-pouch ileoanal anastomosis. Arch Surg 2000;135:347.

Mowschenson PM, Critchlow JF, Peppercorn MA. Ileoanal pouch operation: long-term outcome with or without diverting ileostomy. Arch Surg 2000;135:463.

Reilly WT, Pemberton JH, Wolff BG, et al. Randomized prospective trial comparing ileal pouch–anal anastomosis performed by excising the anal mucosa to ileal pouch–anal anastomosis performed by preserving the anal mucosa. Ann Surg 1997;225:666.

Sullivan ES, Garnjobst WM. Advantage of initial transanal musocal stripping in ileo-anal pull-through procedures. Dis Colon Rectum 1982;25:170.

Thompson-Fawcett MW, Warren BF, Mortensen NJ. A new look at the anal transitional zone with reference to restorative proctocolectomy and the columnar cuff. Br J Surg 1998;85:1517.

49 Abdominoperineal Proctectomy for Benign Disease

INDICATIONS

Inflammatory bowel disease, including ulcerative colitis and Crohn's colitis with intractable rectal involvement that precludes restorative proctocolectomy

PREOPERATIVE PREPARATION

See Chapter 48.

PITFALLS AND DANGER POINTS

Operative damage to or interruption of pelvic autonomic nerves in male patients, leading to sexual impotence or failure of ejaculation

Pelvis sepsis, especially in patients who have perineal fistulas

Inadequate management of perineal wound, resulting in a chronic perineal draining sinus

OPERATIVE STRATEGY

Abdominoperineal proctectomy is not a cancer operation. Resection should be conservative, and every attempt should be made to avoid damage to adjacent structures.

Transection of the hypogastric sympathetic nerve trunks that cross over the anterior aorta causes ejaculatory failure in men. Beyond the aortic bifurcation these nerves diverge into two bundles going toward the region of the right and left hypogastric arteries, where they join the inferior hypogastric plexus on each side. According to Lee et al. (1973) the *parasympathetic* sacral autonomic outflow is interrupted if the lateral ligaments are divided too far lateral to the rectum or if the nerve plexus between the rectum and prostate is damaged. Parasympathetic nerve damage results in failure of erection. Proper strategy requires that the mesentery in the region of the rectosigmoid be divided along a line just adjacent to the colon, leaving considerable fat and mesentery in the presacral space to protect the hypogastric nerves. The remainder of the pelvic dissection should be carried out as close to the rectum as possible, *especially in the region of the lateral ligaments and prostate*.

So long as there are no multiple perineal fistulas, it is generally possible to achieve primary healing of the perineum *if deadspace between the closed levators and the peritoneal pelvic floor is eliminated*. Because there is no need for radical excision of the pelvic peritoneum, preserve as much of it as possible and mobilize additional pelvic peritoneum from the lateral walls of the pelvis and the bladder. If there is sufficient peritoneum to permit the pelvic peritoneal suture line to come down easily into contact with the reconstructed levator diaphragm, close this layer. Otherwise it is much better to leave the pelvic peritoneum entirely unsutured to permit the small bowel to fill this space. To aid in preventing perineal sinus formation due to chronic low-grade sepsis, insert closed-suction catheters into the presacral space and instill an antibiotic solution postoperatively.

Lyttle and Parks (1977) advocate *preservation of the external sphincter muscles*. They begin the perineal dissection with an incision near the dentate line of the anal canal and continue the dissection in the intersphincteric space between the internal and external sphincters of the anal canal. Thus the rectum is cored out of the anal canal, leaving the entire levator diaphragm and external sphincters intact. We have used this technique and found that it causes less operative trauma, minimizes deadspace, and may further reduce the incidence of damage to the prerectal nerve plexus.

OPERATIVE TECHNIQUE

Abdominal Incision and Position

With the patient positioned on Lloyd-Davies leg rests, thighs abducted and slightly flexed, make a midline incision from the mid-epigastrium to the pubis (see Fig. 45-3a). If the patient has previously undergone subtotal colectomy with ileostomy and mucous fistula, free the mucous fistula from its attachments to the abdominal wall. Ligate the lumen with umbilical tape and cover it with a sterile rubber glove.

Mesenteric Dissection

Divide the mesentery between sequentially applied Kelly clamps along a line *close to the posterior wall* of the rectosigmoid. Continue the line of dissection well into the presacral space. This leaves a considerable amount of fat and mesentery behind to cover the bifurcation of the aorta and sacrum **(Fig. 49–1)**. The fat and mesentery prevent injury to the hypogastric nerve bundles, which travel from the preaortic area down the promontory of the sacrum toward the hypogastric vessels on each side to join the hypogastric plexuses on each side (see Figs. 45-4, 45-6).

Rectal Dissection

Incise the pelvic peritoneum along the line where the peritoneum joins the rectum, preserving as much peritoneum as possible. Accomplish this first on the right and then on the left side (see Fig. 45-5). Note the location of each ureter (see Fig. 45-6). Divide the posterior mesentery to the mid-sacral level. The posterior wall of rectum can now be seen, as at this point the blood supply of the rectum comes from the lateral wall of the pelvis. Elevate the rectum from the distal sacrum by blunt dissection and with Metzenbaum scissors incise Waldeyer's fascia close to the rectum. Draw the rectum in a cephalad direction and place the peritoneum of the rectovesical or rectouterine pouch on stretch. This peritoneum can now be divided easily with Metzenbaum scissors. Division of the lateral ligament can also be accomplished with good hemostasis by inserting a right-angle clamp underneath the ligament and dividing the overlying tissue with electrocautery (see Fig. 45-9).

With cephalad traction on the rectum and a Lloyd-Davies retractor holding the bladder forward, divide

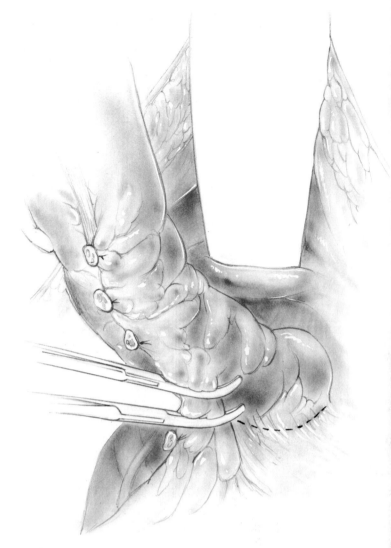

Fig. 49-1

Denonvilliers' fascia at the level of the proximal portion of the prostate (see Fig. 45-11b). Keep the dissection *close to the anterior rectal wall*, which should be bluntly separated from the body of the prostate. In female patients, the dissection separates the rectum from the vagina. When the dissection has continued beyond the tip of the coccyx posteriorly and the prostate anteriorly, initiate the perineal dissection.

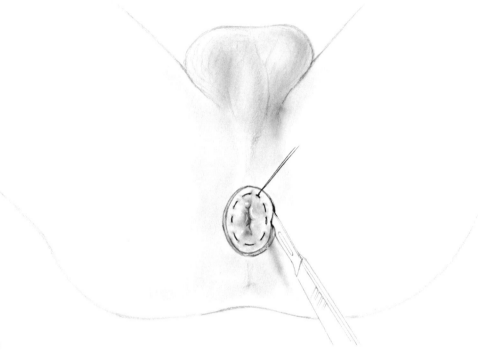

Fig. 49-2

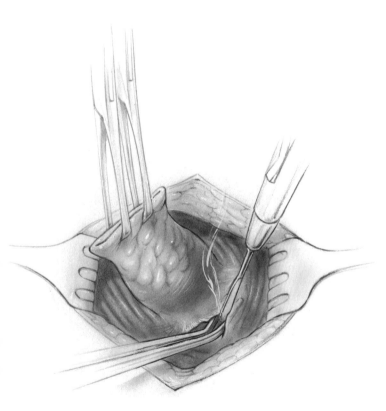

Fig. 49-3

Perineal Incision

Close the skin of the anal canal with a heavy purse-string suture **(Fig. 49–2)**. Then make an incision circumferentially in the skin just outside the sphincter muscles of the anus. Carry the dissection down *close* to the outer margins of the external sphincter to the levator muscles **(Fig. 49–3)**. The inferior hemorrhoidal vessels are encountered running toward the rectum overlying the levator muscles. Occlude these vessels by electrocautery. After the incision has been deepened to the levators on both sides, expose the tip of the coccyx. Transect the anococcygeal ligament by electrocautery and enter the presacral space posteriorly. The fascia of Waldeyer, which attaches to the anterior surfaces of the lower sacrum and coccyx and to the posterior rectum, forms a barrier that blocks entrance into the presacral space from below even after the anococcygeal ligament has been divided. If this fascia is elevated from the sacral periosteum by forceful blunt dissection in the perineum, venous bleeding and damage to the sacral neural components of the nervi erigentes may occur. Consequently, divide this *sharply* from above (Fig. 45-10) or below before an attempt is made to enter the presacral space from below.

Division of Levator Diaphragm

From the perineal approach, insert the left index finger into the opening to the presacral space and place

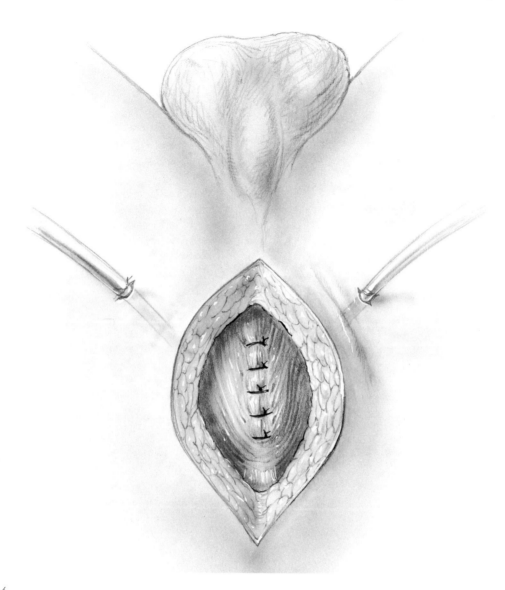

Fig. 49-4

it in the groove between the rectum and the levator muscles. Use electrocautery to divide the levators close to the rectum on either side. Then deliver the specimen from the presacral space down through the posterior perineum, so the anal canal is attached only anteriorly. Visualize the prostate gland. Using electrocautery, transect the puborectalis and rectourethralis muscles close to the anterior rectal wall. Carry this dissection down to the level of the prostate and remove the specimen.

Closure of Pelvic Floor

Insert one or two large (6 mm) plastic catheters through the skin of the perineum and the levator muscles into the presacral space for closed-suction drainage. Alternatively, these drains may be brought up from the presacral space into the pelvis and out through puncture wounds of the abdominal wall.

Close the defect in the levator diaphragm using interrupted sutures of 2-0 PG after thoroughly irrigating the pelvis with an antibiotic solution and achieving perfect hemostasis **(Fig. 49–4)**. Close the skin with subcuticular sutures of 4-0 PG. Attach the catheters to suction for the remainder of the procedure while an assistant closes the peritoneum of the pelvic floor with continuous 2-0 PG sutures using the abdominal approach.

Ileostomy

Choose a suitable site and construct a terminal ileostomy as described in Chapter 50 (if not already performed during a previous operation).

Abdominal Closure

After checking the integrity of the peritoneal pelvic suture line and making certain it is contiguous with the pelvic floor, irrigate the abdominal cavity and pelvis. Approximate the abdominal wall with interrupted sutures using the modified Smead-Jones technique.

POSTOPERATIVE CARE

See Chapter 46.

COMPLICATIONS

See Chapter 46.

REFERENCES

Lee JF, Maurer VM, Block GE. Anatomic relations of pelvic autonomic nerves to pelvic operations. Arch Surg 1973; 107:324.

Lyttle JA, Parks AG. Intersphincteric excision of the rectum. Br J Surg 1977;64:413.

O'Bichere A, Wilkinson K, Rumbles S, et al. Functional outcome after restorative panproctocolectomy for ulcerative colitis decreases an otherwise enhanced quality of life. Br J Surg 2000;87:802.

50 End-Ileostomy

INDICATIONS

An end-ileostomy is generally done in conjunction with a subtotal or total colectomy for inflammatory bowel disease. Continent alternatives have been developed (see References).

Occasionally a temporary end-ileostomy and mucous fistula of the distal end of the bowel is constructed after resection of a gangrenous segment of intestine or a perforated cecal lesion, when primary anastomosis is contraindicated.

PITFALLS AND DANGER POINTS

Devascularization of an excessive amount of terminal ileum, with resultant necrosis and stricture formation

Ileocutaneous fistula resulting from a too-deep stitch in the seromuscular layer of the ileum when fashioning the ileostomy

OPERATIVE STRATEGY

Prevention of peristomal skin excoriation (due to escape of small bowel contents underneath the faceplate of the ileostomy appliance) requires formation of a permanently protruding ileostomy. Properly performed, the ileostomy resembles the cervix of the uterus. A permanent protrusion of 2.0 cm is desirable, which allows for the likelihood that an underweight patient accumulates a subcutaneous layer of fat following successful surgery for colitis. To prevent herniation of the small bowel, close the gap between the cut edge of the ileum and the lateral abdominal wall when fashioning a permanent ileostomy.

OPERATIVE TECHNIQUE

Preoperative Selection of Ileostomy Site

Apply the face-plate of an ileostomy appliance tentatively to various positions in the right lower quadrant of the patient to make sure it does not come into contact with the costal margin or the antero-superior spine when the patient is in a sitting position. The face-plate should not extend beyond the mid-rectus line or the umbilicus. During emergency operations, when an ileostomy has not been contemplated, the site for the ileostomy should be placed approximately 5 cm to the right of the midline and about 4 cm below the umbilicus.

Incision

Because ileostomy generally is not the main part of the contemplated operation, a midline incision has already been made. Now make a circular incision in the previously selected site in the right lower quadrant and excise a circle of skin the diameter of a nickel (2 cm) **(Fig. 50–1)**. The incision then spontaneously stretches to the proper diameter. Make a linear incision down to the anterior rectus fascia and insert retractors to expose the fascia. Do not excise a core of subcutaneous fat unless the patient is significantly obese.

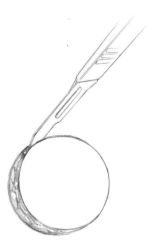

Fig. 50–1

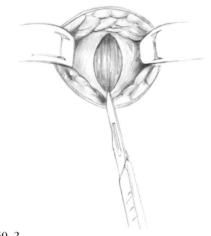

Fig. 50-2

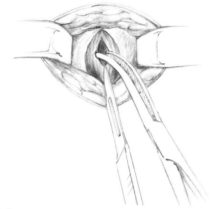

Fig. 50-3

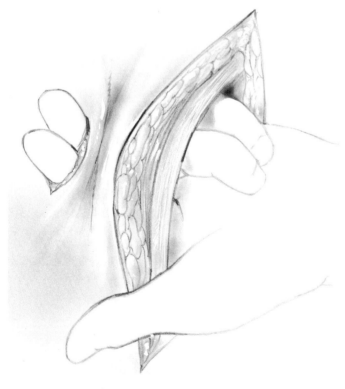

Fig. 50-4

Make a longitudinal 2 cm incision in the fascia, exposing the rectus muscle **(Fig. 50–2)**. Separate the muscle fibers with a Kelly hemostat **(Fig. 50–3)** and make a longitudinal incision in the peritoneum. Then dilate the opening in the abdominal wall by inserting two fingers **(Fig. 50–4)**.

Fashioning the Ileal Mesentery

At least 6–7 cm of ileum is required beyond the point at which the ileum meets the peritoneum if a proper ileostomy of the protruding type is to be made. More length may be required in the obese patient. If the entire mesentery is removed from this length of ileum, necrosis of the distal ileal mucosa takes place in many patients. Consequently, the portion of the ileum that passes through the abdominal wall must retain a sufficient width of mesentery to ensure vascularity. The "marginal" artery can be visualized in the mesentery within 2 cm of the ileal wall. Preserve this segment of vasculature while carefully dividing the mesentery. Complete removal of the mesentery is well tolerated at the distal 2–3 cm of the ileum.

Closure of Mesenteric Gap

Insert a Babcock clamp into the abdominal cavity through the opening made for the ileostomy. Grasp the terminal ileum with the clamp and gently bring it through this opening, with the mesentery placed in a cephalad direction **(Fig. 50–5)**. Place no sutures between the ileum and the peritoneum or the rectus fascia **(Fig. 50–6)**.

Using a continuous 2-0 PG suture, suture the cut edge of the ileal mesentery to the cut edge of the paracolic peritoneum. This maneuver completely obliterates the mesenteric defect **(Fig. 50–7)**.

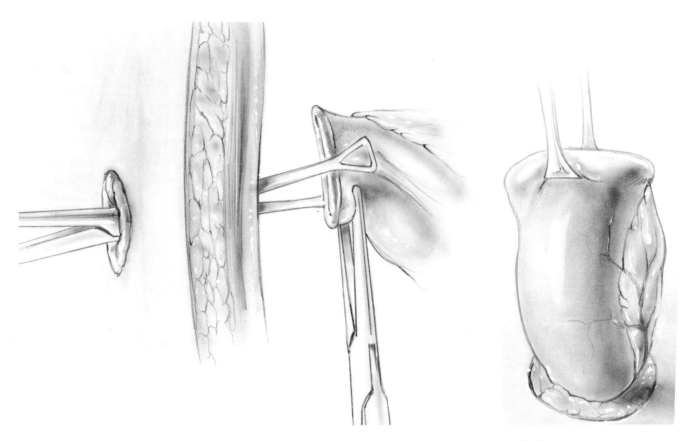

Fig. 50-5

Fig. 50-6

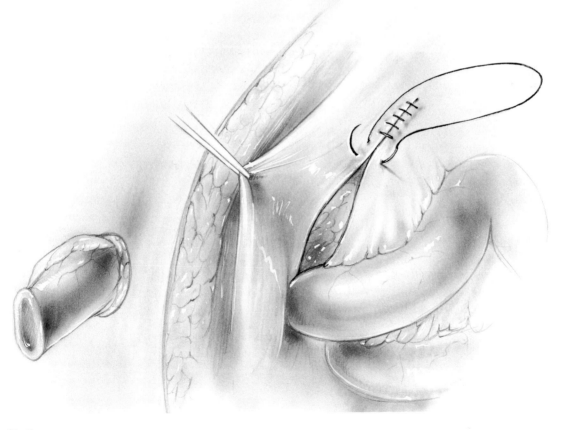

Fig. 50-7

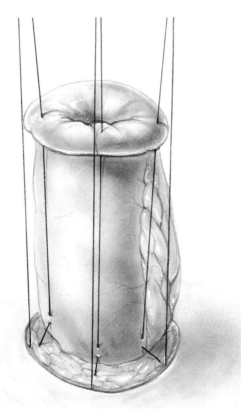

Fig. 50-8

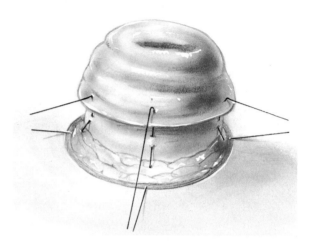

Fig. 50-9

Mucocutaneous Fixation of Ileostomy

Construct a "cervix" by inserting interrupted 4-0 PG sutures through the full thickness of the terminal ileum; then, using the same needle, take a shallow seromuscular bite of the lateral wall of the ileum, which is situated opposite the level of the skin. Complete the suture by taking a bite of the subcuticular layer of skin **(Fig. 50–8)**. Temporarily hold the stitch in a hemostat and place identical stitches in each of the other quadrants of the ileostomy. After all the sutures have been inserted tighten them gently to evert the ileum **(Fig. 50–9)**. Then tie the sutures. Place one additional suture of the same type between each of the four quadrant sutures, completing the mucocutaneous fixation.

POSTOPERATIVE CARE

Nasogastric suction may be required, depending on the nature of the primary procedure.

Prescribe perioperative antibiotics.

Apply a Stomahesive disk to the ileostomy in the operating room; place an ileostomy bag over the disk.

Instruct the patient in ileostomy care.

COMPLICATIONS

Early problems

   Occasional necrosis of the distal ileum (although rare when good technique is used)

   Peristomal infection or fistula

Late problems

   Prolapse of ileostomy

   Stricture of ileostomy

   Obstruction of ileostomy due to food fiber

   Peristomal skin ulceration

REFERENCE

Dozois RR. Alternative to Conventional Ileostomy. Chicago, Year Book, 1985.

51 Loop Ileostomy

INDICATIONS

Loop ileostomy is performed when temporary diversion of the fecal stream is required. It may be used to protect a tenuous colon anastomosis or as part of the initial treatment of severe inflammatory bowel disease.

In some patients loop ileostomy is easier to construct than end-ileostomy. It allows better preservation of the blood supply to the stoma.

PITFALLS AND DANGER POINTS

If the ileum is not transected at the proper point, to make the proximal stoma the dominant one, total fecal diversion is not accomplished.

See Chapter 50.

OPERATIVE STRATEGY

Properly performed, this technique is a good method for achieving temporary but complete diversion of the intestinal contents. Because the entire mesentery is preserved, the blood supply to the stoma is optimized. Closure can be accomplished by a local plastic procedure or by local resection and anastomosis.

OPERATIVE TECHNIQUE

If a loop ileostomy is being performed as a primary procedure, a midline incision beginning at the umbilicus and proceeding caudally for 8–10 cm is adequate. Identify the distal ileum and the segment selected for ileostomy by applying a single marking suture to that segment of the ileum that will form the *proximal* limb of the loop ileostomy.

Select the proper site in the right lower quadrant (see Chapter 50) and excise a nickel-size circle of skin. Expose the anterior rectus fascia and make a 2 cm longitudinal incision in it (see Fig. 50-1). Separate the rectus fibers with a large hemostat and make a similar vertical incision in the peritoneum (see Figs. 50-2, 50-3). Then stretch the ileostomy orifice by inserting two fingers (see Fig. 50-4).

After this step has been accomplished, insert a Babcock clamp through the aperture into the abdominal cavity. Arrange the ileum so the proximal segment emerges on the cephalad side of the ileostomy. Then grasp the ileum with the Babcock clamp and deliver it through the abdominal wall with the aid of digital manipulation from inside the abdomen. The proximal limb should be on the cephalad surface of the ileostomy.

Confirm that there is no tension whatever on any distal anastomosis **(Fig. 51–1)**. Position the ileum so the afferent or proximal limb of ileum enters the stoma from its cephalad aspect and the distal ileum leaves the stoma at its inferior aspect. To ensure that the proximal stoma dominates the distal stoma and completely diverts the fecal stream, transect the anterior half of the ileum at a point 2 cm distal to the

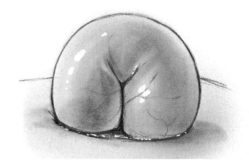

Fig. 51-1

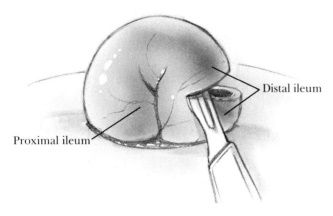

Fig. 51-2

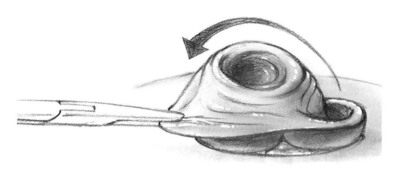

Fig. 51-3

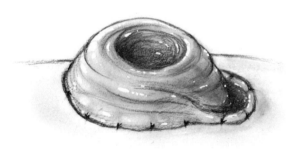

Fig. 51-4

apex of the loop **(Fig. 51–2)**. Then evert the ileostomy **(Fig. 51–3)**. Insert interrupted atraumatic sutures of 4-0 PG to approximate the full thickness of the ileum to the subcuticular portion of the skin. The end result should be a dominant proximal stoma

that compresses the distal stoma **(Fig. 51–4)**. We do not suture the ileum to the peritoneum or fascia.

To minimize contamination of the abdominal cavity, it is possible to deliver the loop of ileum through the abdominal wall and then pass a small catheter around the ileum and through the mesentery to maintain the position of the ileum. Division of the ileum and suturing of the ileostomy may be postponed until the abdominal incision has been completely closed. After suturing the ileum to the subcutis, remove the catheter.

Close the abdominal wall with interrupted No. 1 PDS sutures by the modified Smead-Jones technique described in Chapter 3. Close the skin with interrupted fine nylon or skin staples. Then mature the loop ileostomy as described above if this step has not already been done.

POSTOPERATIVE CARE

See Chapter 50.

COMPLICATIONS

See Chapter 50.

REFERENCES

Beagley MJ, Poole G, Peat BG, Rees MJ. The use of temporary laparoscopic loop ileostomy in lumbosacral burns. Burns 2000;26:298.

Flati G, Talarico C, Carboni M. An improved technique for temporary diverting ileostomy. Surg Today 2000;30: 104.

Fonkalsrud EW, Thakur A, Roof L. Comparison of loop versus end ileostomy for fecal diversion after restorative proctocolectomy for ulcerative colitis. J Am Coll Surg 2000;190:418.

Hasegawa H, Radley S, Morton DG, Keighley MR. Stapled versus sutured closure of loop ileostomy: a randomized controlled trial. Ann Surg 2000;231:202.

Lane JS, Kwan D, Chandler CF, et al. Diverting loop versus end ileostomy during ileoanal pullthrough procedure for ulcerative colitis. Am Surg 1998;64:979.

Turnbull R, Weakley FL. Surgical treatment of toxic megacolon: ileostomy and colostomy to prepare patients for colectomy. Am J Surg 1971;122:325.

52 Cecostomy

Surgical Legacy Technique

INDICATIONS

Cecostomy is an alternative to resection when there is impending perforation of the cecum secondary to a colonic obstruction or ileus. Colonoscopic decompression is a better alternative for cases of pseudo-obstruction. Cecostomy is used only when other methods have failed.

PREOPERATIVE PREPARATION

Perioperative antibiotics

Nasogastric suction

Fluid resuscitation

PITFALLS AND DANGER POINTS

Cecostomy may fail to produce adequate decompression.

Limited exploration through a small incision may miss an area of perforation elsewhere.

Fecal matter may spill into the peritoneal cavity.

OPERATIVE STRATEGY

There are two kinds of cecostomy. A simple tube cecostomy is constructed in a manner analogous to a Stamm gastrostomy (see Chapter 32). Even a large tube is easily plugged by fecal debris, and this kind of cecostomy primarily allows decompression of gas and liquid. The main advantage of tube cecostomy is that when the cecostomy is no longer needed removing the tube frequently results in spontaneous closure. The skin-sutured cecostomy described here provides more certain decompression but requires formal closure. In the attempt to avoid fecal contamination of the abdominal cavity during this operation, the cecum is sutured to the external oblique aponeurosis before being incised.

OPERATIVE TECHNIQUE

Skin-Sutured Cecostomy

Incision

Make a transverse incision about 4–5 cm long over McBurney's point and carry it in the same line through the skin, external oblique aponeurosis, the internal oblique and transversus muscles, and the peritoneum. Do not attempt to split the muscles along the line of their fibers.

Exploration of Cecum

Rule out patches of necrosis in areas beyond the line of incision by carefully exploring the cecum. To accomplish this without the danger of rupturing the cecum, insert a 16-gauge needle attached to an empty 50 cc syringe, which releases some of the pressure. After this has been accomplished, close the puncture wound with a fine suture. Elevate the abdominal wall with a retractor to expose the anterior and lateral walls of the cecum. If the exposure is inadequate, make a larger incision. If a necrotic patch of cecum can be identified, use this region as the site for the cecostomy and excise it during the procedure.

Cecal Fixation

Suture the wall of the cecum to the external oblique aponeurosis with a continuous 4-0 PG suture on a

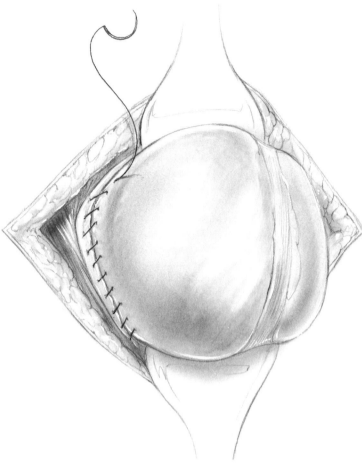

Fig. 52-1

fine needle to prevent any fecal spillage from reaching the peritoneal cavity **(Fig. 52–1)**. If the incision in the external oblique aponeurosis is longer than 4-5 cm, narrow it with several PG sutures. Narrow the skin incision also to the same length with several fine PG subcuticular sutures.

Mucocutaneous Suture

Make a transverse incision in the anterior wall of the cecum 4 cm long **(Fig. 52–2)** and aspirate liquid stool and gas. Then suture the full thickness of the cecal wall to the subcuticular layer of the skin with a continuous or interrupted suture of 4-0 PG on an atraumatic needle **(Fig. 52–3)**. Place a properly fitted ileostomy bag over the cecostomy at the conclusion of the operation.

Tube Cecostomy

The abdominal incision and exploration of the cecum for a tube cecostomy are identical to those done for a skin-sutured cecostomy. Insert a purse-string suture in a circular fashion on the anterior wall of the cecum using 3-0 atraumatic PG. The diameter of the circle should be 1.5 cm. Insert a second purse-string suture outside the first, using the same suture material. Then make a stab wound in the middle of the purse-string suture; insert a 36F soft-rubber tube into the suture and for about 5-6 cm into the ascending colon. Tie the first purse-string suture around the rubber tube; then tie the second purse-string suture so as to invert the first. It is helpful if several large side-holes have been cut first in the distal 3-4 cm of the rubber tube.

Select a site about 3 cm above the incision for a stab wound. Bring out the rubber tube through this stab wound and suture the cecum to the peritoneum around the stab wound. Use four interrupted 3-0 PG atraumatic sutures to keep the peritoneal cavity free of any fecal matter that may leak around the tube.

Close the abdominal incision in a single layer by

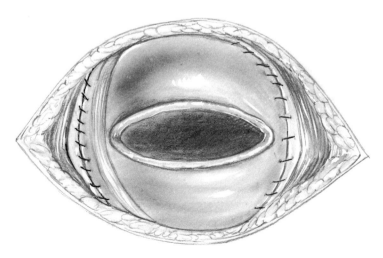

Fig. 52-2

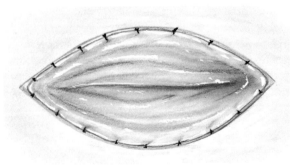

Fig. 52-3

the modified Smead-Jones technique using interrupted 1-0 PDS sutures. Do not close the skin wound; insert several 4-0 nylon interrupted skin sutures, which will be tied 3–5 days after operation.

POSTOPERATIVE CARE

Manage the skin-sutured cecostomy in the operating room by applying an adhesive-backed ileostomy-type disposable plastic appliance to it. The tube cecostomy requires repeated irrigation with saline to prevent it from being plugged by fecal particles. It may be removed after the tenth postoperative day if it is no longer needed.

COMPLICATIONS

The major postoperative complication of this procedure is peristomal sepsis, as the possibility of bacterial contamination of the abdominal incision cannot be completely eliminated. Nevertheless, peristomal sepsis is much less common than one would anticipate with an operation of this type.

REFERENCE

Duh QY, Way LW. Diagnostic laparoscopy and laparoscopic cecostomy for colonic pseudoobstruction. Dis Colon Rectum 1993;36:65.

53 Transverse Colostomy

INDICATIONS

Relief of obstruction due to lesions of the left colon

Diversion of fecal stream

Complementary to left colon anastomosis (see also Chapter 51)

PREOPERATIVE PREPARATION

Before performing a colostomy for colonic obstruction, confirm the diagnosis by barium enema, colonoscopy, or computed tomography (CT) of the abdomen.

Use a preoperative flat radiograph of the abdomen to identify the position of the transverse colon relative to a fixed point, such as a coin placed over the umbilicus.

Apply fluid resuscitation.

Place a nasogastric tube.

Prescribe perioperative antibiotics.

PITFALLS AND DANGER POINTS

Performing colostomy in error for diagnoses such as fecal impaction or pseudo-obstruction

Be certain the "ostomy" is, in fact, being constructed in the transverse colon, not in the redundant sigmoid colon, jejunum, or even the gastric antrum.

With advanced colonic obstruction, be aware of the possibility of impending cecal rupture for which transverse colostomy is an inadequate operation unless the cecum is seen to be viable.

OPERATIVE STRATEGY

Impending Rupture of Cecum

For routine cases of left colon obstruction, with the diagnosis confirmed by barium enema radiography, the colon may be approached through a small transverse incision in the right rectus muscle. This incision should be made for the colostomy alone; the rest of the abdominal cavity does not have to be explored. Exceptions to this policy should be made for patients with a sigmoid volvulus, those suspected to have ischemic colitis or perforation, and those in whom an advanced obstruction threatens cecal rupture.

When impending rupture is suspected, direct visual inspection of the cecum is mandatory. This may be accomplished with a midline laparotomy incision or a transverse right lower quadrant incision made over the cecum. Cecal necrosis or perforation mandates resection, usually with ileostomy and mucous fistula.

Diversion of Fecal Stream

Contrary to widespread medical opinion, it is not necessary to construct a double-barreled colostomy with complete transection of the colon to divert the stool from entering the left colon. We agree with Turnbull and Weakley (1967) that if a 5 cm longitudinal incision is made on the antimesenteric wall of the transverse colon and is followed by immediate maturation, fecal diversion is accomplished even in the absence of a supporting glass rod. The long incision in the colon permits the posterior wall to prolapse, resulting in functionally separate distal and proximal stomas.

OPERATIVE TECHNIQUE

Incision

Make a transverse incision over the middle and lateral thirds of the upper right rectus muscle (**Fig. 53–1**). Ideally the length of the skin incision equals the length of the longitudinal incision to be made in the colon (5–6 cm). To accomplish this it is necessary to identify the level at which the transverse colon crosses the path of the right rectus muscle. It may be done on a preoperative flat radiograph of the abdomen, followed by confirmation using percussion of the upper abdomen in the operating room. Make the transverse incision sufficiently long to accomplish accurate identification of the transverse colon. The incision will be partially closed, leaving a 5 cm gap to accommodate the colostomy.

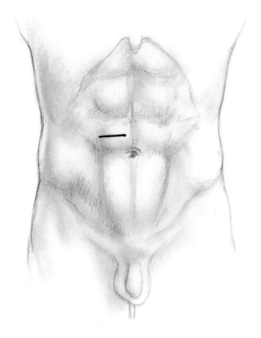

Fig. 53–1

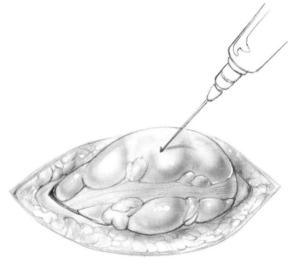

Fig. 53–2

When the transverse colostomy is to precede a subsequent laparotomy for removal of colon pathology, begin the transverse incision 2 cm to the right of the midline and extend it laterally. If this is done, the colostomy does not prevent the surgeon from using a long midline incision for the second stage of the operation.

After the skin incision is made, incise the anterior rectus fascia with a scalpel. Insert a Kelly hemostat between the muscle belly and the posterior rectus sheath. Incise the rectus muscle transversely over the hemostat with coagulating electrocautery for a distance of 6 cm. Then enter the abdomen in the usual manner by incising the posterior rectus sheath and peritoneum.

Identification of Transverse Colon

Even though the transverse colon is covered by omentum, in the average patient the omentum is thin enough that the colon can be seen through it. Positive identification can be made by observing the taenia. Divide the omentum for 6–7 cm over the colon. If colon is not clearly visible, extend the length of the incision.

Exteriorize the omentum and draw it in a cephalad direction; its undersurface leads to its junction with the transverse colon. At this point make a window in the overlying omentum so the transverse colon may protrude through the incision. Then replace the omentum into the abdomen.

Immediate Maturation of Colostomy

In patients who undergo operations for colon obstruction, the transverse colon is often so tensely distended it is difficult to deliver the anterior wall of the colon from the abdominal cavity without causing damage. To solve this problem, apply two Babcock clamps 2 cm apart to the anterior wall of the transverse colon. Insert a 16 gauge needle attached to a low-pressure suction line into the colon between the Babcock clamps (**Fig. 53–2**). After gas has been allowed to escape through the needle, the colon can be exteriorized easily.

The incision in the abdominal wall should be about 6 cm long. If it is longer than 6 cm, close the lateral portion with interrupted No. 1 PDS sutures of the Smead-Jones type. Shorten the skin incision with interrupted 4-0 nylon skin sutures as needed.

Make a 5- to 6-cm longitudinal incision along the anterior wall of the colon, preferably in the taenia (**Fig. 53–3**). Aspirate the bowel gas. Irrigate the op-

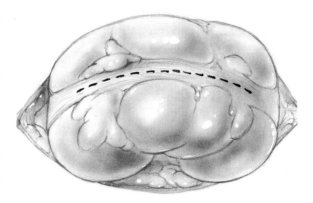

Fig. 53–3

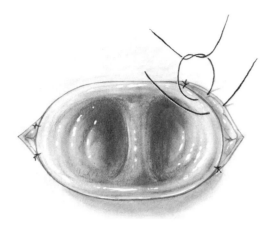

Fig. 53-4

erative field with 0.1% kanamycin solution. Then suture the full thickness of the colon wall to the *subcuticular* layer of the skin with 4-0 PG sutures, either interrupted or continuous **(Fig. 53–4)**. Attach a disposable ileostomy or colostomy bag to the colostomy.

Modification of Technique Using a Glass Rod

We prefer not to interrupt the suture line between the colon and skin by use of a glass rod. In markedly obese patients who have a short mesentery, a mod-

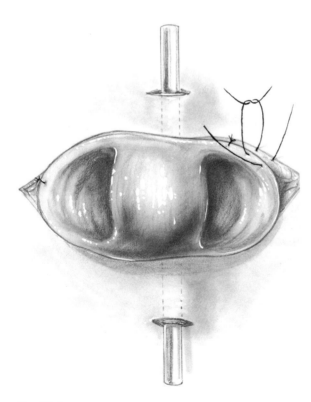

Fig. 53-5

ified glass rod technique may be used to prevent retraction while keeping the colocutaneous suture line intact. Make a stab wound through the skin at a point about 4 cm caudal to the midpoint of the proposed colostomy. By blunt dissection pass a glass or plastic rod between the subcutaneous fat and the anterior rectus fascia, proceeding in a cephalad direction. Pass the rod deep to the colon and have it emerge from a second stab wound 4 cm cephalad to the colostomy **(Fig. 53–5)**. This technique permits the subcutaneous fat to be protected from postoperative contamination by stool and greatly simplifies application of the colostomy bag.

An alternative to the solid rod is a thick Silastic tube, 6 mm in diameter, such as a nonperforated segment of a closed-suction drain tube. We prefer this method because it produces minimal inflammatory tissue response. However, because this tube is soft, it must be fixed to the skin of the two stab wounds with nylon sutures.

POSTOPERATIVE CARE

In the operating room apply a plastic disposable adhesive-type colostomy bag.

Apply nasogastric suction until the colostomy functions.

COMPLICATIONS

Peristomal sepsis is surprisingly uncommon. Treatment requires local incision and drainage. Massive sepsis would require moving the colostomy to another site.

Prolapse of the defunctionalized limb is fairly common when a loop colostomy is allowed to remain for months or years. It is managed by resection of the colostomy with restoration of gastrointestinal continuity or conversion to an end-colostomy. Careful tacking of both limbs at the peritoneal level helps prevent this complication but renders mobilization and subsequent closure more difficult.

REFERENCES

Abcarian H, Pearl RK. Stomas. Surg Clin North Am 1988; 68:1295.

Bergren CT, Laws HL. Modified technique of colostomy bridging. Surg Gynecol Obstet 1990;170:453.

Doberneck RC. Revision and closure of the colostomy. Surg Clin North Am 1991;71:193.

Fitzgibbons RJ Jr, Schmitz GD, Bailey RT Jr. A simple technique for constructing a loop enterostomy which allows immediate placement of an ostomy appliance. Surg Gynecol Obstet 1987;164:78.

Gooszen AW, Geelkerken RH, Hermans J, Lagaay MB, Gooszen HG. Temporary decompression after colorectal surgery: randomized comparison of loop ileostomy and loop colostomy. Br J Surg 1998;85:76.

Kyzer S, Gordon PH. Hidden colostomy. Surg Gynecol Obstet 1993;177:181.

Majno PE, Lees VC, Goodwin K, Everett WG. Siting a transverse colostomy. Br J Surg 1992;79:576.

Morris DM, Rayburn D. Loop colostomies are totally diverting in adults. Am J Surg 1991;161:668.

Ng WT, Book KS, Wong MK, Cheng PW, Cheung CH. Prevention of colostomy prolapse by peritoneal tethering. J Am Coll Surg 1997;184:313.

Turnball RB Jr, Weakly FL. Atlas of Intestinal Stomas. St. Louis, Mosby, 1967.

54 Closure of Temporary Colostomy

INDICATIONS

A temporary colostomy should be closed when it is no longer needed. Anastomotic healing and absence of a distal obstruction should be demonstrated by contrast studies. Suitably prepared patients may undergo colostomy closure as early as 2-3 weeks after surgery.

PREOPERATIVE PREPARATION

Barium colon enema radiography to demonstrate patency of distal colon

Nasogastric tube

Routine mechanical and antibiotic bowel preparation (saline enemas to cleanse the inactivated left colon segment may be required as well)

Perioperative systemic antibiotics

PITFALLS AND DANGER POINTS

Suture-line leak

Intraabdominal abscess

Wound abscess

OPERATIVE STRATEGY

To avoid suture-line leakage, use only healthy, well vascularized tissue for colostomy closure. Adequate lysis of the adhesions between the transverse colon and surrounding structures allows a sufficient segment of transverse colon to be mobilized, avoiding tension on the suture line. If necessary, the incision in the abdominal wall should be enlarged to provide exposure. If the tissue in the vicinity of the colostomy has been devascularized by operative trauma, do not hesitate to resect a segment of bowel and perform an end-to-end anastomosis instead of a local reconstruction. Proper suturing or stapling of healthy colon tissue and minimizing fecal contamination combined with perioperative antibiotics helps prevent formation of abscesses.

Infection of the operative incision is rather common following colostomy closure, owing in part to failure to minimize the bacterial inoculum into the wound. Another phenomenon that contributes to wound infection is retraction of subcutaneous fat that occurs around the colostomy. This can produce a gap between the fascia and the epidermis when the skin is sutured closed, creating deadspace. Avoid this problem by leaving the skin open at the conclusion of the operation.

OPERATIVE TECHNIQUE

Incision

Occlude the colostomy by inserting small gauze packing moistened with povidone-iodine solution. Make an incision in the skin around the colostomy 3-4 mm from the mucocutaneous junction (**Fig. 54-1**). Continue this incision parallel to the mucocutaneous junction until the entire colostomy has been encircled. Applying three Allis clamps to the lips of the defect in the colon expedites this dissection and helps prevent contamination. Deepen the incision by scalpel dissection until the seromuscular coat of colon can be identified. Then separate the serosa and surrounding subcutaneous fat by Metzenbaum scissors dissection (**Fig. 54-2**). Perform this dissection with meticulous care to avoid trauma

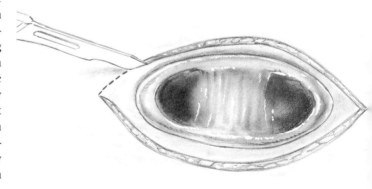

Fig. 54-1

502

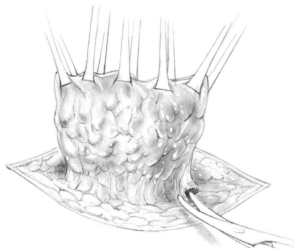

Fig. 54-2

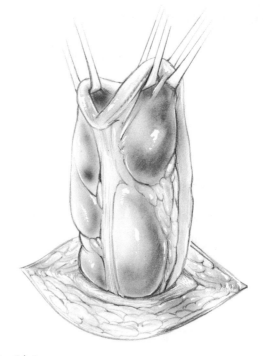

Fig. 54-3

to the colon wall. Continue down to the point where the colon meets the anterior rectus fascia.

Fascial Dissection

Identify the fascial ring and use a scalpel to dissect the subcutaneous fat off the anterior wall of the fascia for a width of 1-2 cm until a clean rim of fascia is visible all around the colostomy. Then dissect the colon away from the fascial ring until the peritoneal cavity is entered.

Peritoneal Dissection

Once the peritoneal cavity has been identified, it is often possible to insert an index finger and gently dissect the transverse colon away from the adjoining peritoneal attachments. Using the index finger as a guide, separate the remainder of the colon from its attachments to the anterior abdominal wall. This can often be accomplished without appreciably enlarging the defect in the abdominal wall. However, if any difficulty whatever is encountered while freeing the adhesions between the colon and peritoneum, extend the incision laterally by dividing the remainder of the rectus muscle with electrocautery for a distance adequate to accomplish the dissection safely.

Closure of Colon Defect by Suture

After the colostomy has been freed from all attachments for a distance of 5-6 cm **(Fig. 54-3)**, detach the rim of skin from the colon. Carefully inspect the wall of the colon for injury. A few small superficial patches of serosal damage are of no significance so long as they are not accompanied by devascularization. In most cases, merely freshening the edge of

the colostomy by excising a rim of 3-4 mm of scarred colon reveals healthy tissue.

The colon wall should now be of relatively normal thickness. In these cases the colostomy defect, which resulted from a longitudinal incision in the transverse colon at the initial operation, should be closed in a transverse direction. Initiate an inverting stitch of 4-0 PG on an atraumatic curved needle at the caudal margin of the colonic defect and pursue it as a continuous Connell or continuous Cushing suture to the midpoint of the defect **(Fig. 54-4)**. Then initiate a second suture of the same material on the cephalad margin of the defect and continue it also to the midpoint; terminate the suture line here (Fig.

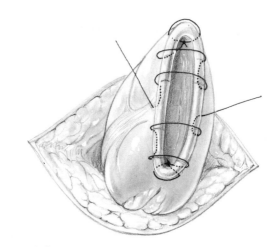

Fig. 54-4

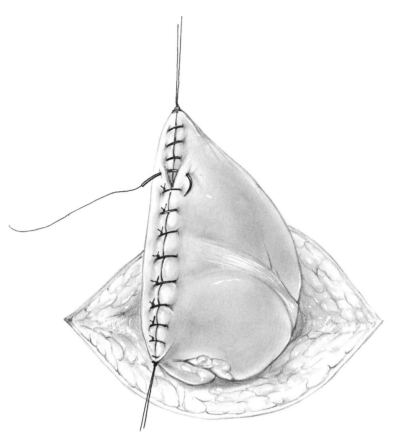

Fig. 54-5

54-4). Invert this layer with another layer of interrupted 4-0 silk atraumatic seromuscular Lembert sutures **(Fig. 54–5)**. Because of the transverse direction of the suture line, the lumen of the colon is quite commodious at the conclusion of the closure. There should be no tension whatever on this suture line. Finally, irrigate the operative field and reduce the colon into the abdominal cavity.

Closure of Colonic Defect by Staples

If the colon wall is not so thick that compressing it to 2 mm produces necrosis, stapling is an excellent method for closing the colon defect. Align the defect so the closure can take place in a transverse direction. Place a single guy suture to mark the midpoint of the transverse closure **(Fig. 54–6)** and apply Allis clamps to approximate the colon staple line with the bowel wall in eversion.

Carry out stapling by triangulation with two applications of the 55 mm linear stapling device, rather than attempting a single application of a 90 mm device. This minimizes the chance of catching the back wall of the colon in the staple line. First, apply the stapler across the everted mucosa supported by the Allis clamps on the caudal aspect of the defect and

the guy suture. Fire the staples and use Mayo scissors to excise the redundant everted mucosa flush with the stapler. Leave the guy suture at the midpoint of the closure intact.

Make the second application of the 55 mm linear stapler with the device positioned deep to the Allis clamps on the cephalad portion of the defect **(Fig. 54–7)**. It is important to position the guy suture to include the previous staple line in this second line of staples, ensuring that no gap exists between the two staple lines. Then fire the staples. Remove any redundant mucosa by excising it with Mayo scissors flush with the stapler. Lightly electrocoagulate the everted mucosa. Carefully inspect the integrity of the staple line to ensure that proper B formation has taken place. It is important, especially with stapling, to ascertain that no tension is exerted on the closure.

Resection and Anastomosis of Colostomy

Whenever the tissue is of inadequate quality for simple transverse closure, enlarge the incision in the abdominal wall and resect a segment of colon. Mobilize a sufficient section of the right transverse colon, occasionally including the hepatic flexure. Dissect the omentum off the transverse colon proximal and distal to the defect. After the proximal and distal segments of the colon have been sufficiently mobilized and the traumatized tissue excised, an end-to-end anastomosis can be constructed by the usual two-layer suture technique (see Figs. 44-18 through 44-26) or the staple technique (see Figs. 44-35 through 44-38).

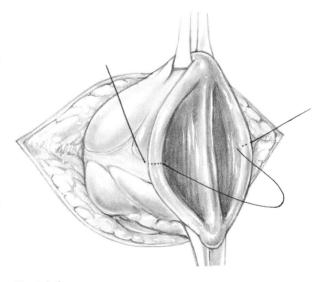

Fig. 54-6

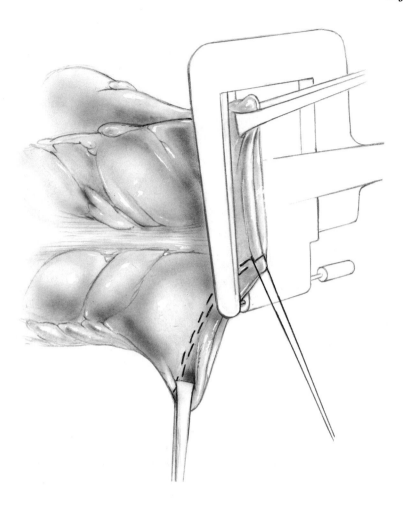

Fig. 54–7

Closure of Abdominal Wall

Irrigate the area with a dilute antibiotic solution and apply an Allis clamp to the midpoint of the abdominal wall on the caudal and cephalad aspects of the wound. Then close the incision by the modified Smead-Jones technique (see Chapter 3).

Management of Skin Wound

Frequently the colostomy can be closed without enlarging the skin incision, which was no longer than 5-6 cm. There is a high incidence of wound infection following primary closure of the skin. In such cases we simply insert loosely packed gauze into the subcutaneous space, which we allow to heal by granulation and contraction. If desired, several interrupted vertical mattress sutures of nylon may be inserted, but do not tie them until the eighth or tenth postoperative day. Keep the subcutaneous tissue separated with moist gauze packing and approximate the skin by previously placed sutures or tape strips when healthy granulation tissue has formed.

POSTOPERATIVE CARE

Apply nasogastric suction if necessary.

Systemic antibiotics are not continued beyond the perioperative period unless there was serious wound contamination during surgery.

COMPLICATIONS

Wound infection

Abdominal abscess

Colocutaneous fistula

REFERENCES

Doberneck RC. Revision and closure of the colostomy. Surg Clin North Am 1991;71:193.

Renz BM, Feliciano DV, Sherman R. Same admission colostomy closure (SACC): a new approach to rectal wounds: a prospective study. Ann Surg 1993;218:279.

Sola JE, Buchman TG, Bender JS. Limited role of barium enema examination preceding colostomy closure in trauma patients. J Trauma 1994;36:245.

55 Operations for Colonic Diverticulitis (Including Lower Gastrointestinal Bleeding)

INDICATIONS

Elective

    Recurrent diverticulitis

    Colovesical fistula

Urgent

    Diverticular abscess or phlegmon unresponsive to medical management

    Complete colon obstruction

    Suspicion of coexistent carcinoma

Emergent

    Spreading or generalized peritonitis

    Massive hemorrhage

PREOPERATIVE PREPARATION

See Chapter 42.

OPERATIVE STRATEGY

This operation is applicable to elective surgery for diverticular disease and may be used during emergency surgery for lower gastrointestinal bleeding. In the latter case, it is crucial to localize the bleeding source before surgery.

The operative technique for resecting the left colon and for the anastomosis is similar to that described for left colectomy for carcinoma but with a number of important exceptions.

1. Because there is no need to perform a high lymphovascular dissection in the absence of cancer, the mesentery may be divided at a point much closer to the bowel unless the mesentery is so inflamed and edematous it cannot hold ligatures.

2. In most cases it is not necessary to elevate the rectum from the presacral space, as this area is rarely the site of diverticula. The anastomosis can be done at the promontory of the sacrum.

3. Though it is important to remove the greatest concentration of diverticula, in elderly patients it is not necessary to perform an extensive colectomy just because there are some innocent diverticula in the ascending or transverse colon. The site selected for anastomosis should be free of diverticula and gross muscle hypertrophy.

4. Primary anastomosis should be performed only if the proximal and distal bowel segments selected for anastomosis are free of cellulitis and of marked muscle hypertrophy. If an abscess has been encountered in the pelvis, so that the anastomosis would lie on the wall of an evacuated abscess cavity, it is wise to delay the anastomosis for a second-stage operation.

OPERATIVE TECHNIQUE

Primary Resection and Anastomosis

Incision

Make a midline incision from the upper epigastrium to the pubis.

Liberation of Sigmoid and Left Colon

Initiate the dissection in the region of the upper descending colon by incising the peritoneum in the paracolic gutter. Then insert the left hand behind the colon (**Fig. 55–1**) in an area above the diverticulitis to elevate the mesocolon. Continue the incision in the paracolic peritoneum down to the descending colon and sigmoid to the brim of the pelvis.

At this point, to safeguard the left ureter from damage, it is essential to locate it in the upper portion of the dissection, where the absence of inflammation simplifies its identification. Then trace the

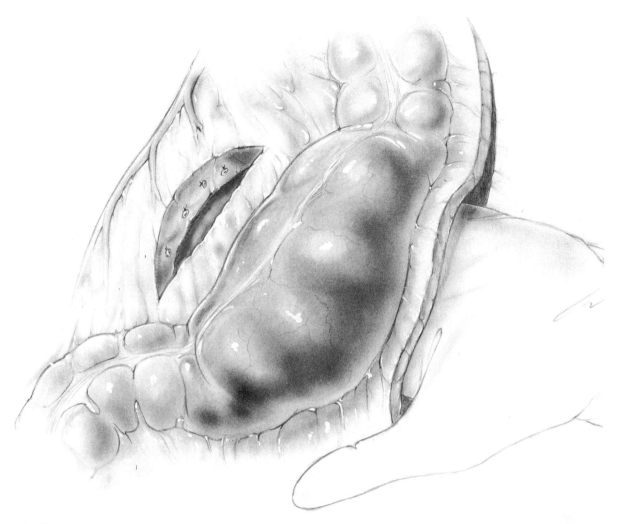

Fig. 55–1

ureter down into the pelvis. It may have to be dissected off an area of fibrosis in the sigmoid. When this dissection has been completed, the sigmoid is free down to the promontory of the sacrum.

Division of Mesocolon

In elective cases the mesentery generally can be divided serially between Kelly hemostats at a point no more than 4-6 cm from the bowel wall (Fig. 55-1). Initiate the line of division at a point on the left colon that is free of pathology. This sometimes requires liberation of the splenic flexure and distal transverse colon. Continue the dissection to the rectosigmoid. Remove the specimen after applying Allen clamps.

Anastomosis

Perform an open-type anastomosis in one or two layers or by stapling as described in Chapter 44 (see Figs. 44-12 through 44-38). In rare cases it is necessary to make the anastomosis at a lower level, where the ampulla of the rectum is significantly larger in diameter than the proximal colon. In that case a side-to-end Baker anastomosis is preferable, as described in Chapter 45 (see Figs. 45-12 through 45-22).

Abdominal Closure

In the absence of intraabdominal or pelvic abscesses, close the abdomen in the useful fashion (see Chapter 3). Intraperitoneal drains are not needed.

Primary Resection with End-Colostomy and Mucous Fistula

If it is decided to delay the anastomosis for a second stage, it is not necessary to excise every bit of inflamed bowel, as this frequently requires a Hartmann pouch at the site of the rectosigmoid transaction and makes the second stage more difficult than if a mucous fistula can be constructed. In almost every case, proper planning of the operation permits exteriorization of the distal sigmoid as a mucous fistula, which can be brought out through the lower margin of the midline incision after a De Martel clamp or stapled closure is secured **(Fig. 55–2)**. Divide the mesocolon to preserve the vascularity of the mucous fistula. Then bring out an uninflamed area of the descending colon as an end-colostomy through a separate incision in the lateral portion of the left rectus muscle and excise the intervening diseased colon. The second stage of this operation—removal of the colostomy and mucous fistula and anastomosis of the descending colon to the rectosigmoid—may be carried out after a delay of several weeks.

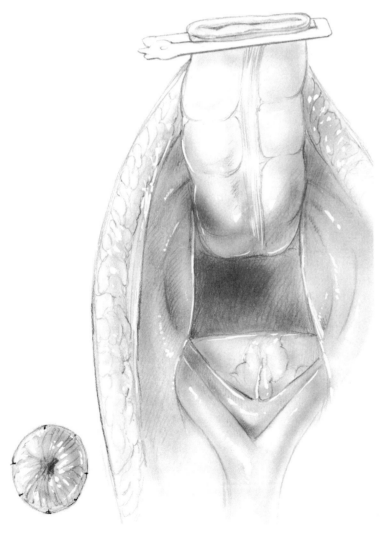

Fig. 55-2

Emergency Sigmoid Colectomy with End-Colostomy and Hartmann's Pouch

Indications

For patients suffering generalized or spreading peritonitis secondary to perforated sigmoid diverticulitis, a conservative approach with diverting transverse colostomy and local drainage is associated with a mortality rate of more than 50%. Immediate excision of the perforated bowel is necessary to remove the septic focus. Following this excision the preferred procedure is a mucous fistula and end-colostomy. However, if excising the perforated portion of the sigmoid leaves an insufficient amount of distal bowel with which to form a mucous fistula, Hartmann's operation is indicated. It is not wise to attempt to create a mucous fistula by extensive presacral dissection in the hope of lengthening the distal segment, as it only opens new planes to potential sepsis.

Preoperative Preparation

Preoperative preparation primarily involves rapid resuscitative measures using intravenous fluids, blood, and antibiotics, as some patients are admitted to the hospital in septic shock. Complete colon preparation may not be possible, although many patients are given a modified dose of GoLYTELY for colonic cleansing. Nasogastric suction and bladder drainage with a Foley catheter should be instituted.

Operative Technique

Incision and Liberation of Left Colon
The steps for incision and liberation of the left colon are identical to those described above. It is essential to find the proper retromesenteric plane by initiating the dissection above the area of maximal inflammation. Once this has been achieved, with the left hand elevate the sigmoid colon and the diseased mesocolon (generally the site of a phlegmon) so the left paracolic peritoneum may be incised safely (Fig. 55-1). Again, it is essential to identify the left ureter in the upper abdomen to safeguard it from damage. Sometimes a considerable amount of blood oozes from the retroperitoneal dissection, but it can often be controlled by moist gauze packs while the dissection continues. After the left colon has been liberated, divide the mesentery serially between hemostats, as above.

Hartmann's Pouch
Often with acute diverticulitis the rectosigmoid is not involved to a great extent in the inflammatory

process. Mesenteric dissection should be terminated at this point. If the rectosigmoid is not excessively thick, occlude it by applying a 55/4.8 mm linear stapler. Place an Allen clamp on the specimen side of the sigmoid and divide the bowel flush with the stapler. After the stapling device is removed there should be slight oozing of blood through the staples, which is evidence that excessively thickened tissue has not been necrotized by using the stapling technique on it **(Fig. 55–3)**.

If the tissue is so thick that compression to 2 mm by the stapling device would result in necrosis, the technique is contraindicated. The rectal stump should then be closed by a continuous layer of locked sutures of 3-0 PG. Invert this layer with a second layer of continuous 3-0 PG Lembert sutures. Suture the apex of the Hartmann pouch to the pelvic fascia near, or if possible higher than, the promontory of the sacrum to prevent retraction low into the pelvis, which would make a secondary anastomosis more difficult.

End-Colostomy

Use an uninflamed area of the left colon for an end-colostomy. In a patient who is desperately ill, the colostomy may be brought out through the upper portion of the midline incision if it can save time. Otherwise, bring it out through a transverse incision over the lateral portion of left rectus muscle. The incision should admit two fingers. Bring out the cut end of the colon and immediately suture it with 4-0 PG, either interrupted or continuous, to the subcuticular layer of the skin incision.

Wound Closure

Any rigid abscess cavities that cannot be excised should be managed by insertion of sump drains. If no rigid abscess walls have been left behind, the abdomen should be copiously irrigated and closed in the usual fashion without drainage. The skin can be managed by delayed primary closure.

REFERENCES

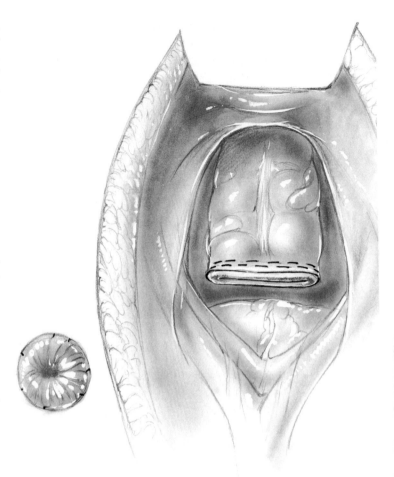

Fig. 55-3

Bergamaschi R, Arnaud JP. Intracorporeal colorectal anastomosis following laparoscopic left colon resection. Surg Endosc 1997;11:800.

Bouillot JL, Aouad K, Badawy A, Alamowitch B, Alexandre JH. Elective laparoscopic-assisted colectomy for diverticular disease: a prospective study in 50 patients. Surg Endosc 1998;12:1393.

Eng K, Ranson JH, Localio SA. Resection of the perforated segment: a significant advance in the treatment of diverticulitis with free perforation of abscess. Am J Surg 1977;133:67.

Smadja C, Sbai Idrissi M, Tahrat M, et al. Elective laparoscopic sigmoid colectomy for diverticulitis: results of a prospective study. Surg Endosc 1999;13:645.

Wexner SD, Moscovitz ID. Laparoscopic colectomy in diverticular and Crohn's disease. Surg Clin North Am 2000;80:1299.

56 Ripstein Operation for Rectal Prolapse

INDICATIONS

Complete prolapse of the rectum

PREOPERATIVE PREPARATION

Mechanical and antibiotic bowel preparation

Sigmoidoscopy

Barium colon enema

Foley catheter in bladder

Perioperative antibiotics

PITFALLS AND DANGER POINTS

Excessive constriction of the rectum by mesh, which may result in partial obstruction or, rarely, erosion of mesh into the rectal lumen

Disruption of suture line between mesh and presacral space

Presacral hemorrhage

OPERATIVE STRATEGY

The Ripstein operation uses permanent polypropylene mesh to fix the rectum to the presacral fascia, thereby restoring the normal posterior curve of the rectum and eliminating intussusception and prolapse. This operation is indicated only in patients who are not also suffering from significant constipation. Constipated patients do better with resection of the redundant sigmoid colon and colorectal anastomosis with sutures attaching the lateral ligaments of the rectum to the sacral fascia. For extremely poor-risk patients with rectal prolapse, a Thiersch operation (see Chapter 63) or perineal resection (see References) may be performed.

To prevent undue constriction of the rectum when the mesh is placed around it, *leave sufficient room to pass two fingers behind the rectum* after the mesh has been fixed in place. The success of the Ripstein operation is *not predicated on any degree of constriction* of the rectum. It suffices if the mesh simply prevents the rectum from advancing in an anterior direction away from the hollow of the sacrum.

The site on the rectum selected for placing the mesh is important. The upper level of the mesh should be 5 cm below the promontory of the sacrum, which requires opening the rectovesical or rectouterine peritoneum. In most cases the lateral ligaments of the rectum need not be divided. Avoid damage to the hypogastric nerves in the presacral area, especially in male patients, in whom nerve transection produces retrograde ejaculation.

OPERATIVE TECHNIQUE

Incision

A midline incision between the umbilicus and pubis provides excellent exposure in most patients. In young women the operation is accompanied by im-

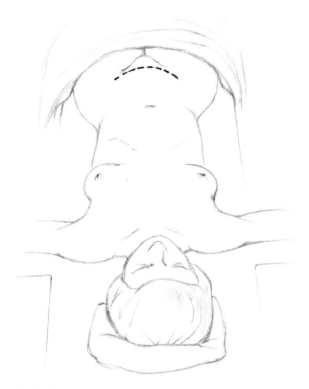

Fig. 56–1

proved cosmetic results if it is performed through a Pfannenstiel incision. Place the 12- to 15-cm long Pfannenstiel incision just inside the public hairline, in the crease that goes from one anterior superior iliac spine to the other **(Fig. 56–1)**. With the scalpel, divide the subcutaneous fat down to the anterior rectus sheath and the external oblique aponeurosis. Divide the anterior rectus sheath in the line of the incision about 2 cm above the pubis **(Fig. 56–2)**. Extend the incision in the rectus sheath laterally in both directions into the external oblique aponeurosis. Apply Allis clamps to the cephalad portion of this fascial layer and bluntly dissect it off the underlying rectus muscles almost to the level of the umbilicus **(Fig. 56–3)**. Separate the rectus muscles in the midline, exposing the preperitoneal fat and peritoneum. Grasp the fat and peritoneum in an area sufficiently cephalad to the bladder to not endanger that organ. Incise the peritoneum, open the abdominal cavity, and explore it for coincidental pathology. A moderate Trendelenburg position is helpful.

Incision of Pelvic Peritoneum

Retract the small intestine in a cephalad direction. Make an incision in the pelvic peritoneum beginning at the promontory of the sacrum and proceed along the left side of the mesorectum down as far as the cul-de-sac. Identify the left ureter.

Make a second incision in the peritoneum on the right side of the mesorectum, where the mesorectum meets the pelvic peritoneum. Extend this incision also down to the cul-de-sac and identify and preserve the right ureter. Join these two incisions by dividing the peritoneum at the depth of the rectovesical or rectouterine pouch using Metzenbaum scissors (see Figs. 45–4 through 45–6). Frequently, the cul-de-sac is deep in patients with rectal prolapse. Further dissection between the rectum and the prostate or vagina is generally not necessary.

Presacral Dissection

For rectal prolapse the rectum can be elevated with ease from the hollow of the sacrum. Enter the presacral space via a Metzenbaum dissection, a method similar to that described for anterior resection (see Chapter 45). Take the usual precautions to avoid damage to the presacral veins. Inspect the presacral area for hemostasis, which should be perfect before the procedure is continued.

Application of Mesh

Fit a section of Prolene mesh measuring 5 × 10 cm or 5 × 12 cm into place overlying the lower rectum.

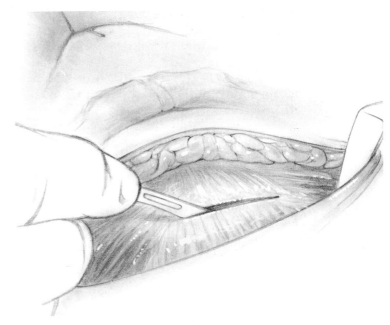
Fig. 56–2

The upper margin of the mesh should lie over the rectum at a point 4-5 cm below the sacral promontory. Using a small Mayo needle, insert three interrupted sutures of 2-0 Prolene or Tevdek into the right margin of the mesh and attach the mesh to the sacral periosteum along a line about 1-2 cm to the

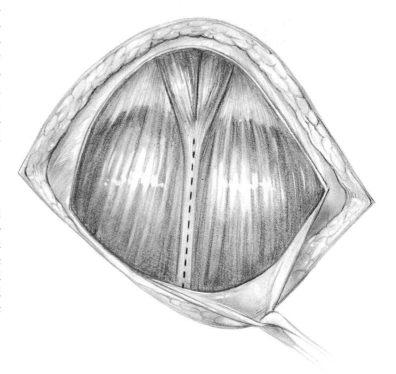
Fig. 56–3

right of the mid-sacral line. Use the same technique to insert three interrupted sutures in the left lateral margin of the mesh and through the sacral fascia and periosteum **(Fig. 56–4a)**. Tie none of these sutures yet, but apply a hemostat to each of them temporarily. After all six sutures have been inserted, have the assistants draw them taut. Then insert two fingers between the rectum and sacrum to check the tension of the mesh, thereby ensuring that there will be no constriction of the rectum **(Fig. 56–4b)**. Now tie all six sutures. Use additional sutures of 4-0 atraumatic Prolene or Tevdek to attach both the proximal and distal margins of the mesh to the underlying rectum, so there is no possibility of the rectum sliding forward underneath the mesh.

Because there is a significant incidence of severe constipation and narrowing of the lumen by the mesh, Nicosia and Bass described fixation of the mesh to the presacral fascia using sutures or a fascial stapler. The mesh is then *partially* wrapped around and sutured to the rectum, leaving the anterior third of the rectal circumference free to dilate as necessary **(Figs. 56–5, 56–6)**.

Closure of Pelvic Peritoneum

Irrigate the pelvic cavity. Close the incision in the pelvic peritoneum with a continuous suture of 2-0 atraumatic PG **(Fig. 56–7)**.

Wound Closure

To close the Pfannenstiel incision, grasp the peritoneum with hemostats and approximate it with a continuous 2-0 atraumatic PG suture. Use several sutures of the same material loosely to approximate the rectus muscle in the midline. Close the transverse incision in the rectus sheath and external oblique aponeurosis with interrupted sutures of atraumatic 2-0 PG. Close the skin with a continuous 4-0 PG subcuticular suture.

Generally, no pelvic drains are necessary. If hemostasis is not perfect, bring a 6 mm Silastic catheter out from the presacral space through a puncture wound in the lower abdomen and attach it to a closed-suction device (Fig. 56–5).

POSTOPERATIVE CARE

Nasogastric suction is not necessary.

COMPLICATIONS

Most patients who have a complete prolapse have suffered from years of *constipation*. They may have to continue the use of laxatives, although in some cases there is a definite improvement in the patient's bowel function following the operation.

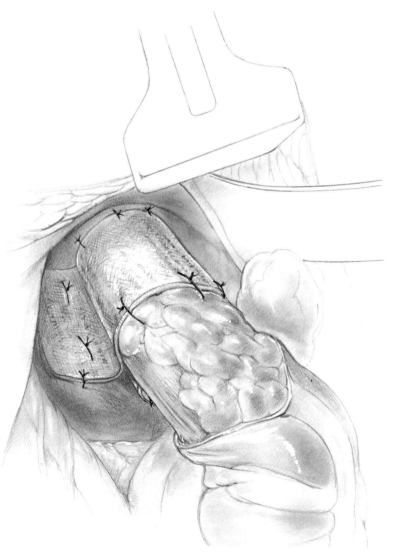

Fig. 56–4a

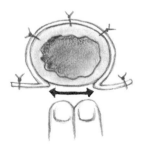

Fig. 56–4b

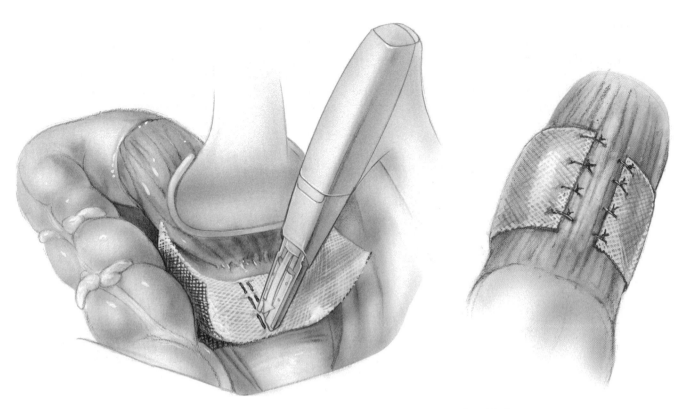

Fig. 56-5

Fig. 56-6

Fecal incontinence—the result of many years of dilatation of the anal sphincters due to repeated prolapse—is also common among these patients. Correction of the prolapse does not automatically eliminate incontinence. This condition is alleviated over time in more than 30% of patients who are placed on a regimen of high fiber and muscle-strengthening exercises, occasionally supplemented with biofeedback.

REFERENCES

Corman ML. Rectal prolapse: surgical techniques. Surg Clin North Am 1988;68:1255.

Cuschieri A, Shimi SM, Vander Velpen G, Banting S, Wood RA. Laparoscopic prosthesis fixation rectopexy for complete rectal prolapse. Br J Surg 1994;81:138.

Eu KW, Seow-Choen F. Functional problems in adult rectal prolapse and controversies in surgical treatment. Br J Surg 1997;84:904.

Jacobs LK, Lin YJ, Orkin BA. The best operation for rectal prolapse. Surg Clin North Am 1997;77:49.

McKee RF, Lauder JC, Poon FW, Aitchison MA, Finlay IG. A prospective randomized study of abdominal rectopexy with and without sigmoidectomy in rectal prolapse. Surg Gynecol Obstet 1992;174:145.

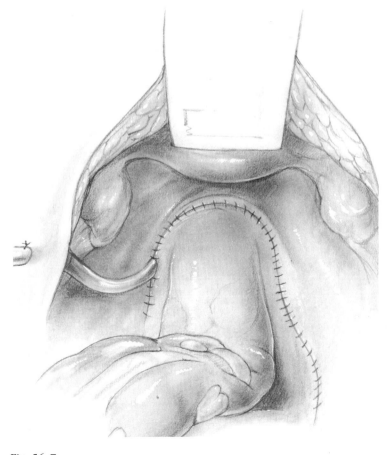

Fig. 56-7

Nicosia JF, Bass NM. Use of the fascial stapler in proctopexy for rectal prolapse. Dis Colon Rectum 1987;30: 900.

Prasad ML, Pearl RK, Abcarian H, et al. Perineal proctectomy, posterior rectopexy, and postanal levator repair for the treatment of rectal prolapse. Dis Colon Rectum 1986;29:547.

Ripstein CB. Surgical care of massive rectal prolapse. Dis Colon Rectum 1965;8:34.

Roberts PL, Schoetz DJ Jr, Coller JA, Veidenheimer MC.

Ripstein procedure: Lahey Clinic experience. Arch Surg 1988;123:554.

Tobin SA, Scott IH. Delorme operation for rectal prolapse. Br J Surg 1994;81:1681.

Watts JD, Rothenberger DA, Buls JG, et al. The management of procidentia, 30 years experience. Dis Colon Rectum 1985;28:96.

Yoshioka K, Hyland G, Keighley MR. Anorectal function after abdominal rectopexy: parameters of predictive value in identifying return of continence. Br J Surg 1989;76:64.

Part VI
Anus, Rectum, and Pilonidal Region

57 Concepts in Surgery of the Anus, Rectum, and Pilonidal Region

Amanda M. Metcalf

Successful management of anorectal disease depends on a clear understanding of what symptoms can be attributed to various conditions.[1,2] In addition, consideration must be given to the impact of other aspects of colorectal physiology on function and healing. The perianal skin and lower aspect of the anal canal is richly innervated by sensory fibers. External hemorrhoids are venous plexuses located below the dentate line and covered with squamous epithelium. Internal hemorrhoids are submucosal vascular tissue containing blood vessels, smooth muscle, and connective tissue that are normally located above the dentate line. They are covered with transitional epithelium. Chronic straining is thought to cause excessive engorgement of the vascular cushions and disruption of the smooth muscle and connective tissue. This disruption allows the vascular cushions and the overlying mucosa to slide down

the anal canal and prolapse during straining. Repetitive straining promotes further prolapse.

Internal hemorrhoids are classified by their extent of prolapse down the anal canal during straining. Second-degree internal hemorrhoids are those that prolapse down the anal canal during straining and spontaneously reduce. Third-degree internal hemorrhoids prolapse with straining and require manual reduction. Fourth-degree hemorrhoids cannot be reduced.

The pressure generated in the anal canal to keep it closed during periods of inattention or sleep is called the resting anal tone. Approximately half of the normal resting anal tone is contributed by the internal anal sphincter, which is a continuation of the circular muscle of the rectum (**Fig. 57–1**). The lower edge of the internal sphincter and the groove between the internal and external sphincter can be

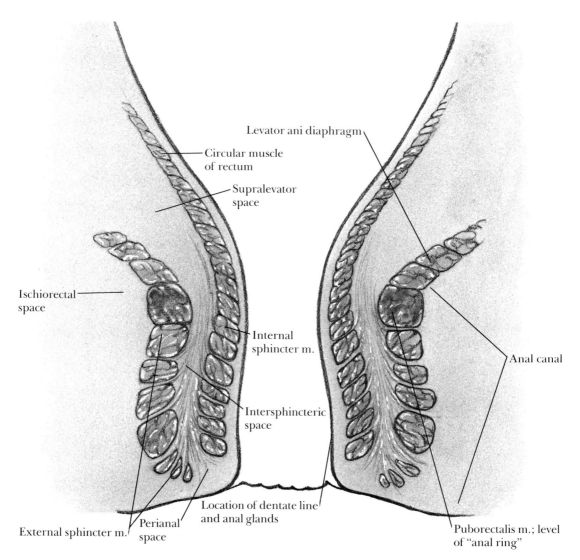

Levator ani diaphragm

Circular muscle
of rectum

Supralevator
space

Ischiorectal
space

Internal
sphincter m.

Intersphincteric
space

Anal canal

Location of dentate line
and anal glands

External sphincter m.   Perianal
space

Puborectalis m.; level
of "anal ring"

Fig. 57-1

palpated approximately 1 cm below the dentate line. The remainder of the resting anal tone is provided by the external sphincter muscles and the puborectalis. The external anal sphincters encircle the lower portion of the anal canal, and the puborectalis surrounds the posterior and lateral portions of the upper anal canal. The puborectalis, which is continuous with the levator ani muscles that form the pelvic diaphragm, is best palpated posteriorly and is often referred to as the anorectal ring.

The maximum pressure that can be generated in the anal canal is produced by the voluntary contraction of the external sphincters and the puborectalis. It is called the maximum voluntary squeeze and can be maintained for only a short time. Contraction of the striated sphincteric mechanism is also caused as a reflex in response to coughing or sneezing. Continence depends on the interaction between the anal sphincters, the type of challenge (solid, liquid, gas), and the compliance of the rectum. The compliance of the rectum can be thought of as its ability to act as a reservoir. Decreased compliance of the rectum produces urgent calls to stool at low intrarectal volumes. Common causes of decreased rectal compliance include radiation proctitis, inflammatory bowel disease, rectal resection, and irritable bowel syndrome. Patients with incontinence often have abnormalities in more than one area. Patients with a sphincter injury may have a good control of formed stool but be incontinent with liquid stool. Subtle abnormalities in sphincter function and continence may be unmasked by anal surgery. This can occur even with procedures that are usually not associated with changes in continence, such as a partial lateral internal sphincterotomy. Therefore it is extremely important to determine any abnormalities in bowel function that would predispose individuals to impaired continence postoperatively. Historical information regarding bowel habits and symptoms of minor sphincter dysfunction such as seepage, pruritus, or incontinence of flatus should be noted and documented.

Anal fissures are posterior or anterior midline epithelial defects or ulcers in the anal canal. Anal fissures are caused by the trauma of defecation and should never extend above the level of the dentate line or out onto the anal verge. The biomechanics of the anal canal are such that most fissures occur in the midline posteriorly or, less commonly, anteriorly. Painful anal fissures are associated with spasm of both the internal and external sphincters. Despite this spasm, it should be possible to see an anal fissure by gently spreading the skin of the anal verge and lower anal canal. Decreased resting anal tone in association with an anal fissure or an anal fissure in a patient with diarrhea suggests the diagnosis of Crohn's disease. Other possibilities are viral infection, such cytomegalovirus or herpes in an immunocompromised host. In either of these situations, the ulcer commonly appears unusually broad or deep. Current theory regarding the etiology of typical anal fissures is that the spasm of the sphincteric mechanism results in decreased blood flow to the lining of the anal canal, and that the resultant relative ischemia produces poor healing.

Perianal infections may present as obviously indurated, erythematous areas adjacent to the anus. They may also present more subtly with complaints of discomfort in the perineum or buttock and minimal physical findings. Most perianal infections are caused by enteric flora and originate in anal glands. Perianal infections caused by skin organisms are more likely to be manifestations of other processes such as folliculitis or hidradenitis suppurativa. The anal glands thought to be the origin of most perianal infections empty into the anal crypts at the level of the dentate line. The function of these glands is obscure. Only a small proportion of the anal glands traverse the internal sphincter into the intersphincteric space and can therefore serve as a source of infection. Infection in the intersphincteric space can spread directly caudad to the perianal skin or can penetrate the external sphincter or puborectalis to produce infection in the ischiorectal fossa. Midline anal glands posteriorly towad the coccyx can produce horseshoe abscesses, as potential perianal spaces communicate posteriorly.

Fistulas that result from perianal abscesses have been classified according to their relation to the sphincteric mechanism by Parks and others (1976).

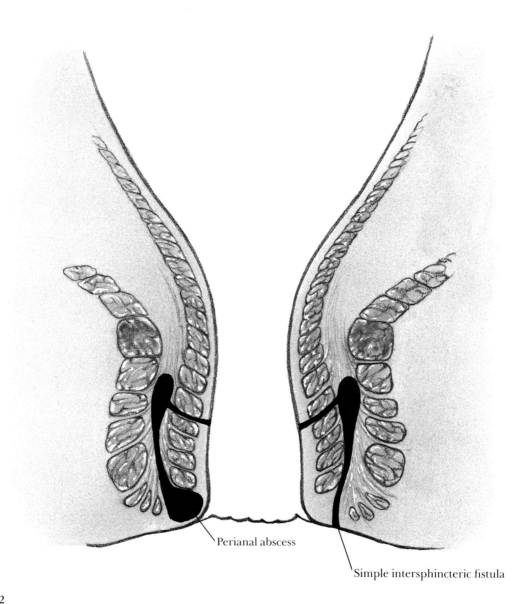

Perianal abscess

Simple intersphincteric fistula

Fig. 57-2

A type 1 fistula is intersphincteric **(Fig. 57–2)** and extends from its origin through the intersphincteric space to the perianal skin. A type 2 fistula is transsphincteric **(Fig. 57–3)** and extends through the external sphincter into the ischiorectal space to the skin of the buttocks. A type 3 fistula is supras-

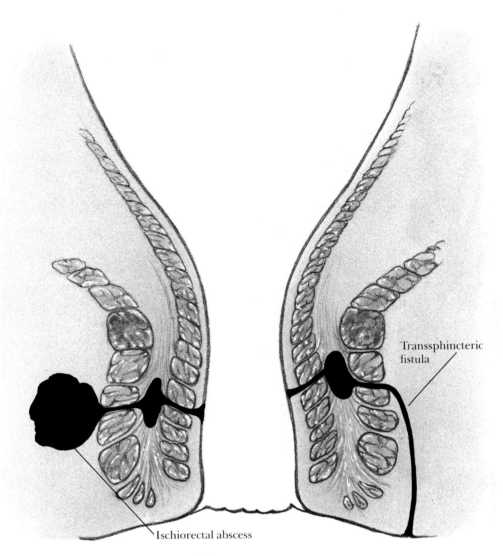

Fig. 57-3. Transphincteric fistula and ischiorectal abscess.

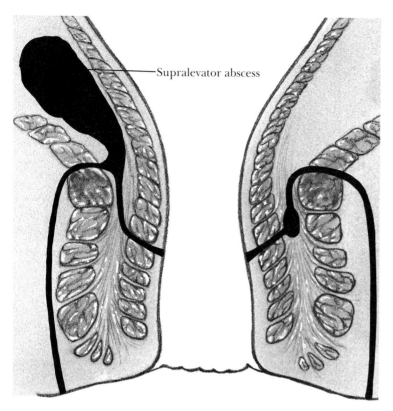

Fig. 57–4. Suprasphincteric fistulas.

unless the patient is coagulopathic or the internal hemorrhoids are grade 3 or larger. In general, internal hemorrhoids cause an unpleasant pressure sensation while they are prolapsed, which resolves with reduction of the prolapse. Internal hemorrhoids that do not prolapse should not cause pain. The amount of hemorrhoidal prolapse a patient has is best assessed while the patient is on the commode. The patient is asked to strain on the commode; and then, while still straining, is asked to lean forward to allow the examiner to visualize the perineum.

Irritation of the perianal skin produces an itching or burning sensation. These symptoms are independent of any underlying venous plexuses or redundant skin and are therefore not a symptom of external hemorrhoids. Internal hemorrhoids contribute to these symptoms only when they are chronically prolapsed and in this state increase perianal moisture. Chronically prolapsed internal he-

phincteric **(Fig. 57–4)**. It travels cephalad in the intersphincteric space, encircles the puborectalis, and then perforates the levator ani, continuing to the perianal skin. A type 4 fistula is extrasphincteric **(Fig. 57–5)**. Only rarely related to cryptoglandular infection, it usually originates from an intraabdominal source that has caused an infection in the pelvis. Conditions that could cause this type of fistula include diverticulitis, Crohn's disease, and foreign body perforation of the rectum. Fistulas caused by cryptoglandular infection therefore always surround a portion of the internal sphincter and a variable portion of the external sphincter. Because there is a relative deficiency of sphincter muscle anteriorly owing to the absence of the puborectalis, anterior fistulas encompass a relatively larger percentage of the sphincter mechanism than do posterior fistulas.

CLINICAL CONDITIONS: SYMPTOMS AND MANAGEMENT CONCEPTS

The most common symptom of *internal hemorrhoids* is painless rectal bleeding. The bleeding can vary in quantity and frequency, but generally the quantity is fairly predictable for a given patient. It is not usually of significant amount to produce anemia

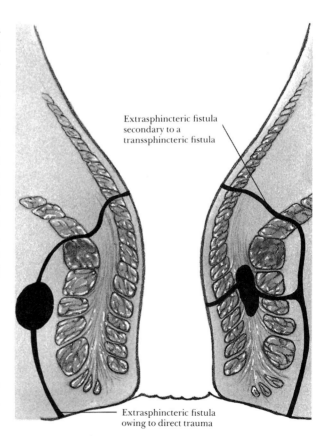

Fig. 57–5. Extrasphincteric fistulas.

morrhoids should be readily visible at the anal orifice.

External hemorrhoids become engorged with blood during a Valsalva maneuver. They cause pain only when they become thrombosed. When thrombosed, they appear as firm, painful, bluish skin-covered masses on the anal verge. Although discomfort is maximal for the first 48–72 hours, residual discomfort persists for 7 days, and the "lump" may take several weeks to resolve. Within the first 72 hours of occurrence, excision of the thrombosed hemorrhoid relieves more pain than it causes. The converse is true after this time interval. As previously discussed, discomfort from internal hemorrhoids occurs when they remain prolapsed after straining. If internal hemorrhoids are acutely prolapsed and not reduced, they cause engorgement and edema of the external hemorrhoidal complex on the ipsilateral side. Eventually, both components may thrombose and appear as firm, painful, nonreducible masses, the inner covered with mucosa and the outer with squamous epithelium. When thrombosis has already occurred, treatment should be dictated by the time interval since onset: If less than 72 hours, hemorrhoidectomy is reasonable; if more than 72 hours, conservative management with stool softeners and analgesics is appropriate.

Over the years many treatments have been proposed for symptomatic internal hemorrhoids and have enjoyed brief surges of popularity. Among the nonsurgical techniques, only rubber band ligation has truly withstood the test of time.

Hemorrhoid banding is the treatment of choice for prolapsing symptomatic internal hemorrhoids. It is easily performed in the outpatient setting, requires no anesthetic, and is associated with few complications. With this technique, a strangulating rubber band is placed on the redundant rectal mucosa above the hemorrhoid. This procedure not only removes some of the redundant mucosa but also produces fixation of residual mucosa to the submucosa in the region of the banding. The residual vascular cushion in this location is fixed in the anal canal and does not prolapse with straining.

Hemorrhoidectomy should be reserved for patients who have failed banding, have large grade 3 or grade 4 hemorrhoids, or have smaller hemorrhoids associated with other anal pathology that requires operative intervention.

Anal fissures usually cause painful rectal bleeding. Reducing the anal canal pressure medically or by dividing a portion of the internal sphincter increases anal canal blood flow and promotes healing of the anal fissure. Medical therapy of an anal fissure should almost always precede surgical therapy. Stool bulking agents such as psyllium seed or methylcellulose in quantities sufficient to provide bulky soft stools reliably are the mainstays of medical therapy. Stool softeners and other laxatives should be avoided, as the resultant stool is so soft it does not dilate the anal canal. Dilute nitroglycerine ointment (0.2%) applied to the anus before and after bowel movements has been advocated by some as an adjunct to bulking agents to decrease pain and promote healing. Persistence of a painful anal fissure for 6 weeks on good medical therapy or development of a complication such as infection constitute an indication for surgical therapy. Surgical therapy is not indicated for a painless anal fissure.

Perianal abscesses require surgical drainage unless spontaneous rupture has produced adequate drainage. Because most perianal infections caused by cryptoglandular infections result in an anal fistula, it is helpful to drain the abscess through an incision as close to the anus as possible. This minimizes the length of a subsequent fistulotomy wound. Small abscesses that are easily visible on inspection and are not associated with systemic signs or symptoms can often be drained under local anesthesia. Ischiorectal fossa abscesses that present with ill-defined areas of induration and are associated with fever and leukocytosis are probably best drained under regional or general anesthesia. Whatever technique is used, it is imperative to have close follow-up examinations of the patient to document resolution of the problem. This is especially true in patients with diabetes, who are prone to developing necrotizing fasciitis in an incompletely drained perianal abscess.

A *fistula-in-ano* can be diagnosed by failure of the drainage wound to heal completely or by abscess recurrence after apparently complete healing. A recurrent abscess may occur years after the original infection. A typical fistula tract can often by palpated subcutaneously as a fibrous cord between the external opening and the anal orifice. The origin of the fistula in the anal canal (primary opening) is most easily found when there is an active external (secondary) opening. If the site of the primary opening cannot be identified, a fistulotomy should not be performed. A fistulotomy always impairs sphincter function to some degree. Because the puborectalis is not present anteriorly, an anterior fistulotomy is more likely to result in a perceptible alteration in continence than a posterior fistulotomy of an equivalent amount of muscle. The amount of sphincter division that can be tolerated by the patient depends on the baseline sphincter function, the usual consistency of their stools, and the compliance of their rectum. A young patient with infrequent predictable stools tolerates far more sphincter division than does the elderly patient with irritable bowel syndrome and frequent erratic stools. No patient is continent if the entire anorectal ring is divided, regardless of his or her bowel habits. A history of diarrhea in association with a perianal fistula mandates preoperative evaluation for inflammatory bowel disease.

Delayed wound healing after anal surgery can be frustrating to both patient and surgeon. The single best agent to promote healing in the anal canal without stenosis after anal surgery is a bulky, soft, formed stool. Psyllium seed preparations or methylcellulose-based agents should be prescribed postoperatively for most patients. The use of constipating analgesics should be minimized. Altered bowel consistency, whether too hard or too loose, delays wound healing. Delayed wound healing is also seen in patients who have undergone irradiation, have diabetes or inflammatory bowel disease, or who have compromised immune systems.

Pilonidal disease is not an anorectal disease in the purest sense. Its association with anorectal disease is only by proximity. Pilonidal disease is a term used to describe infections that originate in the gluteal cleft. It is currently thought to be an acquired rather than a congenital disorder. The precise sequence of events is debated, but there is agreement that the shape of the gluteal cleft and its effect on loose hair in this region leads to penetration of hair underneath the skin. This leads to formation of chronic subcutaneous abscesses that contain hair. Multiple infectious episodes create multiple openings along the midline and lateral to it that can mimic other anal conditions. The variety of operations that have been described for this condition suggest that there is no solitary infallible procedure for cure. Current trends are toward less radical surgery. Avoidance of a midline wound, removal of the foreign material from the abscess cavity, and removal of hair in the region of the gluteal cleft by shaving or tweezing seem to be important elements for obtaining a healed wound.

REFERENCES

Beck DE, Wexner SD. Fundamentals of Anorectal Surgery, 2nd ed. Philadelphia, Saunders, 1998.

Gordan PH, Nivatvongs S. Principles and Practice of Surgery for Colon, Rectum and Anus, 2nd ed. St. Louis, Quality, 1999.

Parks AG, Hardcastle JD, Gordon PH. A classification of fistula-in-ano. Br J Surg 1976;63:1.

58 Rubber Band Ligation of Internal Hemorrhoids

INDICATIONS

Symptomatic (bleeding or prolapsed) internal hemorrhoids situated above the area in the anal canal, which is innervated by sensory nerves

PITFALLS AND DANGER POINTS

Applying a rubber band in an area supplied by sensory nerves

OPERATIVE STRATEGY

To avoid postoperative pain, apply the rubber band to a point *at least 5-6 mm above the dentate line*. In some patients a margin of 5-6 mm is not sufficient to avoid pain. These patients can be identified by pinching the mucosa at the site of the proposed application of the band. If the patient has pain when the mucosa is pinched, apply the band at a higher level where the mucosa is not sensitive or abandon the rubber-banding procedure.

If the patient has severe pain after the rubber band has been applied, remove the rubber band immediately using fine-tipped forceps and sharp pointed scissors. If this removal is delayed until several hours after the application, surrounding edema often makes the procedure difficult if not impossible without anesthesia and without causing bleeding.

OPERATIVE TECHNIQUE

Perform sigmoidoscopy to rule out other possible sources of rectal bleeding. With the patient in the knee-chest position, insert a fenestrated anoscope (e.g., Hinkel-James type) that permits the internal hemorrhoid to protrude into the lumen of the anoscope. A lighted anoscope is a great convenience. Inspect the circumference of the anal canal. Try to identify the hemorrhoid that caused the bleeding. If this is not possible, identify the largest internal hemorrhoid. Insert the curved Allis tissue forceps into the anoscope and pinch the mucosa around the base of the hemorrhoid to identify an insensitive area. Ask the assistant to hold the anoscope in a steady position. Now inspect the McGivney rubber band applicator. Be sure that two rubber bands have been inserted into their proper position on the drum of the applicator. Ask the patient to strain. With the left hand pass the drum up to the *proximal* portion of the hemorrhoid. Insert the angled tissue forceps through the drum.

When grasping the rectal mucosa, be sure to grasp it along the cephalad surface of the hemorrhoid at point A (not point B) in **Figure 58–1**. If this is done, the rubber band does not encroach on the sensitive tissue at the dentate line. Draw the mucosa into the drum and simultaneously press the drum

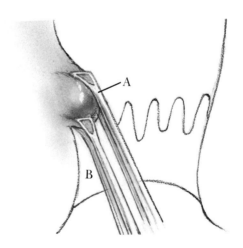

Fig. 58-1

525

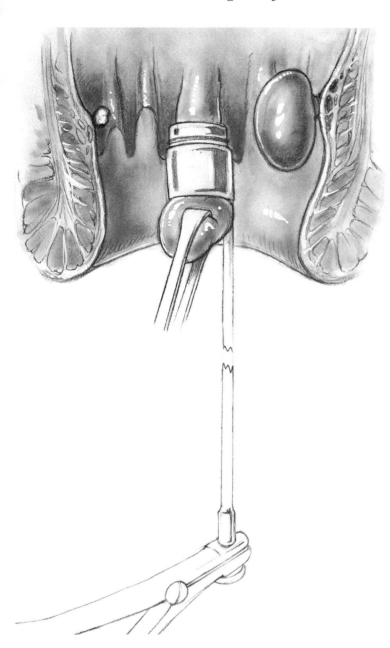

Fig. 58-2

against the wall of the rectum **(Fig. 58–2)**. When the McGivney applicator is in the proper position, compress the handle of the applicator. Remove the tissue forceps and the McGivney applicator from the anoscope. The result should be a round purple mass of hemorrhoid about the size of a cherry and strangulated by the two rubber bands at its base.

Tchirkow et al. (1982) recommended injecting 1–2 ml of a local anesthetic (we use 0.25% bupivacaine or lidocaine with epinephrine 1:200,000), using a 25-gauge needle, into the banded hemorrhoid. This maneuver appears to lessen some of the post-

operative discomfort and may accelerate sloughing of the strangulated mass.

Nivatvongs and Goldberg (1982) advocate applying the band to redundant rectal mucosa just proximal to the hemorrhoid. Insert the slotted anoscope and ask the patient to strain. The redundant rectal mucosa just *proximal to the hemorrhoid* bulges into the slot of the anoscope. Apply the band to this mucosa as detailed above.

In general, only one hemorrhoid is treated at each office visit. Have the patient return in about 3 weeks for the second application. Rarely are more than three applications necessary. Applying two or three bands at one sitting often causes significant discomfort.

POSTOPERATIVE CARE

Inform the patient that postoperatively he or she may feel a vague discomfort in the area of the rectum accompanied by mild tenesmus, especially for 1–2 days after the procedure. Prescribe mild non-constipating analgesic medication. Apprehensive patients do well if this medication is supplemented by a tranquilizer such as diazepam.

Warn the patient prior to the procedure that on rare occasions sometime between the 7th and 10th postoperative days, when the slough separates, there may be active bleeding into the rectum. A serious degree of bleeding requiring hospitalization occurs in no more than 1–2% of cases.

Prescribe a stool softener such as Colace. For constipated patients, Senokot-S (two tablets nightly) helps to keep the stool soft and stimulates colonic peristalsis.

Patients may return to their regular occupation when they so desire.

COMPLICATIONS

Sepsis. Even though tens of thousands of patients have undergone hemorrhoid banding safely, there are reports in the literature of at least nine patients with serious postoperative pelvirectal sepsis, five of whom died (Clay et al., 1986; O'Hara; Russell and Donohue, 1980; Shemesh et al., 1987). The typical patient suffering postbanding sepsis complains of rectal pain and urinary retention on the third of fourth postoperative day. The physical examination and leukocyte count at this time may be normal. Blood cultures in all nine cases were found to be normal. During the next day or two edema of the rectum, perineum, or lower abdominal wall may develop and can be confirmed by computed tomography (CT).

Proctoscopic examination at this stage demonstrates marked edema of the rectum and necrosis at the sites of banding; fever and leukocytosis are also notable at this time, and death is not far off. At autopsy, marked rectal and pelvic edema, sometimes phlegmonous, is common, occasionally accompanied by a small rectal or pelvic abscess. Shemesh et al. theorized that following band ligation transmural ischemic necrosis of the tissue enclosed in the band allowed egress of bowel bacteria into the surrounding pelvic soft tissues. Although the blood cultures were all negative in the reported cases, postmortem bacterial cultures revealed coliform bacteria and, in one case, *Clostridium perfringens, Clostridium sporogenes*, and *Bacteroides* (O'Hara).

All the patients who survived this complication were treated as soon as they presented with pain and urinary symptoms. Intensive, early treatment with intravenous antibiotics aimed at clostridia, other anaerobes, and gram-negative rods is essential. Patients who undergo banding must be told that if they experience urinary symptoms, fever, or pain 1–4 days after the procedure they must promptly return to the surgeon for hospital admission to receive immediate antibiotic treatment, even if physical signs at that time are negligible.

Pain. If *severe* pain occurs upon application of the band, remove the band promptly before the patient leaves the office. Treat a *mild* degree of vague discomfort with medication.

Bleeding. If the patient sustains a mild degree of blood spotting in the stool when the slough separates a week or 10 days after the banding, treat it expectantly. If the patient has lost more than a few hundred milliliters, admit the patient to the hospital for proctoscopy. Suction out all the clots and identify the bleeding point. In some cases the bleeding point can be grasped with Allis tissue forceps and a rubber band again applied to the area. Alternatively, under general or local anesthesia, use either electrocautery or a suture to control the bleeding.

REFERENCES

Barron J. Office ligation treatment of hemorrhoids. Dis Colon Rectum 1963;6:109.

Clay LD III, White JJ Jr, Davidson JT, et al. Early recognition and successful management of pelvic cellulitis following hemorrhoidal banding. Dis Colon Rectum 1986;29:579.

Lee HH, Spencer RJ, Beart RW Jr. Multiple hemorrhoidal bandings in a single session. Dis Colon Rectum 1994;37:37.

Nivatvongs S, Goldberg SM. An improved technique of rubber band ligation of hemorrhoids. Am J Surg 1982;144:379.

O'Hara VS. Fatal clostridial infection following hemorrhoidal banding. Dis Colon Rectum 1980;23:570.

Rudd WWH. Ligation of hemorrhoids as an office procedure. Can Med Assoc J 1973;108:56.

Russell TR, Donohue JH. Hemorrhoidal banding: a warning. Dis Colon Rectum 1985;28:291.

Shemesh EL, Kodner IJ, Fry RD, et al. Severe complication of rubber band ligation of internal hemorrhoids. Dis Colon Rectum 1987;30:199.

Tchirkow G, Haas PA, Fox TA Jr. Injection of a local anesthetic solution into hemorrhoidal bundle following rubber band ligation. Dis Colon Rectum 1982;25:62.

59 Hemorrhoidectomy

INDICATIONS

Persistent bleeding or protrusion

Symptomatic second- and third-degree (combined internal-external) hemorrhoids

Symptomatic hemorrhoids combined with mucosal prolapse

Strangulation of internal hemorrhoids

Early stage of acute thrombosis of external hemorrhoid

CONTRAINDICATIONS

Portal hypertension

Inflammatory bowel disease

Anal malignancy

PREOPERATIVE PREPARATION

Advise patients to discontinue aspirin and other nonsteroidal antiinflammatory agents.

A sodium phosphate packaged enema (Fleet) is adequate cleansing for most patients.

Sigmoidoscopy, colonoscopy, or both are done as indicated by the patient's symptoms.

Routine preoperative blood coagulation profile (partial thromboplastin time, prothrombin time, platelet count) in performed.

Preoperative shaving of the perianal area is preferred by some surgeons but is not necessary.

PITFALLS AND DANGER POINTS

Narrowing the lumen of the anus, thereby inducing anal stenosis

Trauma to sphincter

Failing to identify associated pathology (e.g., inflammatory bowel disease, leukemia, portal hypertension, coagulopathy, squamous carcinoma of the anus)

Failure to manage postoperative bowel function

OPERATIVE STRATEGY

Avoiding Anal Stenosis

The most serious error when performing hemorrhoidectomy is failure to leave adequate bridges of mucosa and anoderm between each site of hemorrhoid excision. If a minimum of 1.0–1.5 cm of viable anoderm is left intact between each site of hemorrhoid resection, the risk of developing anal stenosis is minimized. Preserving viable anoderm is much more important than is removal of all external hemorrhoids and redundant skin.

One method of preventing anal stenosis is to insert a large anal retractor, such as the Fansler or large Ferguson, after resecting the hemorrhoids. If the incisions in the mucosa and anoderm ("closed hemorrhoidectomy") can be sutured with the retractor in place, anal stenosis should not occur if good bowel function is maintained postoperatively.

Achieving Hemostasis

Traditionally, surgeons have depended on mass ligature of the hemorrhoid "pedicle" for achieving hemostasis. This policy ignores the fact that small arteries penetrate the internal sphincter and enter the operative field. Also, numerous vessels are divided when incising the mucosa to dissect the pedicle. In fact, the concept of a "pedicle" as being the source of a hemorrhoidal mass is large erroneous. A hemorrhoidal mass is not a varicose vein situated at the termination of the portal venous system. It is a vascular complex with multiple channels fed by many small vessels. Therefore it is important to control bleeding from each vessel as it is transected during the operation. A convenient method for accomplishing this goal is careful, accurate application of coagulating electrocautery. As pointed out by Goldberg and associates (1980), much of the bleeding comes from the mucosal incision. Therefore it is well to achieve perfect hemostasis before suturing the defect following hemorrhoid excision.

Associated Pathology

Even though hemorrhoidectomy is a minor operation, a complete history and physical examination are necessary to rule out important systemic diseases such as leukemia. Leukemic infiltrates in the rectum can cause severe pain and can mimic hemorrhoids and anal ulcers. Operating erroneously on an undiagnosed acute leukemia patient is fraught with the dangers of bleeding, failure to heal, and sepsis. Crohn's disease must also be ruled out by history, local examination, and sigmoidoscopy, as well as biopsy in doubtful situations.

Another extremely important condition sometimes overlooked during the course of hemorrhoidectomy is squamous cell carcinoma of the anus. It may resemble nothing more than a small ulceration on what appears to be a hemorrhoid. Any hemorrhoid that demonstrates a break in the continuity of the overlying mucosa should be suspected of being a carcinoma, as should any ulcer of the anoderm, except for the classic anal fissure located in the posterior commissure. Before scheduling hemorrhoidectomy, biopsy all ulcerations and atypical lesions of the anal canal.

OPERATIVE TECHNIQUE

Closed Hemorrhoidectomy

Local Anesthesia

Choosing an Anesthetic Agent
A solution of 0.5% lidocaine (maximum dosage 80 ml) or 0.25% bupivacaine (maximum dosage 80 ml), combined with epinephrine 1:200,000 and 150–300 units of hyaluronidase is effective and has extremely low toxicity. Because perianal injection of these agents is painful, premedicate the patient 1 hour before the operation with an intramuscular injection of some combination of narcotic and sedative (e.g., Demerol and a barbiturate, or Innovar, 1–2 ml). Alternatively, give diazepam in a dose of 5–10 mg intravenously just before the perianal injection.

Techniques of Local Anesthesia
With the technique originally introduced by Kratzer (1974), the anesthetic agent is placed in a syringe with a 25-gauge needle. The needle should be at least 5 cm in length. Initiate the injection at a point 2–3 cm lateral to the middle of the anus. Inject 10–15 ml of the solution in the *subcutaneous* tissues surrounding the right half of the anal canal including the area of the anoderm at the anal verge. Warn the patient that this injection may be quite painful. Repeat this maneuver through a needle puncture site to the left of the anal canal. After placing a slotted anoscope in the anal canal, insert the needle into the tissues just underneath the anoderm and into the plane between the submucosa and the internal sphincter 3–4 cm deep into the anal canal **(Fig. 59–1)**. If the injection creates a wheal in the mu-

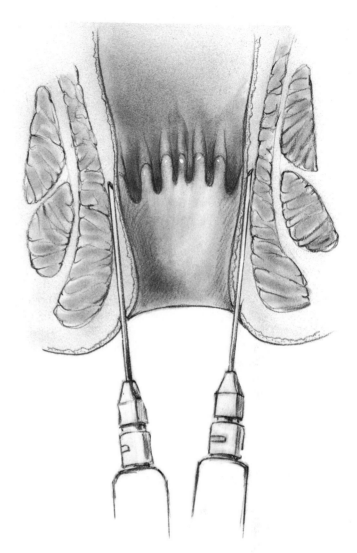

Fig. 59-1

cosa similar to that seen in the skin after an intradermal injection, the needle is in a too-shallow position. An injection into the proper submucosal plane produces no visible change in the overlying mucosa. Inject 3–4 ml of anesthetic solution during the course of withdrawing the needle. Make similar injections in each of the four quadrants until the subdermal and submucosal tissues of the anal canal have been surrounded with anesthetic agent. It should require no more than 30–40 ml of anesthetic solution. Satisfactory relaxation of the sphincters is achieved without the need to inject solution directly into the muscles or to attempt to block the inferior hemorrhoidal nerve in the ischiorectal space. Wait 5–10 minutes for complete relaxation and anesthesia.

In 1982, Nivatvongs described a technique to minimize pain. It consisted, first, of inserting a small anoscope into the anal canal. Make the first injection into the *submucosal* plane 2 mm *above* the dentate line. Because of the difference in sensory innervation of the mucosa above the dentate line, injection here does not produce acute pain. Inject 2–3 ml of anesthetic solution and then an equal amount of solution in each of the remaining three quadrants of the anus. Remove the anoscope and insert a well lubricated index finger into the anal canal. Use the tip of the index finger to massage the anesthetic agent from the submucosal area down into the tissues underneath the anoderm. Repeat this maneuver with respect to each of the four injection sites. By spreading the anesthetic agent distally, this maneuver serves to anesthetize the highly sensitive tissues of the anoderm just distal to the dentate line. When this has been accomplished, make another series of injections 2 mm *distal* to the dentate line. Inject 2–3 ml of solution underneath the anoderm and the subcutaneous tissues in the perianal region through four sites, one in each quadrant of the anus. Then use the index finger again to massage the tissues of the anal canal to spread the anesthetic solution circumferentially around the anal and perianal area. In some cases additional anesthetic agent is necessary for complete circumferential anesthesia. An average of 20–25 ml of solution is required. Nivatvongs stated that this technique provides excellent relaxation of the sphincters and permits operation such as hemorrhoidectomy to be accomplished without general anesthesia. For a lateral sphincterotomy, it is not necessary to anesthetize the entire circumference of the anal canal when using this technique. Inject only the area of the sphincterotomy.

Intravenous Fluids

Because local anesthesia has few systemic effects, it is not necessary to administer a large volume of intravenous fluid during the operation. If large volumes of fluid are administered intraoperatively, the bladder becomes rapidly distended. In the presence of general anesthesia or even heavy sedation during local anesthesia, the patient is not sufficiently alert to have the desire to void. By the time the patient is alert, the bladder muscle has been stretched and may be too weak to empty the bladder, especially if the patient also has anal pain and some degree of prostatic hypertrophy. This can cause postoperative urinary retention, requiring catheterization. All of this can be prevented by avoiding general anesthesia and heavy premedication and by limiting the dosage of intravenous fluids to 100–200 ml during and after hemorrhoidectomy.

Positioning the Patient

We prefer to place the patient in the semiprone jackknife position with either a sandbag or rolled-up sheet under the hips and a small pillow to support the feet. It is not necessary to shave the perianal area; if the buttocks are hirsute, shave this area. Then apply tincture of benzoin. When this solution has dried, apply wide adhesive tape to the buttock and attach the other end of the adhesive strap to the operating table. In this fashion lateral traction is applied to each buttock, affording excellent exposure of the anus.

Incision and Dissection

Gently dilate the anal canal so it admits two fingers. Insert a bivalve speculum such as the Parks retractor or a medium-size Hill-Ferguson retractor. One advantage of using the medium Hill-Ferguson retractor is that it approximates the diameter of the normal anal canal. If the defects remaining in the mucosa and anoderm can be sutured closed with the retractor in place following hemorrhoid excision, no narrowing of the anal canal occurs. Each of the hemorrhoidal masses can be identified by rotating the retractor and applying countertraction to the skin of the opposite wall of the anal canal. Generally, three hemorrhoidal complexes are excised: one in the left midlateral position, another in the right anterolateral position, and the third in the right posterolateral location. Avoid placing incisions in the anterior or posterior commissures. Grasp the most dependent portion of the largest hemorrhoidal mass in a Babcock clamp. Then make an incision in the anoderm outlining the distal extremity of the hemorrhoid **(Fig. 59–2)** using a No. 15 (Bard Parker) scalpel. If the hemorrhoidal mass is unusually broad (>1.5 cm), do not excise all of the anoderm and mucosa overlying

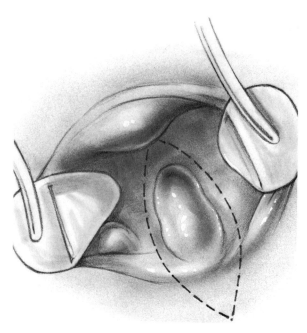

Fig. 59-2

the hemorrhoid. If each of the hemorrhoidal masses is equally broad, excising all of the anoderm and mucosa overlying each of the hemorrhoids results in inadequate tissue bridges between the sites of hemorrhoid excision. In such a case incise the mucosa and anoderm overlying the hemorrhoid in an elliptical fashion. Then initiate a submucosal dissection using small, pointed scissors to elevate the mucosa and anoderm from the portion of the hemorrhoid that remains in a submucosal location. Carry the dissection of the hemorrhoidal mass down to the internal sphincter muscle **(Fig. 59–3)**. After incising the mucosa and anoderm, draw the hemorrhoid away from the sphincter, using blunt dissection as necessary, to demonstrate the lower border of the internal sphincter. This muscle has whitish muscle fibers that run in a transverse direction. A thin bridge of fibrous tissue is often seen connecting the substance of the hemorrhoid to the internal sphincter. Divide these fibers with a scissors. Dissect the hemorrhoidal mass for a distance of about 1-2 cm above the dentate line where it can be divided with the electrocoagulator **(Fig. 59–4)**. Remove any residual internal hemorrhoids from underneath the adjacent mucosa. Achieve complete hemostasis, primarily with careful electrocoagulation. It is not necessary to clamp and suture the hemorrhoidal "pedicle," although many surgeons prefer to do so **(Fig. 59–5)**. It is helpful to remove all the internal hemorrhoids, but we do not attempt to extract fragments of ex-

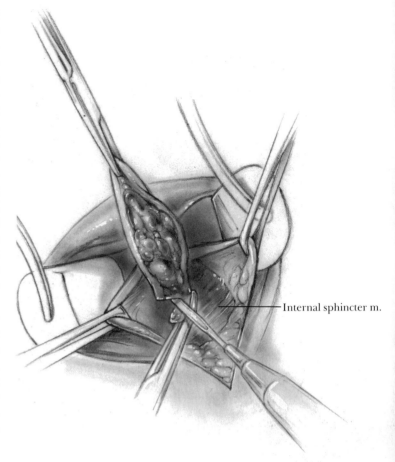

Internal sphincter m.

Fig. 59-4

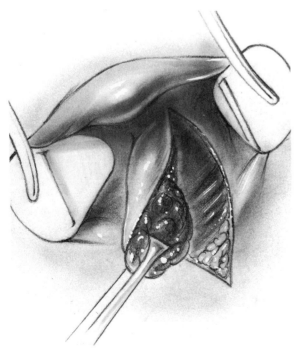

Fig. 59-3

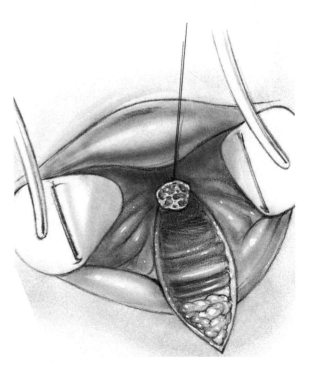

Fig. 59-5

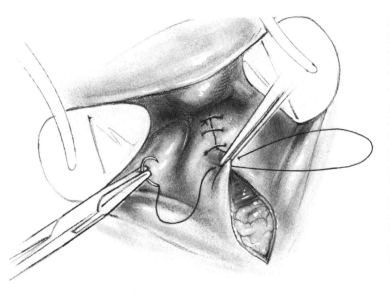

Fig. 59-6

ternal hemorrhoids from underneath the anoderm, as this step does not appear necessary. Most of these small external hemorrhoids disappear spontaneously following interna hemorrhoidectomy.

After complete hemostasis has been achieved, insert an atraumatic 5-0 Vicryl suture into the apex of the hemorrhoidal defect. Tie the suture and then close the defect with a continuous locking suture taking 2- to 3-mm bites of mucosa on each side **(Fig. 59–6)**. Also include a small bit of the underlying internal sphincter muscle with each pass of the nee-

dle. This maneuver serves to force the mucosa to adhere to the underlying muscle layer and thereby helps prevent mucosal prolapse and recurrent hemorrhoids. Continue the suture line until the entire defect has been closed. Now repeat the same dissection for each of the other two hemorrhoidal masses. Close each of the mucosal defects by the same technique **(Fig. 59–7)**. Be certain not to constrict the lumen of the anal canal. The rectal lumen should admit a Fanster or a large Ferguson rectal retractor after the suturing is completed. To avoid anal stenosis remember that the ellipse of mucosa-anoderm excised with each hemorrhoidal mass must be relatively narrow. Also remember that if the tissues are sutured under tension, the suture line will undoubtedly break down.

A few patients have some degree of anal stenosis in addition to hemorrhoids. Under these conditions, rather than forcibly dilating the anal canal at the onset of the operation, perform a partial lateral internal sphincterotomy to provide adequate exposure for the operation. This is also true for patients who have a concomitant chronic anal fissure.

For surgeons who prefer to keep the skin unsutured for drainage, modify the above operative procedure by discontinuing the mucosal suture line at the dentate line, leaving the defect in the anoderm unsutured. It is also permissible not to suture the mucosal defects at all after hemorrhoidectomy (see above).

Radical Open Hemorrhoidectomy

Incision

Radical open hemorrhoidectomy is restricted to patients who no longer have three discrete hemorrhoidal masses but in whom all of the hemorrhoids and prolapsing rectal mucosa seem to have coalesced into an almost circumferential mucosal prolapse. For these patients the operation excises the hemorrhoids, both internal and external, the redundant anoderm, and prolapsed mucosa from both the left and right lateral portions of the anus, leaving 1.5 cm bridges of intact mucosa and anoderm at the anterior and posterior commissures. With the patient in the prone position, as described above for closed hemorrhoidectomy, outline the incision on both sides of the anus as shown in **Figure 59–8**.

Excising the Hemorrhoidal Masses

Elevate the skin flap together with the underlying hemorrhoids by sharp and blunt dissection until the lower border of the internal sphincter muscle has been unroofed **(Fig. 59–9)**. This muscle can be identified by its transverse whitish fibers. Now elevate

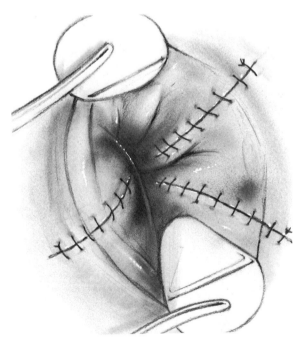

Fig. 59-7

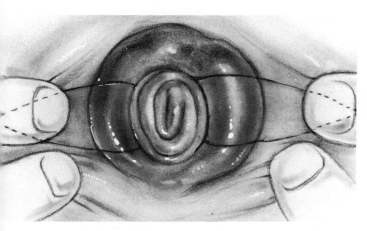

Fig. 59-8

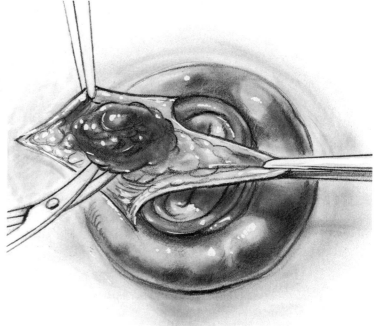

Fig. 59-10

the anoderm above and below the incision to enucleate adjacent hemorrhoids that have not been included in the initial dissection **(Fig. 59–10)**. This maneuver permits removal of almost all the hemorrhoids and still allows an adequate bridge of anoderm in the anterior and posterior commissures.

After the mass of hemorrhoidal tissue with overlying mucosa has been mobilized to the level of the normal location of the dentate line, amputate the mucosa and hemorrhoids with electrocautery at the level of the dentate line. This leaves a free edge of rectal mucosa. Suture this mucosa to the underlying internal sphincter muscle with a continuous 5-0 atraumatic Vicryl suture, as illustrated in **Figure**

59–11, to recreate the dentate line at its normal location. Do not bring the rectal mucosa down to the area that is normally covered by anoderm or skin, as it would result in continuous secretion of mucus, which would irritate the perianal skin.

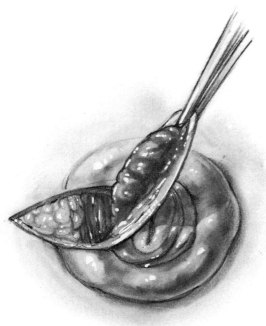

Fig. 59-9

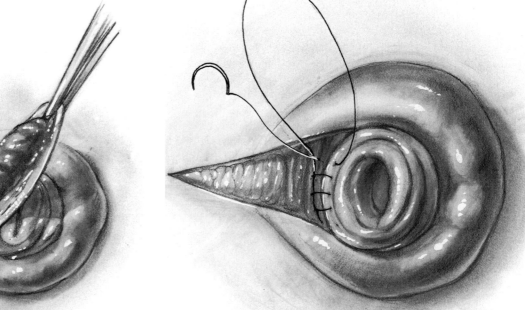

Fig. 59-11

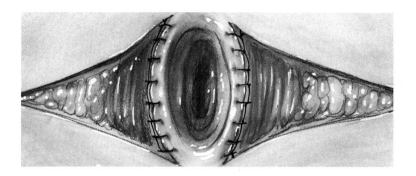

Fig. 59-12

Execute the same dissection to remove all of the hemorrhoidal tissue between 1 and 5 o'clock on the right side and reattach the free cut edge of rectal mucosa to the underlying internal sphincter muscle, as depicted in **Figure 59–12**. There may be some redundant anoderm together with some external hemorrhoids at the anterior or posterior commissure of the anus. Do not attempt to remove every last bit of external hemorrhoid as it would jeopardize the viability of the anoderm in the commissures. Unless viable bridges, about 1.5 cm each in width, are preserved in the anterior and posterior commissures, the danger of a postoperative anal stenosis far outweighs the primarily cosmetic ill effect of leaving behind a skin tag or an occasional external hemorrhoid.

Ensure that hemostasis is complete using electrocautery and occasional suture-ligatures of fine PG or chromic catgut. Some surgeons also insert a small piece of rolled-up Gelfoam into the anus at the completion of the procedure. This roll, which should not be more than 1 cm in thickness, serves to apply gentle pressure and to encourage coagulation of minor bleeding points that may have been overlooked. The Gelfoam need not be removed, as it dissolves when the patient starts having sitz baths postoperatively. Apply a sterile dressing to the perianal area.

Anal packing with anything more substantial than the 1 cm roll of soft Gelfoam should not be necessary, as hemostasis with electrocautery should be meticulous. Large gauze or other rigid packs are associated with increased postoperative pain and urinary retention.

POSTOPERATIVE CARE

Encourage ambulation the day of operation.

Prescribe analgesic medication preferably of a nonconstipating type such as Darvocet.

Prescribe Senokot-S, Metamucil, or mineral oil while the patient is in the hospital. After discharge, limit the use of cathartics because passage of a well formed stool is the best guarantee the anus will not become stenotic. In patients with severe chronic constipation, dietary bran and some type of laxative or stool softener is necessary following discharge from the hospital.

Order warm sitz baths several times a day, especially following each bowel movement.

Discontinue intravenous fluids as soon as the patient returns to his or her room and initiate a regular diet and oral fluids as desired.

If the patient was hospitalized for the hemorrhoidectomy, he or she is generally discharged on the first or second postoperative day. Most patients tolerate hemorrhoidectomy in the ambulatory outpatient setting.

COMPLICATIONS

Serious bleeding during the postoperative period is rare if complete hemostasis has been achieved in the operating room. However, if bleeding is brisk, the patient should probably be returned to the operating room to have the bleeding point suture-ligated. Most patients who experience major bleeding after discharge from the hospital have experienced a minor degree of bleeding before discharge. About 1% of patients present with hemorrhage severe enough to require reoperation for hemostasis, generally 8–14 days following operation. If the bleeding is slow but continues or if no bleeding site is identified, the patient should be evaluated for coagulopathy, including that caused by platelet dysfunction.

If for some reason the patient is not returned to the operating room for the control of bleeding, it is possible to achieve at least temporary control by inserting a 30 ml Foley catheter into the rectum. The Foley balloon is then blown up, and downward traction is applied to the catheter. Reexploration of the anus for surgical control of bleeding is far preferable.

Infection occurs but is rare.

Skin tags follow hemorrhoidectomy in 6–10% of cases. Although no treatment is required, for cosmetic purposes a skin tag may be excised under local anesthesia as an office procedure when the operative site has healed completely.

REFERENCES

Corman ML. Hemorrhoids. In Colon and Rectal Surgery, 3rd ed. Philadelphia, Lippincott, 1993, pp 54–115.

Ferguson JA, Heaton JR. Closed hemorrhoidectomy. Dis Colon Rectum 1959;2:176.

Goldberg SM, Gordon PH, Nivatvongs, S. Essentials of Anorectal Surgery. Philadelphia, Lippincott, 1980.

Kratzer GL. Improved local anesthesia in anorectal surgery. Am Surg 1974;40:609.

Mazier WP. Hemorrhoids, fissures, and pruritus ani. Surg Clin North Am 1994;74:1277.

Nivatvongs S. An improved technique of local anesthesia for anorectal surgery. Dis Colon Rectum 1982;25:259.

Thomson WHF. The nature of hemorrhoids. Br J Surg 1975;162:542.

60 Anorectal Fistula and Pelvirectal Abscess

INDICATIONS

Drainage of anorectal abscess is indicated *as soon as the diagnosis is made*. There is no role for conservative management because severe sepsis can develop and spread before fluctuance and typical physical findings appear. This is especially true in diabetic patients.

Recurrent or persistent drainage from a perianal fistula calls for repair.

Weak anal sphincter muscles are a relative *contraindication* to fistulotomy, especially in the unusual cases in which the fistulotomy must be performed through the anterior aspect of the anal canal. Absence of the puborectalis muscle in the anterior area of the canal causes inherent sphincter weakness in this location. This category of case is probably better suited for treatment by inserting a seton or by an advancement flap, especially in women.

PREOPERATIVE PREPARATION

Cathartic the night before operation and saline enema on the morning of operation

Preoperative anoscopy and sigmoidoscopy

Colonoscopy, small bowel radiography series, or both when Crohn's enteritis or colitis is suspected

Antibiotic coverage with mechanical bowel preparation if an advancement flap is contemplated

PITFALLS AND DANGER POINTS

Failure to diagnose anorectal sepsis and to perform early incision and drainage

Failure to diagnose or control Crohn's disease

Failure to rule out anorectal tuberculosis or acute leukemia

Induction of fecal incontinence by excessive or incorrect division of the anal sphincter muscles

OPERATIVE STRATEGY

Choice of Anesthesia

Because palpation of the sphincter mechanism is a key component of the surgical procedure, a light general anesthetic is preferable to a regional anesthetic.

Localizing Fistulous Tracts

Goodsall's Rule

When a fistulous orifice is identified in the perianal skin posterior to a line drawn between 3 o'clock and 9 o'clock, the internal opening of the fistula is almost always found in the posterior commissure in a crypt approximately at the dentate line. Goodsall's rule also states that if a fistulous tract is identified anterior to the 3 o'clock/9 o'clock line, its internal orifice is likely to be located along the course of a line connecting the orifice of the fistula to an imaginary point exactly in the middle of the anal canal. In other words, a fistula draining in the perianal area at 4 o'clock in a patient lying prone is likely to have its internal opening situated at the dentate line at 4 o'clock. There are exceptions to this rule. For instance, a horseshoe fistula may drain anterior to the anus but continue in a posterior direction and terminate in the posterior commissure.

If the external fistula opening is more than 3 cm from the anal verge, be suspicious of unusual pathology. Look for Crohn's disease, tuberculosis, or other disease processes such as hidradenitis suppurativa or pilonidal disease.

Physical Examination

First, attempt to identify the course of the fistula in the perianal area by palpating the associated fibrous tract. Second, carefully palpate the region of the dentate line. The site of origin is often easier to feel than it is to see. Next, insert a bivalve speculum into the anus and try to identify the internal opening by gentle probing at the point indicated by Goodsall's rule. If the internal opening is not readily apparent, do not make any false passages. The most accurate method for identifying the direction of the tract is gently to insert a blunt malleable probe, such as a lacrimal duct probe, into the fistula with the index finger in the rectum. In this fashion it may be possible to identify the internal orifice by palpating the probe with the index finger in the anal canal.

Injection of Dye or Radiopaque Material

On rare occasions injection of a blue dye may help identify the internal orifice of a complicated fistula. Some surgeons have advocated the use of milk or hydrogen peroxide instead of a blue dye. These agents allow one to perform multiple injections without the extensive tissue staining that follows the use of blue dye. Injection of a radiopaque liquid followed by radiographic studies can be valuable for the extrasphincteric fistulas leading high up into the rectum, but it does not appear to be helpful for the usual type of fistula.

Endorectal sonography and computed tomography (CT) or magnetic resonance imaging (MRI) fistulography are more modern techniques for evaluating complex fistulas. However, they do not reveal enough detail to identify the site of origin of the fistula precisely.

Preserving Fecal Continence

As mentioned in the discussion above, the puborectalis muscle (anorectal ring) must function normally to preserve fecal continence following fistulotomy. Identify this muscle accurately before dividing the anal sphincter muscles during the course of a fistulotomy. Use local anesthesia with sedation or general anesthesia for the fistulotomy. If the fistulous tract can be identified with a *probe preoperatively*, the surgeon's index finger in the anal canal can identify the anorectal ring without difficulty, especially if the patient is asked to tighten the voluntary sphincter muscles.

If there is any doubt about the identification of the anorectal ring (the proximal portion of the anal canal), do not complete the fistulotomy; rather, insert a heavy silk or braided polyester ligature through the remaining portion of the tract. Tie the ligature loosely with five or six knots without completing the fistulotomy. When the patient is examined in the awake state, it is simple to determine whether the upper border of the seton has encircled the anorectal ring or there is sufficient puborectalis muscle (1.5 cm or more) above the seton to complete the fistulotomy by dividing the muscles enclosed in the seton at a later stage. If no more than half of the external sphincter muscles in the anal canal have been divided, fecal continence should be preserved in patients with formed stools and a normally compliant rectum. An exception would be those patients who had a weak sphincter muscle prior to operation.

Fistulotomy Versus Fistulectomy

When performing surgery to cure an anal fistula, most authorities are satisfied that incising the fistula along its entire length constitutes adequate therapy. Others have advocated excision of the fibrous cylinder that constitutes the fistula, leaving only surrounding fat and muscle tissue behind. The latter technique leaves a large open wound, however, which takes much longer to heal. Moreover, much more bleeding is encountered during a fistulectomy than a fistulotomy. Hence there is no evidence to indicate that excising the wall of the fistula has any advantages.

Combining Fistulotomy with Drainage of Anorectal Abscess

For patients with an acute ischiorectal abscess, some have advocated that the surgical procedure include a fistulotomy simultaneous with drainage of the abscess. After the pus has been evacuated, a search is made for the internal opening of the fistulous tract and then the tract is opened. This combination of operations is contraindicated for two reasons. First, many of our patients who undergo simple drainage of an abscess never develop a fistula. It is likely that the internal orifice of the anal duct has become occluded before the abscess is treated. These patients do not require a fistulotomy. Second, acute inflammation and edema surrounding the abscess make accurate detection and evaluation of the fistulous tract extremely difficult. There is great likelihood that the surgeon will create false passages that may prove so disabling to the patient that any time saved by combining the drainage operation with a fistulotomy is insignificant. We presently drain many anorectal abscesses in the office under local anesthesia, in part because this method removes the temptation to add a fistulotomy to the drainage procedure.

OPERATIVE TECHNIQUE

Anorectal and Pelvirectal Abscesses

Perianal Abscess

When draining an anorectal abscess it is important to excise a patch of overlying skin so the pus drains freely. The typical perianal abscess is located fairly close to the anus, and often drainage can be performed under local anesthesia. Packing is rarely necessary and may impede drainage.

A Malecot catheter can be placed in the cavity and sewn in place in patients with recurrent abscesses or Crohn's disease in whom continued problems may be anticipated. After 10 days, ingrowth of tissue keeps the Malecot in place without sutures. This serves as a temporizing procedure prior to fistulotomy in patients without Crohn's disease. It may be used as a permanent solution for the difficult Crohn's patient with perianal fistula disease.

Ischiorectal Abscess

The ischiorectal abscess is generally larger than the perianal abscess, develops at a greater distance from the anus, and may be deep-seated. Fluctuance on physical examination may be a late sign. Early drainage under general anesthesia is indicated. Make a cruciate incision over the apex of the inflamed area close to the anal verge so any resulting fistula is short. Excise enough of the overhanging skin to permit free drainage and evacuate the pus. Explore the abscess for loculations.

Intersphincteric Abscess

Many physicians fail to diagnose an intersphincteric abscess until the abscess ruptures into the ischiorectal space and forms an ischiorectal abscess. A patient who complains of persistent anal pain should be suspected of harboring an intersphincteric abscess. This is especially true if, on inspecting the anus with the buttocks spread apart, the physician can rule out the presence of an anal fissure. Examination under anesthesia may be necessary to confirm the diagnosis. Digital examination in the unanesthetized patient may indicate at which point in the anal canal the abscess is located. Parks and Thomson (1973) found that 61% of the intersphincteric abscesses occurred in the posterior quadrant of the anal canal. In half their patients a small mass could be palpated in the anal canal with the index finger inside the canal and the thumb just outside. Occasionally an internal opening draining a few drops of pus is identified near the dentate line. A patient may have both an anal fissure and an intersphincteric abscess.

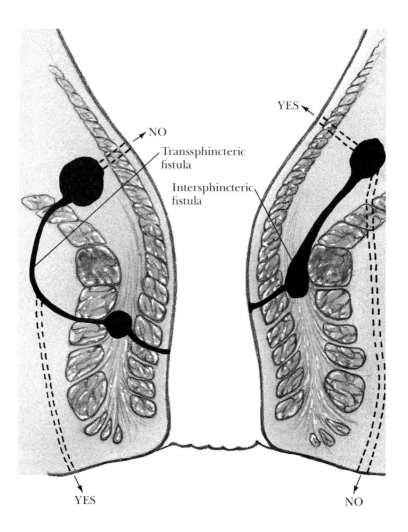

Fig. 60–1

Under local or general anesthesia, carefully palpate the anal canal. Then insert a bivalve speculum and inspect the circumference of the anus to identify a possible fissure or an internal opening of the intersphincteric abscess. After identifying the point on the circumference of the anal canal that is the site of the abscess, perform an internal sphincterotomy by the same technique as described in Chapter 61 for an anal fissure. Place the internal sphincterotomy directly over the site of the intersphincteric abscess. Explore the cavity, which is generally small, with the index finger. If the abscess has been properly unroofed, simply reexamine the area daily with an index finger for the first week or so postoperatively. Uneventful healing can be anticipated unless the abscess has already penetrated the external sphincter muscle and created an undetected extension in the ischiorectal space.

Pelvirectal Supralevator Abscess

An abscess above the levator diaphragm is manifested by pain (gluteal and perineal), fever, and leukocytosis; it often occurs in patients with diabetes or other illnesses. Pus can appear in the supralevator space by extension upward from an inter-

sphincteric fistula, penetration through the levator diaphragm of a transsphincteric fistula, or direct extension from an abscess in the rectosigmoid area. When there is obvious infection in the ischiorectal fossa secondary to a *transsphincteric* fistula, manifested by local induration and tenderness, make an incision at the dependent point of the ischiorectal infection **(Fig. 60–1)**. The incision must be large enough to explore the area with the index finger. It may be necessary to incise the levator diaphragm from below and to enlarge this opening with a long Kelly hemostat to provide adequate drainage of the supralevator abscess. After thoroughly irrigating the area, insert gauze packing.

In pelvirectal abscesses arising from an *intersphincteric* fistula, one is often able to palpate the fluctuant abscess by inserting the index finger high up in the rectum. Aspirate the region of fluctuation under general anesthesia. If pus is obtained, make an incision in the rectum with electrocautery and drain the abscess through the rectum (Fig. 60-1).

Under no condition should one drain a supralevator abscess through the rectum if the abscess has its origin in an *ischiorectal* space infection **(Fig. 60–2)**, an error that could result in a high extrasphincteric fistula. Similarly, if the supralevator sep-

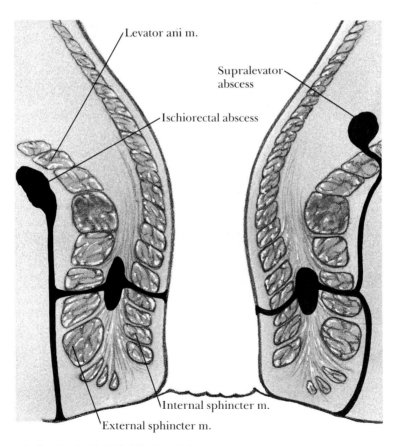

Fig. 60-2. Transsphincteric fistulas (with high blind tracks).

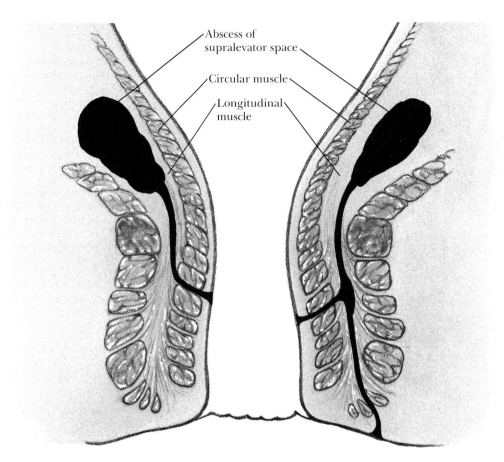

Fig. 60-3. High intersphincteric track fistulas (with supralevator abcesses).

sis has arisen from an intersphincteric abscess, draining the supralevator infection through the ischiorectal fossa also leads to a high extrasphincteric fistula, and this error should also be avoided **(Fig. 60–3)**.

Anorectal Fistula

Intersphincteric Fistula

Simple Low Fistula

When dealing with an unselected patient population, simple low fistula occurs in perhaps half of all patients presenting with anorectal fistulas. Here the injected anal gland burrows distally in the intersphincteric space to form either a perianal abscess or a perianal fistula, as illustrated in Figure 57-2. Performing a fistulotomy here requires only division of the internal sphincter and overlying anoderm up to the internal orifice of the fistula approximately at the dentate line. This divides the distal half of the internal sphincter, rarely producing any permanent disturbance of function.

High Blind Track (Rare)

With a high blind track fistula the mid-anal infection burrows in a cephalad direction between the circular internal sphincter and the longitudinal muscle fibers of the upper canal and lower rectal wall to form a small *intramural* abscess above the levator diaphragm **(Fig. 60–4)**. This abscess can be palpated by digital examination. The infection will probably heal if the primary focus is drained by excising a 1 × 1 cm square of internal sphincter at the site of the internal orifice of this "fistula." Parks et al. (1976) stated that even if the entire internal sphincter is divided while laying open this high blind track by opening the internal sphincter from the internal orifice of the track to the upper extension of the track, little disturbed continence develops because the edges of the sphincter are held together by the fibrosis produced as the track develops.

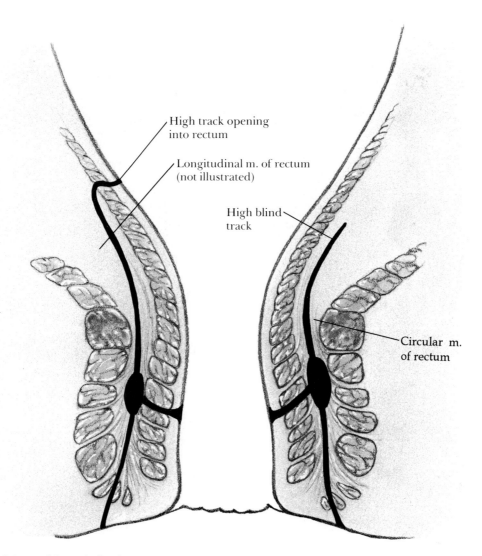

High track opening
into rectum

Longitudinal m. of rectum
(not illustrated)

High blind
track

Circular m.
of rectum

Fig. 60-4. High intersphincteric fistulas.

High Track Opening into Rectum (Rare)

With a high track opening into the rectum, a probe inserted into the internal orifice continues upward between the internal sphincter and the longitudinal muscle of the rectum. The probe opens into the rectum at the upper end of the fistula (Fig. 60-4). If by palpating the probe the surgeon recognizes that this fistula is quite superficial and is located deep only to the circular muscle layer, the tissue overlying the probe can be laid open without risk. On the other hand, if the probe goes deep to the *external* sphincter muscle prior to reentering the rectum (see Fig. 57-5), it constitutes a type of extrasphincteric fistula that is extremely difficult to manage (see below). If there is any doubt about the true nature of this type of fistula, refer the patient to a specialist.

High Track with No Perineal Opening (Rare)

An unusual intersphincteric fistula is the high track fistula with no perineal opening. The infection begins in the mid-anal intersphincteric space and burrows upward in the rectal wall, reentering the lower rectum through a secondary opening above the

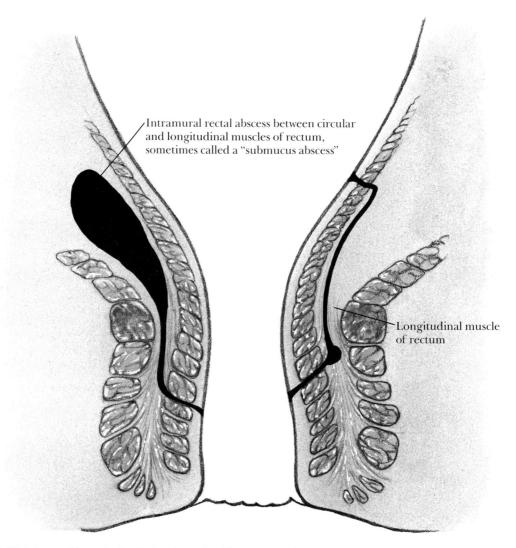

Fig. 60-5. High intersphincteric fistula (or abscess) with no perineal openings.

anorectal ring **(Fig. 60–5)**. There is no downward spread of the infection and no fistula in the perianal skin. To treat this fistula it is necessary to lay the track open from its internal opening in the mid-anal canal up into the lower rectum. Parks and associates emphasized that the lowermost part of the track in the mid-anal canal must be excised because it contains the infected anal gland, which is the primary source of the infection. Leaving it behind may result in a recurrence. If a fistula of this type presents in the acute phase, it resembles a "submucous abscess," but this is an erroneous term because the infection is indeed deep not only to the mucosa but also to the circular muscle layer (Fig. 60-5). This type of abscess is drained by incising the overlying mucosa and circular muscle of the rectum.

High Track with Pelvic Extension (Rare)

With a high track fistula with pelvic extension the infection spreads upward in the intersphincteric space, breaks through the longitudinal muscle, and enters the pelvis (supralevator) (Fig. 60-3). To treat it, open the fistulous track by incising the internal sphincter together with the overlying mucosa or anoderm up into the rectum for 1-3 cm. Drain the pelvic collection through this incision, with the drain exiting into the rectum.

High Track Secondary to Pelvic Disease (Rare)

As mentioned above, the intersphincteric plane "is a natural pathway for infection from the pelvis to follow should it track downward" (Parks et al.). This type of fistula **(Fig. 60–6)** does not arise from anal disease and does not require perianal surgery. Treatment consists of removing the pelvic infection by abdominal surgery.

Transsphincteric Fistula

Uncomplicated Fistula

As illustrated in Figure 57-3, the fairly common uncomplicated transsphincteric fistula arises in the intersphincteric space of the mid-anal canal, with the infection then burrowing laterally directly through the external sphincter muscle. There it may form either an abscess or a fistulous track down through the skin overlying the ischiorectal space. If a probe is passed through the fistulous opening in the skin and along the track until it enters the rectum at the internal opening of the fistula, all of the overlying tissue may be divided without serious functional disturbance because only the distal half of the internal sphincter and the distal half of the external sphincter has been transected. Occasionally one of these fistulas crosses the external sphincter closer to the puborectalis muscle than is shown here. In this case, if there is doubt that the entire puborectalis can be left intact, the external sphincter should be divided in two stages. Divide the distal half during the first stage and insert a seton through the remaining fistula, around the remaining muscle bundle. Leave it intact for 2–3 months before dividing the remainder of the sphincter.

High Blind Track

The fistula with high blind track burrows through the external sphincter, generally at the level of the mid-anal canal. The fistula then not only burrows downward to the skin but also in a cephalad direction to the apex of the ischiorectal fossa (Fig. 60–2).

Occasionally it burrows through the levator ani muscles into the pelvis. Parks et al. pointed out that when a probe is passed into the external opening, it generally goes directly to the upper end of the blind track and that the internal opening in the mid-anal canal may be difficult to delineate by such probing. Occasionally there is localized induration in the mid-anal canal to indicate the site of the infected anal gland that initiated the pathologic process. Probing this area should reveal the internal opening. By inserting the index finger into the anal canal, one can often feel, above the anorectal ring, the induration that is caused by the supralevator extension of the infection. The surgeon can often feel the probe in the fistula with the index finger. The probe may feel close to the rectal wall. Parks emphasized that it is dangerous to penetrate the wall of the rectum with this probe or to try to drain this infection through

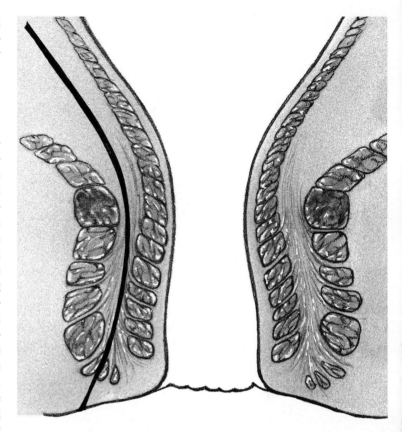

Fig. 60-6. High intersphincteric track fistula (*secondary to pelvic sepsis*).

the upper rectum. If it is done, an extrasphincteric fistula would be created with grave implications for the patient. The proper treatment for this type of fistula, even with a supralevator extension, is to transect the mucosa, internal sphincter, external sphincter, and perianal skin from the mid-anal canal down to the orifice of the track in the skin of the buttock. The upper extension heals with this type of drainage.

Suprasphincteric Fistula (Extremely Rare)

The suprasphincteric fistula originates, as usual, in the mid-anal canal in the intersphincteric space, where its internal opening can generally be found. The fistula extends upward in the intersphincteric plane above the puborectalis muscle into the supralevator space, where it often causes a supralevator abscess. The fistula then penetrates the levator diaphragm and continues downward in the ischiorectal space to its external orifice in the perineal skin (Fig. 57-4). This type of supralevator infection must not be drained through an incision in the rectum. Parks and Stitz (1958) recommended an internal sphincterotomy from the internal opening of the fistula distally and excision of the abscess in the intersphincteric space, if present. They then divide the lower 30–50% of the external sphincter muscle and continue this incision laterally until the lower portion of the fistulous track has been opened down to its external opening in the skin. This maneuver leaves the upper half of the external and internal sphincter muscles and the puborectalis muscle intact. Insert a seton of heavy braided nylon through the fistula as it surrounds the muscles. Tie the seton with five or six knots but keep the loop in the seton loose enough so it does not constrict the remaining muscles at this time. Insert a drain into the supralevator abscess, preferably in the intersphincteric space between the seton and the remaining internal sphincter muscle. Once adequate drainage has been established, remove this drain, as the heavy seton prevents the lower portion of the wound from closing prematurely. Parks does not remove these setons for at least 3 months. It is often necessary to return the patient to the operating room 10–14 days following the initial operation to examine the situation carefully and to ascertain that no residual pocket of infection has remained undrained. Examination under anesthesia may be necessary on several occasions before complete healing has been achieved. In most cases, after 3 months or more has passed the supralevator infection has healed completely, and it is not necessary to divide the muscles enclosed in the seton. In these cases simply remove the seton and permit the wound to heal spontaneously. If after 3–4 months there is lingering infection in the upper reaches of the wound, it is possible to divide the muscles contained in the seton because the long-standing fibrosis prevents significant retraction and the muscle generally heals with restoration of fecal continence.

Alternatively, an advancement flap to close the internal opening of the fistula may save these patients multiple operations. It also avoids sphincter division.

Extrasphincteric Fistula (Extremely Rare)

Secondary to Transsphincteric Fistula

In an unusual situation, a transsphincteric fistula, after entering the ischiorectal fossa, travels not only downward to the skin of the buttocks but also in a cephalad direction, penetrating the levator diaphragm into the pelvis and then through the entire wall and mucosa of the rectum (Fig. 57–5). If this fistula were to be completely laid open surgically, the entire internal and entire external sphincter together with part of the levator diaphragm would have to be divided. The result would be total fecal incontinence. The proper treatment here consists of a temporary di-

verting colostomy combined with simple laying open of the portion of the fistula that extends from the mid-anal canal to the skin. After the defect in the rectum heals, the colostomy can be closed.

The extrasphincteric fistula may also be treated by fashioning an advancement flap. With this procedure it is often unnecessary to create a temporary colostomy.

Secondary to Trauma

A traumatic fistula may be caused by a foreign body penetrating the perineum, the levator ani muscle, and the rectum. A swallowed foreign body such as a fish bone may also perforate the rectum above the anorectal ring and be forced through the levator diaphragm into the ischiorectal fossa. An infection in this space may then drain out through the skin of the perineum to form a complete extrasphincteric fistula. In either case, treatment consists of removing any foreign body, establishing adequate drainage, and sometimes performing a temporary colostomy. It is not necessary to divide any sphincter muscle because the anal canal is not the cause of the patient's pathology.

Secondary to Specific Anorectal Disease

Conditions such as ulcerative colitis, Crohn's disease, and carcinoma may produce unusual and bizarre fistulas in the anorectal area. They are not usually amenable to local surgery. The primary disease must be remedied, often requiring total proctectomy.

Secondary to Pelvic Inflammation

A diverticular abscess of the sigmoid colon, Crohn's disease of the terminal ileum, or perforated pelvic appendicitis may result in perforation of the levator diaphragm, with the infection tracking downward to the perineal skin. To make the proper diagnosis, a radiographic sinogram is performed by injecting an aqueous iodinated contrast medium into the fistula. This procedure may demonstrate a supralevator entrance into the rectum. Therapy for this type of fistula consists of eliminating the pelvic sepsis by abdominal surgery. There is no need to cut any of the anorectal sphincter musculature.

Technical Hints for Performing Fistulotomy

Position

We prefer the prone position, with the patient's hips elevated on a small pillow. The patient should be under regional or local anesthesia with sedation.

Exploration

In accordance with Goodsall's rule, search the suspected area of the anal canal after inserting a Parks bivalve retractor. The internal opening should be located in a crypt near the dentate line, most often in the posterior commissure. If an internal opening has been identified, insert a probe to confirm this fact. Then insert a probe into the external orifice of the fistula. With a simple fistula, in which the probe goes directly into the internal orifice, simply make a scalpel incision dividing all of the tissues superficial to the probe. A grooved directional probe is helpful for this maneuver.

With complex fistulas the probe may not pass through the entire length of the track. In some cases gentle maneuvering with variously sized lacrimal probes may be helpful. If these maneuvers are not successful, Goldberg and associates suggested injecting a dilute (1:10) solution of methylene blue dye into the external orifice of the fistula. Then incise the tissues over a grooved director along that portion of the track the probe enters easily. At this point it is generally easy to identify the probable location of the fistula's internal opening. For fistulas in the posterior half of the anal canal, this opening is located in the posterior commissure at the dentate line. If a patient has multiple fistulas, including a horseshoe fistula, the multiple tracks generally enter into a single posterior track that leads to an internal opening at the usual location in the posterior commissure of the anal canal. In patients with multiple complicated fistulas, fistulograms obtained by radiography or magnetic resonance imaging help delineate the pathology.

Marsupialization

When fistulotomy results in a large gaping wound, Goldberg and associates suggested marsupializing the wound to speed healing: Suture the outer walls of the laid-open fistula to the skin with a continuous absorbable suture. Curet all of the granulation tissue away from the wall of the fistula that has been laid open.

POSTOPERATIVE CARE

Administer a bulk laxative such as Metamucil daily. For the first bowel movement, an additional stimulant, such as Senokot-S (two tablets) may be necessary.

The patient is placed on a regular diet.

For patients who have had operations for fairly simple fistulas, warm sitz baths two or three times daily may be initiated beginning on the first postoperative day, after which no gauze packing may be necessary.

For patients who have complex fistulas, light general anesthesia may be required for removal of the first gauze packing on the second or third postoperative day.

During the early postoperative period, check the wound every day or two to be sure that healing takes place in the depth of the wound before any of the more superficial tissues heal together. Later check the patient once or twice weekly.

When a significant portion of the external sphincter has been divided, warn the patient that for the first week or so there will be some degree of fecal incontinence.

In the case of the rare types of fistula with high extension and a deep wound, Parks and Sitz recommended that the patient be taken to the operating room at intervals for careful examination under anesthesia.

Perform a weekly anal digital examination and dilatation, when necessary, to avoid an anal stenosis secondary to the fibrosis that takes place during the healing of a fistula.

COMPLICATIONS

Urinary retention

Postoperative hemorrhage

Fecal incontinence

Sepsis including cellulitis and recurrent abscess

Recurrent fistula

Thrombosis of external hemorrhoids

Anal stenosis

REFERENCES

Eisenhammer S. A new approach to the anorectal fistulous abscess based on the high intermuscular lesion. Dis Colon Rectum 1976;19:487.

Garcia-Aguilar J, Belmonte C, Wong WD, Goldberg SM, Madoff RD. Anal fistula surgery: factors associated with recurrence and incontinence. Dis Colon Rectum 1996;39:723.

Goldberg SM, Gordon PH, Nivatvongs S. Essentials of Anorectal Surgery. Philadelphia, Lippincott, 1980.

Kodner IJ, Mazor A. Shemesh EI, et al. Endorectal advancement flap repair of rectovaginal and other complicated anorectal fistulas. Surgery 1993;114:682.

McCourtney JS, Finlay IG. Setons in the surgical management of fistula in ano. Br J Surg 1995;82:448.

Parks AG, Stitz RW. The treatment of high fistula-in-ano. Dis Colon Rectum 1958;106:595.

Parks AG, Thomson JPS. Intersphincter abscess. BMJ 1973; 2:337.

Parks AG, Hardcastle JD, Gordon PH. A classification of fistula-in-ano. Br J Surg 1976;63:1.

Rosen L. Anorectal abscess-fistulae. Surg Clin North Am 1994;74:1293.

61 Lateral Internal Sphincterotomy for Chronic Anal Fissure

INDICATIONS

Painful chronic anal fissure not responsive to medical therapy

PREOPERATIVE PREPARATION

Many patients with anal fissure cannot tolerate a preoperative enema because of excessive pain. Consequently, a mild cathartic the night before operation constitutes the only preoperative care necessary.

PITFALLS AND DANGER POINTS

Injury to external sphincter

Inducing fecal incontinence by overly extensive sphincterotomy

Bleeding, hematoma

OPERATIVE STRATEGY

Accurate identification of the lower border of the internal sphincter is essential to successful completion of an internal sphincterotomy. Insert a bivalve speculum (e.g., Parks retractor) into the anal and open the speculum for a distance of about two fingerbreadths to place the internal sphincter on stretch. Feel for a distinct groove between the subcutaneous external sphincter and the lower border of the tense internal sphincter. This groove accurately identifies the lower border of the internal sphincter. Optionally, the surgeon may make a radial incision through the mucosa directly over this area to identify visually the lower border of the internal sphincter (we have not found this step necessary).

OPERATIVE TECHNIQUE

Anesthesia

A light general or local anesthesia is satisfactory for this procedure.

Closed Sphincterotomy

Place the patient in the lithotomy position. (The prone position is also satisfactory.) Insert a Parks retractor with one blade placed in the anterior aspect and the other in the posterior aspect of the anal canal. Open the retractor about two fingerbreadths. Now, at the right or left lateral margin of the anal canal, palpate the groove between the internal and external sphincter. Once this has been clearly identified, insert a No. 11 scalpel blade into this groove **(Fig. 61–1)**. During this insertion keep the flat portion of the blade parallel to the internal sphincter. When the blade has reached the level of the dentate line (about 1.5 cm), rotate the blade 90° so its sharp edge rests against the internal sphincter muscle **(Fig. 61–2)**. Insert the left index finger into the anal canal opposite the scalpel blade. Then, with a gentle sawing motion transect the lower portion of the internal sphincter muscle. There is a gritty sensation while the internal sphincter is being transected, followed by a sudden "give" when the blade has reached the mucosa adjacent to the surgeon's left index finger. Remove the knife and palpate the area of the sphincterotomy with the left index finger. Any remaining muscle fibers are ruptured by lateral pressure exerted by this finger. In the presence of bleeding, apply pressure to this area for at least 5 minutes. It is rarely necessary to make an incision in the mucosa to identify and coagulate a bleeding point.

An alternative method of performing the subcutaneous sphincterotomy is to insert a No. 11 scalpel blade between the mucosa and the internal sphincter. Then turn the cutting edge of the blade so it faces laterally; cut the sphincter in this fashion. This approach has the disadvantage of possibly lacerating the external sphincter if excessive pressure is applied to the blade. Do not suture the tiny incision in the anoderm.

Open Sphincterotomy

For an open sphincterotomy a radial incision is made in the anoderm just distal to the dentate line and is carried across the lower border of the internal sphincter in the midlateral portion of the anus. Then the lower

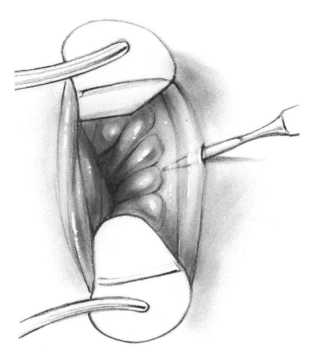

Fig. 61-1

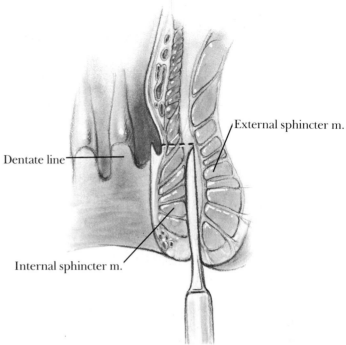

External sphincter m.

Dentate line

Internal sphincter m.

Fig. 61-2

border of the internal sphincter and intersphincteric groove are identified. The fibers of the internal sphincter have a whitish hue. Divide the lower portion of the internal sphincter up to a point level with the dentate line. Achieve hemostasis with electrocautery, if necessary. Leave the skin wound and apply a dressing.

Removal of the Sentinel Pile

If the patient has a sentinel pile more than a few millimeters in size, simply excise it with a scissors. Leave the skin defect unsutured. Nothing more elaborate need be done.

If in addition to the chronic anal fissure the patient has symptomatic internal hemorrhoids that require surgery, hemorrhoidectomy may be performed simultaneously with the lateral internal sphincterotomy. If the patient has large internal hemorrhoids, and hemorrhoidectomy is not performed simultaneously, the hemorrhoids may prolapse acutely after sphincterotomy, although it is not common.

POSTOPERATIVE CARE

Apply a simple gauze dressing to the anus and remove it the following morning.

Discharge the patient the same day. Generally, there is dramatic relief of the patient's pain promptly after sphincterotomy.

Have the patient continue taking the bulk laxative (e.g., psyllium) that was initiated prior to surgery.

Prescribe a mild analgesic in case the patient has some discomfort at the operative site.

COMPLICATIONS

Hematoma or bleeding (rare)

Perianal abscess (rare)

Flatus and fecal soiling

Some patients complain that they have less control over the passage of flatus following sphincterotomy than they had before operation, or they may have some fecal soiling of their underwear; but generally these complaints are temporary, and the problems rarely last more than a few weeks.

REFERENCES

Abcarian H. Surgical correction of chronic anal fissure: results of lateral internal sphincterotomy vs fissurectomy—midline sphincterotomy. Dis Colon Rectum 1980;23:31.

Eisenhammer S. The evaluation of the internal anal sphincterotomy operation with special reference to anal fissure. Surg Gynecol Obstet 1959;109:583.

Mazier WP. Hemorrhoids, fissures, and pruritus ani. Surg Clin North Am 1994;74:1277.

Notaras MJ. The treatment of anal fissure by lateral subcutaneous internal sphincterotomy: a technique and results. Br J Surg 1971;58:96.

62 Anoplasty for Anal Stenosis

INDICATIONS

Symptomatic fibrotic constriction of the anal canal not responsive to simple dilatation

PREOPERATIVE PREPARATION

Preoperative saline enema

PITFALLS AND DANGER POINTS

Fecal incontinence

Slough of flap

Inappropriate selection of patients

OPERATIVE STRATEGY

Some patients have a tubular stricture with fibrosis involving mucosa, anal sphincters, and anoderm. This condition, frequently associated with inflammatory bowel disease, is not susceptible to local surgery. In other cases of anal stenosis, elevating the anoderm and mucosa in the proper plane frees these tissues from the underlying muscle and permits formation of sliding pedicle flaps to resurface the denuded anal canal subsequent to dilating the stenosis.

Fecal incontinence is avoided by dilating the anal canal gradually to two or three fingerbreadths and performing, when necessary, a lateral internal sphincterotomy. Patients with mild forms of anal stenosis may respond to a simple internal sphincterotomy if there is no loss of anoderm.

OPERATIVE TECHNIQUE

Sliding Mucosal Flap

Incision

With the patient under local or general anesthesia, in the prone position, and with the buttocks retracted laterally by means of adhesive tape, make an incision at 12 o'clock. This incision should extend from the dentate line outward into the anoderm for about 1.5 cm and internally into the rectal mucosa for about 1.5 cm. The linear incision is then about 3 cm in length. Elevate the skin and mucosal flaps for about 1.0–1.5 cm to the right and to the left of the primary incision. Gently dilate the anus (**Fig. 62–1**).

Internal Sphincterotomy

Insert the bivalved Parks or a Hill-Ferguson retractor into the anal canal after gently dilating the anus. Identify the groove between the external and internal sphincter muscles. If necessary, incise the distal portion of the internal sphincter muscle, no higher than the dentate line (**Fig. 62–2**). This should permit dilatation of the anus to a width of two or three fingerbreadths.

Advancing the Mucosa

Completely elevate the flap of rectal mucosa. Then advance the mucosa so it can be sutured circumferentially to the sphincter muscle (**Fig. 62–3**). This suture line should fix the rectal mucosa near the normal location of the dentate line. Advancing the

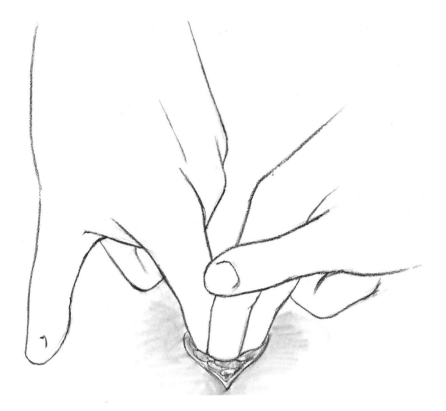

Fig. 62-1

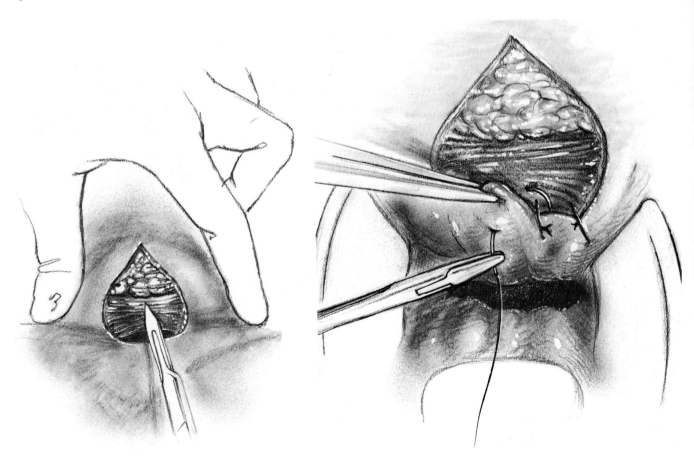

Fig. 62-2

Fig. 62-3

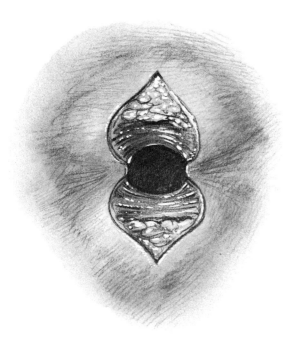

mucosa too far results in an ectropion with annoying chronic mucus secretion in the perianal region. Use fine chromic catgut or PG for the suture material. It is not necessary to insert sutures into the perianal skin. In a few cases of severe stenosis it may be necessary to repeat this process and create a mucosal flap at 6 o'clock **Figs. 62–4, 62–5)**.

Hemostasis should be complete following the use of accurate electrocautery and fine ligatures. Insert a small Gelfoam pack into the anal canal.

Sliding Anoderm Flap

Incision

After gently dilating the anus so a small Hill-Ferguson speculum can be inserted into the anal canal, make a vertical incision at the posterior commissure, beginning at the dentate line and extending upward in the rectal mucosa for a distance of about 1.5 cm.

Fig. 62-4

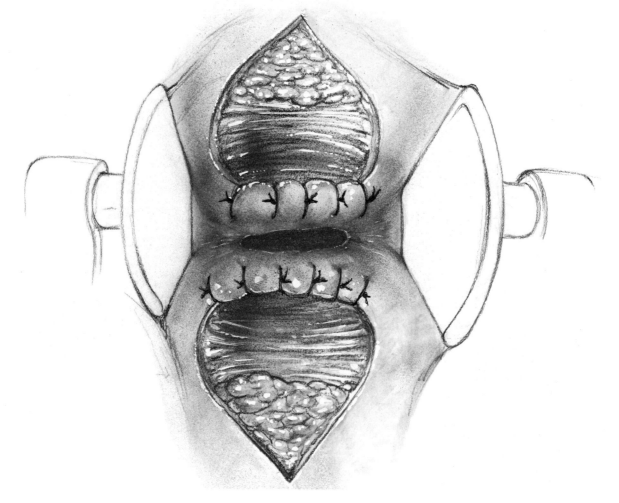

Fig. 62-5

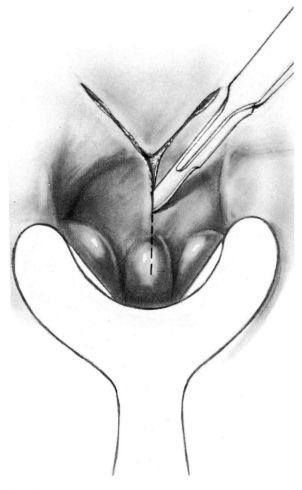

Fig. 62-6

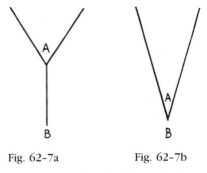

Fig. 62-7a   Fig. 62-7b

Advancing the Anoderm

Using continuous sutures of 5-0 atraumatic Vicryl, advance the flap of anoderm so point A meets point B (Fig. 62-7b; **Fig. 62–8**) and suture the anoderm to the mucosa with a continuous suture that catches a bit of the underlying sphincter muscle. When the suture line has been completed, the original Y incision in the posterior commissure resembles a V (Fig.

Then make a Y extension of this incision on to the anoderm as in **Figure 62–6**. Be certain the two limbs of the incision in the anoderm are separated by an angle of at least 90° (angle A in **Fig. 62–7a**). Now by sharp dissection, gently elevate the skin and mucosal flaps for a distance of about 1–2 cm. Take special care not to injure the delicate anoderm during the dissection. When the dissection has been completed, it is possible to advance point A on the anoderm to point B on the mucosa (**Fig. 62–7b**) without tension.

Internal Sphincterotomy

In most cases enlarging the anal canal requires division of the distal portion of the internal sphincter muscle. This may be performed through the same incision at the posterior commissure. Insert a sharp scalpel blade in the groove between the internal and external sphincter muscles. Divide the distal 1.0–1.5 cm of the internal sphincter. Then dilate the anal canal to width of two or three fingerbreadths.

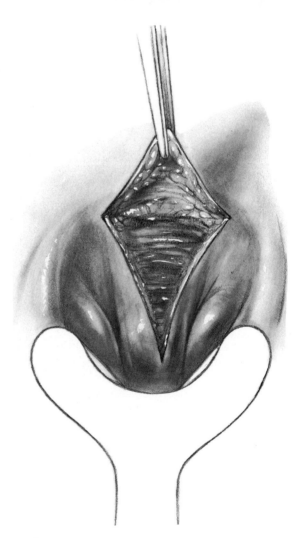

Fig. 62-8

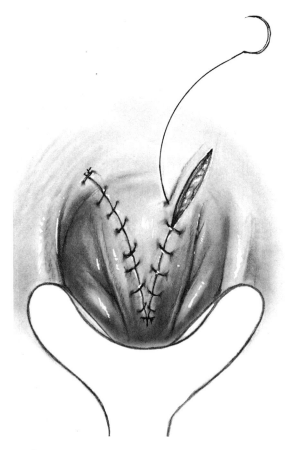

Fig. 62-9

62-7b; **Fig. 62–9**). Insert a small Gelfoam pack into the anal canal.

POSTOPERATIVE CARE

Remove the gauze dressings from the anal wound. It is not necessary to mobilize the Gelfoam because it tends to dissolve in sitz baths, which the patient should start two or three times daily on the day following the operation.

A regular diet is prescribed.

Mineral oil (45 ml) is taken nightly for the first 2–3 days. Thereafter a bulk laxative, such as Metamucil, is prescribed for the remainder of the postoperative period.

Discontinue all intravenous fluids in the recovery room if there has been no postanesthesia complication. This practice reduces the incidence of postoperative urinary retention.

COMPLICATIONS

Urinary retention

Hematoma

Anal ulcer and wound infection (rare)

REFERENCE

Khubchandani IT. Anal stenosis. Surg Clin North Am 1994; 74:1353.

63 Thiersch Operation for Rectal Prolapse

Surgical Legacy Technique

INDICATIONS

The Thiersch operation is indicated in poor-risk patients who have prolapse of the full thickness of rectum (see Chapter 56). Other perineal operations, including the Delorme procedure, are excellent alternatives in poor-risk patients and have largely supplanted this legacy procedure.

PREOPERATIVE PREPARATION

Sigmoidoscopy (barium colon enema) is performed.

Because many patients with rectal prolapse suffer from severe constipation, cleanse the colon over a period of a few days with cathartics and enemas.

Initiate an antibiotic bowel preparation 18 hours prior to scheduled operation, as for colon resection (see Chapter 42).

PITFALLS AND DANGER POINTS

Tying the encircling band too tight so it causes obstruction

Wound infection

Injury to vagina or rectum

Fecal impaction

OPERATIVE STRATEGY

Selecting Proper Suture or Banding Material

Lomas and Cooperman (1972) recommended that the anal canal be encircled by a four-ply layer of polypropylene mesh. The band is 1.5 cm in width, so the likelihood it would cut through the tissues is minimized. Labow and associates (1980) used a Dacron-impregnated Silastic sheet (Dow Corning No. 501-7) because it has the advantage of elasticity.

Achieving Proper Tension of the Encircling Band

Although some surgeons advocate that the encircling band be adjusted to fit snugly around a Hegar dilator, we have not found this technique satisfactory. Achieve proper tension by inserting an index finger into the anal canal while the assistant adjusts the encircling band so it fits snugly around the finger. If the band is too loose, prolapse is not prevented.

OPERATIVE TECHNIQUE

Fabricating the Encircling Band of Mesh

Although Lomas and Cooperman preferred Marlex

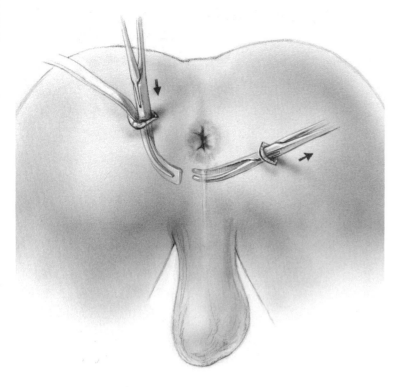

Fig. 63-1

mesh, we believe that Dacron-impregnated Silastic mesh is preferable because of its elasticity. Cut a rectangle of Silastic mesh 1.5 × 20.0 cm. Cut the strip so it is elastic along its longitudinal axis. **Figure 63–1**

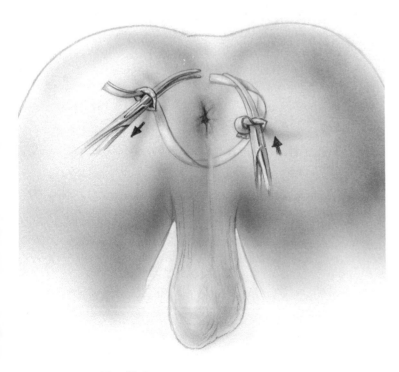

Fig. 63-2

and subsequent drawings illustrate Lomas and Cooperman's technique of using a tight roll of Marlex; we now use a 1.5 cm strip elasticized Silastic. Except for the nature of the mesh, the surgical technique is unchanged.

Incision and Position

This operation may be done with the patient in the prone jackknife or the lithotomy position, under general or regional anesthesia. We prefer the prone position. Make a 2 cm radial incision at 10 o'clock starting at the lateral border of the anal sphincter muscle and continue laterally. Make a similar incision at 4 o'clock. Make each incision about 2.5 cm deep.

Inserting the Mesh Band

Insert a large curved Kelly hemostat or a large right-angle clamp into the incision at 4 o'clock and gently pass the instrument around the external sphincter muscles so it emerges from the incision at 10 o'clock. Insert one end of the mesh strip into the jaws of the hemostat and draw the mesh through the upper incision and extract it from the incision at 4 o'clock. Then pass the hemostat through the 10 o'clock incision around the other half of the circumference of the anal canal until it emerges from the 4 o'clock incision. Insert the end of the mesh into the jaws of the hemostat and draw the hemostat back along this path **(Fig. 63–2)** so it delivers the end of the mesh band into the posterior incision. At this time the entire anal canal has been encircled by the band of mesh, and both ends protrude through the posterior incision. During this manipulation be careful not to penetrate the vagina or the anterior rectal wall. Also, do not permit the mesh to become twisted during its passage around the anal canal. Keep the band flat.

Adjusting Tension

Apply a second sterile glove on top of the previous glove on the left hand. Insert the left index finger into the anal canal. Apply a hemostat to each end of the encircling band. Ask the assistant to increase the tension gradually by overlapping the two ends of mesh. When the band feels snug around the index finger, ask the assistant to insert a 2-0 Prolene suture to maintain this tension. After the suture has been inserted, recheck the tension of the band. Then remove the index finger and remove the contaminated glove. Insert several additional 2-0 Prolene interrupted sutures or a row of 55 mm linear staples to approximate the two ends of the mesh and amputate the excess length of the mesh band. The patient should now have a 1.5 cm wide band of mesh encircling the external sphincter muscles at the midpoint of the anal canal with sufficient tension to be snug around an index finger in the rectum **(Fig. 63–3)**.

Closure

Irrigate both incisions thoroughly with a dilute antibiotic solution. Close the deep perirectal fat with interrupted 4-0 PG interrupted sutures in both incisions. Close the skin with interrupted or continuous subcuticular sutures of the same material **(Fig. 63–4)**. Apply collodion over each incision.

POSTOPERATIVE CARE

Prescribe perioperative antibiotics.

Prescribe a bulk-forming laxative such as Metamucil plus any additional cathartic that may be necessary to prevent fecal impaction. Periodic Fleet enemas may be required.

Initiate sitz baths after each bowel movement and two additional times daily for the first 10 days.

COMPLICATIONS

If the patient develops a *wound infection* it may not be necessary to remove the band. First, open the incision to obtain adequate drainage and treat the patient with antibiotics. If the infection heals, it is not necessary to remove the foreign body.

Some patients experience *perineal pain* following surgery, but it usually diminishes in time. If the pain is severe and unrelenting, the mesh must be removed. If removal can be postponed for 4–6 months, there may be enough residual perirectal fibrosis to prevent recurrence of the prolapse.

REFERENCES

Kuijpers HC. Treatment of complete rectal prolapse: to narrow, to wrap, to suspend, to fix, to encircle, to plicate or to resect? World J Surg 1992;15:826.

Labow S, Rubin RJ, Hoexter B, et al. Perineal repair of rectal procidentia with an elastic sling. Dis Colon Rectum 1980;23:467.

Lomas ML, Cooperman H. Correction of rectal procidentia by use of polypropylene mesh (Marlex). Dis Colon Rectum 1972;15:416.

Oliver GC, Vachon D, Eisenstat TE, Rubin RJ, Salvati EP. Delorme's procedure for complete rectal prolapse in severely debilitated patients: an analysis of 41 cases. Dis Colon Rectum 1994;37:461.

Williams JG, Rothenberger DA, Madoff RD, Goldberg SM. Treatment of rectal prolapse in the elderly by perineal rectosigmoidectomy. Dis Colon Rectum 1992;35:830.

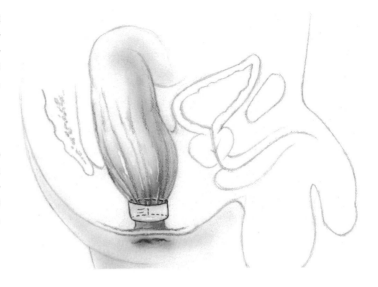

Fig. 63–3

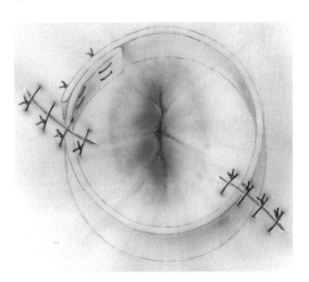

Fig. 63–4

64 Operations for Pilonidal Disease

INDICATIONS

Recurrent symptoms of pain, swelling, and purulent drainage

PITFALLS AND DANGER POINTS

Unnecessarily radical excision

OPERATIVE STRATEGY

Acute Pilonidal Abscess

If an adequate incision can be made and all of the granulation tissue and hair are removed from the cavity, a cure is accomplished in a number of patients with acute abscesses.

Marsupialization

During marsupialization a narrow elliptical incision is used to unroof the length of the pilonidal cavity. Do not excise a significant width of the overlying skin—only enough to remove the sinus pits. If this is accomplished, one can approximate the lateral margin of the pilonidal cyst wall to the subcuticular layer of the skin with interrupted sutures. At the conclusion of the procedure, no subcutaneous fat is visible in the wound. Healing of exposed subcutaneous fat tends to be slow. On the other hand, the fibrous tissue lining the pilonidal cyst contracts fairly rapidly, producing approximation of the marsupialized edges of skin over a period of only several weeks. There is no need to excise a width of skin more than 0.8–1.0 cm. Conservative skin excision is followed by more rapid healing. Of course, all granulation tissue and hair must be curetted away from the fibrous lining of the pilonidal cyst.

Excision with Primary Suture

Allow several months to pass after an episode of acute infection to minimize the bacterial content of the pilonidal complex. Successful accomplishment of primary healing requires that the pilonidal cyst be encompassed by excision of a narrow strip of skin that includes the sinus pits and a patch of subcutaneous fat not much more than 1 cm in width. If this can be achieved without entering the cyst, closing the relatively shallow, narrow wound is not difficult. Perform the dissection with electrocautery. Hemostasis must be perfect to ensure complete excision of the cyst and any sinus tracts without unnecessary contamination of the wound. If this technique has been successful, postoperative convalescence is quite short.

It is not necessary to carry the dissection down to the sacrococcygeal ligaments to ensure successful elimination of the pilonidal disease. In essence, the surgeon is simply excising a chronic granuloma surrounded by a fibrous capsule and covered by a strip of skin containing the pits that constituted the original portal of entry of infection and hair into the abscess.

Primary healing requires good wound architecture. If a large segment of subcutaneous fat is excised, simply approximating the skin over a large deadspace may result in temporary healing, but eventually the wound is likely to separate. Unless the surgeon is willing to construct extensive sliding skin flaps or a Z-plasty, excision with primary closure should be restricted to patients in whom wide excision is not necessary.

OPERATIVE TECHNIQUE

Although it is possible to excise the midline sinus pits and to evacuate the pus and hair through this incision under local anesthesia, often the abscess points in an area away from the gluteal cleft and complete extraction of the hair prove to be too painful to the patient. Consequently, in most cases simply evacuate the pus during the initial drainage procedure and postpone a definitive operation until the infection has subsided.

Infiltrate the skin overlying the abscess with 1% lidocaine containing 1:200,000 epinephrine. Make a

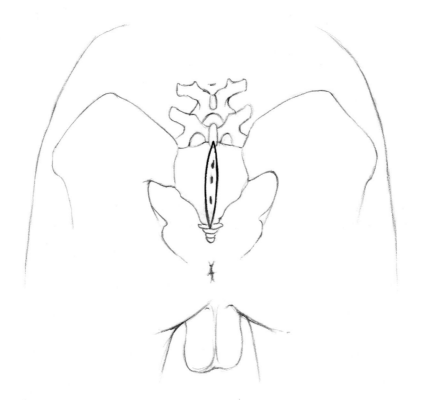

Fig. 64-1

scalpel incision of sufficient size to evacuate the pus and necrotic material. Whenever possible, avoid making the incision in the midline. If it is possible to extract the loose hair in the abscess, do so; otherwise, simply insert loose gauze packing.

Marsupialization

First described by Buie in 1944, marsupialization begins by inserting a probe or grooved director into the sinus. Then incise the skin overlying the probe with a scalpel. Do not carry the incision beyond the confines of the pilonidal cyst. If the patient has a tract leading in a lateral direction, insert the probe into the lateral sinus and incise the skin over it. Now excise no more than 1–3 cm of the skin edges on each side to include the epithelium of all of the sinus pits along the edge of the skin wound **(Fig. 64–1)**. This maneuver exposes a narrow band of subcutaneous fat between the lateral margins of the pilonidal cyst and the epithelium of the skin. Achieve complete hemostasis by carefully electrocauterizing each bleeding point.

After unroofing the pilonidal cyst, remove all granulation tissue and hair, if present, using dry gauze, the back of a scalpel handle, or a large curet to wipe clean the posterior wall of the cyst **(Fig. 64–2)**. Then approximate the subcuticular level of

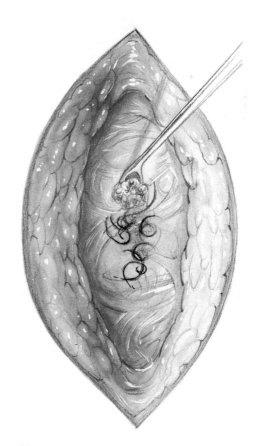

Fig. 64-2

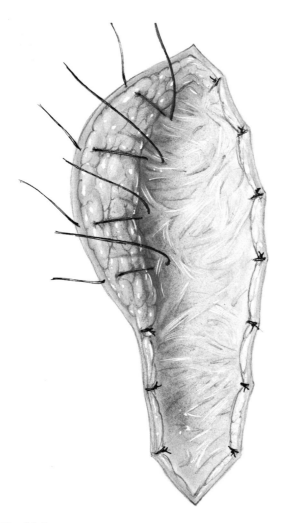

Fig. 64–3

the patient in the prone position with a pillow under the hips and the legs slightly flexed.

Apply adhesive strapping to each buttock and retract each in a lateral direction by attaching the adhesive tape to the operating table. Before scrubbing, in preparation for the surgery insert a sterile probe into the pilonidal sinus and gently explore the dimensions of the underlying cavity to confirm that it is not too large for excision and primary suture.

After shaving, cleansing, and preparing the area with an iodophor solution, make an elliptical incision only of sufficient length and width to encompass the underlying pilonidal sinus and the sinus pits in the gluteal cleft (Fig. 64-1). In properly selected patients this requires excising a strip of skin no more than 1.0-1.5 cm in width. Deepen the incision on each side of the pilonidal sinus **(Fig. 64–4)**. Use elec-

the skin to the lateral margin of the pilonidal cyst with interrupted sutures of 3-0 or 4-0 PG **(Fig. 64–3)**.

Ideally, at the conclusion of this procedure there is a fairly flat wound consisting of skin attached to the fibrous posterior wall of the pilonidal cyst, with no subcutaneous fat visible. In the rare situation where the pilonidal cyst wall is covered by squamous epithelium, the marsupialization operation is just as effective as in most cases where the wall consists only of fibrous tissue. We usually perform this operation with the patient in the prone position with the buttocks retracted laterally by adhesive straps under local anesthesia, as Abramson advocated for his modification of the marsupialization operation.

Pilonidal Excision with Primary Suture

For pilonidal excision with primary suture, use regional, general, or local field block anesthesia. Place

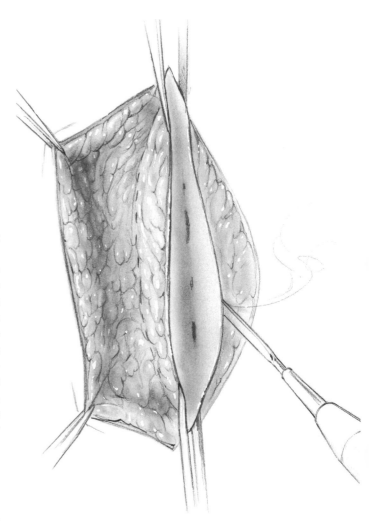

Fig. 64-4

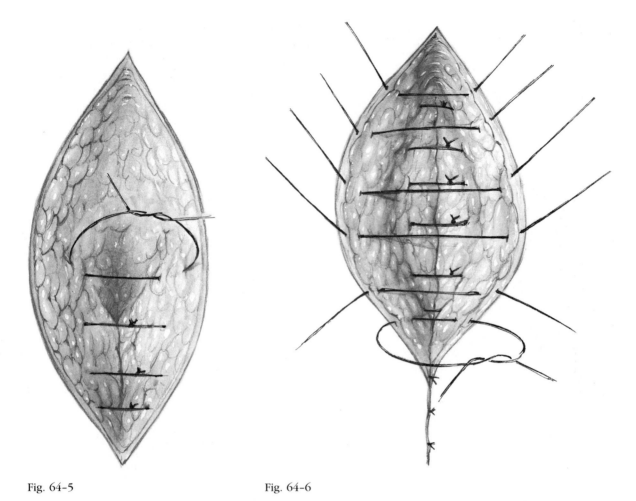

Fig. 64-5   Fig. 64-6

trocautery for this dissection to achieve complete hemostasis. Otherwise, the presence of blood prevents the accurate visualization necessary to avoid entering one of the potentially infected pilonidal tracts. Dissect the specimen away from the underlying fat without exposing the sacrococcygeal periosteum or ligaments. Remove the specimen and check for complete hemostasis. The specimen should not measure more than 5.0 × 1.5 × 1.5 cm. It should be possible to approximate the subcutaneous fat with interrupted 3-0 or 4-0 PG sutures without tension **(Fig. 64–5)**. Insert interrupted subcuticular sutures of 4-0 PG **(Fig. 64–6)** or close the skin with interrupted nylon vertical mattress sutures. Avoid leaving any deadspace in the incision. If at some point during the operation the pilonidal cyst has been opened inadvertently, irrigate the wound with a dilute antibiotic solution and complete the operation as planned unless frank pus has filled the wound. In the latter case, simply leave the wound open and insert gauze packing without any sutures.

The patient must remain inactive to encourage primary healing.

Excision of Sinus Pits with Lateral Drainage

For Bascom's (1980) modification of Lord and Millar's (1965) operation, only the sinus pits **(Fig. 64–7)**

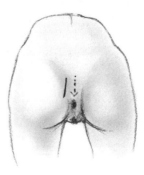

Fig. 64-7

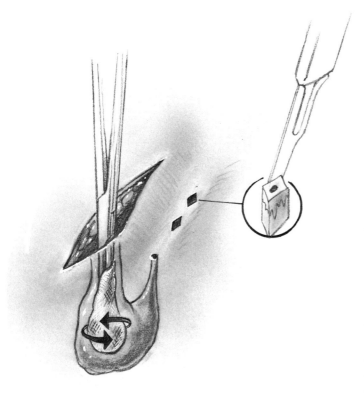

Fig. 64–8a

are excised in the mid-gluteal cleft. This may be accomplished with a pointed No. 11 scalpel blade **(Fig. 64–8a)** or with the dermatologist's round skin biopsy punches. The latter, available in diameters as large as 5 mm, are simply cork-borers whose ends have been sharpened to a cutting edge. Most of the pits are simply epithelial tubes going down toward the pilonidal cyst for a distance of a few millimeters. Leave unsutured the resulting wounds from the pit excisions.

Insert a probe into the underlying pilonidal cavity to determine its dimensions. Then make a vertical incision parallel to the long axis of the pilonidal cavity. Make this incision about 1.5 cm lateral to the mid-gluteal cleft **(Fig. 64–8b)**. Open the pilonidal cyst through this incision. Curet out all of the granulation tissue and hair. Achieve complete hemostasis with the electrocoagulator. A peanut gauze dissector is also useful for this step. Bascom did not insert drains or packing. Occasionally three or more enlarged follicles (pits) are so close together in the mid-gluteal cleft that individual excision of each follicle is impossible. In this case Bascom simply excised a narrow strip of skin encompassing all of the pits. If the skin defect in the cleft exceeded 7 mm, he sutured it closed. The lateral incision is always left open. In patients who have lateral extensions of their pilonidal disease, each lateral sinus pit is excised. Bascom found that occasionally there was an ingrowth of der-

mal epithelium into the subcutaneous fat, forming an epithelial tube resembling a thyroglossal duct remnant. These structures resemble pieces of macaroni, and Bascom advised excising these epithelial tubes through the lateral incision.

POSTOPERATIVE CARE

Following drainage of an *acute pilonidal abscess*, remove the gauze packing the next day and have the patient shower daily to keep the gluteal cleft clean and free of any loose hair. Shave the skin for a distance of about 5 cm around the mid-gluteal cleft weekly. In some cases it is possible to use a depilatory cream to achieve the same result. Otherwise, hair finds its way into the pilonidal cavity and acts as a foreign body, initiating a recurrent infection.

Following *excision and primary suture*, remove the gauze dressing on the second day and leave the wound exposed. Initiate daily showering especially after each bowel movement. Observe the patient closely two or three times a week in the office. If evidence of a localized wound infection appears, open this area of the wound and administer appropriate antibiotics, treating the condition the same way you would treat an infection in an abdominal incision. If the infection is extensive, it is then necessary to lay open the entire incision. With good wound architecture, infection is uncommon. Also shave or apply a depilatory cream to the area of the mid-gluteal cleft for the first two to three postoperative weeks or until the wound is completely healed.

If the patient has undergone *pit excision and lateral drainage*, postoperative care is limited to daily showers and weekly observation by the surgeon to remove any hairs that may have invaded the wound. Bascom applied Monsel's solution to granulation tissue. All of his patients have been operated in the ambulatory outpatient setting. No matter what the operative procedure, patients with pilonidal disease require instruction always to avoid accumulation of loose hair in the mid-gluteal cleft. Daily showering with special attention to cleaning this area should prevent recurrence.

COMPLICATIONS

Infection may follow the primary suture operation.

Hemorrhage has been reported by Lamke et al. (1974) Of the patients treated by wide excision and packing, 10% experienced postoperative hemorrhage requiring blood transfusion and reoperation. This complication is easily preventable by meticulous electrocoagulation of each bleeding point in the operating room. It is rare following primary suture or marsupialization operations.

Among patients followed for a number of years, pilonidal disease *recurs* in 15% whether treated by primary suture, excision and packing, or marsupialization. Even the radical excision operation does not seem to prevent recurrence. Consequently, it appears that in most cases recurrence is caused by poor hygiene, permitting hair to drill its way into the skin of the mid-gluteal cleft, rather than by inadequate surgery. Most recurrences are in the midline.

There may be a *failure to heal*. Some patients, especially those who have had a radical excision of pilonidal disease that leaves a large midline defect bounded by sacrococcygeal periosteum in its depths and subcutaneous fat around its perimeter, endure healing failure for a period as long as 2 years (Bascom). In some cases it is due to inadequate postoperative care in which the bridging of unhealed cavities has taken place or in which loose hair has found its way into the cavity and produced reinfection. Occasionally, even when postoperative care is conscientious in these patients, there is protracted healing of the residual wound.

REFERENCES

Abramson DJ. A simple marsupialization technique for treatment of pilonidal sinus; long-term follow-up. Ann Surg 1960;151:261.

Allen-Mersh TG. Pilonidal sinus: finding the right track for treatment. Br J Surg 1990;77:123.

Bascom J. Pilonidal disease: origin from follicles of hairs and results of follicle removal as treatment. Surgery 1980;87:567.

Buie LA. Jeep disease (pilonidal disease of mechanized warfare). South Med J 1944;37:103.

Holm J, Hulten L. Simple primary closure for pilonidal disease. Acta Chir Scand 1970;136:537.

Lamke LO, Larsson J, Nylen B. Results of different types of operation for pilonidal sinus. Acta Chir Scand 1974;140:321.

Lord PH, Millar DM. Pilonidal sinus: a simple treatment. Br J Surg 1965;52:298.

Patey DH, Scarff RW. Pathology of postanal pilonidal sinus: its bearing on treatment. Lancet 1946;2:484.

Surrell JA. Pilonidal disease. Surg Clin North Am 1994;74:1309.

Part VII
Hepatobiliary Tract

65 Concepts in Hepatobiliary Surgery

Michael Edye
Elliot Newman
H. Leon Pachter

CHOLELITHIASIS

Laparoscopic cholecystectomy has become the method of choice when gallbladder removal is necessary. The rapidity with which this technique has become dominant is truly astonishing. In 1988 it was thought that, at best, only 30–40% of patients would be suitable candidates. Exponential improvement in both optics and equipment followed, and now 98–99% of all elective cholecystectomies are performed laparoscopically. Laparoscopic cholecystectomy has proven to be quite safe, although the incidence of common duct injury (0.5–0.7%) appears to remain about twice that of open cholecystectomy. Our own database consists of more than 2000 consecutive cases treated from 1990 to 1999 without mortality. Included in this cohort of patients were both elective and emergent referrals. As experience accrued coupled with refinement of the instruments used, laparoscopic cholecystectomy was extended to patients with cirrhosis, extensive previous upper abdominal surgery, acute and gangrenous cholecystitis, Mirizzi syndrome, and choledocholithiasis. Dedicated laparoscopic surgeons can achieve results in the modern era of anesthesia and intensive care at least equivalent, and often superior, to open methods. At times, however, inflammatory changes are so severe the laparoscopic approach should be abandoned and conversion to open cholecystectomy undertaken without the slightest hesitation.

Diagnosis of Gallstones

Most patients treated electively are diagnosed by history, physical examination, and upper abdominal sonogram. The presence, size, number, and mobility of stones must be documented in addition to the thickness of the gallbladder wall and the measured diameter of the common duct. The rare carcinoma of the gallbladder should also be excluded during this examination. The presence of adjacent fluid and a sonographic Murphy's sign are good evidence of acute inflammation. A hepatobiliary (HIDA) scan

may be useful in the intensive care unit (ICU) patient with a difficult abdomen to examine and known gallstones. A patent cystic duct virtually rules out acute cholecystitis. The use of cholecystokinin to stimulate gallbladder emptying may be useful in patients with typical biliary colic but no demonstrable radiographic gallstones. If pain is experienced after injection of cholecystokinin or the ejection fraction of tracer is well below the lower limit of normal, the test is considered positive. Although such patients are frequently referred to surgeons, a full upper gastrointestinal (GI) workup should be done *before* surgery to avoid prompt postoperative recurrence of symptoms.

Gallbladder as an Unrecognized Source of Sepsis

Hospitalized patients on medical services, severely injured or burned patients, and patients during the immediate postoperative period after a variety of surgical procedures who develop shock or sepsis should undergo evaluation of their gallbladder as part of the workup. Acute gangrenous cholecystitis can complicate the period after chest, cardiac, or abdominal surgery; and cholecystectomy may have to be performed promptly. Percutaneous image-guided cholecystostomy may be a life-saving temporizing alternative. Antibiotic treatment alone is generally not sufficient; these patients are frequently already on broad-spectrum antibiotics, and antibiotic therapy does not alleviate gangrenous cholecystitis.

Choice of Operation: Open Versus Laparoscopic

In experienced hands successful laparoscopic removal is possible in most patients regardless of the pathology encountered. If a difficult cholecystectomy is anticipated, the procedure should commence with a diagnostic laparoscopy to determine by inspection and laparoscopic palpation if continuing laparoscopically is wise. Acute cholecystitis that has been present for a week or more with a palpable mass falls into this category. There can be two parts to the difficulty: First, exposing the gallbladder in the phlegmonous mass of omentum and colon can be difficult especially if the attack is more than 2 weeks old. Second, exposure of the gallbladder–cystic duct junction is difficult because of induration of the gallbladder wall and the presence of a large stone impacted in the infundibulum. If a laparoscopic approach is chosen, it may be prudent, as with open surgery, to take down the gallbladder from the fundus first and work one's way to the cystic duct–common duct junction by keeping the dissection as close to the gallbladder wall as possible.

In patients with chronic liver disease (see below) the liver is often shrunken and rigid. The usual retraction techniques using the fundus of the gallbladder do not work, and exposure of the hepatobiliary triangle is difficult. Varices in adhesions, omentum, hepatoduodenal ligament, and gallbladder add to the bleeding potential of this operation.

Carcinoma of the gallbladder is best treated by open cholecystectomy with excision of a wedge of liver tissue and regional lymph nodes where appropriate [1]. Trocar site recurrences have been reported after laparoscopic cholecystectomy, reflecting this tumor's propensity for implantation.

Should Operative Cholangiography Be Done?

Intraoperative cholangiography (IOC) does not prevent ductal injury, but it *may* serve to identify that the structure that has been cannulated is not the cystic duct. If the surgeon recognizes it on the radiograph, the lesion can be repaired appropriately. This usually means conversion to laparotomy and the assistance of a surgeon experienced in repair of biliary tract injuries.

A technique that may aid in limiting bile duct injuries during the laparoscopic approach is taking down the gallbladder *from the fundus down* and performing operative cholangiography as the last step of the dissection [2]. By staying close to the gallbladder wall no blood vessel of significant size is encountered until the cystic artery is reached. Branches from this vessel traveling onto the gallbladder wall are then divided between clips, ties, or electrocoagulation depending on size. The next structure encountered is the cystic duct. In this way the ductal system is approached from the peripheral aspect, the hepatobiliary triangle is opened away from the hepatoduodenal ligament containing the common duct, and no early dissection can take place

near the common bile duct. It is at this point, not earlier in the exposure, that cholangiography is performed. This technique is similar to that used for decades during open cholecystectomy. It is the best method that has emerged for avoiding ductal injury during laparoscopic cholecystectomy. If nothing remains to be divided, and the duct is visually and radiographically intact, there is no possibility of ductal injury. Although this exposure is the reverse of what is currently taught, it nevertheless merits consideration as a safe and effective method for limiting bile duct injuries.

Cholangiography demonstrates the length of the cystic duct remnant; outlines the lumen of the common duct to identify stones and patency of the papilla, the diameter of the common duct, and the intrahepatic anatomy; and remains as a permanent record of the state of the common duct at the time of surgery. When performed routinely, IOC is rapid, adding only 5–10 minutes to the procedure. It can also serve to delineate asymptomatic common duct stones. The chief argument not to perform cholangiography other than time and cost is the possibility of a false-positive study. This possibility is largely avoided by meticulously avoiding air bubbles and the use of real-time video imaging. None of the known complications of biliary surgery (hemorrhage, bile leak, common duct injury, pancreatitis, visceral injury) are increased in incidence if the cholangiogram catheter is sited at the point where the cystic duct would otherwise have been divided.

Cholecystocholangiography is favored by some for eliminating the possibility of causing ductal injury. Technically it is less desirable because stones can propagate downstream, and the method is impractical in patients with acute cholecystitis when a stone is impacted in the infundibulum. If the cystic duct is so tiny that insertion of the cholangiography catheter is technically not feasible, there is virtually no possibility that stones have passed into the common duct and the study can be eliminated.

Preoperative endoscopic retrograde cholangiography (ERC) is superfluous for surgeons experienced in clearance of the common duct by laparoscopic techniques except in the following instances: persisting jaundice (as part of a workup to rule out malignant bile duct obstruction); suppurative cholangitis; and gallstone pancreatitis that does not rapidly resolve. Is cholangiography necessary if patients have undergone ERC prior to cholecystectomy? In our database are 31 patients who had undergone preoperative ERC. In one-third of these patients (5/15) whose duct was said to be free of stones, recurrent or residual stones were seen on the IOC. One-half (8/16) of patients whose duct was said to have been cleared of stones at the time of ERC had recurrent or residual stones. Thus preoperative ERC is no argument for avoiding IOC.

Special Circumstances

Pregnancy

Symptomatic cholelithiasis during pregnancy is common and is best managed by accurate sonographic diagnosis and symptomatic care including a low-fat diet with the aim of deferring cholecystectomy until the postnatal period. Crescendo attacks of biliary colic or choledocholithiasis require more urgent attention. Cholecystectomy can be performed safely during the middle trimester. If common duct exploration is necessary it can be performed without radiography, and the duct can usually be cleared successfully by transcystic choledocholescopic techniques. The fetus should be evaluated preoperatively by an obstetric consultant, usually with sonography and fetal heart monitoring. Advice regarding the use of tocolytics should be sought at the later stages of the second trimester. At operation, open insertion of the first cannula to eliminate the chance of perforating the uterus with a Veress needle or trocar should be standard practice. CO_2 insufflation pressures just sufficient to provide a comfortable operating field reduce the tendency to CO_2 absorption. Ventilation should be adjusted by the anesthetist to keep the PCO_2 around 40 mm Hg or less. These measures ensure that fetal physiology is minimally affected by the procedure and reduces the risks of long-term ill effects. Prompt surgery by the most experienced operator available serves the expectant mother best.

Radiography is safe after the first trimester, but it is still standard practice to shield the uterus with a lead screen placed between the x-ray source and the uterus. Scatter is minimal and has no effect on the fetus at this age. Reevaluation by sonogram and fetal heart monitoring in the recovery room prior to discharge is necessary to complete the documentation of fetal health. If cholecystectomy has been deferred until the end of pregnancy, it is wise if possible to wait until the second or third postnatal month to avoid the period of known physiologic hypercoagulability.

Cirrhosis

Chronic liver disease complicates the overall management of gallstones, and laparoscopic cholecystectomy offers a safer approach than open cholecystectomy. The mortality associated with open cholecystectomy in cirrhotic patients may be as high as 25–50%. By reducing the size of the abdominal wall and intraabdominal wounds, by performing accurate hemostasis, and with aggressive supportive care, excellent results from laparoscopic cholecystectomy can be obtained in cirrhotic patients. Symptomatic cholelithiasis can present in a number of settings. Acute cholecystitis in the pretransplant patient, if not rapidly responsive to aggressive antibiotic therapy, should undergo prompt cholecystectomy. The ability to complete the procedure laparoscopically is determined by the size and location of intraabdominal varices and the relation of the gallbladder to the liver. A deeply intrahepatic gallbladder in a profoundly nodular, hard, contracted liver can defy even the most skilled laparoscopist. This finding alone should prompt conversion to an open approach, perhaps with the help of an experienced hepatic or liver transplant surgeon. Moreover, sound surgical judgment may dictate the need for a cholecystostomy under these circumstances.

Preoperatively, vitamin K and fresh frozen plasma should be administered to lower the prothrombin time to less than 14–15 seconds. If thrombocytopenia is present, platelet infusions should be given liberally.

Avoid drains and T-tubes unless strictly necessary. Ascites leaks through the drain tract long after the drain has been removed. Healing around the T-tube is extremely slow, and the risk of bile peritonitis is high in cirrhotic patients. If a T-tube is employed, leave it in place for 3–4 weeks or more.

The chief technical difficulties when operating on these patients are (1) dense vascular adhesions to the gallbladder and liver; (2) a rigid nodular liver that cannot be retracted by conventional laparoscopic means; and (3) liver parenchyma that bleeds profusely.

Ultrasonic dissecting shears can be used to great effect for dividing structures behind the gallbladder, which bleed profusely. The liver should be retracted via the epigastric port using the flat shaft of a smooth, round-tipped laparoscopic instrument, literally levering the liver up from Morrison's pouch. The gallbladder is removed fundus first. There should be no hesitation in leaving the infundibulum suture-ligated in a mass if dissection in the hepatobiliary triangle becomes difficult. In the face of a markedly inflamed, thickened gallbladder that is partly intrahepatic, the peritoneal aspect of the gallbladder wall should be excised, leaving wall adherent to the liver in situ. Electrocoagulation or an argon beam can be used to ablate the remaining mucosa. The cystic duct orifice should be suture-ligated with an absorbable purse-string suture.

Previous Abdominal Surgery

Rarely, prior abdominal surgery precludes a laparoscopic approach to cholecystectomy. It is wise to position the first cannula in a nonscarred site using the open technique. Only enough adhesions necessary to expose the right upper quadrant and elevate the liver should be taken down, which allows adequate exposure for the rest of the procedure. Lysis of adhesions is ideally performed using an angled scope oriented to look up to the abdominal wall.

Patients with Known Coagulopathy

By reducing the overall surgical wound size, the risk of postoperative hemorrhage in patients who are anticoagulated or who have a coagulopathy is markedly reduced. The use of conical tipped trocars or radially expanding cannulas rather than trocars with a cutting blade, reduces the chance of lacerating an abdominal wall vessel.

Hemophiliacs should be observed in hospital for 48 hours after surgery as delayed hemorrhage is possible. Undue abdominal pain with a falling hematocrit should prompt aggressive factor VIII replacement and a return to the operating room to evacuate the hemoperitoneum. Commonly, no discrete bleeding point is found. Do not forget to inspect the deep aspect of each port puncture carefully for the presence of clot, as it is a common source of postoperative intraabdominal hemorrhage.

Complications

Bile Duct Injuries

The "Achilles heel" of laparoscopic cholecystectomy appears to be inadvertent injury to the common bile duct (CBD) or common hepatic duct. Bile duct injuries seem to be a persistent and inherent problem associated with the technique. These injuries can occur at any given instance but most commonly are noted to happen when patients present acutely, rendering precise identification of ductal anatomy difficult at best [3–5].

Misidentification of the cystic duct is the most frequent culprit, but ill-advised use of cautery in the vicinity of the common bile duct may also lead to serious ductal damage without actually severing the duct. The usual injury is division of the bile duct somewhere between the cystic duct and the duodenum, with excision of a length of duct that includes the confluence of cystic and common hepatic ducts. The proximal line of injury can reach as high as the confluence of the right and left hepatic ducts in the porta hepatis.

The mechanism of injury is failure to recognize that

the structure being dissected is not the cystic duct but the CBD or an aberrant right hepatic duct. The CBD (misidentified as the cystic duct) is clipped and severed, most often below the cystic duct–CBD junction. The specimen is retracted cephalad. To remove the specimen, the biliary tree must be severed again, resulting in clipping of the common hepatic duct. Depending on the degree of traction the CBD is at times severed just at or above the bifurcation of the main right and left hepatic ducts. The resultant defect varies, but loss of 10–20 mm of duct has been reported.

Prevention of Common Bile Duct

The goal of any laparoscopic surgeon is to avoid injury to major biliary ductal structures. A number of strategies have been suggested to achieve this goal, including use of an angled laparoscope. The most important dictum is that *no structure should be divided until its identity has been anatomically confirmed*. This is done by creating an ample window between the cystic duct and common hepatic duct. No other biliary ductal structure is likely to be encountered in this region. Fundus-down dissection (described above) with IOC as the last stage shows the best promise for limiting ductal injuries. By staying close to the gallbladder it is often possible to avoid ligating the main trunk of the cystic artery. The dissection cones down to a single tubular structure, the cystic duct, which is then cannulated for cholangiography, or divided, depending on the surgeon's preference. This concept of defensive cholecystectomy is not new but is germane given the potential for disorientation during laparoscopy.

Bile Leak after Cholecystectomy

The prevalence of accessory ducts is around 1–4%. These ducts leak bile if divided sharply and not ligated. Careful removal of the gallbladder with magnification in a bloodless field identifies most of the small structures frequently close to the cystic duct. Routine drainage of the gallbladder bed after uneventful open cholecystectomy has not proven to be beneficial, and there is no reason to believe that it would be during laparoscopic cholecystectomy. Drainage is warranted in the following circumstances.

Severe acute cholecystitis with significant bile and stone spillage requiring irrigation

Denuded hepatic parenchyma

After placement of a T-tube in the common duct

Following complicated CBD exploration

Many bile leaks are due to insecure closure of the cystic duct. The endoscopic biliary surgeon must have a variety of closure techniques. Clips should be reserved for only the most normal cystic duct, 3–4 mm in diameter, with a pliable wall. Larger or thicker ducts should be ligated with an absorbable No. 0 PG pretied loop. If the cystic duct stump is short, suture-ligature is the safest option. Stacking multiple clips across a dilated cystic duct is to be condemned. Do not use clips on cystic ducts that are small (<2 mm), large (>5 mm), short, inflamed, thickened, or stretched (after transcystic CBD exploration) or in patients with poor healing due to cirrhosis, renal failure, or chronic steroid therapy. The latter conditions are associated with fragile tissue quality; clips are more likely to cut through or fracture, inevitably leading to a bile leak.

Deep Vein Thrombosis Prophylaxis

Mechanical thromboembolic prophylaxis in the form of calf/thigh compression is now commonly employed. Laparoscopic surgery appears to predispose to an increased likelihood of deep venous thrombosis (DVT) because of the head-up position, positive intraabdominal pressure, and reduced venous return. Patel and colleagues (1996) performed lower limb duplex Doppler examinations before and after laparoscopic cholecystectomy. Using accepted Doppler criteria for the presence of DVT, they found 11 postoperative DVTs in 19 patients studied. None was clinically apparent [6]. Despite the alarming potential for venous thrombosis we have been impressed by the dearth of clinically apparent DVTs in patients undergoing laparoscopic cholecystectomy electively and emergently. We know of only one pulmonary embolus suffered by a patient following cholecystectomy in our database of 2000 cases. If patients receive mechanical prophylaxis and are ambulated early, thromboembolic complications can be expected to be rare.

CHOLEDOCHOLITHIASIS

Diagnosis

Common bile duct stones are generally diagnosed preoperatively by a combination of ultrasonography and blood tests. Elevation of serum alkaline phosphatase, gamma glutamine transferase, or both suggests biliary obstruction. A history of fluctuating jaundice is particularly suggestive of stones. Incomplete obstruction may not cause the serum bilirubin to rise, and clinical jaundice is generally not noted until the bilirubin reaches 3 mg/dl. Occasionally, asymptomatic CBD stones are found during routine IOC (more frequently in elderly patients with longstanding calculus biliary tract disease).

Management of Choledocholithiasis

Stones in the CBD almost always originate in the gallbladder as calculi that are small enough to traverse the cystic duct. The stone may then pass uneventfully through the ampulla, lodge transiently at the ampulla, or remain free-floating in the lumen of the CBD. Clinically, stones in the CBD may cause biliary pancreatitis or obstructive jaundice (with or without suppurative cholangitis), or they may be clinically silent. Silent free-floating stones grow slowly as material continues to precipitate on the stone. In time, both the stone and the CBD enlarge. The incidence of choledocholithiasis increases with age, and occasionally stones are found in the CBD months or years after an apparently successful procedure for calculous biliary tract disease.

There are three basic procedural approaches to CBD stones, and the choice must be individualized according to the time of discovery (before, during, or after cholecystectomy), patient circumstances, and local expertise. Such procedures are endoscopic retrograde cholangiography with papillotomy and stone removal, laparoscopic common duct exploration (transcystic or via choledochotomy), and open common duct exploration. Laparoscopic common duct exploration at the time of laparoscopic cholecystectomy has emerged as the most cost-effective approach for routine management.

Ductal Drainage Procedures

Ductal drainage procedures—transduodenal sphincteroplasty and choledochoduodenostomy—are performed when it is likely that retained or residual stones will cause postoperative problems. This situation is more likely to occur if large numbers of stones are retrieved at the initial procedure or if stones recur after apparently successful ductal clearance.

Transduodenal Sphincteroplasty Versus Choledochoduodenostomy

The transduodenal approach to the common duct is occasionally required when an impacted stone cannot be removed from above. Fashioning this approach into a sphincteroplasty allows formal, controlled drainage to be performed. This technique should be part of the armamentarium of any surgeon working around the biliary tract. It is occasionally used for patients with ampullary stenosis. Careful workup with biliary manometry and exclusion of malignancy are required.

Both transduodenal sphincteroplasty and choledochoduodenostomy create a sutured anastomosis between the distal bile duct and the duodenum. The choice of procedure is based partially on the size of the duct and the ease with which (generally open) common duct exploration was performed. If an impacted stone has necessitated transduodenal exploration for removal, a transduodenal sphincteroplasty is a natural option. Similarly, it is a better option for a relatively small duct. A large duct is easily managed by choledochoduodenostomy. Transduodenal sphincteroplasty carries a risk of posterior leakage and pancreatitis. The risk of either complication can be minimized by careful technique, as described in Chapters 66–76.

BENIGN STRICTURES AND DUCTAL INJURIES

Most bile duct strictures are iatrogenic. The unfortunate ductal strictures and injuries that follow laparoscopic cholecystectomy are usually seen in patients whose CBD is small in caliber and in relatively young patients. An excellent surgical result is required to attain a normal life expectancy. Failure of repair may result in secondary biliary fibrosis, cholangitis, liver abscess, or other complications. The best chance for an excellent outcome is at the time of the first repair. Prompt recognition of injury and referral to a surgeon or center with expertise managing these problems helps maximize the chance of success.

The Bismuth classification provides a common terminology that is in widespread use [7].

Bismuth 1: low stricture with hepatic duct stump > 2 cm

Bismuth 2: mid-common hepatic duct stricture with stump < 2 cm

Bismuth 3: hilar stricture with no residual hepatic duct but with intact hepatic confluence

Bismuth 4: destruction of hilar confluence with left and right ducts completely separated

Bismuth 5: involvement of aberrant right sectoral duct alone or including the common duct

Injuries during laparoscopic cholecystectomy are frequently Bismuth 2 or 5, commonly with excision of a segment of duct. When the injury is recognized during cholecystectomy, experienced assistance should be sought. The duct is tiny, and primary repair is not advisable. It may be necessary to temporize by placing a tube for drainage and refer the patient for definitive repair. Generally choledochojejunostomy or hepaticojejunostomy is required.

Bismuth type 3 and 4 strictures require exploration of the hilum. Good ductal tissue proximal to the injury must be identified for anastomosis; otherwise the stricture recurs. Occasionally the liver must be split or partially resected or the left hepatic duct approached in the umbilical fissure to attain adequate exposure of normal ducts [8].

PERIAMPULLARY AND BILE DUCT MALIGNANCIES

Periampullary Malignancies

Duodenal, distal bile duct, and pancreatic cancer can all cause obstruction of the CBD, which is generally diagnosed by endoscopic retrograde cholangiopancreatography (ERCP) with biopsy or brushing or occasionally by choledochoscopy. Radical resection with pancreaticoduodenectomy is the preferred management wherever possible. Local excision of periampullary villous adenomas or small distal bile duct malignancies is an alternative to radical resection in selected patients (particularly the frail elderly). The resulting defect is managed much as a sphincteroplasty. Reapproximation of the pancreatic duct to duodenal mucosa may be required.

Hepatic Duct Bifurcation (Klatskin) Tumors

Tumors at the hepatic duct bifurcation (Klatskin tumors) represent a difficult challenge technically. The proximity of these lesions to hepatic inflow vessels of the hepatic artery and portal vein render most of these lesions unresectable. Modern preoperative imaging has vastly improved the ability to determine resectability and avoid unnecessary explorations. At the turn of this century patients with hilar cholangiocarcinoma are best evaluated with duplex ultrasonography and magnetic resonance imaging (MRI) with MR cholangiography. These imaging modalities are noninvasive and have been shown to be highly accurate for assessing local extent of disease, vascular involvement, and the presence or absence of distant disease [9,10]. The goal of the management of hepatic bifurcation tumors is curative surgery, as defined by negative margins of resection grossly and microscopically. It has been clear in multiple series that achieving negative histologic margins is associated with improved survival [11–14]. What has also become evident in these series is that the ability to achieve negative histologic margins of resection correlates with partial hepatectomy with or without associated caudate lobe resection in addition to bile duct resection [11]. Therefore anyone embarking on surgery for hilar cholangiocarcinoma must be prepared to perform an associated hepatectomy and, furthermore, do so liberally as it is the best way to guarantee a negative microscopic surgical margin.

LIVER RESECTION

Maximizing Safety During Major Liver Resection

Controlling inflow with particular attention to the segmental vasculature decreases blood loss and allows anatomic resection and sparing of liver parenchyma. It is also generally good practice to control the major hepatic veins outside the liver parenchyma before embarking on the parenchymal resection. This is easily accomplished on the right side; and although more difficult on the left side, it can be done there as well. If this is not possible, knowledge of the intraparenchymal course of the major hepatic veins is critical, as it facilitates control of these vessels intraparenchymally and thereby decreases blood loss.

One other useful adjunct to major liver resection that can help decrease blood loss is the monitoring and maintenance of low central venous pressure during mobilization and resection [15]. This technique requires good communication between the surgical and anesthesia teams. Moreover, although seemingly counterintuitive to the management of these patients (i.e., a low central pressure is dangerous in a case with the potential for blood loss, and it is better to have these patients "tanked up"), in fact this approach allows easier, safer control of vascular structures during liver mobilization and resection and ultimately lowers blood loss. By careful anatomic resection and expert intraoperative anesthetic management, mortality associated with major liver resection in experienced centers is now less than 5% for the noncirrhotic liver [16].

REFERENCES

1. Fong Y, Jarnagin W, Blumgart LH. Gallbladder cancer: comparison of patients presenting initially for definitive operation with those presenting after prior noncurative intervention. Ann Surg 2000;232:557.

2. Kato K, Kasai S, Matsuda M, et al. A new technique for laparoscopic cholecystectomy: retrograde laparoscopic cholecystectomy: an analysis of 81 cases. Endoscopy 1996;28:356.

3. Fletcher DR, Hobbs MST, Tan P, et al. Complications of cholecystectomy: risks of the laparoscopic approach and protective effects of operative cholan-giography; population based study. Ann Surg 1999; 229:449.

4. Russell JC, Walsh SJ, Mattie AS, et al. Bile duct injuries, 1989-1993: a statewide experience. Connecticut Laparoscopic Cholecystectomy Registry. Arch Surg 1996; 131:382.

5. Stewart L, Way LW. Bile duct injuries during laparoscopic cholecystectomy: factors that influence the results of treatment. Arch Surg 1995;130:1123.

6. Patel MI, Hardman DT, Nicholls D, et al. The incidence of deep venous thrombosis after laparoscopic cholecystectomy. Med J Aust 1996;164:652.

7. Bismuth H. Postoperative strictures of the bile duct. In Blumgart LH (ed) The Biliary Tract. Clinical Surgery International, vol 5. Edinburgh, Churchill Livingstone, 1982, pp 209-218.

8. Matthews JB, Blumbart LH. Benign biliary strictures. In Blumgart LJ (ed) Surgery of the Liver and Biliary Tract, 2nd ed, vol 1. Edinburgh, Churchill Livingstone, 1994, pp 865-894.

9. Hann LE, Fong Y, Shriver CD, et al. Malignant hepatic hilar tumors: can ultrasonography be used as an alternative to angiography with CT arterial portography for determination of unresectability? J Ultrasound Med 1996;15:37.

10. Lee MG, Lee HJ, Kim MH, et al. Extrahepatic biliary disease: 3D MR cholangiopancreatography. Radiology 1997;202:663.

11. Miyazaka M, Ito H, Nakagawa K, et al. Aggressive surgical approaches to hilar cholangiocarcinoma: hepatic or local resection? Surgery 1998;123:131.

12. Nagino M, Nimura Y, Kamiya J, et al. Segmental liver resection for hilar cholangiocarcinoma. Hepatogastroenterology 1998;45:7.

13. Burke E, Jarnigan WR, Hochwald SN, et al. Hilar cholangiocarcinoma patterns of spread, the importance of hepatic resection for curative operation, and a presurgical clinical staging system. Ann Surg 1998; 228:385.

14. Chamberlain RS, Blumgart LH. Hilar cholangiocarcinoma: a review and commentary. Ann Surg Oncol 2000;7:55.

15. Melendez JA, Arslan V, Fischer ME, et al. Perioperative outcomes of major hepatic resections under low central venous pressure anesthesia: blood loss, blood transfusion, and the risk of postoperative renal dysfunction. J Am Coll Surg 1998;187:620.

16. Cunningham J, Fong Y, Shriver C, et al. One hundred consecutive hepatic resections: blood loss, transfusion, and operative technique. Arch Surg 1994;129: 1050.

66 Cholecystectomy

INDICATIONS

Symptomatic cholelithiasis, when laparoscopic cholecystectomy is not feasible

Acute cholecystitis, both calculous and acalculous

Chronic acalculous cholecystosis and cholesterosis, when accompanied by symptoms of gallbladder colic

Carcinoma of gallbladder

Trauma

Incidental removal during laparotomy for another indication, either for technical reasons or gallstones

Failed laparoscopic cholecystectomy ("conversion")

PREOPERATIVE PREPARATION

Diagnostic confirmation of gallbladder disease

Perioperative antibiotics

Nasogastric tube for patients with acute cholecystitis or choledocholithiasis

PITFALLS AND DANGER POINTS

Injury to bile ducts

Injury to hepatic artery or portal vein

Hemorrhage from cystic or hepatic artery, or from liver bed

Injury to duodenum or colon

OPERATIVE STRATEGY

Anomalies of the Extrahepatic Bile Ducts

Anomalies, major and minor, of the extrahepatic bile ducts are quite common. A surgeon who is not aware of the variational anatomy of these ducts is much more prone to injure them during biliary surgery. The most common anomaly is a right segmental hepatic duct that drains the dorsal caudal segment of the right lobe. This segmental duct may drain into the right hepatic duct, the common he-

patic duct **(Fig. 66–1a)**, the cystic duct **(Fig. 66–1b)**, or the common bile duct (CBD) **(Fig. 66–1c)**. Division of this segmental duct may result in a postoperative bile fistula that drains as much as 500 ml of bile per day. Ligation, rather than preservation, is the appropriate management if a small segmental duct is injured.

Important cystic duct anomalies **(Fig. 66–2)** include the entrance of the cystic duct into the right hepatic duct (Fig. 66-2e), a low entrance of the cystic duct that occasionally joins the CBD rather close to the ampulla (Fig. 66-2c), and a cystic duct that enters the left side of the CBD (Fig. 66-2f).

Another extremely important anomaly of which the surgeon should be aware is the apparent entrance of the right main hepatic duct into the cystic duct. The latter duct, in turn, joins the left hepatic

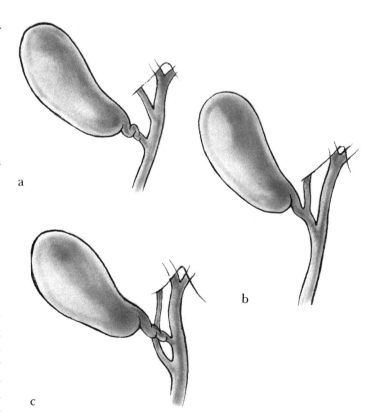

Fig. 66-1. Anomalous segmental right hepatic ducts.

572

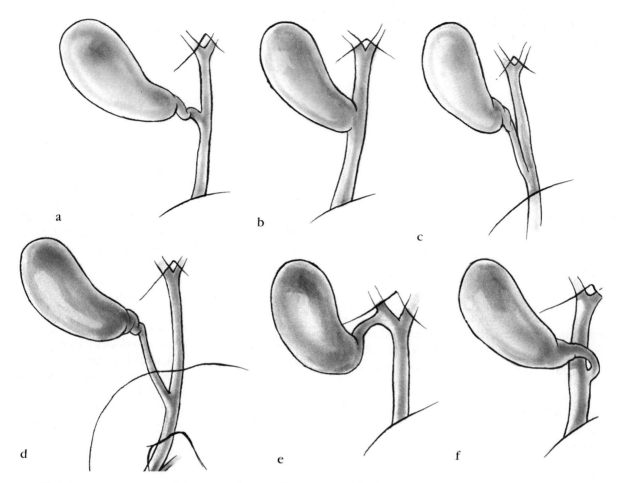

Fig. 66–2. Variations in entry of the cystic duct into the common bile duct.

duct to form the CBD, as illustrated in **Figure 66–3**. In this case, dividing and ligating the cystic duct at its apparent point of origin early in the operation results in occluding the right hepatic duct. If the technique described in the next section is carefully followed, this accident can be avoided.

Avoiding Injury to the Bile Ducts

Most serious injuries of the bile ducts are not caused by congenital anomalies or unusually severe pathologic changes. In most cases iatrogenic trauma results because the surgeon who mistakenly ligates and divides the CBD thinks it is the cystic duct. It is important to remember that the diameter of the normal CBD may vary from 2 to 15 mm. It is easy to clamp, divide, and ligate a small CBD as the first step in cholecystectomy under the erroneous impression that it is the cystic duct. The surgeon who makes this mistake must also divide the common hepatic duct before the gallbladder is freed from all its attachments. This leaves a 2- to 4-cm segment of common and hepatic duct attached to the specimen

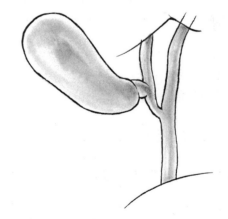

Fig. 66–3. Anomalous entry of the right hepatic duct into the cystic duct.

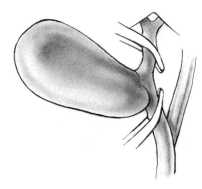

Fig. 66-4

(Fig. 66–4). Because this is the most common cause of serious duct injury, *we never permit the cystic duct to be clamped or divided until the entire gallbladder has been dissected free down to its junction with the cystic duct*. Division of the cystic duct is always the last step in the cholecystectomy. When the back wall of the gallbladder is being dissected away from the liver, it is important carefully to dissect out each structure that may enter the gallbladder from the liver. Generally, there are only a few minor blood vessels that may be divided by sharp dissection and then occluded by electrocoagulation. Any structure that resembles a bile duct must be carefully delineated by sharp dissection. In no case should the surgeon apply a hemostat to a large wad of tissue running from the liver to the gallbladder, as it may contain the common hepatic duct.

Rarely, an anomalous bile duct enters the gallbladder directly from the liver bed. Such ducts should be suture-ligated or clipped to avoid postoperative bile drainage.

Ligating the Hepatic Artery Inadvertently

Careful dissection prevents injury or inadvertent ligature of one of the hepatic arteries. However, if one of these vessels should be ligated accidentally, this complication is not ordinarily fatal because hepatic viability can usually be maintained by the remaining portal venous flow and by arterial collaterals, such as those from the undersurface of the diaphragm. This is true only if the patient has normal hepatic function and there has been no jaundice, hemorrhage, shock, trauma, or sepsis. Generally, based on findings from experimental work on animals, antibiotics are administered in cases of this type, although the need for antibiotic therapy has not been firmly established in humans.

Although hepatic artery ligation generally has a low mortality rate, it is not zero. Consequently, if a major lobar hepatic artery or the common hepatic artery has been inadvertently divided or ligated, end-to-end arterial reconstruction may be performed if local factors are favorable. For other branches of the hepatic artery, arterial reconstruction is not necessary. Variations in the anatomy of the hepatic arteries are shown in **Figure 66–5**.

Avoiding Hemorrhage

In most cases hemorrhage during the course of cholecystectomy is due to inadvertent laceration of the cystic artery. Often the stump of the bleeding vessel retracts into the fat in the vicinity of the hepatic duct, making accurate clamping difficult. If the bleeding artery is not distinctly visible, do not apply any hemostats. Rather, grasp the hepatoduodenal ligament between the index finger and thumb of the left hand and compress the common hepatic artery. This measure temporarily stops the bleeding. Now check whether the exposure is adequate and if the anesthesiologist has provided good muscle relaxation. If necessary, have the first assistant enlarge the incision appropriately. After adequate exposure has been achieved, it is generally possible to identify the bleeding vessel, which is then clamped and ligated. Occasionally the cystic artery is torn off flush with the right hepatic artery. If so, the defect in the right hepatic artery must be closed with a continuous vascular suture such as 6-0 Prolene. On rare occasions it is helpful to occlude the hepatoduodenal ligament by applying an atraumatic vascular clamp. It is safe to perform this maneuver for as long as 15–20 minutes.

The second major cause of bleeding during the course of a cholecystectomy is hemorrhage from the gallbladder bed in the liver. Bleeding occurs when the plane of dissection is too deep. This complication may be prevented if the plane is kept between the submucosa and the "serosa" of the gallbladder. If this layer of fibrous tissue is left behind on the liver, there is no problem controlling bleeding. With this plane intact, it is easy to see the individual bleeding points and to control them by electrocoagulation. Occasionally, a small artery requires a suture-ligature or a hemoclip for hemostasis. With proper exposure, hemostasis should be perfect. On the other hand, when this fibrous plane has been removed with the gallbladder and liver parenchyma is exposed, the surface is irregular and the blood vessels retract into the liver substance, making electrocoagulation less effective. Blood may ooze from a large area. In this case, apply a layer of topical hemostatic agent to the bleeding surface and cover it with a dry gauze pad; use a retractor to apply pressure to the gauze pad. After 15 minutes carefully remove the gauze pad. The topical hemostatic agent may then be carefully removed or left in place.

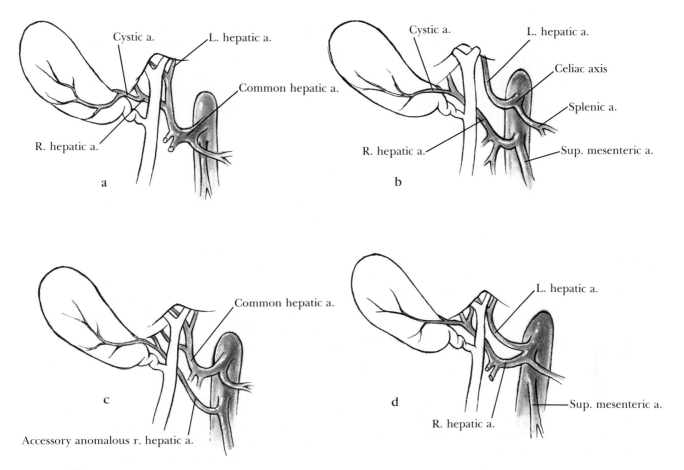

Fig. 66–5. Variations in the anatomy of the hepatic arteries.

Cystic Duct Cholangiography

Cystic duct cholangiography is useful for detecting CBD stones and delineating biliary anatomy. The major advantage of cystic duct cholangiography is that it has eliminated previously "routine" CBD exploration. Because addition of CBD exploration to a simple open cholecystectomy may result in a higher mortality rate, the use of routine cystic duct cholangiography appears valuable. It has the additional virtue of delineating the anatomy of the bile ducts, which helps prevent inadvertent injury. When cholangiography is used routinely, it requires only 5–10 minutes of additional operating time; over time the surgical and radiology teams gain expertise with the technique, making the results more accurate.

Modifications in Operative Strategy Due to Acute Cholecystitis

Decompressing the Gallbladder

Tense enlargement of the gallbladder due to cystic duct obstruction interferes with exposure of adjacent vital structures. Insert a trocar or an 18-gauge needle attached to suction and aspirate bile or pus from the gallbladder, allowing the organ to collapse. After the trocar has been removed, close the puncture site with a purse-string suture or a large hemostat.

Sequence of Dissection

Although there is sometimes so much edema and fibrosis around the cystic and common ducts that the gallbladder must be dissected from the fundus down, in most patients an incision in the peritoneum overlying the cystic duct near its junction with the CBD reveals that these two structures are not intimately involved in the acute inflammatory process. When this is the case, identify and encircle (but do not ligate) the cystic duct with 4-0 silk sutures and dissect out the cystic artery.

If the cystic artery is not readily seen, make a window in the peritoneum overlying Calot's triangle just cephalad to the cystic duct. Next, insert the tip of a Mixter right-angle clamp into this window and elevate the tissue between the window and the liver on the tip of this clamp. This maneuver improves exposure of this area. By carefully dissecting out the contents of this tissue, one can generally identify the cystic artery. Ligate it with 2-0 silk and divide the artery. When this can be done early in the operation, there is less bleeding during liberation of the fundus of the gallbladder.

Dissecting the Gallbladder Away from the Liver

Use a scalpel incision on the back wall of the gall-bladder and carry it down to the mucosal layer of the gallbladder. If part of the mucosa is necrotic, dissect around the necrotic area so as not to lose the proper plane. If it has not been possible to delineate the proper plane and the dissection inadvertently is between the outer layer of the gallbladder and the hepatic parenchyma, complete the dissection quickly and apply a topical hemostatic agent to the oozing liver bed. Then apply a moist gauze pad and use a retractor over the gauze pad to maintain exposure while the dissection is being completed. If the cystic artery has not been ligated in the previous step, it is identifiable as it crosses from the region of the common hepatic duct toward the back wall of the gallbladder.

Management of the Cystic Duct

Cholangiography

Cholangiography is performed in patients with acute obstructive cholecystitis to exclude the presence of common duct stones and to delineate anatomy. If the cystic duct is not patent, perform cholangiography through a small scalp vein needle inserted directly into the CBD.

Occasionally, the cystic duct is so inflamed it is easily avulsed from its junction with the CBD. If this accident occurs, suture the resulting defect in the CBD with a 5-0 Vicryl suture. If the cystic duct has been avulsed and its orifice in the CBD cannot be located, simply insert a sump or closed-suction catheter to a point deep to the CBD in the right renal fossa after obtaining a cholangiogram.

When to Abandon Cholecystectomy and Perform Cholecystostomy

If at any time during the course of dissecting the gall-bladder such an advanced state of fibrosis or inflammation is encountered that continued dissection may endanger the bile ducts or other vital structures, all plans for completing the cholecystectomy should be abandoned. Convert the operation to a cholecystostomy (see Chapter 68). If a portion of the gall-bladder has already been mobilized or removed, it is possible to perform a partial cholecystectomy and to insert a catheter into the gallbladder remnant. Then sew the remaining gallbladder wall around the catheter. Place additional drains in the renal fossa. Remove the gallbladder remnant at a later date, after the inflammation has subsided. Meanwhile, the pus has been drained out of the gallbladder.

The need to abandon cholecystectomy for a lesser

procedure occurs in no more than 1% of all cases of acute cholecystitis if the surgeon has experience with this type of surgery. Less experienced surgeons should not hesitate to perform a cholecystostomy when they believe that removing the gallbladder may damage a vital structure.

OPERATIVE TECHNIQUE

Incision

We prefer to make a subcostal incision for almost all cholecystectomies because of the excellent exposure afforded in the region of the gallbladder bed and cystic duct. It is important to start the incision at least 1 cm to the left of the linea alba. Then incise in a lateral direction roughly parallel to and 4 cm below the costal margin **(Fig. 66–6a)**. Continue for a variable distance depending on the patient's body build. This incision divides the ninth intercostal nerve, which emerges just lateral to the border of the rectus muscle. Cutting one intercostal nerve produces a small area of hypoesthesia of the skin but no muscle weakness. If more than one intercostal nerve is divided, the abdominal musculature sometimes bulges.

In a thin patient with a narrow costal arch, a Kehr hockey-stick modification is useful **(Fig. 66–6b)**. This incision starts at the tip of the xiphoid, pro-

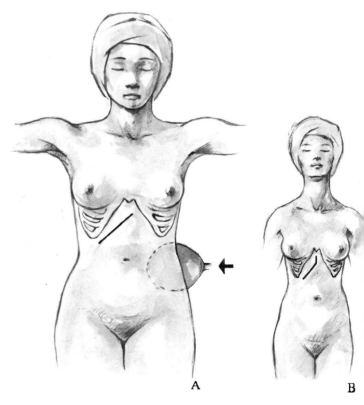

A   B

Fig. 66-6

ceeds down the midline for 3–4 cm, and then curves laterally in a direction parallel to the costal margin until the width of the right belly of the rectus muscle has been encompassed. If a midline incision is utilized, excellent exposure often requires that the incision be continued 3–6 cm below the umbilicus.

When the liver and gallbladder are high under the costal arch and this anatomic configuration interferes with exposure, or when necessary in obese patients, add a Kehr extension (up the midline to the xiphoid) to a long subcostal incision and divide the falciform ligament. This vertical extension of the incision often markedly improves exposure. Also, apply an Upper Hand or Thompson retractor to the costal arch and draw it upward.

After the incision has been made, the entire abdomen is thoroughly explored. Then direct attention to the gallbladder, confirming the presence of stones by palpation. Check the pancreas for pancreatitis or carcinoma and palpate the descending duodenum for a possible ampullary cancer.

Dissecting the Cystic Duct

Expose the gallbladder field by applying a Foss retractor to the inferior surface of the liver just medial to the gallbladder and a Richardson or a Balfour self-retaining retractor to the costal margin. Alternatively, affix a Thompson retractor to the operating table; then attach a blade to the Thompson retractor and use it to elevate and pull the right costal margin in a cephalad direction. Apply a gauze pad over the hepatic flexure and another over the duodenum. Occasionally, adhesions between omentum, colon, or duodenum and the gallbladder must be divided prior to placing the gauze pads. Have the first assistant retract the duodenum away from the gallbladder with the left hand. This move places the CBD on stretch.

Place a Kelly hemostat on the fundus of the gallbladder. With traction on the gallbladder, slide Metzenbaum scissors underneath the peritoneum that covers the area between the wall of the gallbladder and the CBD (**Fig. 66–7**). Expose the cystic duct by

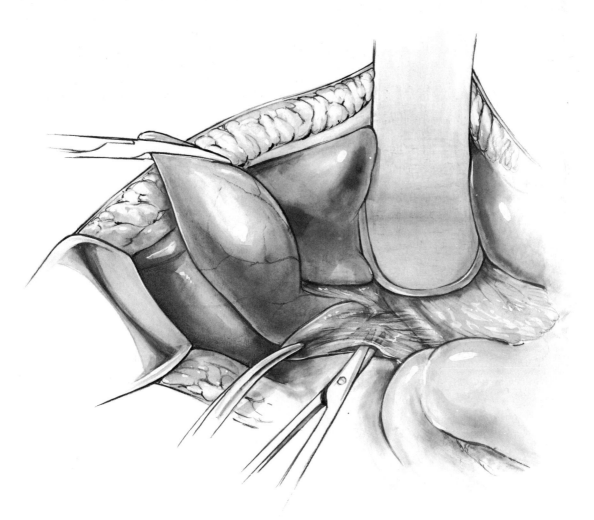

Fig. 66-7

alternately sliding Metzenbaum scissors underneath the peritoneum to define the plane and then cutting along the gallbladder wall. If the inferior surface of the gallbladder is dissected free and elevated, this plane of dissection must lead to the cystic duct, provided the plane hugs the surface of the gallbladder. The cystic duct can be easily delineated by inserting a right-angle Mixter clamp behind the gallbladder. Apply a temporary ligature of 4-0 silk to the cystic duct with a single throw to avoid inadvertently milking calculi from the gallbladder into the CBD. Do not injure the cystic duct by strangulating it with this ligature because this structure, on occasion, proves to be a small CBD, not the cystic duct. If you do not elect to obtain a cholangiogram, proceed to ligating and dividing the cystic artery. Otherwise, at this point in the operation perform cystic duct cholangiography.

Cystic Duct Cholangiography

We routinely perform cholangiography during cholecystectomy. There are two major impediments to catheterizing the cystic duct: (1) the internal diameter may be too small for the catheter; and (2) the valves of Heister frequently prevent passage of

the catheter or needle even for the 4–5 mm necessary to properly secure the catheter tip with a ligature. Although the valves may be disrupted by insertion of a malleable probe or a pointed hemostat, this maneuver sometimes results in shredding the cystic duct. A method that facilitates intubating the cystic duct is isolation of the proximal portion of the duct, including its junction with the gallbladder. Here the duct is large enough to permit introduction of the catheter at a point *proximal* to the valves of Heister, simplifying the entire task.

After the cystic duct has been isolated, continue the dissection proximally until the infundibulum of the gallbladder has been freed. The diameter at this point should be 4–5 mm. Then milk any stones up out of the cystic duct into the gallbladder and ligate the gallbladder with a 2-0 silk ligature **(Fig. 66–8a)**. Pass another 2-0 ligature loosely around the cystic duct. Make a small transverse scalpel incision in the ampulla of the gallbladder near the entrance of the cystic duct.

At this point attach a 2 meter length of plastic tubing to a 50 ml syringe that has been filled with a 1:1 solution of Conray/saline. Then check to see that the entire system—the syringe, 2 meters of plastic tubing, cholangiogram catheter—is *absolutely free*

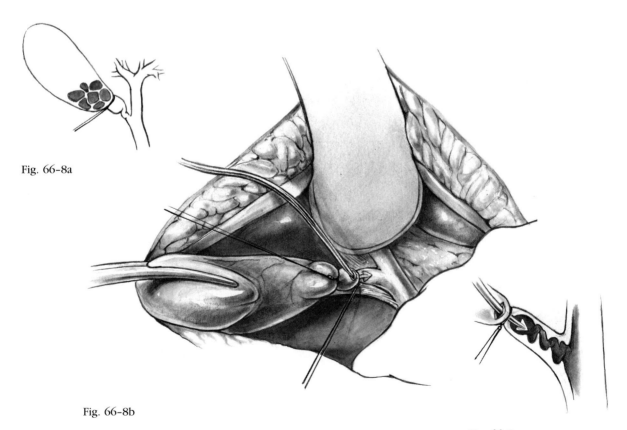

Fig. 66–8a

Fig. 66–8b

Fig. 66–8c

of air bubbles. Pass the catheter into the incision and then into the cystic duct for a distance of 5 mm **(Fig. 66–8b)**. Tie the previously placed 2-0 ligature just above the bead at the termination of the cholangiogram catheter **(Fig. 66–8c)**. Under no condition attempt to aspirate bile into the system, as this maneuver often results in aspirating air bubbles into the tubing. Some surgeons prefer a ureteral or intravenous catheter over the Taut cholangiogram catheter to intubate the cystic duct.

Elevate the left side of the patient about 10 cm above the horizontal table to prevent the image of the CBD from being superimposed on the vertebral column with its confusing shadows. This is done by having the anesthesiologist inflate a previously positioned rubber balloon under the left hip and flank (Fig. 66–6a); alternatively, two folded sheets may be placed underneath the patient's left hip and flank.

Now stand behind a portable lead shield covered with a sterile sheet. If a C-arm fluoroscopy unit is available, make the injection under fluoroscopic control. If not, follow the procedure described here and record two exposures in sequence. After the film and x-ray tube have been positioned, slowly inject no more than 4 ml of contrast medium for the first exposure. Although x-ray film is then put into position and a second exposure recorded after an additional injection of 4–6 ml. When radiographing a hugely dilated bile duct, as much as 30–40 ml may be required in *fractional* doses. On rare occasions, spasm in the region of the ampulla of Vater does not permit passage of contrast medium into the duodenum unless a small dose of nitroglycerin is administered intravenously. We have found nitroglycerin to be superior to intravenous glucagon (1 mg) for relieving sphincter spasm. If the duodenum is still not visualized, choledochotomy and exploration are indicated.

While waiting for the films to be developed, continue with the next step in the operation, ligating and dividing the cystic artery, without removing the cannula from the cystic duct. Ensure objectivity by *requesting the radiologist to provide immediate interpretation of the cholangiographic films*. Inspect the films yourself as well.

When cystic duct cholangiography is performed prior to instrumentation of the CBD and ampulla, dye almost always enters the duodenum if there is no CBD or ampullary pathology. When T-tube cholangiography is performed after completing the bile duct exploration, spasm often prevents visualization of the terminal CBD and ampulla. This problem can be averted by routine cholangiography prior to choledochotomy, even if you have already decided to explore the CBD.

Common Errors of Operative Cholangiography

Injecting too much contrast material. When a large dose of contrast material is injected into the ductal system, the duodenum is frequently flooded with dye, which may obscure stones in the distal CBD.

Dye too concentrated. Especially when the CBD is somewhat enlarged, the injection of concentrated contrast material can mask the presence of small radiolucent calculi. Consequently, dilute the contrast material 1:2 with normal saline solution when the CBD is large.

Air bubbles. Compulsive attention is necessary to eliminate air bubbles from the syringe and the plastic tubing leading to the cystic duct. Also, never try to aspirate bile into this tubing, as the ligature fixing the cystic duct around the cholangiography cannula may not be airtight and air may be sucked into the system and later injected into the CBD. It may then be impossible to differentiate between an air bubble and a calculus.

Poor technical quality. If the radiograph is not of excellent quality, there is a greater chance of a false-negative interpretation. It is useless to try to interpret a film that is not technically satisfactory. One technical error is easily avoided by elevating the left flank of the patient about 8–10 cm so the image of the bile ducts is not superimposed on the patient's vertebral column (Fig. 66–6a). Especially in obese patients, it is important to be sure that all the exposure factors are correct by using a scout film prior to starting the operation. Using an image-enhancing film-holder with a proper grid also improves technical quality. If the *hepatic ducts* have not been filled with contrast material, repeat the radiography after injecting another dose into the cystic duct. Otherwise hepatic duct stones are not visualized. It is sometimes helpful to administer morphine sulfate, which induces sphincter spasm. Dye injected into the cystic duct then fills the hepatic ducts.

Performing cystic duct cholangiography routinely serves to familiarize the technicians and the surgical team with all of the details necessary to provide superior films. It also shortens the time required for this step to 5–10 minutes.

Sphincter spasm. Spasm of the sphincter of Oddi sometimes prevents passage of contrast medium into the duodenum. Although this outcome is far more frequent after CBD exploration with instrumentation of the ampulla, it does occur on rare occasions during cystic duct cholangiography. We have found that giving nitroglycerin intravenously seems to be more effective than using intravenous glucagon to relax the sphincter. Simultaneous with sphincter relaxation, there is generally a mild drop in the patient's blood pressure. At this time inject the contrast medium into the CBD. Nitroglycerin is also useful when performing completion cholangiography when the CBD exploration has been completed.

Failing to consult with the radiologist. It is not reasonable for the operating surgeon to be the only physician responsible for interpreting the cholangiographic films. The surgeon tends to be overoptimistic, tends to accept poor technical quality, and is responsible for an excessive number of false-negative interpretations. Always have a consultation with a radiologist familiar with this procedure before forming a final conclusion concerning the cholangiogram.

Ligating the Cystic Artery

Gentle dissection in the triangle of Calot reveals the cystic artery, which may cross over or under the common or right hepatic duct on its way to the gallbladder. It frequently divides into two branches, one anterior and one posterior. Confirmation of the identity of this structure is obtained by tracing the artery up along the gallbladder wall and demonstrating the lack of any sizable branch going to the liver. Often the anterior branch of the cystic artery can be seen running up the medial surface of the gallbladder. Tracing this branch from above down to its point of origin leads to the cystic artery. Ligate this artery in continuity after passing a 2-0 silk ligature around it with a Mixter right-angle hemostat **(Fig. 66–9)**. Apply a hemoclip to the gallbladder side of the vessel and transect the cystic artery, preferably leaving a 1 cm stump of artery distal to the ligature **(Fig. 66–10)**. If there is fibrosis in Calot's triangle and the artery is not evident, pass a Mixter clamp underneath these fibrotic structures. While the first assistant exposes the structures by elevating the Mixter clamp, the surgeon can more easily dissect out the artery from the surrounding scar tissue. If the cystic artery is torn and hemorrhage results, control it by inserting the left index finger into the foramen of Winslow and compressing the hepatic artery between the thumb and forefinger until the exact source of bleeding is secured by a clamp or a suture.

Dissecting the Gallbladder Bed

In no case during cholecystectomy is the cystic duct transected or clamped prior to complete mobilization of the gallbladder. Mobilization may be done by taking advantage of the incision in the peritoneum overlying Calot's triangle as described above and simply continuing this peritoneal dissection from below upward along the medial border of the gallbladder. Insert a Mixter clamp underneath the peritoneum while the first assistant

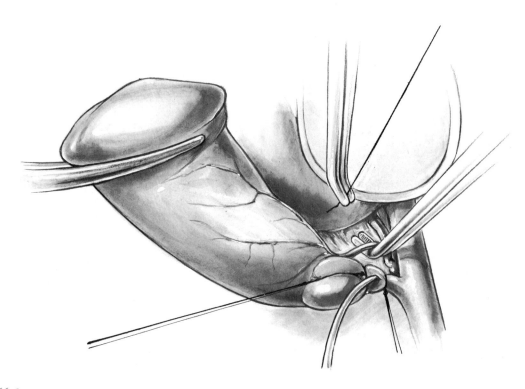

Fig. 66–9

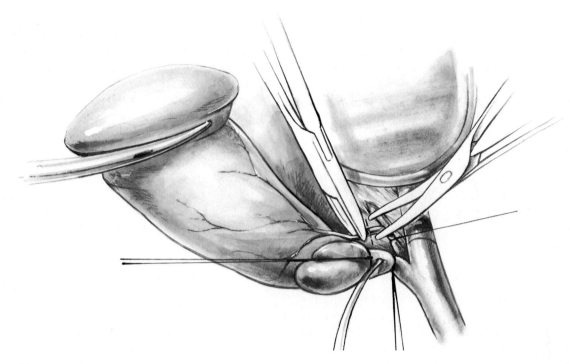

Fig. 66-10

makes an incision using electrocautery **(Fig. 66–11)**. Alternatively, make a scalpel incision in the superficial layer of the gallbladder wall across its fundus. Use electrocautery to dissect the mucosal layer of the gallbladder away from the serosal layer, *leaving as much tissue as possible on the liver side*. This leaves a shiny layer of submucosa on the gallbladder. Tiny vessels coming from the liver to the gallbladder can be identified and individually controlled with electrocautery. When the plane of dissection is deep to the serosa, raw liver parenchyma presents itself. Oozing from raw liver is difficult to control with electrocoagulation. In this case, either prolonged pressure with moist gauze or application of a small sheet of Surgicel to the raw liver surface can provide excellent hemostasis after 10-15 minutes of local compression.

As the dissection proceeds down along the liver, do not apply any hemostats, as the vessels in this plane are small. Near the termination of this dissection along the posterior wall of the gallbladder, a bridge of tissue is found connecting the gallbladder ampulla with the liver bed. Instruct the assistant to pass a Mixter clamp through the opening in Calot's

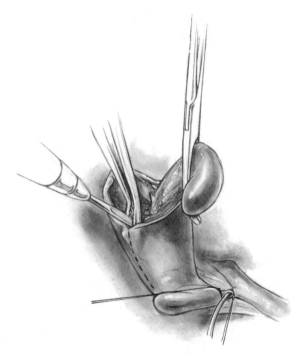

Fig. 66-11

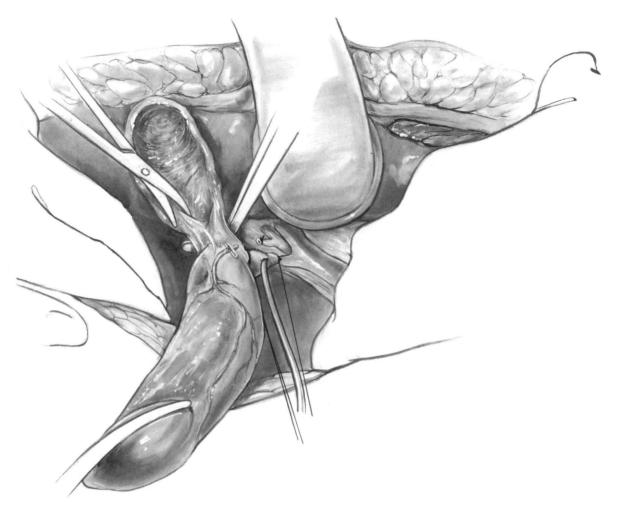

Fig. 66-12

triangle that had been made when the cystic artery was ligated **(Fig. 66–12)**. This clamp elevates the bridge of tissue, and the surgeon dissects out its contents by carefully nibbling away at it with Metzenbaum scissors to rule out the possibility that it contains the common hepatic duct. In cases where excessive fibrosis has prevented identification and ligature of the cystic artery, there is generally, at this stage of the dissection, no great problem identifying this vessel coming from the area near the hilus of the liver toward the back wall of the gallbladder.

With the gallbladder hanging suspended only by the cystic duct, dissect the duct down to its junction with the common hepatic duct. Exact determination of the junction between the cystic and hepatic ducts is usually not difficult after electrocoagulating one or two tiny vessels that cross over the acute angle between the two ducts. Rarely, a lengthy

cystic duct continues distally toward the duodenum for several centimeters.

The cystic duct may even enter the CBD on its *medial* aspect near the ampulla of Vater. In these cases it is hazardous to dissect the cystic duct down into the groove between the duodenum and pancreas; it is preferable to leave a few centimeters of duct behind. The anatomy may be confirmed by cholangiography. In general, clamp and divide the cystic duct at a point about 1 cm from its termination **(Fig. 66–13a)**. Transfix the cystic duct stump with a 3-0 PG suture-ligature **(Fig. 66–13b)**. *Never clamp or divide the cystic duct except as the last step during a cholecystectomy.*

Achieve complete hemostasis of the liver bed with electrocautery **(Fig. 66–14)**. If necessary, use suture-ligatures. In unusual cases, leave a sheet of topical hemostatic agent in the liver bed to control venous oozing.

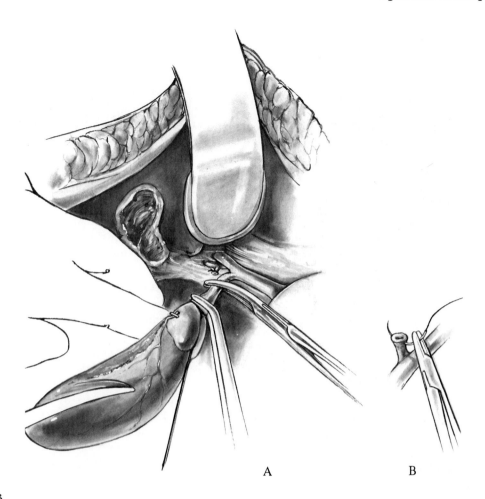

A   B

Fig. 66-13

Palpating the CBD

Prior to terminating the operation, especially if cholangiography has not been performed, it is essential to palpate the CBD properly to reduce the possibility of overlooked calculi. This is done by inserting the index finger into the foramen of Winslow and palpating the entire duct between the left index finger and thumb. Because a portion of the distal CBD is situated between the posterior wall of the duodenum and the pancreas, *it is necessary to insert the index finger into the potential space posterior to the pancreas and behind the second portion of the duodenum*. It is not necessary to perform a complete Kocher maneuver. Gently insinuate the left index finger behind the CBD and continue in a caudal direction behind the pancreas and the duodenum. In this fashion, with the index finger behind the second portion of the duodenum and the thumb on

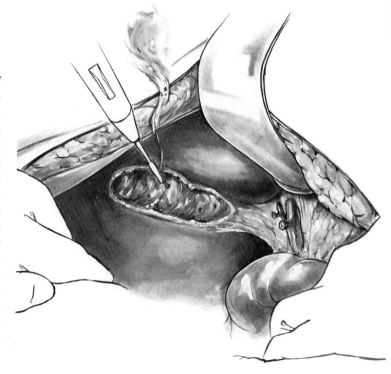

Fig. 66-14

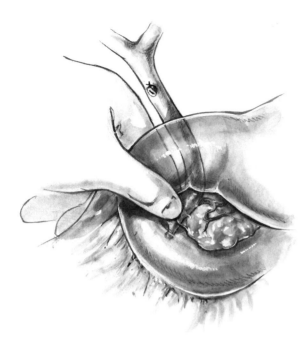

Fig. 66-15

its anterior wall, carcinomas of the ampulla and calculi in the distal CBD can be detected **(Fig. 66–15)**. Do not use force if the index finger does not pass easily; rather, proceed to a formal Kocher maneuver.

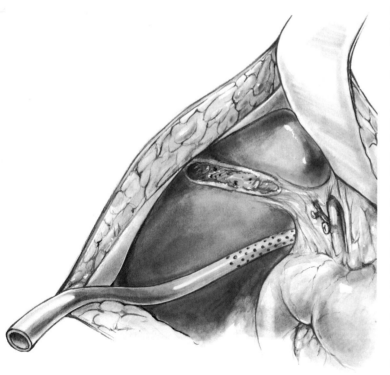

Fig. 66-16

Drainage and Closure

We insert a flat Silastic Jackson-Pratt closed-suction catheter following cholecystectomy only in cases of acute cholecystitis. Bring the catheter out from the renal fossa through a puncture wound just lateral to the right termination of the subcostal incision **(Fig. 66–16)**. There is abundant evidence that a patient who has undergone a technically precise and uncomplicated simple cholecystectomy does not require insertion of any type of drain.

Do not reperitonealize the liver bed, as this step serves no useful purpose. Close the abdominal wall in routine fashion (see Chapter 3). We use No. 1 PDS suture material for this step.

POSTOPERATIVE CARE

After an uncomplicated cholecystectomy, nasogastric suction is not necessary. In patients with acute cholecystitis, paralytic ileus is not uncommon, so nasogastric suction may be necessary for 1–3 days.

After uncomplicated cholecystectomy, antibiotics are not required except in the older age group (> 70 years). Elderly patients have a high incidence of bacteria in the gallbladder bile and so should be given perioperative antibiotics prior to and for two or three doses after operation. Following cholecystectomy for acute cholecystitis, administer antibiotics for 4–5 days, depending on the Gram stain of the gallbladder bile sampled in the operating room. Unless there is a significant amount of bilious drainage, remove the drain on approximately the fourth postoperative day.

COMPLICATIONS

Bile leak. Minor drainage of bile may follow interruption of some small branches of the bile ducts in the liver bed. This does not occur if the outer layer of the gallbladder serosa is left behind on the liver bed. On rare occasions a duct of significant size may enter the gallbladder, but we have never encountered such an instance. Bile drainage of 100–200 ml occurs if the surgeon has inadvertently transected an anomalous duct draining the dorsal caudal segment of the right lobe. If this complication is diagnosed by a sinogram radiograph, expectant therapy may result in gradual diminution of drainage as the track becomes stenotic. Endoscopic radiographic cholangiopancreatography (ERCP) and papillotomy or nasobiliary drainage may hasten resolution.

If there is any infection in the area drained by the duct, recurrent cholangitis or liver abscess may occur. In this case, permanent relief may eventually necessitate resecting the segment of the liver drained by the transected duct. If the volume of bile drainage exceeds 400 ml/day, suspect transection of the hepatic or the common bile duct.

Jaundice. Postcholecystectomy jaundice is usually due to ligature of the CBD or an overlooked CBD stone. If other causes are ruled out, ERCP is indicated to identify the obstruction.

Hemorrhage. If the cystic artery has been accurately ligated, postoperative bleeding is rare. Occasionally, oozing from the liver bed continues postoperatively and may require relaparotomy for control.

Subhepatic and hepatic abscesses. Following cholecystectomy these two complications are seen primarily in cases of acute cholecystitis. Postoperative abscesses are rare in patients whose surgery was for chronic cholecystitis unless a bile leak occurs. Treatment by percutaneous computed tomography-guided catheter drainage is usually successful.

REFERENCES

Morgenstern L, Wong L, Berci G. Twelve hundred open cholecystectomies before the laparoscopic era: a standard for comparison. Arch Surg 1992;127:400.

Olsen DO. Mini-lap cholecystectomy. Am J Surg 1993;165:400.

Roslyn JJ, Binns GS, Hughes EFX, et al. Open cholecystectomy: a contemporary analysis of 42,474 patients. Ann Surg 1993;218:129.

Smadja C, Blumgart LH. The biliary tract and the anatomy of biliary exposure. In Blumgart LH (ed) Surgery of the Liver and Biliary Tract, 2nd ed. Edinburgh, Churchill Livingstone, 1994.

Steiner CA, Bass EB, Talamini MA, Pitt HA, Steinberg EP. Surgical rates and operative mortality for open and laparoscopic cholecystectomy in Maryland. N Engl J Med 1994;330:403.

67 Laparoscopic Cholecystectomy

INDICATIONS

Confirmed diagnosis of symptomatic gallstones

Acute or chronic cholecystitis

CONTRAINDICATIONS

Prior major surgery of the upper abdomen

Cirrhosis and bleeding disorders (relative contraindications)

PREOPERATIVE PREPARATION

Ultrasonography demonstrating the presence of gallbladder calculi

Perioperative antibiotics initiated prior to the induction of anesthesia

Insertion of a nasogastric tube

Insertion of a Foley catheter (optional)

In patients whose common bile duct measures >7 mm on ultrasonography examination and whose liver chemistry profile shows abnormalities, endoscopic radiographic cholangiopancreatography (ERCP) is indicated for detection of possible common bile duct (CBD) calculi. If calculi are present and a skilled operator is available, endoscopic papillotomy with extraction of the stones is advisable. Subsequent to this procedure, a delay of 2-3 days permits the surgeon to rule out the complication of postpapillotomy acute pancreatitis prior to performing laparoscopic cholecystectomy. For a team skilled at laparoscopic choledocholithotomy, preoperative ERCP may not be necessary.

OPERATIVE STRATEGY

Avoiding Bleeding

Meticulous hemostasis is essential for laparoscopic cholecystectomy, not only to avoid blood loss but because bleeding impairs the visibility necessary to perform this operation safely and with precision.

Careful use of electrocautery can accomplish this end.

Cautery Versus Laser

Despite the extensive early publicity concerning the use of lasers for laparoscopic cholecystectomy, randomized prospective studies have shown no advantage of lasers, and most surgeons now use electrocautery. Some anecdotal reports suggest an increased danger of injury to vital structures with the use of lasers. Great care must be exercised with any source of energy, especially in the triangle of Calot, as there have been reports of lengthy strictures of the common and hepatic ducts presumably due to careless application of the laser or electrocautery in this area. When employing cautery near the bile ducts, use a hook cautery and elevate the tissues above any underlying structures in Calot's triangle before applying energy. This practice minimizes damage to the bile ducts.

Preventing Bile Duct Damage

As discussed under Complications at the conclusion of this chapter, most serious bile duct injuries result from the surgeon's mistaking the CBD for the cystic duct, resulting in transection of the CBD and occasionally excision of the CBD and most of the common hepatic duct. During laparoscopic cholecystectomy, cephalad retraction of the gallbladder fundus results in abnormal displacement of the usual pathway of the common and hepatic ducts. Normally the CBD and common hepatic duct are aligned essentially in a straight line ascending from the duodenum to the liver. However, with forceful cephalad retraction of the gallbladder fundus, the CBD appears to run in a straight line with the cystic duct directly into the gallbladder, as illustrated in **Figure 67–1**. In this situation, the common hepatic duct appears to join this straight line at a right angle. It is dangerous to initiate the dissection in the region of the bile ducts, as it may lead to the mistake of assuming that the CBD is indeed the cystic duct. A dissection proceeding in an ascending direction toward the gallbladder may very well transect the common hepatic duct.

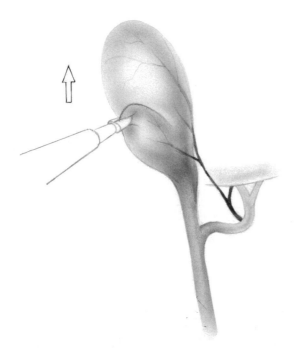

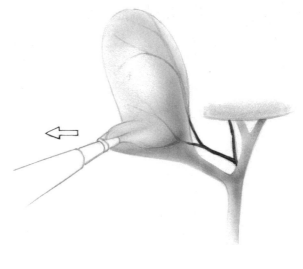

Fig. 67-2a

Fig. 67-1

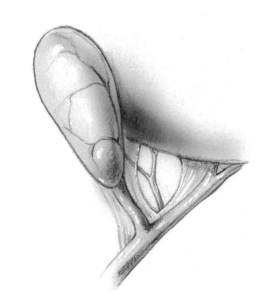

Fig. 67-2b

Two precautions must be taken to avoid this error. First, always initiate the dissection on the gallbladder and remove all areolar tissue in a downward direction so the dissection continuously proceeds from the gallbladder ampulla downward toward the cystic duct. Second, after the gallbladder ampulla and infundibulum have been cleared of areolar tissue and fat, retract these structures laterally toward the patient's right, as seen in **Figure 67–2a**. This helps restore the normal anatomy of the common and hepatic ducts and serves to open up the triangle of Calot and the space between the cystic and common hepatic ducts.

The final essential component of a technique that avoids damaging the common bile duct is *creating a window behind the gallbladder near the termination on the cystic duct* by dissecting the gallbladder away from the liver. Then, having exposed the posterior surface of the gallbladder, continue to clear the posterior walls of the infundibulum and the cystic duct until there is a 3- to 4-cm window of empty space behind the cystic duct, infundibulum, and gallbladder ampulla **(Fig. 67–2b)**. If the continuum between gallbladder, infundibulum, and cystic duct is clearly identified after elevating the structures, one can then be assured of the identity of the cystic duct. If by mistake one had initiated the dissection by freeing up the CBD caudal to its junction with the cystic duct, as the dissection proceeded cephalad toward the gallbladder the common hepatic duct would be encountered joining the cystic

duct on its medial aspect (Fig. 67–1). This approach puts the hepatic and common ducts at risk of major injury.

Ensuring Good Exposure

Because excellent visibility is essential to prevent unnecessary damage, do not hesitate to install an additional cannula and use a retractor to depress the transverse colon or to elevate the liver when necessary.

Intraoperative Cholangiography

Many experienced laparoscopic surgeons believe that an intraoperative cholangiogram, obtained as soon as the cystic duct is identified, is an excellent means for ascertaining the exact anatomy of the biliary tree. This confirms identification of the cystic duct and detects an anomalous hepatic duct in time to avoid operative trauma.

Conversion to Open Cholecystectomy

Whenever there is any doubt about the safety of a laparoscopic cholecystectomy, whether because of inflammation, scarring, poor visibility, equipment deficiencies, or any other reason, *do not hesitate to convert* the operation to an open cholecystectomy. Every patient's preoperative consent form should acknowledge the possibility that an open cholecystectomy may be necessary for the patient's safety. *Conversion to open cholecystectomy is not an admission of failure but an expression of sound judgment by a surgeon who gives first priority to the safe conduct of the operation. Because conversion is generally required only in difficult cases, it is essential that the laparoscopic surgeon be familiar with the material in Chapter 66 on the open cholecystectomy even though most cholecystectomies are performed laparoscopically.*

PITFALLS AND DANGER POINTS

Be aware that some patients have a *short cystic duct*, which increases the risk of bile duct damage by misidentification. Again, if the dissection is initiated to free the posterior wall of the gallbladder and its infundibulum, expose the common hepatic duct behind the gallbladder early during the dissection (**Fig. 67–3**). This should prevent misidentification of the anatomy. If one suspects the presence of a short cys-

tic duct but is not certain, perform intraoperative cholecystocholangiography by injecting contrast material into the gallbladder with a long needle.

There may be *damage to aorta, vena cava, iliac vessels, or bowel during trocar insertion* (see Chapter 8). There may also be *damage to the common or hepatic duct* due to misidentification.

Bleeding may be due to avulsion of the posterior branch of the cystic artery that has not been properly identified.

OPERATIVE TECHNIQUE

The room setup, entry into the peritoneal cavity, and first steps for any laparoscopic procedure are described in Chapter 8.

Initial Inspection of the Peritoneal Cavity

Plan the initial trocar site either just above or below the umbilicus in a natural skin crease. Gain access to the abdomen via a closed (Veress needle) or open (Hassan cannula) technique. Some surgeons prefer a 30° angled laparoscope for biliary surgery, but the operation can comfortably be performed with a straight (0°) laparoscope.

Insert the laparoscope into the cannula. Inspect the organs of the pelvis and posterior abdominal wall. Look for unexpected pathology and evidence of trauma that might have been inflicted during needle insertion to the vascular structures or the bowel. If no evidence of trauma is seen, aim the telescope at the right upper quadrant and make a preliminary observation of the upper abdominal organs and gallbladder.

Insertion of Secondary Trocar-Cannulas

A second 10- to 11-mm cannula is inserted in the epigastrium at a point about one-third the distance between the xiphoid process and the umbilicus. It generally is placed just to the right of the midline to avoid the falciform ligament. With a finger, depress the abdominal wall in this general area and observe with the telescope to define the exact location at which to insert the trocar. Make a 1 cm transverse skin incision at this point and insert the trocar-cannula under direct vision by aiming the telescope-camera at the entry point of the trocar. Apply even pressure with no sudden motions. Serious injuries of the liver and other organs have been reported following vigorous insertions of the trocar. As soon as the cannula has entered the abdominal cavity, re-

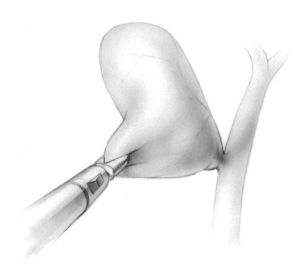

Fig. 67–3

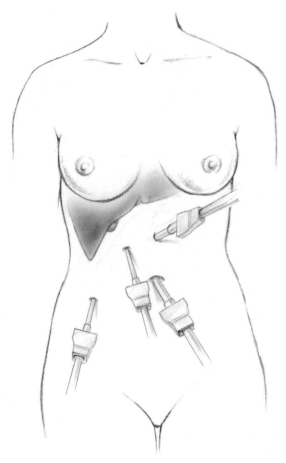

Fig. 67–4

move the trocar; this site constitutes the main operating port.

Establish two secondary ports, one in the mid-clavicular line about 2–3 cm below the costal margin and the other in the anterior axillary line at a point about level with the umbilicus. These two 5 mm ports are mainly used for grasping and retraction.

Insert a trocar in each of these ports after making a 5 mm skin incision. Observe and control the entry of these trocars carefully by watching the television monitor. The objective is to position the ports so the surgeon can manipulate the dissecting instruments at a point in front of and roughly at right angles to the telescope. **Figure 67–4** illustrates a typical arrangement of cannulas.

Dissecting the Gallbladder to Expose the Cystic Duct

To expose the gallbladder, elevate the head of the table to a 30° reverse Trendelenburg position. Apply suction to the nasogastric tube as necessary to deflate the stomach. Sometimes moderate upward rotation of the right side of the operating table is

also helpful for improving exposure. Insert a grasping forceps through the right lateral port and grasp the upper edge of the gallbladder. Push the gallbladder in a cephalad direction anterior to the liver. Utilizing the mid-clavicular port, have the assistant insert a second grasping forceps to grasp the gallbladder fundus and apply countertraction while the surgeon uses an appropriate dissecting forceps inserted through the upper midline port.

The first objective is to expose the gallbladder fundus by dissecting away any adherent omentum and other structures. Then grasp the areolar tissue and fat overlying the fundus with a grasping forceps **(Fig. 67–5)**, apply a burst of coagulating current, and pull the tissue in a caudad direction. While this is being done, the assistant's grasping forceps draws the ampulla of the gallbladder gently toward the patient's right, as illustrated in Figure 67-2. Hook electrocautery or electrified scissors can also be used to divide the peritoneal layers that cover the infundibulum of the gallbladder and cystic duct. Use the hook dissector to liberate the lower portion of the gallbladder from its attachment to the liver, both laterally and medially. *Create a large window of space behind the gallbladder, the infundibulum, and the cystic duct* (Fig. 67-2). The dissection should continuously be directed from the gallbladder downward toward the cystic duct. Always consider that the CBD and hepatic ducts may be closer to the gallbladder than you think, especially in patients who have a short cystic duct (Fig. 67-3). Concentrating on the lower portion of the gallbladder and infundibulum is much safer than initiating the dissection behind what you *think* is the cystic duct but that may indeed be the CBD.

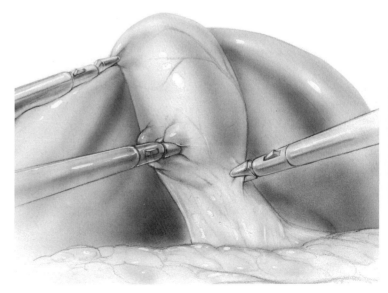

Fig. 67–5

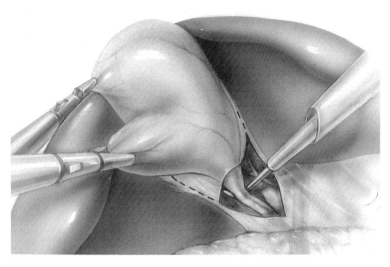

Fig. 67-6

After dissecting on both sides of the cystic duct by manipulating the ampulla from right to left, pass a right-angled Maryland dissector or a hook behind the cystic duct and free up several centimeters so there is *complete exposure of the continuum of the posterior cystic duct going up to the infundibulum and the lower portion of the gallbladder* (**Fig. 67–6**).

Cystic Duct Cholangiogram

When certain that the cystic duct has been identified, apply an endoscopic clip to the area of the infundibulum of the gallbladder and use scissors to make an incision in the cystic duct just below the clip (**Fig. 67–7**). For cholangiography we prefer a balloon-tipped catheter of the type made by the Arrow Company. Test the balloon and insert the

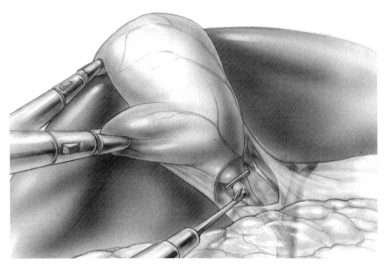

Fig. 67-7

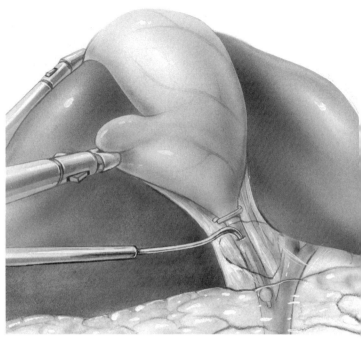

Fig. 67-8

catheter into the upper midline or mid-clavicular port. Adjust the curvature of the catheter tip by pushing or withdrawing the catheter through its curved plastic catheter-holder. Thread the catheter into the cystic duct incision for no more than 1 cm (**Fig. 67–8**), a point marked by two black lines on the catheter body. Inflate the balloon and tentatively inject some contrast material to determine that leakage does not take place. Do not insert the catheter too far into the cystic duct; otherwise, it enters the CBD, and the balloon occludes the CBD at the point of injection, resulting in an image of the distal CBD only from the catheter tip to the ampulla of Vater. This image cannot prove that the common hepatic duct is intact. In this case, back out the catheter for a short distance and repeat the cholangiogram. Use C-arm fluoroscopy to monitor the injection. If fluoroscopy is not available, obtain two plain radiographs. Inject 4 ml of contrast material for the first film and an additional 8 ml for the second. *If the proximal ducts do not fill, assume a CBD injury and convert to open laparostomy.*

If the cholangiogram demonstrates satisfactory filling of the hepatic duct and CBD as well as the duodenum, remove the catheter and continue to the next step, which is dividing the cystic duct as described below. If the cholangiogram demonstrates a calculus in the CBD, perform a laparoscopic CBD exploration if the technology and skill are available (see References). Otherwise, one has the choice of performing an open cholecystectomy and choledocholithotomy or scheduling the patient for a post-operative endoscopic papillotomy for stone extraction. If the stone is exceedingly large (approaching 2 cm) an open choledocholithotomy is preferable. This is also the case if the patient has a large number of stones or has had a previous Billroth II gastrectomy, making endoscopic papillotomy an unlikely choice.

There need be no hesitation on the part of the surgeon to proceed to open cholecystectomy and choledocholithotomy. This is a safe operation that generally accomplishes complete clearing of the CBD in one procedure. Such clearance may take the endoscopist several attempts to accomplish by endoscopic papillotomy. Remember also that endoscopic papillotomy for CBD extraction is associated with 1% mortality. One advantage of the open choledocholithotomy in patients who have 10–20 calculi is the ability to incorporate into the operation a biliary-enteric bypass, such as choledochoduodenostomy. Because endoscopic papillotomy is feasible in only about 90% of patients owing to anatomic variability or periampullary diverticula, it may be helpful to insert a guidewire through the opening in the cystic duct and pass it down the CBD into the duodenum. Duodenal placement can be confirmed by an abdominal radiograph. In the presence of this guidewire, endoscopic papillotomy can be performed in almost 100% of patients.

In cases where passage of the cholangiogram catheter is obstructed by the valves of Heister, the obstruction may be corrected by inserting the tip of the scissors into the cystic duct. Keep the scissors closed upon entering the duct and then open them with mild force to dilate the valves.

Removing the Gallbladder

Remove the cholangiogram catheter and apply another endoscopic clip on the gallbladder side of the incision **(Fig. 67–9)**. Then apply two clips on the distal portion of the cystic duct. Divide the cystic duct with scissors.

During dissection of the cystic duct, the cystic artery is generally identified slightly cephalad to the cystic duct. Whenever this structure has been clearly identified, elevate it with either a Maryland dissector or a hook so at least 1 cm is dissected completely from surrounding structures. Then apply one endoscopic clip above and two clips below, and divide the artery with scissors **(Fig. 67–10)**. Note that the point at which the cystic artery divides into its anterior and posterior branches can be somewhat variable. When you think you have divided the main cystic artery, you may have divided only the anterior

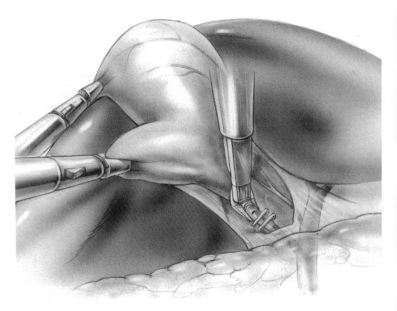

Fig. 67-9

branch. Be alert during the latter part of the dissection for a posterior branch that must often be clipped and divided when the infundibulum of the gallbladder is freed. If this branch is small enough, it may be handled by electrocautery instead of clipping.

Now continue to dissect the gallbladder away from the liver. This can be done with electrocautery using either a hook or a spatula dissection. Divide the peritoneum between the gallbladder and the liver on each side of the gallbladder. Then continue the dissection on the posterior wall of the gallbladder. The first assistant maneuvers the two grasping forceps to expose various aspects of the gallbladder

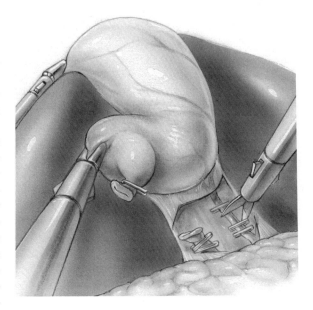

Fig. 67-10

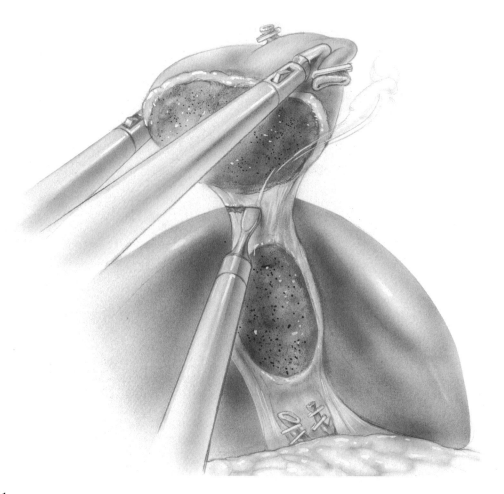

Fig. 67-11

and applies countertraction for the surgeon. Some
surgeons utilize a two-handed technique: dissection
with the right hand and manipulating the medial
grasping forceps with the left hand.

Before the gallbladder is totally free of its attachment to the liver, carefully inspect the liver bed for
bleeding points. Irrigate the area. If there are any
bleeding points in the liver bed, they can be occluded by applying a suction-electrocoagulator.

Finally, elevate and divide the gallbladder from its
final attachment to the liver **(Fig. 67–11)**. Leave the
gallbladder in position over the dome of the liver being held in the lateral port grasper.

Remove the laparoscope from the umbilical cannula and place it through the upper midline sheath.
Insert a large claw grasper through the umbilical cannula. Pass the claw along the anterior abdominal wall
to reach the gallbladder over the dome of the liver.
Follow the action with the camera. The claw grasps
the gallbladder at its neck. Then pull the gallbladder
into the umbilical cannula as far as it will go. Now
remove the cannula together with the gallbladder.
As soon as the neck of the gallbladder is seen out-

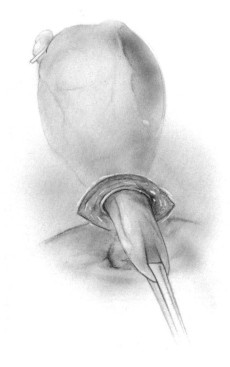

Fig. 67-12

extract it from the abdomen while observing the action on the video monitor **(Fig. 67–15)**. If the gallbladder is too large to pass through the umbilical incision, the incision can be enlarged somewhat by inserting a large hemostat and stretching the width of the incision. Alternatively, the incision may be lengthened by several millimeters in both directions using the scalpel until the gallbladder can be removed. Sometimes an endoscopic retrieval bag is useful, particularly if the gallbladder is inflamed.

In the patient with a small gallbladder, do not move the telescope from the umbilical port. Rather, pass the claw grasper through the epigastric port and draw the gallbladder through the epigastric incision.

If the laparoscope has been transferred to the epigastric port, return it to the umbilical cannula and make a last inspection of the abdominal viscera, pelvis, and gallbladder bed. If there are any signs of retroperitoneal hematomas in the region of the aorta, vena cava, or iliac vessels, assume that there has been major injury to these vessels and perform a laparotomy if necessary to rule out this possibility. Remember, even with disposable trocars that have plastic shields, forceful collision of the shielded trocar with the vena cava may result in perforation of this vessel. Bleeding from the great vessels consti-

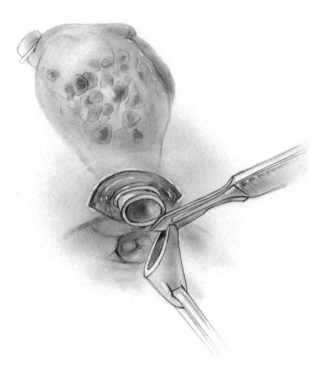

Fig. 67-13

side the umbilicus **(Fig. 67–12)** make an incision in the gallbladder **(Fig. 67–13)** and insert a suction device to aspirate bile **(Fig. 67–14)**. Apply a Kelly hemostat to the neck of the gallbladder and gradually

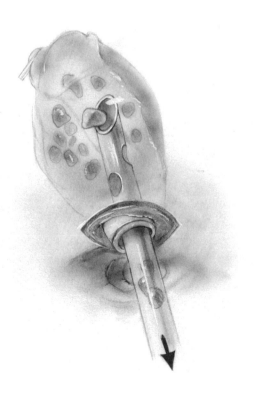

Fig. 67-14

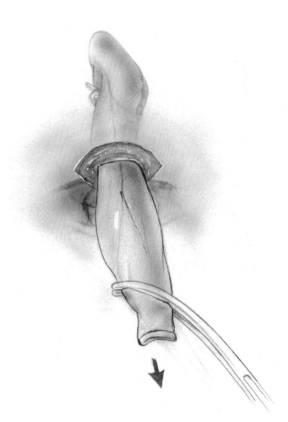

Fig. 67-15

tutes the main cause of the rare fatality that follows laparoscopic cholecystectomy. Carefully observe the withdrawal of each cannula to ascertain the absence of bleeding in each case. Finally, permit the escape of carbon dioxide from the abdominal cavity and remove the final cannula. Insert sutures of heavy Vicryl in the two 10 mm incisions in the midline of the abdomen. The 5 mm incisions do not require closure. Close the skin with sterile adhesive tape or subcuticular sutures.

POSTOPERATIVE CARE

Remove the nasogastric or orogastric tube and urinary catheter (if placed) before the patient leaves the recovery room. Mild pain medication may be necessary. Ambulate the patient as soon as he or she awakens. A regular diet may be ordered unless the patient is nauseated.

Discharge patients a day or two following surgery. They may resume full activity by the end of 1 week.

COMPLICATIONS

Needle or Trocar Damage

Retroperitoneal bleeding from damage to one of the great vessels during insertion of the initial trocar can be fatal. A retroperitoneal hematoma noted during laparoscopy requires open exploration for great vessel injury.

Bowel injury can result from introducing the Veress needle or a trocar, especially if the trocar is passed through adherent bowel. Careful inspection of the abdomen by laparoscopy after inserting the initial trocar and again before terminating the operation is essential if these injuries are to be detected early and then repaired.

Insufflation-Related Complications

See Chapter 8.

Bile Duct Damage; Excision of Common and Hepatic Ducts

The classic laparoscopic biliary injury includes resection of large sections of the CBD and the common hepatic duct together with the cystic duct and the gallbladder **(Fig. 67–16)**. Injury results from mistaking the CBD for the cystic duct and applying clips to the CBD. The CBD is then dissected in a cephalad direction as though it were the cystic duct with transection of the proximal hepatic ductal system with or without clip ligation.

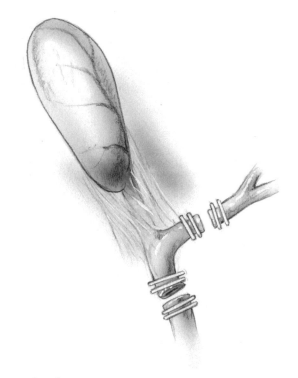

Fig. 67–16

Significant leakage of bile into the operative field is a danger sign that should not be ignored. Inadequate visualization of the surgical field often contributes to these errors and to significant bleeding.

If, in fact, a surgeon divides the common bile duct by mistake, there is certainly no excuse for failing to detect this error when the dissection encounters the common hepatic duct. As seen in Figure 67–16 (modified from Davidoff et al. (1992)), if one dissects the proximal divided end of the CBD in a cephalad direction, it is not possible to remove the gallbladder without transecting the common hepatic duct. With proper surgical dissection, it should be obvious that the presence of this duct indicates that the operative strategy is wrong and requires an immediate course correction.

Rossi et al. (1992) described the repair of laparoscopic bile duct injuries in 11 patients referred to Lahey Clinic. They found that fibrosis or scarring in Calot's triangle was an important factor contributing to the injury in many of their cases. Their conception of the mechanism of injury is illustrated in **Figure 67–17**. The cystic duct is densely adherent to the common hepatic duct for several centimeters above the junction of the cystic and common ducts. This injury does not occur if the dissection is initiated at the distal gallbladder and if the posterior portion of the gallbladder infundibulum is dissected away from the liver before dissecting the cystic duct. Dissection should always progress from the gallbladder to-

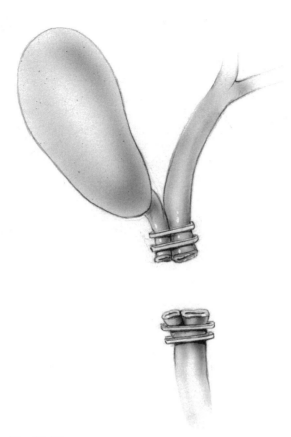

Fig. 67-17

ward the cystic duct, completely freeing the entire circumference of the fundus, the infundibulum of the gallbladder, and the cystic duct.

Davidoff and associates described a variant of the classic CBD injury. It is illustrated in **Figure 67–18**. Here, clips were applied to the CBD just below its junction with the cystic duct, but the transection took place across the distal portion of the cystic duct. In this case the patient will have a total biliary fistula into the peritoneal cavity. These authors also described two patients who presented 4-6 weeks after surgery with jaundice and extensive strictures of their common and hepatic ducts. They hypothesized that this pathology resulted from thermal injury in the region of Calot's triangle by laser or electrocoagulation.

The CBD may also be injured when the clip applied to the proximal portion of the cystic duct also encompasses the right hepatic duct. Fibrosis in Calot's triangle may contribute to this injury by placing the right hepatic duct in close proximity to the cystic duct. This injury may be avoided if the surgeon properly dissects the gallbladder infundibulum and cystic duct from above down prior to applying the clips.

In summary, prevention of damage to the bile ducts requires good visibility (sometimes facilitated by use of a 30° angled laparoscope); lateral traction on the fundus and infundibulum of the gallbladder

to separate the cystic duct from the common hepatic duct; directing the dissection from the distal gallbladder downward toward the cystic duct rather than the reverse; using electrocautery with caution; applying routine cholangiography early in the operation; and converting to open cholecystectomy whenever there is any doubt concerning the safety of the laparoscopic cholecystectomy. A satisfactory intraoperative cholangiogram must show intact bile ducts from the right and left hepatic ducts down to the duodenum. When there is doubt concerning which duct to use for the cholangiogram, a cholecystocholangiogram may be obtained by injecting 30-40 ml of contrast material directly into the gallbladder.

Bile Leak

Leakage of bile into the right upper quadrant following laparoscopic cholecystectomy does not necessarily indicate an injury to the bile duct. It may simply mean that the occluding clips have slipped off the cystic duct or that a minor accessory bile duct is leaking. Symptoms generally develop a few days after laparoscopic cholecystectomy and consist of generalized abdominal discomfort, anorexia, fatigue, and sometimes jaundice. Sonography can reveal the presence of fluid in the subhepatic space. A HIDA scan demonstrates the presence of bile outside the biliary tree, and ERCP demonstrates the point of leak-

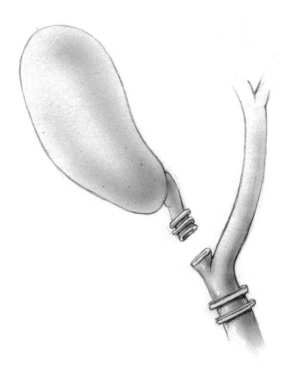

Fig. 67-18

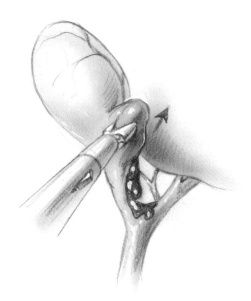

Fig. 67-19

age. In the absence of obstruction in the CBD, these leaks generally heal spontaneously. Healing may be expedited by percutaneous insertion of a drainage catheter into the right upper quadrant and insertion of a stent into the CBD following endoscopic papillotomy. Of course, major ductal injury requires surgical reconstruction, generally by the hepaticojejunostomy Roux-en-Y procedure.

Intraoperative Hemorrhage from Cystic Artery

Occasionally brisk bleeding results when the cystic artery is cut or torn. It is generally a minor complication during open cholecystectomy because grasping the hepatic artery between two fingers in the foramen of Winslow (Pringle maneuver) ensures prompt if temporary control of bleeding. With laparoscopic cholecystectomy, however, losing 30–40 ml of blood may be serious because the blood obscures visibility through the laparoscope.

Frequently it is possible to control cystic artery bleeding by grasping the gallbladder ampulla near the bleeding vessel and pushing the ampulla firmly against the liver **(Fig. 67–19)**. If this maneuver successfully controls the bleeding, insert one or more additional cannulas for suction and retraction and attempt to localize and clip the bleeding vessel. It is not worth spending much time on occluding this bleeder laparoscopically because making a subcostal incision affords an opportunity to localize and control the bleeder quickly with no risk.

REFERENCES

Bauer TW, Morris JB, Lowenstein A, et al. The consequences of a major bile duct injury during laparoscopic cholecystectomy. J Gastrointest Surg 1998;2:61.

Branum G, Schmitt C, Bailie J, et al. Management of major biliary complications after laparoscopic cholecystectomy. Ann Surg 1993;217:532.

Davidoff AM, Pappas TN, Murray EA, et al. Mechanisms of major biliary injury during laparoscopic cholecystectomy. Ann Surg 1992;215:196.

Gadacz TR. Update on laparoscopic cholecystectomy, including a clinical pathway. Surg Clin North Am 2000; 80:1127.

Hannan EL, Imperato PJ, Nenner RP, et al. Laparoscopic and open cholecystectomy in New York State: mortality, complications, and choice of procedure. Surgery 1999;125:223.

Rossi RL, Schirmer WJ, Braasch LW, et al. Laparoscopic bile duct injuries: risk factors, recognition, and repair. Arch Surg 1992;127:596.

Soper NJ, Brunt LM. The case for routine operative cholangiography during laparoscopic cholecystectomy. Surg Clin North Am 1994;74:953.

Strasberg SM, Callery MP, Soper NJ. Laparoscopic surgery of the bile ducts. Gastrointest Endosc Clin North Am 1996;6:81.

Strasberg SM, Hertl M, Soper NJ. An analysis of the problem of biliary injury during laparoscopic cholecystectomy. J Am Coll Surg 1995;180:101.

68 Cholecystostomy

SURGICAL LEGACY TECHNIQUE

INDICATIONS

Cholecystostomy may be performed in patients suffering from acute cholecystitis when cholecystectomy may be hazardous for technical reasons, or when cholecystectomy has been attempted and is too technically difficult. Computed tomography (CT)-guided percutaneous catheter drainage may be the most pragmatic method for managing acute cholecystitis in poor-risk patients. Rarely, it is not possible for technical reasons, and open or laparoscopic (see References) cholecystostomy is an option in these cases.

CONTRAINDICATION

Patients with acute cholangitis owing to common bile duct (CBD) obstruction

PREOPERATIVE PREPARATION

Appropriate antibiotics

PITFALLS AND DANGER POINTS

Overlooking acute purulent cholangitis
Overlooking gangrene of the gallbladder
Postoperative bile leak

OPERATIVE STRATEGY

When Is Cholecystostomy Inadequate?

Cholecystostomy does not provide adequate drainage for an infected bile duct. In most cases it is not difficult to differentiate acute cholecystitis from acute cholangitis. When a patient with acute cholangitis does not respond immediately to antibiotic treatment, prompt drainage of the CBD is lifesaving. Undrained acute purulent cholangitis is often rapidly fatal. When performing cholecystostomy, one must be alert not to overlook this disease of the bile duct.

Gangrene of the gallbladder is another complication of acute cholecystitis, for which cholecystostomy is an inadequate operation. The gangrene may occur in the deep portion of the gallbladder fundus, where it may be hidden by adherent omentum or bowel. It is easy to overlook a patch of necrosis when operating through a small incision under local anesthesia. When a necrotic area is found in the gallbladder, it is preferable to perform a complete cholecystectomy; if this operation is impossible for technical reasons, a partial cholecystectomy around a catheter with removal of the gangrenous patch can be done **(Fig. 68–1)**.

Choice of Anesthesia

Because of the danger of overlooking disease of the CBD and gangrene or perforation of the gallbladder, it is preferable to perform the cholecystostomy through an adequate incision under general anes-

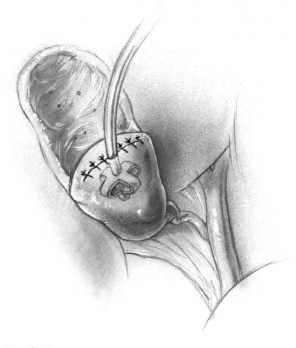

Fig. 68-1

597

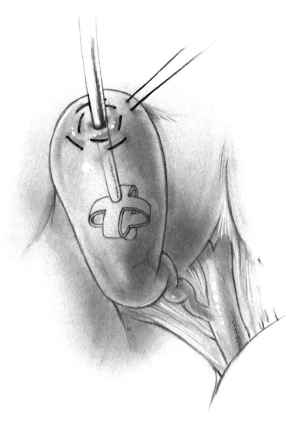

Fig. 68-2

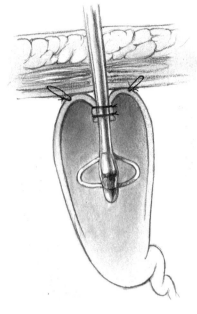

Fig. 68-3

thesia. With modern anesthesia and monitoring techniques, it is safe for most poor-risk patients to undergo a biliary operation under general anesthesia. Otherwise, perform percutaneous catheter drainage of the gallbladder.

Preventing Bile Leaks

One distressing complication that occasionally follows cholecystostomy is leakage of bile around the catheter into the free peritoneal cavity, resulting in bile peritonitis. This complication can generally be avoided by using a large catheter and suturing the gallbladder around the catheter **(Fig. 68–2)**. It is important also to suture the fundus of the gallbladder to the peritoneum around the exit wound of the drainage catheter **(Fig. 68–3)**. Adequate drainage is also necessary in the vicinity of the gallbladder.

OPERATIVE TECHNIQUE

Incision

Under general anesthesia, make a subcostal incision at least 10-12 cm in length. Find the plane between the adherent omentum and the inflamed gallbladder. Once this plane is entered, the omentum can gen-

erally be freed from the gallbladder wall by gentle blunt dissection. Continuing in this plane, inspect the gallbladder and its ampulla.

Emptying the Gallbladder

After ascertaining that there is no perforation of the gallbladder or any patch of gangrene, empty the gallbladder with a 16-gauge needle or a suction trocar inserted into the tip of the gallbladder. Perform an immediate Gram stain. Enlarge the stab wound in the gallbladder. Attempt to remove the gallbladder calculi with pituitary scoops and Randall stone forceps. It may be necessary to compress the gallbladder ampulla manually to milk stones up toward the fundus. After flushing the gallbladder with saline, insert a 20F straight or Pezzar catheter 3-4 cm into the gallbladder. Close the defect in the gallbladder wall with two inverting purse-string sutures of 2-0 PG suture material (Fig. 68-2). If the gallbladder wall is unusually thick, it may be necessary to close the gallbladder around the catheter with interrupted Lembert sutures.

If the patient is in satisfactory condition, attempt cholangiography through the gallbladder catheter. It is not always possible to extract a stone that is impacted in the cystic duct. This circumstance eliminates the possibility of obtaining a cholangiogram by this route.

Now make a stab wound through the abdominal wall close to the fundus of the gallbladder. Draw the catheter through the abdominal wall and suture the fundus of the gallbladder to the peritoneum alongside the stab wound (Fig. 68-3). Make a stab wound and insert two closed-suction catheters: one in the vicinity of the cholecystostomy and one in the right renal fossa.

Close the abdominal incision in routine fashion as described in Chapter 3. We use No. 1 PDS sutures for this closure.

POSTOPERATIVE CARE

Connect the cholecystostomy catheter to a sterile plastic collecting bag for gravity drainage.

Continue antibiotic treatment for the next 7–10 days. Until bacterial culture and sensitivity studies have been reported on the gallbladder bile, use antibiotics that are effective against gram-negative bacteria, enterococci, and anaerobes.

Employ nasogastric suction if necessary.

Measure the daily output of bile and replace with an appropriate dose of sodium.

Do not remove the gallbladder drainage catheter for 12–14 days. Obtain a cholangiogram before removing the catheter.

COMPLICATIONS

Bile peritonitis

Subhepatic, subphrenic, or intrahepatic abscess

Septicemia

Patients with acute cholecystitis generally respond promptly to adequate drainage of the infection. If the patient shows persistent signs of sepsis and bacteremia, it is likely that this complication stems from an undrained focus of infection. It may be an obstructed CBD with cholangitis or a subhepatic, *intrahepatic*, or subphrenic abscess. Endoscopic retrograde cholangiopancreatography (ERCP) and CT scanning may be helpful for detecting these complications.

REFERENCES

Berber E, Engle KL, String A, et al. Selective use of tube cholecystostomy in acute cholecystitis. Arch Surg 2000;135:341.

Borzellino G, deManzoni G, Ricci F, et al. Emergency cholecystostomy and subsequent cholecystectomy for acute gallstone cholecystitis in the elderly. Br J Surg 1999;86:1521.

Davis CA, Landercasper J, Gundersen LH, Lambert PJ. Effective use of percutaneous cholecystomy in high-risk surgical patients: techniques, tube management, and results. Arch Surg 1999;134:727.

Johnson AB, Fink AS. Alternative methods for management of the complicated gallbladder. Semin Laparosc Surg 1998;5:115.

69 Common Bile Duct Exploration

SURGICAL LEGACY TECHNIQUE

INDICATIONS

Multiple alternatives have largely superseded open common bile duct (CBD) exploration. Endoscopic retrograde cholangiopancreatography (ERCP) with sphincterotomy provides access to the common duct for extraction of stones and biliary decompression. Laparoscopic transcystic common duct exploration or laparoscopic choledochotomy are alternatives when common duct stones are found at laparoscopic cholecystectomy. Open CBD exploration is still occasionally needed when these methods are not available or fail. The principles of access to the CBD described here are used during the performance of advanced biliary tract surgery and must be thoroughly understood.

Chills, fever, and jaundice prior to operation (in more than 90% of cases CBD exploration reveals calculi)

Palpation of a calculus in the CBD

Acute suppurative cholangitis

Positive finding of a calculus on routine cystic duct cholangiography, preoperative ERCP, or percutaneous transhepatic cholangiogram

Access to the CBD is sometimes required during the course of other procedures in this region (e.g., to delineate the course of the CBD during a difficult ulcer operation). The principles delineated here apply in those situations as well. Adequate cholangiography can prove or disprove the presence of stones in many situations that formerly were listed as relative indications for CBD exploration.

PREOPERATIVE PREPARATION

Computed tomography (CT) or sonography is used. Generally ERCP is performed as the next diagnostic maneuver when dilated ducts are seen.

Correct abnormalities of the serum prothrombin preoperatively with injections of vitamin K.

When CBD exploration is planned, the patient should receive perioperative intravenous antibiotics beginning 1 hour prior to operation. To ensure an adequate antibacterial blood level, repeat the dose in 3 hours, during the operation. We use either a third- or fourth-generation cephalosporin or a penicillin-aminoglycoside combination.

PITFALLS AND DANGER POINTS

Injuring the bile ducts

Creating a false passage into the duodenum when probing the CBD; damaging the ampulla or pancreas; inducing postoperative pancreatitis

Perforating a periampullary duodenal diverticulum

Sepsis

Failing to remove all of the biliary calculi

OPERATIVE STRATEGY

Avoiding Postoperative Pancreatitis

Postoperative acute pancreatitis can be lethal. Use routine cholangiography to minimize the number of unnecessary CBD explorations. Explore the distal duct with delicacy and meticulous care to avoid trauma to the ampulla or pancreas, which may induce pancreatitis.

CBD Perforations

Another *serious and often fatal error* is to perforate the distal CBD and penetrate the pancreas with an instrument such as the metal Bakes dilator. When the surgeon experiences any difficulty negotiating the ampulla with an instrument, duodenotomy and direct exposure of the ampulla are preferable to repeated blunt trauma from above. Using a 10F Coude or whistle-tipped rubber catheter, rather than a metal dilator, lessens the risk of ampullary trauma and postoperative acute pancreatitis. Never forcefully dilate the sphincter of Oddi; this procedure serves no useful purpose, and the trauma to the ampulla not only increases the risk of postoperative acute pancreatitis it produces lacerations and hematomas of the ampulla.

If an instrument has perforated the distal CBD and the head of the pancreas, it may be detected when the CBD is irrigated with saline by noting saline leakage from the posterior surface of the pancreas. The perforation may also be detected by cholangiography. This type of trauma, which leads to bile flow directly into the head of the pancreas, often causes fatal pancreatitis. For this reason, when this complication is identified divide the CBD just above its entry into the pancreaticoduodenal sulcus; transfix the distal end of the duct with a suture and anastomose the proximal cut end of the CBD to a Roux-en-Y segment of jejunum. When this procedure is carried out, diverting the bile from the traumatized pancreas may prove lifesaving. Also insert a closed-suction drain behind the pancreatic head to remove any leaking pancreatic secretions.

If the CBD has been perforated at an accessible point proximal to the head of the pancreas, suture the laceration with 5-0 PG or PDS. If the laceration is not accessible, simply insert a large-caliber T-tube into the CBD for decompression proximal to the laceration. Then place a closed-suction catheter drain down to the region of the laceration.

Locating and Removing Biliary Calculi

To avoid overlooking biliary calculi, obtain a cystic duct cholangiogram before exploring the CBD. Be sure that the radiograph clearly shows the hepatic ducts and the distal CBD. If the hepatic ducts cannot be seen because the dye runs into the duodenum, administer morphine to induce spasm of the ampulla; alternatively, open the CBD, insert an 8F Foley catheter into the proximal CBD, and use this device to obtain a radiograph of the intrahepatic radicles. This cholangiogram can provide an estimate of size, number, and location of calculi.

Always perform a Kocher maneuver before exploring the CBD. It permits the surgeon to place the fingers of the left hand behind the ampullary region with the thumb on top of the anterior wall of the duodenum. This allows the instrument to be directed more accurately while palpating its distal tip.

Once the CBD has been opened, the safest, most effective device for extracting stones is the pituitary scoop with a malleable handle. Available with various size cups, this device can be bent to the exact curvature required to pass through the CBD down to the ampulla. By delicate maneuvering, the surgeon can remove most stones with the scoop. Also, it is often easy to palpate a stone against this metallic instrument.

Other methods that are helpful for retrieving stones are the Randall stone forceps, the Fogarty balloon, and thorough saline irrigation. On rare occasions a Dormia basket can retrieve a stone that is otherwise inaccessible. Choledochoscopy, discussed below, is another excellent means for helping to identify residual biliary calculi in the operating room.

When the ampullary region contains an impacted stone that cannot be removed with minimal trauma by the usual methods, *do not hesitate to perform a sphincteroplasty for the purpose of extracting the stone* under direct vision. Otherwise, excessive trauma to the ampullary region may cause serious postoperative acute pancreatitis.

A completion cholangiogram through the T-tube after the exploration has been concluded is the final maneuver required to minimize the number of stones overlooked at operation. It is important to use a T-tube that is 16F or larger following choledocholithotomy. Otherwise, the track remaining when the T-tube is removed may not be large enough to admit the instruments required to remove residual stones by Burhenne's method. Even small ducts admit a 16F T-tube if the tube is trimmed by the technique described below (see Fig. 69-5, p. 606).

OPERATIVE TECHNIQUE

Cholangiography

If for some reason the cystic duct is not a suitable route for cholangiography, insert a 21-gauge scalp vein needle into the CBD. Aspirate bile to confirm that the needle is in the duct lumen. Use a structure to fix the needle to the CBD. Attach a 2 meter length of sterile plastic tubing filled with the proper contrast medium. The remaining details of cholangiography are the same as those described in Chapter 66.

Kocher Maneuver

After the gallbladder has been removed and it is determined that CBD exploration is indicated, perform a Kocher maneuver (see Figs. 11-14 through 11-16) by incising the lateral peritoneal attachments along the descending duodenum. Then incise the layer of avascular fibrous tissue that attaches the posterior duodenum to Gerota's fascia and to the foramen of Winslow. Elevate the duodenum and head of the pancreas by sharp and blunt dissection in the areolar plane until the inferior vena cava is seen. With the left index and middle fingers situated behind the pancreas and duodenum and the thumb applied to the anterior wall of the duodenum, palpate the distal CBD and the ampulla. Pay special attention to the ampullary region so as not to overlook a small ampullary carcinoma, which is often felt as a hard protrusion into the lumen from the back wall of the duodenum. An adequate Kocher maneuver allows the surgeon to palpate the distal duct and head of pancreas and makes it possible to straighten the distal duct by gentle downward traction.

Choledochotomy Incision

Incise the peritoneum overlying in CBD to identify the duct's anterior wall. Select an area for the choledochotomy preferably distal to the entrance of the cystic duct. Insert two guy sutures of 4-0 PG or PDS, one opposite the other on the anterior wall of the duct. If there are any obvious blood vessels located in this area, transfix them with 5-0 PG or PDS suture-ligatures or apply careful electrocautery. Use a No. 15 scalpel blade to make a short incision in the anterior wall of the CBD while the assistant holds up the guy sutures. Then use Potts angled scissors to enlarge the incision in both directions. Pay attention to the possibility that the cystic duct may share a wall with the CBD for a distance of 2 cm or more. If the incision is made in the vicinity of this common wall, it is possible to open the cystic duct instead of the CBD, which would cause considerable confusion. It is even possible to make an incision along the common wall and not encounter the lumen of either the cystic duct or the CBD and to expose the portal vein. If the anteromedial aspect of the CBD is used for the choledochotomy incision, this problem is avoided.

Exploring the CBD

As soon as the CBD has been opened, take a sample of the bile for bacteriologic culture and Gram stain. During passage of the instruments, maintain the left hand behind the duodenum and head of pancreas. Gentle downward traction can be used to straighten the distal duct, and the sense of touch facilitates passing the instruments through the ampulla.

Using the left thumb and index finger, milk down any possible stones from the common hepatic duct into the choledochotomy incision. Perform the same maneuver on the distal CBD. This maneuver often delivers several calculi into the choledochotomy. Take care not to push stones up into the intrahepatic biliary tree where subsequent extraction may be difficult.

Pass a pituitary scoop of the appropriate size up into the right and left main hepatic ducts to remove any possible calculi (**Fig. 69–1**). Then, with the left index finger placed behind the ampulla, use the right hand to pass a pituitary scoop down to the region of the ampulla and remove any calculi encountered with this maneuver. It is helpful simultaneously to palpate with the left index finger behind the distal CBD while the scoop is being passed. Avoid excessive trauma to the ampulla. A Randall stone forceps (**Fig. 69–2**) may be inserted into the CBD for the purpose of removing stones, but we have not found this instrument to be particularly valuable compared to the pituitary scoop. Following these maneuvers, use a small, straight catheter to irrigate both the hepatic ducts and the distal CBD with normal saline solution (**Fig. 69–3**).

Now try to pass a 10F Coude tipped catheter through the ampulla. Inject saline through the catheter. The saline is seen to flow back out through the choledochotomy so long as the catheter is in the duct. When the catheter passes into the duodenum, the flow of saline ceases. If metal Bakes dilators are used instead to determine the patency of the ampulla, perform this maneuver with great delicacy as it is easy to perforate the distal CBD and to make a

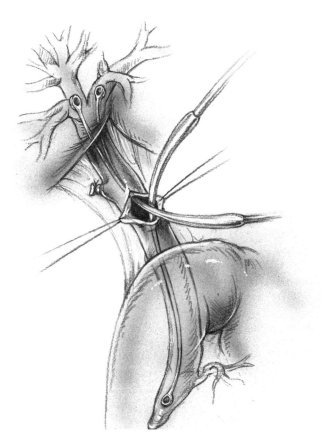

Fig. 69-1

If an impacted stone in the distal CBD cannot be removed in a nontraumatic fashion by these various maneuvers, do not hesitate to perform a sphincteroplasty (see Chapter 71). This choice is safer than traumatizing the ampulla.

Choledochoscopy

We believe that choledochoscopy is an integral part of the CBD exploration. This procedure can detect and retrieve stones or detect and biopsy ductal tumors, in some cases when all other methods have failed. Both rigid and flexible fiberoptic choledochoscopes are available. The rigid right-angle choledochoscope (Storz Endoscopy), which contains a Hopkins rod-lens system that is illuminated by a fiberoptic channel, gives the best image quality. It is simpler to operate and less expensive than the flex-

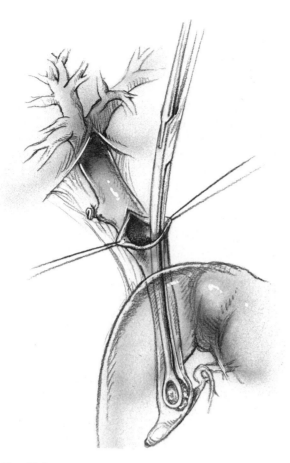

Fig. 69-2

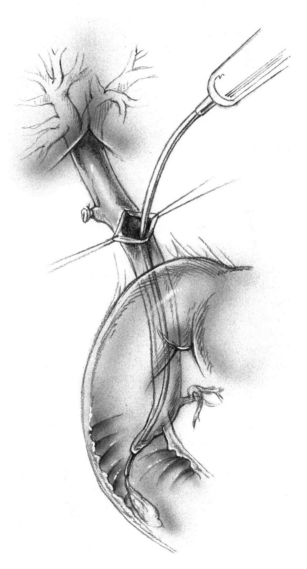

false passage through the head of the pancreas. It is not necessary to pass any instrument larger than a No. 3 Bakes dilator through the ampulla.

If there appears to be a calculus in the distal end of the CBD and it is not easily removed by means of the scoop, insert a biliary Fogarty catheter down the CBD into the duodenum. Blow up the balloon, which helps identify the ampulla by affording a sense of resistance as the catheter is pulled back. Gradually deflate the balloon as the catheter is withdrawn until it traverses the ampulla. As soon as the balloon is inside the CBD, reinflate and withdraw it. This occasionally removes a stone that has been overlooked. Repeat the same maneuver in the right and left hepatic ducts. It is for retrieval of hepatic duct stones that the Fogarty catheter has its greatest usefulness.

Another maneuver that occasionally removes a stone is use of a 16F rubber catheter. Cut most of the flared proximal end of the catheter off and insert this end down the CBD to make contact with the stone. Amputate the tip of the catheter and attach a syringe to the catheter's distal tip; apply suction while simultaneously withdrawing the catheter. The suction sometimes traps the calculus in the end of the catheter, after which it is easily removed.

Fig. 69-3

ible fiberoptic endoscopes. Both rigid and flexible choledochoscopes must be sterilized by ethylene oxide gas, precluding repeated utilization of the same scope on the same day. Although flexible instruments have a higher initial cost, more expensive upkeep, shorter life-span, much greater susceptibility to damage, and somewhat inferior optical properties, they have one important advantage over the rigid scopes: The flexible scope can be passed for greater distances up along the hepatic radicles for extraction of an otherwise inaccessible stone in this location. Similarly, the flexible scope can be passed right down to the ampulla and in about one-third of cases into the duodenum to rule out the presence of stones in the distal ampulla. Even if the scope does not enter the duodenum, when it is passed down to the ampullary orifice and the flow of saline enters the duodenum without refluxing back up into the CBD it constitutes good evidence that the distal duct is free of calculi. The rigid scopes are not generally of sufficient length to accomplish this mission. Another area in which the flexible scope is occasionally useful is extraction of retained calculi via the T-tube track subsequent to CBD exploration.

Because of their lower cost and greater durability, the rigid scopes have been adopted more widely than have the flexible scopes despite the handicap mentioned above. The horizontal arm of the Storz choledochoscope comes in two lengths: 40 and 60 mm. The vertical limbs of the two models are identical. The cross section of the horizontal limb, which must pass into the bile duct is 5×3 mm, approximately the diameter of a No. 5 Bakes dilator. If the CBD does not admit a No. 5 dilator, choledochoscopy by this technique is contraindicated.

Rigid and flexible choledochoscopes operate in a liquid medium, which requires that a continuous stream of sterile saline under pressure be injected into the sidearm of the scope. The saline then flows into the bile ducts. By crossing the two guy sutures over the choledochotomy incision, the CBD can be maintained in a state of distension by the flow of saline, providing optimal visualization. If the CBD is large enough, a metal instrument channel can be attached to the choledochoscope. Through this channel can be passed a flexible biopsy punch, a flexible forceps (7F size), a Dormia stone basket, or a Fogarty biliary catheter (5F caliber).

To use the choledochoscope, stand on the left side of the patient. Make the choledochotomy incision as far distal in the CBD as possible, and insert the choledochoscope toward the hepatic duct **(Fig. 69–4)**. Initiate the flow of saline, and cross over the two guy sutures to reduce the loss of saline from the choledochotomy incision. Enclose the 1 liter bag of

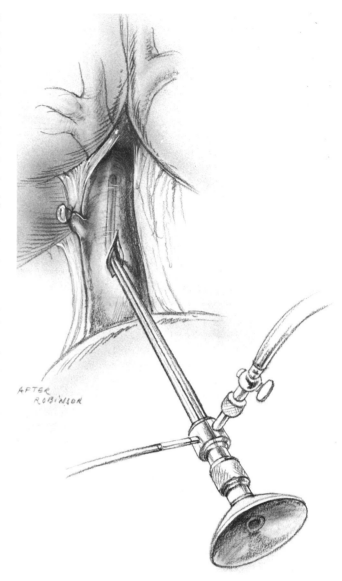

AFTER
ROBINSON

Fig. 69–4

sterile saline in a pressure pump (Fenwall) and use sterile intravenous tubing to connect the bag of saline to three-way stopcock. Insert the stopcock into the saline channel on the side of the choledochoscope.

Pass the horizontal limb of the scope up the common hepatic duct; the bifurcation of the right and left ducts is soon seen. Occasionally the first branch of the right main duct opens into the bifurcation so it resembles a trifurcation. Generally the left duct appears to be somewhat larger and easier to enter than the right. By properly directing the scope, it is possible to see into the orifices of many of the secondary and tertiary ducts. Withdraw the scope until the bifurcation is again seen and then pass the instrument into the right main duct using the same technique.

Before passing the scope down into the distal CBD, be sure the duodenum has been completely Kocherized. By placing slight traction with the left hand on the region of the ampulla, the surgeon helps elongate and straighten the course of the CBD. This step is important because the scope then visualizes the duct with clear focus to infinity. What the surgeon really wants to learn from the choledochoscopy is whether there are residual calculi between the scope and the ampulla. It requires exact knowledge of the appearance of the ampulla, which has been described as an inverted cone with a small orifice that opens and closes intermittently to permit the passage of saline. However, we have found that using these landmarks as the only criterion for identifying the ampulla may lead to error. Occasionally, this type of error permits a stone in the distal CBD to go undetected. Consequently, we believe there are only two positive methods for identifying the distal termination of the CBD. One is passage of the 60 mm choledochoscope through a patulous ampulla (rarely possible). When it is possible and if the duodenum is inflated with saline, one can see quite clearly the duodenal mucosa, which is markedly different from the smooth epithelium of the CBD. If the duodenum is not filled with saline, the mucosa is not seen. If the scope does not pass into the duodenum spontaneously, make no attempt to pass it forcibly. A second method for positively identifying the termination of the CBD is to pass a Fogarty balloon catheter alongside the choledochoscope into the duodenum. Inflate the balloon and draw back on the catheter. By following the catheter with a choledochoscope down to the region of the balloon one can be more certain that the entire CBD has been visualized and that there are no residual calculi.

Occasionally, the view of the distal CBD is impeded by what appear to be shreds of fibrin or ductal mucosa, which may hang as a partially obscuring curtain across the lumen of the duct. Despite some of these difficulties while interpreting choledochoscopic observations, this procedure does indeed detect stones that were missed by all other methods. In the hands of an experienced observer, choledochoscopy is probably the most accurate single method for detecting CBD stones. Calculi are easily identified. It may at first be confusing to find that a calculus 3 mm in diameter looks as big as a chunk of coal through the magnifying lens system. It is important to note that the Storz-type choledochoscope achieves a clear focus at distances of about 5 mm to infinity, and that any object within 0–5 mm of the tip of the scope is not in focus.

If stones are seen, remove the choledochoscope and extract the stones by the usual means. If this is not possible, reinsert the choledochoscope and use a flexible alligator forceps, a Fogarty catheter, or the Dormia stone basket, *all under direct visual control of the choledochoscope.*

If a suspicious mucosal lesion is identified, insert a flexible biopsy punch and obtain a sample. Sometimes an ampullary or distal bile duct carcinoma is diagnosed in this manner. Bile duct cancers can be multicentric, and a second lesion may be found in the common duct or the hepatic duct. Under direct visual control, accurate biopsy is not difficult through the choledochoscope.

Routine CBD exploration and removal of calculi is accompanied by a 3% incidence of retained stones. Choledochoscopy decreases the incidence of residual stones to 0–2%. Using choledochoscopy routinely during CBD exploration adds no more than 10 minutes to the procedure and, in our experience, occasionally detects a stone that has been missed by all other modalities. Because it appears to be devoid of dangerous complications, we have adopted choledochoscopy as a part of routine CBD exploration. We have experienced one complication that was possibly related to the saline flush under pressure during choledochoscopy, namely, a mild case of postoperative pancreatitis. However, we have no data to indicate that the incidence of postoperative pancreatitis is increased by the use of choledochoscopy.

Sphincterotomy for Impacted Stones

Perform a complete Kocher maneuver down to the third part of the duodenum and insert a folded gauze pad behind the duodenum and the head of the pancreas. Pass a stiff catheter or a No. 4 Bakes dilator into the choledochotomy incision and down to the distal CBD. Do not pass it into the duodenum. By palpating the tip of the catheter or the Bakes instrument through the anterior wall of the duodenum, ascertain the location of the ampulla. Make a 4 cm incision in the lateral wall of the duodenum opposite the ampulla. Insert small Richardson retractors to expose the ampulla. Often the impacted stone is not in the lumen of the CBD but partially buried in the duct wall. This permits the Bakes dilator to pass beyond the stone and distend the ampulla. If this is the case, make a 10 mm incision with a scalpel through the anterior wall of the ampulla down to the metal instrument at 11 o'clock, a location far away from the entrance of the pancreatic duct. A 10 mm incision allows the dilator to enter the duodenum. Remove the Bakes dilator through the choledochotomy incision and explore the distal CBD through the sphincterotomy incision. Use the smallest size pituitary scoop. Often the stone can be easily removed in this fashion. If the papillotomy incision must be extended a significant distance to provide adequate exposure, a complete sphincteroplasty should be undertaken, which is described in Chapter 71. If the sphincterotomy is less than 10 mm in length, it is generally not necessary to suture the mucosa of the CBD to that of the duodenum. Rather, if there is no bleeding, leave the papillotomy undisturbed after the impacted stone has been removed. Repair the duodenotomy by the same technique as described following sphincteroplasty (see Chapter 71). Then insert the T-tube into the CBD incision.

Checking for Ampullary Stenosis

Before completing the CBD exploration, the diameter of the ampulla of Vater may be calibrated by passing a catheter or a Bakes dilator. If a 10F rubber catheter passes through the ampulla, no further calibration is necessary. If this device is too soft, try a Coude tipped catheter. If the catheters fail to pass, insert the left hand behind the region of the ampulla and pass a No. 3 Bakes dilator gently through the ampulla. Failure to pass through the ampulla with ease is more often due to pushing the instrument in

the wrong direction than to an ampullary stenosis. In the absence of malignancy, we have found it rare to be unable to pass a catheter or dilator through the ampulla using gentle manipulation. If the pre-exploration cystic duct cholangiogram showed dye passing through the duodenum, failing to pass a 3 mm instrument through the ampulla is not by itself an indication for sphincteroplasty or biliary-intestinal bypass.

In any case, never use excessive force when passing these instruments. Penetration of the intrapancreatic portion of the CBD may produce fatal complications, especially if the damage is not recognized during the operation.

Insertion of the T-Tube

Although it is possible in some cases to avoid draining the CBD following stone removal, we believe that a T-tube should be inserted routinely to decompress the CBD and to facilitate cholangiography 7–8 days following surgery. Do not use a silicone T-tube, as this substance is nonreactive. Consequently, there may be no well organized tract from the CBD to the outside, and bile peritonitis may occur when the silicone tube is removed. Use a 16F rubber tube to facilitate extraction of any residual stones post-

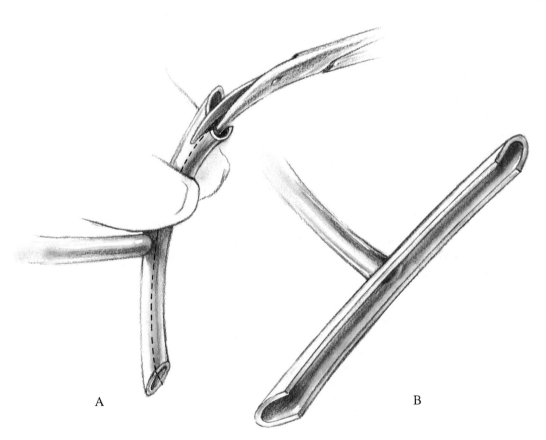

A   B

Fig. 69–5

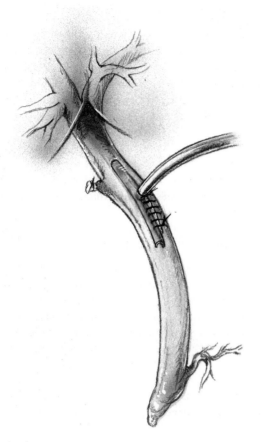

Fig. 69-6

operatively through the T-tube track. If the duct is small, excise half the circumference from the horizontal limb of the 16F tube as illustrated in **Figures 69–5a** and **69–5b**. After inserting the T-tube, close the choledochotomy incision with a continuous 4-0 atraumatic PG or PDS suture **(Fig. 69–6)**. Make this closure snug around the T-tube to avoid leakage during cholangiography and subsequent leakage of bile.

Completion Cholangiogram

Eliminate the air in the long limb of the T-tube by inserting the long cholangiogram catheter that was used for the cystic duct cholangiogram down into the vertical limb of the T-tube for its full distance. Then gradually inject the contrast medium into this limb while simultaneously removing the plastic catheter. This maneuver fills the vertical limb with contrast material and displaces the air. Then attach the T-tube directly to a long plastic connecting tube, which in turn is attached to a 30 ml syringe.

Elevate the left flank about 10 cm above the horizontal operating table. Stand behind a lead screen covered with sterile sheets and obtain the cholangiogram by injecting 4 ml of diluted contrast medium

for the first radiograph and an equal amount for the second and third pictures. Fluoroscopy with a C-arm (if available) allows the surgeon to watch the flow of contrast and facilitates the procedure. We use a mixture of one part Conray and one or two parts saline. The larger the duct, the more dilute is the solution.

If the contrast material has not entered the duodenum, repeat the sequence after giving nitroglycerin intravenously. If the contrast material still does not enter the duodenum but the radiograph is otherwise negative, discontinue the study. Severe sphincter spasm often follows ampullary instrumentation and cannot be overcome during completion cholangiography.

Drainage and Closure

Bring the T-tube out through a stab wound near the anterior axillary line. Place a closed-suction drain through a separate stab wound and bring it down near the CBD. Place omentum over the CBD and under the incision. Suture the T-tube to the skin, leaving enough slack between the CBD and the abdominal wall to allow for some abdominal distension. Close the abdominal wall in the usual fashion.

POSTOPERATIVE CARE

Attach the T-tube to a sterile plastic bag. Permit it to drain freely by gravity until cholangiography is performed through the T-tube in the radiology department on postoperative day 5. Do not permit contrast material to be injected into the T-tube under pressure, as it may produce pancreatitis or bacteremia. Injection by gravity flow is preferable. If the cholangiogram is negative and shows free flow into the duodenum, clamp the T-tube. Unclamp it if the patient experiences any abdominal pain, nausea, vomiting, shoulder pain, or leakage of bile around the T-tube. Remove the T-tube on postoperative day 21.

Following choledocholithotomy, continue antibiotics for at least 3 days, depending on the results of the Gram stain, the bacteriologic studies, and the patient's clinical response. Continue nasogastric suction for 1–3 days. Remove the closed-suction drain 4–7 days following surgery unless there has been significant bilious drainage.

Observe the patient carefully for possible development of postoperative acute pancreatitis by determining the serum amylase levels every 3 days. If there is significant elevation, continue nasogastric suction and intravenous fluids. Some patients with postoperative acute pancreatitis do not have pain or significantly elevated serum amylase, but they do have intolerance for food, with frequent vomiting after nasogastric suction has been discontinued. In these cases a sonogram or CT scan showing an enlarged pancreas is enough to confirm the diagnosis. In general, do not feed the patient following biliary tract surgery if the serum amylase level is significantly elevated or if there is any other strong suspicion of acute pancreatitis, as this complication may be serious.

COMPLICATIONS

Bile Leak and Bile Peritonitis

T-Tube displacement. The T-tube is fixed at two points: (1) the CBD and (2) the point on the skin where the T-tube is sutured in position. Enough slack must be left in the long limb of the T-tube between the CBD and the skin so an increase in abdominal distension does not result in the tube being drawn out of the CBD. Occasionally, the T-tube is inadvertently partially withdrawn from the CBD even before the abdominal incision is closed. When bile leaks around the choledochotomy incision, bilious drainage from the drain track alongside the T-tube is noted. If this leak occurs during the first few days following the operation, upper abdominal pain and tenderness may appear, indicating bile peritonitis. A localized bile leak is fairly well tolerated in the postoperative patient who has adequate drainage, whereas when bile spreads diffusely over a large part of the abdominal cavity it may produce generalized bile peritonitis if the bile is infected. Diffuse abdominal tenderness generally demands either immediate laparotomy for replacement of the T-tube or insertion of an ERCP stent into the CBD.

Ductal injury. When a completion cholangiogram through the T-tube is obtained in the operating room, a *major* ductal injury is apparent on the film, whereas an injury to an *accessory* duct may not be. If the latter manifests by continuous drainage of small to moderate amounts of bile along the drain tract and the cholangiogram is persistently normal, remove the T-tube and insert a small Foley catheter into the drain tract. Two weeks after surgery perform cholangiography through this catheter after the balloon has been inflated. The most frequently injured anomalous bile duct is that which drains the dorsal caudal segment of the right lobe.

Postoperative Acute Pancreatitis

Acute pancreatitis following choledocholithotomy accounts for about half the postoperative fatalities.

It is often caused by instrumental trauma to the ampullary region owing to excessive zeal when dilating the ampulla or when extracting an impacted stone. In the latter case, if the impacted stone cannot be removed with ease through the choledochotomy incision, approach it via a duodenotomy and papillotomy. Treatment of acute pancreatitis calls for prolonged nasogastric suction, fluid replacement, and respiratory support when indicated. Antibiotics are probably also indicated.

Frequent determinations of the serum amylase level in patients following choledocholithotomy are necessary because some patients with postoperative pancreatitis do not complain of an unusual degree of pain. Their only symptom may be abdominal distension and vomiting unless shock and hypoxia supervene. The mortality rate following postoperative acute pancreatitis is reported to be quite high, approaching 30–50%. Total parenteral nutrition is indicated because many of these patients require 3–6 weeks of nasogastric suction before the amylase returns to normal, at which time food may be given by mouth. Premature feeding in these cases may cause a severe, even fatal exacerbation.

Increasing Jaundice

After choledocholithotomy in the jaundiced patient, it is common for the serum bilirubin concentration to increase by 4–6 mg/dl during the first postoperative week. This does not mean that the patient necessarily has a CBD obstruction. Rather, imposition of major surgery and anesthesia on the liver already damaged by a period of ductal obstruction temporarily aggravates the hepatic dysfunction. By postoperative days 10–12, the bilirubin level has peaked and has started on its way down toward normal, unless there is another cause for the postoperative jaundice, possibly a blood clot or an overlooked carcinoma in the main hepatic duct. Obstruction of the distal CBD by a retained stone does not produce postoperative jaundice if the T-tube is functioning properly. Obtain a routine cholangiogram through the T-tube by postoperative day 7. It can clarify the cause of the persistent jaundice.

Hemorrhage

Intraabdominal hemorrhage. Intraabdominal hemorrhage often manifests as red blood coming through the drainage track. If it is not accompanied by systemic symptoms or abdominal signs, one may suspect that the bleeding arises from a blood vessel in the skin or the abdominal wound. Bleeding of sufficient magnitude to require one or more blood transfusions invariably originates from the operative area. The cause may be a defective ligature on the cystic artery or oozing from the liver or some intraabdominal blood vessel. These patients require prompt reexploration through the same incision, complete evacuation of the blood clots, and identification of the bleeding point.

Hemobilia. Bleeding through the T-tube indicates hemobilia. It may arise from intrahepatic trauma during attempts to extract an intrahepatic calculus. Generally, expectant therapy is sufficient in any vitamin K deficiency has been corrected preoperatively. In case of persistent hemobilia, perform hepatic arteriography, as iatrogenic trauma to a specific branch of the hepatic artery during the hepatic duct exploration may be the source of bleeding. This is a rare complication, with a reported incidence of less than .1%. Treatment consists of transcatheter embolization in the angiography suite. If open exploration is required, a T-tube cholangiogram plus the hepatic arteriogram may help the surgeon identify the appropriate vessel to ligate.

Residual CBD Stone

Early postoperative treatment. Most often a residual CBD stone is detected when postoperative T-tube cholangiography is performed. When this study is read as positive for calculi by the radiologist, carefully review the films. Request a repeat study to rule out the possibility that the shadow is due to an air bubble. Shadows that are odd in shape may not be calculi but may be due to residual blood clot or debris. There is no need for early operative intervention aimed at removing a residual CBD stone so long as the T-tube is draining well. This is true because the nonoperative methods of extracting calculi are extremely effective and have a low complication rate. Also, some of the radiographic shadows, interpreted as calculi, may indeed be artifacts that disappear without treatment.

If the radiographic evidence is convincing and a stone less than 1 cm in diameter is seen in the lower portion of the CBD, a saline flush with or without heparin solution may be indicated if tolerated by the patient. This should not be performed before the 12th postoperative day. Infuse 1000 ml of normal saline with 5000 units of heparin through the T-tube over a 24-hour period, provided it does not produce excessive pain. If the calculus completely blocks the distal CBD, this technique is contraindicated. Repeat this therapy every day for 4–5 days if tolerated. Then repeat the cholangiogram. If the radiographic appearance of the stone shows a reduction in size, repeat the series of saline flushes the following week. Otherwise, send the patient home with the T-tube

in place. If the stone is not obstructing and the patient tolerates clamping of the T-tube, keep the tube clamped. Prescribe a choleretic such as Decholin to dilute the bile. Otherwise, have the patient inject 30–60 ml of sterile saline into the T-tube daily. Ask the patient to return to the hospital about 6 weeks following operation.

Subsequent postoperative treatment. When the patient returns for examination 6 weeks after the operation, repeat the T-tube cholangiography to confirm the persistence of the residual stone because in a number of cases the calculus spontaneously passes into the duodenum. The simplest, safest method for extracting residual calculi is that described by Burhenne. With this method it is necessary that the long arm of the T-tube be at least the size of a 14–16F catheter. After cholangiography is completed and confirms the presence of stones, remove the T-tube and insert a flexible catheter that can be manipulated, such as the one available from Medi-Tech. With a continuous flow of contrast medium through the catheter, insert the device down the T-tube track until the CBD has been entered. Then, directing the tip of the catheter toward the calculus, insert a Dormia stone basket device through the Medi-Tech catheter. Under fluoroscopic control, trap the stone in the stone basket and withdraw the basket, the stone, and the catheter through the T-tube track. Experienced radiologists such as Burhenne have reported a success rate better than 90% with this technique. If the stone is quite large, it may not fit into the T-tube track. Large stones are not commonly left behind by competent surgeons, so almost all residual stones can be removed by this technique. It is even possible to cannulate the right and the left hepatic ducts to remove stones. Another method for accomplishing the same end is to pass a flexible fiberoptic choledochoscope into the CBD via the T-tube track.

If these methods have failed, endoscopic papillotomy by ERCP should be tried *if an expert is available.* Experience endoscopists have reported performing ERCP-papillotomy and extraction of retained stones with 1–2% mortality. If expertise with this technique is not available, a stone blocking the flow of bile to the CBD requires relaparotomy and choledochotomy for removal. A CBD stone that is not symptomatic when the T-tube is clamped presents a more difficult problem. Some surgeons elect to remove the T-tube, continue to observe the patient, and reserve reoperation for patients who later become symptomatic. Alternatively, it may well be argued that it is safer to perform an elective operation to remove the stone than an urgent procedure in the presence of cholangitis. In most cases elective choledocholithotomy is indicated (see Chapter 70).

REFERENCES

Allen B, Shapiro H, Way LW. Management of recurrent and residual common duct stones. Am J Surg 1981;142:41.

Berci G, Shore JM, Morgenstern L, et al. Choledochoscopy and operative fluorocholangiography in the prevention of retained bile duct stones. World J Surg 1978;2:411.

Burhenne HJ. Complications of nonoperative extraction of retained common duct stones. Am J Surg 1976;131:260.

Crawford DL, Phillips EH. Laparoscopic common bile duct exploration. World J Surg 1999;23:343.

Cuschieri A, Kimber C. Common bile duct exploration via laparoscopic choledochotomy. In Scott-Conner CEH (ed) The SAGES Manual: Fundamentals of Laparoscopy and GI Endoscopy. New York, Springer-Verlag, 1999, pp 178–187.

Dsendes A, Burdiles P, Diaz JC. Present role of classic open choledochostomy in the surgical treatment of patients with common bile duct stones. World J Surg 1998; 22:1167.

Heiken TJ, Birkett DH. Postoperative T-tube tract choledochoscopy. Am J Surg 1992;163:28.

Jones DB, Soper NJ. The current management of common bile duct stones. Adv Surg 1996;29:271.

Park AE, Mastrangelo MJ Jr. Endoscopic retrograde cholangiopancreatography in the management of choledocholithiasis. Surg Endosc 2000;14:219.

Petelin JB. Laparoscopic common bile duct exploration: transcystic duct approach. In Scott-Conner CEH (ed) The SAGES Manual: Fundamentals of Laparoscopy and GI Endoscopy. New York, Springer-Verlag, 1999, pp 127–177.

Phillips EH. Controversies in the management of common duct calculi. Surg Clin North Am 1994;74:931.

Rosenthal RJ, Rossi RL, Martin RF. Options and strategies for the management of choledocholithiasis. World J Surg 1998;22:1125.

Soravia C, Meyer P, Mentha G, Ambrosetti P, Rohner A. Flushing technique in the management of retained common bile duct stones with a T tube in situ. Br J Surg 1992;79:149.

Thompson JE Jr, Bennion RS. The surgical management of impacted common bile duct stones without sphincter ablation. Arch Surg 1989;124:1216.

70 Secondary Choledocholithotomy

SURGICAL LEGACY TECHNIQUE

INDICATIONS

Retained or recurrent common bile duct (CBD) stones subsequent to previous cholecystectomy that cannot be removed by endoscopic retrograde cholangiopancreatography (ERCP)

See Chapter 69

PREOPERATIVE PREPARATION

Generally, ultrasonography has demonstrated ductal dilatation and may show CBD stones.

Most retained stones are currently extracted endoscopically. It is only the failed cases that come to surgery. If ERCP was performed, these films can help guide the surgical approach.

Computed tomography (CT) of the abdomen is often performed to exclude other causes of jaundice, such as pancreatic cancer.

Obtain a copy of the operative report and any cholangiograms, as for any reoperative surgery.

Give vitamin K if necessary to restore the prothrombin time to normal.

Perform routine measures to prepare a patient for major surgery.

Perioperative antibiotics are indicated.

PITFALLS AND DANGER POINTS

Trauma to adherent duodenum, colon, or liver

Trauma to CBD hepatic artery or the portal vein

OPERATIVE STRATEGY

If the patient's first operation was not followed by any significant collection of bile, blood, or pus in the right upper quadrant, secondary choledo- cholithotomy is not generally a difficult dissection. On the other hand, occasionally the right upper quadrant is obliterated by dense adhesions requiring a carefully planned sequential dissection. First, dissect the peritoneum of the anterior abdominal wall completely free from underlying adhesions. Carry this dissection to the right as far as the posterior axillary line, which exposes the lateral portion of the right lobe of the liver and the hepatic flexure of the colon.

The strategy now is to free the inferior surface of the liver from adherent colon and duodenum. Approach this from the lateral edge of the liver and proceed medially. After 3–6 cm of the undersurface of the lateral portion of the liver has been exposed, start to dissect the omentum and colon away form the anterior border of the undersurface of the liver. The dissection now goes from lateral to medial and from anterior to posterior. If this dissection becomes difficult and there is a risk of perforating the duodenum or colon, enter the right paracolic gutter and incise the paracolic peritoneum at the hepatic flexure. Placing the left hand behind the colon gives the surgeon entry into a virgin portion of the abdomen, which aids in freeing the colon from the liver. The maneuver uncovers the descending portion of duodenum, also in virgin territory. Perform a Kocher maneuver and bring the left hand behind the duodenum, which helps guide the dissection toward the CBD. If the foramen of Winslow is accessible at this point, inserting the finger into this foramen permits palpation of the hepatic artery with the thumb against the forefinger. The CBD can be found to the right of the pulsation of the hepatic artery.

Now, resume the lateral to medial and anterior to posterior dissection until the undersurface of the liver has been cleared down to the CBD and the hepatic artery. It is not necessary to free the undersurface of the liver for a large area medial to the CBD for adequate exposure.

OPERATIVE TECHNIQUE

Incision

Use a subcostal incision (see Chapter 66) if the previous operation was performed laparoscopically. If the patient has had a previous open subcostal incision, we prefer a long vertical midline incision. If the patient has previously been operated on through a vertical incision, a long subcostal incision, about two fingerbreadths below the costal margin, is preferred. Placing the incision at a site away from the previous operative field makes it easier for the surgeon to enter the abdominal cavity expeditiously. Once the peritoneum and falciform ligament have been identified, free the abdominal wall from all underlying adhesions over the entire right side of the upper abdomen.

Freeing Subhepatic Adhesions

In the usual case, initiate the dissection on the right lateral edge of the liver, clearing its undersurface from right to left. If this dissection goes easily, it may be a simple matter to use Metzenbaum scissors to divide filmy adhesions by the techniques described in Chapter 38. When it is difficult to differentiate colon or duodenum from scar tissue, identify the ascending colon in the right gutter. Incise the paracolic peritoneum and slide the left hand behind the ascending colon. Liberate the hepatic flexure up to the undersurface of the liver, and then free the colon from the liver.

If similar difficulties are encountered when identifying or dissecting the duodenum, perform a Kocher maneuver and slide the left hand behind the duodenum, dissecting this organ away from the renal fascia, vena cava, and aorta. Now start dissecting the omentum, colon, and duodenum from the undersurface of the liver, going from anterior to posterior until the hepatoduodenal ligament has been reached. Confirm the identity of the hepatoduodenal ligament by inserting the left index finger into the foramen of Winslow and palpating the hepatic artery, which should be just to the left of the CBD. Confirm the position of the CBD, if necessary, by aspirating bile with a 25-gauge needle and syringe.

Exploring the CBD

After the CBD has been identified, a cholangiogram may be obtained by inserting a 21-gauge scalp vein needle into the duct and starting cholangiography. The technique for CBD exploration is no different from that described in Chapter 69. Choledochoscopy and postexploratory cholangiography should be included in the operative procedure.

Draining the CBD

Insert a 16F T-tube trimmed as in Figure 69–5, and close the choledochotomy with 5-0 Vicryl sutures, continuous or interrupted. The indications for sphincteroplasty or biliary-intestinal bypass are discussed in Chapter 71. That the common duct is thick-walled or dilated does not itself constitute an indication for additional surgery other than choledocholithotomy. The abdomen is drained and closed as in Chapter 69. Postoperative care and complications are similar to those discussed in Chapter 69.

71 Sphincteroplasty

SURGICAL LEGACY TECHNIQUE

INDICATIONS

Failed previous surgery for common bile duct (CBD) stasis with sludge, primary, or recurrent stones

Doubt that all CBD stones have been removed; hepatic duct stones that cannot be removed

Ampullary or pancreatic duct orifice stenosis with recurrent pain or pancreatitis (rare)

PREOPERATIVE PREPARATION

Perioperative antibiotics

Vitamin K in the jaundiced patient

Endoscopic retrograde cholangiopancreatography (ERCP) to identify CBD calculi or ampullary stenosis and to visualize the pancreatic duct

PITFALLS AND DANGER POINTS

Trauma to the pancreatic duct or pancreas resulting in postoperative pancreatitis

Postoperative duodenal fistula secondary to a leak from sphincteroplasy or duodenotomy suture line

Postoperative hemorrhage

OPERATIVE STRATEGY

Protecting the Pancreatic Duct

Make the incision in the ampulla on its superior wall at about 10 or 11 o'clock. After making the initial incision about 5-6 mm in length, locate the orifice of the pancreatic duct. In 80% of cases it can be identified at about 5 o'clock where it enters the ampulla just proximal to the ampulla's termination. Wearing telescopic lenses with a magnification of about 2.5× for this operation helps a great deal. If the orifice of the pancreatic duct cannot be identified, inject secretin to stimulate flow of the watery pancreatic secretion and facilitate identification of the ductal orifice. Insert a lacrimal probe or a No. 2 Bakes dilator into the orifice

to confirm that it is indeed the pancreatic duct. Some surgeons prefer to insert a 6F or 8F pediatric feeding tube into the duct to protect it while suturing the sphincteroplasty. We agree with Jones that keeping a tube in the duct is not necessary if one keeps the ductal orifice in view during the suturing process.

When the indication for sphincteroplasty is ampullary stenosis, abdominal pain, or recurrent pancreatitis, it is essential to add a "ductoplasty" of the pancreatic ductal orifice by incising the septum that forms the common wall between the distal pancreatic duct and the ampulla of Vater. After the pancreatic duct's orifice has been enlarged, it should freely admit a No. 3 Bakes dilator.

Preventing Hemorrhage

The long sphincterotomy incision used for sphincteroplasty cuts across the anterior wall of the distal CBD and the back wall of the duodenum for a distance of 1.5–2.0 cm. This "blind" incision may lacerate an anomalous retroduodenal or an anomalous right hepatic artery arising from the superior mesenteric artery and crossing in this region. It is important to *palpate the area behind the ampulla to detect pulsation of an anomalous artery*. If such a vessel is behind the ampulla, sphincteroplasty by the usual technique may be contraindicated. We are aware, by anecdote, of two patients who died subsequent to a classic sphincteroplasty by the Jones technique owing to massive postoperative hemorrhage despite reexploration. In one case, autopsy demonstrated laceration of an anomalous right hepatic artery. The laceration had apparently been temporarily controlled by the 5-0 interrupted silk sutures that had been used to fashion the sphincteroplasty.

Using Jones's technique, initially small straight hemostats grasp 3–4 mm of tissue on either side of the contemplated ampullary incision. The tissue between the hemostats is then divided. Next, a 5-0 silk suture is inserted behind each of the two hemostats, and two additional hemostats are inserted. The sphincterotomy incision is lengthened, and silk sutures again are placed behind each hemostat. In this way it is possible to divide a large anomalous vessel partially and achieve temporary control, first by the hemostat and then by the 5-0 silk suture. During the postoperative period the artery may escape from the 5-0 stitch, and serious hemorrhage may follow. Although hemorrhage is a rare complication, it appears prudent to omit this prior application of hemostats. By first making a 3- to 4-mm incision with Potts scissors, one should become immediately aware of any laceration of a major vessel at a time when proper reparative measures can be effectively undertaken. Otherwise, inflammation that occurs 5–6 days after the operation may make accurate identification of the anatomy difficult during any relaparotomy for hemorrhage. For this reason, we recommend making the incision first for a short distance, next inserting sutures, then lengthening the incision and inserting additional sutures sequentially until the proper size sphincteroplasty has been achieved.

Avoiding Duodenal Fistula

Leakage from the duodenum can occur from the apex of the sphincteroplasty because at this point the CBD and duodenum no longer share a wall. Here accurate suturing is necessary to reapproximate the incised CBD to the back wall of the duodenum.

A second potential source of leakage is the suture line closing the duodenotomy. A longitudinal duodenotomy is preferred because it may be extended in either direction if the situation requires more exposure. Close this longitudinal incision in the same direction in which the incision was originally made. Otherwise, distortion of the duodenum takes place, and linear tension on the suture line may impair successful healing. Precise insertion of sutures, one layer in the mucosa and another in the seromuscular layer, can be accomplished without narrowing the duodenum. Leaks from incisions in the second portion of the duodenum cause serious if not lethal consequences; therefore take special care when resuturing the duodenotomy incision.

OPERATIVE TECHNIQUE

Incision and Exploration

Make a long right subcostal or midline incision, free any adhesions, and perform a routine abdominal exploration. If satisfactory preoperative ERCP has not been accomplished, perform cholangiography.

Kocher Maneuver

Perform a complete Kocher maneuver and gently elevate the duodenum up almost to the level of the anterior abdominal wall, facilitating exposure of the ampulla (see Figs. 78-2, 78-3). Place the left hand behind the head of the pancreas and elevate it fro the flimsy attachments to the vena cava and posterior abdominal wall. Place a gauze pack behind the pancreatic head.

CBD Exploration

Make an incision in the anterior wall of the CBD as close to the duodenum as possible because, if for some reason sphincteroplasty is not feasible, it may prove desirable to perform a choledochoduodenostomy. For the latter operation, an incision in the distal portion of the CBD allows the surgeon to make an anastomosis to the duodenum under less tension than an incision made at a higher level. If CBD exploration for calculi is indicated, follow the procedure described in Chapter 69. Then pass a No. 4 Bakes dilator into the CBD down to, but not through, the ampulla of Vater. Palpating the tip of the dilator through the anterior duodenal wall facilitates placement of the duodenal incision accurately with reference to the location of the ampulla.

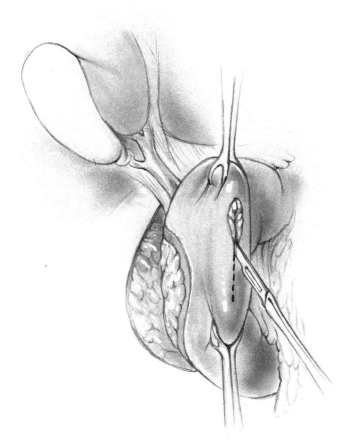

Fig. 71-1

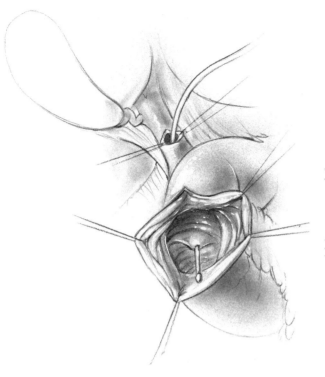

Fig. 71-2

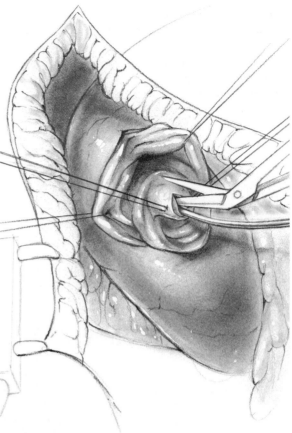

Fig. 71-3

Duodenotomy and Sphincterotomy

Make a 4 cm scalpel incision along the antimesenteric border of the duodenum **(Fig. 71–1)**. Center this incision at the estimated location of the ampulla, as judged by palpating the tip of the Bakes dilator **(Fig. 71–2)**. Control bleeding points by careful electrocoagulation and an occasional 5-0 PG suture. Achieve exposure of the ampulla by inserting appropriately sized Richardson retractors at the proximal and distal extremities of the duodenal incision.

Make a 5 mm incision at 10 or 11 o'clock along the anterior wall of the ampulla using a scalpel blade against the large Bakes dilator impacted in the ampulla or Potts scissors with one blade inside the ampulla **(Fig. 71–3)**. Insert one or two 5-0 Vicryl sutures on each side of the partially incised ampulla **(Fig. 71–4)**. Place small hemostats on the tails of the tied sutures and use them to apply gentle traction.

Identify the orifice of the pancreatic duct, which enters the back wall of the ampulla at about 5 o'clock near its termination. If the exposure of this portion of the ampulla is inadequate, extend the sphincterotomy by another 3-4 mm and insert an additional suture on each side. If the ductal orifice still has not been located, inject secretin (1 unit/kg body weight) intravenously to stimulate the flow

of pancreatic juice into the duodenum. Verify the location of the ductal orifice by inserting either a lacrimal probe or a No. 2 Bakes dilator. Then make a mental note to avoid traumatizing this area by inaccurate dissecting or suturing. Continue the sequence of incising the ampulla for about 3 mm at a time and inserting interrupted sutures **(Fig.**

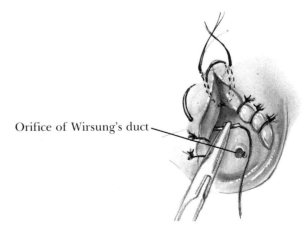

Orifice of Wirsung's duct

Fig. 71-4

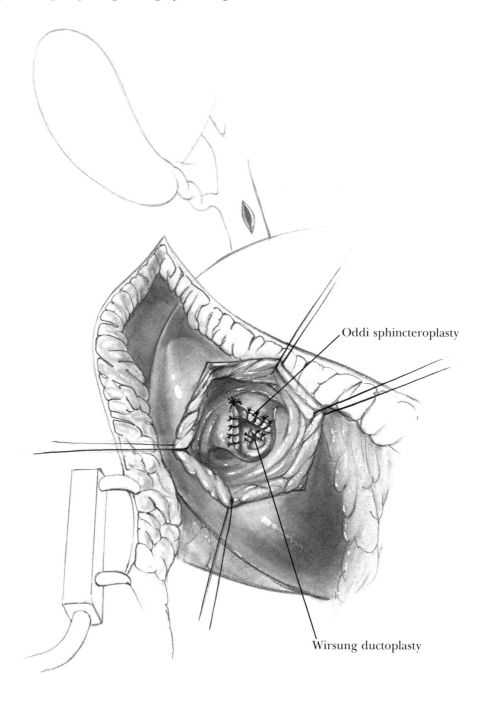

Oddi sphincteroplasty

Wirsung ductoplasty

Fig. 71-5

71–5). To incise the entire sphincter of Oddi, the sphincterotomy must be almost 2 cm in length. Additionally, if residual calculi are possible and the CBD is large, the length of the sphincterotomy incision should at least equal the diameter of the CBD. Biopsy any area suspicious for cancer and obtain a frozen section evaluation.

It is important to insert a figure-of-eight suture at the apex of the sphincterotomy to minimize the possibility of leakage. Carefully inspect the sutures at the

conclusion of this step. They should be close together, and bleeding should be completely controlled.

When the indication for sphincteroplasty is recurrent pancreatitis or recurrent abdominal pain, pancreatography is a vital part of the operation unless this step has been done preoperatively by means of ERCP. Insert a suitable plastic tube such as an angiocath or a ureteral or small whistle-tip rubber catheter into the pancreatic duct. Use only 2–3 ml of diluted Conray or Hypaque and make the injection without pressure. Most patients with chronic recurrent pancreatitis have multiple areas of narrowing and dilatation of the pancreatic duct, making sphincteroplasty a useless therapeutic procedure. If the pancreatic duct is dilated and the ductal orifice is narrowed so it does not admit a No. 3 Bakes dilator, enlarging this orifice by ductoplasty may prove beneficial, although this combination of conditions occurs only rarely.

Ductoplasty for Stenosis of the Pancreatic Duct Orifice

Magnify the orifice of the pancreatic duct by wearing telescopic lenses. Insert Potts scissors into the pancreatic duct orifice and incise the septum, which constitutes the common wall between the anterior surface of the pancreatic duct and the posterior wall of the ampulla. Sometimes the orifice is too narrow to admit the blade of the Potts scissors. In that case, insert a metal probe into the ductal orifice and cut the anterior wall of the duct by incising for 3-4 mm using a scalpel against the metal of the probe. Then complete the incision with Potts scissors. Generally, an 8- to 10-mm incision permits easy passage of a No. 3 Bakes dilator into the pancreatic duct.

Insert several 3-0 PG sutures to maintain the approximation of the pancreatic duct to the mucosa of the ampulla (Fig. 71-5). We do not insert any type of stent through the pancreatic ductoplasty.

Closing the Duodenotomy

Close the duodenal incision longitudinally in two layers by the usual method of inverting the mucosa with a continuous Connell, Cushing, or seromucosal suture. Close the seromuscular layer by carefully inserting interrupted 4-0 silk Lembert sutures.

When the diameter of the duodenum appears narrower than usual, include only the protruding mucosa in the first layer; make no attempt to invert the serosa with this suture line. For the second layer, insert interrupted Lembert sutures that take small, accurate bites of the seromuscular coat, including submucosa. If this is done with precision, closing the longitudinal incision does not narrow the duodenum. Cover the duodenotomy with omentum.

Cholecystectomy

If the gallbladder has not been removed at a previous operation, a sphincteroplasty produces increased stasis of gallbladder bile, which may lead to stone formation. Consequently, perform a cholecystectomy.

Abdominal Closure and Drainage

After irrigating the operative site and the incision with a dilute antibiotic solution, drain the area of the sphincteroplasty with a closed-suction plastic catheter (4-5 mm diameter) brought out through a puncture wound in the upper abdomen. Be careful to avoid contact between the catheter and the duodenal suture lines. Suture the tip of the catheter in the proper location with fine catgut.

Place an indwelling 14F T-tube into the CBD for drainage and close the CBD around the T-tube using a 5-0 PG suture. Then close the abdominal wall in the usual fashion.

POSTOPERATIVE CARE

Continue nasogastric suction for a few days or until evidence of peristalsis is present with the passage of flatus.

Monitor the serum amylase level every 2 days.

Continue perioperative antibiotics for 24 hours. If the bile is infected, continue the antibiotics for 7 days.

Perform cholangiography on the 7th postoperative day and remove the T-tube on the 14th postoperative day if the radiograph shows satisfactory flow into the duodenum without leakage.

Remove the closed-suction drain by the 7th postoperative day unless there is bilious or duodenal drainage.

COMPLICATIONS

Duodenal fistula. A suspected duodenal fistula can often be confirmed by giving the patient methylene blue dye by mouth and looking for the blue dye in the closed-suction catheter or by performing T-tube cholangiography. For minor duodenal fistulas where there is neither significant systemic toxicity nor abdominal tenderness, it is possible that a small leak will heal when managed by continuing the closed-suction drainage supplemented by systemic antibiotics and intravenous alimentation.

A major *leak* from the duodenum is a life-threatening complication. If systemic toxicity is not controlled by conservative management, relaparotomy is indicated. Resuturing the duodenum generally fails because of the local inflammation. In this situation, insert a sump-suction catheter into the duodenal fistula. Isolate the fistula by performing a Billroth II gastrectomy with vagotomy. Divert the bile from the duodenum by dividing the CBD and anastomosing the proximal cut end of the duct to a Roux-en-Y segment of jejunum so bile drains into the efferent limb of the jejunum distal to the gastrojejunostomy.

REFERENCES

Eckhauser FE, Knol JA, Raper SE, Mulholland M. A simplified and reliable method for transduodenal sphincteroplasty. Surg Rounds 1991;595.

Jones SA. The prevention and treatment of recurrent bile duct stones by transduodenal sphincteroplasty. World J Surg 1978;2:473.

Moody FG. Surgical applications of sphincteroplasty and choledochoduodenostomy. Surg Clin North Am 1981; 61:909.

Moody FG, Vecchio R, Calaguig R, Runkel N. Transduodenal sphincteroplasty with transampullary septectomy for stenosing papillitis. Am J Surg 1991;161:213.

Nussbaum MS, Warner BW, Sax HC, Fischer JE. Transduodenal sphincteroplasty and transampullary septotomy for primary sphincter of Oddi dysfunction. Am J Surg 1989;157:38.

72 Choledochoduodenostomy

SURGICAL LEGACY TECHNIQUE

INDICATIONS

Common bile duct (CBD) stasis with sludge or primary or recurrent stones (only if the bile duct is more than 1.5 cm in diameter)

Doubt that all CBD stones have been removed (only if CBD is >1.5 cm in diameter)

Constriction of distal CBD because of chronic pancreatitis (see Chapter 70)

CONTRAINDICATIONS

CBD diameter <1.5 cm

Acute inflammation or excessive fibrosis in duodenal wall

Carcinoma of the pancreatic head (Hepaticojejunostomy Roux-en-Y is our preferred bypass procedure for pancreatic carcinoma obstructing the CBD. It is a safer operation, and the anastomosis is not obstructed by the advancing growth of the malignancy.)

PREOPERATIVE PREPARATION

Perioperative antibiotics

Vitamin K in jaundiced patients

Nasogastric tube

PITFALLS AND DANGER POINTS

Anastomotic stoma too small, resulting in postoperative recurrent cholangitis

Diameter of CBD too small

Anastomotic leak, duodenal fistula

Postoperative "sump" syndrome

OPERATIVE STRATEGY

Size of Anastomotic Stoma

As the anastomotic stoma after choledochoduodenostomy permits passage of food from the duodenum into the CBD, it is important that the anastomosis be large enough to permit the food to pass back freely into the duodenum. Otherwise, food particles partially obstruct the anastomotic stoma and produce recurrent cholangitis. If the surgeon constructs an anastomosis with a stoma 2.5 cm or more in diameter, postoperative cholangitis is rare. The size of the stoma may be estimated postoperatively by an upper gastrointestinal barium radiographic study.

Obviously, if the diameter of the CBD is small, a large anastomotic stoma is difficult to achieve. Transduodenal sphincteroplasty (see Chapter 71) is a better option for the patient with a small CBD.

Location of the Anastomosis

There are several alternative locations for incisions in the CBD and duodenum. If postoperative anastomotic leakage is to be prevented, it is vitally important that these incisions be made in tissues of satisfactory quality and that there be no tension on the anastomosis.

A problem occurs when the surgeon has made one incision in the CBD in the vicinity of the cystic duct for the CBD exploration and a second (duodenal) incision opposite the ampulla for an impacted ampullary calculus. Under these conditions, even with an extensive Kocher maneuver, it may not be possible to approximate these two incisions by suturing because there is too much tension on the anastomosis. In this situation a Roux-en-Y choledochojejunostomy or a sphincteroplasty is preferable. When the possibility of a choledochoduodenostomy is anticipated prior to the CBD exploration, make the incision in the CBD near the point where it enters the sulcus between the pancreas and the duodenum. This facilitates constructing the anastomosis described in this chapter.

When the incision in the CBD has been made in a more proximal location, test the mobility of the duodenum after performing a Kocher maneuver. If the duodenum is easily elevated to the region of the CBD incision, a choledochoduodenostomy by the method illustrated in Figures 72–6 and 72–7 is acceptable. There must be no tension on the anastomosis.

Preventing the Sump Syndrome

Sporadic reports have appeared describing the accumulation of food debris or calculi in the terminal portion of the CBD following choledochoduo-denostomy. Such an accumulation produces inter-mittent cholangitis and has been called the "sump syndrome." Several techniques have been advocated to prevent it. All are more complex than the tech-nique described here.

In the simplest variation, the CBD is divided and the distal portion oversewn. The proximal portion is anastomosed to the duodenum to create an end-to-side, rather than a side-to-side, choledochoduo-denostomy. Alternatively, the proximal CBD may be anastomosed to a Roux-en-Y limb of jejunum. This construction completely prevents food from enter-ing the CBD and provides the lowest incidence of sump syndrome.

OPERATIVE TECHNIQUE

Incision

A right subcostal or a midline incision from the xiphoid to a point 5 cm below the umbilicus is suit-able for this operation. Divide any adhesions and ex-plore the abdomen. Perform a complete Kocher maneuver. If the diameter of the CBD is less than 1.5 cm, do *not* perform a choledochoduodenostomy.

Choledochoduodenal Anastomosis

Free the peritoneum over the distal CBD. Make an incision on the anterior wall of the CBD for a dis-tance of at least 2.5 cm. This incision should termi-nate close to the point where the duodenum crosses the distal CBD. Make another incision of equal size along the long axis of the duodenum at a point close to the CBD **(Fig. 72–1)**. Insert the index finger into the duodenum and palpate the ampulla of Vater to be certain a carcinoma of the ampulla has not been overlooked.

Place guy sutures at the midpoints of the lateral and medial margins of the CBD incision. Apply trac-tion to these guy sutures in opposite directions to open up the choledochotomy incision **(Fig. 72–2)**. One layer of interrupted 4-0 Vicryl sutures is used for this anastomosis. Insert the first stitch of the poste-rior layer approximating the midpoint of the duode-nal incision to the distal margin of the choledo-chotomy. Tie the stitch with the knot inside the lumen. Insert additional stitches that go through the full thickness of the duodenum and the CBD **(Fig. 72–3)** until the entire posterior layer has been com-pleted. Cut all of the sutures except the most lateral and most medial stitches. Approximate the proximal margin of the choledochotomy with the same suture material to the midpoint of the anterior layer of the duodenum and tie this stitch so it inverts the mucosa

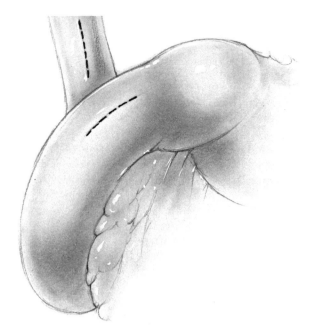

Fig. 72-1

of the duodenum **(Fig. 72–4)**. Continue to insert in-terrupted through-and-through sutures until the an-terior layer has been completed **(Fig. 72–5)**. This anastomosis should be completed without tension.

Alternative Method of Anastomosis

In some cases the surgeon elects to perform a choledochoduodenal anastomosis after making a

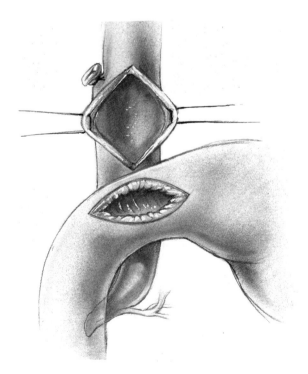

Fig. 72-2

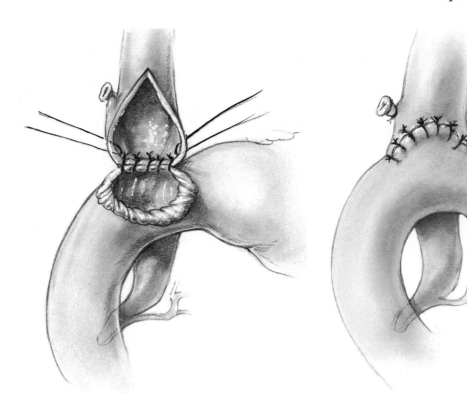

Fig. 72-3

Fig. 72-5

choledochotomy incision in a location too far proximal on the CBD to accomplish the anastomosis by the above technique. In this case, enlarge the choledochotomy so it measures at least 2.5 cm in length.

Next, perform a thorough Kocher maneuver to increase the mobility of the duodenum. Then move the duodenum toward the choledochotomy incision and determine which portion of the duodenum is most suitable for a side-to-side anastomosis *without*

tension. If tension cannot be avoided, perform a Roux-en-Y anastomosis.

Make an incision in the duodenum parallel to the choledochotomy and approximately equal in length **(Fig. 72–6)**. Approximate the posterior layer with

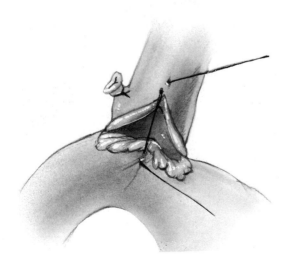

Fig. 72-4

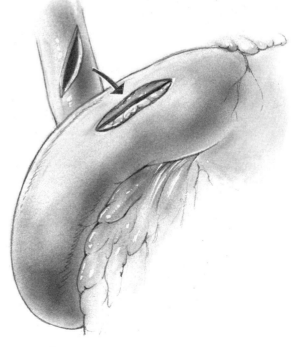

Fig. 72-6

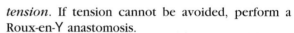

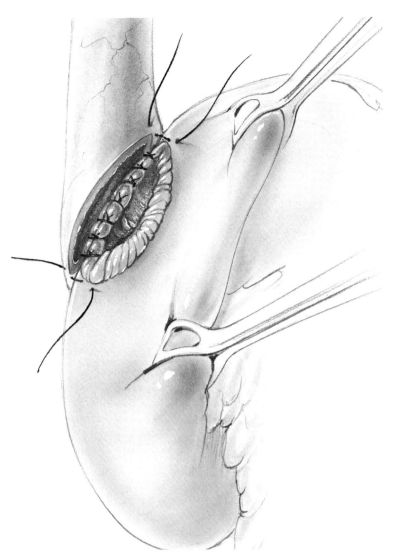

Fig. 72-7

Drainage and Closure

As bile has an extremely low surface tension, there is a tendency for a small amount of this substance to leak out along the suture holes during the first day or two following a biliary tract anastomosis. For this reason, insert a closed-suction drainage catheter through a puncture wound in the right upper quadrant and bring the catheter to the general vicinity of the anastomosis.

POSTOPERATIVE CARE

Continue nasogastric suction if necessary.

Leave the closed-suction drain in place for 5–7 days.

COMPLICATIONS

Duodenal fistula (see Chapter 71)

Subhepatic abscess

Late development of cholangitis owing to the anastomotic stoma being too small

Late development of "sump" syndrome

REFERENCES

Akiyama H, Ikezawa H, Kamcya S, et al. Unexpected problems of external choledochoduodenostomy: fiberscopic examination in 15 patients. Am J Surg 1980;140:660.

Bismuth H, Franco D, Coriette MB, et al. Long term results of Roux-en-Y hepaticojejunostomy. Surg Gynecol Obstet 1978;146:161.

Degenshein GA. Choledochoduodenostomy: an 18 year study of 175 consecutive cases. Surgery 1974;76:319.

Escudero-Fabre A, Escallon A Jr, Sack J, et al. Choledochoduodenostomy: analysis of 71 cases followed for 5 to 15 years. Ann Surg 1991;213:635.

Kraus MA, Wilson SD. Choledochoduodenostomy: importance of common duct size and occurrence of cholangitis. Arch Surg 1980;115:1212.

McSherry CK, Fischer MG. Common bile duct stones and biliary-intestinal anastomoses. Surg Gynecol Obstet 1981;153:669.

Schein CJ, Gliedman ML. Choledochoduodenostomy as an adjunct to choledocholithotomy. Surg Gynecol Obstet 1981;152:797.

Tanaka M, Ikeda S, Yoshimoto H. Endoscopic sphincterotomy for the treatment of biliary sump syndrome. Surgery 1983;93:264.

White TT. Indications for sphincteroplasty as opposed to choledochoduodenostomy. Am J Surg 1973;126:165.

interrupted sutures and tie them **(Fig. 72–7)**, with the knots inside the lumen. Leave the tails of the most cephalad and most distal sutures long, but cut all other sutures. Bisect the anterior layer of the anastomosis and insert a 4-0 PG Lembert suture to approximate the midpoint of the CBD incision to the midpoint of the duodenal incision. Tie this suture so the duodenal mucosa is inverted. Insert additional sutures of the same type to complete the approximation. The knots are on the outside surface of the anastomosis for the anterior layer. Because the CBD is quite large in these cases and the duodenal wall is free of pathology, no T-tube or other stent is necessary.

73 Roux-en-Y Biliary-Enteric Bypass

INDICATIONS

Biliary reconstruction after major ductal injury.

Common bile duct obstruction due to nonresectable tumor, chronic pancreatitis, or surgical trauma

PREOPERATIVE PREPARATION

Perioperative antibiotics

Vitamin K in jaundiced patients

PITFALLS AND DANGER POINTS

Devascularizing the jejunal segment by inaccurate division of the mesentery

OPERATIVE STRATEGY

Choice of Bypass

An isoperistaltic Roux-en-Y segment of jejunum provides a safe way to drain the extrahepatic biliary tract. There are several ways to construct the anastomosis to the bile duct. Side-to-end or side-to-side choledochojejunostomy is equivalent and has the advantage of simplicity. Circumferential dissection of the common bile duct (CBD) is not required, and an anastomosis is rapidly constructed between the side of the CBD and the Roux limb of jejunum. Either the end of the Roux limb (as shown in Figs. 73–3 through 73–5) or the side may be used. Because the mesentery of the jejunum tethers the Roux loop, the loop tends to curl in such a manner that the antimesenteric border lies comfortably in apposition to the CBD. This type of anastomosis is commonly performed for palliation of carcinoma of the pancreas, when endoscopic stenting fails or is not technically feasible.

End-to-side or end-to-end choledochojejunostomy eliminates the blind segment of distal CBD and the potential for debris, food, and calculi to ac-cumulate, causing the sump syndrome. It requires circumferential dissection of the CBD. The anastomosis is commonly performed for operative strictures or injuries.

Preserving Vascular Supply to the Jejunal Loop

Creating a Roux-en-Y loop requires precise division of the jejunal mesentery to preserve the blood supply to both segments of jejunum. In most cases the marginal artery of the jejunum is divided immediately distal to the artery supplying the second arcade. By dividing only one or two additional arcade vessels, sufficient jejunum can be mobilized to reach the hepatic duct without tension. The jejunum is passed through an incision in the avascular portion of the transverse mesocolon, generally to the right of the middle colic artery. This dissection must be done carefully and is facilitated by transilluminating the jejunal mesentery by means of a spotlight or a sterilized fiberoptic illuminator.

Create the Roux limb early, as soon as it is decided to proceed with this bypass. Then wrap both ends in a moist laparotomy pad and return them to the abdomen. This allows time for any ischemic regions to manifest. If the end of either segment turns dusky, resect the darkened portion back to pink, bleeding intestine.

When a Roux-en-Y biliary-intestinal bypass is performed for carcinoma of the pancreas, carefully evaluate the root of the small bowel mesentery before dividing it. Some pancreatic tumors extend deeply into this mesentery, making it impossible to separate the jejunal blood supply for the Roux-en-Y segment. This operation is contraindicated in these few cases, and some other type of bypass must be considered. Under these conditions, anastomosing the gallbladder to the side of a loop of jejunum may prove adequate palliation for the short life expectancy of these patients. Many of these patients are better managed by endoscopic biliary stents rather than operative bypass.

OPERATIVE TECHNIQUE

Incision and Biopsy

If there has been a previous operation on the biliary tract that utilized a subcostal incision, make a long midline incision. If the previous incision was vertical, make a long subcostal incision and enter the abdomen. In secondary cases the first effort is to free the peritoneum of the anterior abdominal wall from all its underlying adhesions as far lateral as the midaxillary line. Then continue to free the structures as described in Chapter 70.

With primary operations for carcinoma of the pancreas, make a long midline incision from the xiphoid to a point 6–7 cm below the umbilicus. This incision is good for a bypass or for partial or total pancreatectomy. Conduct the usual exploration to arrive at an accurate diagnosis. In patients with inoperable pancreatic carcinoma take biopsy specimens from areas of obvious carcinoma with a scalpel or biopsy a metastatic lymph node. When these steps are not possible, we have generally been successful in confirming the diagnosis of carcinoma by inserting a syringe with a 22-gauge needle into the hardest part of the pancreas. As soon as the needle enters the suspicious area, apply suction and plunge the needle for 1 cm distances in two directions. Then release the plunger of the syringe so no further suction is being applied. Remove the syringe and the needle. Pass it promptly to the cytopathologist, as *immediate* fixation is necessary for an accurate cytologic diagnosis. This method has provided us with a higher percentage of positive diagnoses of carcinoma of the pancreas than the tissue techniques. The cytologist's report should not take more than 10–15 minutes.

Which Type of Bypass?

For carcinoma of the pancreas, evaluate the local extent of disease and its probable future encroachment on the common duct, cystic duct, and root of the jejunal mesentery. If extensive disease limits access to the common duct or involves the root of the mesentery, a dilated Courvoisier gallbladder may be simply anastomosed to an omega loop of jejunum. Ascertain that the cystic duct–common duct juncture is high enough above the tumor that this bypass remains patent.

If access to the common duct is good, a choledochojejunostomy or hepaticojejunostomy is preferred. Remove the gallbladder, if present. This ac-

complishes two things: It significantly improves access to the CBD, and it prevents subsequent cholecystitis due to bile stasis and bacterial contamination. A cholangiogram, obtained through the cystic duct, may help operative planning and is easy to obtain. With operations performed for stricture, the site of the stricture determines the level of the anastomosis.

Creating the Roux-en-Y Jejunal Limb

Once it is decided to proceed with a Roux-en-Y bypass, divide the jejunum and its mesentery. Inspect the proximal jejunal mesentery and look for the first two branches from the superior mesenteric artery to the jejunum just beyond the ligament of Treitz. Identify the marginal artery at a point 2 cm beyond its junction with the second jejunal branch, which is generally about 15 cm from the ligament of Treitz. Make a light scalpel incision over the jejunal mesentery from the jejunum across the marginal artery and into the avascular area of the mesentery. Divide the mesentery in a distal direction until the third vessel is encountered. Divide and ligate this vessel and continue the incision in the mesentery down to the fourth vessel. This most often does not require division **(Fig. 73–1)**.

Clean the mesenteric margin of the jejunum and divide between Allen clamps or with a cutting linear gastrointestinal stapler. Tentatively pass the liberated limb of jejunum up toward the hepatic duct to determine whether sufficient mesentery has been dissected. If this is so, expose the right portion of the transverse mesocolon. Find an avascular area, generally to the right of the middle colic vessels and make a 2- to 3-cm incision through the mesocolon. Pass the liberated limb of jejunum through the incision in the mesocolon. It may be necessary to free some of the omentum from the area of the hepatic flexure to permit free passage of the jejunum up to the hepatic duct. The end of the jejunum should reach the proximal portion of the common hepatic duct with no tension whatever.

Place both ends of the jejunum in a moist laparotomy pad and return them to the abdomen. Reassess the color and blood supply before making the anastomosis. Do not hesitate to resect a dusky portion at either end.

Side-to-end Choledochojejunostomy or Hepaticojejunostomy

Remove the Allen clamp or staple line by incising adjacent jejunum with electrocautery. If the jejunal

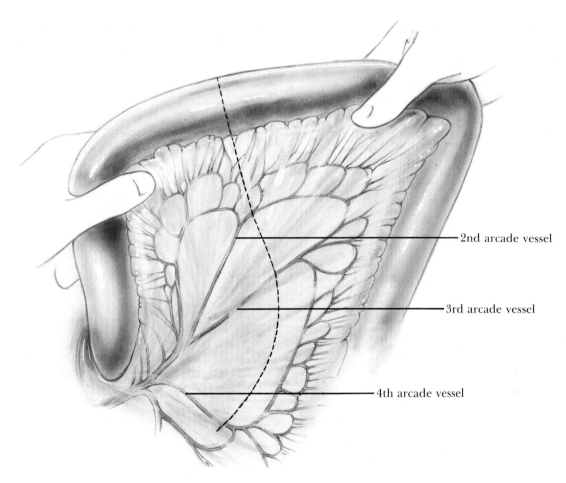

2nd arcade vessel

3rd arcade vessel

4th arcade vessel

Fig. 73–1

mucosa protrudes more than 2 mm beyond the incised seromuscular layer, amputate it flush with the seromuscular incision or use a continuous suture of 5-0 PG in an over-and-over fashion to approximate the mucosa to the cut end of the seromuscular layer.

This step is advisable because the hepaticojejunal anastomosis is performed with one layer of sutures. Clean the mesenteric border of the jejunum for a distance of about 5 mm from its cut end.

In cases of carcinoma, expose the proximal por-

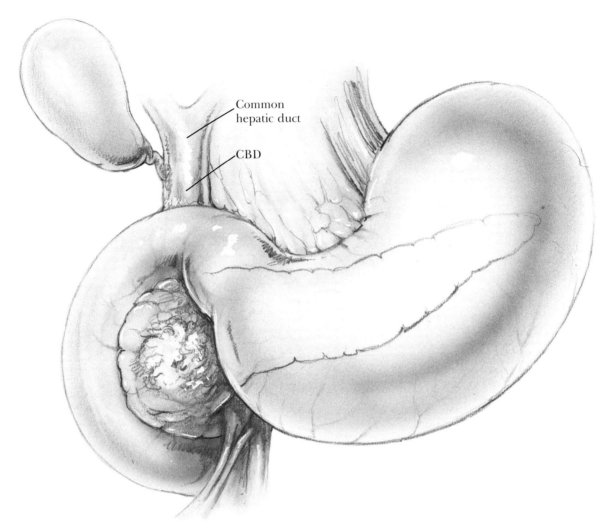

Fig. 73-2

tion of the hepatic duct **(Fig. 73–2)** to place the anastomosis as far from the tumor as possible because pancreatic and CBD malignancies grow upward along the wall of the CBD. Placing the anastomosis at a distance generally avoids occlusion of the anastomosis by further growth of the malignancy. In the case of benign disease, the anastomosis may be made at any convenient location along the dilated hepatic or CBD. Incise the layer of peritoneum overlying the duct. Then make a 2.5- to 3.5-cm longitudinal incision in the anterior wall of the hepatic duct and evacuate the bile.

Only one layer of seromucosal sutures is necessary for this anastomosis **(Fig. 73–3)**. Each bite of the suture material should encompass 4 mm of the jejunum and the full thickness of the hepatic duct. Place the sutures about 4 mm apart. Initiate the anastomosis by inserting the first 5-0 PG or PDS suture at the caudal end of the anastomosis, which corre-

sponds with the mesenteric border of the jejunum. Tie the suture and tag it with a hemostat. Then insert the most cephalad stitch and tag it with a hemostat. Complete the right side of the anastomosis with interrupted 5-0 sutures by the technique of successive bisection (see also Figs. 4-19, 4-20). Do not tie any of these sutures but tag each with a hemostat. After all the sutures have been placed, tie them and complete the right-hand side of the anastomosis **(Fig. 73–4)**. All of the mucosa should have been inverted. If there is any difficulty inverting this mucosa, it is permissible to use an accurate Lembert-type stitch on the jejunum and a through-and-through stitch on the CBD. Cut all the tails of the sutures except the most proximal and distal stitches, which are retained as guy sutures. Then retract the jejunum somewhat toward the patient's right. Now initiate the left half of the anastomosis by bisecting the area between the proximal and distal stitches.

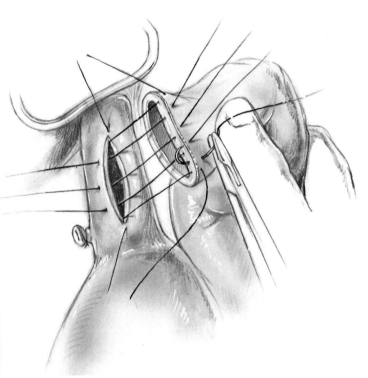

Fig. 73–3

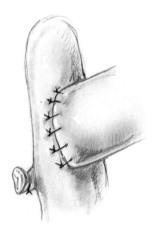

Fig. 73–4

Insert the first stitch at this point **(Fig. 73–5)**. If the hepatic duct is large, it is permissible to tie these sutures as they are inserted. If the duct is small enough to cause concern that you may catch the opposite wall of the bile duct while inserting stitches, do not tie any of them until all of the sutures have been inserted. The bile duct can then be easily inspected prior to tying the stitches. Constructing this anastomosis with continuous sutures is also acceptable.

After all the sutures are tied, it is evident that a large end-to-side anastomosis has been accomplished with little difficulty. All the knots are tied outside the lumen of the anastomosis in this case, although the use of synthetic absorbable suture material makes it of no importance whether the knots are inside or outside the lumen. We see no indication at this time for the use of nonabsorbable sutures in the bile ducts. We have not used a stent, catheter, or T-tube in any of the Roux-en-Y biliary-jejunal anastomoses unless they were done for posttraumatic or iatrogenic bile duct strictures.

To perform a side-to-side choledochojejunostomy or hepaticojejunostomy, close the end of the jejunum by applying a 55/3.5 mm linear stapler. Cut the excess jejunum off flush with the stapler. If the jejunum was divided with the linear cutting stapler and the end has retained its viability, it may be possible simply to use this staple line. Lightly cauterize

the mucosa. It is not necessary to invert the staple line with sutures. Using 5-0 PG or PDS suture material, insert through-and-through sutures on the posterior layer and tie the knots inside the lumen. On the anterior layer of this anastomosis, the knots are tied outside the lumen with mucosa being inverted. Again, a Lembert suture may be used if necessary because there is little danger of inverting too much jejunum when only one layer of sutures is used and the duct is large.

If an anastomosis is contemplated between the divided cut end of the hepatic duct and the side of

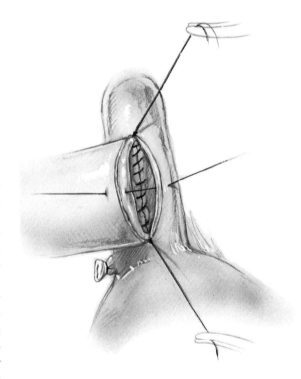

Fig. 73–5

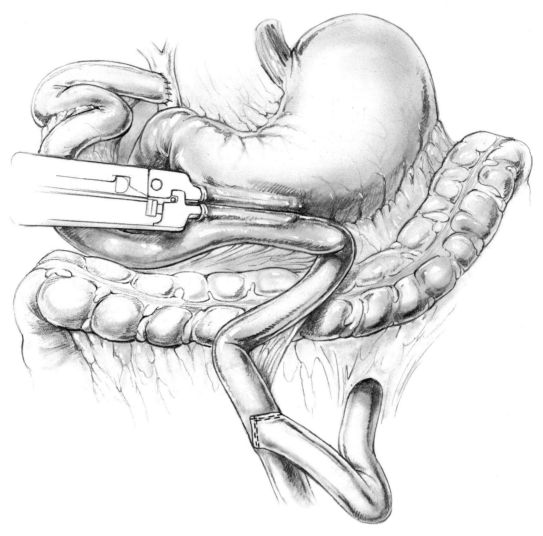

Fig. 73-6

the jejunum, accomplish oblique division of the hepatic duct. This converts the anastomosis from a circular to an elliptical shape and has the effect of enlarging the diameter of the anastomotic stoma.

In cases of bile duct strictures, it is imperative to dissect out and remove the portion of the bile duct that consists largely of scar tissue and has no mucosa, so the anastomosis is constructed with normal, unscarred duct. Make an incision on the antimesenteric side of the jejunum. This incision should be a millimeter or two larger than the diameter of the transected hepatic duct. Use 5-0 PG or PDS to place interrupted sutures and create the posterior suture line first. Excise any redundant protruding jejunal mucosa to facilitate a one-layer anastomosis. Take a bite of hepatic duct and then of jejunum, encompassing only 2–3 mm of tissue with each bite, but penetrate the entire wall of the bile

duct and the jejunum. Tie the knots on the inside of the lumen for the posterior half of the anastomosis. For the anterior half of the anastomosis, insert the sutures so the knots are tied outside the lumen, spaced 3–4 mm apart. After the anastomosis has been completed, inspect the back side and the anterior wall for possible imperfections. To avoid linear tension on the anastomosis by gravity, insert a few seromuscular sutures into the jejunum and attach the jejunum to the undersurface of the liver or to adjacent peritoneum.

Gastrojejunostomy

Because patients with pancreatic carcinoma may develop duodenal obstruction before succumbing to their malignancy, we generally invest a few additional minutes to perform a stapled side-to-side gastrojejunostomy. This anastomosis is created 60 cm distal to the hepaticojejunostomy.

Pass the jejunal limb antecolic and lay it in a comfortable position adjacent to the greater curvature of the gastric antrum. Divide and ligate the branches of the gastroepiploic arcade along the greater curvature of the antrum so a 5- to 7-cm area is free.

Use electrocautery to make a stab wound on the greater curvature aspect of the stomach and on the antimesenteric side of the jejunum. Insert the linear cutting stapling device in a position where it does not transect any blood vessels. Lock the device (**Fig. 73–6**). Fire the stapler and remove it. Inspect the suture line for bleeding, which should be controlled with cautious electrocoagulation or 3-0 PG suture-ligatures. Then grasp the two ends of the staple line with Allis clamps and apply additional Allis clamps to the gap between stomach and jejunum. Then close this gap with a single application of a 55/4.8 mm linear stapler. With Mayo scissors amputate the redundant tissue and lightly electrocoagulate the mucosa. Remove the stapling device and inspect the anastomosis for any possible defects or bleeding (see Figs. 28-5, 28-6).

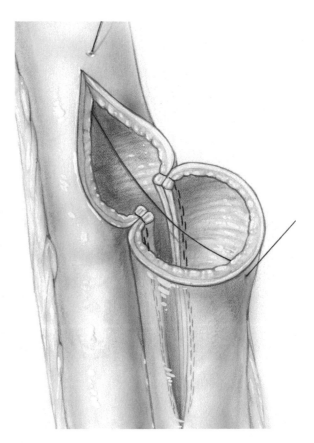

Fig. 73–8

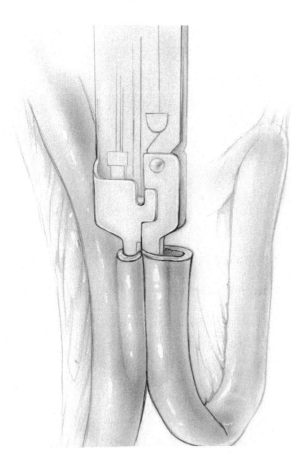

Fig. 73–7

Stapling the Roux-en-Y Jejunojejunostomy

At a point 10–15 cm distal to the gastrojejunostomy, align the proximal cut end of the jejunum with the descending limb of jejunum, as depicted in **Figure 73–7**. It is important to have the cut end of the proximal jejunum facing in a cephalad direction, thereby facilitating construction of the stapled anastomosis. Make a 1.5 cm longitudinal incision with electrocautery on the antimesenteric border of the descending limb of jejunum 10–15 cm distal to the gastrojejunostomy. Remove the Allen clamp from the proximal end of the jejunum and insert the cutting linear stapling device, one limb into the stab wound and the other limb into the open end of jejunum (Fig. 73-7). Lock the stapler, fire it, and remove it. Inspect the staple line for bleeding.

Place a guy suture at the midpoint of the remaining defect approximating the descending limb of jejunum with the proximal open end of jejunum as in **Figure 73–8**. Apply Allis clamps to the anterior and posterior terminations of the staple line

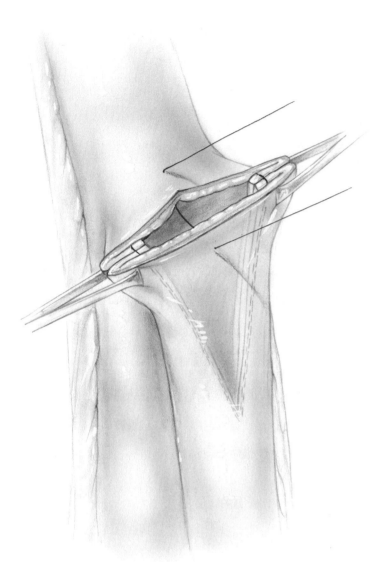

Fig. 73–9

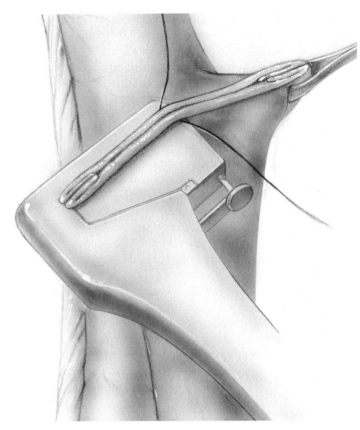

Fig. 73-10

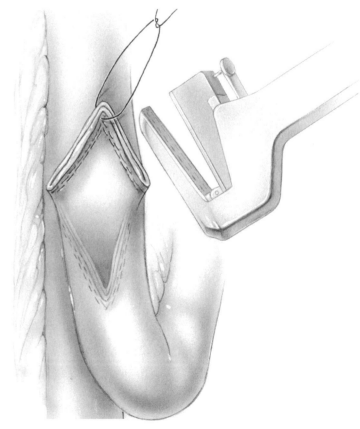

Fig. 73-11

(Fig. 73–9). Close the remaining defects with additional Allis clamps and close the defect by triangulation in the usual manner **(Figs. 73–10, 73–11)**.

Closure of Mesenteric Gaps

Using 4-0 PG or other suture material, place interrupted sutures to attach the transverse mesocolon to the limb of jejunum, which has been brought up to the incision in the mesocolon. This maneuver eliminates any gaps through which small bowel might herniate. Use the same technique to close the gaps in the mesentery of the jejunum in which the Roux-en-Y jejunojejunostomy has been constructed.

Abdominal Closure and Drainage

Close the abdomen in routine fashion. Because bile has extremely low surface tension, a small amount of bile may escape from the anastomosis during the first couple of days following the operation. For this reason, insert a closed-suction drainage catheter through a puncture wound in the lateral abdominal wall. Bring the catheter up to the region of the hepaticojejunostomy.

POSTOPERATIVE CARE

Continue nasogastric suction for 1–2 days.

Acid-reducing therapy with H$_2$-blocking agents or proton pump inhibitors is prudent.

Remove the closed-suction drain after drainage has essentially ceased.

COMPLICATIONS

Bile leak. Although occasionally bile drainage persists for as long as 5–7 days, it invariably ceases in our experience and has never constituted a significant problem following the Roux-en-Y anastomosis.

Stenosis of the anastomosis. Late stenosis of the anastomosis, signaled by cholangitis or jaundice, may occur. Patients should be followed with periodic checks of liver chemistry tests (bilirubin, alkaline phosphatase, γ-glutamyl transferase) to detect this complication early. Sometimes endoscopic or transhepatic dilatation is feasible.

Cholangitis. Cholangitis is rare following a Roux-en-Y hepaticojejunostomy unless the anastomosis becomes stenotic. In patients who have had multiple hepatic duct calculi, there may be transient cholangitis while a calculus is in transit from the hepatic duct down to the hepaticojejunostomy.

Postoperative duodenal ulcer. Patients with chronic pancreatitis already have minimal flow of alkaline pancreatic juice into the duodenum; thus with all the bile diverted into the Roux-en-Y hepaticojejunostomy, there may be an increased tendency for duodenal ulcer formation. These patients should be warned to return for prompt medical attention if they develop symptoms of peptic ulceration. Alternatively, hepaticojejunoduodenostomy **(Fig. 73–12)** may be performed in patients known to have an ul-

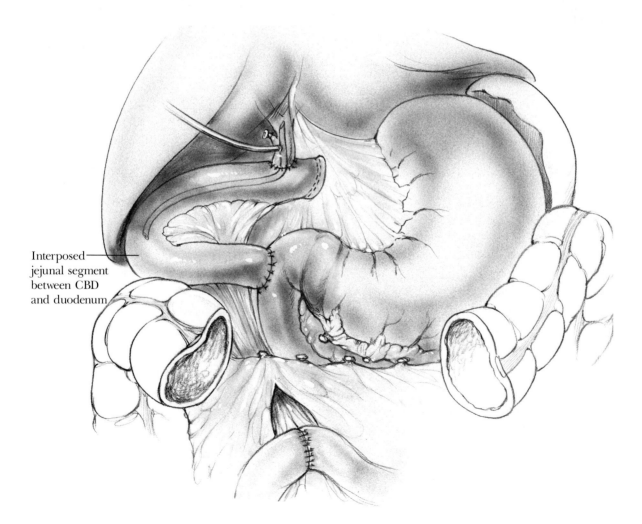

Interposed jejunal segment between CBD and duodenum

Fig. 73-12

cer diathesis, although it is rarely needed with the current methods of treating duodenal ulcer disease.

Delayed gastric emptying. Following choledochojejunostomy with or without concomitant gastrojejunostomy, 10–20% of patients develop delayed gastric emptying. All of our patients with this problem responded to a period of nasogastric suction, sometimes with the assistance of bethanecol or metoclopramide.

REFERENCES

Andersen JR, Sorensen SM, Kruse A, Rokkjaer M, Matzen P. Randomized trial of endoscopic endoprosthesis versus operative bypass in malignant obstructive jaundice. Gut 1989;30:1132.

Bismuth H, Franco D, Corlette MB, et al. Long-term results of Roux-en-Y hepaticojejunostomy. Surg Gynecol Obstet 1978;146:161.

Blievernicht SW, Neifeld JP, Terz JJ, et al. The role of prophylactic gastrojejunostomy for unresectable periampullary carcinoma. Surg Gynecol Obstet 1980;151:794.

Dayton MT, Traverso LI, Longmire WP Jr. Efficacy of the gallbladder for drainage in biliary obstruction: comparison of malignant and benign disease. Arch Surg 1980;115:1086.

Stoker J, Lameris JS, Jeekel J. Percutaneously placed Wallstent endoprosthesis in patients with malignant distal biliary obstruction. Br J Surg 1993;80:1185.

Tocchi A, Mazzoni G, Liotta G, et al. Management of benign biliary strictures: biliary enteric anastomosis versus endoscopic stenting. Arch Surg 2000;135:153.

Wheeler ES, Longmire WP Jr. Repair of benign stricture of the common bile duct by jejunal interposition choledochoduodenostomy. Surg Gynecol Obstet 1978;146:260.

74 Transduodenal Diverticulectomy

INDICATIONS

Perforation

Hemorrhage

PREOPERATIVE PREPARATION

Perioperative antibiotics

PITFALLS AND DANGER POINTS

Injury to pancreas, resulting in postoperative acute pancreatitis

Injury to distal common bile duct (CBD)

OPERATIVE STRATEGY

The strategy of managing patients operated on for perforation depends on the degree of surrounding inflammation. If the neck of the diverticulum is free of inflammation, it may be possible to accomplish primary closure of the neck of the sac with interrupted sutures. More often, leakage of duodenal content through a perforated periampullary diverticulum produces a violent inflammatory reaction. One cannot expect primary suture of the duodenal wall to be secure under these conditions. Consequently, as a lifesaving measure it may be necessary to divert both bile and gastric contents and to insert multiple suction drains to the area of perforation.

In elective cases *where the diverticulum is free of inflammation*, the technique of transduodenal diverticulectomy described here works well. The sac of the diverticulum is inverted through an incision in the second portion of the duodenum. The diverticulum is excised, and the defect in the duodenal wall is closed from inside the lumen.

An alternative technique involves dissecting the duodenal diverticulum from surrounding pancreas and duodenal wall down to its neck near the ampulla. The terminal CBD must be identified as it enters the posterior wall of the duodenum. Place a catheter in the CBD. Then transect the diverticulum at its neck and repair the defect in the duodenal wall. This technique may be facilitated by inflating the duodenal diverticulum with air injected through a nasogastric tube. It requires meticulous dissection of the pancreas away from its attachments to the posterior duodenal wall. As the pancreas is dissected away from the duodenum, the terminal portion of the CBD and the diverticulum may be exposed. This dissection is tedious and sometimes difficult. It carried a greater risk of inducing postoperative acute pancreatitis than does the transduodenal approach.

OPERATIVE TECHNIQUE

Incision

Make a midline incision from the xiphoid to a point about 5 cm below the umbilicus or, alternatively, a long subcostal incision.

Kocher Maneuver

Incise the lateral peritoneal attachments of the descending duodenum and mobilize the duodenum and the head of the pancreas as shown in Figures 11-14 to 11-16. Place a gauze pad behind the head of the pancreas to elevate the duodenum.

Duodenotomy and Diverticulectomy

Make a 4- to 5-cm longitudinal incision near the antimesenteric border of the descending duodenum

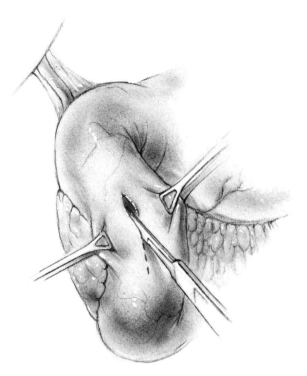

Fig. 74-1

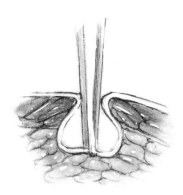

Fig. 74-3

(Fig. 74–1). Identify the ampulla by palpation or visualization **(Fig. 74–2)**. If there is any difficulty identifying the ampulla in this fashion, do not hesitate to make an incision in the CBD and pass a Coude catheter gently down to the ampulla through the CBD incision. Identify the orifice of the periampullary diverticulum, and insert forceps into the diverticulum. Grasp the mucosal wall of the diverticulum **(Fig. 74–3)** and gently draw the mucosa into

the lumen of the duodenum until the entire diverticulum has been inverted into the lumen of the duodenum **(Figs. 74–4, 74–5)**. Transect the neck of the diverticulum about 2-3 mm from its junction with the duodenal wall.

Inspect the bed of the diverticulum through the orifice in the duodenum to check for bleeding. Then close the duodenal wall by suturing the seromuscular layer with interrupted 4-0 PG and invert this layer into the lumen of the duodenum. Close the defect in the mucosa with inverting sutures of interrupted 5-0 PG **(Fig. 74–6)**. This provides a two-layered closure of the diverticulum, performed from inside the duodenum.

Close the duodenotomy incision in two layers. Use interrupted or continuous inverting sutures of 5-0 PG for the mucosal layer and interrupted 4-0 atraumatic silk Lembert sutures for the seromuscular coat.

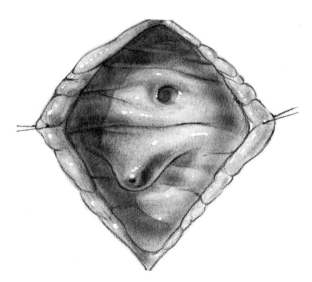

Fig. 74-2

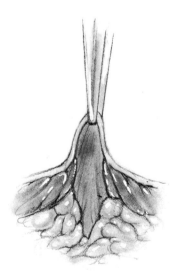

Fig. 74-4

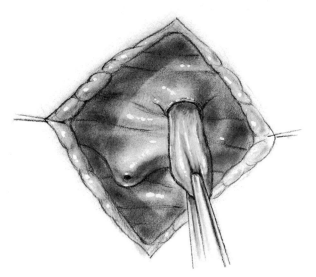

Fig. 74-5

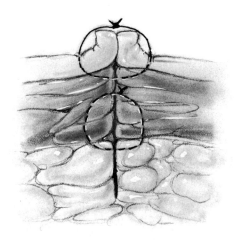

Fig. 74-6

Closure and Drainage

Bring a closed-suction drain out from the region of
the head of the pancreas through a puncture wound
in the right upper quadrant of the abdomen. Close
the abdominal wall in routine fashion.

POSTOPERATIVE CARE

Continue nasogastric suction for 3–5 days.

Give the patient perioperative antibiotics.

Check postoperative levels of serum amylase to detect postoperative pancreatitis.

COMPLICATIONS

Acute pancreatitis

Duodenal leakage

REFERENCES

Afridi SA, Fichtenbaum CJ, Taubin H. Review of duodenal
  diverticula. Am J Gastroenterol 1991;86:935.

Androulakis J, Colborn GL, Skandalakis PN, Skandalakis LJ,
  Skandalakis JE. Embryology and anatomic basis of duodenal surgery. Surg Clin North Am 2000;80:171.

Duarte B, Nagy KK, Cintron J. Perforated duodenal diverticulum. Br J Surg 1992;79:877.

Eggert A, Teichmann W, Wittmann DH. The pathologic
  implication of duodenal diverticula. Surg Gynecol Obstet 1982;154:62.

Iida F. Transduodenal diverticulectomy for periampullary
  diverticula. World J Surg 1979;3:103.

Lobo DN, Balfour TW, Iftikhar SY, Rowlands BJ. Periampullary diverticula and pancreaticobiliary disease. Br
  J Surg 1999;86:588.

Lotveit T, Skar V, Osnes M, Juxtapapillary duodenal diverticula. Endoscopy 1988;20(suppl 1):175.

Manny J, Muga M, Eyal Z. The continuing clinical enigma
  of duodenal diverticulum. Am J Surg 1981;142:396.

Thompson NW. Transduodenal diverticulectomy for peri-
  ampullar diverticula: invited commentary. World J Surg
  1979;3:135.

75 Operations for Carcinoma of Hepatic Duct Bifurcation

INDICATIONS

Carcinoma of hepatic duct bifurcation

PREOPERATIVE PREPARATION

Computed tomography (CT) scan

Percutaneous transhepatic cholangiography (PTC) to demonstrate the proximal extent of the tumor

Perioperative antibiotics

Nasogastric tube

PITFALLS AND DANGER POINTS

Trauma to liver during transhepatic intubation at laparotomy

Trauma to portal vein or hepatic artery during tumor excision at hilus

Failure to achieve adequate drainage of bile

OPERATIVE STRATEGY

Resection

Resection of malignant tumors at the bifurcation of the hepatic duct is safe when the surgeon can demonstrate that there is no invasion of the underlying portal vein or liver tissue and if the proximal extent of the tumor does not reach the secondary divisions of the hepatic ducts. Resecting hepatic parenchyma is generally not necessary unless it facilitates exposure of the ducts for anatomosis.

Patients who do not meet these criteria of resectability should undergo transhepatic intubation of the ducts and not resection. Most of these cases should be identified before surgery and be stented by the interventional radiologist or endoscopist.

Avoiding hemorrhage during the operation depends on careful dissection of the common hepatic duct and the tumor away from the bifurcation of the portal vein. This is best done by dividing the common bile duct (CBD), mobilizing the gallbladder, and elevating the hepatic duct together with the tumor to expose the portal vein and its bifurcation. In borderline cases, remove the gallbladder and make a preliminary assessment regarding invasion of the portal vein by dissecting underneath the common hepatic duct toward the tumor before dividing the CBD. This dissection may be facilitated if a radiologist has passed percutaneous transhepatic catheters into both the right and left main ducts. Because bifurcation of the common hepatic duct occurs outside the liver in almost all cases, palpation of these catheters helps identify the position of the ducts.

Dilating Malignant Strictures of the Hepatic Duct Bifurcation

When the tumor is nonresectable, dilatation and stenting may provide good palliation. With improved endoscopic and radiographic methods of determining resectability and passing stents, operative intubation is rarely needed. This procedure is included for its occasional use in difficult circumstances.

Most tumors of the hepatic duct involve the bifurcation. When nonoperative stenting is not feasible, these tumors may be dilated and stented in the operating room after they are found to be nonresectable. Silastic stents are fashioned, preferably so they are 6 mm outer diameter and fairly thick-walled to prevent the tumor from occluding them. Because it is desirable to catheterize both the right and left hepatic ducts, two such stents are required. These two stents rarely fit into the CBD, so it is generally necessary to perform a Roux-en-Y hepaticojejunostomy to permit the two stents to enter the jejunum and drain the bile in this fashion. If the occlusion of the left hepatic duct cannot be dilated from below, it is often possible to identify the left hepatic duct above the tumor and pass a stent through an incision in the hepatic duct above the tumor.

OPERATIVE TECHNIQUE

Resection of Bifurcation Tumors

Incision

In most cases a midline incision from the xiphocostal angle to a point about 5–8 cm below the umbilicus

636

is suitable. It is helpful to apply a Thompson or an Upper Hand retractor to the right costal margin to improve the exposure at the hilus of the liver.

Determination of Operability

Perform a cholecystectomy by the usual technique. Incise the layer of peritoneum overlying the common hepatic duct beginning at the level of the cystic duct stump and progressing cephalad. Unroof the peritoneum overlying the hepatic artery so the common hepatic duct and the common hepatic artery have been skeletonized **(Fig. 75–1)**. Now dissect along the lateral and posterior walls of the common hepatic duct near the cystic stump and elevate the hepatic duct from the underlying portal vein. Try to continue the dissection along the anterior wall of the portal vein toward the tumor so a judgment can be made as to whether the tumor has invaded the portal vein. A more accurate determination is made later during the dissection after the CBD has been divided and elevated. If there are no signs of gross invasion, identify the anterior wall of the tumor and try to palpate the Ring catheters if they have been placed in the right and the left hepatic ducts prior to operation. This maneuver gives the surgeon some idea of the cephalad extent of the tumor. Frequently, this judgment can be made based on the preoperative transhepatic cholangiogram. If the tumor has grossly invaded the hepatic parenchyma, it may be considered a relative contraindication to resection. Operative ultrasonography may be a useful adjunct.

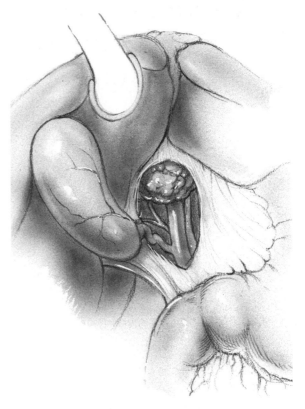

Fig. 75-1

For a final determination of the advisability of resecting the tumor, divide the CBD **(Fig. 75–2)** distal to the cystic duct stump. Oversew the distal end

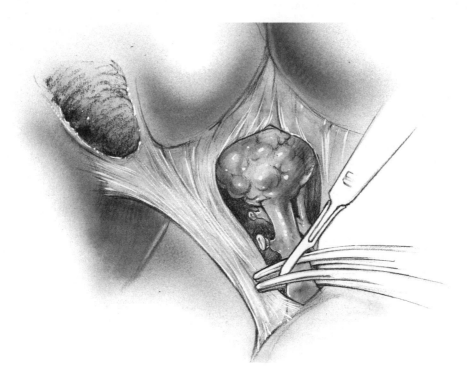

Fig. 75-2

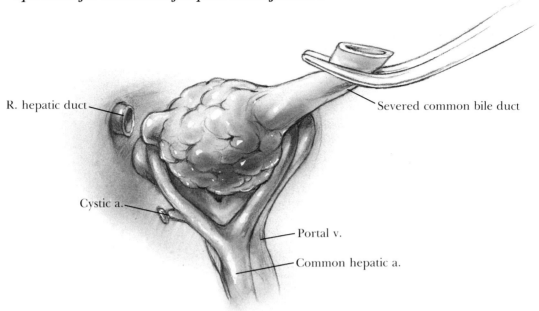

R. hepatic duct

Severed common bile duct

Cystic a.

Portal v.

Common hepatic a.

Fig. 75-3

of the CBD with continuous 4-0 PG suture material. Dissect the proximal stump of the CBD off the underlying portal vein by proceeding in a cephalad direction **(Fig. 75–3)**. Skeletonize the portal vein and sweep any lymphatic tissue toward the specimen. Carefully identify the bifurcation of the portal vein behind the tumor.

Perform this portion of the dissection with great caution because lacerating a tumor-invaded portal vein bifurcation produces hemorrhage that is difficult to correct if one side of the laceration consists of tumor. During this dissection, pay attention also to the common hepatic and the right hepatic arteries that course behind the tumor. Bifurcation tumors occasionally invade or adhere to the right hepatic artery.

After demonstrating that the tumor is clear of the underlying portal veins and hepatic arteries, continue the dissection along the posterior wall of the tumor. The right and left hepatic ducts and even secondary branches can often be identified without resecting hepatic parenchyma. It is sometimes difficult to determine the proximal extent of the tumor by palpation. If preoperative catheters have been placed, palpate the right and left ducts for the presence of the catheters. After adequate exposure has been obtained, transect the ducts and remove the tumor **(Fig. 75–4)**. Perform frozen-section examination of the proximal portions of the right and left ducts in the specimen to determine if the tumor has been completely removed. If the report is positive for tumor, determine whether removing a reasonable additional length of duct is feasible. If this ad-

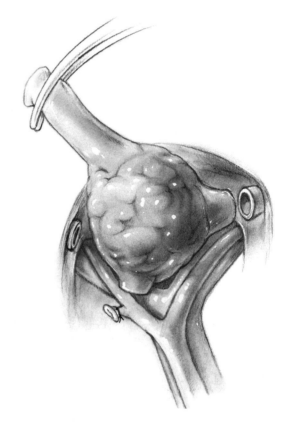

Fig. 75-4

ditional duct is resected, it may be necessary to anastomose three or four hepatic ducts to the jejunum. Although some adjacent hepatic parenchyma may be left attached to the duct during blunt dissection, it may be necessary to perform a major hepatic resection for some tumors at the bifurcation. Insert Silastic tubes into each severed duct by one of the techniques described below.

Anastomosis

Construct a Roux-en-Y jejunal limb as described in Chapter 73 and bring the closed end of jejunum to the hilus of the liver. Make an incision in the antimesenteric border of the jejunum equal to the diameter of the open left hepatic duct. Anastomose the end of the left hepatic duct to the side jejunum with a single layer of interrupted 5-0 PG or PDS sutures. Perform the same type of anastomosis between the right hepatic duct and a second incision in the jejunum. Pass each Silastic catheter through the anastomosis into the jejunum so it projects for a distance of 5–6 cm into the jejunum **(Fig. 75–5)**. These catheters may then be left in as stents. If no Ring catheters were placed before surgery, pass a small Silastic tube across each biliary enteric anastomosis as a stent and bring these tubes out through a jejunostomy.

Drainage and Closure

At the site where the Silastic tube enters the left hepatic duct at the dome of the liver, insert a mattress suture of 3-0 PG into the liver capsule to minimize the possibility of bile draining around the tube at this point. Tie the two tails of this suture around the Silastic tube to anchor it in place. Perform an identical maneuver at the point where the second tube enters the anterior surface of the right lobe of the liver. Then make a puncture wound through the abdominal wall in the right upper quadrant. Pass the Silastic tube through this puncture wound, leaving enough slack to compensate for some degree of abdominal distension. Suture the Silastic tube to the skin securely using 2-0 nylon. Perform an identical maneuver to pass the other Silastic tube that exits from the liver through a puncture wound in the left upper quadrant of the abdominal wall. In addition, place closed-suction drains near each of the exist wounds in the right and left lobes of the liver and bring them through abdominal stab wounds. Place a third closed-suction drain at the hilus of the liver near the hepaticojejunal anastomoses. Close the abdominal incision in routine fashion.

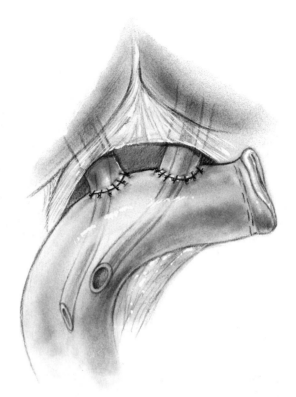

Fig. 75-5

Intubation of Hepatic Duct Without Resecting Tumor

Incision

Make a midline incision from the xiphoid to a point 4–5 cm below the umbilicus.

Dilating the Malignant Structure

Identify the common hepatic duct below the tumor. Make a 1.5- to 2.0-cm incision in the anterior wall of the duct. If the patient has previously undergone percutaneous transhepatic catheterization of the right and left hepatic ducts and if both catheters have passed into the CBD, use these catheters to draw Silastic tubes into each hepatic duct. In the absence of intraductal catheters, pass a Bakes dilator into the common hepatic duct and try to establish a channel leading into the right hepatic duct. After the channel has been established, dilate the passageway by sequentially passing No. 3, 4, 5, and 6 Bakes dilators if possible. Once this has been achieved, pass a Silas-

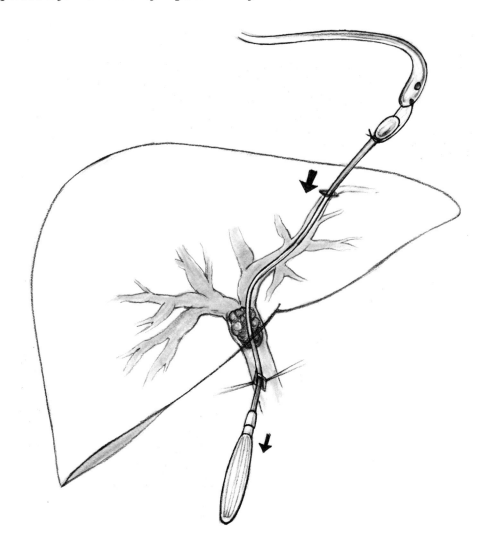

Fig. 75–6

tic catheter into the right hepatic duct by the technique shown in **Figure 75–6**.

Try to identify the channel leading from the common hepatic duct into the left hepatic duct with a No. 2 or 3 Bakes dilator **(Fig. 75–7)**. If this channel cannot be established, try to identify the left hepatic duct just above the tumor. Having accomplished this, incise the duct and pass a Silastic tube through the duct and out the parenchyma of the liver on the anterior surface of the left lobe. It is necessary to anastomose a Roux-en-Y limb of jejunum to this opening in the left hepatic duct. Pass the Silastic tube through the anastomosis into the jejunum.

As previously discussed, the CBD may be too small to accommodate two Silastic tubes, and a Roux-en-Y hepaticojejunostomy to the divided right and left hepatic ducts may be needed. Then pass each tube down into the jejunum for a distance of at least 6 cm **(Fig. 75–8)**. Perform the end-to-side jejunojejunostomy for completing the Roux-en-Y

anastomosis at a point 60–70 cm distal to the hepaticojejunostomy using the method illustrated in Chapter 73.

Other Intubation Techniques

There are many techniques aimed at minimizing trauma when passing a tube through the liver into the hepatic ducts. It is helpful to keep the hole in Glisson's capsule as small as possible to minimize leakage of bile around the tube. If the patient has already undergone preoperative transhepatic catheterization of the hepatic duct, and if the point at which this catheter penetrates the liver capsule is in a satisfactory location, one may suture a urologic filiform to the end of the intraductal catheter. Then by withdrawing the catheter through the liver, the filiform is brought through the opening in the liver capsule. Urologic filiform-followers may then be attached to the end of the filiform so the path of the catheter

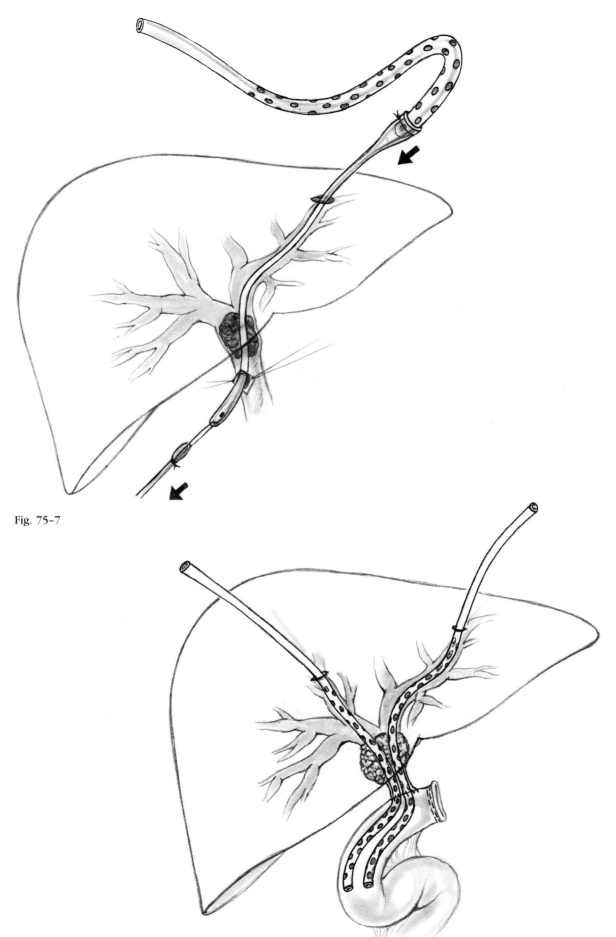

Fig. 75-7

Fig. 75-8

can be dilated about 6 mm. The Silastic tube can then be inserted into the open end of the follower from below and sutured securely in place. By withdrawing the follower, the Silastic tube catheter can be brought through the liver with minimal trauma and then out through the skin.

In the absence of an intraductal catheter, pass a No. 2 or 3 Bakes bile duct dilator through the cut end of the right or left hepatic duct. Pass the dilator through the duct until it reaches a point about 1.0–1.5 cm from Glisson's capsule in an appropriate location on the anterior surface of the liver. The tip of the dilator can frequently be felt under the capsule of the liver. Then make a tiny incision in the capsule and push the metal dilator through the hepatic parenchyma. Suture the tip of the 10F straight rubber catheter to the Bakes dilator (Fig. 75–6). This step may be simplified if a small hole has been drilled in the tip of the Bakes dilator to accept the suture. After drawing the Bakes dilator downward, the catheter is led into the hepatic duct at the hilus of the liver. Then insert a Silastic tube, 6 mm in outer diameter, into the flared open end of the French catheter and suture it securely in this location (Fig. 75–7). By drawing the catheter out of the hepatic duct at the hepatic hilus, the Silastic tube moves to the proper location. Make certain that holes have been punched in the Silastic tube prior to its insertion. These holes should be situated above and below the site of the tumor, so bile can flow into the catheter above and exit from the catheter below the tumor. A convenient source of this Silastic multiperforated tubing is a round Jackson-Pratt drain.

Bring the Silastic catheters out through puncture wounds in the abdominal wall. Then insert closed-suction drains into the sites from which the catheters exit from the right and left hepatic lobes. Place one drain to the hilus of the liver.

POSTOPERATIVE CARE

Attach the Silastic catheters to plastic bags for gravity drainage. Leave them in place until there is no bile drainage along any of the closed-suction drains. Then occlude the Silastic catheters with a stopcock. Instruct the patient to irrigate each catheter twice daily with 25 ml of sterile saline. The nylon suture fixing the catheter to the skin must be replaced approximately every 4–6 weeks.

Instruct the patient to return to the radiology department every 3 months to have the catheters replaced, as sludge tends to occlude the openings over time. The catheters are replaced by passing a sterile guidewire through the Silastic tube; the Silastic tube is then removed with sterile technique and replaced with another tube of the same type. Remove the wire and obtain a cholangiogram to confirm that the tube has been accurately placed. Then suture the tube to the skin. If the patient develops cholangitis, it may be necessary to replace the tube earlier than 3 months. Remove the closed-suction drains when there is no further drainage of bile.

Continue perioperative antibiotics until the closed-suction drains have been removed. Maintain nasogastric suction for 3–5 days. Prescribe an H_2-blocker or proton pump inhibitor intravenously to lower the incidence of postoperative gastric "stress" bleeding. Maintain this regimen until the patient has resumed a regular diet.

Modern methods of brachytherapy permit insertion of radioactive pellets into the Silastic catheters in such fashion that a large dose of radiation can be administered precisely to the bed of the tumor postoperatively. The range of radiation is limited to a precise, shallow depth.

COMPLICATIONS

Sepsis, subhepatic or subphrenic. Cholangitis generally does not occur unless something obstructs the drainage of bile. If the ducts draining only one lobe of the liver have been intubated, leaving the opposite hepatic duct completely occluded but not drained, cholangitis or even a liver abscess frequently appears over time. Consequently, in the presence of a tumor at the bifurcation of the hepatic duct that occludes both right and left hepatic ducts, drainage of each duct is necessary. If drainage of both ducts cannot be accomplished in the operating room, request the radiologist to insert a catheter into the undrained duct percutaneously via the transhepatic route after operation. Routine replacement of the Silastic tubes at intervals of 2–3 months prevents most cases of postoperative cholangitis.

Bile may *leak* around the Silastic tube early if the puncture wound in Glisson's capsule is larger than the diameter of the Silastic tube. If leakage occurs late during the postoperative course, attempt to replace the tube around which the bile is leaking with a tube of somewhat larger diameter. If leakage occurs during the immediate postoperative course, check the position of the Silastic tubes by performing cholangiography to ascertain that none of the side holes in the tubes is draining freely into the peritoneal cavity.

Upper gastrointestinal *hemorrhage* may occur after procedures that divert bile from the duodenum. Patients should be alerted to this possibility and treated promptly with antacid therapy and cimetidine.

REFERENCES

Adson MA, Farnell MB. Hepatobiliary cancer: surgical consideration. Mayo Clin Proc 1981;56:686.

Braunum G, Schmitt C, Baillie J, et al. Management of major biliary complications after laparoscopic cholecystectomy. Ann Surg 1993;217:532.

Cameron JL, Broe P, Zuidema GD. Proximal bile duct tumors: surgical management with Silastic transhepatic biliary stents. Ann Surg 1982;196:412.

Cameron JL, Gayler BW, Zuidema GD. The use of Silastic transhepatic stents in benign and malignant biliary strictures. Ann Surg 1978;188:332.

Gerhards MF, van Gulik TM, Bosma A, et al. Long-term survival after resection of proximal bile duct carcinoma (Klatskin tumors). World J Surg 1999;23:91.

Hart MJ, White TT. Central hepatic resections and anastomosis for stricture or carcinoma at the hepatic bifurcation. Ann Surg 1980;192:299.

Iwatsuki S, Todo S, Marsh JW, et al. Treatment of hilar cholangiocarcinoma (Klatskin tumors) with hepatic resection or transplantation. J Am Coll Surg 1998;187:358.

Launois B, Terblanche J, Lakehal M, et al. Proximal bile duct cancer: high resectability rate and 5-year survival. Ann Surg 1999;230:266.

Lillemoe KD. Current status of surgery for Klatskin tumors. Curr Opin Gen Surg 1994;161.

Liu CL, Lo CM, Lai EC, Fan ST. Endoscopic retrograde cholangiopancreatography and endoscopic endoprosthesis insertion in patients with Klatskin tumors. Arch Surg 1998;133:293.

Millikan KW, Gleason TG, Deziel DJ, Doolas A. The current role of U tubes for benign and malignant biliary obstruction. Ann Surg 1993;218:621.

Polydorou AA, Cairns SR, Dowsett JF, et al. Palliation of proximal malignant obstruction by endoscopic endoprosthesis insertion. Gut 1991;32:685.

Tartarchuk JW, White TT. A new instrument for inserting a U-tube. Am J Surg 1979;137:425.

Taschieri AM, Elli M, Danelli PG, et al. Third segment cholangio-jejunostomy in the treatment of unresectable Klatskin tumors. Hepatogastroenterology 1995;42:597.

76 Hepatic Resection

INDICATIONS

Isolated liver metastases

Symptomatic benign liver lesions

Primary hepatic malignancies

Parasitic or bacterial infections, hepaticolithiasis, and trauma (infrequent indications)

The major *contraindications* to hepatic resections are hepatic insufficiency and advanced stage of malignancy.

PREOPERATIVE PREPARATION

Prescribe mechanical and antibiotic bowel preparation.

Correct coagulopathy, if present.

Provide adequate blood and blood product support.

Correct malnutrition.

Defer resection temporarily for diffuse fatty infiltration of the liver and attempt to improve nutritional parameters.

PITFALLS AND DANGER POINTS

Hemorrhage from hepatic or portal veins or hepatic arteries

Air embolism from hepatic venous injury

Injury to the bile ducts, with postoperative obstruction or fistula

Portal or hepatic vein compromise with subsequent ischemia or postsinusoidal portal hypertension

Dr. David M. Nagorney authored this chapter in the previous edition. The current version was informed by Dr. Nagorney's previous contribution.

Prolonged vascular inflow occlusion leading to refractory liver ischemia

Injury to the diaphragm, inferior vena cava, or intestine (especially after prior gastric, hepatobiliary, or colon surgery)

OPERATIVE STRATEGY

Anatomic Basis for Liver Resection

There are three major hepatic veins: left, right, and middle. Each delineates a plane (termed a hepatic scissura) that divides the liver into functional anatomic units **(Fig. 76–1)**.

The middle hepatic vein defines the main scissura. This anatomic plane divides the liver into two roughly equal units, the left and right liver. The terms left and right liver are used to avoid confusion with older terminology in which left and right hepatic lobes were defined by surface anatomy, rather than deep anatomy. The location of this plane can be approximated by a plane running through the gallbladder fossa anterior to the left margin of the inferior vena cava posteriorly. In modern terminology, a right hepatic lobectomy consists of removing all of the right liver, and left hepatic lobectomy removes the entire left liver.

The portal pedicles contain major branches of the hepatic artery, portal vein, and bile ducts running together. These pedicles interdigitate with the hepatic veins. The territory served by the portal pedicles and their major branches define the sectors and segments of the liver **(Fig. 76–2;** see also Fig. 76-1).

Segments 1-4 comprise the left liver and segments 5-8 the right liver. Each segment has an identifiable portal pedicle. Segmental hepatic venous drainage is variable and anatomically separate from the portal pedicles because of the manner in which the hepatic veins interdigitate with and cross these portal pedicles inside the liver (Fig. 76-1).

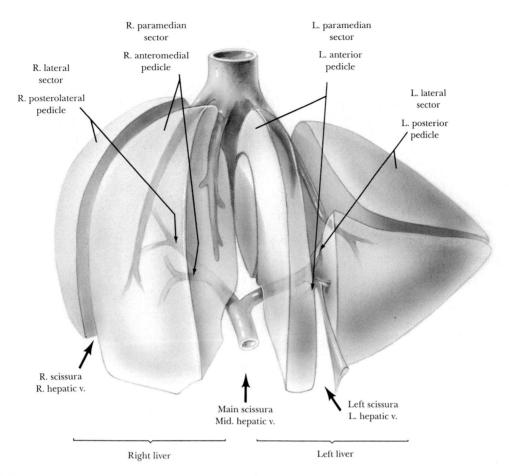

R. paramedian sector

R. anteromedial pedicle

L. paramedian sector

L. anterior pedicle

R. lateral sector

R. posterolateral pedicle

L. lateral sector

L. posterior pedicle

R. scissura
R. hepatic v.

Main scissura
Mid. hepatic v.

Left scissura
L. hepatic v.

Right liver

Left liver

Fig. 76-1

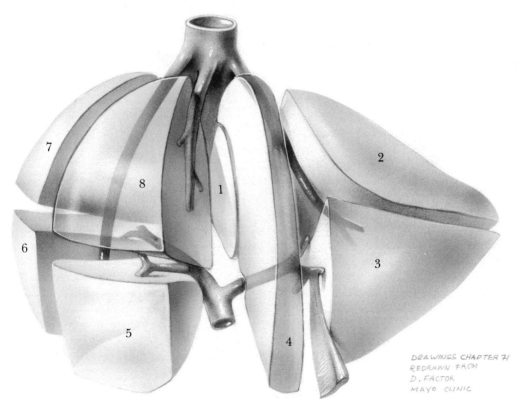

7

8

1

2

6

3

5

4

DRAWINGS CHAPTER 71
REDRAWN FROM
D. FACTOR
MAYO CLINIC

Fig. 76-2

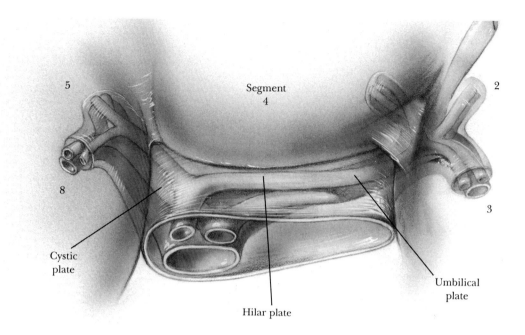

Fig. 76-3

Extent of Resection

At the hilum the portal pedicles branch into the right and left pedicles **(Fig. 76–3)**. A continuation of peritoneum termed the cystic plate covers the right pedicle, and the left pedicle is invested by the umbilical plate. This peritoneum fuses with Glisson's capsule, and the falciform ligament attaches at the cephalad aspect of the umbilical plate. Adequate exposure of this area requires upward mobilization of segment 4 and incision of Glisson's capsule.

Extent of Resection

The need to achieve a clean resection with an adequate margin must always be balanced against the need to preserve an adequate mass of functioning liver parenchyma. Because the liver has a remarkable capacity for regeneration, patients without underlying liver disease can tolerate resection of up to six of the eight liver segments. The situation is far different when resection is contemplated in the setting of acute or chronic liver disease. Careful preoperative assessment and judicious treatment of the underlying liver disease are needed. Hence patients with known chronic liver disease or cirrhosis are best evaluated in centers performing orthotopic liver transplantation.

Excise benign lesions completely whenever possible. The specific resection strategy (enucleation versus wedge versus formal anatomic resection) depends on the size, location, and relation to the tumor of the major afferent and efferent vasculature and bile ducts. Enucleation is effective for encapsulated or sharply demarcated lesions. Wedge resections are typically subsegmental and performed without reference to anatomic boundaries. These nonanatomic resections generally are undertaken for peripheral liver masses that are not adjacent to the hilus or hepatic veins. Wedge resections are easiest for small (<4 cm) tumors arising within anterior liver segments 3–6. Formal anatomic resection should be considered for large or deeply seated lesions or those with indistinct margins, such as hepatic adenomas or some cavernous hemangiomas. This resection may be a standard right or left anatomic lobectomy, or it may be tailored along segmental boundaries in such a manner as to maximize residual functioning hepatic mass and preserve vital vascular and ductal structures to the liver remnant.

Malignant hepatic tumors, primary or metastatic, require resection with a margin of normal liver. Ideally, a 1- to 2-cm margin is preferred to reduce the risk of recurrence. Protect the afferent and efferent vasculature of the anticipated postresection liver remnant scrupulously to prevent postoperative liver failure. Use preoperative imaging studies to exclude patients with multicentric tumor arising in both lobes and those with distant disease. Additional intraoperative findings that preclude resection are peritoneal metastases, extensive regional lymph node involvement, unexpected pulmonary metastases discovered during a thoracoabdominal approach, or malignant thromboses extending into the main portal vein or inferior vena cava. Formal anatomic resection is preferred for malignancies unless the malignancy is small and located peripherally. Intraoperative ultrasonography is a useful adjunct.

Anatomic Liver Resections

Resection of a single liver segment or multiple contiguous segments requires identification and ligation of the segmental vasculobiliary pedicle and parenchymal division through anatomic intersegmental planes. Resection along intraoperatively defined anatomic boundaries is the major difference between nonanatomic wedge resections and anatomic segmental resections. In general, anatomic resections are preferable for primary malignancies because they remove segmental intraportal metastases and enhance preservation of function in adjacent segments in cirrhotic livers.

Resection of segments 2 and 3 is commonly termed left lateral lobectomy. It consists of removing the hepatic parenchyma to the left of the falciform ligament. This deceptively easy resection is fraught with hazard, as the left hepatic vein is large and may be encountered in the plane of dissection. A second danger comes from recurring or feedback branches of the vasculobiliary pedicle to segment 4, which must be preserved. Maintaining the plane of dissection 1–2 cm to the left of the falciform ligament is crucial for safe resection.

Lobar resections have also been termed right and left hemihepatectomy, lobectomy, or hepatectomy. Lobar resections are actually polysegmental resections based on the main right or left vasculobiliary pedicles. Operative risk of significant blood loss is reduced by ligation of the appropriate lobar hepatic artery and portal vein branch prior to parenchymal transection. Subsequent ligation of the corresponding hepatic vein, if technically possible, further reduces operative blood loss. Ligation of the respective bile duct is deferred until it is unequivocally identified (Starzl et al. 1980, 1982).

Major lobar resections may be extended anatomically or nonanatomically. Anatomic extensions are performed by removing the liver segments adjacent to the principal plane. For example, a right hepatectomy (polysegmentectomy of 5–8) may be extended anatomically to include segment 4 (polysegmentectomy of 4–8); or a left hepatectomy (polysegmentectomy of 1–4) can be extended anatomically to include segments 5 and 8 (polysegmentectomy of 1–5 and 8). Anatomic extensions imply formal ligation of the appropriate segmental pedicle and transection of the liver along intersegmental planes other than the principal plane. Nonanatomic extensions are self-explanatory.

Principles of Safe Liver Resection

Liver resection can be conceptualized as involving three phases: parenchymal transection, vascular control, and identification and preservation of the bile duct to the liver remnant. The order in which these phases are performed varies. For simple enucleations and wedge resections, only parenchymal transection is required. For major anatomic resections, vascular control is obtained first. The parenchyma is then divided, and the bile ducts are divided only when the surgeon has ascertained the precise anatomy and ensured that drainage to the remnant is preserved.

Parenchymal Transection

Embedded in the soft liver parenchyma are vascular and ductal structures of greater mechanical strength. Most methods of parenchymal transection use this difference in tissue strength to surgical advantage. Conceptually, the surgeon simply disrupts the parenchyma along the planned transection plane to expose bile ducts and vessels for ligation. Because all branches of the portal pedicle are enveloped by extensions of the vasculobiliary sheath, the portal veins are less fragile than branches of the hepatic vein. Disruption of the small hepatic veins (<1–2 mm) during parenchymal transection is common. Hemorrhage from small hepatic veins is easily controlled by parenchymal compression, electrocautery, or a suture-ligation.

Liver parenchyma can be disrupted by compression methods such as finger fracture, contact methods [Cavitron ultrasonic aspirator (CUSA), waterjet], or thermal methods (electrocautery or laser). Each method has its advantages and disadvantages. Although the zone of parenchymal damage adjacent to the transection plane varies among these methods, the clinical significance of these microscopic zones of devitalized parenchyma is negligible unless the transection results in major damage to the vasculature of the liver remnant and significant regional ischemia occurs. We prefer finger fracture for small wedge resections and CUSA for large parenchymal transections.

The first step is always to score the capsule of the liver along the line of the planned transection with electrocautery. Parenchymal transection is most conveniently begun at a free edge, where the liver is relatively thin.

Finger fracture simply involves pinching and compressing about 1 cm of liver parenchyma between thumb and forefinger. A pill-rolling back-and-fourth motion of thumb and finger while squeezing the liver disrupts normal liver easily yet preserves most vascular and ductal structures. As the fracture plane develops, the surgeon and first assistant work together to compress the parenchyma on both sides of the developing cleft and to open the cleft to expose the deeper portions. The inside part of a pool-tip sucker can be used as an adjunct to finger fracture. The CUSA is more precise but somewhat slower **(Fig. 76–4)**. It should be set to disrupt rather than cauterize, and in this mode it functions as a mechanical disruptor with suction. It is particularly useful for delicate dissection in the region of the hilum.

Typically, any structures >2 mm require ligation. Near-circumferential exposure of intraparenchymal structures optimizes secure ligation. Intraparenchymal portal pedicle branches and hepatic veins can be ligated between fine silk sutures, metal clips, or a combination of the two. Avulsion of small hepatic vein branches from a major hepatic vein can be par-

ticularly troublesome. Hemorrhage from the orifice of an avulsed hepatic vein branch of an exposed major hepatic vein is best controlled by a fine vascular suture material (5-0 or 6-0 Prolene) while carefully maintaining blood flow through the main hepatic vein. If bleeding results from a small hepatic vein without exposure of its major hepatic vein, a single figure-of-eight suture ligature is adequate. Conceptualize a transection plane during parenchymal transection. Transection along the plane without deviation results in a reduced risk of hemorrhage and elimination of partial devascularization of the adjacent liver segment at the interface.

Vascular Control

Safe major hepatic resection primarily depends on avoiding and controlling hemorrhage. Early during the dissection obtain circumferential access to the hepatoduodenal ligament. This permits total hepatic vascular inflow occlusion (Pringle maneuver) to control hemorrhage from the high-pressure afferent vasculature at any time during resection. Control he-

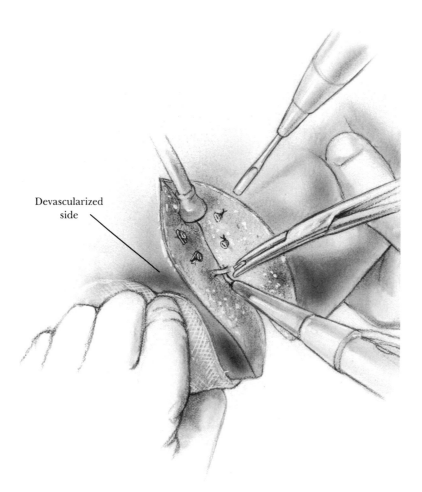

Devascularized side

Fig. 76-4

morrhage from the low-pressure hepatic venous system temporarily by digital pressure, parenchymal compression, or packing.

Exposure of the hepatic veins at the junction of the inferior vena cava requires complete division of the ligamentous attachments to the liver. In particular, the retrocaval ligament bridging segments 6 and 7 must be completely divided to expose the right hepatic vein. Approach the hepatic veins only after controlling the afferent vessels. If tumor obscures the hepatic venous anatomy at its junction with the inferior vena cava, consider total hepatic vascular isolation to permit safe exposure and control. Circumferentially expose the inferior vena cava above (infradiaphragmatic) and below (suprarenal) the liver and apply large vascular clamps. No lumbar veins enter the retrohepatic inferior vena cava. Ligation of the right adrenal vein combined with infra- and suprahepatic inferior vena cava clamping and inflow vascular occlusion of the hepatoduodenal ligament results in total hepatic vasculature isolation. The hepatic veins can then be exposed in a controlled fashion (Delva and associates).

Preservation of Bile Ducts

Bile duct injury is a potential source of major morbidity following hepatic resection. Identify the ductal confluence unequivocally before ligating any major lobar branches during formal or extended lobectomy. If ductal anatomy is in question, two options exist. First, major lobar branches can always be clearly identified by deferring ductal ligation until parenchymal transection exposes the major ducts at the level of the hilar plate. With the surrounding parenchyma transected, the major ducts can be traced from the parenchyma to the confluence and ligated or preserved accordingly. Parenchyma around the major ducts can be excised by CUSA if necessary. Division of the ducts within the parenchyma and probe cannulation distally allows unequivocal confirmation of patency of the ductal confluence. Alternatively, a choledochotomy permits cannulation of the proximal ducts with Bakes dilators or other intraluminal devices, which in turn allows tactile and visual identification of the major ducts for appropriate management.

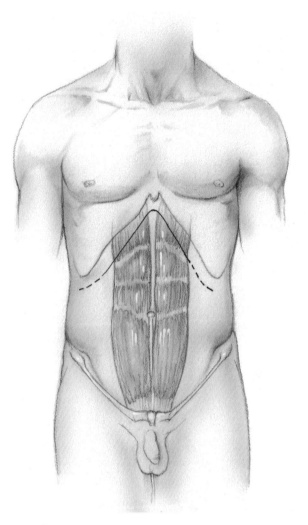

Fig. 76-5

OPERATIVE TECHNIQUE

Incision and Exposure

A bilateral subcostal incision affords wide exposure for most hepatic resections **(Fig. 76–5)**. We use a vertical midline extension with a partial or complete sternotomy if necessary for additional exposure in difficult situations. Some surgeons prefer a right thoracic extension for this purpose.

For limited resections of segments 2 through 6, a vertical midline incision may provide sufficient ex-

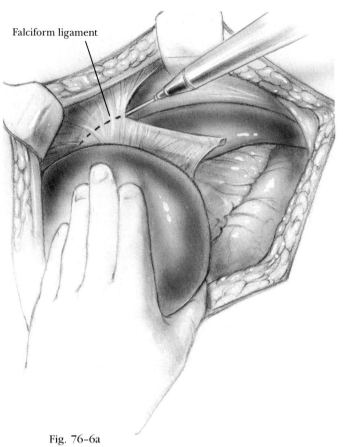

Falciform ligament

Fig. 76-6a

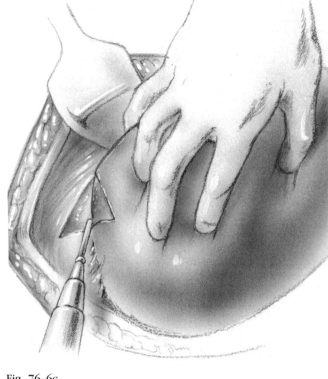

Fig. 76-6c

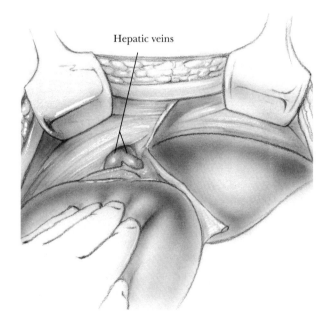

Hepatic veins

Fig. 76-6b

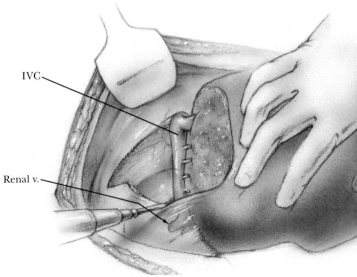

IVC

Renal v.

Fig. 76-6d

posure. Tumor involving segments 7 and 8 or extended lobar resections are approached more safely through a bilateral subcostal incision with an upper midline extension if necessary.

Divide any perihepatic adhesions. Fully mobilize the liver by dividing the ligamentous attachments (**Fig. 76–6a-d**). Divide the gastrohepatic omentum and expose the foramen of Winslow for inflow vascular occlusion. Use an Upper Hand or Thompson retractor to elevate the rib cage cephalad, and place additional retractors as needed to retract the hollow viscera caudally.

Wedge (Nonanatomic, Subsegmental, or Peripheral) Resection

For a wedge resection, after mobilizing the liver, place laparotomy pads posteriorly between the liver and diaphragm to enhance exposure by anterior displacement. Estimate the planned margin of resection by palpation and score the liver capsule with cautery to outline the margin. Transect the parenchyma with cautery, finger fracture, or CUSA (Fig. 76-4). Clip or ligate bile ducts or vessels >2 mm. After obtaining local bile stasis and hemostasis, close the abdomen. Drainage is generally not necessary for simple wedge resections within a single segment or adjacent segments unless concurrent biliary tract disease is present.

Anatomic Unisegmental and Polysegmental Resections

For anatomic uni- or polysegmental resections, define the segmental location of the tumor with intraoperative ultrasonography. Identify the portal pedicle(s) supplying the segment(s). These structures must be ligated for accurate anatomic segmental resection. They may be accessed by proximal dissection from the hilar bile ducts and vasculature to the appropriate pedicle or by direct rapid parenchymal transection along an estimated intersegmental plane with ultrasound guidance. Dissection from the hilus is most applicable for anterior segments 3-6. The parenchymal transection approach is more appropriate for ligation of the posterior segmental pedicles to segments 7 and 8. Both approaches are greatly facilitated by using temporary vascular inflow occlusion to reduce hemorrhage and using CUSA for rapid exposure of the pedicle through the intervening parenchyma. Alternatively, methylene blue injection of the segmental or portal pedicle using ultrasound guidance can provide accurate segmental or sectoral definition. Once the appropriate portal venous branch is injected, segmental boundaries are defined by parenchymal staining, and resection proceeds according to the defined boundaries. Although precise,

this approach is more technically demanding and requires expertise in operative ultrasonography.

To approach anterior liver segments 3, 4, 5, and 8 for resection, mobilize the liver and incise the hilar plate. Identify the appropriate lobar pedicle. Dissection proceeds proximally until the segmental pedicle is exposed. Confirm accurate segmental pedicle identification by ultrasonography. Temporarily occlude the pedicle to (1) outline the segmental boundaries with cautery, (2) ensure that the tumor is included within the segmental demarcation, and (3) confirm that the pedicle provides adequate margins. If appropriate, ligate the segmental pedicle with a silk suture. Transect the parenchyma by cautery, finger fracture, or CUSA. Use temporary inflow vascular occlusion during dissection of the pedicle and parenchymal transection as needed. Few vessels or ducts require ligation if the resection is truly along intersegmental planes. Hepatic veins do require ligation, and they are individually ligated with silk. If the margins are narrow, extend the resection either nonanatomically into contiguous liver segments or anatomically by adjacent segmentectomy. After securing bile stasis and hemostasis, place a single suction drain in the resection bed and close the abdomen.

Polysegmentectomy is performed in a manner similar to unisegmentectomy except that each segmental pedicle is ligated sequentially before extending the parenchymal transection. Once all appropriate pedicles are ligated, the contiguous liver segments are removed en bloc.

Resection of Segments 2 and 3 (Left Lateral Lobectomy)

For a left lateral lobectomy, mobilize the left lobe of the liver by dividing the left triangular ligament (Figs. 76-6a, 76-6b). Take care to avoid the left hepatic vein. Identify and separately ligate the vasculobiliary pedicles to segments 2 and 3. Seek and preserve any recurring or feedback structures that drain and supply segment 4 (Fig. 76-3). Divide the parenchyma, taking care to remain to the left of and preserve the left hepatic vein by remaining well to the left of the falciform ligament.

Anatomic Right Hepatectomy (Right Hepatic Lobectomy)

For right hepatic lobectomy, fully mobilize the liver and perform cholecystectomy to enhance exposure of the hilar vasculature. First ligate the right hepatic artery, which generally traverses the triangle of Calot. Excise the pericholedochal lymph nodes to further expose the bile duct, portal vein, and hepatic artery. Incise the right lateral aspect of the hepatoduodenal

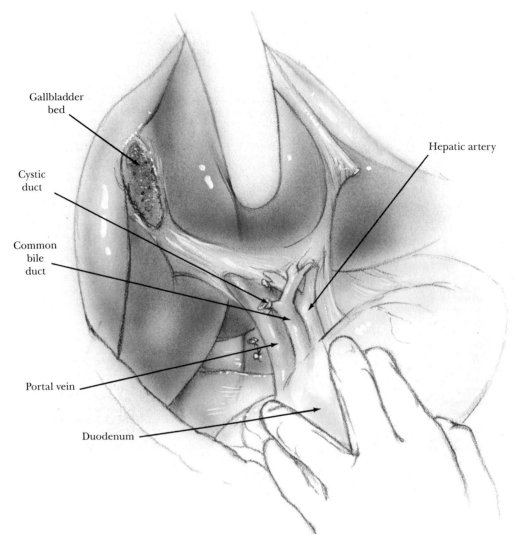

Gallbladder bed

Cystic duct

Common bile duct

Hepatic artery

Portal vein

Duodenum

Fig. 76-7

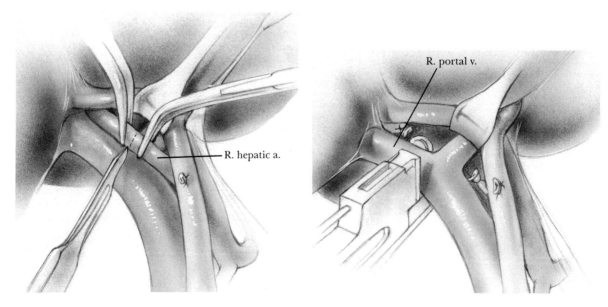

R. hepatic a.

R. portal v.

Fig. 76-8a

Fig. 76-8b

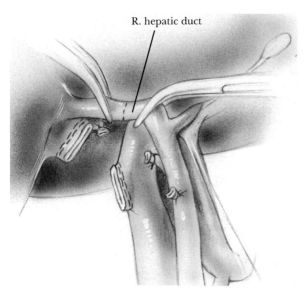

R. hepatic duct

Fig. 76–8c

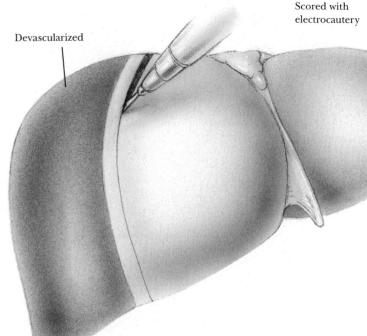

Devascularized

Scored with electrocautery

Fig. 76–9

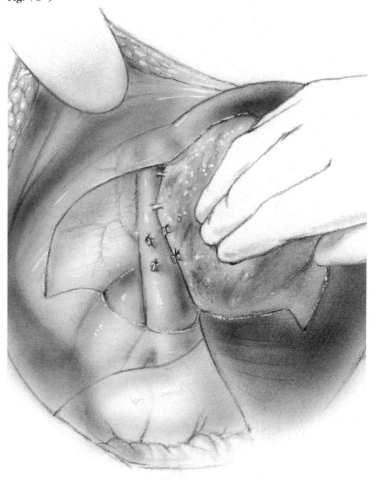

Fig. 76–10

ligament longitudinally just posterior to the bile duct **(Fig. 76–7)**. The hepatic arteries are always found lateral to the common hepatic duct, at the point where they enter the liver parenchyma. Ligate lymphatic vessels around the hepatic arteries before dividing them to reduce postoperative lymph drainage. Temporarily occlude the right hepatic artery while palpating the artery to the opposite lobe to ensure patency of the arterial supply to the liver remnant. Having confirmed this, double-ligate the right hepatic artery with heavy silk and divide it **(Fig. 76–8a)**.

Retract the bile duct anteriorly with a vein retractor to expose the portal vein bifurcation. Expose the right portal vein from the right of the hepatoduodenal ligament. The two major branches of the right portal vein (anterior and posterior) may arise separately without a common trunk, resulting in a portal vein trifurcation. Free the right portal vein branch from surrounding lymphoareolar tissue and ligate it with a vascular stapler or a running vascular suture after division between clamps **(Fig. 76–8b)**. Do not use a simple ligature because dislodgement risks life-threatening hemorrhage. The bile duct to the right lobe may be ligated and divided at this time if the anatomy is clear **(Fig. 76–8c)**, or this step may be deferred until further dissection has been completed. A clear line of vascular demarcation along the principal liver plane between lobes confirms appropriate and complete lobar ligation **(Fig. 76–9)**.

After the afferent vessels are controlled, approach the hepatic veins. Multiple small short hepatic veins between the inferior vena cava and segments 1, 6, and 7 must be ligated as the liver is retracted anteriorly and to the left **(Fig. 76–10)**. Ligation starts infrahepatically and proceeds cephalad. Occasionally a large, right inferior hepatic vein enters the inferior vena cava from the posterior aspect of segment 6. Staple or suture closure for secure ligation is preferred.

To expose the main right hepatic vein, divide the retrocaval ligament bridging segments 1 and 7 (**Fig. 76–11**). A moderate-sized vein frequently traverses the ligament and requires ligation. Then dissect the main right hepatic vein from the inferior vena cava and liver. Unless a large tumor precludes access, transect the right hepatic vein with a vascular stapler (McEntee and Nagorney, 1991) and ligate the paren-chymal side with a running vascular suture before parenchymal transection (**Fig. 76–12**). Alternatively, ligate the right hepatic vein as the final step of a formal lobectomy after parenchymal transection.

Transect the parenchyma on the line of vascular demarcation along the principal plane by finger fracture, cautery, or CUSA (**Fig. 76–13**). Clip bile ducts or vessels on the resection side of the liver and ligate them on the remnant side to reduce artifact image distortion on postoperative follow-up computed tomography (CT) scans. Ligate the middle hepatic vein during the parenchymal phase as encountered. As the hilus is approached, the bile ducts to the lobe being resected are exposed. Again, ligation is performed only when patency of the remaining lobar

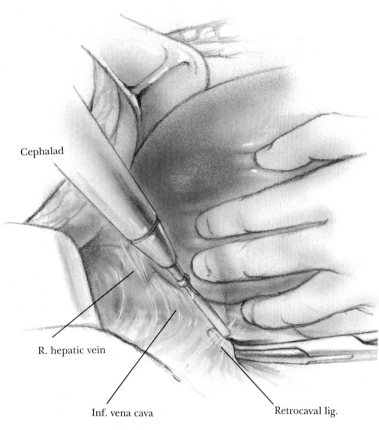

Cephalad

R. hepatic vein

Inf. vena cava

Retrocaval lig.

Fig. 76–11

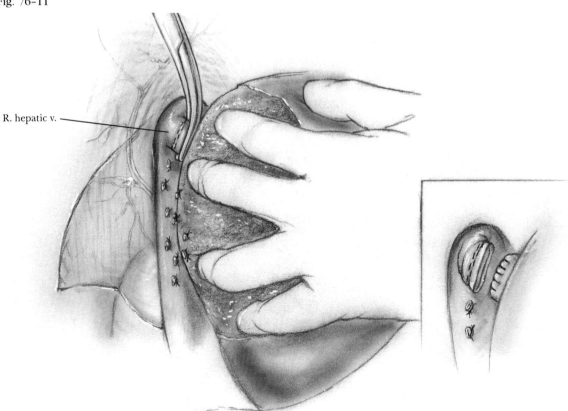

R. hepatic v.

Fig. 76–12

Middle hepatic v.

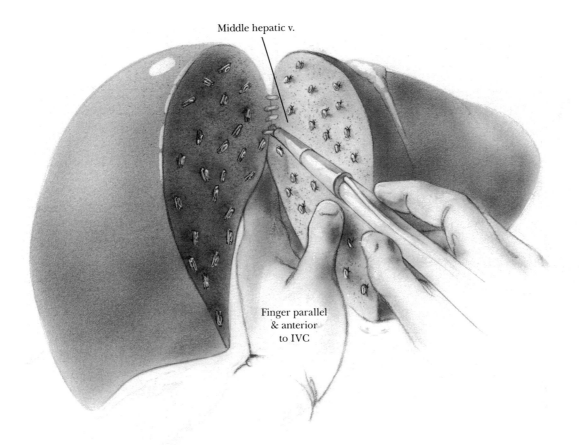

Finger parallel
& anterior
to IVC

Fig. 76-13

duct can be ensured. Look for the smaller ducts to segment 1 posterior to the main ductal confluence and ligate them if encountered. Next, transect the parenchyma of the caudate process, or that liver substance between the posterior aspect of the portal vein and the inferior vena cava, to expose the anterior surface of the inferior vena cava. Continue parenchymal transection along the principal plane until the main hepatic veins are encountered. If the major hepatic vein has been ligated, simply remove the lobe. If not, clamp or divide the hepatic veins with a vascular stapler. Use inflow vascular occlusion during parenchymal transection to reduce intraoperative hemorrhage if necessary.

Obtain hemostasis and bile stasis but avoid large interlocking parenchymal liver sutures. **Figure 76–14** shows the appearance of the hepatic remnant after right hepatic lobectomy. A suction drain is placed adjacent to the transected liver surface and bought out dependently through the abdominal wall. Occasionally the divided falciform is reapproximated to prevent torsion of the liver remnant and postoperative vascular compromise. The omentum is not attached to the parenchyma. The abdomen is closed in standard fashion.

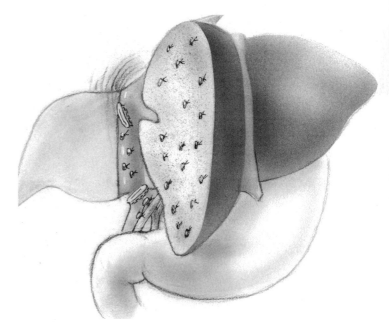

Fig. 76-14

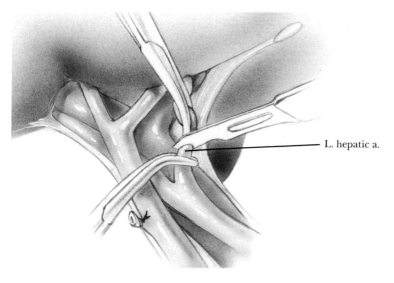

Fig. 76-15a

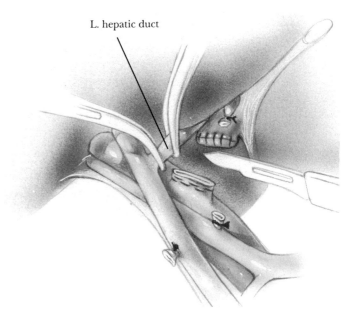

Fig. 76-15c

hepatic omentum. Confirm the patency of the arterial supply to the right liver by temporarily occluding the left hepatic artery before clamping, ligating, and dividing the vessel (Fig. 76-15a).

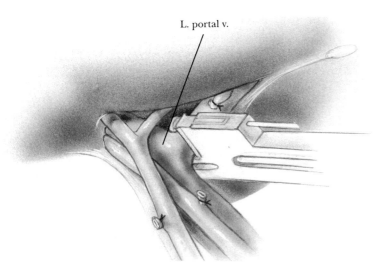

Fig. 76-15b

Anatomic Left Hepatectomy (Left Hepatic Lobectomy)

For anatomic left hepatectomy, in a manner analogous to that used for the anatomic right hepatic lobectomy first identify and divide the left hepatic artery and portal vein. After division of the gastrohepatic omentum, approach the left hepatic artery through the lesser sac via the left lateral aspect of the hepatoduodenal ligament. The main left hepatic artery is generally found just inferior to the base of the round ligament as it enters the left lobe between segments 3 and 4 **(Fig. 76-15)**. An accessory left hepatic artery, arising from the left gastric artery, always courses through the gastrohepatic omentum and is often divided during division of the gastro-

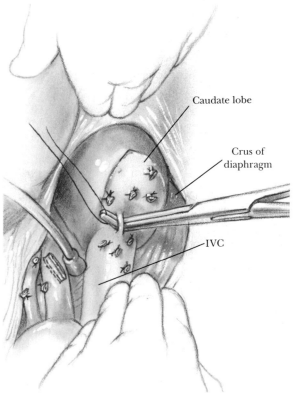

Fig. 76-16

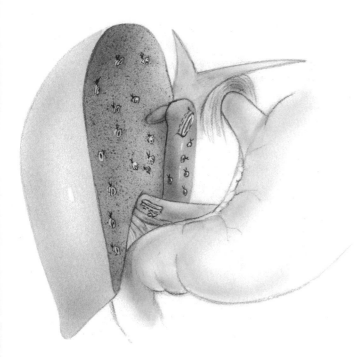

Fig. 76-17

While retracting the bile duct with a vein retractor, identify the left portal vein at the left aspect of the hepatoduodenal ligament. The main left portal vein branch always bifurcates from the right main branch at approximately 90° and courses anterolaterally. Divide it with a vascular stapler (Fig. 76-15b) or running suture as previously described. Note the developing line of transection, as the left liver lobe should now be completely devascularized. If the ductal anatomy is clear, double-ligate and divide the left hepatic duct (Figure 76-15c); if the anatomy is in doubt, defer this step until later in the dissection.

The main left hepatic vein frequently joins the middle hepatic vein. In contrast to right hepatic lobectomy, postpone ligation of the main left hepatic vein until parenchymal transection is complete because extrahepatic exposure is generally not feasible. Ligate the short, direct, hepatic veins between the inferior vena cava and segment 1 (caudate lobe) initially from the right of the hepatoduodenal ligament until segment 1 is mobilized inferiorly **(Fig. 76–16)**. As the veins are ligated and divided, segment 1 can be retracted anteriorly, and the remainder of the hepatic veins between the inferior vena cava and caudate lobe can be divided safely. Division of the retrocaval ligament from the left side of the inferior vena cava allows complete mobilization of segment 1.

The remainder of the resection proceeds much as previously described. The completed operative field is shown in **Figure 76–17**.

POSTOPERATIVE CARE

Postoperative care requires appropriate fluid administration, using colloids in addition to crystalloid to reduce postoperative weight gain and maintain adequate urine output. Mild acidosis and coagulation abnormalities are common and need not be treated unless symptomatic. Nasogastric intubation is continued overnight to prevent the risk of aspiration. Epidural analgesia postoperatively markedly improves pulmonary function and pain control.

COMPLICATIONS

The major complications of hepatic resection are hemorrhage, biliary fistula, intraabdominal infection, and liver failure. All complications are best treated by careful intraoperative prophylaxis. Hemostasis is secured meticulously, as is bile stasis. Hepatic insufficiency is treated as clinically indicated. Hepatic failure may require orthotopic liver transplantation.

REFERENCES

Chang YE, Huang TL, Chen CL, et al. Variations of the middle and inferior hepatic vein: applications in hepatectomy. J Clin Ultrasound 1997;25:175.

Couinaud C. Surgical Anatomy of the Liver Revisited. Paris, C. Couinaud, 1989.

Delattre JP, Avisse C, Flament JB. Anatomic basis of hepatic surgery. Surg Clin North Am 2000;80:345.

Delva E, Camus Y, Nordlinger B, et al. Vascular occlusions for liver resections. Ann Surg 1989;209:211.

McEntee GP, Nagorney DM. Use of vascular staplers in major hepatic resections. Br J Surg 1991;40:78.

Putnam CW. The surgeon at work: techniques of ultrasonic dissection in resection of the liver. Surg Gynecol Obstet 1983;157:475.

Scheele J, Stangl R. Segment oriented anatomical liver resections. In Blumgart LH (ed) Surgery of the Liver and Biliary Tract, 2nd ed. New York, Churchill Livingstone, 1994, pp 1557-1578.

Schroder T, Hasselgren P-O, Brackett K, et al. Techniques of liver resection: comparison of suction, knife, ultrasonic dissector, and contact neodymium-YAG laser. Arch Surg 1987;122:1166.

Smadja C, Blumgart LH. The biliary tract and the anatomy of biliary exposure. In Blumgart LH (ed) Surgery of the Liver and Biliary Tract, 2nd ed. New York, Churchill Livingstone, 1994, pp 11-24.

Starzl TE, Koep LJ, Weil R III, et al. Right trisegmentectomy for hepatic neoplasms. Surg Gynecol Obstet 1980;150:208.

Starzl TE, Shaw BW Jr, Waterman PNI, et al. Left hepatic trisegmentectomy. Surg Gynecol Obstet 1982;21:155.

Part VIII
Pancreas

77 Concepts in Surgery of the Pancreas

William H. Nealon

CARCINOMA OF THE PANCREAS

Diagnosis

The standard description of a patient above the age of 55 with a complaint of "painless jaundice" belies the significant pain that develops as carcinoma of the pancreas progresses. Because some patients first come to medical attention with advanced disease, the presence or absence of pain should never be used to eliminate this diagnosis. Early symptoms consist of dyspepsia and weight loss. Jaundice is often initially absent. Recognition of jaundice frequently triggers the use of abdominal ultrasonography or computed tomography (CT). Since the last edition of this text, there has been considerable development in the area of imaging of the pancreas.

Imaging

In the past, *abdominal ultrasonography* did not yield sufficient detail to evaluate pancreatic carcinoma routinely. It was useful for documenting hepatic metastasis, but overlying gas in the intestine made clear evaluation of the pancreas problematic. Similarly, early-generation *CT scans* of the abdomen could define a mass effect in the head of the pancreas but were unable clearly to delineate the boundary between a carcinoma and the surrounding desmoplastic reaction that is characteristic of this disease. Fortunately, new generation *spiral CT* scanners can now clearly define the boundaries of a carcinoma in the midst of the otherwise enlarged head of the pancreas. This single development has greatly enhanced our ability to define exact sizes of tumors preoperatively and greatly facilitates CT-directed fine-needle and core biopsies of a pancreatic cancer, which may be necessary prior to operation. Thus, even though a patient may have had a conventional CT scan before coming to the surgeon, it is advised that a spiral CT scan be obtained to provide additional and more precise information regarding the tumor.

Endoscopic ultrasonography (EUS) is now being used to evaluate carcinoma of the pancreas. There are a number of advantages for this modality and certain limitations. The added detail in the images obtained with the proximity of the probe to the pancreas has been considerable. Abnormal lymph nodes may be identified and biopsied even when not significantly enlarged. The accuracy of these biopsies has been established at 80–90% [1]. Similarly, identification of vascular structures, particularly the superior mesenteric artery and the splenic vein, portal vein, and superior mesenteric vein, is excellent with EUS. Clear planes between structures can normally be identified; hence invasion into the walls of any of these structures is clearly delineated using EUS. All layers of the intestinal wall can be demarcated and any invasion into one of these layers identified. The actual pancreatic tumor may be biopsied as well. The biopsy device can be easily seen with the linear probe, and biopsies obtained using simultaneous EUS have a high likelihood of yielding a confirmatory diagnosis. It has not yet reached the point where one could say that EUS would replace the spiral CT scan as a form of evaluation, but for local and regional disease one might argue that EUS gives comparable or superior information. The one limitation worth mentioning with EUS is failure to evaluate the liver fully. The decision regarding resectability of the carcinoma of the pancreas depends on a number of issues, but clearly hepatic metastasis is an important one. Thus in the absence of another form of imaging, the EUS is unlikely to give a full evaluation of resectability.

Mesenteric arteriography, routinely used in the past to evaluate vascular involvement, has been abandoned by most experienced pancreatic surgeons in favor of less invasive methods. The spiral CT scan shows the vascular anatomy clearly and is now established as the more appropriate imaging technique for evaluating the resectability of carcinoma of the pancreas.

Magnetic resonance imaging (MRI) and *magnetic resonance cholangiopancreatography* (MRCP) are related technologies that have gained attention since the last edition. Clear anatomic features of the main pancreatic duct (MPD) and the common bile duct (CBD) allow stones and tumors to be easily defined with MRCP. Vascular anatomy can be delineated with *MR angiography* (MRA). If the signal weighting is altered, an adequate view of the liver and of peripancreatic lymph nodes can be obtained. These studies can be obtained quickly and noninvasively. Although no data have yet been developed to establish its superiority, one might argue that this procedure is capable of defining all of the necessary features to establish both diagnosis and resectability. If one flaw exists regarding this modality, it is that the fine anatomy of the MPD and the CBD may be less clear than that obtainable with EUS or endoscopic retrograde cholangiopancreatography (ERCP). Finally, specialized MR studies are not yet universally available.

There has been controversy about ERCP for evaluating patients with carcinoma of the pancreas. This lesion originates in the ducts, so it should not be surprising that 94–96% of patients with this diagnosis have an abnormal pancreatogram. If preoperative biliary drainage is desired, ERCP can help accomplish it. Unfortunately, there are no data to suggest the therapeutic value of this strategy. Prospective studies of preoperative transhepatic cholangiographic drainage failed to show an advantage, and some complications (hemorrhage, bile leak, cholangitis) arose from the procedure [2]. It is our opinion that preoperative drainage of the biliary tree is unnecessary and may have a negative impact on the outcome of operative therapy. In reality many of these patients are referred from gastroenterology specialists, who have often placed a stent in the bile duct prior to referring the patient for resection. In some regards, such stent placement may be unavoidable if ERCP is performed. During ERCP the instrument traverses the (contaminated) intestinal tract before injecting contrast into an obstructed bile duct, placing the patient immediately at risk for cholangitis. Once this entity is recognized the endoscopist has no choice but to place a stent to prevent the development of cholangitis. We believe that ERCP, if used at all, should be implemented within 24 hours of operation, so any information that helps with the diagnosis is obtained when the risk of sepsis is extremely low. The procedure is of potential value in patients in whom the diagnosis is equivocal or if choledocholithiasis is suspected, as choledocholithiasis can be diagnosed and treated by ERCP by simply adding endoscopic sphincterotomy and stone extraction. Again I stress that it is our belief that preoperative biliary decompression is unnecessary and probably increases the complications in these patients.

Percutaneous transhepatic cholangiography (PTC) may establish a diagnosis and an access point for biliary decompression but is rarely needed in current practice. PTC was initially favored by many because of its relative ease in patients with dilated intrahepatic biliary trees, and the technique remains an option. Its applicability to the management of pancreatic carcinoma has become negligible for two main reasons: (1) ERCP gives adequate access to the biliary tract in most cases where it is needed; and (2) preoperative biliary decompression is not uniformly favored. PTC is a highly invasive procedure that is associated with a risk of bleeding or bile leak. It is difficult to use in patients with small or even normal intrahepatic biliary systems. In this case, ERCP would be the better choice. When obstructive jaundice is diagnosed by PTC, a transhepatic stent must be placed to avoid bile leak and bile peritonitis.

Finally, it should be stressed that for an experienced pancreatic surgeon *tissue documentation of the diagnosis of pancreatic carcinoma is not considered mandatory*. In major centers as many as half of the resections in these patients are performed without the benefit of tissue confirmation [3]. This should not convey the message that pancreaticoduodenectomy is an operation undertaken lightly. A mass in the head of the pancreas, obstructive jaundice, weight loss, and nonspecific dyspeptic symptoms in a patient over the age of 55 form a constellation of signs and symptoms highly suspicious for the diagnosis of carcinoma of the pancreas. In this situation, I believe that one must have rather compelling reasons not to proceed to resection. The distinction between cancer and chronic pancreatitis is almost always clear; and when there is controversy, tissue confirmation is increasingly available.

Preoperative biopsies are required in patients who are enlisted for *neoadjuvant chemoradiation*. This modality has been primarily championed by the investigators at M. D. Anderson Cancer Center in Houston [4]. Patients undergo 8–12 weeks of therapy before operation. The diagnosis must be confirmed by fine-needle aspiration or core biopsy under CT or EUS guidance before initiating therapy. Because of the delay prior to operative therapy, patients enlisted in this program also routinely undergo biliary decompression. Thus patients enlisted in neoadjuvant chemoradiation require two treatment modalities not routinely used when operation is performed first.

Determination of Resectability

Many of the same modalities used for diagnosis can also be employed to determine resectability. Three categories of factors determine resectability: local invasion of the tumor into contiguous structures that should be preserved (e.g., vascular structures); tumor spread in the abdomen to sites remote from the primary tumor; and hepatic metastasis. Each is discussed separately.

Vascular Invasion

Invasion, encasement, or obliteration of the superior mesenteric artery or the celiac trunk precludes resection. Invasion into the portal vein or the superior mesenteric vein/splenic vein confluence may or may not represent an unresectable lesion because resection and reconstruction of the portal vein is an established modality. A segmental resection of part of the circumference of the vein with a patch graft or complete vein resection can be performed. These operative procedures are longer in duration than conventional pancreaticoduodenectomy, and blood loss is higher. Survival appears to be considerably better with segmental resection and the patch graft than with complete resection of the vein, possibly reflecting the extent of invasion required to proceed to complete vein resection versus a simple patch graft [5]. As previously mentioned, vascular invasion may be judged by spiral CT, MRA, or EUS.

Tumor Extension Remote from the Primary Tumor

Local extension may be paraaortic disease, extension into the colon or stomach, or carcinomatosis. Spiral CT, EUS, MRI, or laparoscopy may define this entity, but often it is established only at laparotomy.

Hepatic Metastasis

Spiral CT scan and MRI may be helpful for detecting hepatic metastases; ERCP and PTC are not. *Transabdominal ultrasonography* sometimes demonstrates hepatic metastases more clearly than routine spiral CT. We have had considerable success with the *portal enhanced CT scan*. This imaging modality involves celiac arteriography performed simultaneously with the CT scan of the liver. As many as 25% of hepatic metastases are not seen by conventional or spiral CT scan but are clearly delineated on portal enhanced CT scans [6]. Perhaps more important, a single hepatic metastasis may be seen on a spiral CT scan, when in fact a much larger number of undetected metastases may be seen on the portal enhanced CT scan. This invasive procedure provides no additional information regarding the pancreas.

Resectability may be further evaluated intraoperatively. Using laparoscopic or mini-laparotomy techniques, it is possible to utilize intraoperative ultrasonography or laparoscopic ultrasonography to evaluate the resectability of the tumor. Sadly, with all the modalities previously mentioned, the rate of finding an unresectable tumor at the time of exploration is still 40-50%. One can only hope that EUS and some of the other recently developed modalities can lower this rate, but all major reports on management of carcinoma of the pancreas continue to report this high rate of unresectability at the time of exploration.

To reduce this rate, Warshaw is credited with proposing *laparoscopy* even before the overwhelming developments in laparoscopic applications for general surgeons. Warshaw and colleagues recommend lavage of the peritoneal cavity to permit cytologic evaluation and visual evaluation of the peritoneal cavity [7]. This modality also permits biopsy. Peritoneal seeding or small peripheral hepatic metastases are recognized immediately upon visual or tactile inspection, whereas they may have eluded all other imaging modalities. If they are seen at laparoscopy or mini-laparotomy, palliation can be achieved without operation in most patients.

Treatment

Neoadjuvant Chemoradiation

Because neoadjuvant chemoradiation requires a separate set of standards for the approach, I present this subject first. Neoadjuvant chemoradiation has been proposed to improve overall survival, although no data have yet confirmed it. Thirty-five percent of patients enlisted in such a program are found to have advanced disease and therefore are unacceptable for resection after they have completed their 8-12 weeks of neoadjuvant chemoradiation. It is the opinion of these investigators that this is advantageous because these patients clearly would have had poor outcomes after operative intervention had they undergone operation prior to their neoadjuvant care. If we accept this proposal, one would expect that the outcomes would be better for those who undergo resection because the patients with more advanced disease have been eliminated. Unfortunately, this has not been the case. Patients are generally offered a course of combined radiotherapy and 5-fluorouracil (5FU)-base chemotherapy or radiotherapy and gemcitabine-based chemotherapy. Patients are reevaluated after their course of therapy to determine the resectability of their lesion [8].

Down-staging of Carcinoma

Down-staging is a relatively new concept applicable to patients with carcinoma that is unresectable by current standards. The theory behind this practice is that aggressive combined chemotherapy and irradiation may be sufficiently effective to clear those areas in which a lesion was deemed unresectable and thereby down-stage the disease to a level that is considered resectable. Several centers have evaluated this concept. Unfortunately, success rates have rarely exceeded 10%, and long-term outcomes have not proved favorable [9].

Carcinoma of the Body and Tail of the Pancreas

Whereas at the time of the last edition of this book the historically dismal outcomes for carcinoma of the body and tail of the pancreas were thought to preclude considering resection in this subgroup, it is now considered acceptable to at least evaluate these patients. A large series from the Memorial Sloan-Kettering Cancer Center in New York suggested that the outcomes were not particularly favorable but were essentially not different from the outcomes for resection in the head of the gland [10]. Resectability criteria are essentially the same in this subgroup. Evaluation for local and locoregional spread and for liver metastasis is required before considering resection. It is generally believed that the absence of jaundice permits this disease to progress much farther before diagnosis, which may well explain why the overall outcomes have been less favorable in this group of patients. Many of the lesions are unresectable at the time of diagnosis.

Operative Management

Surgical resection provides the only hope for cure of this disease. Most patients are treated with a *pylorus-preserving pancreaticoduodenectomy*. A number of important margins are considered in this resection. As a routine, the bile duct is divided above the cystic duct entry and the common hepatic duct is a margin, which is sent for frozen section analysis. The body of the pancreas is typically divided at or slightly to the left of the area that overlies the portal vein and the superior mesentery vein/splenic vein confluence. The duodenum is divided just past the pylorus. Each of these margins should be sent for frozen section pathologic analysis during the operative procedure; a report of positive margins is an indication for further resection. Perhaps the most problematic margin is that at the uncinate process as it abuts the superior mesenteric artery. This and the radial margin of the uncinate process extending down into the retroperitoneum are commonly found to be unexpectedly involved in tumor at final pathology. In some regard, these margins are not cor-

rectable because we would not consider resecting the superior mesenteric artery, and a deeper dissection into the retroperitoneum is not considered reasonable because of the proximity of the vena cava and the aorta.

Total pancreatectomy has been proposed to treat cancer of the pancreas. It appears to be a rare patient whose lesion is considered resectable yet requires total pancreatectomy. In most cases resection of the body and tail with a distal pancreatectomy or resection of the head and body with a pancreaticoduodenectomy are sufficient to achieve cure. There are no data to suggest that total pancreatectomy enhances survival [10]. Multicentricity of carcinoma of the pancreas is rarely described.

Essentially all pancreatic surgeons agree that a *truncal vagotomy is not necessary* after pancreaticoduodenectomy. As many as 65% of patients complain of delayed gastric emptying early after Whipple resection, a concern that dictates omitting vagotomy, which might potentiate the problem. It was hoped that this complication would be less common when the pylorus is preserved. Unfortunately, pylorus-preserving pancreatic head resection is still associated with a reasonable rate of delayed gastric emptying. Some surgeons routinely employ a prokinetic agent during the immediate postoperative period after this procedure. Fortunately, long-term delayed gastric emptying is reported far less frequently. Pharmacologic acid suppression may be necessary.

Complications

Any pancreatic resection carries an associated risk of *pancreatic fistula*. In the past, this complication was considered to be the cause of the high mortality rate associated with these resections. Pancreaticoduodenectomy adds the risk of bile and gastrointestinal anastomotic leakage. Because of the rich vascular anatomy in the area of the head of the pancreas, *major bleeding* can also occur. Somewhat less recognized are the *vascular accidents* seen with this procedure. The dissection planes include the superior mesenteric vein, portal vein, common hepatic artery, and superior mesenteric artery. In a worst case scenario it is possible to interrupt completely the vascular supply to the liver (portal vein and hepatic artery) or the vascular supply or venous drainage to the intestine (superior mesenteric artery and portal vein). Thus necrosis of the liver and necrosis of intestine are known risks of this procedure.

Most pancreatic surgeons now place closed-suction drainage in the area of the pancreaticojejunostomy and the hepaticojejunostomy. Some believe this practice is responsible for the higher rate of reported pancreatic fistula than was seen in the past. This might be viewed with alarm were it not for the fact that the overall mortality for this procedure has now reached well below 5% and in capable hands may be 2–3%. In this regard, there appears to be conflicting data for the high rates of pancreatic fistula and low mortality rates. Most believe that the correlation of pancreatic fistula to mortality in the past was related to the coexistence of abdominal sepsis. Abdominal sepsis in the presence of the pancreatic fistula can be devastating because the microorganisms activate pancreatic enzymes and convert a benign pancreatic fistula to a lethal complication. There is consensus that pancreatic fistulas are far more common when the texture of the pancreas is essentially normal and soft; it is consequently poorly prepared to hold a stitch. With chronic pancreatitis or pancreatic carcinoma, the parenchyma is firm and holds sutures quite well. Technical faults may account for some of these fistulas. It should be stressed that a well drained pancreatic fistula in most series is a relatively meaningless complication, and spontaneous closure of such fistulas can be anticipated in more than 98% of patients.

Bile fistula may be more lethal than pancreatic fistula. Controlled bile fistula should be a fairly benign event when managed with closed-suction drainage. Spontaneous closure again should be anticipated in more than 98% of patients. An uncontrolled bile fistula, however, can result in bile peritonitis and sepsis and may represent an extremely morbid complication.

Dehiscence of the gastrointestinal anastomoses represents the least frequent of all complications. Prevent this problem by following the normal precepts of intestinal anastomotic technique.

Prevention of *vascular accidents* depends entirely on recognition of these structures, particularly the hepatic artery and the superior mesenteric artery. Each of these vessels may be unintentionally ligated. For that reason clear dissection of these structures is recommended. Unfortunately, superior mesenteric vein and portal vein injuries may occur simply because of dense adhesion to these structures due to chronic pancreatitis or to invasion of these structures by carcinoma.

ISLET CELL TUMORS

Islet cell tumors, which are rare, are well known to be diagnostically elusive. Their clinical presentation may be subtle; and localization of the tumor once the endocrinopathy has been defined is even more challenging. A number of modalities are utilized. Ultrasonography or spiral CT scans comprise a good initial approach. As with other potentially malignant lesions of the pancreas, ultrasonography is more effective for evaluating the liver for metastatic lesions; and spiral CT scanning is much more effect for evaluating the pancreas. Unfortunately, neither of these modalities is typically associated with significant success. Selective venous sampling (portal and splenic veins and venous tributaries from the pancreas), sometimes combined with the use of secretagogues such as secretin, has been used in the past with varying success.

The innovation of a radioisotope scan using *octreotide* as the marker has had some success for detecting all known islet cell tumors. It has been known for years that immunocytochemistry evaluation of islet cell tumors routinely yields the presence of various other islet cell products in addition to the primary one associated with the endocrinopathy in individual patients. In other words, a patient with an insulinoma is likely to have somatostatin and possibly glucagon or gastrin in the islets present within the insulinoma. In view of the added specificity of octreotide scanning, most recommend that it be performed early in the diagnostic workup of patients with suspected islet cell tumors.

The role of EUS and of laparoscopic ultrasonography remains uncertain. These modalities may reveal lesions not found using conventional imaging techniques. An advantage for both procedures is their ability to access the duodenal wall, which is the most common site of extrapancreatic gastrinoma.

Finally, one may be left with the challenge of establishing the location of these tumors intraoperatively and here *intraoperative ultrasonography* continues to play a major role. The so-called gastrinoma triangle is bounded by a vertical line drawn between the pylorus and the third portion of the duodenum. The apex of the triangle is the hilum of the liver, which is a reasonable starting point for assessing the possible locations of this entity. For all other islet cell tumors the primary site is almost always within the pancreatic parenchyma. In this regard, we simply advise careful evaluation of the uncinate process and the inferior border of the pancreas as the superior mesenteric vein progresses underneath it. Each of these sites is somewhat remote until adequate dissection has been performed.

Where possible, we recommend enucleation in almost all patients. If there is any evidence of extension beyond the capsule or if lymph node involvement (and certainly hepatic involvement) is evident, one must consider the malignant character or these lesions and undertake more extensive resection. It is important to realize that gastrinoma metastatic to the liver may be present in a patient for decades. We also advocate resection when lesions are strongly suspected in a particular location but are not easily defined in the operating room. In this case, a formal resection is preferable to blind excavation of the pancreas. One exception to the operative approach to islet cell tumors is when a gastrinoma is associated with multiple endocrine neoplasia type I. These patients have multiple sites of gastrinoma, and it is the general consensus that complete resection of each of these multiple lesions is unreasonable.

CHRONIC PANCREATITIS

Diagnosis

The diagnosis of chronic pancreatitis depends on a combination of episodic or daily moderate to severe upper abdominal pain radiating to the back associated with structural or functional derangements in the pancreas. Such derangements distinguish this entity from recurring acute pancreatitis or from acute relapsing pancreatitis. The functional derangements are endocrine or exocrine.

Endocrine dysfunction is reflected in insulin-dependent diabetes. This form of diabetes has been termed pancreatogenic diabetes or type III diabetes. Interesting studies have evaluated the differences between this form of diabetes and standard insulin-dependent diabetes known as type I diabetes. Vascular and neuropathic complications appear to be less common with pancreatogenic diabetes. *Exocrine insufficiency* presents clinically as pancreatic malabsorption, commonly manifested by fat malabsorption and steatorrhea. Both endocrine and exocrine dysfunction may be treated with replacement therapy even after near-complete loss of function. Much has been made of the challenging form of glucose hemostasis seen with end-stage chronic pancreatitis whereby glucose levels may fluctuate between a level as high as 900 mg/dl and, after insulin injection, as low as 30 mg/dl. This is attributed to the absence of the modulating effects of glucagon. These functional abnormalities may help establish the diagnosis.

Delineating *structural derangements* in the pancreas has become the mainstay for the diagnosis of chronic pancreatitis. For years the simple presence of calcification on an abdominal radiograph was the extent of the imaging capabilities. With the introduction of abdominal ultrasonography, some additional definition was obtainable. Abdominal CT scans greatly furthered this imaging detail. Conventional CT scanning is variable in its ability to define the main pancreatic duct. The nearly simultaneous development of ERCP offered the opportunity to define all of the fine details of ductal structure. In addition, coexistent abnormalities in the bile duct can be evaluated. By combining the spiral CT scan with ERCP, one may define sequentially the structural abnormalities associated with this disease.

The earliest abnormalities are known as *secondary ductular ectasia*. This entity suggests abnormalities seen only in the side branches of the main pancreatic duct with no significant abnormalities in the main pancreatic duct. Defining this specific abnormality remains the domain of ERCP, and none of the more advanced imaging has yet to compare with this sort of precision. EUS may prove competitive in this area, but as yet this subtle early structural change in chronic pancreatitis is seen only by ERCP.

Calcification in the parenchyma of the pancreas occurs in approximately 60% of patients with chronic pancreatitis. There is a greater prevalence of this finding in certain geographic areas, as there is clearly clustering of this disease in specific areas. It should be mentioned that it has been repeatedly observed that this disease may have differing presentations in different geographic areas. A *dominant mass* associated with chronic pancreatitis appears to be far more common in middle Europe than in the United States. Surgical management of this disease has been affected by this characteristic, and resectional therapy is correspondingly more routine in Europe. The variant of chronic pancreatitis with nondilated ducts, the so-called "small duct variant" of chronic pancreatitis, appears to be more common in Great Britain; and resectional therapy predominates there. Dilated ducts with a variably significant mass and head of the pancreas appears to be more common in the United States. Thus U.S. reports tend to include more of a mix of drainage procedures and resectional therapy.

After the initial signs of secondary ductular ectasia, the next anatomic abnormalities are associated with the *main pancreatic duct*. Typically, there is irregularity of the duct with areas of narrowing and areas of dilatation. In some, the main pancreatic duct may dilate to as much as 30 mm in diameter, whereas others may never be significantly dilated. Some may have such significant dilatation that it is interpreted as cystic structures within the pancreas. A mass effect is common and may reach the extreme of a mass in the head of the pancreas measuring 10 cm in diameter. The term dominant mass in the head of the pancreas is generally reserved for patients with a mass >5 cm in diameter. Segmental chronic pancreatitis may be seen in patients who have ductal obstruction from prior episodes of acute pancreatitis complicated by ductal disruption or in those who sustained injury to their pancreas after trauma. At some point in the development of this disease, some element of *narrowing of the common bile duct* may also be anticipated. This abnormality is found in 30-50% of patients with chronic pancreatitis. Significant dilatation of the common bile duct coexists with markedly elevated alkaline phosphatase levels and normal bilirubin. Only rarely does a patient with chronic pancreatitis present with true obstructive jaundice and significantly elevated serum bilirubin levels. This is one important means by which chronic pancreatitis can be distinguished from carcinoma of the pancreas, a distinction that has historically been considered challenging.

Pseudocysts are often associated with chronic pancreatitis. They are not significantly different from pseudocysts associated with acute pancreatitis and are not in themselves managed differently. It is our belief, however, that the approach to an incidentally found pseudocyst unassociated with a discrete episode of acute pancreatitis should include a review and determination of the coexistence of chronic pancreatitis. Many data, including our own, have shown that a patient presenting with abdominal pain and a pseudocyst and who has coexisting chronic pancreatitis experiences persistent pain after simple draining of a cyst. We advocate simultaneous management of the chronic pancreatitis and the cyst to achieve a successful outcome.

Thus from the point of view of imaging, the secondary ductular ectasia and defined changes in the ductular anatomy of the main pancreatic duct and of bile duct are by far best evaluated by ERCP. One should mention that MRCP has gained considerable attention as an alternative. It appears from early evaluations that many features are similar and that this procedure may well serve as an alternative if locally available. Although the fine detail of the main pancreatic duct is not as well seen, the general information is comparable. Information is gained about the common bile duct, and the study may be performed quickly and noninvasively. Spiral CT scanning provides considerably more detailed information regarding the main pancreatic duct than does conventional CT scan. It is also able to define the biliary tree in cross section, which can be helpful for defining biliary dilatation. Interestingly, the presence of calcification in the pancreas is found in an additional 10-15% of patients when evaluated by CT scanning compared to conventional radiography.

EUS also holds promise as a means of obtaining more precise detail of the parenchyma of the pancreas and of ductular abnormalities. Evaluating perioperative fluid collections is most clearly performed using spiral CT, MRCP, and EUS. It should be mentioned that it is rarely necessary to use all of these measures. We have obtained data suggesting that the associated ductal anatomy and communication or noncommunication with a pseudocyst may be helpful for establishing a treatment strategy; thus we advocate routine use of preoperative ERCP. The presence of ductal disruption or of communication between the cyst and the main pancreatic duct are aspects particularly helpful when choosing lesions best treated by percutaneous or endoscopic drainage. Laparoscopic and intraoperative ultrasonography should be included in the armamentarium of a pancreatic surgeon and can be helpful in the management of chronic pancreatitis and the cystic structures associated with chronic pancreatitis. A pseudocyst that is obvious on preoperative imaging may not be as obvious at operation.

To provide some insight into sequencing an evaluation, we currently apply spiral CT as a first modality and then ERCP immediately prior to operation. In general, the spiral CT scan provides information regarding masses in the pancreas and cystic structures surrounding the pancreas, and ERCP provides precise details of the ductal anatomy. It is sometimes necessary to perform a biopsy to confirm or disprove a possible diagnosis of carcinoma of the pancreas. EUS with simultaneous biopsies certainly offers this capability, as does CT-directed fine-needle aspiration.

Medical Management

The typical patient with chronic pancreatitis generally requires a period of intensive medical therapy before any consideration for surgery. Narcotic dependence is common owing to the chronic abdominal pain present in 95% of patients. This is complicated by the alcohol dependence or abuse that usually causes the disease. Nutritional depletion is common owing to exocrine or endocrine failure or to severe postprandial pain. Thus the immediate steps required are an evaluation of the nutritional status and the pancreatic functional status. Supplementing with insulin or enzymes is a significant first step. Textbooks could be written on the nuances of managing the narcotics needs of these patients, who have the challenging combination of chronic pain syndromes superimposed on a personality pre-disposed to addiction as reflected in their alcohol dependence.

Two kinds of abdominal pain are commonly seen with this disease. *Unrelenting abdominal pain* may occur daily, requiring chronic narcotic use. *Episodes of exacerbation* of pain unassociated with enzyme elevations or other signs may nonetheless be mistaken for an episode of acute pancreatitis. Some patients have daily pain without exacerbations; many have both; and certain patients have intermittent attacks only.

Octreotide, the somatostatin analog, has been investigated as an alternative to narcotics for pain management. Unfortunately, the studies using this modality were mixed at best, and there is no consensus on the use of this agent for this purpose [11]. *Anticholinergic medications* have been evaluated in the past without success. For years, oral enzyme supplements were used based on the theory that lack of digestive enzymes in the intestine results in the feedback signaling to cholecystokinin (CCK)-containing cells in the jejunum, which cause chronic stimulation of the pancreas and ongoing pain. Administration of enzyme supplements would theoretically reverse this feedback and reduce the CCK levels circulating in the blood, reduce chronic stimulation of the pancreas, and so reduce the pain associated with this disease. All clinical studies have failed to show an improvement using this mechanism; in practice, many still employ enzymes in the hope of reducing or abolishing the chronic unrelenting abdominal pain. We do not advocate this modality.

Finally, one may include *endoscopy* under the category of medical management. It should be noted that recent articles suggest that endoscopic placement of pancreatic ductal stents may ameliorate or abolish the pain associated with chronic pancreatitis. No prospective analysis has been performed, and suggestions have been made about the possible complications of these procedures, including stent failure and infectious complications in the pancreas. This entity continues to be explored. It can be viewed only as a temporary measure unless one wishes to replace the stents at intervals throughout this person's life. It is possible that successful pain relief by a stent may predict the success of operative decompression.

Surgical Management

One may infer from the data presented in the prior section that medical management has not been met with significant success; therefore most regard surgical management as the only reasonable option for patients sufficiently troubled by this disease. The indications for surgery are severe, unrelenting abdominal pain, in most cases resulting in narcotic dependence. Hence one would expect that in most cases it results in significant alteration of life style and quality of life based on the chronic pain and the narcotics requirements. The need for intermittent hospitalization is another important indicator supporting the use of invasive, potentially lethal treatments.

It is our belief that patients must be advised at the outset that some form of detoxification of their narcotic use is necessary after operation. The practitioner must be especially careful when evaluating drug-seeking behavior in regard to the patient's abdominal pain. Even in patients without addictive personalities, the chronic requirement of narcotics is likely to result in some element of dependence; and the success of the operative procedure can be established only after the patient has been completely weaned from narcotic usage.

Choice of Operation

In general terms the operative procedures for chronic pancreatitis include *resection, drainage* or *decompression*, and *nerve ablation*. The primary goal of each of these operative procedures is pain relief. *Pancreaticoduodenectomy*, typically performed as pylorus-preserving resection of the pancreatic head, is the classic resection. Indications for pancreaticoduodenectomy are the symptoms previously described combined with a dominant mass in the head of the pancreas. Resection is further indicated in any patient in whom there remains the suspicion of malignancy based on imaging studies or the relatively inaccurate CA 19-9 tumor marker. Resection is also considered reasonable after failure of a previous drainage procedure and is advocated in patients with a so-called small duct variance of chronic pancreatitis.

A variation of the classic Whipple resection known as the *duodenum-preserving pancreatic head resection* has been devised. This procedure was designed and has been championed by Hans Beger from Ulm, Germany; and further data have accrued through the work of Marcus Buchler in Berne, Switzerland [12]. In prospective studies, both the conventional Whipple operation and the duodenum-preserving pancreatic head resection achieve long-lasting pain relief in 75–95% of patients. The specific advantages suggested for duodenum preservation including enhanced nutritional status and better gastric emptying. The body of the pancreas is divided in a manner similar to that for the Whipple resection, and pancreatic tissue is excavated from the C-loop of the duodenum, preserving the floor of this dissection plane and leaving a small remnant of pancreas along the edges of the duodenum. Reconstruction is performed by placing a Roux limb of jejunum over the excavated head of the pancreas and similarly into the remnant of the body and tail of the pancreas after it has been divided.

This innovation forms the basis for a number of modifications that appear to be intermediary between drainage procedures and resections. They include the so-called Frey procedure, in which more limited excavation of the head of the pancreas is combined with longitudinal drainage of the main pancreatic duct. No division of the body of the pancreas is performed during this procedure [13]. After Frey's original description many have explored the effectiveness of the procedure, and the results have been favorable. The indications for this modification include a dilated main pancreatic duct throughout the gland associated with the mass and the head of the pancreas. A more recent innovation by Izbicki focuses on small duct disease treated with a V-shaped excavation along the body of the pancreas down to the main pancreatic duct [14]. The concept behind this procedure is to extract the inflammatory tissue surrounding the duct and created an operative equivalent of a Puestow-type drainage procedure. Unfortunately, the only data available regarding this procedure are those developed by Izbicki, who reported a high level of persistent pain relief after this procedure with apparent preservation of function. One important precept of surgery for chronic pancreatitis is that preservation of the pancreatic parenchyma is a goal, and all efforts to preserve function while providing adequate pain relief are desirable. Near-total or 95% pancreatectomy is almost never utilized, and we have no enthusiasm for this procedure.

Drainage Procedures

The classic drainage procedure is the *Puestow procedure*. In view of the prior discussion of the modifications of resection, it should be noted that the Puestow procedure is in fact just such a modification. It was developed as a modification of the Duval procedure: resection of the tail of the pancreas and Roux-en-Y jejunal drainage of the distal duct. Puestow modified the Duval procedure by combining resection of the tail of the pancreas with a longitudinal incision along the main pancreatic duct. This procedure has been evaluated extensively in clinical series and achieves 85-95% clearance of pain. Many give credit to Partington and Rochell for modifying the Puestow procedure by simply excluding resection of the tail of the pancreas, but the

true innovation was addition of a longitudinal incision along the pancreatic duct [15].

The Puestow procedure allows no loss of parenchymal tissue and provides persistent relief of pain. We have recently shown that the rate at which patients with chronic pancreatitis continue to lose function appears to be significantly delayed after the drainage procedure. Thus we suggest that the advantages of the Puestow-type drainage procedure are preservation of parenchyma and some protection from the inevitable loss of function seen with this disease. Mortality and morbidity rates for this procedure are also considerably lower than those for resective procedures, particularly the Whipple resection. Mortality rates of less than 1% and morbidity rates of less than 10% have been achieved with the Puestow procedure [16]. These figures compare favorably with the 2-5% mortality rate and the 25-40% morbidity rate associated with the Whipple resection.

The indication for operation is a dilated duct. Successful outcomes appear to be limited to ducts >6 mm in diameter. The diameter of a normal pancreatic duct is 2-3 mm. Ducts that have been less dilated have been associated with a higher failure rate in terms of achieving pain relief. It is conceivable that the rate improves when the modification previously described by Izbicki is used.

Biliary Decompression

Biliary stenosis and dilatation occur in 30-50% of patients with chronic pancreatitis. The problems vary from obvious narrowing seen by an imaging study with normal blood chemistries to a massively dilated common bile duct associated with significant elevations in the serum alkaline phosphatase levels (often above 1000 U/dl). Because the narrow area of the common bile duct is elongated, extending well beyond the wall of the duodenum, neither sphincterotomy nor long-term stenting is generally useful. There is some concern that prolonged obstruction of the bile duct results in ongoing fibrosis of the liver and finally leads to biliary cirrhosis. We generally reserve consideration of a simultaneous biliary drainage procedure for patients with significant dilatation of the common bile duct (>10 mm in diameter) associated with a chronically elevated alkaline phosphatase level (>400 U/dl). Although the purported advantage of biliary bypass is protecting the patient from biliary cirrhosis, the risk of developing biliary cirrhosis in this setting is not known. Supporting evidence comes from a study in which liver biopsies were done before and after biliary decompression in patients with chronic pancreatitis. Regression in hepatic fibrosis was noted [17]. Further support comes from the possibility that the chronic abdominal pain associated with chronic pancreatitis is due in part to biliary obstruction, and relieving this obstruction may also alleviate some of the pain.

Nerve Ablation

The concept of nerve ablation for chronic pancreatitis has been present for decades. In its first incarnation, *operative celiac ganglionectomy* was proposed. The success rates for this procedure was relatively low, and it was supplanted by percutaneous *chemical ablation of the celiac ganglion* with alcohol. When performed somewhat blindly, this procedure had an exceedingly low success rate. *CT* or *EUS guidance* achieves somewhat higher success rates. The relative indications for proceeding with nerve ablation have never been adequately established, but certainly this modality is ideal for patients who are not surgical candidates or who have failed resective procedures. We have had some successes with attempting repeat nerve ablation when the initial nerve ablation has failed.

Division of the thoracic sympathetic chain has also been suggested as a possible method for relieving abdominal pain associated with chronic pancreatitis. This method was further evaluated after the development of thoracoscopic techniques. Unfortunately, no large series have evaluated the success rates for this modality, and in general there is no enthusiasm for it.

CYSTIC LESIONS OF THE PANCREAS

Pseudocysts of the pancreas occur with both acute and chronic pancreatitis. As stated previously, it is our belief that this distinction is vital for proper management of patients with these lesions. Failure to recognize the coexistence of chronic pancreatitis may result in persistence of pain after treatment of an obvious pseudocyst. We therefore advocate combined decompression of the cyst and the main pancreatic duct when appropriate. We have developed data sufficient to establish a grading system for pancreatic pseudocysts [18]. In general, patients may be placed in three categories. First, patients may present with obvious chronic pancreatitis and a cystic structure. Second, some patients present with an episode of moderate to severe acute pancreatitis with peripancreatic fluid collections that finally coalesce into a pseudocyst. Finally, patients may present at an intermediate stage where the date of onset of the cyst is not apparent, and during workup for abdominal pain the patient is found to have the

cyst in the pancreas. The importance of these three categories is that patients associated with a clear episode of acute pancreatitis have an approximately 80% rate of spontaneous resolution. In contrast, patients with a known diagnosis of chronic pancreatitis have only a 4% spontaneous resolution rate. Thus operative intervention in our experience may proceed fairly promptly in patients with known chronic pancreatitis, whereas a minimum 4-week observation period is reasonable in patients with a cyst associated with acute pancreatitis because of the likelihood of spontaneous resolution. Patients in the intermediate stage are evaluated for the possibility of coexisting chronic pancreatitis. The rate of spontaneous resolution in this group is approximately 35%.

There is an area of pseudocyst management in which several proper treatment modalities overlap. In general, the choices include operative decompression of a cyst, percutaneous decompression of the cyst by interventional radiologists, and endoscopic transluminal decompression of a pseudocyst or endoscopic endoluminal transpapillary decompression of the cyst by placing a stent in the main pancreatic duct. Long-term success rates for percutaneous endoscopic and endoluminal decompression have been approximately 70%. These data are comparable to the known operative success rates for external drainage of pseudocysts established decades ago, which typically were about 70% as well. Although some endoscopic and some interventional studies have reported slightly higher success rates, long-term follow-up has been scant.

Infectious complications have been common after percutaneous or endoscopic drainage procedures. This is not altogether surprising, as many cysts contain solid or semisolid material that is unlikely to be adequately drained through passive drainage with relatively small catheters. It poses a risk for secondary infection after being exposed to microorganisms via drainage tubes. Despite this problem, we support the use of these alternative nonoperative methods when appropriate. We have explored the possibility of predicting who is best suited for each of these modalities based on the anatomy of the main pancreatic duct and the presence or absence of communication with the cyst.

The options for providing operative drainage include cystgastrostomy and Roux-en-Y cyst jejunostomy. Resection of the pancreatic pseudocyst is also an option and is generally reserved for cysts in the body and tail of the pancreas. At all times we favor obtaining an intraoperative frozen section biopsy specimen of the wall of the cyst to rule out the presence of a cystic neoplasm. An overall operative mortality rate of less than 3% should be achieved for pseudocyst drainage. Although many have reported morbidity rates of about 30%, our rates have been much lower when a Roux-en-Y cyst stage jejunostomy is done.

With regard to *cystic neoplasms*, the presence of a cystadenoma in a cyst surrounding the pancreas has been recognized as a possibility for decades. More recently, the important distinction between serous and mucinous adenomas has been established. The premalignant potential of serous adenomas is considered to nil. In contrast, mucinous adenoma is a recognized premalignant lesion. These lesions are more common in women, and cystadenocarcinoma is more common in older women. Patients with recognized mucinous adenomas are candidates for resection at all times.

Preoperative establishment of this diagnosis depends on a number of features. It is possible to aspirate fluid and measure mucin levels in the fluid. In addition, several investigators have suggested measuring tumor markers including carcinoembryonic antigen (CEA), CA 19-9, and pancreatitis-associated peptide (PAP). The presence of mucin is confirmatory, but the markers are not. Cytology may also be undertaken, and some studies have looked at CA 72-4 in cyst fluid levels. They concluded that pancreatic cysts with high serum CA 19-9 levels, positive cytology, or high CA 72-4 levels in the fluid should be considered for resection.

Accompanying the recent interest in cystic neoplasms of the pancreas has been a relative explosion in the variety of diagnoses. *Mucinous ductal ectasia* was recently defined, for example. A retrospective evaluation was performed at the Mayo Clinic in which lesions previously presumed to be conventional ductal adenocarcinoma were identified by retrospective analysis as mucinous ductal ectasia-associated ductal adenocarcinoma. This lesion is associated with massive dilatation of the ducts and ductules, significant dilatation of the ampulla, and thick viscous pancreatic fluid. This lesion has been recognized as premalignant, and resection is indicated whenever it is diagnosed. The term *intraductal papillary mucinous tumor of the pancreas* was subsequently established. Seeming to extend from this diagnosis are the cystic papillary neoplasms of the pancreas. Although rare, these entities must be considered in patients with cystic lesions of the pancreas, particularly in patients without a clear history of pancreatitis. I would caution that even with a reasonable suspicion for pancreatitis, these lesions may be present; and unfortunately, aspiration of the fluid may yield high levels of pancreatic enzymes, excluding this test as a means of distinguishing neoplasms from cysts associated with pancreatitis. Each

of these lesions is considered to be premalignant, and resection is recommended.

REFERENCES

1. Mertz HR, Sechopoulos P, Delbeke D, Leach SD. EUD, PET, and CT scanning for evaluation of pancreatic adenocarcinoma. Gastrointest Endosc 2000;52:376-71.

2. Pitt HA, Gomes AS, Lois JF, Mann LL, Deutsch LA, Longmire WP Jr. Does preoperative percutaneous biliary drainage reduce operative risk or increase hospital cost? Ann Surg 1985;201:545-53.

3. Schirmer WJ, Rossi RL, Braasch JW. Common difficulties and complications in pancreatic surgery. Surg Clin North Am 1991;71:1391-1417.

4. Breslin TM, Janjan NA, Lee JE, et al. Neoadjuvant chemoradiation for adenocarcinoma of the pancreas. Front Biosci 1998;3:E193-203.

5. Bold RJ, Charnsangavej C, Cleary KR, Jennings M, Madray A, et al. Major vascular resection as part of pancreaticoduodenectomy for cancer: radiologic, intraoperative, and pathologic analysis. J Gastrointest Surg 1999;3:233-43.

6. Vogel SB, Drane WE, Ros PR, Kerns SR, Bland KI. Prediction of surgical resectability in patients with hepatic colorectal metastases. Ann Surg 1994;219:508-516.

7. Jimenez RE, Warshaw AL, Fernandez-Del Castillo C. Laparoscopy and peritoneal cytology in the staging of pancreatic cancer. J Hepatobiliary Pancreat Surg 2000; 7:15-20.

8. Jessup JM, Steele G, Mayer R Jetal. Neoadjuvant therapy for unresectably pancreatic adenocarcinoma. Arch Surg 1993;128:559-564.

9. Mehta VK, Fisher G, Ford J, et al. Preoperative chemoradiation for marginally resectable adenocarcinoma of the pancreas. Gastro Intest Surg 2001;5:27-35.

10. Karpoff HM, Klimstra DS, Brennan MF, Conlon KC. Results of total pancreatectomy for adenocarcinoma of the pancreas. Arch Surg 2001;135:44-8.

11. Uhl W, Anghelacopoulos SE, Friess H, Buchler MW. The role of octreotide and somatostatin in acute and chronic pancreatitis. Digestion 1999;60:23-31.

12. Beger HG, Schlosser W, Friess HM, Buchler MW. Duodenum-preserving head resection in chronic pancreatitis changes the natural course of the disease: a single-center 26-year experience. Ann Surg 1999;230: 512-23.

13. Frey CF. The surgical management of chronic pancreatitis: the Frey procedure. Adv Surg 1999;32:41-85.

14. Izbicki Jr, Bloechle C, Broering DC, et al. Extended drainage versus resection in surgery for chronic pancreatitis: a prospective randomized trial comparing the longitudinal pancreaticojejunostomy combined with local pancreatic head excision with the pylorus-preserving pancreatoduodenectomy. Ann Surg 1998; 228:771-9.

15. Partington PF, Rochelle RE. Modified Puestow procedure for retrograde drainage of the pancreatic duct. Ann Surg 1960;152:1037–1042.

16. Izbicki JR, Bloechle C, Knoefel WT, Rogiers C, Kuechler T. Surgical treatment of chronic pancreatitis and quality of life after operation. Surg Clin North Am 1999;79:913–944.

17. Hammel P, Couvelard A, O'Toule Dital. Regression of liver fibrosis after biliary drainage in patients with chronic pancreatitis and stenosis of the common bile duct. N Engl J Med 2001;344:418–423.

18. Nealon WH, Walser E. Preoperative ERCP can direct choice of modality for treating pancreatic pseudocysts (surgery is percutaneous drainage). Paper presented at 35th Annual Meeting of the Pancreas Club, May 20, 2001; Atlanta, GA.

78 Partial Pancreatoduodenectomy

INDICATIONS

Carcinoma of ampulla, head of pancreas, distal bile duct, or duodenum

Select patients with chronic pancreatitis and intractable pain whose disease is limited to the head of the pancreas (see Chapter 77)

CONTRAINDICATIONS

Distant metastases (liver or peritoneal surfaces)

Distant lymph node metastases (celiac axis)

More than minimal invasion of portal vein, superior mesenteric vessels, or root of small bowel mesentery

In the absence of a surgical team experienced in pancreatoduodenectomy, when a patient suffering from obstructive jaundice has been found to have operable ampullary or pancreatic cancer refer the patient to an appropriate center of expertise.

PREOPERATIVE PREPARATION

Correct hypoprothrombinemia with vitamin K.

Accomplish nutritional rehabilitation, if necessary.

Perform diagnostic procedures. Selective use of computed tomography (CT), endoscopic retrograde cholangiopancreatography (ERCP), magnetic resonance imaging (MRI), endoscopic ultrasonography (EUS), and preoperative laparoscopy helps with accurate staging and minimizes nontherapeutic laparotomy for cancer of the pancreas.

Prescribe perioperative antibiotics.

Preoperative biliary decompression, formerly advocated, has not been shown to be beneficial and is rarely employed.

PITFALLS AND DANGER POINTS

Intraoperative hemorrhage

Trauma to or inadvertent ligation of superior mesenteric artery or vein, an anomalous hepatic artery, or the portal vein

Failure of pancreaticojejunal anastomosis with leakage

Failure of choledochojejunal anastomosis with leakage (rare)

Postoperative hemorrhage

Postoperative sepsis

Postoperative acute pancreatitis

Postoperative marginal ulcer with bleeding

OPERATIVE STRATEGY

The operation may be conceptualized as consisting of three stages: assessment of pathology to determine resectability, resection, and reconstruction. Standard pancreaticoduodenectomy, described first, includes a gastric resection. Pylorus-preserving pancreaticoduodenectomy avoids this resection, decreasing the operating time and producing a more physiologic result. This procedure is described second.

Assessment of Pathology to Determine Resectability

Better preoperative staging has decreased the probability of finding unexpected peritoneal metastases at laparotomy. Obvious disease outside the surgical field precludes resection; if none is found, the pancreas is mobilized to determine if local invasion (most commonly into the portal vein) precludes resection. Full mobilization is performed before committing to resection.

A generous Kocher maneuver is performed to confirm that the pancreas is not adherent to the inferior vena cava. The lesser sac is entered and the stomach elevated to display the pancreas. The most hazardous part of the operation occurs next, when the pancreas is gently elevated from the portal vein.

Avoiding and Managing Intraoperative Hemorrhage

The greatest risk of major intraoperative hemorrhage occurs when the surgeon is dissecting the portal vein away from the neck of the pancreas. This is especially true when an inexperienced pancreatic surgeon has misjudged the resectability of a carcinoma of the pancreas. In this case, while injudiciously trying to separate the portal vein from an invading carcinoma one can produce a major laceration of the portal vein before achieving sufficient exposure to effect a repair. Freeing the portal vein is the most dangerous step in this operation.

Temporary control of hemorrhage is generally possible in this situation if the surgeon compresses the portal and superior mesenteric veins against the tumor by passing the left hand behind the head of the pancreas. An experienced assistant then divides the neck of the pancreas anterior and just to the left of the portal vein. In some cases it is necessary to isolate and temporarily occlude the splenic, inferior mesenteric, superior mesenteric, coronary, and portal veins to achieve proximal and distal control. If tumor has indeed invaded the portal vein, a patch or a segment of vein may have to be excised to be replaced by a saphenous vein patch or, in some cases, a vein graft. An end-to-end anastomosis of the portal vein to the superior mesenteric vein is possible when the segment to be resected is short. To replace longer segments of resected portal vein, interpose a saphenous vein graft. Ligating the portal vein is often fatal unless the superior mesenteric vein is preserved and is free to drain *into the intact splenic and then into the short gastric veins.*

Avoiding Postoperative Hemorrhage

Postoperative hemorrhage is a preventable and potentially lethal complication. It stems from one of four major causes: (1) gastric stress ulcers or gastritis; (2) marginal ulcer; (3) digestion of the retroperitoneal blood vessels by combined leakage of both bile and pancreatic juice; or (4) inadequate ligature of the innumerable blood vessels divided during surgery.

Gastric stress ulcers or gastritis. After surgery, use an H_2-blocker or proton pump inhibitor to maintain the gastric pH at ≥ 5.0. Follow the protocol in the intensive care unit for surgical patients who are at risk of developing stress bleeding.

Marginal Ulcer

With the standard pancreaticoduodenectomy, the incidence of marginal ulcer is decreased by performing an adequate antrectomy and/or adding truncal vagotomy. This is less of a concern with current methods of pharmacological control of ulcer diathesis. Preservation of the pylorus may reduce the incidence of postoperative ulcers.

Hemorrhage secondary to the digestion of retroperitoneal tissues by activated pancreatic juice is best prevented by observing the operative strategy

(outlined below) aimed at minimizing the chance of pancreaticojejunal anastomotic leak. Hemorrhage that results from a ligature slipping off the gastroduodenal or right gastric artery is a result of careless operative technique. During pancreatectomy carefully *skeletonize* each of these two arteries prior to ligating them. Use nonabsorbable ligature material and *always leave an adequate stump of vessel distal to the ligature* to prevent slipping. The same principles apply to the branches of the portal and superior mesenteric veins.

Avoiding Leakage from the Pancreaticojejunal Anastomosis

Failure of the pancreaticojejunal anastomosis has in our experience been the most common serious technical complication of pancreatoduodenectomy. Failure of the anastomosis is more common in patients who have carcinoma of the distal portion of the common bile duct (CBD) or the duodenum because many of these patients do not develop obstruction of the pancreatic duct, which is frequently accompanied by some degree of pancreatitis. Both obstruction and pancreatitis produce thickening of the pancreatic duct and the pancreatic parenchyma.

In the absence of this thickening, sewing a small thin-walled duct to the jejunum produces a high failure rate. When a small duct and soft pancreatic parenchyma are encountered, some surgeons believe that total pancreatectomy is the safest alternative, even though it produces postoperative diabetes. This option is rarely needed. If the patient has a soft pancreas and a pancreatic duct that is not markedly enlarged, do not try to construct a duct-to-mucosa anastomosis. Rather, invaginate the pancreatic remnant into the lumen of the jejunum for a depth of at least 2 cm with two layers of sutures, as described later in the chapter. When the remaining pancreas is thickened with fibrosis and the duct has been markedly enlarged by the chronic obstruction, careful construction of an anastomosis between the pancreatic duct and the jejunal mucosa has a high likelihood of success. Rossi and Braasch insert a small catheter into the pancreatic duct in most patients and then lead the catheter through a puncture wound in the wall of the jejunum and out through the abdominal wall to drain the pancreatic secretions away from the healing anastomosis into a drainage bag. When we use this type of drainage, we leave the catheter in at least 2 weeks.

If leakage of pancreatic juice occurs, it is important to have adequate drains in the area of the anastomosis. Leakage of pure pancreatic juice that has not been activated does not damage the surrounding tissues, and the pancreatocutaneous fistula generally closes spontaneously without damaging the patient. On the other hand, if leakage from the pancreaticojejunostomy is accompanied by simultaneous seepage of bile into the same region, the pancreatic enzymes become activated and begin to digest the surrounding retroperitoneal tissues, leading to sepsis and bleeding—complications that constitute the chief causes of death following pancreatoduodenectomy. Consequently, make every attempt to divert the flow of bile from the area of the pancreaticojejunostomy, allowing an adequate length of jejunum to separate these anastomoses. This may help prevent the bile from refluxing up into the pancreaticojejunal anastomosis.

Treating a Pancreatic Fistula by Removing the Pancreatic Stump

When a patient suffers a pancreatocutaneous fistula that leaks clear pancreatic juice, only expectant therapy is necessary. If the clear, watery secretion turns green after a few days, indicating bile admixture, the situation is much more serious. A major leak of bile and pancreatic juice is associated with a high mortality rate. If the patient's condition begins to deteriorate despite adequate drainage, serious consideration should be given to exploration and removing the remnant of pancreas together with the spleen. Under certain conditions converting the Whipple operation to a total pancreatectomy constitutes a life-saving operation. Trede and Schwall reported success with this reoperation.

Avoiding Trauma to an Anomalous Hepatic Artery Arising from the Superior Mesenteric Artery

About 18-20% of individuals have an anomaly in which the common hepatic artery or right hepatic artery arises from the superior mesenteric artery, generally running posterior to the pancreas into the hepatoduodenal ligament. Such a vessel is encountered in the operative field and may be injured. Sometimes this anomaly is identified on preoperative imaging studies. In 1% of the cases in the anatomic study, the common hepatic artery arose from the superior mesenteric and passed *through* the head of the pancreas on its way to the liver; in this case pancreaticoduodenectomy necessitates dividing and ligating this vessel. The adequacy of the collateral circulation determines the effect on hepatic perfusion and ultimately on liver function.

Proper anatomic dissection of the superior mesenteric vessels away from the superior uncinate

process *with alert palpation of the posterior pancreas* allows the surgeon to identify this anomaly if it is not demonstrated on preoperative studies.

OPERATIVE TECHNIQUE

Standard pancreaticoduodenectomy

Incision

Make a midline incision from the xiphoid to a point 10 cm below the umbilicus. In stocky patients with a broad subcostal arch, a bilateral subcostal incision is an excellent alternative.

Evaluation of Pathology: Confirmation of Malignancy

If no tissue diagnosis has been obtained preoperatively, attempt to confirm the diagnosis by biopsy or fine-needle aspiration cytology (FNAC). Divide the omentum between hemostats to expose the anterior surface of the pancreatic head **(Fig. 78–1)**. If a stony-hard area of tumor is visible on the anterior or pos-

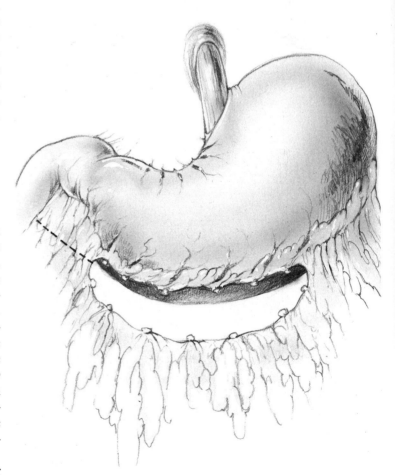

Fig. 78-1

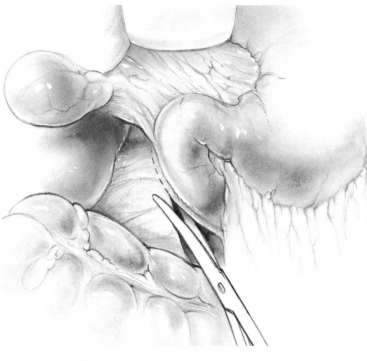

Fig. 78-2

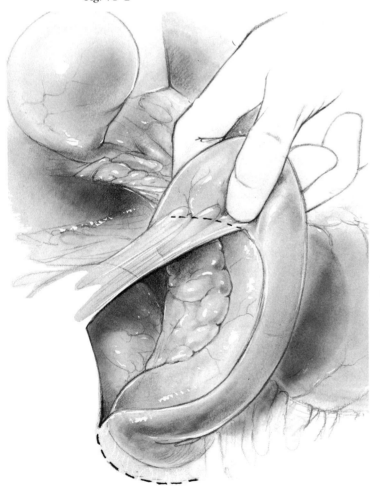

Fig. 78-3

terior surface of the pancreas, shave the surface of the tumor with a scalpel or remove a wedge of tissue. If the tumor appears to be deep, perform FNAC by inserting a 22-gauge needle into the tumor. Use a 10 ml syringe containing 4–5 ml of air. Aspirate and then expel the sample on a sterile slide; spray the slide *promptly* with a fixation solution and submit the slide for immediate cytologic study. In most cases we have found FNAC both safe and accurate.

If the results are not confirmatory for cancer, perform a biopsy by passing a cutting biopsy needle through both walls of the duodenum on its way to the pancreas. This technique helps avoid a postoperative pancreatic fistula. When lesions of the distal common duct are suspected, obtain a tissue sample by passing a small curet through a cholodochotomy incision and scrape the region of the suspected malignancy. Choledochoscopy is an excellent means for obtaining a biopsy of common duct tumors. If a tumor is palpable in the region of the ampulla, make a longitudinal or oblique duodenotomy incision over the mass and excise a sample under direct vision. Close the duodenotomy. Discard all instruments that have come into contact with the tumor during the biopsy and redrape the field. Occasionally it is necessary to proceed without confirmation of malignancy.

If malignancy has *not* been confirmed and there is not excellent preoperative radiographic visualization of the CBD, perform operative cholangiography or choledochoscopy to rule out an impacted common duct stone as the cause of the patient's jaundice. Next, evaluate the lesion for operability. Check for metastatic involvement of the liver, the root of the small bowel mesentery, and the celiac axis lymph nodes. Metastasis to a lymph node along the gastrohepatic or gastroduodenal artery adjacent to the malignancy does not contraindicate resection.

Determination of Resectability; Dissection of Portal and Superior Mesenteric Veins

Perform an extensive Kocher maneuver by incising the peritoneal attachment **(Fig. 78–2)** along the lateral portion of the descending duodenum. Divide the lateral duodenal ligament to the point where the superior mesenteric vein crosses the transverse duodenum **(Fig. 78–3)**. Avoid excessive upward traction on the duodenum and pancreas, as it may tear the superior mesenteric vein. Liberate the duodenum superiorly as far as the foramen of Winslow.

If the head of the pancreas is replaced by a relatively bulky tumor, it may be difficult to expose the superior mesenteric vein. In such cases, after divid-

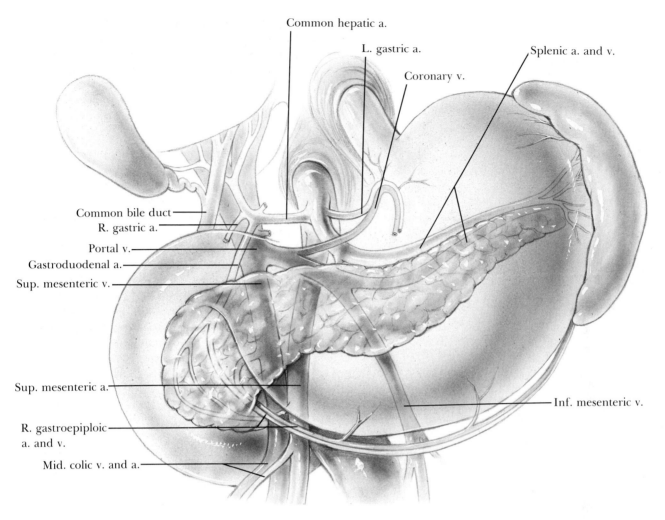

Common hepatic a.

L. gastric a.

Coronary v.

Splenic a. and v.

Common bile duct

R. gastric a.

Portal v.

Gastroduodenal a.

Sup. mesenteric v.

Sup. mesenteric a.

R. gastroepiploic a. and v.

Mid. colic v. and a.

Inf. mesenteric v.

Fig. 78-4

ing the omentum to expose the anterior surface of the pancreas, identify the middle colic vein and trace it to its junction with the superior mesenteric vein **(Fig. 78–4)**. Although this junction may be hidden from view by the neck of the pancreas, one can generally identify the superior mesenteric vein without difficulty by following the middle colic vein. Gentle dissection is important in this area as there are often large fragile branches joining both the middle colic and the superior mesenteric veins with the inferior pancreaticoduodenal vein. If these branches

are torn, control of bleeding behind the neck of the pancreas is difficult.

Gross invasion of the vena cava or the superior mesenteric vein contraindicates resection. Identify the hepatic artery medial to the lesser curvature of the stomach after incising the filmy avascular portion of the gastrohepatic omentum. Incise the peritoneum overlying the common hepatic artery and sweep the lymph nodes toward the specimen. Continuing this dissection toward the patient's right reveals the origin of the gastroduodenal artery. Dissect

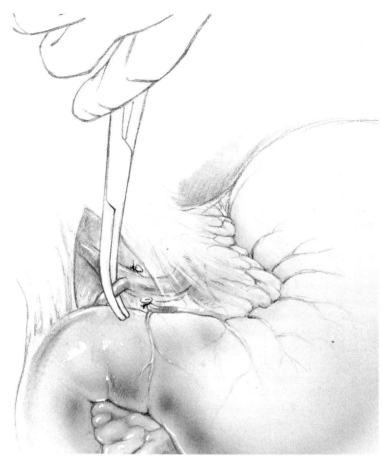

Fig. 78-5

this artery free using a Mixter clamp **(Fig. 78–5)** and divide the vessel between two ligatures of 2-0 silk, leaving about 1 cm beyond the proximal tie to prevent the possibility of the ligature slipping off. Continue the dissection just deep and slightly medial to the divided gastroduodenal artery and identify the anterior aspect of the portal vein **(Fig. 78–6)**. In the presence of carcinoma near the head of the pancreas there are often numerous small veins superficial to the portal vein. *Do not use hemostatic clips in this area* because they would be inadvertently wiped away during the subsequent dissection and manipulation. Individually divide and ligate each vessel with 3-0 or 4-0 silk ligatures.

After identifying the shiny surface of the portal vein, gently free this vein from the overlying pancreas using a peanut sponge dissector. If there is no invasion of the portal vein by tumor, there is no attachment between the anterior wall of the portal vein and the overlying pancreas; thus a finger can be passed between this vein and the neck of the pancreas **(Fig. 78–7)**. Maximize the distance from the tumor by staying slightly on the left, rather than the right, as this dissection is performed. Occasionally, this is easier to accomplish by inserting the finger from below the pancreas between the superior mesenteric vein and the overlying gland. With one finger inserted between the neck of the pancreas

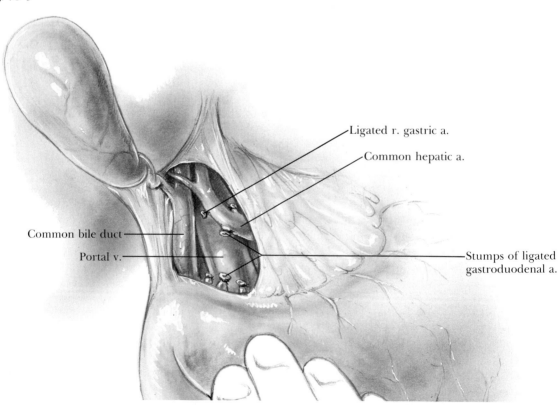

Ligated r. gastric a.

Common hepatic a.

Common bile duct

Portal v.

Stumps of ligated gastroduodenal a.

Fig. 78-6

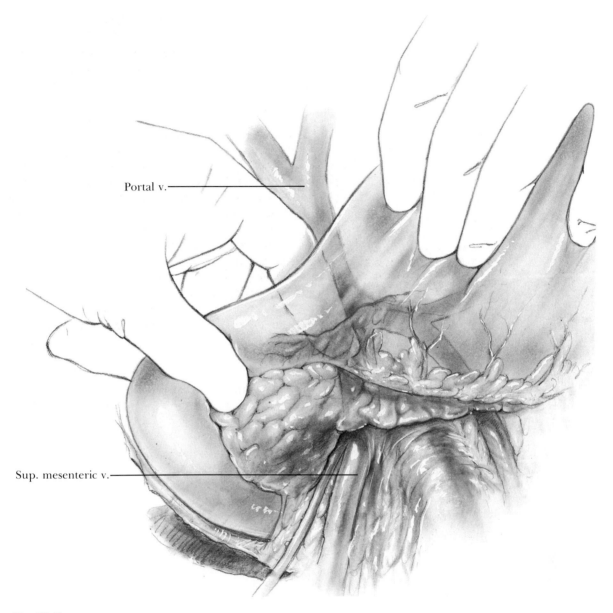

Portal v.

Sup. mesenteric v.

Fig. 78-7

and the superior mesenteric vein, pass the other hand behind the head of the pancreas and try to determine if the tumor has invaded the uncinate process, the posterior side of the portal vein, or the superior mesenteric vessels. If all of the above conditions have been fulfilled, the tumor is probably resectable; and one may proceed now with pancreatectomy. Execute this dissection carefully, as it is the most hazardous during the entire procedure. If the tumor has invaded the portal vein and the finger dissection produces laceration of the vein, controlling the hemorrhage is extremely difficult. (See discussion above under Operative Strategy.)

Continue the dissection of the hepatic artery by dividing and ligating the right gastric artery. Incise the peritoneum over the common hepatic artery as far as the porta hepatis. Unroof and expose the CBD and sweep the lymphatic tissue from the porta hepatis down to the specimen, thereby skeletonizing the hepatic artery and CBD.

Cholecystectomy

Perform a cholecystectomy in the usual manner (see Chapter 66 and Fig. 79-12). Encircle the common hepatic duct just proximal to the point where it is joined by the cystic duct. Apply an occluding temporary ligature or clamp to the hepatic duct and divide it distal to the ligature or clamp, sweeping lymphatic tissue toward the specimen.

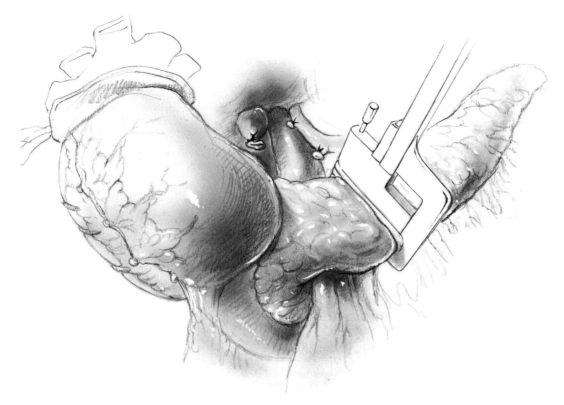

Fig. 78–8a

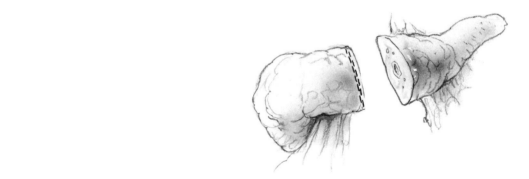

Fig. 78–8b

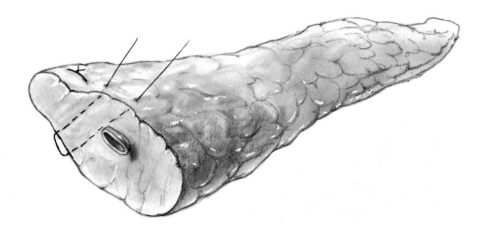

Fig. 78–9

Vagotomy and Antrectomy

Proceed with vagotomy (if desired) and antrectomy (see Chapters 25 and 29; see also Fig. 79-11). Swing the divided stomach to the right to expose the body of the pancreas fully.

Division of Pancreas

In patients with periampullary or distal CBD tumors there may be no obstruction of the pancreatic duct. Place the line of division of the pancreas 3 cm to the left of the superior mesenteric vessels. This leaves a remnant of pancreatic tail that is suitable for implanting into the open end of the jejunum when the pancreatic duct is too small for a good anastomosis. If this method is elected, carefully free the neck and body of the pancreas from the underlying splenic vein by working from above and from below. A few small branches from the pancreas to the splenic vein may require division.

After the neck and body of the pancreas have been elevated, apply a 35/3.5 mm linear stapler across the pancreas **(Fig. 78–8a)**. Fire the stapling device and divide the pancreas *to the left* of the stapling device **(Fig. 78–8b)**. Identify the pancreatic

duct and insert a plastic catheter into the duct to prevent its being occluded by sutures **(Fig. 78–9)**.

In patients who have an ampullary carcinoma that obstructs the pancreatic duct, the thickened, dilated duct together with the secondary pancreatitis produced by this obstruction makes both the duct and the pancreas suitable for accurate suturing. The same technique of division is used. Generally, it is necessary to suture-ligate a superior and an inferior pancreatic artery in the pancreatic stump.

Dissection of Uncinate Process

Retract the cut, stapled end of pancreas and the divided stomach toward the patient's right, exposing the anterior surface of the superior mesenteric and portal veins **(Fig. 78–10)**. Two or three arterial branches of the superior mesenteric artery pass deep to the superior mesenteric vein and into the head of the pancreas and are generally easy to identify. Divide and ligate each with 3-0 silk. Several branches from the pancreas drain into the superior mesenteric vein from the patient's right. These too are divided and ligated. The superior mesenteric vein may now be gently retracted to the patient's left, revealing the superior mesenteric artery. The uncinate process

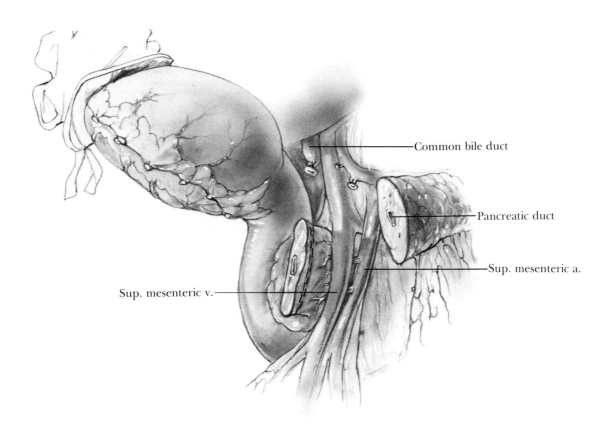

Fig. 78-10

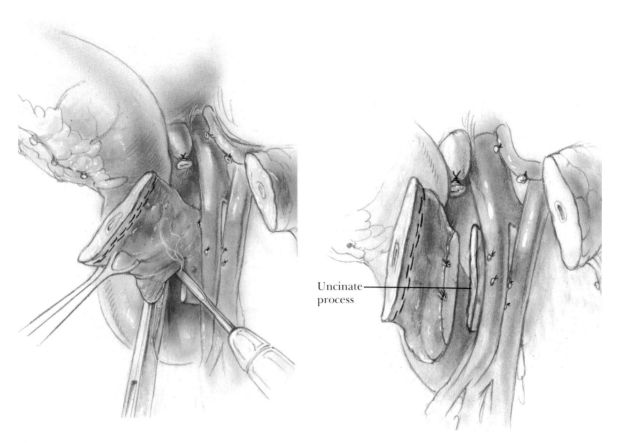

Fig. 78-11

Uncinate process

Fig. 78-12

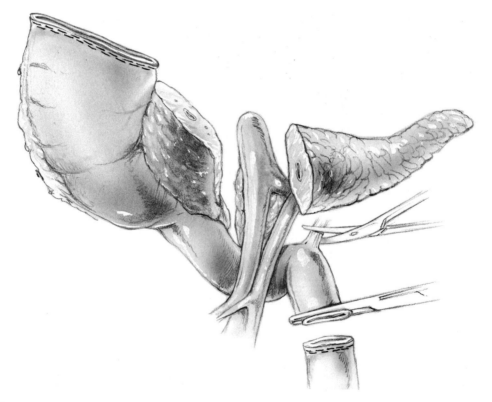

Fig. 78-13

may terminate at this point in some fibroareolar tissue. Divide it under direct vision. More often a tongue of uncinate process is attached to the posterior surface of the superior mesenteric artery. First pass the left hand behind the uncinate process *to check again that there is no major anomalous hepatic artery* coming from the superior mesenteric. Use electrocautery to divide the uncinate process **(Figs. 78–11, 78–12)**. Another convenient method is to apply a 55/3.5 mm linear stapler across the uncinate process prior to dividing it. Be certain to avoid injuring the superior mesenteric vein and artery. At the end of this dissection the gastric antrum, duodenum, and head of the pancreas are attached only at the duodenojejunal junction **(Fig. 78–13)**.

It is possible to save 10–12 minutes of operating time by applying a cutting linear stapler across the fourth portion of duodenum and dividing the duodenum, thereby releasing the specimen from all of its attachments. The proximal and distal segments of divided duodenum are thus closed by staples, which avoids the need to divide the proximal jejunal mesentery and free the duodenojejunal junction from the ligament of Treitz. The stomach, hepatic duct, and pancreas can each then be anastomosed end-to-side to the jejunum. Most surgeons do free the duodenojejunal junction from the ligament of Treitz, divide the mesentery in this region, and divide the jejunum a few centimeters beyond the ligament of Treitz. This procedure is described in the next section.

Dissection and Division of Proximal Jejunum

Expose the ligament of Treitz under the transverse mesocolon and divide it so the duodenojejunal junction is completely free. Serially clamp, divide, and ligate each of the mesenteric branches from the superior mesenteric vessel to the proximal 6–8 cm of the jejunum. This maneuver releases the proximal jejunum. Unless it is planned to implant the pancreatic tail into the open end of jejunum, apply a 55/3.5 mm linear stapling device across the proximal jejunum and fire it (see Fig. 79–14). Then using a scalpel divide the jejunum flush with the stapler. Lightly electrocoagulate the everted mucosa and remove the stapling device (see Fig. 79–15). It is not necessary to invert this staple line with a row of sutures. Remove the specimen.

Pancreaticojejunal Duct-to-Mucosa Anastomosis

Pass 12–13 cm of proximal jejunum through the aperture in the transverse mesocolon. Construct an end-

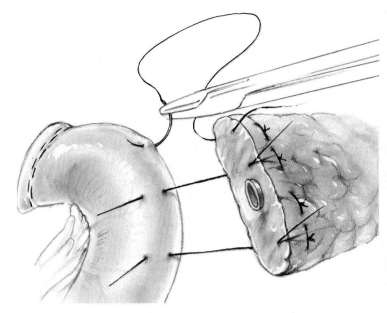

Fig. 78-14

to-side pancreaticojejunostomy along the antimesenteric aspect of the jejunum, beginning at a point about 3 cm from the staple line. Use interrupted 4-0 Prolene stitches to suture the posterior capsule of the pancreas to the seromuscular layer of jejunum **(Fig. 78–14)**. Then make a small incision slightly larger than the diameter of the pancreatic duct **(Fig. 78–15)**. Approximate the pancreatic duct to the full thickness of the jejunal wall using interrupted 6-0 Prolene or

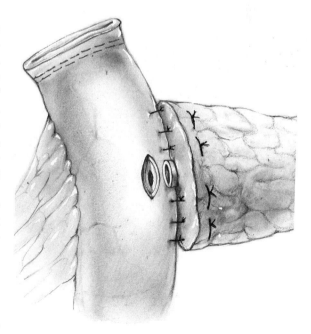

Fig. 78-15

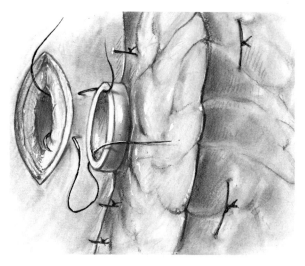

Fig. 78–16

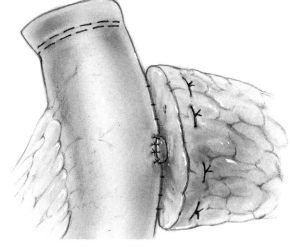

Fig. 78–17

PDS sutures **(Fig. 78–16)**. Wearing telescopic lenses with 2.5× magnification is helpful for ensuring an accurate anastomosis. After the posterior half of this anastomosis has been completed, insert an 8–10F pediatric feeding tube into the pancreatic duct. Thread the long end of the catheter into the jejunum. Make no holes in the catheter on the jejunal side of the anastomosis. The catheter is brought out from the jejunum about 10 cm beyond this anastomosis and passed through a stab wound in the abdominal wall for drainage to the outside. Insert a 4-0 silk purse-string suture around the hole in the jejunum through which the catheter exits. Then complete the duct-to-jejunum anastomosis with 6-0 Prolene or PDS sutures

(Fig. 78–17). Carefully buttress the remainder of the pancreas into the anterior wall of jejunum with additional 4-0 sutures **(Fig. 78–18)**. It is important to suture the catheter to the pancreas by means of a single 5-0 PG stitch; otherwise it is easily dislodged during subsequent steps of the operation. Also suture the jejunostomy site to the stab wound of the abdominal wall if possible.

Pancreaticojejunal Anastomosis by Invagination

An alternative method for anastomosing pancreas to jejunum is to invaginate 2–3 cm of the pancreatic

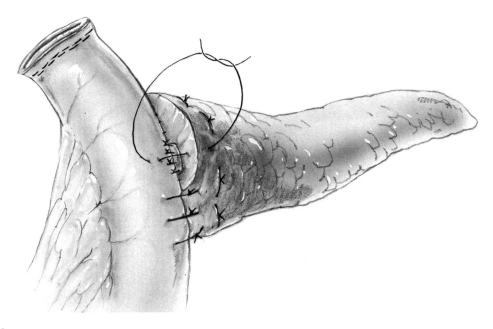

Fig. 78–18

stump into the lumen. First insert a catheter into the pancreatic duct as described above. Suture the catheter into the duct with fine PG. Pass 3 cm of the pancreatic stump into the open proximal end of the jejunum, which is easily accomplished by inserting guide sutures at the superior and inferior margins of the anastomosis. Use 4-0 Prolene and insert the needle into the superior aspect of the jejunum 3 cm away from its proximal margin **(Fig. 78–19a)**.

Using the same needle, take a bite of the superior margin of the pancreas. Then return the same suture from the lumen out through the open end of the jejunum, emerging 3 cm from the cut edge. Place an identical suture at the inferior margin of the jejunum and pancreas. By putting traction on these two sutures, the pancreas can be brought into the open end of the jejunum. If the jejunum does not accommodate the pancreas because the pancreatic stump is too large, inject glucagon (1 mg) intravenously to relax the jejunum. If the jejunum still cannot accommodate the pancreatic stump after

glucagon injection, utilize the techniques described below where the pancreatic stump is invaginated into the jejunum through an incision in the jejunum along its antimesenteric margin. Bring the catheter out of the jejunum through a small stab wound 6–8 cm distal to the pancreaticojejunal anastomosis. If an external drainage catheter is not used, insert a short segment (4–5 cm) of catheter into the pancreatic duct so about 1–2 cm projects beyond the cut edge of the duct. This helps prevent some of the sutures used to create the anastomosis from encompassing the duct and thereby occluding it. This tube is ejected into the intestinal stream spontaneously at a later date. Now insert additional 4-0 Prolene sutures to fix the cut edge of the pancreas to the circumference of the jejunum **(Fig. 78–19b)**. If the sutures are inserted but not tied, this step can be accomplished under direct vision to avoid damage to the pancreatic duct. When the sutures have been inserted, the pancreas is readjusted in its new location inside the jejunal lumen, and each of the

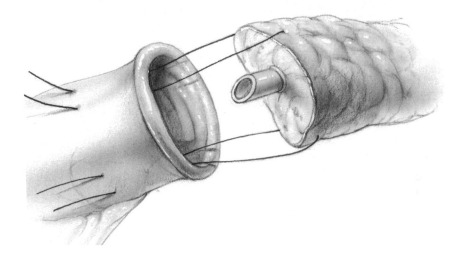

Fig. 78–19a

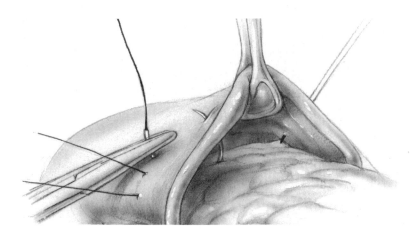

Fig. 78–19b

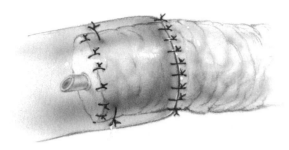

Fig. 78-20

sutures is tied. A second layer of Lembert sutures is inserted from the proximal cut edge of the jejunum to the periphery of the pancreas in such fashion that the jejunal mucosa is inverted **(Fig. 78–20)**.

Another method for intussuscepting the pancreatic stump into the jejunum is described beginning with **Figure 78–21**. Using interrupted 4-0 Prolene or silk, insert Lembert-type stitches to approximate the pancreas to the jejunum at a point 2.5 cm from their proximal margins, as shown. After completing this seromuscular layer of sutures, insert a second

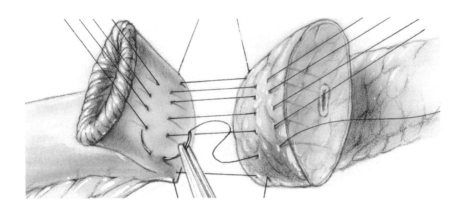

Fig. 78-21

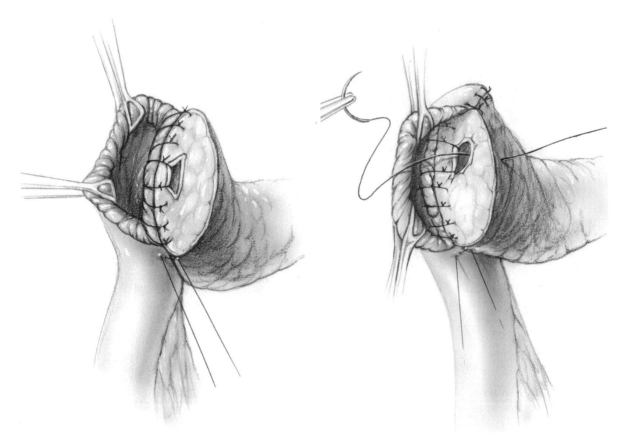

Fig. 78-22   Fig. 78-23

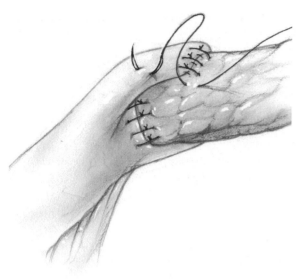

Fig. 78-24

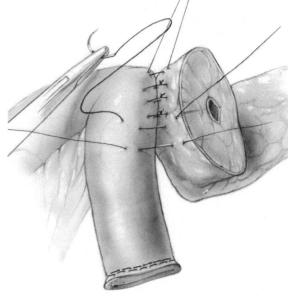

Fig. 78-26

layer, approximating the proximal margin of the pancreas to the full thickness of jejunum, as demonstrated in **Figure 78–22**. If the pancreatic duct is large enough, include the posterior wall of the pancreatic duct in the suture line as shown. The first layer in the anterior suture line is demonstrated in **Figure 78–23**. Use Lembert sutures to invert the mucosa of the jejunum into the parenchyma of the pancreas. The final anterior row of sutures between the seromuscular coat of jejunum to the pancreas completes the intussusception of the pancreas into the jejunum, as shown in **Figures 78–24** and **78–25**.

When the stump of the pancreas is too large to be invaginated into the lumen of the jejunum even after administration of glucagon, another method may be employed. As shown in **Figure 78–26**, close the cut end of the jejunum with a 55/3.5 mm linear stapling device. This need not be inverted by a layer of sutures. Approximate the cut edge of the pancreas to the antimesenteric border of the jejunum to

complete an end-to-side anastomosis, leaving 1–2 cm of jejunum hanging freely beyond the anastomosis. Insert 4-0 sutures of the Lembert type, approximating the seromuscular coat of the jejunum to the pancreas. The pancreatic sutures should be inserted about 1.5 cm away from its cut edge. When this layer is complete, make an incision along the antimesenteric border of the jejunum slightly shorter than the diameter of the pancreas, as seen in **Figure 78–27**. Then insert sutures between the posterior edge of

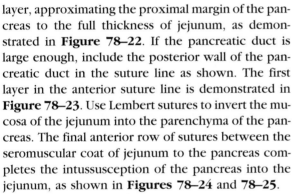

Fig. 78-25

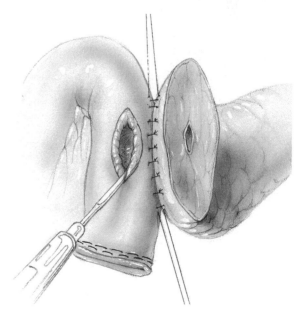

Fig. 78-27

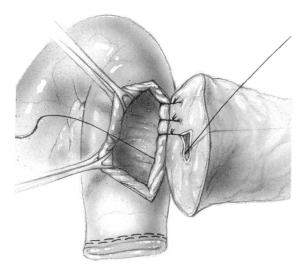

Fig. 78-28

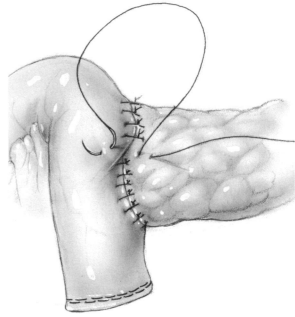

Fig. 78-30

the pancreas, taking the full thickness of the jejunum in interrupted fashion to constitute the second posterior layer. If the pancreatic duct is large enough, include the posterior wall of the pancreatic duct in the sutures **(Fig. 78–28)**. Again, use interrupted 4-0 sutures to approximate the anterior edge of the pancreas to the full thickness of the jejunum, as in **Figure 78–29**. The final anterior layer of sutures complete the invagination of the pancreas by approximating the anterior wall of the pancreas to the seromuscular coat of the jejunum, as in **Figure 78–30**.

Hepaticojejunal Anastomosis

Before anastomosing the hepatic duct to jejunum, make a tiny stab wound in the anterior wall of the hepatic duct about 3 cm proximal to its cut end. Insert a Mixter clamp into the hepatic duct through

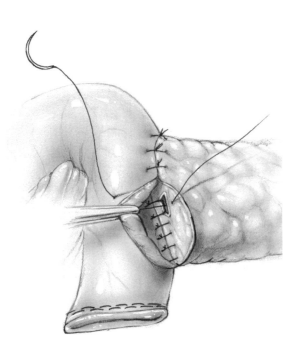

Fig. 78-29

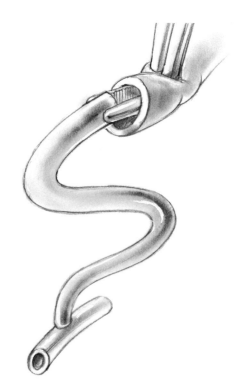

Fig. 78-31

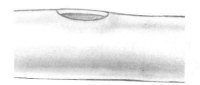

Fig. 78–33

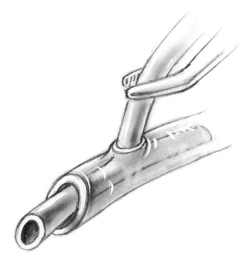

Fig. 78–32

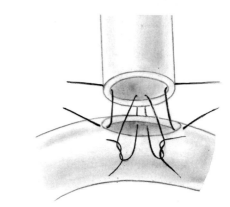

Fig. 78–34

the stab wound. Grasp the *long arm* of a 16F or 18F T-tube **(Fig. 78–31)** and draw it through the stab wound **(Fig. 78–32)**. The purpose of this T-tube is to drain bile to the outside until the pancreaticojejunostomy has completely healed.

Make an incision on the antimesenteric border of the jejunum **(Fig. 78–33)** about 15–20 cm distal to the pancreaticojejunostomy. The jejunal incision should be approximately equal to the diameter of the hepatic duct. Use one layer of interrupted 5-0 PDS or PG sutures to approximate the full thickness of hepatic duct to the full thickness of jejunum **(Fig. 78–34)**. Tie the knots of the posterior layer of sutures in the lumen. The anterior knots are placed on the serosal surface of the hepaticojejunal anastomosis. On the jejunal side of the anterior layer use a seromucosal-type stitch (see Fig. 4-13). Leave only 3-4 mm of space between sutures **(Fig. 78–35)**. We have not found it necessary to insert two layers of sutures. If the diameter of the hepatic duct is small, enlarge the ductal orifice by making a small Cheatle incision in the anterior wall of the duct.

Gastrojejunostomy

Identify the proximal jejunum and bring it to the gastric pouch in an antecolic fashion. Place the antimesenteric border of jejunum in apposition with the posterior wall of the residual gastric pouch for the gastrojejunal anastomosis. Leave 10-20 cm between the hepaticojejunostomy and the gastric anastomosis. Insert a guy stitch approximating the antimesenteric wall of the jejunum to the greater curvature of the stomach at a point about 3 cm proximal to the previously placed staple line. Then, with electrocautery make small stab wounds in the posterior wall of the stomach and the jejunum. Insert the linear cut-

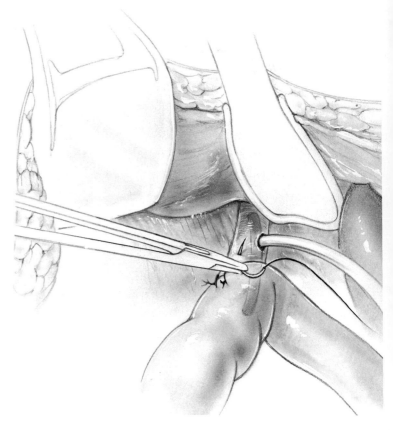

Fig. 78–35

ting stapling device, one fork in the gastric lumen and one in the jejunum (see Fig. 29–44). Be certain there is no extraneous tissue between the walls of the stomach and the jejunum. After locking the stapler, insert a single Lembert stitch to approximate the stomach and jejunum at the tip of the stapler; then fire and remove it. Carefully inspect the staple line for bleeding, which should be corrected by cautious electrocoagulation or insertion of 4-0 PG sutures. Apply Allis clamps to the anterior and posterior terminations of the staple line. Use additional Allis clamps to close the remaining aperture in the gastrojejunal anastomosis. Apply a 55 mm linear stapler deep to the line of Allis clamps and fire the staples. (The details of this technique are described in Chapter 29.)

Close the defect in the mesocolon at the region of Treitz's ligament by means of continuous and interrupted sutures of 4-0 PG around the jejunum and its mesentery. Try to isolate the hepaticojejunal anastomosis from the pancreatic anastomosis by suturing the free edge of the omentum to the remaining

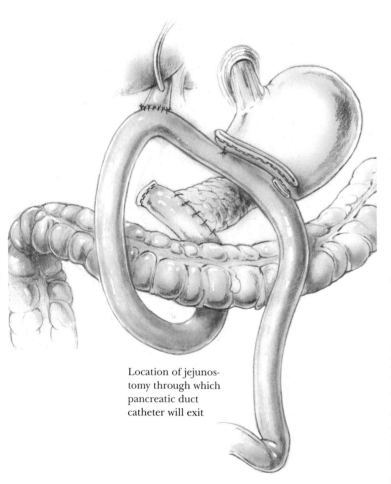

Location of jejunostomy through which pancreatic duct catheter will exit

Fig. 78–36

hepatoduodenal ligament overlying the hepatic duct. Intermittently during the entire operation a dilute antibiotic solution is used to irrigate the operative field. **Figure 78–36** illustrates the completed operation.

Insertion of Drains

Insert a closed-suction drain through a stab wound in the right upper quadrant down to the vicinity of the hepaticojejunostomy. Allow the T-tube to exit through a separate stab wound in the right upper quadrant.

Bring the pancreatic catheter through a tiny stab wound in the antimesenteric wall of the jejunum about 10 cm distal to the pancreatic anastomosis. Place a 4-0 silk purse-string suture around this tiny stab wound; then make a stab wound in the appropriate portion of the abdominal wall, generally in the right upper quadrant, and bring the catheter through this stab wound. If feasible, fix the jejunum to the abdominal wall around the catheter's exit point using four sutures of interrupted 3-0 PG, one suture to each quadrant. This prevents intraperitoneal leakage of jejunal contents. Connect this catheter to a plastic collecting bag. Alternatively, bring the catheter through a stab wound in the *proximal* jejunum as depicted in Figure 78–39. Through stab wounds in the left upper quadrant, insert Jackson-Pratt closed-suction drains and place them in the vicinity of the pancreaticojejunostomy and subhepatic spaces.

Needle-Catheter Jejunostomy

Consider performing a needle-catheter jejunostomy during all pancreatoduodenectomies. If the patient should suffer from delayed gastrointestinal function due to leakage of one of the anastomoses, jejunal feedings are superior to total parenteral nutrition.

Closure

Close the abdominal wall using No. 1 PDS sutures in the usual fashion.

Partial Pancreatoduodenectomy with Preservation of Stomach and Pylorus

The important steps of partial pancreatoduodenectomy are identical with the standard Whipple pancreatoduodenectomy except that the pylorus, 2 cm of duodenum, and all of the vagus nerve branches are preserved. In the hope of reducing the risk of marginal ulceration, we place the duodeno-jejunal anastomosis closer to the biliary and pancreaticojejunal anastomoses than is the case with the Whipple operation.

Included in this operative description is a method for bringing the pancreatic catheter to the abdominal wall through a tiny stab wound near the closed proximal end of the jejunal segment (Fig. 78-39). This has the important advantage that the length of the catheter between the pancreatic duct and the abdominal wall is much less than that described for the Whipple operation (above).

Operative Technique

Follow the procedure described in the first part of this chapter with the following exceptions.

1. Do not perform a vagotomy.
2. Dissect the posterior wall of the duodenum off the head of the pancreas for a distance of 2.5 cm after dividing and ligating the gastroduodenal and right gastric arteries as described above.
3. Apply the cutting linear stapling device to the duodenum at a point about 2.5 cm distal to the pylorus. Fire the stapling device. This transects the duodenum and staples closed the proximal and distal ends of the divided duodenum.
4. *Be careful to avoid injuring the gastroepiploic arcade* in the greater omentum along the greater curvature of the stomach, as much of the blood supply to the proximal duodenum now comes from the intact left gastroepiploic artery down to the pylorus. Beyond this point the duodenum is fed by the intramural circulation. Additional blood supply comes from the left gastric artery along the lesser curve of the stomach.
4. Anastomose the end of the duodenum to the antimesenteric side of the jejunum at a point about 20 cm distal to the hepaticojejunal anastomosis.

Bring the jejunum fairly directly from the hepaticojejunostomy to the duodenum for an end-to-side duodenojejunal anastomosis in the supramesocolic space.

5. The first step when preparing for the anastomosis is to apply several Allis clamps to the line of staples closing the duodenum. Then excise the staple line with scissors, leaving the duodenum wide open. Observe the cut duodenum for adequacy of bleeding. Although pulsatile flow is not generally seen and the duodenum may be somewhat cyanotic, fairly brisk oozing of red blood is an indication of satisfactory circulation.
6. Do not place the anastomosis close to the pylorus because the close proximity of the suture line to the pylorus interferes with pyloric function and results in gastric retention. Insert a layer of 4-0 interrupted silk Lembert sutures to approximate the posterior seromuscular coat of the duodenum to the antimesenteric border of the jejunum. After this has been done, make an incision in the antimesenteric border of the jejunum. Obtain hemostasis with absorbable sutures or electrocoagulation. Then begin the mucosal layer. Use 5-0 atraumatic Vicryl suture material and place the first stitch in the middle of the posterior layer of the anastomosis. Run a continuous locked stitch from this point to the left-hand termination of the posterior layer. Take relatively small bites through the full thickness of duodenum and jejunum. If the bites are small, the continuous suture does not act as a purse string to narrow the anastomosis.
7. Insert a second 5-0 PG suture adjacent to the first one at the midpoint of the posterior layer. Run this stitch in a continuous locked fashion toward the patient's right. Accomplish closure of the first anterior layer of the anastomosis using the same

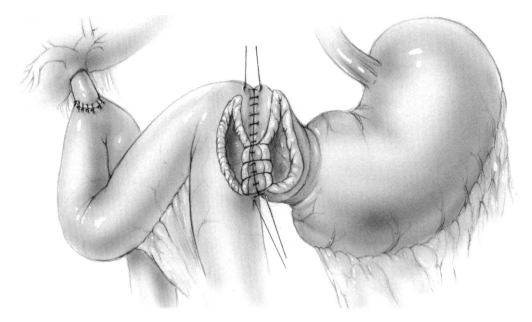

Fig. 78-37

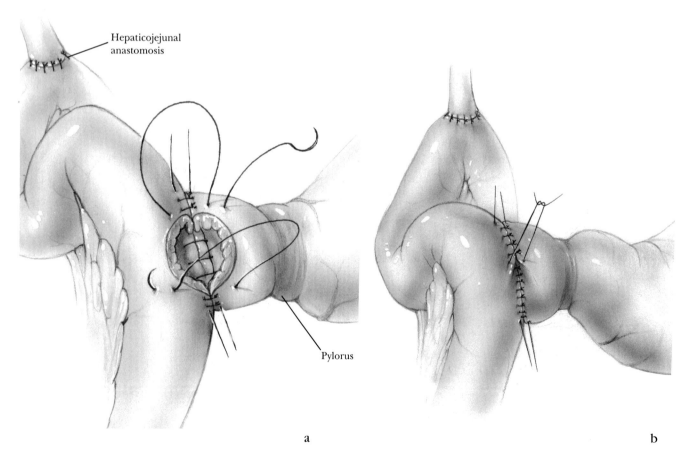

Hepaticojejunal anastomosis

Pylorus

a

b

Fig. 78-38

5-0 PG as a Connell, a Cushing, or a seromucosal stitch **(Fig. 78–37)**. Terminate this layer by tying the ends of the two continuous PG sutures to each other in the middle of the anterior layer. Complete the anterior layer of the anastomosis by inserting interrupted 4-0 silk Lembert seromuscular sutures **(Fig. 78–38)**. **Figure 78–39** illustrates the method of draining the pancreatic duct. Insert the pediatric feeding tube into the pancreatic duct after completing the posterior layers of the pancreaticojejunostomy. Suture the catheter to the pancreas with a 3-0 PG stitch; then bring it through a puncture wound in the proximal jejunum. Close the jejunal puncture wound around the catheter with a 4-0 silk purse-string suture. Bring the catheter through a puncture

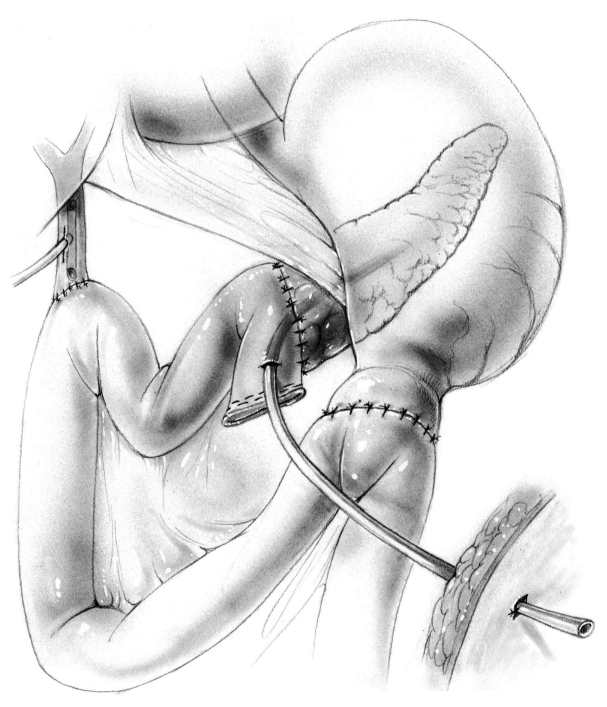

Fig. 78–39

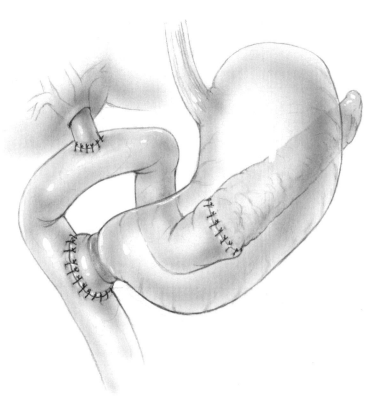

Fig. 78-40

wound of the abdominal wall to the left of the midline incision and transfix it to the skin with a suture. In most cases it is possible to suture the jejunum to the parietal peritoneum around the puncture wound through which the catheter exits.

Figure 78-40 illustrates the end result of this operation without a catheter in the pancreatic duct but with the pancreatic stump invaginated into the jejunal lumen. Insert a closed-section drainage catheter near the pancreatic anastomosis. Bring the catheter out through a puncture wound in the upper abdominal wall.

Complications

Delayed gastric emptying. This complication occurs if the duodenojejunal suture line abuts the pyloric sphincter muscle and thus interferes with this sphincter's proper functioning. Most cases of delayed gastric emptying subsequent to a pancreatoduodenectomy are due to leakage from the pancreaticojejunal or hepaticojejunal anastomoses or intraperitoneal sepsis rather than some intrinsic disorder of gastric function. Evacuation of intraperitoneal collections or abscesses accelerates the return to normal gastric emptying. Most of these abscesses

can be evacuated by percutaneous CT-guided insertion of drainage catheters.

Pyloroduodenal ulcer. Superficial ulceration may follow impairment of the duodenal blood supply. Peptic ulcer of the duodenum or jejunum may occur if the gastric acidity following the operation is permitted to fall below pH 4–5. With bile diverted into the T-tube and all the pancreatic juice draining to the outside via the pancreatic duct catheter, one of our patients developed gastric pH 1 postoperatively while receiving cimetidine 100 mg per hour intravenously. The patient bled from a superficial pyloroduodenal ulcer that healed when the pancreatic secretions were injected into the nasogastric tube together with antacids. During the early postoperative period it is important to administer enough H$_2$-blocker to raise the gastric pH to 5.0.

POSTOPERATIVE CARE

Perioperative antibiotics, which were initiated prior to the operation, are repeated by the intravenous route every 4 hours during the procedure and then every 6 hours for four doses postoperatively. If the bile was infected prior to surgery, administer antibiotics until the infection is suppressed.

Maintain the gastric pH at or above 5.0 with parenteral agents. Test the intragastric pH on the sample of gastric juice aspirated through the nasogastric tube every 2 hours. Administer additional antacid, if necessary, in doses sufficient to maintain the desired pH.

Intravenous fluids should be administered in sufficient quantities to ensure normal urine output. Hemodynamic monitoring is helpful in older cardiac patients. Some of our patients have required 8 liters of isotonic fluid or more on the day of operation to maintain cardiovascular homeostasis even in the absence of significant blood loss. Because it is an extensive operation, one can expect considerable sequestration of fluids into the "third space." By the third postoperative day there is frequently a brisk diuresis, at which time intravenous fluids should be limited in volume.

Initiate enteral feedings by way of the jejunostomy catheter after the operation is completed and continue these feedings until the patient is able to take a full diet by mouth.

Leave the T-tube and the pancreatic catheter in place for 21 days. If there has been no drainage of pancreatic juice or bile by the seventh or eighth day, mobilize and slowly remove the latex drains. Remove the Jackson-Pratt drain on day 8–10 unless significant amounts of fluid are being aspirated.

A clear, watery secretion draining from the operative site represents a pancreatocutaneous fistula, which will probably heal with the passage of time. Somatostatin analog therapy may decrease the incidence and severity of this problem. If this leak of pancreatic juice becomes complicated by an admixture of bile and pus, the pancreatic enzymes are activated and start digesting tissues in the vicinity of the anastomosis. This complication can be serious and even fatal. Initially, attempt conservative therapy by continuous irrigation of the anastomotic site through the catheter using sterile saline containing appropriate dilute antibiotics. A dosage of 1-2 liters per day seems appropriate. If, despite this management, the patient's condition continues to deteriorate, relaparotomy to remove the remaining tail of the pancreas together with the spleen may prove life-saving.

COMPLICATIONS

Leakage from pancreatic anastomosis.

Leakage from biliary anastomosis.

Postoperative sepsis.

Acute pancreatitis.

Hepatic failure.

Postoperative hemorrhage. In our experience sepsis and hemorrhage are most often the result of leakage from the pancreaticojejunal anastomosis. In some cases this is due to the development of acute pancreatitis in the pancreatic tail. As discussed above, the only solution to this vicious cycle is sometimes surgical removal of the residual pancreas.

Postoperative gastric bleeding. If the gastric pH is kept elevated by antacid therapy, bleeding due to gastric ulceration is rare.

Thrombosis of the superior mesenteric artery or vein. Although we have never encountered this complication, thrombosis can occur. It can be prevented by dissecting these two vital structures with care and precision.

Gastric bezoar. We have had two patients who developed gastric phytobezoars following pancreatoduodenectomy with vagotomy. Each was treated with gastric lavage and medication, which included papain and cellulose, with satisfactory results.

When *undrained collections* are identified on the CT scan, ask the interventional radiologist to insert a CT-guided percutaneous drain

REFERENCES

Cameron JL. Whipple or pylorus preservation? A critical reappraisal and some new insights into pancreaticoduodenectomy. Ann Surg 2000;231:301.

Cameron JL, Crist DW, Sitzman JV, et al. Factors influencing survival after pancreaticoduodenectomy for pancreatic cancer. Am J Surg 1991;161:120.

Earnhardt RC, McQuone SJ, Minasi JS. Intraoperative fine needle aspiration of pancreatic and extrahepatic biliary masses. Surg Gynecol Obstet 1993;177:147.

Grant CS, Van Heerdan JA. Anastomotic ulceration following subtotal and total pancreatectomy. Ann Surg 1979;190:1.

Jimenez RE, Warshaw Al, Rattner DW, et al. Impact of laparoscopic staging in the treatment of pancreatic cancer. Arch Surg 2000;135:414.

Lin PW, Lin YJ. Prospective randomized comparison between pylorus-preserving and standard pancreaticoduodenectomy. Br J Surg 1999;86:603.

Rossi RL, Braasch JW. Techniques of pancreaticojejunostomy in pancreatoduodenectomy. Probl Gen Surg 1985;2:306.

Sohn TA, Yeo CJ, Cameron JL, Pitt HA, Lillemoe KD. Do preoperative biliary stents increase postpancreaticoduodenectomy complications? J Gastrointest Surg 2000;4:267.

Trede M, Schwall G. The complications of pancreatectomy. Ann Surg 1988;207:39.

Tsao JI, Rossi RL, Lowell JA. Pylorus-preserving pancreatoduodenectomy: is it an adequate cancer operation? Arch Surg 1994;129:405.

Tyler DS, Evans DB. Reoperative pancreaticoduodenectomy. Ann Surg 219:211–221.

Yeo CJ, Cameron JL, Sohn TA, et al. Pancreaticoduodenectomy with or without extended retroperitoneal lymphadenectomy for periampullary adenocarcinoma: comparison of morbidity and mortality and short-term outcome. Ann Surg 1999;229:613.

Yeo CJ, Cameron JL, Sohn TA, et al. Six hundred fifty consecutive pancreaticoduodenectomies in the 1990's: pathology, complications, and outcomes. Ann Surg 1997;226:248.

79 Total Pancreatoduodenectomy

INDICATIONS

Carcinoma of the pancreas (see Chapter 77)

CONTRAINDICATIONS

Distant metastases

Absence of an experienced surgical team

Patient who lacks alertness and intelligence to manage diabetes

Invasion of portal or superior mesenteric vein

PREOPERATIVE PREPARATION

See Chapter 78.

OPERATIVE STRATEGY

Complete omentectomy is generally performed as part of a total pancreatectomy. Division of the splenic, short gastric, right gastric, and gastroduodenal arteries leaves the gastric pouch dependent on the left gastric artery for its blood supply. For this reason, do not divide the left gastric artery at its

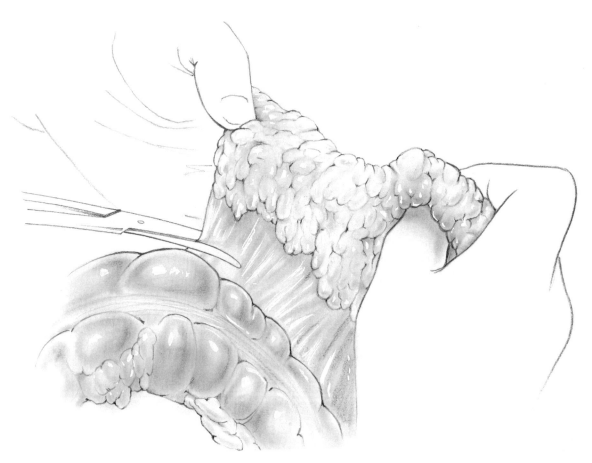

Fig. 79-1

point of origin from the celiac axis. Rather, divide it along the lesser curvature distal to the point where the branches to the proximal stomach and esophagus arise. This chapter concentrates on the additional features necessary to complete the pancreatic resection and should be read in conjunction with Chapter 78.

OPERATIVE TECHNIQUE

Incision

Except for extremely stocky patients, we use a long midline incision from the xiphoid to a point 10 cm below the umbilicus.

Evaluation of Pathology, Determination of Resectability, Initial Mobilization

The technique followed here is identical to that described in Figures 78-2 through 78-7, except that the omentum is detached from the transverse colon and is removed with the specimen (**Figs. 79–1, 79–2**).

Splenectomy and Truncal Vagotomy

With the stomach and omentum retracted in a cephalad direction, identify the splenic artery along the superior surface of the pancreas. Open the peritoneum over the splenic artery at a point 1-2 cm

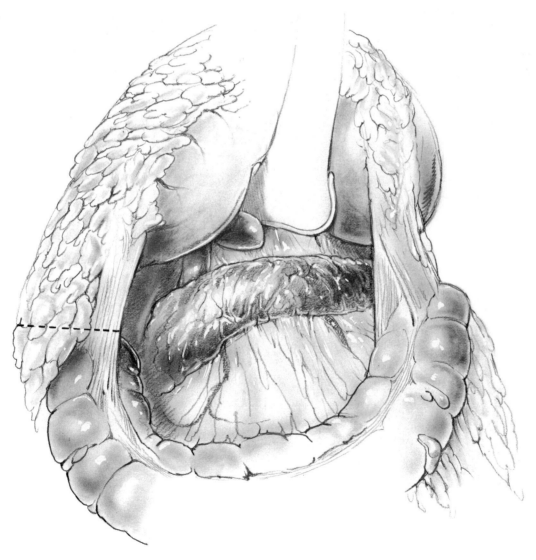

Fig. 79-2

distal to its origin at the celiac axis. With a right-angle Mixter clamp, free the posterior surface of the artery and apply a 2-0 silk ligature **(Fig. 79–3)**. Ligate the vessel but do not divide it at this point.

Apply a Thompson retractor to the left costal margin to improve the exposure of the spleen. Make an incision in the avascular lienophrenic fold of the peritoneum **(Figs. 79–4a, 79–4b)**. Electrocoagulate any bleeding vessels. Elevate the tail of the pancreas together with the spleen. Divide the attachments between the lower pole of the spleen and the colon.

Expose the posterior surface of the spleen and identify the splenic artery and veins at this point. If there is any bleeding, ligate these vessels. Insert moist gauze pads into the bed of the elevated spleen.

At this time remove the Thompson retractor from the left costal margin and place it in the region of the sternum. Apply traction in a cephalad and anterior direction, exposing the abdominal esophagus. Incise the peritoneum over the abdominal esophagus. Use a peanut-gauze dissector to separate the crus of the diaphragm from the esophagus **(Fig.**

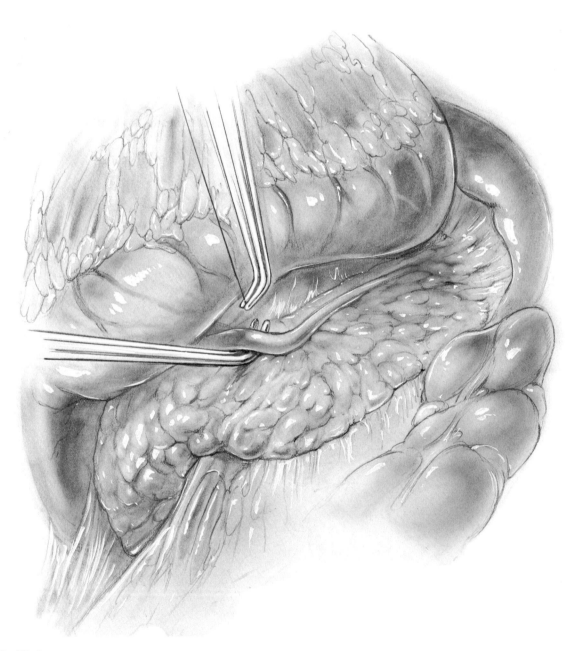

Fig. 79–3

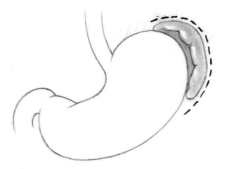

Fig. 79-4a

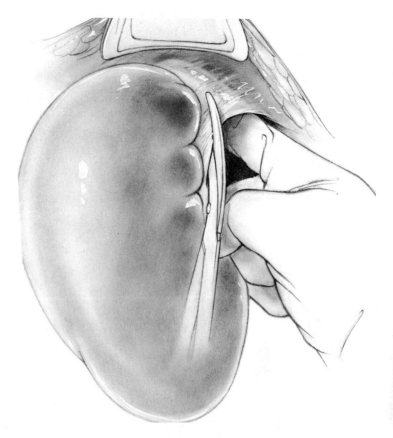

Fig. 79-4b

79–5) and perform a truncal vagotomy as described in Chapter 25.

Mobilizing the Distal Pancreas

Identify the proximal short gastric vessel, and insert the left index finger underneath the gastrophrenic ligament. Apply a hemostatic clip to the distal portion of the vessel. Ligate the gastric side of the vessel with 2-0 or 3-0 silk and divide it **(Fig. 79–6)**. Con-

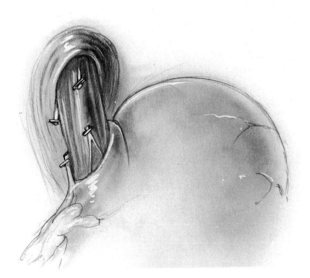

Fig. 79-5

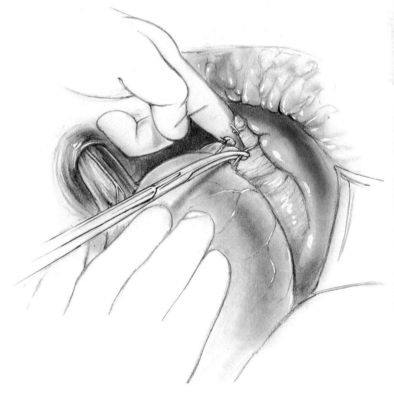

Fig. 79-6

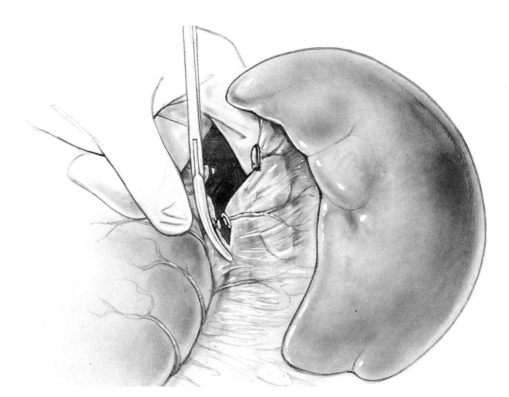

Fig. 79-7

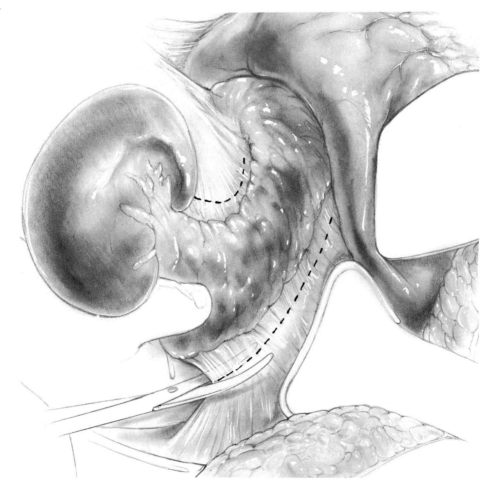

Fig. 79-8

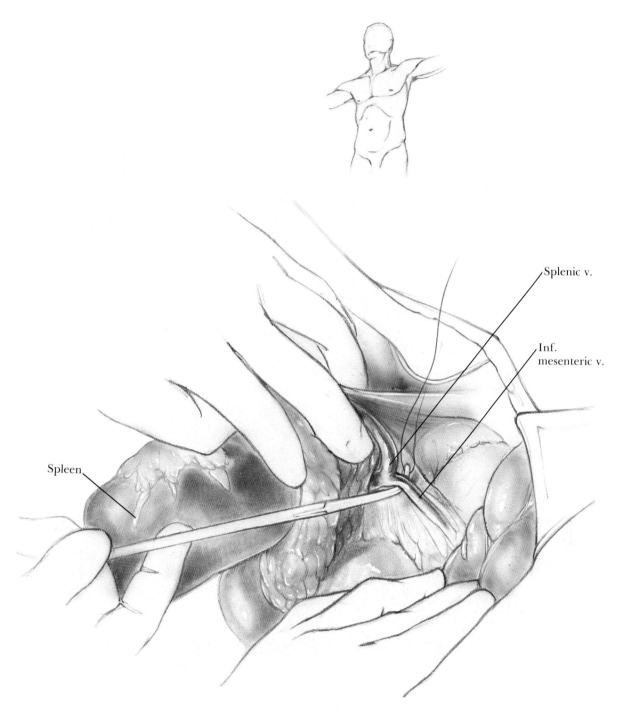

Fig. 79-9

tinue the dissection in this manner until all of the short gastric vessels have been divided **(Fig. 79–7)**.

Now redirect attention to the tail and body of the pancreas, which is covered by a layer of posterior parietal peritoneum. Incise this avascular layer first along the superior border of the pancreas and then again along the inferior border of the pancreas after elevating the tissue with an index finger **(Fig. 79–8)**. As the pancreas is elevated from the posterior abdominal wall, follow the posterior surface of the splenic vein to the point where the inferior mesenteric vein enters; then divide this vessel between 2-0 silk ligatures **(Fig. 79–9)**. Follow the splenic artery to its point of origin, where the previous ligature can be seen. Double-ligate the proximal stump of the splenic artery and apply a similar ligature to the distal portion of the splenic artery. Divide between these ties. Carefully dissect the junction of the splenic and portal veins away from the posterior wall of the pancreas. After 2 cm of the terminal portion of the splenic

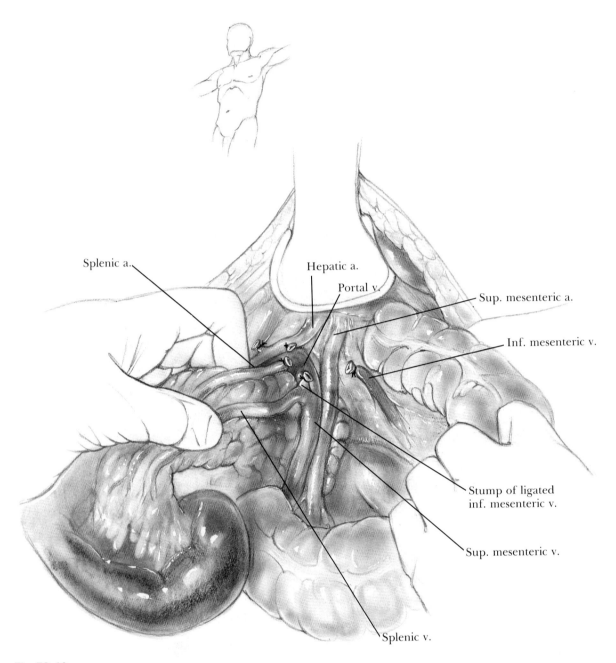

Splenic a.

Hepatic a.

Portal v.

Sup. mesenteric a.

Inf. mesenteric v.

Stump of ligated
inf. mesenteric v.

Sup. mesenteric v.

Splenic v.

Fig. 79-10

vein has been cleared **(Fig. 79–10)**, divide the splenic vein between 2-0 silk ligatures.

Antrectomy

Divide the stomach as previously described **(Fig. 79–11)**.

Cholecystectomy and Division of the Hepatic Duct

The hepatic duct, portal vein, and hepatic artery have already been stripped of overlying peritoneum and lymph nodes. At this time, divide and ligate the cystic artery. Remove the gallbladder by dissecting

it out of the liver bed from above down **(Fig. 79–12)**. Obtain complete hemostasis in the liver bed with electrocautery. Ligate the cystic duct. Divide it and remove the gallbladder.

Dissect the hepatic duct free from the portal vein at a point just above its junction with the cystic duct. Free about 1.5 cm of hepatic duct. Apply a ligature to the distal end and an atraumatic bulldog clamp to the proximal end and divide the duct.

Freeing the Uncinate Process

Retract the spleen, pancreas, and duodenum to the patient's right. Gentle dissection discloses three or four

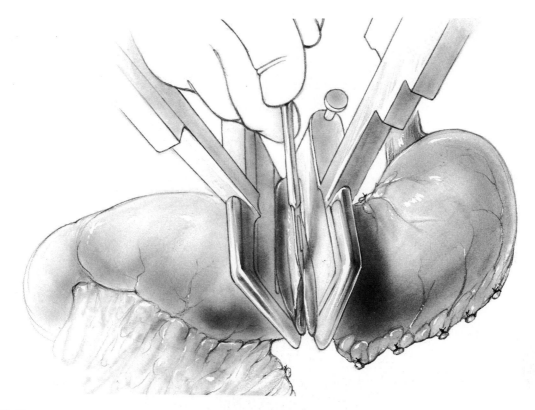

Fig. 79-11

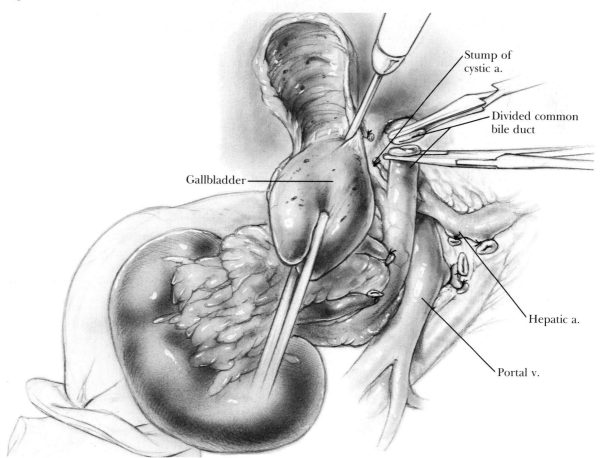

Stump of
cystic a.

Divided common
bile duct

Gallbladder

Hepatic a.

Portal v.

Fig. 79-12

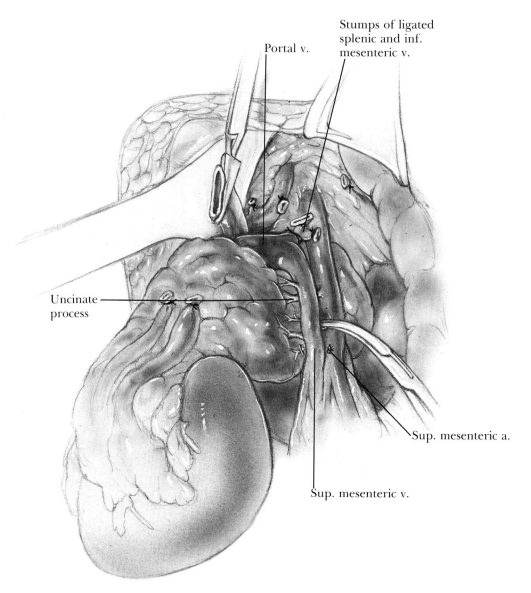

Fig. 79-13

venous branches between the posterior surface of the pancreatic head and the portal-superior mesenteric veins **(Fig. 79–13)**. Ligate each of these vessels with 3-0 silk and divide them. It is now possible gently to retract the portal vein to the right. At this point the su-

perior mesenteric artery can generally be clearly identified. In some cases it is easy to identify several arterial branches that can be dissected free, divided, and individually ligated **(Fig. 79–14)**. Divide the uncinate process as previously described (see Chapter 78).

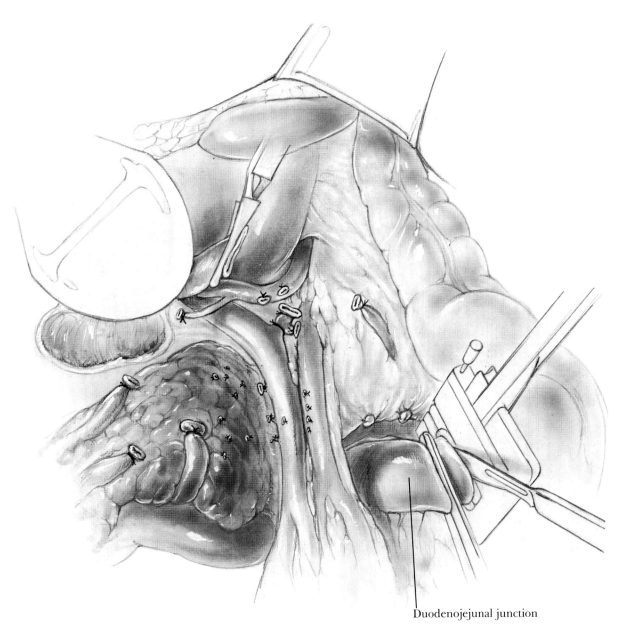

Duodenojejunal junction

Fig. 79-14

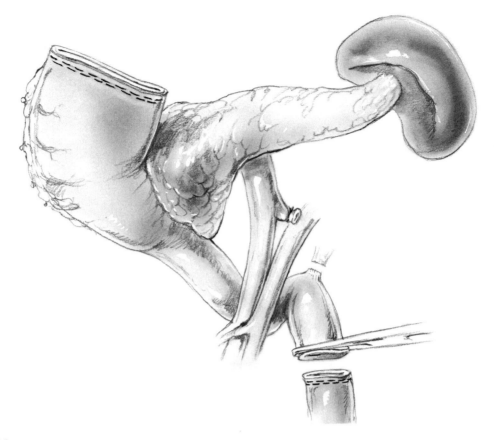

Fig. 79-15

Mobilizing the Duodenojejunal Junction

Expose the ligament of Treitz by elevating the transverse colon. Divide the jejunum as previously described and remove the specimen **(Fig. 79–15**; see also Fig. 79-14).

Hepaticojejunostomy

Reconstruction is simpler because no pancreatic anastomosis is needed. The hepaticojejunostomy is performed first, as described in Chapter 78.

At a point about 50 cm downstream from the hepaticojejunal anastomosis, construct a stapled gastrojejunostomy **(Figs. 79–16, 79–17)**. Bring the T-tube out through a stab wound in the right upper quadrant. Irrigate the entire operative field with a dilute antibiotic solution. Be certain that hemostasis is complete. Insert a large Jackson-Pratt suction-drainage catheter in the right upper quadrant of the operative field and bring it out through a stab wound in the abdominal wall. Close the midline incision in routine fashion. Close the skin with interrupted nylon sutures or staples.

POSTOPERATIVE CARE

The principles of postoperative care described in Chapter 78 apply to total pancreatectomy except there is no possibility of a pancreatic fistula. The suction-drainage catheter is removed sometime after the fourth postoperative day unless a significant amount of drainage persists. The T-tube is left in place for 21 days.

The most important element of postoperative care following total pancreatectomy is regulation of the resulting diabetes. The greatest danger is hypoglycemia due to administration of too much insulin. Perform blood glucose determinations every 3–4 hours for the first few days. Do not try to keep the blood glucose level below 200 mg/dl. Especially during the early postoperative period the diabetes is quite brittle, and an overdose of only a few units of insulin may produce hypoglycemic shock. There is much more danger from hypoglycemia than from diabetic acidosis. Administer regular insulin in doses of 2–5 units every few hours as necessary. Frequently no more than 10–20 units are required per day. After patients begin to eat, they may be switched to one of the longer-acting insulin prod-

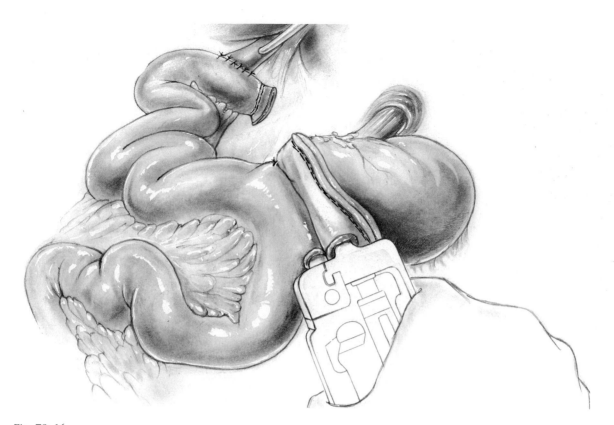

Fig. 79-16

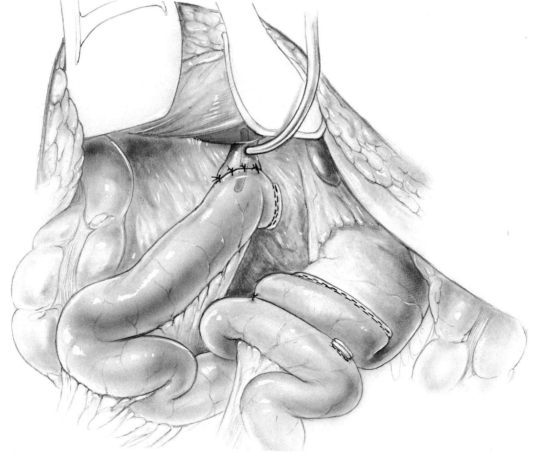

Fig. 79-17

ucts. Patients and their relatives should be carefully instructed about the symptoms of hypoglycemia.

Repeated measurements of the gastric pH are vital to prevent postoperative gastric hemorrhage. Use intravenous H_2-blockers to keep the gastric pH at 5 or above.

A sufficient dose of pancreatic enzymes must be given to prevent steatorrhea. It may require three tablets of Pancrease before each meal.

COMPLICATIONS

Hypoglycemia or hyperglycemia

Postoperative gastric bleeding due to stress ulceration or a marginal ulcer

Postoperative hemorrhage

Postoperative sepsis

Leakage from biliary anastomosis

Mesenteric venous thrombosis

Hepatic failure

REFERENCES

Bakkevold KE, Kambestad B. Morbidity and mortality after radical and palliative pancreatic cancer surgery: risk factors influencing the short-term results. Ann Surg 1993;217:356.

Brooks JR, Brooks DC, Levine JD. Total pancreatectomy for ductal cell carcinoma of the pancreas: an update. Ann Surg 1989;209:405.

Swope TJ, Wade TP, Neuberger TJ, Virgo KS, Johnson FE. A reappraisal of total pancreatectomy for pancreatic cancer: results from US Veterans Affairs hospitals 1987–1991. Am J Surg 1994;168:582.

80 Distal Pancreatectomy

INDICATIONS

Resectable malignant tumors located to the left of superior mesenteric vessels

Benign tumors that cannot be locally excised (e.g., insulinoma)

Pseudocysts of the tail (selected)

Chronic pancreatitis localized to the body and tail

Trauma

PREOPERATIVE PREPARATION

Localization maneuvers are required for small tumors such as insulinomas: computed tomography (CT), magnetic resonance imaging (MRI), angiography, and endoscopic or intraoperative ultrasonography.

Operations for insulinoma require careful monitoring of the blood glucose at frequent intervals prior to and during operation.

In patients suspected of having a gastrinoma the diagnosis should be confirmed by serial serum gastrin levels before and after administration of intravenous secretin.

PITFALLS AND DANGER POINTS

Lacerating splenic or portal vein

OPERATIVE STRATEGY

Choice of Operative Approach

Splenic preservation is feasible in selected patients with benign tumors or stable trauma patients. Careful dissection of the splenic artery and vein are required (see References). Laparoscopic distal pancreatectomy is being performed in some centers.

Avoiding Damage to Blood Vessels

Once the decision has been made to proceed with distal pancreatectomy and splenectomy, locate the splenic artery a few centimeters beyond its origin at the celiac axis. Ligate the vessel in continuity to re-duce the size of the spleen and the volume of blood loss if the splenic capsule is ruptured during the dissection.

The greatest danger when resecting the body and tail of the pancreas arises when a malignancy in the body obscures the junction between the splenic and portal veins. Invasion of the portal vein by the tumor is an indication of inoperability. If elevation of the tail and body of the pancreas together with the tumor should result in a tear at the junction of the splenic and portal veins and this accident occurs before the tumor has been completely liberated, it may be extremely difficult to repair the lacerated portal vein. If an accident of this type should occur, it is necessary to find the plane between the neck of the pancreas and the portal vein and then divide the pancreas across its neck while manually occluding the lacerated vein. With the portal and superior mesenteric veins exposed after the neck of the pancreas has been divided, occluding vascular clamps may be applied and the laceration repaired. This complication can generally be avoided by careful inspection of the tumor after elevating the tail of the pancreas and by observing the area where the splenic vein joins the portal vein. If the tumor extends beyond this junction, it is probably inoperable.

Avoiding Pancreatic Fistula

We have used the 55 mm linear stapling device for years to accomplish closure of the cut end of the remaining pancreas after resecting the body and tail of this organ. When the stapler is used across the neck of a pancreas of average thickness, the staples seem to occlude the cut end of the pancreatic duct successfully; no supplementary sutures are needed to prevent a fistula. If the stapler is not used, be certain to occlude the cut pancreatic duct by inserting a nonabsorbable mattress suture.

OPERATIVE TECHNIQUE

Incision and Exposure

In the average patient a long midline incision from the xiphoid to a point about 6–10 cm beyond the umbilicus provides adequate exposure for mobilizing the spleen and the tail of the pancreas. In an

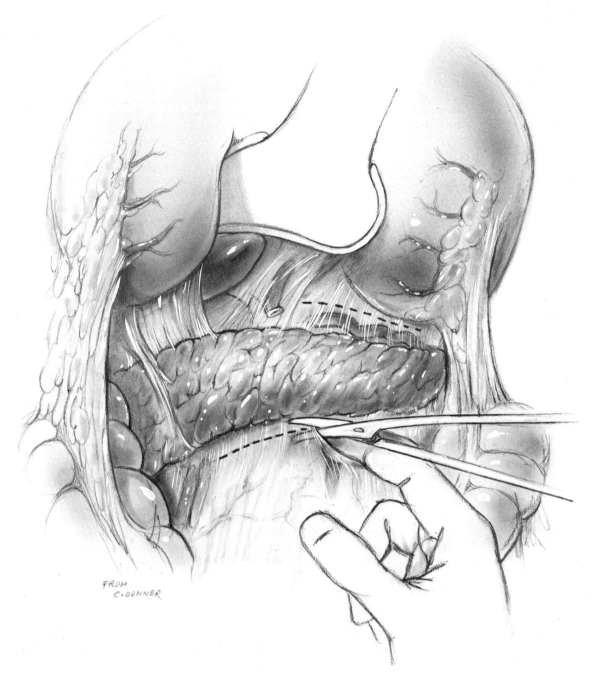

Fig. 80-1

Exploration; Liberating the Omentum

After thoroughly exploring the abdomen, expose the body and tail of the pancreas by liberating the omentum from its attachments to the transverse colon. An alternative method is to divide the omentum between hemostats, which exposed the anterior surface of the pancreas. To palpate the posterior sur-

obese or a highly muscular individual with a wide costal angle, a long transverse or left subcostal incision is a suitable alternative.

face of the pancreas, it is necessary to incise the layer of peritoneum that covers the pancreas and then continues down to the transverse colon, forming one leaflet of the transverse mesocolon. Incise this layer along the inferior border of the tail of the pancreas **(Fig. 80–1)**. The only major blood vessel deep to this layer of peritoneum is the inferior mesenteric vein, which travels from the transverse mesocolon to join the inferior border of the splenic vein just before the splenic vein joins the portal vein. After completing this incision, insert the index finger behind the pancreas and use the fingertip to elevate

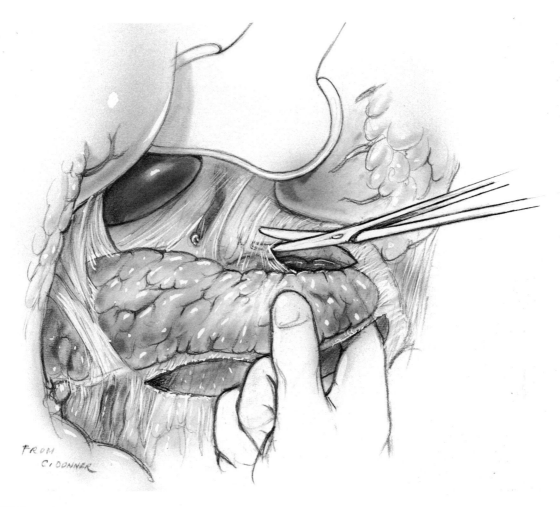

Fig. 80-2

the peritoneum along the superior margin of the pancreas **(Fig. 80–2)**. Incise this layer of peritoneum with scissors, avoiding the sometimes convoluted splenic artery that runs along the superior border of the pancreas deep to the layer of peritoneum. After these two peritoneal incisions have been made, palpate the tail and body of the pancreas between the thumb and forefinger to evaluate the pathology. Intraoperative ultrasonography is a useful adjunct.

If seeking a gastrinoma, perform a Kocher maneuver and palpate the descending duodenum and the head of the pancreas. Some non-beta-cell tumors of the pancreas can be palpated as small projections from the pancreas into the posterior wall of the descending duodenum. Many of the benign tumors can be excised locally or may be shelled out by gentle dissection.

Identifying Splenic Artery

Palpate the splenic artery along the upper border of the neck of the pancreas at a point a few centimeters from its origin. If there is some confusion as to the identity of the artery, occlude it with the fingertip and palpate the hepatoduodenal ligament to determine whether the hepatic artery (rather than the splenic artery) has been occluded. If hepatic artery pulsation is normal, open the peritoneum overlying the splenic artery. Encircle it with a right-angle clamp and ligate it in continuity with 2-0 silk (see Fig. 84-3).

Mobilizing the Spleen and Pancreas

Retract the spleen to the patient's right, placing the splenorenal ligament on stretch. Incise this ligament (see Fig. 85-1) with Metzenbaum scissors or electrocautery. Continue this incision up to the diaphragm and down to include the splenocolic ligament. Now elevate the spleen and the tail of the pancreas from the renal capsule by fingertip dissection. The greater omentum may be attached to the lower portion of the spleen; dissect it away from the spleen. It should now be possible to elevate the spleen and the tail and body of the pancreas up into the incision, leaving the kidney and adrenal gland behind. Cover these structures with a large moist gauze pad.

The spleen remains attached to the greater curvature of the stomach by means of the intact left gastroepiploic and short gastric vessels. Divide each of these structures individually between hemostats and then ligate each with 2-0 silk (see Figs. 84-2, 84-4). Inspection of the posterior surface of the pancreas reveals the splenic vein. Dissecting along the inferior border of the pancreas unroofs the inferior mesenteric vein on its way to join the splenic vein.

Identify, encircle, and divide the inferior mesenteric vein between 2-0 silk ligatures.

Dividing the Splenic Artery and Vein

Gently elevate the splenic vein by sweeping the areolar tissue away from this vessel with a peanut dissector until the junction between the splenic and portal vein is identified. At this point encircle the splenic vein

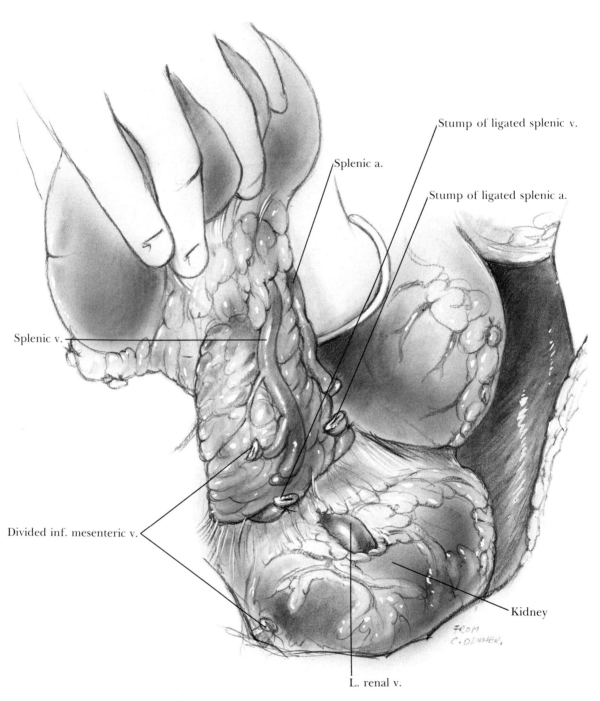

Fig. 80-3

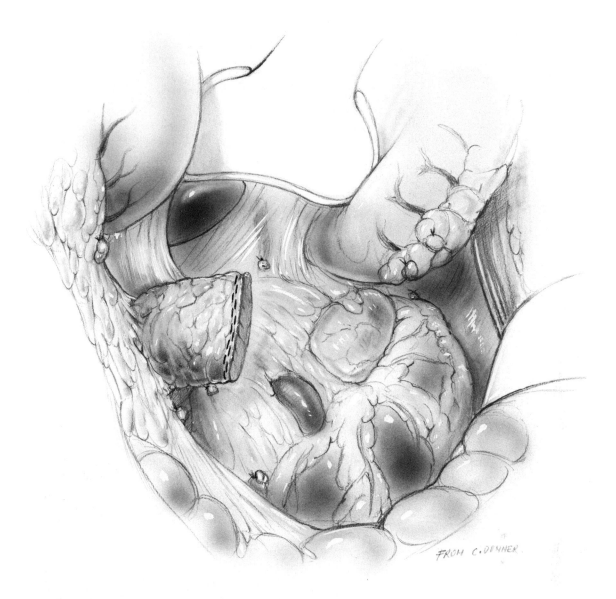

Fig. 80–4

with a right-angle clamp at a point about 2 cm proximal to its junction with the portal vein. Pass two ligatures of 2-0 silk around the splenic vein and tie the ligatures about 1.5 cm apart. Divide the vein between the two ligatures (**Fig. 80–3**) and identify the previously ligated splenic artery. Tie a second ligature around this artery and divide the vessel distal to the two ligatures. This leaves the specimen attached only by the neck of the pancreas in the region of the portal vein.

Dividing the Pancreas

If the pancreas is of average thickness, simply apply a 55 mm linear stapler across the neck of the pancreas. Using 3.5 mm staples in most cases, fire the staples and divide the pancreas flush with the stapler using a scalpel. Remove the specimen. Then remove the stapling device and inspect the cut edge

of the pancreas carefully for bleeding points (**Fig. 80–4**). It is frequently necessary to suture-ligate a superior pancreatic artery near the upper border of the remaining pancreas. We have not found it necessary to identify or suture the pancreatic duct when using a stapled closure of the transected pancreas.

Alternatively, one may occlude the transected pancreas with interlocking interrupted mattress sutures of 3-0 nonabsorbable suture material. If the pancreatic duct is identified, occlude this duct with a separate mattress suture.

Closure and Drainage

Place a flat closed-suction drainage catheter down to the site of the divided pancreas and bring the catheter out through a puncture wound in the abdominal wall. Close the incision in routine fashion after ascertaining that complete hemostasis in the pancreatic and splenic beds has been achieved.

POSTOPERATIVE CARE

Attach the drainage catheter to a closed-suction system. Leave the drain in place 4–6 days. If a pancreatic duct fistula is suspected, leave the drain in place for a longer time. Occasionally check the serum amylase and blood glucose levels to detect postoperative pancreatitis and diabetes.

COMPLICATIONS

If *pancreatic fistula* develops, it generally resolves spontaneously in 3–4 weeks. If it does not resolve during that time, obtain a radiographic sinogram with aqueous contrast medium.

Acute pancreatitis in the residual pancreas is a possible but uncommon complication.

Diabetes mellitus of mild degree sometimes occurs after an extensive distal pancreatectomy.

REFERENCES

Aldridge MC, Williamson RC. Distal pancreatectomy with and without splenectomy. Br J Surg 1991;78:976.

Benoist S, Dugue L, Sauvanet A, et al. Is there a role of preservation of the spleen in distal pancreatectomy? J Am Coll Surg 1999;188:255.

Cuschieri A, Jakimowicz JJ, van Spreeuwel J. Laparoscopic distal 70% pancreatectomy and splenectomy for chronic pancreatitis. Ann Surg 1996;223:280.

Lillemoe KD, Kaushal S, Cameron JL, et al. Distal pancreatectomy: indications and outcomes in 235 patients. Ann Surg 1999;229:698.

Pachter HL, Hofstetter SR, Liang HG, Hoballah J. Traumatic injuries to the pancreas; the role of distal pancreatectomy with splenic preservation. J Trauma 1989;29:1452.

Pachter HL, Pennington R, Chassin JL, et al. Simplified distal pancreatectomy with the autosuture stapler; preliminary clinical observations. Surgery 1979;85:166.

Salky BA. Distal pancreatectomy. In Scott-Conner CEH (ed) The SAGES Manual: Fundamentals of Laparoscopy and GI Endoscopy. New York, Springer-Verlag, 1999, pp 307–313.

Scott-Conner CE, Dawson DL. Technical considerations in distal pancreatectomy with splenic preservation. Surg Gynecol Obstet 1989;168:451.

Warshaw AL, Rattner DW, Fernandez-del Castillo C, Z'graggen K. Middle segment pancreatectomy: a novel technique for conserving pancreatic tissue. Arch Surg 1998;133:327.

White SA, Sutton CD, Weymss-Holden S, et al. The feasibility of spleen-preserving pancreatectomy for end-stage chronic pancreatitis. Am J Surg 2000;179:294.

81 Operations for Pancreatic Cyst

INDICATIONS

Mature pseudocyst > 5 cm seen by ultrasonography or computed tomography (CT).

PREOPERATIVE PREPARATION

Visualize the cyst by sonogram or CT scan with contrast.

Rule out the presence of gallstones or bile duct obstruction by sonography, oral cholecystography, or endoscopic retrograde cholangiopancreatography (ERCP).

Consider angiography of the splenic artery and pancreas for all chronic pseudocysts prior to surgery (CT with contrast may given equivalent information).

Administer perioperative antibiotics.

Insert a nasogastric tube preoperatively.

PITFALLS AND DANGER POINTS

Anastomotic leak

Postoperative hemorrhage

Mistaken diagnosis (cystadenocarcinoma)

Overlooking an associated pseudoaneurysm

OPERATIVE STRATEGY

Avoiding Anastomotic Leakage

Cystogastrostomy or cystoduodenostomy are appropriate only if the cyst is firmly attached to the wall of the stomach or duodenum. The anastomosis is simply completed through the area of attachment. If the cyst is not adherent, perform a Roux-en-Y cystojejunostomy because leakage from this anastomosis is far less dangerous to the patient than is leakage from the stomach or duodenum.

The wall of the pseudocyst must be thick enough for a safe anastomosis, particularly if a cystojejunostomy is performed. If there is doubt about the adequacy of the cyst wall, perform an external drainage operation.

Avoiding Diagnostic Errors

Always palpate the cyst for pulsation before any manipulation. A pulsatile cyst may contain a free rupture of a splenic artery pseudoaneurysm. Aspirate the cyst before opening it to confirm pancreatic juice without blood. Biopsy the cyst wall to rule out cystadenocarcinoma.

Pseudoaneurysm

When arteriography has demonstrated a leaking pseudoaneurysm of the splenic artery in a large pseudocyst, ask the angiographer to perform preoperative occlusion of the splenic artery. Sometimes the area of inflammation extends close to the origin of the splenic artery, making proximal control in the operating room, under emergency conditions, quite difficult. It is preferable to resect a cyst containing a pseudoaneurysm to prevent postoperative rupture and hemorrhage, rather than to drain it.

Jaundiced Patient

Although jaundice in the presence of a pseudocyst may well be the result of extrinsic pressure by the cyst against the distal common bile duct, it is also important to rule out the presence of calculi or periductal pancreatic fibrosis as the cause of bile duct obstruction. Preoperative ERCP is helpful, but performing operative cholangiography after the cyst has been drained determines whether further surgery of the bile duct is necessary. If the jaundice is due to chronic fibrosis in the head of the pancreas, endoscopic stenting or a bypass operation is required. It may be necessary to perform a side-to-side choledochojejunostomy to the defunctionalized limb of the Roux-en-Y distal to the cystojejunostomy.

OPERATIVE TECHNIQUE

External Drainage

Make a long midline incision. Explore the abdomen and identify the pseudocyst. After making an incision in the greater omentum to expose the anterior

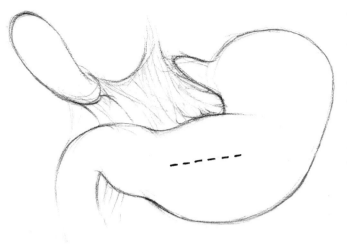

Fig. 81-1

wall of the cyst, insert a needle into the cyst to rule out the presence of fresh blood; then incise the cyst wall and evacuate all of the cyst contents. Take a sample for bacteriologic analysis. If the cyst wall is too thin for anastomosis, insert a soft Silastic catheter and bring it out through an adequate stab wound in the left upper quadrant.

If the cyst wall is thick enough to permit suturing but the contents of the cyst appear to consist of pus and to resemble a large abscess, prepare a Gram stain. Sometimes what appears to be pus is only grumous detritus. If the Gram stain does not show a large number of bacteria, it is still possible to perform an internal drainage operation. Close the abdominal incision in the usual fashion after lavaging the abdominal cavity with a dilute antibiotic solution.

Cystogastrostomy

Make a midline incision from the xiphoid to the umbilicus. Explore the abdomen. If the gallbladder contains stones, perform cholecystectomy and cholangiography. Explore the lesser sac by exposing the posterior wall of the stomach from its lesser curvature aspect. If the cyst is densely adherent to the posterior wall of the stomach, cystogastrostomy is

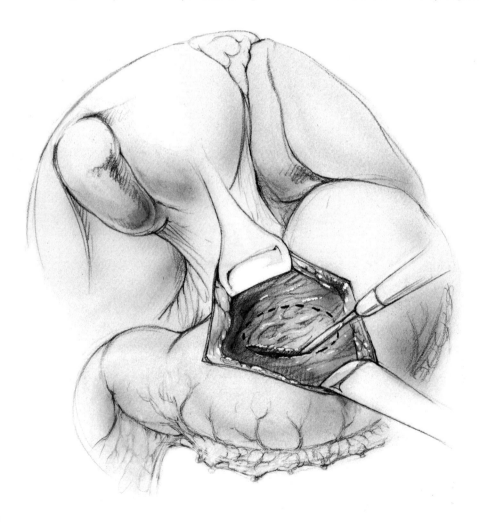

Fig. 81-2

the operation of choice. If the retrogastric mass is pulsatile, consider seriously whether the mass represents an aortic aneurysm or a contained rupture of a splenic artery pseudoaneurysm. Expose the aorta at the hiatus of the diaphragm and prepare a suitable large vascular clamp for emergency occlusion of this vessel should it be necessary. If the surgeon has had no previous experience with this maneuver, he or she should request the presence of a vascular surgeon. A preoperative CT scan should accurately identify the nature of the mass.

Make a 6- to 8-cm incision in the anterior wall of the stomach **(Fig. 81–1)** opposite the most prominent portion of the retrogastric cyst. Obtain hemostasis with electrocautery or ligatures. Then insert an 18-gauge needle through the back wall of the stomach into the cyst and aspirate. If no blood is obtained, make an incision about 3–6 cm in length through the posterior wall of the stomach and carry it through the anterior wall of the cyst. Excise an adequate ellipse of tissue from the anterior wall of the cyst for frozen-section histopathology to rule out the presence of a cystadenoma or cystadenocarcinoma **(Fig. 81–2)**.

Approximate the cut edges of the stomach and cyst by means of continuous or interrupted 3-0 PG sutures **(Fig. 81–3)**. Close the defect in the anterior wall of the stomach by applying four or five Allis clamps and then perform a stapled closure using the 90 mm stapler. If the gastric wall is not thickened, use 3.5 mm staples. Lightly electrocoagulate the everted gastric mucosa. Suture-ligate any arterial bleeders with 4-0 PG.

Roux-en-Y Cystojejunostomy

Make a long midline incision and explore the abdomen. Check the gallbladder for stones. Expose the anterior wall of the cyst by dividing the omentum overlying it. Prepare a segment of jejunum at a point about 15 cm beyond the ligament of Treitz. Divide the jejunal mesentery as illustrated in **Figure 81–4**. Then divide the jejunum between two Allen clamps. Liberate enough of the mesentery of the distal jejunal segment to permit the jejunum to reach the cyst without tension.

Make a small window in an avascular portion of the transverse mesocolon and delivery the distal jejunal segment into the supramesocolic space. Excise a window of anterior cyst wall about 3–4 cm in diameter. Send it for frozen-section histopathologic examination. Perform a one-layer anastomosis between the open end of jejunum and the window in the anterior wall. Insert interrupted 3-0 or 4-0 PG Lembert sutures. Then use 4-0 PG sutures to attach the meso-

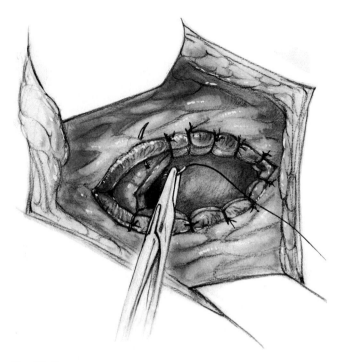

Fig. 81-3

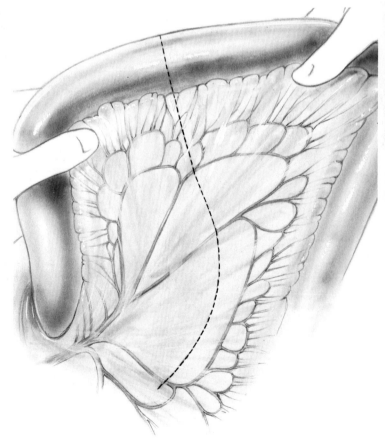

Fig. 81-4

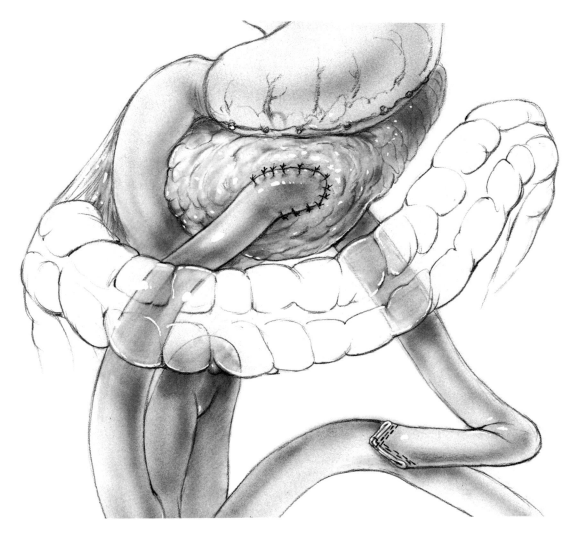

Fig. 81–5

colon to the jejunum at the point where it passes through the mesocolon.

Anastomose the divided proximal end of the jejunum to the antimesenteric border of the descending limb of the jejunum at a point 60 cm beyond the cystojejunal anastomosis. Align the open proximal end of jejunum so its opening points in a cephalad direction. Make a 1.5 cm incision in the antimesenteric border of the descending jejunum using electrocautery (see Fig. 73-7) and complete the Roux-en-Y reconstruction by performing a jejunojejunostomy in the usual manner (see Figs. 73-7 through 73-12).

Use 4-0 PG sutures to close the defect in the jejunal mesentery. The completed cystojejunostomy is illustrated in **Figure 81–5**.

If the cyst wall is of adequate quality, no drains need be used. Close the incision in the usual fashion.

Pancreatic Resection

The techniques of pancreatic resection are described in Chapters 78–80.

POSTOPERATIVE CARE

Apply nasogastric suction for 1–3 days.

Perioperative antibiotics are indicated. If the culture report of the cyst contents comes back positive, administer the appropriate antibiotics for 7 days. In cases of external drainage, administer antibiotics depending on the culture reports.

Use external drainage. Leave the drain in place until the amount of fluid obtained is minimal and a radiographic study with aqueous contrast material shows that the cyst has contracted to the size of the drain. It may be helpful to instill a dilute antibiotic solution into the drain at intervals if the cyst is infected.

COMPLICATIONS

Acute pancreatitis

Persistent fistula following external drainage

Abscess

Postoperative bleeding into gastrointestinal tract (rare if pseudoaneurysms have been excised)

REFERENCES

Adams DB, Harvey TS, Anderson MC. Percutaneous catheter drainage of pancreatic pseudocysts. Am Surg 1991;57:29.

Criado E, De Stefano AA, Weiner TM. Long term results of percutaneous catheter drainage of pancreatic pseudocysts. Surg Gynecol Obstet 1992;175:293.

Fedorak IJ, Rao R, Prinz RA. The clinical challenge of multiple pancreatic pseudocysts. Am J Surg 1994;168:22.

Heider R, Meyer AA, Galanko JA, Behrens KE. Percutaneous drainage of pancreatic pseudocysts is associated with a higher failure rate than surgical treatment in unselected patients. Ann Surg 1999;229:781.

Johnson LB, Rattner DW, Warshaw AL. The effect of size of giant pancreatic pseudocysts on the outcome of internal drainage procedures. Surg Gynecol Obstet 1991;173:171.

Kuroda A, Konishi T, Kimura W, et al. Cystopancreaticostomy and longitudinal pancreaticojejunostomy as a simpler technique of combined drainage operation for chronic pancreatitis with pancreatitis with pancreatic pseudocyst causing persistent cholestasis. Surg Gynecol Obstet 1993;177:183.

Lohr-Happe A, Peiper M, Lankisch PG. Natural course of operated pseudocysts in chronic pancreatitis. Gut 1994;35:1479.

Newell KA, Liu T, Aranha GV, Prinz RA. Are cystagastrostomy and cystjejunostomy equivalent operations for pancreatic pseudocysts? Surgery 1990;108:635.

82 Pancreaticojejunostomy (Puestow) for Chronic Pancreatitis

INDICATIONS

Chronic pancreatitis producing *intractable* pain not responsive to medical treatment, with a dilated (≥5-7 mm) pancreatic duct

PREOPERATIVE PREPARATION

Evaluate hepatic function.

Rule out portal hypertension.

Establish nutritional rehabilitation if necessary.

Order endoscopic retrograde cholangiopancreatography (ERCP).

Rule out biliary calculi by radiography or sonography.

PITFALLS AND DANGER POINTS

Failure to rule out portal hypertension.

Overlooking pancreatic carcinoma. Before deciding on an operative procedure, biopsy suspicious areas. Aspiration cytology in the operating room may be helpful in this situation.

OPERATIVE STRATEGY

Because the dilated pancreatic ducts are thick-walled and fibrotic, pancreaticojejunal anastomosis is a safe procedure. One layer of sutures generally suffices.

OPERATIVE TECHNIQUE

Exposure

Make a midline incision from the xiphoid to a point 4-5 cm below the umbilicus. Separate the greater omentum from the middle of the transverse colon

for a distance sufficient to expose the pancreas. Divide the peritoneal attachments between the pancreas and the posterior wall of the stomach.

Incising the Pancreatic Duct

The main pancreatic duct is generally located about one-third the distance of the cephalad to the caudal margin of the pancreas. If the duct cannot be palpated, inserting a 22-gauge needle and attempting to aspirate pancreatic juice may serve to locate the pancreatic duct. If the duct has not been successfully visualized by preoperative ERCP, perform a ductogram in the operating room by aspirating 2 ml of pancreatic juice with a 22-gauge needle; then inject an equal amount of dilute Hypaque into the duct. If there is suspicion that the common duct is obstructed by chronic pancreatitis, perform cholangiography in the operating room. Once the pancreatic duct has been identified, open it by making an incision along its anterior wall. The incision should open the entire duct from the head to the tail of the pancreas. This may be done with Potts scissors or a scalpel (**Fig. 82–1**). Continue the duct incision farther into the head of the pancreas than is shown here. Secure hemostasis with electrocautery. Occasional bleeding points may require a fine PG suture-ligature. If a stricture of the pancreatic duct is encountered, insert a probe through the strictured area and incise the anterior wall of the duct with a scalpel over the probe. Remove any calculi or debris that may have collected in the ductal system.

Constructing the Roux-en-Y Jejunostomy

Prepare the proximal jejunum for a Roux-en-Y operation as illustrated in Figure 73-1. Select a suitable point about 12-15 cm beyond the ligament of Treitz. After a sufficient amount of mesentery has been divided, apply the 55/3.5 mm linear stapling

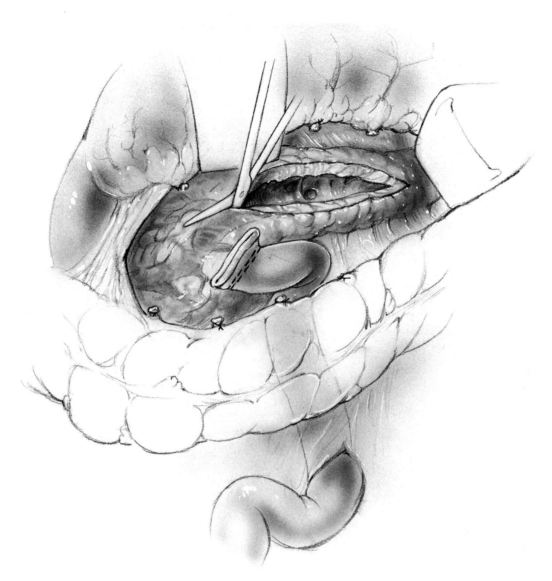

Fig. 82–1

device to the jejunum and fire it. Apply an Allen clamp just proximal to the stapling device. Divide the jejunum flush with the cephalad side of the stapler with a scalpel. Lightly electrocoagulate the everted mucosa and remove the stapler.

Make a 3 cm incision in an avascular area of the transverse mesocolon. Pass the limb of jejunum through this incision and position it side-to-side to the open pancreatic duct. The stapled cut end of the jejunum should be approximated to the tail of the pancreas and the distal jejunum to the head. Now incise the antimesenteric border of jejunum over a

length approximately equal to the incision in the pancreatic duct using a scalpel or electrocautery. Because the fibrotic pancreas accepts sutures easily, one layer of sutures is sufficient. For the posterior layer of the anastomosis, approximate the full thickness of the jejunum to the incision in the pancreatic duct. Use 4-0 PG interrupted sutures. Insert the needle through both the mucosal and seromuscular portions of the jejunal wall. Then pass the needle through the fibrotic parenchyma of pancreas and through the pancreatic duct. Tie the suture with the knot inside the lumen of the pancreatic duct (**Fig.**

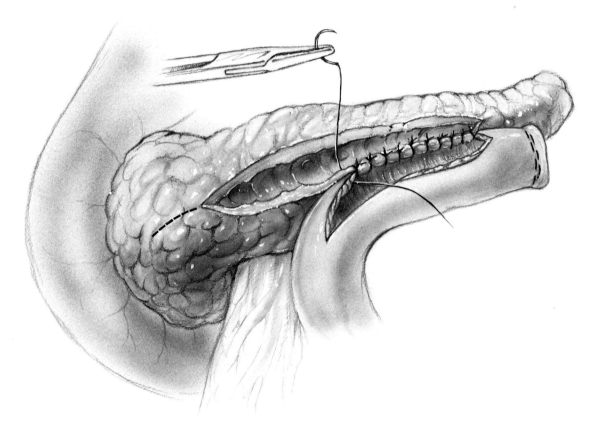

Fig. 82-2

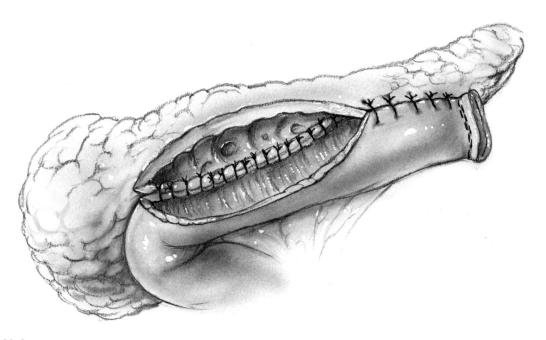

Fig. 82-3

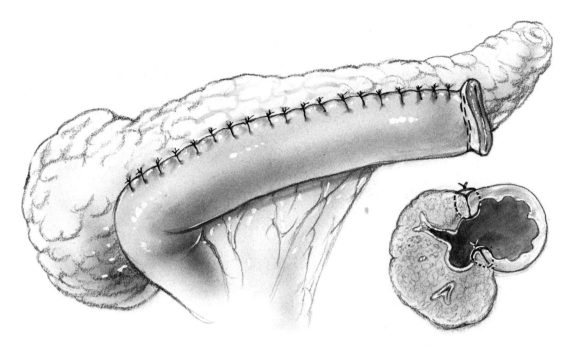

Fig. 82–4a   Fig. 82–4b

82–2). For the anterior layer of the anastomosis use a seromucosal or Lembert stitch on the jejunum. Then pass the needle through the full thickness of the duct including some of the pancreatic parenchyma **(Figs. 82–3, 82–4a, 82–4b)**. Close the defect in the mesocolon by inserting fine interrupted sutures between the mesocolon and the serosa of the jejunum.

At a point at least 60 cm distal to the pancreaticojejunostomy, construct an end-to-side jejunojejunostomy to complete the Roux-en-Y anastomosis. We generally accomplish this anastomosis by stapling as described in Figures 73-7 to 73-12.

If desired, make a puncture wound in the left upper quadrant and insert a Jackson-Pratt closed-suction silicone drainage catheter down to the region of the pancreaticojejunal anastomosis. Close the abdomen in routine fashion.

POSTOPERATIVE CARE

Discontinue nasogastric suction in 1–3 days.
Administer perioperative antibiotics for 24 hours.

COMPLICATIONS

Pancreatic fistula
Abdominal or wound infection

REFERENCES

Drake DH, Fry WJ. Ductal drainage for chronic pancreatitis. Surgery 1989;105:131.

Frey CF, Amikura K. Local resection of the head of the pancreas combined with longitudinal pancreaticojejunostomy in the management of patients with chronic pancreatitis. Ann Surg 1994;220:492.

Izbicki JR, Bloechle C, Broering DC, et al. Extended drainage versus resection in surgery for chronic pancreatitis: a prospective randomized trial comparing the longitudinal pancreaticojejunostomy combined with local pancreatic head excision with the pylorus-preserving pancreatoduodenectomy. Ann Surg 1998;228:771.

Markowitz JS, Rattner DW, Warshaw AL. Failure of symptomatic relief after pancreaticojejunal decompression for chronic pancreatitis: strategies for salvage. Arch Surg 1994;129:374.

Nealon WH, Thompson JC. Progressive loss of pancreatic function in chronic pancreatitis is delayed by main pancreatic duct decompression: a longitudinal prospective analysis of the modified Puestow procedures. Ann Surg 1993;217:458.

Part IX
Spleen

83 Concepts in Splenic Surgery

H. Leon Pachter
Michael Edye
Amber A. Guth

SPLENECTOMY FOR DISEASE

Although the decision to perform splenectomy for hematologic disease is generally made by the treating hematologist, the surgeon must be conversant with the hematologic disorders to ensure that the patient: (1) has been preoperatively immunized with pneumococcal, meningococcal, and (when indicated) *Hemophilus* vaccine; (2) is hematologically optimized for surgery; and (3) is fit for conventional open splenectomy, as laparoscopic splenectomy may require prompt conversion to control hemorrhage.

Common hematologic indications for splenectomy are idiopathic thrombocytopenic purpura (ITP), hereditary spherocytosis, and other forms of hemolytic anemia. Elective splenectomy is also sometimes performed to palliate myelofibrosis or as part of a staging laparotomy for Hodgkin's disease.

Preoperative Evaluation

Standard hematologic parameters are measured. Preoperative radiologic imaging [computed tomography (CT), ultrasonography] do not reliably detect accessory splenic tissue and are rarely indicated during the first operation. When a hematologic disorder recurs owing to a missed accessory spleen, the combined use of damaged red blood cell scintigraphy and CT scanning can be helpful for localizing accessory splenic tissue. Although radiologic embolization has been employed immediately prior to splenectomy to reduce the size and vascularity of the spleen, this approach has not achieved widespread use.

Choice of Surgical Approach: Open Versus Laparoscopic Procedure

The ideal surgical approach for splenectomy would have the following features.

Provide excellent surgical exposure of the splenic hilum, ligaments, and perisplenic tissues

Cause minimal disturbance of the abdominal wall muscles

Permit precise dissection of the splenic vessels and avoid splenic parenchymal injury

Avoid injury to the pancreas, stomach, and adjacent structures

Laparoscopic splenectomy fulfills these criteria in many instances and is rapidly becoming the method of choice for all forms of splenic pathology when the spleen is mildly to moderately enlarged.

If the spleen is significantly enlarged, is the laparoscopic approach truly feasible, or would a generous open incision increase the margin of safety? Massive splenectomy with myelofibrosis in which the spleen is hard, tethered, and supplied by large collateral vessels is not appropriate for minimal access surgery. The surgeon's experience determines the point at which the enlarged spleen is "too large" to remove laparoscopically.

Technical Considerations for Safe Laparoscopic Splenectomy

The spleen develops from buds in the dorsal mesogastrium that subsequently coalesce. This provides the conceptual framework for understanding the layers and contents of the splenic ligaments. The configuration of these ligaments and blood vessels is used to the surgeon's advantage during the laparoscopic approach. Until the surgeon is familiar with mobilizing and handling the organ, it is best that the ligaments of the spleen be left undisturbed until the vessels in the hilum have been divided. Dissection should occur about 10 mm away from the hilum where the vessels are less well fixed and safer to dissect. If the splenic artery is accessible above the pancreas, it can be clipped or tied in continuity. If a stapler is to be used to divide hilar vessels, do not place clips where the stapler is to be positioned to avoid stapler misfires.

Laparoscopic Management of Splenic Cysts

Thick-walled and thin-walled splenic cysts can be unroofed laparoscopically and the cyst wall removed in a retrieval bag. Care must be taken to excise a sufficient portion of the cyst wall to prevent recurrence.

Recurrent Symptoms after Splenectomy for Hematologic Disease

Overlooked *accessory splenic tissue* may hypertrophy, subsequently causing recurrence of the hematologic symptoms for which the splenectomy was initially performed. Some have questioned whether accessory spleens are more likely to be overlooked during laparoscopic splenectomy than open splenectomy [1]. Park et al. reported a 12.3% incidence of accessory splenic tissue in their series of 203 laparoscopic splenectomies, with one patient requiring reexploration for a missed accessory spleen [2]. They attributed this to their ability to visualize the perisplenic tissues better laparoscopically than at open splenectomy. In our experience, the incidence of accessory spleens seen at laparoscopy is 20%, equivalent to the rate generally cited in the literature. A small subset of patients with ITP may ultimately require a subsequent open or laparoscopic procedure to remove an accessory spleen that has caused recurrence of the ITP [3]. It seems unreasonable to impose a major abdominal wound and prolonged hospitalization on the other 80% of patients who do not have accessory spleens.

Splenic implantation is another cause of recurrence. Care must be taken not to fracture the spleen during dissection or to spill splenic tissue during the "morcellation" process. The surgical team must be prepared for an accurate, bloodless splenectomy. All steps should be taken to protect the abdominal cavity from contamination by splenic tissue. This means gentle handling of the spleen and its attachments and use of a strong, impervious extraction bag.

SPLENIC TRAUMA

Splenectomy renders patients susceptible to the lifelong risk of infectious complications. Overwhelming postsplenectomy infection (OPSI) is rare (occurring in only 0.25–5.0% of adult splenectomized patients); but it can occur rapidly and results in a more than 50% mortality rate [4]. Recognition of this syndrome has led to the development and now universal acceptance of splenic preservation as the treatment modality of choice whenever it is safe and feasible.

The importance of splenic preservation has been recognized for more than 20 years. The method of splenic preservation, however, has undergone a remarkable evolution from operative splenorrhaphy to nonoperative management [5]. Advances in modern imaging techniques (CT scanning, ultrasonography) along with technically adept interventional radiologists has established the primacy of the nonoperative approach to splenic trauma [6,7]. Nonetheless, instances arise where operative intervention is required—hence the need for familiarity with techniques such as safe splenectomy, splenorrhaphy, and splenic autotransplantation [8].

When operative intervention has been dictated by a patient's inability to maintain hemodynamic stability despite adequate fluid resuscitation or having sustained multiple injuries, splenectomy should be undertaken without hesitation. When splenectomy is necessary and conditions permit, it seems prudent to use the removed spleen as a source for heterotropic splenic autotransplantation. The benefits derived from heterotopic splenic autotransplantation seem to be, theoretically at least, associated with its ability to restore partially the host's reticuloendothelial function. Whether such partial restoration of reticuloendothelial function is sufficiently protective against specific antigenic challenges is presently unknown. As splenic autotransplantation can be performed with relative ease and has not to date been associated with significant complications, it seems reasonable to continue employing this technique.

In patients with splenic injuries who remain hemodynamically stable but require operative intervention, a variety of techniques can be used to achieve splenic salvage. Included in these techniques is splenorrhaphy, partial splenectomy, mesh splenorrhaphy, topical hemostatic agents, and liberal use of the argon beam laser. The current literature suggests that splenorrhaphy can be achieved in at least 75% of patients with a cumulative success rate of 98%.

Nonoperative Splenic Salvage

In the past splenic salvage was most often achieved (70–75%) by operative splenorrhaphy, partial splenectomy, electrocautery, and the use of adjunctive hemostatic agents. Nonoperative management was, at best, applicable to only 15–20% of patients with blunt injuries. Current data suggest an almost mirror-image reversal, with at least 50–65% of patients with blunt injuries and a small group of select patients with penetrating injuries being managed nonoperatively with success rates exceeding 90%; only 17–20% undergo splenorrhaphy. The most recent data suggest that even splenic injuries are being managed operatively. Splenorrhaphy techniques are detailed in Chapter 85.

Nonoperative Management of Splenic Trauma

An algorithm for nonoperative splenic preservation is given in **Figure 83–1**. The following criteria for nonoperative management have proven safe and effective in our hands.

Hemodynamic stability

CT scan documentation of the injury

No other intraperitoneal or retroperitoneal injuries requiring operative intervention (documented by CT scan)

Limited need for spleen-related transfusions (usually 1 unit)

The almost exponential rise in the number of patients managed nonoperatively since the early 1990s has been a direct result of including the following patients who in the past would have been excluded from nonoperative management: all hemodynamically stable patients regardless of CT grade of splenic injury, patients with intraperitoneal blood accumulation exceeding 250 ml (delineated by CT scan or ultrasonography), patients with pathologically diseased spleens (human immunodeficiency virus, leukemia, mononucleosis), selected patients with isolated stab wounds to the spleen, and neurologically impaired patients.

Prognostic Indicators of Failure of Nonoperative Management

There are certain instances where more active intervention is indicated despite the patient meeting all "conventional" criteria for nonoperative management. Irrespective of the patient's hemodynamic stability, a shattered spleen enveloped by a significant

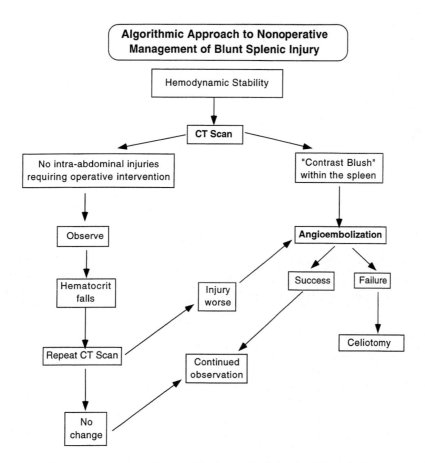

Fig. 83–1. Reproduced, with permission, from Pachter HL, Guth AA, Hofstetter SR, et al. Changing patterns in the management of splenic trauma. Ann Surg 1998;227:708.

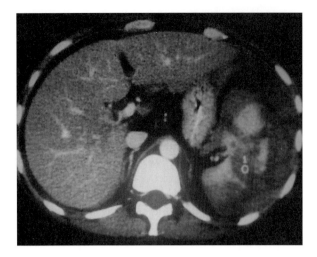

Fig. 83-2

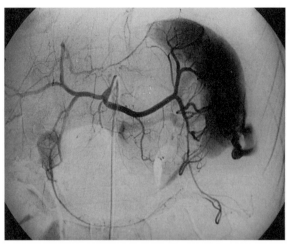

Fig. 83-4. Reproduced, with permission, from Pachter HL, Grau J. The current status of splenic preservation. Adv Surg 2000;34:137.

perisplenic hematoma **(Fig. 83–2)**, in our experience eventually bleeds. It must be remembered that nonoperative management of hepatic and splenic injuries differs greatly. Hepatic injuries rarely rebleed. In contrast, even when bleeding has initially stopped, splenic injuries have a propensity to bleed late. Shattered spleens are particularly vulnerable to this complication. Prompt surgical intervention and expeditious splenectomy, preferably with splenic autotransplantation, is warranted.

Another instance where there is a high degree of sure failure of nonoperative management is when the initial CT scan reveals a "contrast blush." **Figure 83–3** shows a CT scan from a patient who was injured in a motor vehicle collision, demonstrating a contrast "blush" and a large perisplenic hematoma. Such a finding indicates extravasation of contrast material, signifying active bleeding in the splenic parenchyma. One should not be lulled into a false

sense of security by the patient's stable physiologic profile, however, as rapid hemodynamic deterioration can occur at any time. Failure rates of nonoperative management may well be related in part to underestimation of the significance of this finding. The hemodynamically stable patient with CT-demonstrated "contrast blush" should undergo immediate angiographic embolization of the bleeding vessel. **Figure 83–4** shows selective subtraction splenic angiography revealing free extravasation of contrast from the lower pole of the spleen (same patient as in Fig. 83-3). The patient underwent successful angioembolization with a combination of autologous clot and Gelfoam **(Fig. 83–5)**. Angioembolization has become one of the cornerstones in

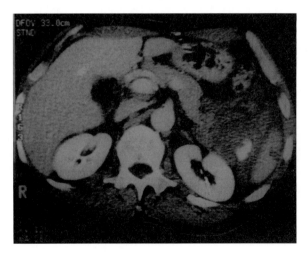

Fig. 83-3

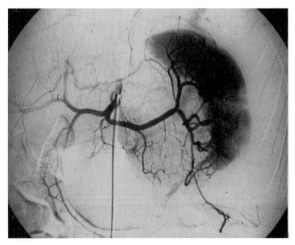

Fig. 83-5. Reproduced, with permission, from Pachter HL, Grau J. The current status of splenic preservation. Adv Surg 2000;34:137.

the successful multidisciplinary approach to the non-operative management of splenic injuries.

Followup Imaging

Most follow-up imaging studies with CT or ultrasonography in patients with stable postobservation courses seem to be superfluous. The role of repeat CT scanning or ultrasonography should be limited to specific circumstances. Imaging may be used as a criterion for moving stable patients out of critical units sooner. All parameters being equal, an ultrasound scan showing at least "no worsening" of the injury allows some patients to move out of the intensive care unit early. Follow-up imaging may also be helpful for determining which patients may return to contact sports, particularly those who initially sustained an American Association for the Surgery of Trauma (AAST) grade III or greater injury. There would be understandable reluctance to allow a patient with a large intrasplenic hematoma to play tackle football without documenting complete resolution of the injury.

In summary, recognition of the pivotal role of the spleen in the immune response has resulted in almost universal policy of avoiding splenectomy when possible. Splenectomy continues to be associated with an increased need for transfusion and excessive perioperative sepsis. Splenic preservation for both blunt injuries and select penetrating injuries has become the accepted treatment protocol of choice. Splenorrhaphy, once the mainstay of splenic preservation, is rarely performed today, having been replaced for the most part by nonoperative observation alone or in conjunction with angioembolization. Nevertheless, operative splenorrhaphy, partial splenectomy, and heterotopic splenic autotransplantation must be in the trauma surgeon's armamentarium.

Laparoscopy for Management of Splenic Trauma

Laparoscopy is another tool available to the trauma surgeon dealing with the diagnosis and management of splenic trauma. Its role in elective splenic surgery is well established, and there is interest in applying the lessons learned to select trauma cases, thereby facilitating splenic salvage while obviating the need for open laparotomy.

The role of diagnostic laparoscopy in the assessment of patients with penetrating thoracoabdominal trauma is well established. Concerns about potentially missed intraperitoneal injuries or the ability to treat discovered injuries has limited the application of diagnostic and therapeutic laparoscopic techniques in this setting. However, multiple case reports have described successful laparoscopic splenic repair and salvage utilizing techniques of intracorporeal suture placement, application of fibrin glue, and absorbable mesh splenorrhaphy.

REFERENCES

1. Gigot JF, Jamar F, Ferrant A, et al. Inadequate dissection of accessory spleens and splenosis with laparoscopic splenectomy: a shortcoming of the laparoscopic approach in hematologic approach in hematologic diseases. Surg Endosc 1998;12:101.

2. Park A, Birgisson G, Mastrangelo MJ, Marcaccio MJ, Witzke DB. Laparoscopic splenectomy: outcomes and lessons learned from over 200 cases. Surgery 2000; 128:660.

3. Velanovich V, Shurafa M. Laparoscopic excision of accessory spleen. Am J Surg 2000;180:62.

4. Lynch AM, Kapila R. Overwhelming postsplenectomy infection. Infect Dis Clin North Am 1996;10:693.

5. Pachter HL, Guth AA, Hofstetter SR, Spencer FC. Changing patterns in the management of splenic trauma: the impact of nonoperative management. Ann Surg 1998; 227:708.

6. Sclafani SJA, Shaftan G, Villalba M, et al. Nonoperative salvage of computed tomography-diagnosed splenic injuries: utilization of angiography for triage and embolization for hemostasis. J Trauma 1995;39:818.

7. Pachter HL, Grau J. The current status of splenic preservation. Adv Surg 2000;34:137.

8. Pister PW, Pachter HL. Autologous splenic transplantation for splenic trauma. Ann Surg 1994;219:225.

84 Splenectomy for Disease

INDICATIONS

Hematologic disorders. Splenectomy may be indicated for patients with hereditary anemias (spherocytosis, elliptocytosis, nonspherocytic hemolytic anemia), primary hypersplenism, and idiopathic thrombocytopenic purpura. Patients with autoimmune hemolytic anemia, secondary hypersplenism, thalassemia, myelofibrosis, chronic lymphatic leukemia, and lymphoma also benefit from splenectomy in selected situations. Splenectomy may be part of the staging procedure for patients with Hodgkin's disease. Because the specific therapy for diseases that require splenectomy is often in a state of flux and many of the conditions are complicated by problems of coagulation, it is important that the indications and timing for surgery be worked out in close cooperation with an experienced hematologist.

Primary splenic tumor.

Splenic abscess.

Splenic cysts, parasitic and nonparasitic.

Gastric varices due to splenic vein thrombosis.

Under unusual circumstances, a large number of other diseases may be benefited by splenectomy, such as Gaucher's disease, sarcoidosis, Felty syndrome, Niemann-Pick's disease, and Fanconi syndrome.

PREOPERATIVE PREPARATION

Consult with an experienced hematologist concerning blood coagulation factors in the patient and arrange for careful cross-matching of an adequate quantity of blood.

Immunize the patient against pneumococcus, meningococcus, and *Hemophilus influenzae* at least 2 weeks prior to surgery.

Perform gastric decompression.

Administer perioperative antibiotics.

Preoperative transcatheter embolization of the splenic artery is a rarely used option in highly selected patients. Splenectomy should be performed promptly after completion of the splenic artery occlusion; otherwise pain, necrosis of the spleen, and sepsis are likely to occur.

PITFALLS AND DANGER POINTS

Intraoperative hemorrhage

Postoperative hemorrhage

Injuring the greater curvature of the stomach

Injuring the pancreas

Postoperative sepsis, especially in immunologically impaired patients

Failure to remove an accessory spleen

OPERATIVE STRATEGY

Choice of Approach: Open or Laparoscopic?

Laparoscopic splenectomy is an excellent alternative for properly selected patients. It is easiest in those with small spleens, such as individuals with idiopathic thrombocytopenic purpura (ITP). Advanced laparoscopy skills are required. The technique is described briefly at the end of Operative Strategy. See References for further technical information.

Avoiding Intraoperative Hemorrhage

First, ensure that exposure is adequate for each step of the operation. Removing a large spleen requires a long incision. It is rarely necessary to perform a thoracic extension. Elevating the left costal margin with a Thompson retractor greatly improves exposure.

Next, meticulously dissect and individually ligate each major vessel to avoid lacerating the splenic vein or a major branch. When performing splenectomy for hematologic disorders, we prefer to isolate the splenic artery as the first step. This frequently allows

732

a large spleen to diminish considerably in size and thus makes the dissection safer.

Patients with portal hypertension, such as with myelofibrosis, have collateral veins in the normally avascular splenophrenic and splenorenal ligaments. These vessels must be individually clamped and ligated.

Preventing Postoperative Hemorrhage

At the conclusion of the splenectomy, it is important to achieve complete hemostasis in the bed of the spleen, especially along the tail of the pancreas, the left adrenal gland, and the posterior abdominal wall. Some of the bleeding points can be controlled by electrocautery; others require clamping. Bleeding from the tail of the pancreas almost always necessitates insertion of fine suture-ligatures on atraumatic needles because the blood vessels tend to retract into the pancreatic tissue. If there is diffuse oozing due to thrombocytopenia or other coagulation deficiencies, administer platelets, fresh frozen plasma, and other coagulation factors as needed *after removing the spleen*. Then continue to observe the operative site until the bleeding stops. Do not simply insert a few drains and close the abdomen, as it often leads to the development of a large hematoma in the left upper quadrant, a major cause of subphrenic abscess.

Avoiding Pancreatic Injury

The greatest risk of injuring the tail of the pancreas occurs when the splenic blood supply is being ligated and divided at the hilus of the spleen. Avoid this by clearly identifying the tail of the pancreas and individually ligating vessels rather than masses of tissue. If each clamp contains only a blood vessel and not other tissue, the pancreas is not crushed by a large hemostat or inadvertently transected.

Avoiding Trauma to the Stomach

During the course of clamping and dividing the short gastric vessels it is easy, especially when a large spleen is being removed, to include the wall of the gastric greater curvature in a hemostat aimed at a short gastric vessel. In other situations the serosa of the stomach may be denuded during the process of dissecting out these blood vessels. In either case, the injury may result in a gastric fistula, which is a serious, life-threatening complication. Consequently, take care to identify clearly each of the vessels and to achieve hemostasis and division of the short gastric vessels without damaging the stomach.

Extra security may be obtained by imbricating the greater curvature with a continuous or interrupted layer of seromuscular Lembert sutures. In this way the ligated stumps of the short gastric vessels and any possibly traumatized gastric wall are inverted together. If the short gastric vessels have been divided with great care under conditions of good visibility and well away from the greater curvature, it may not be necessary to invert this region of the stomach.

Preventing Postoperative Sepsis

Prevent subphrenic abscess by achieving good hemostasis and avoiding injury to adjacent structures. We believe that the use of prophylactic antibiotics administered intravenously at the induction of anesthesia and repeated at intervals for the next 24 hours is an important means to help prevent this complication. This is especially true if there is any danger that the stomach or colon may be entered during a difficult dissection. Routine drainage of the splenic bed appears to increase the incidence of postoperative subphrenic abscess. Selective use of closed-suction drainage in patients with pancreatic injury may be appropriate. Removing the drain within 5 days appears to lower the risk of infection.

Accessory Spleen

Accessory spleens are common and, if overlooked, may in time impair the therapeutic effect of a splenectomy. Seek out and remove accessory spleens before closure.

The most common location of accessory spleen is in the hilus of the spleen and the gastrosplenic, splenocolic, and splenorenal ligaments. Also search the perirenal area, the tail of the pancreas, the small bowel mesentery, and the presacral region for accessory spleens, although these locations are less commonly the site of an accessory spleen than is the area around the splenic hilus.

Laparoscopic Splenectomy

Laparoscopic splenectomy is performed with the patient in the right lateral position. The spleen hangs suspended by its peritoneal attachments, which are divided last. The splenic flexure of the colon is mobilized, and the short gastric vessels are divided to expose the hilum. The splenic artery and vein are ligated or secured with endoscopic vascular staplers. Diaphragmatic attachments are then divided, and the spleen is placed in a large bag. It is morcellated in the bag and sent to the pathologist in small fragments or in the suction cannister.

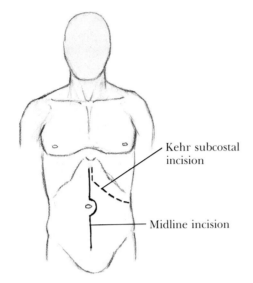

Fig. 84-1

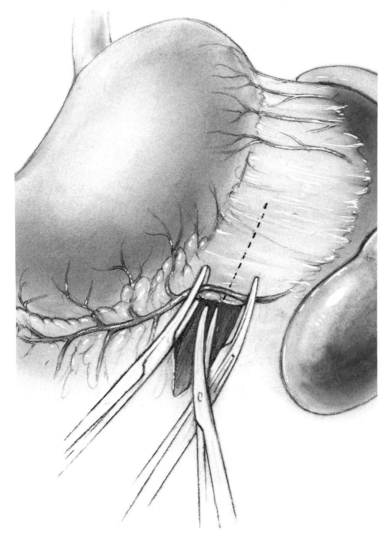

Fig. 84-2

OPERATIVE TECHNIQUE

Incision

In the patient who has a small spleen, as is often the case with ITP, a long left subcostal incision reaching at least to the anterior axillary line provides excellent exposure. In some cases the subcostal incision may be improved by a Kehr extension up the middle to the xiphocostal junction, as illustrated in **Figure 84–1**. A long midline incision may be preferable in patients with marked splenomegaly, especially if the patient has a narrow costal arch. Use electrocautery to incise the abdominal wall. To provide adequate exposure, a midline incision must extend a considerable distance below the umbilicus. Apply a Thompson retractor to elevate the left costal margin and to draw it in a cephalad and lateral direction.

Ligating the Splenic Artery

Incise the avascular portion of the gastrohepatic ligament along the middle of the lesser curvature portion of the stomach and elevate the stomach to expose the upper border of the pancreas. Palpate the splenic artery as it courses along the upper border of the pancreas toward the spleen. If it appears that ligating the splenic artery near the pancreatic tail will be difficult, identify the pancreas behind the lesser curvature of the stomach and incise the peritoneum over the splenic artery where it loops above the body of the pancreas. Carefully pass a blunt-tipped right-angle Mixter clamp around the splenic artery. Temporarily occlude this artery with a vascular clamp or by double-encircling it with a Silastic loop or a narrow umbilical tape fixed in place with a small hemostat.

In most cases approach the splenic artery by opening the gastrocolic omentum outside the gastroepiploic arcade, applying clamps, and dividing and ligating the gastroepiploic vessel **(Fig. 84–2)**. Identify the splenic artery by palpating along the superior border of the pancreatic body or tail. Open the peritoneum over the artery and encircle the artery with a 2-0 silk ligature **(Fig. 84–3)**. Then tie the ligature.

Sometimes identifying the splenic artery requires division of the lower short gastric vessels. If this step has not already been accomplished, identify, clamp, divide, and ligate these structures with 2-0 silk **(Fig. 84–4)**. Continue the division of the short gastric vessels in a cephalad direction so long as the exposure is satisfactory. If the upper short gastric vessel is not long enough to be divided easily at this time, delay it until the spleen has been completely mobilized.

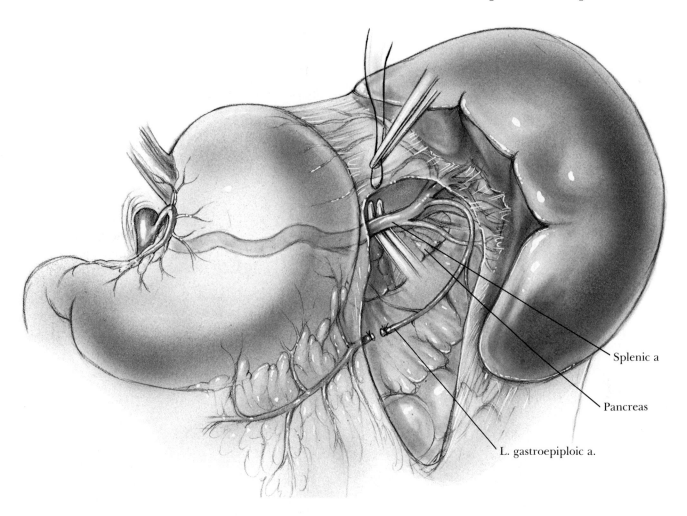

Splenic a

Pancreas

L. gastroepiploic a.

Fig. 84-3

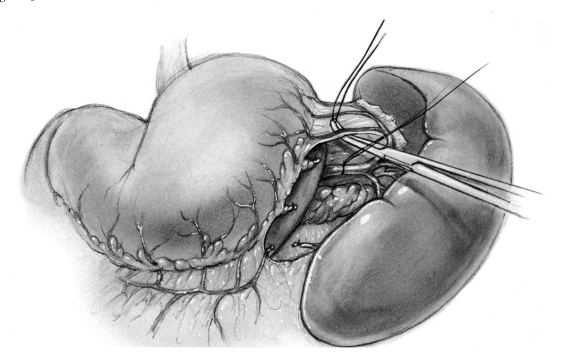

Fig. 84-4

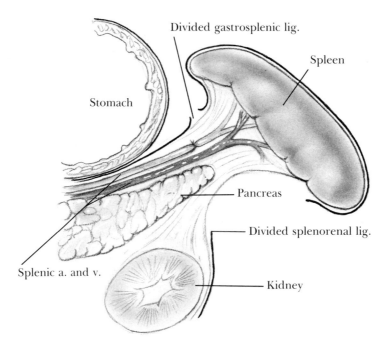

Stomach

Divided gastrosplenic lig.

Spleen

Pancreas

Divided splenorenal lig.

Splenic a. and v.

Kidney

Fig. 84-5

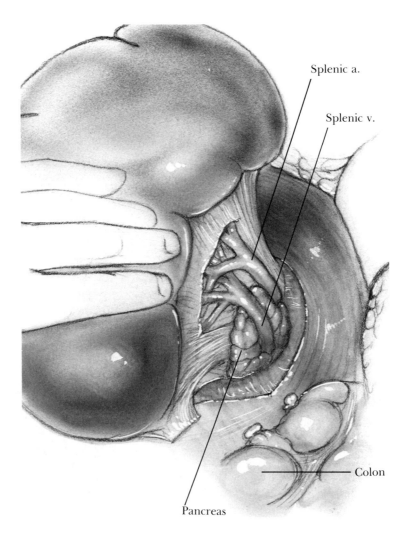

Splenic a.

Splenic v.

Colon

Pancreas

Fig. 84-6

Mobilizing the Spleen

With the left hand, retract the spleen in a medial direction to expose the splenophrenic and splenorenal ligaments, which are generally avascular. Divide the ligaments with Metzenbaum scissors or electrocautery. Only in the presence of portal hypertension is it necessary to ligate a number of bleeding vessels in these ligaments. Insert the left index finger behind the incised splenorenal ligament and continue the incision by both sharp and blunt dissection until the spleen has been freed from the capsule of Gerota and the diaphragm (**Figs. 84–5, 84–6**).

In the same plane, slide the hand behind the posterior surface of the pancreas and elevate the tail of the pancreas and the attached spleen into the abdominal incision. Tearing the splenic capsule by rough maneuvering during this step produces unnecessary bleeding and possible postoperative peritoneal splenosis. Apply a number of moist gauze pads to the bed of the spleen in the posterior abdominal wall.

Slide the index finger behind the splenocolic ligament and divide it, releasing the colon and its attached omentum from the lower pole of the spleen. This dissection leaves the spleen attached only by the splenic artery and vein and perhaps one or two remaining short gastric vessels.

Ligating the Splenic Vessels

With the spleen elevated out of the abdominal cavity, search the posterior aspect of the splenic hilus for the tail of the pancreas. Gently separate the tail of the pancreas from the posterior wall of the splenic artery and vein. Carefully divide and ligate small branches of the splenic vessels entering the tail of the pancreas. Identify the previously ligated splenic artery. Ligate the artery again near the hilus and divide it, leaving a sufficient stump (1 cm). Further dissection reveals the splenic vein, which may be a large structure, or it may have divided into several branches by the time it reaches the splenic hilus. Carefully encircle either the main splenic vein or each of its branches with 2-0 silk ligatures (**Fig. 84–7**). Tie the ligatures, divide the veins between ligatures, and remove the spleen.

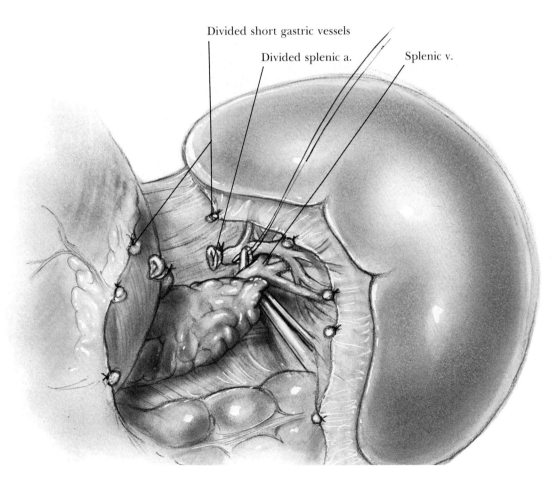

Divided short gastric vessels

Divided splenic a.   Splenic v.

Fig. 84-7

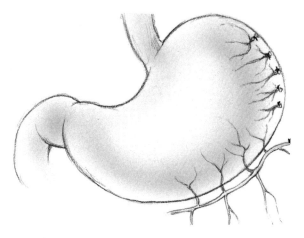

Fig. 84-8

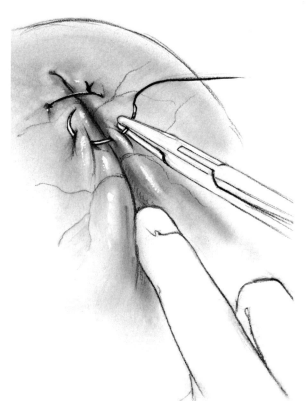

Fig. 84-10

Search for Accessory Spleens

Pack the splenic bed to encourage any minor ooz-ing to stop. Use this time to search the area of the pancreatic tail, kidney, gastrosplenic ligament, omentum, small and large bowel mesentery, and pelvis for accessory spleens. Remove the gauze pads from the splenic bed and accomplish complete he-mostasis utilizing electrocautery and ligatures.

Inverting the Greater Curvature of Stomach

Carefully inspect the greater curvature of the stom-ach. If there is the slightest suspicion of any damage to the tissue in this area, turn in the greater curva-ture together with the ligated stumps of the short gastric vessels. Use continuous or interrupted Lem-

bert sutures of 4-0 atraumatic PG suture material to accomplish this step, which avoids a possible gas-tric fistula **(Figs. 84–8 to 84–11)**.

Abdominal Closure

Irrigate the upper abdomen with a dilute antibiotic so-lution. After aspirating this solution with a suction de-vice, close the abdomen in routine fashion. Do not in-sert any drains unless there has been an injury to the pancreas or complete hemostasis has not been possi-ble. In either case, insert one or two medium-size plas-

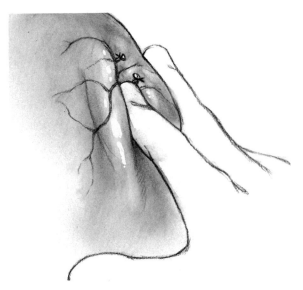

Fig. 84-9

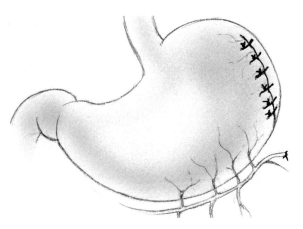

Fig. 84-11

tic closed-suction drains of the Hemovac or Jackson-Pratt type through one or two puncture wounds in the area of the splenic bed and apply suction.

POSTOPERATIVE CARE

Continue nasogastric suction for 1–2 days.

Continue perioperative antibiotics for 24 hours.

Continue steroid medication in patients who were on this therapy prior to and during operation.

Monitor the patient's blood coagulation status and check for postoperative bleeding. Frequently, the platelet count rises postoperatively, but it does not generally require treatment except in patients with myelofibrosis. Patients with this disease have been reported to suffer postoperative portal and mesenteric vein thrombosis.

The leukocyte count may also rise markedly following splenectomy, but it does not necessarily indicate sepsis.

If a patient has undergone total splenectomy, be certain the patient and the family are aware of the risks of overwhelming postsplenectomy sepsis. The patient should wear a Medic-Alert bracelet recording the fact that he or she has undergone splenectomy. If the patient was not immunized preoperatively, administer Pneumovax and meningococcal and *H. influenzae* vaccines. Young children should receive prophylactic penicillin throughout childhood. It is not clear if prophylactic antibiotics are indicated during adult life.

COMPLICATIONS

Bleeding

Subphrenic abscess

Acute pancreatitis

Gastric fistula

Venous thrombosis

REFERENCES

Arregui M, Barteau J, Davis CJ. Laparoscopic splenectomy: techniques and indications. Int Surg 1994;79:335.

Brunt LM, Lander GJ, Quasebarth MA, Whitman ED. Comparative analysis of laparoscopic versus open splenectomy. Am J Surg 1996;172:596.

Delaitre B. Laparoscopic splenectomy: the "hanged spleen" technique. Surg Endosc 1995;9:528.

Farid H, O'Connell TX. Surgical management of massive splenomegaly. Am Surg 1996;62:803.

Irving M. Postoperative complications after splenectomy for hematological malignancies. Ann Surg 1997;225:131.

Rege RV. Laparoscopic splenectomy. In Scott-Conner CEH (ed) The SAGES Manual: Fundamentals of Laparoscopy and GI Endoscopy. New York, Springer-Verlag, 1999, pp 326–335.

85 Operations for Splenic Trauma

INDICATIONS

Nonoperative management is appropriate in many cases of isolated splenic or hepatic trauma (see Chapter 83).

Perform splenectomy if the patient's condition is unstable, there are multiple injuries or gross fecal contamination, the spleen is fragmented beyond repair, or the spleen has been separated from its blood supply. Do not risk the patient's life at any time to preserve an injured spleen, especially in patients over age 50.

Splenorrhaphy or partial splenectomy is indicated in good-risk patients who do not have the above indications for splenectomy.

PREOPERATIVE PREPARATION

Resuscitate the patient by means of adequate fluid and blood replacement.

Insert a nasogastric tube.

If the diagnosis is in doubt, perform computed tomography (CT).

PITFALLS AND DANGER POINTS

Failure to control bleeding

Traumatizing the pancreas

OPERATIVE STRATEGY

Splenectomy

Unlike the technique described for removing the diseased spleen in Chapter 84, initiate the dissection by dividing the splenorenal and splenocolic ligaments as the first step. This permits delivery of the spleen and the tail of the pancreas into the incision. Hemostasis can be maintained by compressing the splenic artery between the thumb and index finger during the rest of the dissection. In the rare case where a giant spleen has been traumatized, it may be advantageous to identify the splenic artery (see Fig. 84-1) and ligate it before delivering the enlarged spleen.

Iatrogenic Injuries

Most spleens injured during dissection may now be salvaged. Commonly, the spleen is injured when the stomach or the transverse colon is retracted away from the spleen, and a small piece of splenic capsule is avulsed. Because the splenic pulp has not been damaged in most of these injuries, it is a simple matter to control the bleeding by applying a topical hemostatic agent, such as oxidized cellulose or Avitene, and then applying pressure with a large gauze pad. Before closing the abdomen, remove the gauze pad carefully and inspect the area for bleeding. This technique is not effective if the injury occurs at the hilus of the spleen.

Splenic Fracture

The splenic artery and vein divide into two to four trunks prior to entering the spleen. The intrasplenic branches generally travel in a horizontal direction. Because most splenic fractures also travel in a transverse direction, often only one or two small blood vessels have been torn. Hemostasis may require only that a hemostatic agent, hemostatic clips, or suture-ligatures be applied; that the laceration be sutured; or that a partial splenectomy be performed. Partial splenectomy is indicated if a portion of the spleen has been separated from its blood supply, which is suggested by cyanotic discoloration of the devascularized segment compared to the remainder of the spleen.

Principles basic to all splenic suturing are adequate exposure combined with *complete mobilization of the spleen* into the abdominal incision. This step is followed by temporary occlusion of the splenic artery by means of a Silastic loop and débridement of the devitalized tissue. Only by dividing the splenorenal and splenocolic ligaments and delivering the spleen together with the tail of the pancreas into the incision can adequate repair of a ruptured spleen be undertaken. The best suture material appears to be 2-0 chromic catgut on an atraumatic straight or curved needle.

After replacing the repaired spleen into its natural bed, always wait 10–15 minutes and reinspect the spleen to be sure the bleeding has indeed been completely controlled. In some cases a narrow pedicle of viable omentum is placed in a fracture and sutured in place with chromic catgut.

After removing a portion of the spleen, it is not necessary to apply sutures to close the cut end of the spleen if good hemostasis can be achieved by means of hemoclips and suture-ligatures in the splenic pulp. When sutures are inserted, they should penetrate the capsule and then be returned as a mattress stitch. When tying the sutures, take care not to tie them so tightly they rupture the capsule. If proper tension is applied to the knot, bolsters of Teflon, omentum, or Surgicel are often not necessary.

OPERATIVE TECHNIQUE

Incision

In the unstable patient, make a midline incision from the xiphoid to a point well below the umbilicus. In the stable patient, a midline incision is suitable for the patient with a narrow costal arch. For the wide-bodied patient, make a long left subcostal incision, dividing the muscular layers with electrocautery to speed the operation. A Kehr extension, which extends up the midline from the medial tip of the subcostal incision and divides the linea alba to the xiphocostal junction, provides excellent exposure. In both the midline and the subcostal incisions, exposure is further enhanced by retracting the left costal margin anterolaterally and in a cephalad direction by means of the Thompson retractor.

Splenectomy

When the spleen is shattered, the hilus has sustained sufficient damage to separate the spleen from its blood supply, or the patient's condition is unstable, emergency splenectomy is the operation of choice. When performing splenectomy for trauma, it is not necessary to isolate and ligate the splenic artery as

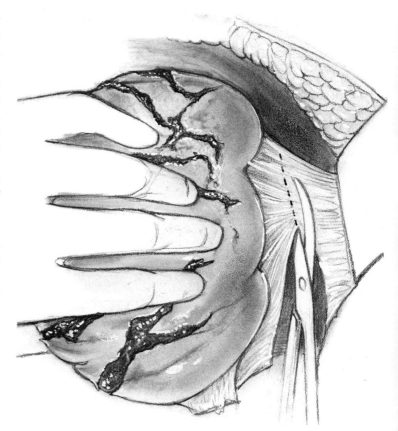

Fig. 85-1

a first step (as described in Chapter 84) unless the traumatized spleen is greatly enlarged owing to a preexisting disease.

Take a position on the patient's right and retract the spleen in a medial direction with the left hand. Create a working space by pulling the spleen gently in a medial direction. Then divide the splenorenal, splenophrenic, and splenocolic ligaments (**Fig. 85–1**). In an emergency situation the experienced surgeon can often perform much of this by blunt finger dissection. After the ligaments have been divided, slide the right hand behind the tail of the pancreas and elevate the tail of the pancreas together with the damaged spleen into the incision. Achieve rapid hemostasis by compressing the splenic artery and vein between the thumb and index finger in the space between the tip of the pancreas and the hilus of the

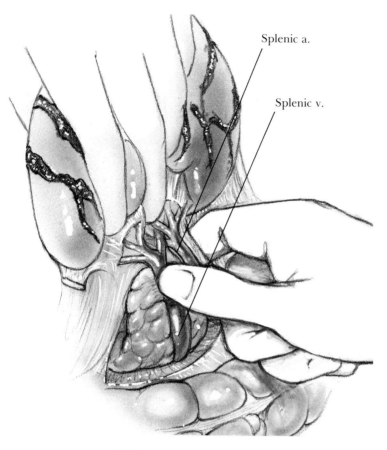

Splenic a.

Splenic v.

Fig. 85-2

spleen **(Fig. 85–2)**. Pack the posterior abdominal wall with moist gauze pads. Expose the posterior aspect of the splenic hilus and identify the splenic artery and vein. It is generally simple to divide these structures between hemostats or ligatures **(Fig. 85–3)**, which controls most of the bleeding. Now deliberately dissect out each of the short gastric vessels and divide each vessel between Adson hemostats. Remove the spleen and then ligate each of the vessels held by hemostats with 2-0 or 3-0 silk. Be sure to apply a second ligature to the splenic artery for added security and to control the minor bleeding points around the tail of the pancreas with fine suture-ligatures. Finally, remove the gauze pads from the splenic bed and achieve complete hemostasis with ligatures and electrocautery. With this technique there need not be any haste to obtain hemostasis because early in the operation the surgeon can control most of the bleeding by finger compression at the hilus of the spleen. This avoids hasty dissection, which may traumatize the tail of the pancreas.

Carefully inspect the greater curvature of the stomach. If there is any suspicion that the stomach wall has been injured during the dissection or the ligation of the short gastric vessels, insert Lembert

sutures to invert this area of stomach as shown in Figures 84-8 to 84-11.

Selecting the Optimal Technique for Splenic Preservation

Avulsion of Capsule; Superficial Injuries

Iatrogenic injury to the spleen during the course of gastric surgery, hiatus hernia repair, or colon resection has constituted the most common single indication for splenectomy in past years. Most of these injuries have involved avulsion of a relatively small patch of splenic capsule. Superficial injuries of this type are best treated by application of topical hemostatic agents (see below) rather than splenectomy. A large subcapsular hematoma, on the other hand, is best treated by incising the capsule, exposing the bleeding points, and applying topical hemostatic agents.

The argon beam coagulator is a noncontact device for applying thermal energy. It is highly affective in controlling minor splenic injuries.

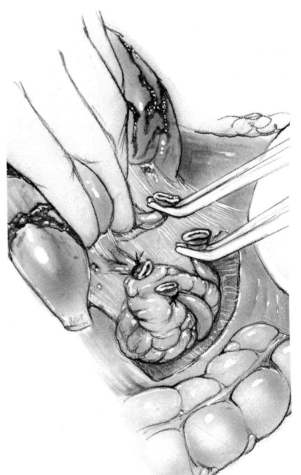

Fig. 85-3

Partial Transverse Fracture

The transverse fracture that does not penetrate the entire thickness of the spleen is a common injury because of the transverse distribution of the splenic blood supply. It is eminently suitable for repair by suturing after hemostasis has been obtained. This technique is described under Splenorrhaphy, below.

Complete Transverse Fracture

When a transverse fracture of the spleen has divided the organ into two or more segments, it is necessary to determine the viability of each segment. This is easily done because the nonviable spleen develops a purple discoloration. Remove the nonviable segments and retain the viable portion of the spleen after achieving hemostasis. Preserving one-third to one-half of the normal spleen is likely to prevent significant diminution of the patient's immune response to infection. The technique for hemisplenectomy is given below. Be sure to identify and ligate the hilar artery that supplied the amputated segment of spleen.

Longitudinal Fracture

Severe blunt injuries may produce a longitudinal fracture in the long axis of the spleen **(Fig. 85–4)**. Because this fracture may lacerate a large number of the transverse branches of the splenic artery and vein, hemostasis is more difficult than is the case with transverse injuries. After controlling the arterial bleeders with hemoclips and suture-ligatures, the residual oozing can generally be managed by inserting a narrow pedicle of viable omentum and fixing it in place with a series of capsular sutures **(Fig. 85–5)**.

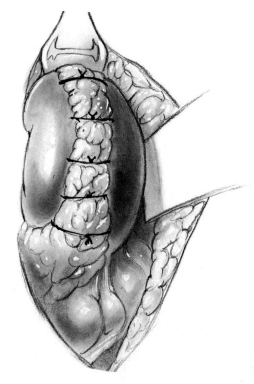

Fig. 85–5

Stellate Fracture

After exploring the depths of the fracture and removing clotted blood, treat the superficial fractures by suturing the capsule. Closing the capsule in this fashion generally controls bleeding from superficial fractures. Alternatively, applying Avitene to the stellate fracture may successfully control all but the arterial bleeders. The efficiency of this topical agent may be enhanced by also inserting capsular sutures. Absorbable mesh wrap is an alternative. Any splenic fracture that significantly involves the hilus of the spleen generally requires partial splenectomy to control hilar bleeding, rather than capsular sutures.

Applying Topical Hemostatic Agents

Most topical hemostatic agents provide a framework for deposition of platelets, which accelerates formation of a blood clot. None of these agents controls rapid bleeding. Consequently, it is necessary to slow down the bleeding from the surface of a damaged spleen by local pressure for a few minutes. If the oozing surface is fairly smooth, apply a double sheet of oxidized cellulose gauze and cover it with a dry gauze pad. Apply even pressure with the gauze pad for 10 minutes. Then gently remove the gauze pad while taking care not to dislodge the sheet of oxidized cellulose, which should now be adherent to the raw surface.

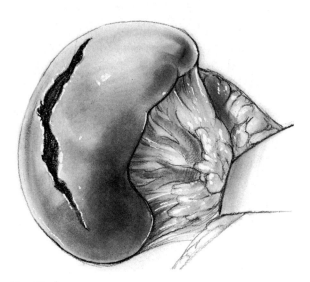

Fig. 85-4

If the bleeding surface is irregular in nature, Avitene is a much better choice than hemostatic sheets. It is highly effective for oozing surfaces due to traumatized capillaries and venous sinusoids. When applying Avitene, make certain to use only absolutely dry instruments. Use a forceps to apply enough Avitene to cover the entire bleeding surface for a thickness of 3–4 mm. Apply the Avitene quickly and cover it with a dry gauze pad. Apply constant pressure for at least 5 minutes. If bleeding breaks through one portion of the Avitene, apply an additional layer of dry Avitene. If bleeding continues to break through, remove the Avitene and pursue further efforts to reduce the rate of bleeding by applying hemostatic clips or suture-ligatures. Rapid bleeding causes the Avitene to gel prematurely, making it useless as a hemostatic agent.

Splenorrhaphy

Mobilizing the Spleen

Do not try to repair the spleen without completely mobilizing the spleen and the tail of the pancreas by the technique described above (Fig. 85–1). Be sure to free any attachments between the spleen and omentum. Adequate exposure may also require division of the lower short gastric vessels. Be careful not to cause further injury to the spleen when dividing the splenic ligaments. Evacuate liquid and clotted blood from the area. Place a large gauze pad against the posterior abdominal wall in the area of the dissection and elevate the spleen and tail of the pancreas into the incision. If any of these maneuvers initiates brisk bleeding, compress the splenic artery and vein between the thumb and index finger at the hilus (Fig. 85–2). Ligate any of the small vessels at the hilus that may have been lacerated by the trauma.

Suturing the Splenic Capsule

For fractures that have not penetrated the full thickness of the spleen, remove devitalized tissue and blood clot from the traumatized areas. Use a narrow-tipped suction device to provide exposure and occlude bleeding arteries by accurately applying small or medium-size hemostatic clips. use 4-0 or 5-0 vascular sutures to control bleeding veins or arteries that have retracted. Control residual oozing of blood from the sinusoids by closing the capsule with interrupted sutures of 2-0 chromic catgut on a medium-size gastrointestinal atraumatic needle, as illustrated in **Figure 85–6**. If necessary, insert these sutures in an interlocking fashion. In other cases, a continuous suture of the same material may prove to be effective. When tying these sutures, take great

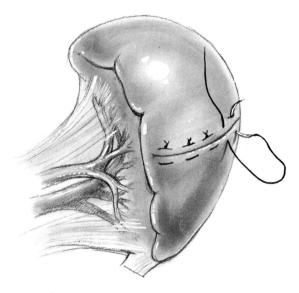

Fig. 85-6

care not to apply force sufficient to tear the delicate splenic capsule. Tie the sutures just tight enough to achieve hemostasis without tearing the spleen. If necessary, use strips or pledgets of Teflon felt, omental pedicle, or even oxidized cellulose gauze; insert the sutures through these pledgets to protect the splenic capsule when the suture is being tied. A linear stapling device may also be used to close the capsule of a small, normal spleen after partial splenectomy.

Absorbable Mesh Wrap

When a spleen is the site of several fractures or the capsule is stripped from a significant part of the surface but the hilum is uninjured, wrapping it with a sheet of PG absorbable mesh after tailoring the mesh and suturing it so it provides even pressure to the damaged spleen may help achieve good hemostasis. Select a large sheet of PG mesh and place it behind the spleen so the edge of the mesh can be gathered around the hilum. Mark the excess, remove it, and cut it to size, leaving at least a 2 cm border all around. With the mesh on a convenient surface away from the operative field, insert a running suture of 2-0 PG around the circumference of the mesh. This suture serves as a purse string to tighten the mesh around the spleen, applying firm, even compression to the splenic pulp without occluding the hilar vessels. Replace the mesh around the spleen. Tie the purse-string suture, taking care not to tighten it around the splenic artery and vein (**Fig. 85–7**). If the mesh is not tight enough, plicate it with additional sutures at a convenient location. Confirm that all bleeding has been controlled and replace the spleen in its bed.

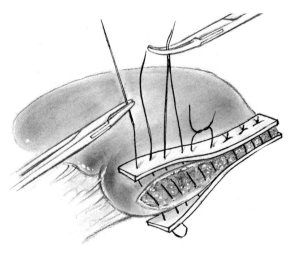

Fig. 85-9

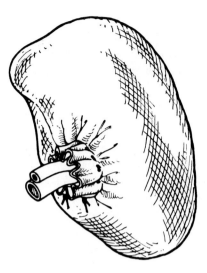

Fig. 85-7. Reprinted, with permission, from Scott-Conner CEH, Dawson DL. Operative Anatomy. Philadelphia, Lippincott, 1993.

Partial Splenectomy

Dividing the Spleen

Temporarily occlude the splenic artery with a Silastic loop. Then aspirate all blood clots from the area of injury, especially at the splenic hilus. Ligate the traumatized vessels at the hilus, preserving the blood supply to the portion of the spleen that is to be retained. Release the splenic artery, observe for a line of demarcation, and mark it with electrocautery along the capsule. Secure the splenic artery again if necessary to limit blood loss.

Use a narrow-tipped suction device to expose the bleeding points in the line of the fracture. Use the suction tip to develop a transverse division of the spleen. Apply small hemostatic clips to bleeding vessels and continue the dissection until the traumatized section of the spleen has been entirely severed. Remove the specimen. Then release the Silastic loop encircling the splenic artery and observe the cut edge of the splenic remnant for hemostasis. Generally, some oozing persists, requiring suturing of the cut end of the spleen. Use 2-0 chromic catgut on an atraumatic needle **(Fig. 85–8)**. Although their use is not often necessary, it is possible to protect the delicate splenic capsule by applying a strip of Teflon felt on the anterior surface of the spleen and a second strip on the posterior surface. Then insert the sutures through the Teflon felt as shown in **Figure 85–9)**. Tie each of these mattress sutures. This maneuver achieves satisfactory hemostasis along the cut edge of the spleen.

Replace the splenic remnant in its natural position after making certain that hemostasis is complete in the posterior abdominal wall and the splenic bed. Use electrocautery along the posterior abdominal wall; but if there are bleeding points in the tail of the pancreas, occlude these bleeding points with 4-0 or 5-0 suture-ligatures.

Do not close the abdominal incision for at least 10-15 minutes so the splenic remnant can be inspected after it has been replaced in the abdomen. Use this time to double-check for other injuries. If there is any bleeding, again deliver the remnant of spleen into the abdominal incision and control the bleeding.

Abdominal Closure and Drainage

Close the abdominal incision in the usual fashion without drainage. If continued hemorrhage or injury

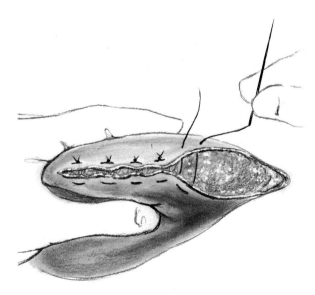

Fig. 85-8

to the pancreas is suspected, place a closed-suction drain in the vicinity of the splenic bed.

POSTOPERATIVE CARE

Administer perioperative antibiotics for 12–24 hours. Observe the patient in an intensive care unit or in another area where vital signs can be carefully monitored for 2–3 days. Follow the vital signs and the hemoglobin or hematocrit to exclude continued bleeding. If a drain was placed, remove it by the second postoperative day.

Keep the patient at bed rest for the first day or two. Thereafter cautiously resume ambulation. Patients who have had a splenorrhaphy or partial splenectomy should avoid vigorous athletic activity for 4–6 weeks.

If a patient has undergone total splenectomy, be certain that the patient and the family are aware of the risks of overwhelming postsplenectomy sepsis. The patient should wear a Medic-Alert bracelet recording the fact that he or she has undergone splenectomy. Administer Pneumovax and vaccines for meningococcus and *Hemophilus influenzae*. Young children should receive prophylactic penicillin throughout childhood. It is not clear if prophylactic antibiotics are indicated during adult life.

COMPLICATIONS

Postoperative bleeding. If proper hemostasis has been attained during the operation, this complication is rare.

Infarction of the splenic remnant.

REFERENCES

Dunham CM, Cornwell EE III, Militello P. The role of the argon beam coagulator in splenic salvage. Surg Gynecol Obstet 1991;173:179.

Fingerhut A, Oberlin P, Cotte JL, et al. Splenic salvage using an absorbable mesh: feasibility, reliability and safety. Br J Surg 1992;79:325.

Uranus S, Kronberger L, Kraft-Kine J. Partial splenic resection using the TA-stapler. Am J Surg 1994;168:49.

Part X

Hernia Repairs, Operations for Necrotizing Fasciitis, Drainage of Subphrenic Abscess

86 Concepts in Hernia Repair, Surgery for Necrotizing Fasciitis, and Drainage of Subphrenic Abscess

Daniel P. Guyton

GROIN HERNIA

We begin with a perspective on one of surgery's most ancient and vexing problems in adults. Inguinal hernia repair now constitutes 35% of all abdominal surgeries submitted to the American Board of Surgery by general surgeons applying for recertification [1]. Rutkow et al., who have a keen interest in socioeconomic issues, reported that nearly 700,000 operations are performed annually [2]. Clearly, this mechanical problem has vast associated medical and economic costs that fuel an interest in this operation that has not abated. Moreover, Smith found 3,100 published citations in the MEDLINE literature search over a 10-year period at the end of the twentieth century dedicated to one aspect or another of groin hernia repair [3]. No wonder surgeons remain bemused and skeptical when a new technique is acclaimed as the ultimate solution. Finally, and again drawing from the American Board of Surgery recertification database, the average number of inguinal hernia repairs performed annually by an individual surgeon was only 35 [1]. This simple fact is important to bear in mind when discussing multiple new and vastly different operative approaches, each of which may have a different learning curve.

Next in this concepts chapter we raise a challenge to one of the most fundamental of all questions regarding inguinal hernia and its treatment: *Should all patients with groin hernia undergo elective repair?*

For generations, the answer to the question regarding elective hernia repair has been an emphatic yes with the exception being patients with significant medical co-morbidities. The intuitive thought behind this dictum was that elective repair under controlled circumstances was far safer than the alternative, that is, to wait and then operate urgently in the face of the potential serious complications of bowel incarceration or strangulation. In particular, with surgery performed on an ambulatory basis and in free-standing hernia centers the operation is associated with low morbidity, making elective repair even more advisable. This thought is so ingrained that few if any studies ever challenged the concept.

One variation of this question is to base the decision for surgery according to symptoms, such as evaluation of cholelithiasis. Indeed, this is the focus of the recently announced joint Veterans Administration, American College of Surgeons, and Northwestern University prospective study. To be conducted over a 2.5-year period, the study design randomizes men on the basis of symptoms. Men with asymptomatic or minimal symptoms of inguinal hernia undergo a period of observation, whereas standard treatment (open repair with mesh) is offered to the symptomatic cohort. An analysis of the medical aspects and associated economic factors with and without repair are evaluated. Hopefully, this landmark study will offer a clearer answer to this question with firm data that allow a thoughtful and perhaps selective decision in the patient's best interest. For the present, however, we remain convinced that most patients should undergo elective repair unless significant medical co-morbidities are present.

Selection of Anesthesia

Elective operation in men or women may be performed under local, attended (regional or epidural), or general anesthesia. Each has its distinct advantages or disadvantages and should be tailored to the comfort of the patient and surgeon. In practice, the choice tends to be based on community experience. Local anesthetics consisting of 1% lidocaine or Marcaine are readily available, easy to use, and well tolerated; they also have a markedly reduced incidence of postoperative headache, nausea, and vomiting. In particular, when administered using a laryngeal mask airway (which does not control the patient's respiration), patient comfort is maximized. A general anesthetic (administered via an endotracheal tube) is preferred when faced with an emergent operation such as incarceration where the bowel may require manipulation. Additionally, a general anesthetic is necessary when the repair is performed laparoscopically. After using all three techniques extensively, I have come to prefer general anesthesia administered via a laryngeal mask airway.

Which Operation for Which Hernia?

Inguinal hernias are broadly classified as direct (i.e., a weakness in the transversalis fascia within Hesselbach's triangle) or indirect (a weakness in the internal inguinal ring associated with a patent processus vaginalis). Usually this distinction is not readily or accurately accomplished preoperatively and is finalized during the operation itself. A femoral hernia occurs through a defect in the femoral canal, lateral to the lacunar ligament and medial to the femoral vein.

In adults the operative repair selected is based on the surgeon's experience and training and should be individualized as much as is feasible. Additionally, hernia repair represents a prime opportunity for each surgeon to analyze his or her individual rates of recurrence, postoperative complications, and resultant disability—key factors consistent with the provision of excellent professional advice.

As implied earlier, the range of operative choices available for groin hernia repair is broad. This chapter reviews primary repair, mesh or tension-free repair, and repair using laparoscopic techniques.

Primary Repair

Primary repair remains the preferred technique in the presence of contamination from incarcerated or strangulated intestine when avoidance of prosthetic mesh is desired. In women, when the round ligament is removed and the residual defect is small, primary repair with interrupted sutures can be readily accomplished without mesh. Usually it can be performed without a great deal of tension. For an adolescent boy, primary suture repair of a weakened internal ring is also appropriate.

Primary repair may be accomplished using the Bassini, McVay, or Shouldice technique. The Bassini

method (which is not described here) is mentioned only for its historical context and relative simplicity. It was the first technique that led to a marked reduction in both operative mortality and recurrence. The basic technique involves opening the transversalis fascia and recreating the floor of the inguinal canal. Bassini accomplished this with interrupted sutures sewing Poupart's ligament to the lateral border of the internal oblique or conjoined tendon. Any peritoneal sac underwent high ligation after opening to ensure the reduction of its contents and to check for a femoral component.

The Shouldice technique, developed at the Shouldice Clinic in Toronto, incorporates complete dissection and reconstruction of the inguinal floor. It is relatively tension-free as the repair utilizes the opened and healthy transversalis fascia imbricated in layers over one another. Four layers of suture are placed to incorporate the transversalis, iliopubic tract, femoral sheath and inguinal ligament. Data from the Shouldice clinic attests to the excellent long-term results coupled with minimal postoperative disability.

McVay's repair is predicated on a detailed study of the anatomy of the inguinal region he performed as a surgical resident. He postulated that the central factor accompanying groin hernia was a weakened posterior floor. To remedy this problem, his method incorporates suturing the transversus abdominis to Cooper's ligament. A transition stitch is placed in the femoral sheath. McVay also popularized the concept of a relaxing incision created in the external oblique aponeurosis at its fusion with the anterior rectus sheath. The purpose was to reduce excessive tension away from the actual repair. This concept of tension and its avoidance is central to all repairs using prosthetic mesh.

Prosthetic Mesh Repair

Currently in the United States mesh repair by the Lichtenstein technique using a precut piece of Marlex mesh or Rutkow's mesh "plug" is increasingly becoming the most popular method. Repair of groin hernias utilizing any type of prosthetic mesh relies on the mesh to first bridge the inguinal defect and then to incite a foreign body reaction with the native tissue. Both are straightforward technically and associated with low postoperative disability and a low (reportedly less than 1%) incidence of recurrence. The common strategy with either method is the concept of minimal tissue dissection, anchoring the mesh with interrupted sutures, and encouraging early ambulation and return to employment. The Lichtenstein repair is remarkably free of postoperative complications, although there have been several reports of "plug" migration into the abdominal cavity leading to small bowel obstruction. Gore-Tex mesh minimizes the foreign body reaction that is useful elsewhere in the body but not in the groin, where a firm scar is welcomed. Gore-Tex also tends to become encapsulated rather than incorporated directly into the adjacent tissue. Absorbable mesh has no role in the repair of inguinal hernia.

Laparoscopic Technique

Inguinal hernia may be repaired laparoscopically. However, of all laparoscopic techniques, repair of groin hernia has the steepest learning curve. The anatomy is new (and often confusing), requiring participation in 40–50 operations before a surgeon becomes experienced. Reported series consistently note a high (approaching 10%) incidence of recurrence during the surgeon's initial operative experience.

Two methods are in wide use: the totally extraperitoneal approach (TEP) and the transabdominal preperitoneal (TAPP) approach. They are based on reconstruction of the weakened posterior abdominal wall. This is the one method of repair where complications can be catastrophic. Yet in the hands of experienced laparoscopic surgeons, excellent results are achieved. Proponents consistently report low disability and early return to work or fully normal activities. As the definition of postoperative disability is expanded, laparoscopic repair may be more widely utilized. This approach may evolve into the preferred technique for bilateral hernias or for a difficult recurrence, although issues of increased resource expenditure remain unresolved.

Repair of Femoral Hernia

The femoral hernia should always be repaired, as there is a high incidence of incarceration that is secondary to the narrow anatomic defect in the femoral canal. When a femoral hernia is diagnosed preoperatively, the surgeon has three operative approaches: low inguinal, high inguinal, or preperitoneal via a low midline incision. We favor a preperitoneal exposure for the following reasons. First, the anatomy is easily and clearly defined, permitting identification and reduction of the sack. The repair is straightforward once this step is accomplished. If the contents are strangulated, conversion to a midline laparotomy is easily completed, obviating the need for two separate incisions.

Occasionally, however, an incarcerated mass may be indistinguishable on physical examination as to the origin (i.e., inguinal or femoral). In these cases a high inguinal incision is best initially. If incarcerated intestine requires resection, it can be a difficult maneuver through a groin incision, as the adjacent mesentery may be shortened, thickened, and inflamed. In this situation, conversion to a midline incision is necessary.

Repair of Recurrent Inguinal Hernia

When faced with a recurrent inguinal hernia in a man, the surgeon must avoid inadvertent transection of the vas deferens and devascularization of the testis. These problems are best avoided using careful slow dissection in a bloodless field. Both the internal inguinal ring and the pubic tubercle should be inspected, as recurrence is common in these regions. Once identified, the recurrence may be easily repaired using the mesh "plug" that is carefully anchored to the usually rigid surrounding tissues. The laparoscopic approach avoids this occasionally difficult exposure.

Repair of Large Ventral Hernias

Large ventral hernias usually require placement of prosthetic mesh as an aid to strengthen the weakened abdominal wall. When it is possible to separate the repair from the abdominal contents, Marlex mesh is preferred because of the same properties we discussed for inguinal hernia repair. When this is not the case, Gore-Tex mesh can be employed. The intestines can adhere to Gore-Tex, and fistulization, a dreaded complication of Marlex, is uncommon.

NECROTIZING FASCIITIS

An unusual but potentially serious and life-threatening complication, necrotizing fasciitis requires early detection, urgent operation, and fearless débridement of any suspected involved tissue. Intraoperative Gram stain and cultures are imperative along with the administration of broad-spectrum antibiotics. Reexploration is often necessary. Temporary closure of the abdominal wall using absorbable mesh can provide an excellent bridge until resolution is complete. We are reluctant to place permanent mesh in the acute situation.

SUBPHRENIC ABSCESS

Most subphrenic abscesses are amenable to image-guided percutaneous drainage. If this technique is technically not feasible or is unsuccessful, an operative approach becomes necessary. The key points emphasized in Chapter 95 (a surgical legacy technique chapter) remain salient.

REFERENCES

1. Ritchie W, Rhodes R, Biesster M. Work loads and practice patterns of general surgeons in the United States, 1995–1997. Ann Surg 1999;230:533.

2. Rutkow I, Robbins A. "Tension-free" inguinal herniorrhaphy: a preliminary report on the "mesh plug" technique. Surgery 1993;114:3.

3. Smith CD. Introduction: inguinal hernia repair. In van Heerden J, Farley D (eds) Operative Techniques in General Surgery. Philadelphia, Saunders, 1999, p 104.

87 Shouldice Repair of Inguinal Hernia

INDICATIONS

All indirect and sliding inguinal hernias should be repaired because of the significant incidence of strangulation.

With the use of local anesthesia, systemic disease is rarely so serious it constitutes a contraindication to operating. Small, nonsymptomatic direct inguinal hernias in elderly patients do not require surgery because they almost never produce strangulation. Direct hernias that produce symptoms, on the other hand, should be repaired.

PREOPERATIVE PREPARATION

Persuade obese patients to lose weight prior to surgery. (Fat interposed between sutured layers of fascia impedes healing.)

PITFALLS AND DANGER POINTS

Injury to femoral vessels during suturing

Injury to bladder (especially with a sliding hernia)

Injury to colon (especially with a sliding hernia)

Injury to deep inferior epigastric vessels with postoperative retroperitoneal bleeding

Injury to ilioinguinal nerve

OPERATIVE STRATEGY

Anesthesia

For inguinal hernia repair, local field block anesthesia is preferred. Patients are ambulatory the afternoon of operation and are able to resume a normal diet the same evening. Overdistension of the anesthetized bladder by intravenous fluids often follows the use of general anesthesia and is a major cause of postoperative urinary retention. Relief requires bladder catheterization, which in some cases of borderline prostatism necessitate prostatectomy after the hernia repair. Urinary retention is avoided with local anesthesia because it does not obtund the patient's sensation of a full bladder or the ability to urinate.

Local anesthesia does not mean that no attention is paid to the patient by anyone other than the operating team. We require that either an anesthesiologist or a nurse sit at the head of the table to monitor vital signs. Although local anesthesia allows us to manage most incarcerated hernias successfully, general anesthesia with endotracheal intubation is indicated whenever strangulation of bowel is suspected.

Avoiding Injury

The *iliac* or *femoral vein* may be injured by blindly inserting a suture too deeply through the iliopubic tract or the inguinal ligament during the lateral portion of the repair. If this should occur, cut the needle off and remove the suture. Then apply pressure to the vein for 5–10 minutes. This maneuver often avoids the need to expose the iliac vein and suture the bleeding point.

Occasionally, serious postoperative *preperitoneal hemorrhage* has been produced by injuring one of the deep inferior epigastric vessels with a deep suture. During the Shouldice technique prevent this problem by completely dissecting the transversalis fascia away from these structures after dividing the external spermatic vessels.

The *bladder* may be injured when attempting to amputate a sac in a sliding inguinal hernia. Overenthusiastic dissection on the medial aspect of an indirect sac for the mistaken notion that the higher the ligation the better may also traumatize the bladder. If a laceration of the bladder has been identified, close the defect by suturing the full thickness of the bladder wall with a continuous 3-0 PG atraumatic suture. Then invert this layer of stitches with a second continuous or interrupted layer of 3-0 PG Lembert-type sutures. Be sure the bladder remains decompressed for the next 8–10 days by means of constant drainage with an adequate indwelling Foley catheter.

Colon and bladder may be injured if the sliding nature of an inguinal hernia is not diagnosed early in the course of operation. Whenever a bulky indirect inguinal hernia is not accompanied by a thin-walled, transparent sac, suspect a sliding component.

All of these inadvertent injuries can be avoided by taking advantage of the extensive exposure that may be attained by a long incision in the transversalis fascia when using the Shouldice method. The deep inferior epigastric vessels and their branches, the iliac vessels, the peritoneum, and in case of a sliding hernia the colon are all easily identified. Visualizing these structures is the best way to prevent damage.

Avoiding Postoperative Wound Infections

Among the patients who suffer a postoperative wound infection, 40–50% develop a recurrent hernia. The rate of infection can be minimized during hernia repair if the entire operation is performed with careful, sharp dissection. Meticulous hemostasis is also important. Irrigate the operative site to remove any blood or debris before closure. Some surgeons add topical antibiotics to the irrigation. Wound infection should be rare after this operation.

OPERATIVE TECHNIQUE

Local Anesthesia

Use a mixture of equal parts of 0.5% Marcaine and 2% Nesacaine. Create a field block by injecting into the subcutaneous tissues along the lines shown in **Figure 87–1a**. Inject also along the line of the incision. A total of 40 ml of anesthetic solution is required.

After making the skin incision and exposing the external oblique aponeurosis, inject another 10 ml just underneath this layer **(Fig. 87–1b)**. Also inject the abdominal musculature along a line 5 cm cephalad to the inguinal canal. This step improves muscle relaxation for the repair. Inject 5 ml around the internal ring **(Fig. 87–2a)**. When the peritoneal sac is exposed, inject 5 ml into the sac **(Fig. 87–2b)** and around the neck of the sac. Not only does this technique of local block eliminate pain, it produces *surprisingly good muscle relaxation*.

Incision

Start the incision in the skin at a point 2.5 cm medial to the anterosuperior spine of the ilium. Continue in an oblique fashion to the point where the external ring adjoins the public tubercle.

Exposure

Clear the external oblique aponeurosis of fat and areolar tissue by sharp scalpel dissection; continue inferiorly beyond the point where the external oblique aponeurosis becomes the inguinal ligament and curves posteriorly in the upper thigh. Expose the external inguinal ring and the spermatic cord emerging from this ring. Secure any bleeding points with 4-0 PG ligatures or electrocautery. Incise the external oblique aponeurosis along the line of its fibers so the incision joins the external inguinal ring at its *cephalad* margin **(Fig. 87–3)**.

Identify the ilioinguinal nerve and dissect it free.

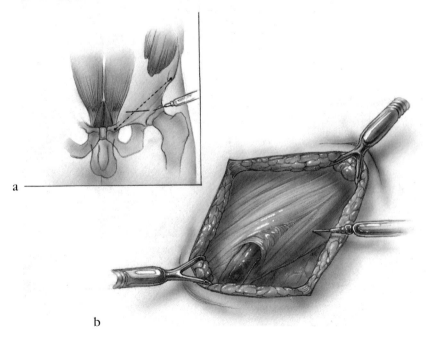

a

b

Fig. 87-1a,b

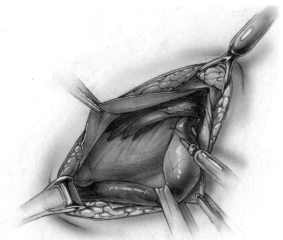

Fig. 87–2a

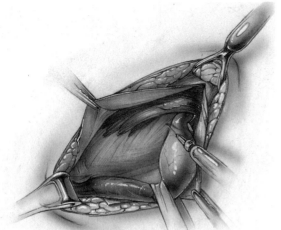

Fig. 87–2b

Occasionally, the ilioinguinal nerve runs with the spermatic cord, in close approximation to the cremaster muscle. Retract the lateral leaflet of the external oblique in a caudal direction and expose its junction with the pubic tubercle. It is important now to elevate the medial leaflet of external oblique aponeurosis from the underlying transversus muscle for a distance of at least 3–4 cm. Retract the medial leaflet cephalad by inserting one fork of the self-retaining Farr retractor underneath this leaflet; the other fork is inserted in the subcutaneous tissue of the lateral skin flap.

Excising Cremaster Muscle

Incise the cremaster muscle sharply in the direction of its fibers before encircling the cord **(Fig. 87–4)**. Then ligate and divide excess cremaster muscle, taking care that no cord structures have inadvertently been included in the ligature. Free the spermatic cord from surrounding attachments at a point medial to the public tubercle. An attempt to encircle the cord lateral to this point may result in traumatizing the structures enclosed in a direct hernia, or it may damage the floor of the inguinal canal. There is much less difficulty freeing the cord from surrounding structures in the medial location. Remember that in patients with a direct hernia the hernial sac remains be-

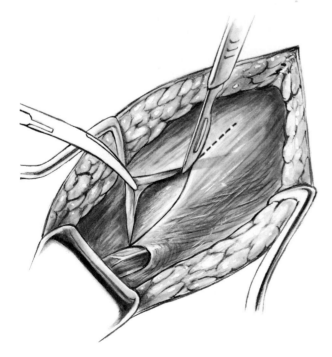

Fig. 87–3

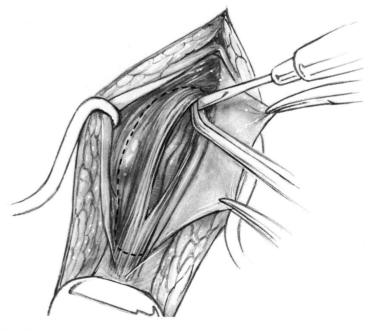

Fig. 87–4

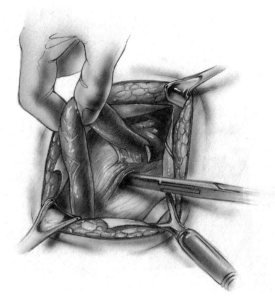

Fig. 87-5

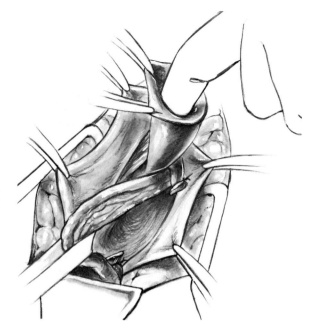

Fig. 87-7

hind when the spermatic cord is elevated from the floor of the canal. Ensure that the posterior genitofemoral nerve and associated structures are included and not injured **(Fig. 87–5)**. Encircle the cord with a latex drain for purposes of traction.

Transect attachments between the spermatic cord and the underlying tissues with electrocautery. Resect lipomas and adipose tissue. To reduce the diameter of the cord, excise the *entire cremaster muscle* from the portion of the spermatic cord that remains in the

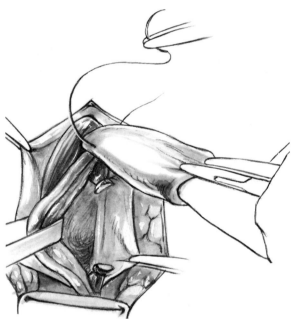

Fig. 87-8a

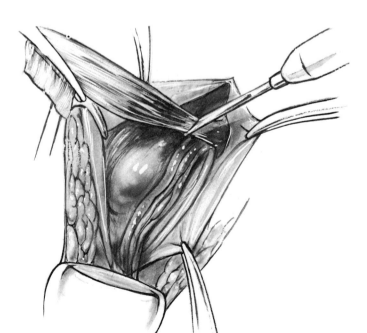

Fig. 87-6

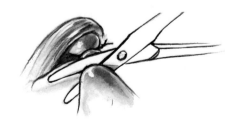

Fig. 87-8b

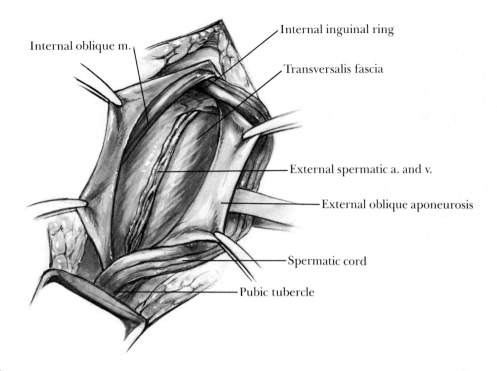

Fig. 87-9

inguinal canal. This minimizes the diameter of the internal inguinal ring when it is reconstructed. Be sure to remove all the cremaster muscle fibers from their attachments to the iliopubic tract, the femoral sheath, and the transversalis fascia **(Fig. 87–6)**. Only after removing all these fibers is there clear visualization of these important structures. Clearly identify the vas deferens and the internal spermatic vessels before resecting the cremaster.

Excising Indirect Sac

At this point, place the left index finger behind the cord near the internal ring and dissect out the cord structures to rule out the presence of an indirect sac in the cord. If the patient has a combined indirect and direct hernia, deal with each sac individually. Simply free the indirect sac to its neck; then explore the sac **(Fig. 87–7)**, transfix it with a single suture-ligature **(Fig. 87–8a)**, and amputate the redundant portion **(Fig. 87–8b)**. It is important to free the neck of the sac from surrounding structures so the stump of the ligated sac can retract into the abdomen. Now remove the hemostat retracting the lateral leaflet of the external oblique aponeurosis. Place the cord and ilioinguinal nerve lateral to this leaflet and replace the hemostat **(Fig. 87–9)**.

Transversalis Dissection

A bulge or weakness in Hesselbach's triangle constitutes the direct "sac." Identify the *external* spermatic

vessels, which branch off the deep inferior epigastric artery and vein and lie superficial to the transversalis fascia (Fig. 87-9). Resect the external spermatic vessels between two ligatures of 2-0 PG: one at their junction with the deep inferior epigastric vessels and the other at the pubic tubercle **(Fig. 87–10)**. Often a small branch of the genitofemoral nerve runs along the floor of the inguinal canal together with the external sper-

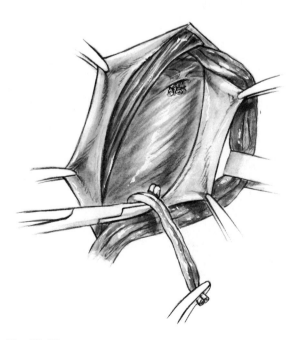

Fig. 87-10

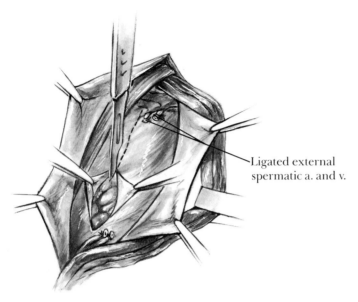

Fig. 87-11

matic vessels. Excise this nerve together with the vessels. These steps clear the entire floor of Hesselbach's triangle. Make a scalpel incision through the bulging attenuated transversalis fascia from the pubic tubercle to a point just medial to the deep inferior epigastric vessels **(Fig. 87–11)**. When lobules of preperitoneal fat bulge through the scalpel incision, extend the incision with Metzenbaum scissors if preferred. If one is in the proper plane of dissection, the deep inferior epigastric vessels have been entirely cleared of areolar tissue; Cooper's ligament is clearly visible laterally, and the preperitoneal fat is easily separated from the deep surface of the transversalis fascia in a cephalad direction **(Fig. 87–12)**. If any branches of the deep inferior epigastric vessels join the deep surface of the transversalis fascia, carefully divide and ligate them so the epigastric vessels can be pushed down away from the repair. Otherwise, retroperitoneal bleeding may be caused by inadvertently piercing these vessels with a needle while suturing the transversalis layer. Excise the attenuated portions of transversalis fascia and apply straight hemostats to the free cut edge of the medial leaflet of the transversalis fascia for purposes of traction. Apply a moist gauze sponge in a sponge-holder to the preperitoneal fat and bladder to push these structures posteriorly.

Shouldice Repair

Layer 1

Anchor the initial stitch (3-0 Tevdek on a C-5 atraumatic needle) by catching the lacunar ligament and pubic periosteum in one bite and the undersurface of the medial flap of transversalis with overlying rectus fascia in the other. Tie this stitch. Apply upward traction on the straight clamps holding the medial leaflet of transversalis fascia; this maneuver reveals a "white line" of fibrous tissue on the undersurface of the transversalis fascia. The "white line" represents the aponeurosis of the transversus muscle as seen through the transversalis fascia. This aponeurosis of

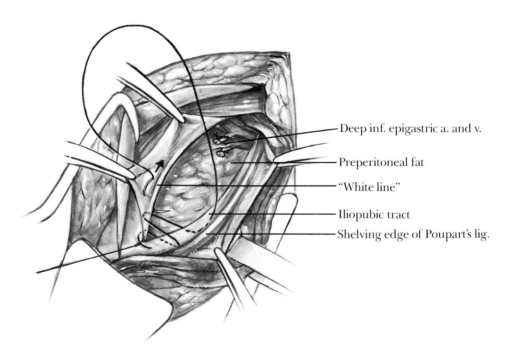

Fig. 87-12

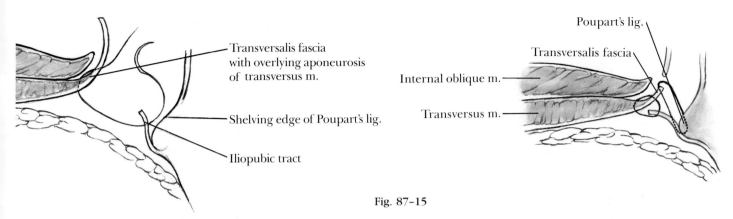

Fig. 87-13

Fig. 87-15

Transversalis fascia
with overlying aponeurosis
of transversus m.

Shelving edge of Poupart's lig.

Iliopubic tract

Poupart's lig.

Transversalis fascia

Internal oblique m.

Transversus m.

the transversus abdominis muscle is thought by Mc-Vay and Halverson and by Nyhus and Condon to be the most important tissue involved in inguinal hernia repair. This arch of aponeurotic tissue becomes muscular as it approaches the internal inguinal ring. Include the "white line" in the continuous stitch that attaches the cut lateral edge of the transversalis fascia to the undersurface of the medial leaf of the transversalis (Fig. 87-12). Insert the needle into the lateral leaflet of transversalis fascia near the point where this layer appears to attach to the inguinal ligament **(Fig. 87–13)**. This condensation of the caudal margin of the transversalis fascia is also termed the iliopubic tract. Be sure to remove all the cremaster muscle fibers that cover the iliopubic tract and femoral sheath. Otherwise it is not possible to identify these structures accurately for proper suturing.

Each stitch should contain 4-6 mm of tissue. Continue the suture in a lateral direction until the newly constructed internal ring has been closed snugly around the spermatic cord so only the tip of a Kelly hemostat fits loosely between the cord and the internal ring.

Layer 2

Excise the attenuated portion of the transversalis fascia and any fatty tissue adherent to the internal oblique muscle layer. Then use the same continuous strand of suture material as in layer 1 and sew the free cut edge of the medial leaflet of transversalis fascia with adjacent internal oblique muscle to the anterior aspect of the iliopubic tract. Include 2-3 mm of the shelving edge of the inguinal ligament in the continuous suture going medially **(Figs. 87–14, 87–15)**. Continue this suture to the pubic tubercle.

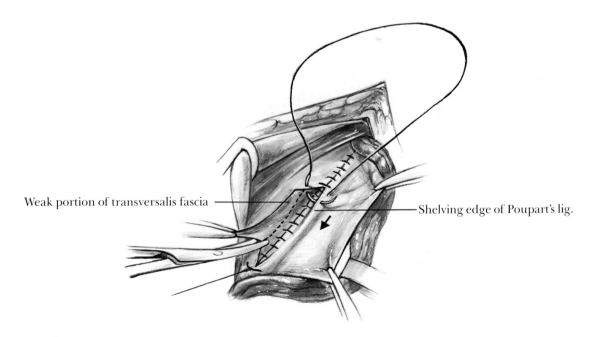

Weak portion of transversalis fascia

Shelving edge of Poupart's lig.

Fig. 87-14

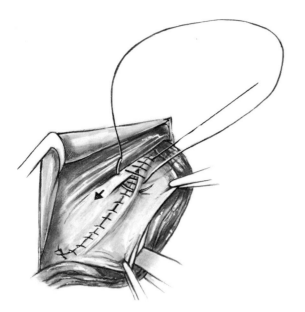

Fig. 87-16

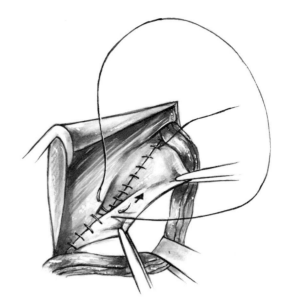

Fig. 87-18

Anchor the last stitch by inserting it into the pubic periosteum. At this point, terminate the suture by knotting it to its tail. A worthwhile modification of the Shouldice technique is to excise the lower 2 cm of the internal oblique muscle to expose the underlying aponeurosis of the transversus muscle. This step is in fact an integral part of McVay's method of hernia repair as shown in Figure 88-1. After accomplishing this step, one can invert the sutures for Shouldice's layer 3 into the transversus aponeurosis instead of into the fleshy, internal oblique muscle.

Layer 3

Use a new strand of 3-0 Tevdek to begin layer 3. Take a bite of internal oblique muscle or "conjoined tendon" and another of the shelving edge of the inguinal ligament and tie the suture, beginning this time at the medial margin of the newly constructed internal ring. If the internal oblique muscle is flimsy, resect the muscle and sew to the underlying aponeu-

rosis of the transversus muscle. Insert this suture continuously in a medial direction **(Figs. 87–16, 87–17)** as far as the pubic tubercle. Do not leave any gap in the suture line near the pubic tubercle as this oversight is a common cause of recurrent hernia adjacent to the pubis.

Layer 4

Use the same continuous suture to create a fourth layer by taking first a bite of internal oblique muscle just cephalad to the previous layer and then a 4 mm bite of the undersurface of external oblique aponeurosis just anterior to the previously inserted layer **(Figs. 87–18, 87–19)**. Continue this suture until it approaches its point of origin at the internal ring, where the suture is terminated by being tied to its tail. Although the classic Shouldice repair calls for the four layers as described, we have frequently found that the width of available external oblique aponeurosis was inadequate to construct the fourth layer. Most often we do three layers and occasion-

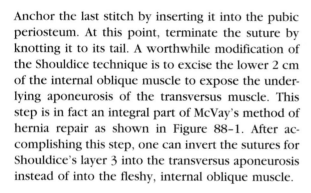

Fig. 87-17

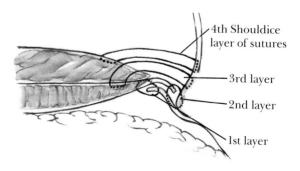

4th Shouldice layer of sutures

3rd layer

2nd layer

1st layer

Fig. 87-19

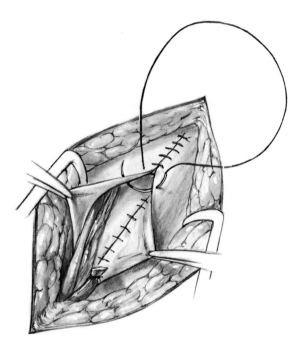

Fig. 87–20

ally two layers. Berliner found no differences in the incidence of recurrence between the two-layer, three-layer, and four-layer Shouldice repairs.

Closure of External Oblique Aponeurosis

Meticulously inspect the cord and obtain complete hemostasis with a combination of fine ligatures and electrocoagulation. Replace the cord in the canal, which is now displaced slightly cephalad. Elevate the medial portion of the external oblique aponeurosis to provide adequate space for the spermatic cord. Close the two leaflets of the external oblique

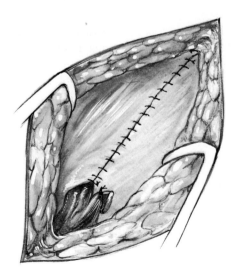

Fig. 87–21

aponeurosis with a continuous 3-0 PG suture **(Fig. 87–20)**. At the new external inguinal ring include in the last bite of this suture the proximal cut edge of the cremaster muscle **(Fig. 87–21)**. This move prevents the testis from descending to an abnormally low point in the scrotum as a consequence of resecting the cremaster muscle. There is no virtue in creating a tight external ring. Rather, allow a 2 cm opening for the spermatic cord.

Approximate Scarpa's fascia with several 4-0 PG sutures. Close the skin with a continuous subcuticular suture of 4-0 PG or PDS supplemented by strips of sterile adhesive to the skin (Steri-Strips).

POSTOPERATIVE CARE

Begin active ambulation the afternoon of the operation. Terminate the intravenous infusion in patients who have undergone local anesthesia when they leave the recovery room. Laxatives may be given on the night of the first postoperative day to avoid patient discomfort at defecation. Generally the patient needs a prescription for pain medication for the first few days.

COMPLICATIONS

Systemic complications of a pulmonary, cardiac, or urologic nature are rare.

Wound infections are rare. Treat them promptly by opening the skin and subcutaneous tissues for adequate drainage and by prescribing appropriate antibiotics.

Hematomas may occur in the wound and are generally treated expectantly. Some degree of superficial ecchymosis may be secondary to injecting agents for local anesthesia.

Testicular swelling is generally due to venous obstruction. Although it is sometimes due to excessive constriction of the newly reconstructed internal ring, it is more often the result of trauma, hematoma, or inadvertent ligature of the internal spermatic veins in the inguinal canal. Although this complication may lead to testicular atrophy or necrosis, in most cases satisfactory results may be anticipated from expectant therapy.

Persistent pain in the area innervated by the ilioinguinal or genitofemoral nerves is a rare but disturbing complication of inguinal hernia repair. Starling and Harms reported on 19 patients with ilioinguinal neuralgia and 17 patients with genitofemoral neuralgia. Most of the pain followed inguinal hernia repair and was attributed to entrapment of the nerve in a stitch or scar tissue. These authors described the diagnostic studies they believed necessary to diagnosis nerve entrapment. In most but not all of their cases, relief of pain was achieved by reexploring the hernia incision and resecting the ilioinguinal nerve. In the case of the genitofemoral nerve, a retroperitoneal lumbar approach was used to transect the genital branch of the genitofemoral nerve.

Recurrent inguinal hernia is possible. See Chapter 91 for a discussion of the incidence, causes, and treatment of this problem.

REFERENCES

Amid PK, Shulman AG, Lichtenstein IL. Local anesthesia for inguinal hernia repair: step-by-step procedure. Ann Surg 1994;220:735.

Berliner SD. Adult inguinal/hernia: pathophysiology and repair. Surg Ann 1983;13:307.

Hay J-M, Boudet M-J, Fingerhut A, et al. Shouldice inguinal hernia repair in the male adult: the gold standard? A multicenter controlled trial in 1578 patients. Ann Surg 1995;222:719.

McVay CB, Halverson K. Inguinal and femoral hernias. In Beahrs RW, Beart RW (eds) General Surgery. Boston, Houghton Mifflin, 1980.

Nyhus LM, Condon RE (eds) Hernia, 4nd ed. Philadelphia, Lippincott, 1995.

Ponka JL. Seven steps to local anesthesia for inguinofemoral hernia repair. Surg Gynecol Obstet 1963; 117:115.

Starling JR, Harms BA. Diagnosis and treatment of genitofemoral and ilioinguinal neuralgia. World J Surg 1989;13:586.

Welsh DRJ, Alexander MAJ. The Shouldice repair. Surg Clin North Am 1993;73:451.

88 Cooper's Ligament (McVay) Repair of Inguinal Hernia

INDICATIONS

Symptomatic direct or indirect inguinal hernia

Femoral hernia

OPERATIVE STRATEGY

The McVay repair uses autogenous tissue to close the floor of the canal. Because the femoral canal is also closed, this is a good repair to use when an associated femoral hernia is found at repair of an inguinal hernia. This repair can succeed only if the fascia is strong. If exploration of the groin reveals tenuous fascia, a prosthetic mesh repair is required (see Chapter 89).

OPERATIVE TECHNIQUE

Incision and Exposure

Make a skin incision over the region of the external inguinal ring and continue laterally to a point about 2 cm medial to the anterosuperior iliac spine. Open the external oblique aponeurosis with an incision along the line of its fibers from the external inguinal ring laterally for a distance of about 5–7 cm (see Fig. 87-3). Mobilize the spermatic cord. Excise the *entire* cremaster muscle from the area of the inguinal canal (see Fig. 87-4) and remove any lipomas of the cord. Explore the cord carefully for the presence of the indirect sac. If a sac is present, dissect it from the cord. Open the sac, explore it, close it at its neck with a suture-ligature, amputate it, and permit the stump to retract into the abdominal cavity. Identify the *external* spermatic vessels at the point where they emerge from the transversalis fascia (see Fig. 87-9). Divide and ligate them at this point, and remove about 4–5 cm of the vessels; ligate them again at the pubic tubercle (see Fig. 87-10).

In patients with an indirect inguinal hernia, identify the margins of the transversalis fascia around the internal inguinal ring. If the internal inguinal ring is only slightly enlarged, close it with several sutures between the healthy transversalis fascia along its cephalad margin and the anterior femoral sheath at its caudal margin. If the hernia has eroded more than 2 cm of posterior inguinal wall, complete reconstruction is necessary. In this case, incise the transversalis fascia with a scalpel beginning at a point just medial to the pubic tubercle (see Fig. 87-11). Carry the incision laterally with a scalpel or Metzenbaum scissors, taking care not to injure the underlying deep inferior epigastric vessels. Continue the incision all the way to the internal inguinal ring. Sweep the preperitoneal fat away from the undersurface of the transversalis fascia. Free the deep inferior epigastric vessels so they may be retracted posteriorly together with the preperitoneal fat. A few small branches may have to be divided and ligated.

Excise the iliopubic tract adjacent to Cooper's ligament. Apply two identifying hemostats to the cephalad cut edge of the transversalis fascia and elevate to expose the aponeurosis of the transversus

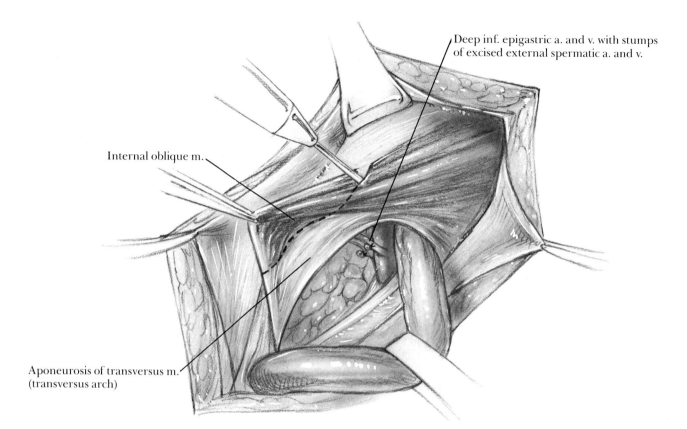

Deep inf. epigastric a. and v. with stumps of excised external spermatic a. and v.

Internal oblique m.

Aponeurosis of transversus m. (transversus arch)

Fig. 88–1

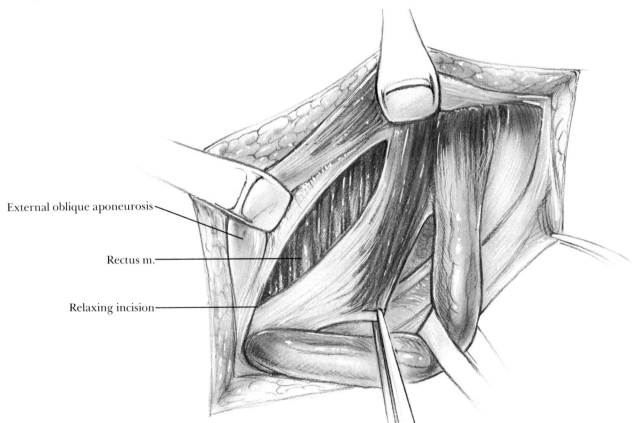

External oblique aponeurosis

Rectus m.

Relaxing incision

Fig. 88–2

muscle. Excise the fleshy portion of the internal oblique muscle overlying the fibrous transversus arch to improve the exposure **(Fig. 88–1)**.

Identify the anterior femoral sheath by gently inserting the back of a scalpel handle between the shelving edge of Poupart's ligament and the femoral sheath overlying the external iliac artery and vein. Then identify the anterior surface of the external iliac vein and artery and retract them gently in a posterior direction with a peanut sponge dissector. This maneuver separates these vessels from the femoral sheath. To see the femoral sheath clearly, be certain to excise 100% of the overlying cremaster muscle fibers.

Making the Relaxing Incision

A relaxing incision is essential to prevent tension on the suture line. Elevate the medial portion of the external oblique aponeurosis and dissect it bluntly away from the internal oblique muscle and from the anterior rectus sheath. Make a 7- to 8-cm incision in the anterior rectus sheath beginning about 1.5 cm above the pubic tubercle and continue the incision in a cephalad fashion just medial to the point where the external oblique aponeurosis fuses with the anterior rectus sheath. This constitutes a vertical line that curves as it continues in a superior direction. The anterior belly of the rectus muscle is exposed as downward traction is applied to the transversus arch **(Fig. 88–2)**.

Inserting Cooper's Ligament Sutures

Suture the transversus arch to Cooper's ligament using atraumatic 2-0 silk or other nonabsorbable suture material **(Fig. 88–3)**. Take substantial bites of both the transversus arch and Cooper's ligament and place the sutures no more than 5 mm apart. Do not tie the sutures until all are in place.

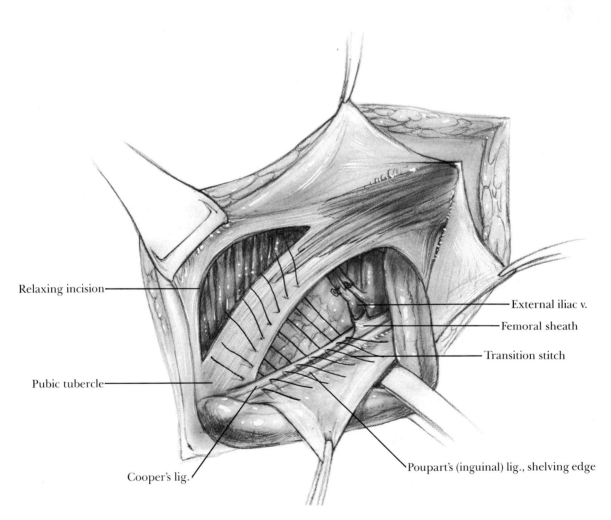

Fig. 88-3

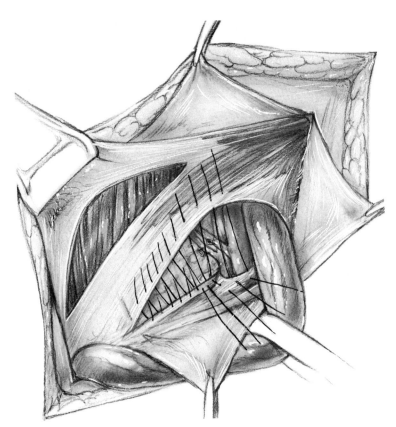

Fig. 88-4

As the suture line progresses laterally, the external iliac vein is approached **(Fig. 88–4)**. At this point insert a "transition suture" **(Fig. 88–5)** that penetrates the transversus arch, Cooper's ligament, and the anterior femoral sheath. Lateral to this suture, sew the transversus arch to the femoral sheath. In his description of Cooper's ligament repair, Rutledge advocated including a bite of the shelving edge of the inguinal ligament together with the anterior femoral sheath. Continue to insert sutures until the internal ring is sufficiently narrowed to admit only a Kelly hemostat alongside the spermatic cord **(Fig. 88–6)**. Do not insert any sutures lateral to the cord. After all the sutures have been inserted, tie each suture proceeding from medial to lateral. Suture the incised anterior rectus sheath down to underlying muscle along the lateral aspect of the relaxing incision with a few 3-0 interrupted silk sutures.

Closing the External Oblique Aponeurosis

Replace the cord in the inguinal canal. Check to ensure complete hemostasis. Close the external

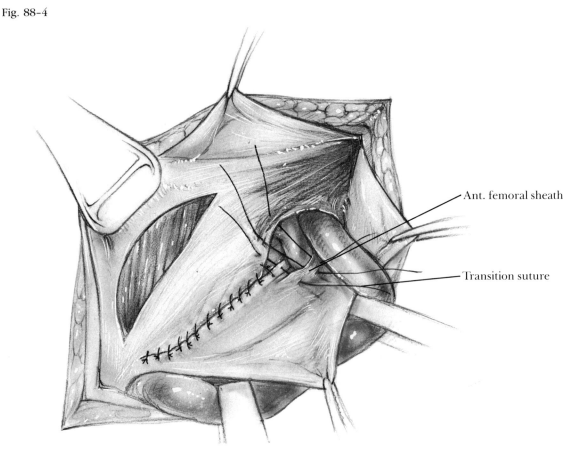

Ant. femoral sheath

Transition suture

Fig. 88-5

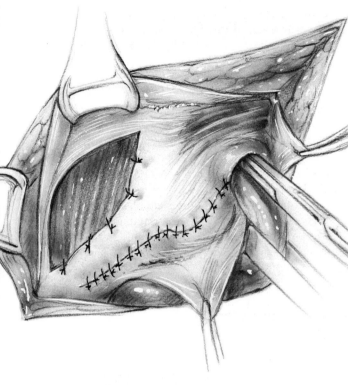

Fig. 88–6

oblique aponeurosis superficial to the cord and complete the wound closure as described in Chapter 87.

POSTOPERATIVE CARE

See Chapter 87.

COMPLICATIONS

See Chapter 87.

REFERENCES

McVay CB, Halverson K. Inguinal and femoral hernias. In Beahrs OH, Beart RW (eds) General Surgery. Boston, Houghton Mifflin, 1980.

Panos RG, Beck DE, Maresh JE, Harford FJ. Preliminary results of a prospective randomized study of Cooper's ligament versus Shouldice herniorrhaphy technique. Surg Gynecol Obstet 1992;175:315.

Rutledge RH. Cooper's ligament repair: a 25 year experience with a single technique for all groin hernias in adults. Surgery 1998;103:1.

89 Mesh Repair of Inguinal Hernia

INDICATIONS

Inadequate fascia for autogenous tissue repair of direct inguinal hernia. We reserve the use of prosthetic mesh for situations where the transversalis fascia and adjacent structures are of insufficient quality for a Shouldice or McVay repair of a direct inguinal hernia.

Recurrent inguinal hernia repair. As discussed in Chapter 91, mesh is frequently used when a recurrent inguinal hernia is approached through the groin.

Prosthetic mesh repairs are used by some surgeons for virtually all inguinal hernias. Advocates of the repair shown here in a modified form cite speed, simplicity, and minimal dissection as major advantages to the surgeon; decreased pain and immediate return to normal activities are advantages to the patient.

PREOPERATIVE PREPARATION

See Chapter 87.

Perioperative antibiotics

PITFALLS AND DANGER POINTS

Failure to identify, reduce, and repair all hernias. A missed indirect hernial sac is a common cause of recurrence (see Chapter 91).

Failure to secure the mesh adequately. Mesh can curl or migrate. When this happens it may fail to produce the desired effect or may be palpable in the subcutaneous tissues of a slender patient.

Infection.

OPERATIVE STRATEGY

This repair is performed through a short incision with minimal dissection. Direct and indirect sacs are identified and reduced. A preformed plug (Per-Fix, Davol Corporation) is used to keep the hernia reduced as a kind of "internal truss." The plug is held in place by the edges of the fascial defect. Most indirect sacs are simply inverted, and the internal ring holds the plug in place. Direct hernial sacs are circumferentially incised to create the fascial ring that anchors the plug.

The plug is reinforced by an onlay patch. The procedure may be done under local or regional anesthesia.

OPERATIVE TECHNIQUE

Incision

Center a small skin line or nearly transverse incision over the medial third of the inguinal ligament and external inguinal ring (see Fig. 87-1a).

Dissection and Identification of Direct and Indirect Sacs

The groin structures are exposed and the external oblique aponeurosis identified as described in earlier chapters. Incise the external oblique aponeurosis in the direction of its fibers, preserving the ilioinguinal nerve (see Fig. 87-3). Encircle the cord and its posterior mesentery (which contains the genitofemoral nerve) (see Fig. 87-5). Perform just enough dissection to encircle the cord. Do not divide the cremaster muscle. Simply incise it in the direction of its fibers to allow careful inspection of the cord structures (see Fig. 87-4).

An indirect sac, if present, is found anteromedial to the cord structures. Trace the cord structures back to the internal ring, with the cord on traction to ensure that the leading edge of any indirect sac is seen. Visualization of the peritoneal lappet, a crescentic thickening of normal peritoneum created by traction on the cord, is positive proof that adequate dissection had been performed.

If an indirect hernia sac is found, separate it from the cord structures all the way to the internal ring. This high dissection allows the sac to be simply inverted into the peritoneum.

Assess the strength of the floor of the inguinal canal by palpation. If a direct hernial defect is present, circumferentially incise the fascial defect with

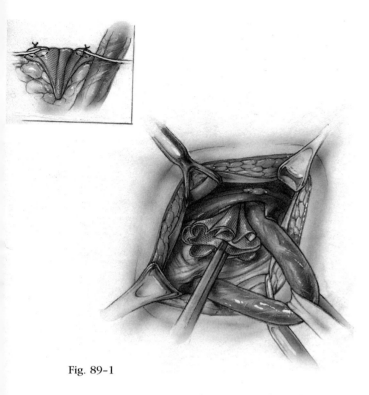

Fig. 89-1

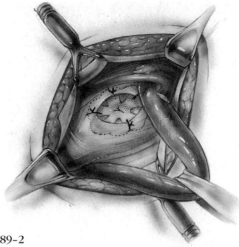

Fig. 89-2

electrocautery and reduce the hernia with the attached portion of sac into the preperitoneal space.

Placement of Plug

Insert the preformed plug, pointed end first, into the internal ring of an indirect hernia or the fascial defect of a direct hernia so the petals unfold under the fascia and anchor it in place **(Fig. 89–1)**. Occasionally, a direct hernial defect is so large two plugs, sutured together side by side, must be used to reduce it. Ask the patient to cough and assess the stability of the plug placement. Anchor the plug with three of four simple interrupted sutures of 3-0 PG placed to the inner aspects of the petals **(Fig. 89–2)**, which allows the plug to expand behind the fascia and buttress the defect.

Placement of onlay patch

Insert the precut patch so it covers the floor of the canal with the cord coming through the hole, and the incision and tails of the mesh extending lateral to the internal ring **(Figs. 89–3, 89–4)**. It should lie

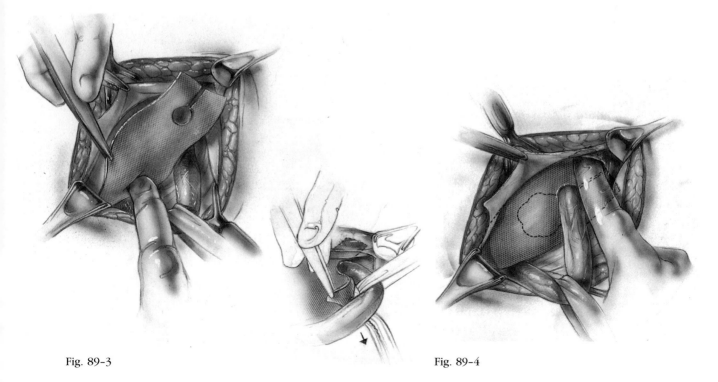

Fig. 89-3

Fig. 89-4

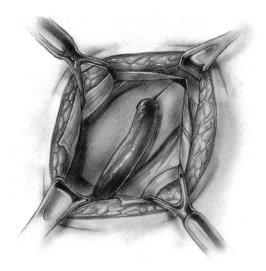

Fig. 89-5

in a flat, stable position covering the floor of the inguinal canal and the plug **(Fig. 89–5)**. Secure it in position with several interrupted sutures of 3-0 PG. Because the plug forms the primary strength layer of this repair, it is necessary to suture the patch in only a few places to ensure that it remains in the proper location until tissue ingrowth occurs. We tend to place sutures medially to the pubic tubercle, laterally to secure the two tails together and tack the lateral part to the aponeurosis of the internal oblique muscle, inferiorly to the inguinal ligament, and superiorly to the conjoint tendon.

Closure

Close the external oblique and remaining layers in the usual fashion.

POSTOPERATIVE CARE

Patients are allowed to lift up to 25 pounds immediately. They may resume heavy manual labor after 2 weeks.

COMPLICATIONS

Infection has been rare in most series.

Mesh migration into adjacent structures (femoral vein, spermatic cord), a theoretic concern, has not proven to be a significant problem. Rutkow and Robbins, in a 1998 review, were unable to find any documented cases.

REFERENCES

Lichtenstein IL, Shulman AG, Amid PK, et al. The tension-free hernioplasty. Am J Surg 1989;157:188.

Robbins AW, Rutkow IM. Mesh plug repair and groin hernia surgery. Surg Clin North Am 1998;78:1007.

Rutkow IM, Robbins AW. The mesh plug technique for recurrent groin herniorraphy: a nine-year experience of 407 repairs. Surgery 1998;124:844.

90 Laparoscopic Inguinal Hernia Repair: Transabdominal Preperitoneal (TAPP) and Totally Extraperitoneal (TEP) Repairs

Muhammed Ashraf Memon
Robert J. Fitzgibbons
Carol E.H. Scott-Conner

INDICATIONS

Inguinal hernia (see Chapter 87). Although the role of this procedure in the management of uncomplicated inguinal hernia is still being elucidated, laparoscopic repair may offer a significant advantage in these special situations:

Recurrent hernia (see Chapter 91). Laparoscopic repair is a logical choice because it avoids the previous surgical field and allows repair to be performed through healthy tissues with potentially better results.

Bilateral hernias. They can be repaired simultaneously without additional incisions or trocar sites.

Incidental herniorraphy during another laparoscopic surgery. Incidental herniorraphy may be performed after completing the primary laparoscopic procedure (e.g., laparoscopic cholecystectomy). It should be considered only if the primary procedure has gone smoothly and did not involve spillage of contaminated material.

PREOPERATIVE PREPARATION

See Chapters 8 and 87.

Insert a Foley catheter or perform immediate preoperative bladder decompression by voiding or inserting a straight catheter.

Prescribe perioperative antibiotics.

PITFALLS AND DANGER POINTS

Missed hernia or inadequate mesh fixation resulting in hernia recurrence

Injury to bladder during the totally extraperitoneal approach

Nerve or major vessel injury

OPERATIVE STRATEGY

There are two general approaches: transabdominal preperitoneal (TAPP) and totally extraperitoneal (TEP). TAPP is the logical choice when inguinal herniorrhaphy is performed after another laparoscopic procedure or when previous preperitoneal dissection limits access to the extraperitoneal space. It offers the additional advantage that the approach and anatomy are familiar to most surgeons, and hernias are readily identified as peritoneal outpouchings. The major disadvantage is penetration of the peritoneal cavity with associated potential for injury or adhesion formation.

The TEP approach avoids entry into the peritoneal cavity and hence minimizes these potential problems; but it requires dissection in the extraperitoneal plane and an excellent understanding of regional anatomy. The TEP approach is contraindicated when previous surgery or radiation therapy may have obliterated the retroperitoneal plane.

Crucial to the success of either approach is accurate identification of anatomy and hernias, accu-

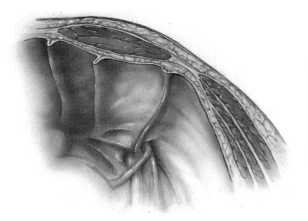

Fig. 90-1

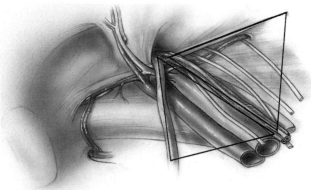

Fig. 90-2

rate placement of mesh, and avoiding injury to adjacent structures. **Figure 90–1** shows the laparoscopic anatomy of the inguinal region. **Figure 90–2** shows two danger areas—the triangle of pain and the triangle of doom—where staple fixation must be avoided. The single most important landmark is the iliopubic tract. If no staples are placed below this structure, major nerves and vessels can be avoided.

When laparoscopic herniorrhaphy follows an unrelated laparoscopic operation on the same patient

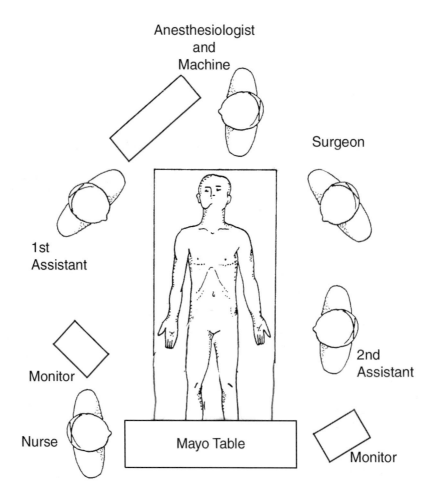

Fig. 90-3

under the same anesthesia, take the time to optimize the working environment for the second procedure. Additional trocars may be required, monitors moved, equipment procured, and other adjustments made. This is time well spent.

OPERATIVE TECHNIQUE

Patient Position and Room Setup: TAPP or TEP

Position the patient supine with arms tucked at the side. Extending the arms on armboards may not allow enough room for the surgeon to operate comfortably in the lower abdomen. The Trendelenburg position allows the bowel to fall away from the pelvis, providing excellent access. A single video monitor at the foot of the operating table adjusted to a comfortable viewing height serves both surgeon and assistants. The surgeon stands on the side opposite the hernia (**Fig. 90–3**).

Although a 30° angled laparoscope is preferred by some surgeons, it is certainly not a necessity. A 0° laparoscope can provide as good a view.

TAPP Approach

Place the first trocar (10-12 mm) at the umbilicus. Place two additional 10- to 12-mm trocars lateral to the rectus sheath on either side at the level of the umbilicus under direct vision (**Fig. 90–4**). Large trocars allow the laparoscope and stapler to be moved

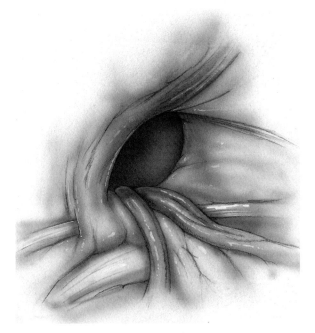

Fig. 90-5a

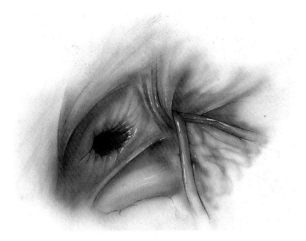

Fig. 90-5b

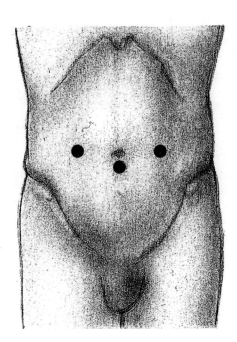

Fig. 90-4

around for optimal dissection, depending on the anatomy. If 5 mm instruments are available, smaller trocars may be used. For a small, unilateral hernia a 5 mm cannula may be substituted for the 10- to 12-mm cannula on the ipsilateral side.

Inspect both inguinal regions. Identify the median umbilical ligament (remnant of the urachus), the medial umbilical ligament (remnant of the umbilical artery), and the lateral umbilical fold (peritoneal reflection over the inferior epigastric artery). If the median umbilical ligament appears to compromise exposure, divide it. A hernia is visible as an outpouching of the peritoneum (**Figs. 90–5a, 90–5b**).

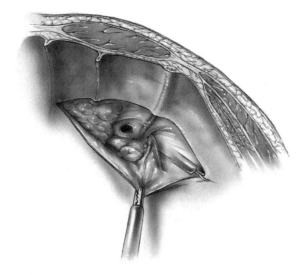

Fig. 90-6

Incise the peritoneum along a line approximately 2 cm above the superior edge of the hernial defect, extending from the median umbilical ligament to the anterosuperior iliac spine. Mobilize the peritoneal flap inferiorly using blunt and sharp dissection **(Fig. 90–6)**. Some surgeons routinely inject local anesthetic (0.25% bupivacaine with epinephrine mixed in an equal amount of normal saline) under the peritoneum before opening it. This makes mobilization of the superior and inferior flaps of peritoneum much easier and provides excellent postoperative pain relief for at least 6 hours.

Expose the inferior epigastric vessels and identify the pubic symphysis and lower portion of the rectus abdominis muscle. Dissect Cooper's ligament to its junction with the femoral vein. Identify the iliopubic tract. Continue the dissection inferiorly, with care to avoid an injury to the femoral branch of the genitofemoral nerve and the lateral femoral cutaneous nerve, which enter the lower extremity just below the iliopubic tract (Fig. 90-2). Complete the dissection by skeletonizing the cord structures. A small indirect hernial sac is easily mobilized from the cord and reduced back into the peritoneal cavity. A large sac may be difficult to mobilize because of dense adhesions between the sac and the cord structures due to the chronicity of the hernia. Undue trauma to the cord may result if an attempt is made to remove the sac in its entirety. In this situation, divide the sac just distal to the internal ring, leaving the distal sac in situ. This is most easily accomplished by opening the sac on the side opposite the cord structures and completing the division from the inside. Dissect the proximal sac away from the cord structures. A direct hernia is easily managed by reducing the sac and preperitoneal fat from the hernial orifice by gentle traction **(Fig. 90–7)**.

Placement of Mesh

Cut a piece of mesh at least 11 × 6 cm (unilateral). The mesh should be able to cover completely the direct, indirect, and femoral spaces. Do not cut a slit for the cord. We prefer to lay the mesh *over* the cord structures, rather than cutting a slit and wrapping the mesh *around* the cord structures. Recurrences have been reported through the orifice created around the new internal ring, even when the mesh has been closed around the cord. A large prosthesis allows intraabdominal pressure to act uniformly over a large area, thereby preventing the mesh from ballooning out through the hernial defect. Roll the mesh longitudinally into a compact cylinder and pass it through one of the trocars. Some surgeons place temporary ties around the cylinder to facilitate handling.

Lie the cylinder at the inferior aspect of the working space and unroll it toward the anterior abdominal wall, smoothing it into place and tucking the corners underneath the peritoneal flap **(Fig. 90–8)**. Take time to lay the mesh carefully over all hernial defects with good overlap. The mesh may be stapled in place or simply placed as an onlay graft. Both techniques are described here.

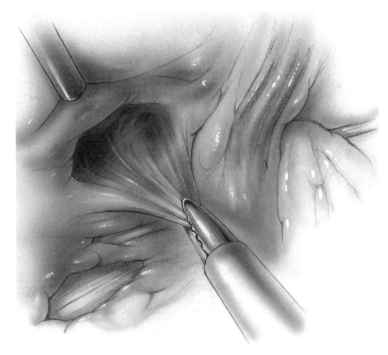

Fig. 90-7

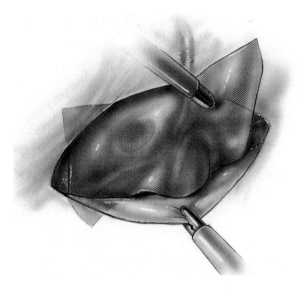

Fig. 90-8

Stapling Technique

Staples or a hernia tacking device may be used to affix the mesh. Begin stapling along the superior border of the prosthesis **(Fig. 90–9)** at the medial aspect of the contralateral pubic tubercle. Place the staples horizontally, progressing laterally along the superior border to the anterosuperior iliac spine. Horizontal staple placement minimizes the chance of injury to the deeper ilioinguinal or iliohypogastric nerves.

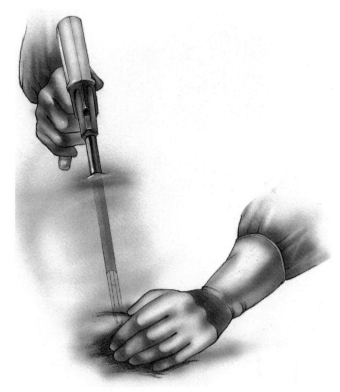

Fig. 90-10

Staple the inferior border to Cooper's ligament medially using a horizontal or vertical orientation depending on the patient's characteristics (i.e., how the staples best attach). Again, the opposite pubic tubercle marks the area to begin placing staples for the inferior border, and stapling is continued over the area of the ipsilateral pubic tubercle to the femoral vein. Do not place staples directly into either pubic tubercle because chronic postoperative pain (osteitis pubis) can result. Always respect the triangles of doom and pain by not placing any staples below the iliopubic tract (Fig. 90-2).

Affix the medial and lateral borders using vertically placed staples, as this is the direction of the lateral cutaneous nerve of the thigh and the femoral branch of the genitofemoral nerve. Lateral to the internal spermatic vessels, place all staples above the iliopubic tract. This avoids neuralgia due to injury to the lateral cutaneous nerve of the thigh or the femoral branch of the genitofemoral nerve (Fig. 90-2).

It is useful to palpate the head of the stapler through the abdominal wall with the nondominant hand, ensuring that stapling is done above the iliopubic tract **(Fig. 90–10)**. It also allows counterpressure to be applied, ensuring better purchase of the staples.

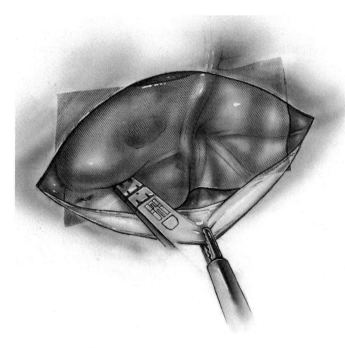

Fig. 90-9

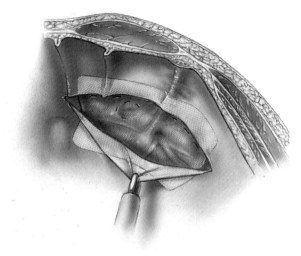

Fig. 90-11

Excise any redundant mesh **(Fig. 90–11)** and close the peritoneal flap over the mesh with staples **(Fig. 90–12)**. The goal is to isolate the mesh prosthesis from intraabdominal viscera. Avoid excessive tension, which could tent the peritoneum over the mesh, creating a potential space into which bowel may herniate. It may be helpful to decrease the pneumoperitoneum before flap closure. Occasionally, it is necessary simply to cover the mesh with the inferior flap, leaving exposed transversalis fascia. Avoid excess gaps between staples, as bowel can herniate or adhere to the mesh through these defects. Inject a long-acting local anesthetic such as bupivacaine into the preperitoneal space before closure to decrease postoperative pain.

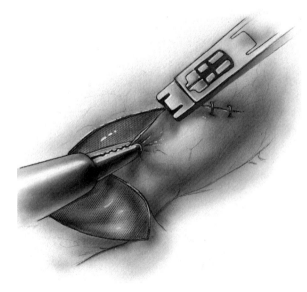

Fig. 90-12

Onlay Graft (Nonstapled) Technique

Simply onlay the mesh in the preperitoneal space created earlier. Make sure the mesh lies perfectly flat with no rolled edges. Excise any redundant mesh and close the peritoneal flaps over the mesh with a continuous simple running intracorporeal suture of 3-0 PG. The goal is to isolate the mesh prosthesis from intraabdominal viscera.

Bilateral Hernias

Bilateral hernias can be repaired using one long transverse peritoneal incision extending from one anterosuperior iliac spine to the other and a single large piece (30.0 × 7.5 cm) of mesh; or it can be done with two peritoneal incisions and two pieces of mesh. We favor the latter approach for the following reasons. First, it is easier to manipulate two small pieces of mesh and tailor them accurately to fit the preperitoneal spaces than a single large piece. Second, there is no potential for damage to a patent urachus if one exists. Finally, there is less concern about interfering with bladder function when two pieces of mesh are used.

TEP Approach

Make the skin incision for the first trocar (10–12 mm) at the umbilicus. Open the anterior rectus sheath on the ipsilateral side and retract the muscle laterally to expose the posterior rectus sheath. Following the incision of the anterior rectus sheath and retraction of the muscle laterally, insert a finger over the posterior rectus sheath and gently develop this space.

Insert a transparent balloon-tipped trocar into this space directed toward the pubic symphysis. Place the laparoscope in the trocar. Under direct vision, inflate the balloon to create an extraperitoneal tunnel or space **(Fig. 90–13)**. Note that dissection in the correct plane mobilizes the bladder downward.

Place two additional trocars in the midline under direct vision: one (5 mm) at the pubic symphysis and the other (10–12 mm) midway between the first and second **(Fig. 90–14)**. Place these trocars by incising the skin with a scalpel followed by blunt dissection with a hemostat under direct vision, rather than using the standard technique, as inadvertent penetration of the narrow preperitoneal space into the peritoneal cavity may result.

Complete the dissection of the preperitoneal space, mesh placement, and stapling in a manner similar to that described for the TAPP procedure **(Fig. 90–15)**. Bilateral hernias can be repaired with the use of a single large prosthesis or two pieces as previously discussed.

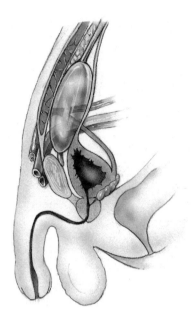

Fig. 90-13

COMPLICATIONS

Vascular injuries. Injury to the inferior epigastric and spermatic vessels are the most common vascular complications. Other vessels at risk include the external iliac, circumflex iliac profunda, and obturator vessels. Use of the open laparoscopic technique for inserting the initial cannula, meticulous dissection, and absolute identification of important landmarks are essential for preventing these injuries.

Urinary retention, urinary infection, hematuria. These are usually secondary to urinary

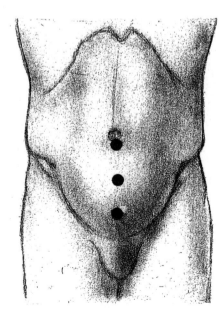

Fig. 90-14

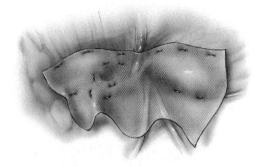

Fig. 90-15

catheterization, extensive preperitoneal dissection, general anesthesia, and administration of large volumes of intravenous fluids. These problems generally respond promptly to the usual treatments.

Bladder injury. This is one of the more common complications of laparoscopic herniorrhaphy. It is seen most commonly in patients with previous "space of Retzius" surgery. Previous surgery in this space (e.g., a prostate operation) should be considered a relative contraindication to laparoscopic hernia repair. If a bladder injury is recognized during hernia repair, it should be repaired immediately laparoscopically or via laparotomy if necessary. Repair the hernia by a conventional anterior approach to avoid placing a foreign body next to the bladder repair. A high index of suspicion is the key to the diagnosis of a missed urinary tract injury. Lower abdominal pain, a distended bladder, dysuria, and hematuria should be promptly investigated. Other signs may include azotemia, electrolyte abnormalities, and ascites. Indwelling catheter drainage alone may suffice for retroperitoneal bladder injuries, but intraperitoneal perforations are best closed laparoscopically or by laparotomy.

Nerve injury. The femoral branch of the genitofemoral nerve, the lateral cutaneous nerve of the thigh, and the intermediate cutaneous branch of the anterior branch of the femoral nerve are at risk of damage during laparoscopic herniorrhaphy because of (1) failure to appreciate the anatomy from the posterior aspect; (2) difficulty visualizing the nerves preperitoneally; (3) the variable course of the nerves in this region; (4) improper staple placement; or (5) extensive preperitoneal dissection. Symptoms of burning pain and numbness usually develop after a variable interval during the postoperative period. If neuralgia is present in the recovery room, immediate reexploration is the best course of action. When the onset of the symptoms is delayed, the condition is usually self-limiting. In most cases nonsteroidal antiinflammatory drugs (NSAIDs) are sufficient. Reexploration and removal of the offending staple is occasionally required.

Vas deferens and testicular complications. Testicular pain may be the result of trauma to the genitofemoral nerve or to the sympathetic innervation of the testis during dissection around the cord structures or during separation of the peritoneum from the cord structures. Testicular swelling may be secondary to narrowing of the deep inguinal ring, ischemia, or interruption of lymphatic or venous vessels resulting from attempts at complete removal of a large indirect inguinal hernial sac. Pain and swelling are usually transient and self-limiting. Transection of the vas deferens and testicular atrophy are seen in about the same incidence as during conventional surgery. The risk of these complications may be significantly decreased if the surgeon avoids excessive tightening of the deep inguinal ring, gently dissects around the cord structures, and does not attempt complete removal of large indirect hernial sacs. Minor cord and testicular complications are treated by supportive care, such as testicular support, limitation of activities, and analgesics. If the vas deferens is transected, the cut ends should be repaired with fine, interrupted sutures unless fertility is not a consideration. There is no treatment for unilateral testicular atrophy. The hypogonadism produced by bilateral testicular atrophy is treated by supplemental testosterone.

Complications related to the mesh. Migration, infection, mass lesions representing palpable mesh, adhesion formation, and erosion of the mesh into intraabdominal organs have been reported following laparoscopic herniorrhaphy. Fixation of the mesh prevents migration. Perioperative prophylactic antibiotics are recommended to prevent mesh infection. Adhesion formation is least likely to occur after the TEP procedure, as the mesh is never in contact with intraabdominal organs unless there are unrecognized peritoneal perforations. Following the TAPP procedure, adequate closure of the peritoneum over the mesh is the most important factor in preventing complications such as bowel herniating through large gaps or becoming adherent to exposed mesh. Minimizing trauma, avoiding infection, sparing the blood supply, and avoiding exposed mesh decreases the incidence of adhesion formation. Mesh complications usually manifest weeks to years after the repair in the form of small bowel obstruction, abscess, or fistula. They may respond to conservative management or may require formal laparotomy.

Recurrence of the hernia. Potential mechanisms for recurrence include missed hernias or failure of the mesh to cover all hernial defects adequately. The latter may occur when the mesh rolls, migrates, is too small, or is improperly secured. We believe that thorough dissection of the preperitoneal space with identification of all the landmarks followed by fixation of a large piece of mesh that adequately covers and overlaps the entire myopectineal orifice without slitting or folding is the best way to avoid recurrence. A repeat laparoscopic repair or a conventional repair (see Chapter 91) is needed to correct the recurrence.

Osteitis. Pelvic or pubic osteitis result from staples placed directly into bone. Placing staples on the anterior and superior portion of Cooper's ligament or avoiding fixing mesh altogether prevents these complications. The diagnosis is essentially one of exclusion. NSAIDs may help.

Wound infection. This may be prevented by using meticulous sterile technique.

REFERENCES

Arregui ME, Navarrete J, Davis CJ, Castro D, Nagan RF. Laparoscopic inguinal herniorrhaphy: techniques and controversies. Surg Clin North Am 1993;73:513.

Camps J, Nguyen N, Annibali R, Filipi CJ, Fitzgibbons RJ Jr. Laparoscopic inguinal herniorrhaphy: current techniques. In Arregui ME, Fitzgibbons RJ Jr, Katkhouda N, McKernan JB, Reich H (eds) Principles of Laparoscopic Surgery: Basic and Advanced Techniques. New York, Springer-Verlag, 1995, pp 400–408.

Colborn GL, Brick WG. Inguinal region. In Scott-Conner CEH, Cuschieri A, Carter FJ (eds) Minimal Access Surgical Anatomy. Philadelphia, Lippincott Williams & Wilkins, 2000, pp 239–266.

Crawford DL, Phillips EH. Laparoscopic repair and groin hernia surgery. Surg Clin North Am 1998;78:1047.

Filipi CJ, Fitzgibbons RJ Jr, Salerno GM. Laparoscopic herniorrhaphy. In Hulka JF, Reich H (eds) Textbook of Laparoscopy, 2nd ed. Philadelphia, Saunders, 1994, pp 313–326.

Fitzgibbons RJ Jr (ed). Nyhus and Condon's Hernia, 5th ed. Philadelphia, Lippincott Williams & Wilkins (in press).

Fitzgibbons RJ Jr, Camps J, Cornet DA, et al. Laparoscopic inguinal herniorrhaphy: results of a multicenter trial. Ann Surg 1995;1:3.

Katkhouda N. Avoiding complications of laparoscopic hernia repair: laparoscopic inguinal herniorrhaphy: current techniques. In Arregui ME, Fitzgibbons RJ Jr, Katkhouda N, McKernan JB, Reich H (eds) Principles of Laparoscopic Surgery: Basic and Advanced Techniques. New York, Springer-Verlag, 1995, pp 435–438.

Lowham AS, Filipi CJ, Fitzgibbons RJ Jr, et al. Mechanisms of hernia recurrence after preperitoneal mesh repair: traditional and laparoscopic. Ann Surg 1997;225:422.

Memon MA, Fitzgibbons RJ Jr. Assessing risks, costs and benefits of laparoscopic hernia repair. Annu Rev Med 1998;49:63.

Memon MA, Fitzgibbons RJ Jr. Laparoscopic inguinal hernia repair: transabdominal preperitoneal (TAPP) and totally extraperitoneal (TEP). In Scott-Conner CEH (ed) The SAGES Manual: Fundamentals of Laparoscopy and GI Endoscopy. New York, Springer-Verlag, 1999, pp 364–378.

Memon MA, Feliu X, Sallent F, Camps J, Fitzgibbons RJ Jr. Laparoscopic repair of recurrent hernias. Surg Endosc 1999;13:807.

Memon MA, Rice D, Donohue JH. Laparoscopic herniorrhaphy. J Am Coll Sug 1997;184:325.

Rosser JB Jr. Laparoscopic Inguinal Hernia Repair: Transabdominal and Balloon-Assisted Extraperitoneal Approaches [CD-ROM]. New York, Springer-Verlag, 1999.

Tetik C, Arregui ME. Prevention of complications of open and laparoscopic repair of groin hernias. In Arregui ME, Fitzgibbons RJ Jr, Katkhouda N, McKernan JB, Reich H (eds) Principles of Laparoscopic Surgery: Basic and Advanced Techniques. New York, Springer-Verlag, 1995, pp 439–449.

91 Operations for Recurrent Inguinal Hernia

INDICATIONS

Strangulation

Incarceration or recent history of incarceration

Symptomatic hernia in good-risk patients

PREOPERATIVE PREPARATION

If the patient suffers from chronic pulmonary disease, make every effort to achieve optimal improvement. Encourage all patients to stop smoking for at least a week before the operation.

Encourage the obese patient to lose weight.

Evaluate elderly male patients for potential prostatic obstruction.

Administer perioperative antibiotics if the use of mesh is anticipated.

Obtain consent for possible orchiectomy in elderly patients.

PITFALLS AND DANGER POINTS

Failing to identify all defects and to tailor the repair to the problem

Injuring internal spermatic artery and vein or iliac artery or vein

Injuring vas deferens

Injuring colon (rare)

Injuring bladder (rare)

Using weak tissues for repair

OPERATIVE STRATEGY

We note here the common causes of recurrence and their prevention. Thorough understanding of this material is essential for anatomic repair of recurrent hernias and helps the surgeon keep the primary recurrence rate low.

Internal Ring Left Too Large

At the conclusion of the repair, the internal ring should admit only the spermatic cord plus 2–3 mm (the tip of a Kelly hemostat). If closure is not adequate, the risk of recurrence is increased. Generally it requires removing both cremaster muscle and any lipomas from the spermatic cord as it passes through the internal ring.

Inadequate closure of the internal ring often follows repair of a large indirect hernia in adults. Simply removing the sac and performing a Bassini-type repair by suturing internal oblique muscle to the inguinal ligament often fails to produce adequate closure of the internal ring.

Defect at Pubic Tubercle

The second most common location of the hernial defect in a recurrent inguinal hernia is the most medial portion of Hesselbach's triangle adjacent to the pubic tubercle. This is often a localized defect measuring no more than 1–2 cm in diameter. The exact cause of this defect is not clear. It may result if the surgeon does not continue the suture line up to and including the pubic periosteum. Tying interrupted sutures (e.g., during a McVay repair) with excessive tension may play a part in the etiology of this type of defect.

Failure to Suture Transversalis Fascia or Transversus Arch

A Bassini repair is apt to fail if performed by suturing internal oblique muscle to the shelving edge of the inguinal ligament. Often these sutures fail to catch transversalis fascia or the aponeurosis of the transversus muscle (transversus arch), which are the strongest structures in the region. With traditional techniques of hernia repair, no attempt was made clearly to identify these structures prior to inserting sutures.

Failure to Excise Sac

Failure to remove the entire indirect sac is an important cause of recurrent hernia. Obviously, if the surgeon fails to remove the sac, hernia recurrence is probable. Even when an obvious direct hernia is found, always explore the cord and remove any indirect sac.

Use of Absorbable Sutures

It was demonstrated long ago that the use of catgut for repairing an inguinal hernia is followed by an excessive rate of recurrence. Nevertheless, a few surgeons persist in using absorbable suture material, which loses most of its tensile strength within several weeks, a length of time inadequate for solid healing of an inguinal hernia repair.

Subcutaneous Transplantation of Cord

A significant number of patients present with recurrent inguinal hernias following a Halsted repair in which the spermatic cord is transplanted into the subcutaneous plane by fashioning a new external ring directly superficial to the internal ring. The superimposition of one ring over the other results in a repair that is weaker than those that preserve the obliquity of the inguinal canal. Following the Halsted repair, a recurrent hernia presents at the point where the spermatic cord exits from the internal-external ring. Generally the two rings appear to have fused, and the hernia protrudes from this common orifice alongside the cord. It is important to recognize this before repairing the recurrence, as the cord is encountered early during the dissection and may be injured.

Femoral Recurrence Following Inguinal Hernia Repair

Several authors (McVay and Halverson; Glassow) have emphasized that following repair of an inguinal hernia 1–3% of patients later develop a femoral hernia on the same side. When operating to repair an inguinal hernia, the surgeon should inspect and palpate the cephalad opening of the femoral canal in search of a small femoral hernia. The normal femoral canal does not admit the surgeon's fingertip. The only circumstances in which this step might be omitted is when a young patient presents with a simple indirect hernia and no weakness of the floor of the inguinal canal.

If a femoral hernia is detected, it should be repaired simultaneously with the inguinal hernia repair. McVay's technique using Cooper's ligament automatically repairs any femoral defect by suturing the transversus arch to Cooper's ligament and the femoral sheath. Glassow recommended exposing the inferior opening of the femoral canal in the groin and repairing it with a few sutures from the lower approach. He then completed the inguinal repair by the Shouldice technique. A "plug" of Marlex mesh may be inserted into the femoral hernial ring from above or below to repair the femoral hernia.

Infection

Infection is rare in modern practice. When it occurs, the risk of subsequent recurrence may be as high as 40%.

Recurrent Indirect Inguinal Hernia

For every repair of an indirect hernia, free the sac above the internal ring after excising the entire cremaster muscle. Remove it and carefully identify the margins of the internal ring. To do this, it is necessary to delineate the transversalis fascia, which forms the medial margin of the internal ring. It is also important to differentiate weak from strong transversalis fascia. After identifying the lateral edge of the transversalis fascia as it joins the internal ring, one can insert the index finger behind the transversalis layer and evaluate the strength of the inguinal canal's floor.

Although in infants and young children it is rarely necessary to reconstruct the internal ring following removal of the sac, in adults the indirect hernia has often reached sufficient width to erode the adjacent transversalis fascia and to leave an internal ring with a diameter of 2–4 cm. When this has occurred, we prefer to perform a Shouldice repair similar to that done for the direct inguinal hernia.

During both indirect and direct hernia repairs in the adult patient, remove all of the cremaster muscle and adipose tissue surrounding the spermatic cord. If the diameter of the spermatic cord is narrowed, the aperture of the internal inguinal ring can also be narrowed, leaving an insignificant defect in the floor of the inguinal canal for a possible recurrent hernia.

Direct Inguinal Hernia

Successful repair of a direct hernia requires meticulous dissection and exposure of the transversalis fascia, the aponeurosis of the transversus muscle, and the lateral condensation of the transversalis fascia near the inguinal ligament (iliopubic tract and femoral sheath) prior to suturing the transversus arch-transversalis fascia to the iliopubic tract and the inguinal ligament. Excellent results have been reported following appropriate use of the Shouldice and McVay repairs and for the various techniques utilizing prosthetic mesh. During any direct inguinal repair, the anatomic structures named above must be carefully dissected and evaluated for areas of weakness. Any weakened areas must be excised, and only strong tissues employed for suturing or for the floor must be replaced with prosthetic mesh.

Choice of Approach

A major decision required before surgery is whether to use an anterior (groin) approach or a preperitoneal (usually laparoscopic) approach. This choice determines the instruments, room setup, and choice of anesthesia. The preperitoneal approach described here as Legacy material is occasionally useful if an anterior approach must be abandoned because of excessive scarring.

Anesthesia

Many groin operations for a recurrent inguinal hernia can be performed under local anesthesia without undue difficulty. Patients who have had previous operations for a recurrent hernia and have accumulated a great deal of scar tissue are preferably operated on with general anesthesia. General anesthesia is also needed for the preperitoneal (open or laparoscopic) approach.

Selecting the Optimal Technique for Repair of Recurrent Inguinal Hernia

There is no single best approach to a recurrent hernia. Obtain the previous operative record and determine what repair was done originally; then make an educated guess as to the probable mechanism and location of the recurrence. The occasional missed indirect inguinal hernia or the direct hernia with a virgin floor may be repaired in a manner similar to that used for primary repair. However, most recurrent hernias are more complex, with scarring and lack of good fascia to approximate without tension. The simplest, most secure way to repair these recurrent hernias is to bridge the gap with prosthetic mesh tailored to overlap good fascia by at least 3 cm and sutured in place. The repair must be individualized, and frequently the decision is made only after the anatomic defect has been exposed and identified.

A preperitoneal approach, whether open (as described by Nyhus) or laparoscopic, allows dissection in virgin planes. The defect is closed, again, after placing a large sheet of prosthetic mesh. This may be the best approach if mesh was placed at the primary operation.

Technique of Dissection

When the anterior inguinal approach has been selected, remember that the patient may have undergone the previous repair by the Halsted technique. Anticipate the possibility of encountering the spermatic cord in the subcutaneous layer of the dissection. Therefore soon after the skin incision is made, elevate the cephalad skin flap and direct the dissection so the anterior surface of the external oblique aponeurosis is exposed at a point 3–5 cm above the inguinal canal. This is virgin territory that has not been involved in previous surgery. Carefully direct the dissection in a manner that does not expose the external oblique aponeurosis inferiorly until the subcutaneous spermatic cord or the reconstructed external ring has been exposed. In the absence of a previous Halsted repair, continue the dissection beyond the previous suture line of the external oblique aponeurosis until the junction of the inguinal ligament and the upper thigh has been exposed. If one does encounter the spermatic cord in a subcutaneous location, meticulous dissection is necessary to preserve the fragile spermatic veins. In the absence of a previous Halsted repair, incise the external oblique aponeurosis with caution to avoid traumatizing the cord.

Avoiding Testicular Complications

In the elderly patient with a large recurrent hernia, the repair can be simplified if the patient is willing preoperatively to accept a simultaneous orchiectomy. In most series of recurrent hernia repairs, 10–15% of patients undergo simultaneous orchiectomy. In younger patients and in those in whom the surgeon wishes to minimize the risk of having a testicular complication, the preperitoneal approach offers a sound alternative to dissection in a previous operative field. Otherwise, take the time to perform meticulous dissection of the spermatic vessels and vas. Sometimes the spermatic veins have been spread apart by a large hernia, increasing their vulnerability to operative trauma.

When the anterior inguinal approach through the previous incision has been selected for repair of a recurrent hernia in a young man, occasionally preserving the spermatic cord seems impossible. In this situation it is advisable to abandon the anterior approach and to extend the skin incision so the medial skin flap can be elevated for a distance of 3–5 cm. Continue the operation by an incision through the abdominal wall using the preperitoneal approach of Nyhus. After dissecting the peritoneum and the sac away from the posterior abdominal wall in the inguinal region, insert a prosthetic mesh. This approach helps avoid testicular complications.

OPERATIVE TECHNIQUE

Inguinal Approach

Incision and Exposure

Enter the operative site through the old incision. It may be cosmetically advantageous to excise the previous scar. Then dissect the skin flap in a cephalad direction. Be aware of the possibility that at the previous operation the surgeon may have transplanted the spermatic cord into a subcutaneous location. Be careful not to injure the cord during this dissection. After the skin flap has been dissected for a distance of about 2–3 cm, carry the dissection down to the aponeurosis of the external oblique muscle. Accomplish this in an area that is superior to the region of the previous surgery. Now dissect all subcutaneous fat off the anterior surface of the aponeurosis, proceeding in an inferolateral direction until the inguinal ligament and the subcutaneous inguinal ring have been cleared.

Repairing Recurrent Hernia Following Previous Halsted Operation Without Opening the Inguinal Canal

If the spermatic cord was transplanted into the subcutaneous plane at the previous operation, the subcutaneous and deep inguinal rings are now superimposed, one directly on the other. In this case the inguinal region is generally quite strong except for a single defect that represents an enlarged common external-internal ring through which the spermatic cord passes together with the hernial sac. In these patients it is often difficult to separate the external oblique aponeurosis from the deeper structures, a step that is necessary before accomplishing either a Shouldice or a McVay repair. Instead of incising the external oblique aponeurosis in the region between the hernial defect and the pubic tubercle in these patients, it may be more prudent to remove the hernial sac and then narrow the enlarged common ring with several heavy sutures.

To accomplish this, carefully identify and dissect the spermatic cord free from surrounding structures and isolate the hernial sac. Open it and insert the in-

dex finger to verify that the floor of the inguinal canal is indeed strong. Dissect the sac away from any attachments at its neck. Close the sac with a single suture-ligature of 2-0 PG. Alternatively, use a purse-string suture. Amputate the sac and permit the stump to retract into the abdominal cavity. Dissect areolar tissue, fat, and cremaster from the margins of the hernial defect. Close the defect medial to the point of exit of the spermatic cord using 2-0 Tevdek or Prolene on an atraumatic needle. In effect, the needle penetrates (at the medial margin of the ring) 5–6 mm of the external oblique aponeurosis, the underlying internal oblique, and the transversalis fascia. At the lateral margin of the repair the needle pierces the external oblique aponeurosis and the shelving edge of the inguinal ligament. Narrow the ring to the extent that a Kelly hemostat can be passed into the revised inguinal ring alongside the spermatic cord. Making the ring any smaller increases the risk of testicular complications.

Inevitably, these sutures must be tied with some tension, which threatens the success of any hernia repair. Therefore it is preferable when possible to insert an appropriately sized plug of Marlex mesh into the ring. Stabilize the plug with sutures as described in Figure 92–7. This method obliterates the defect *with no tension* on the tissues. If the hernial defect is large (>3 cm in diameter), apply a patch consisting of a layer of Marlex or Prolene mesh to cover the defect. Suture the mesh to the edge of the hernial defect using large bites of interrupted or continuous 2-0 atraumatic Prolene. Leave an opening for exit of the spermatic cord along the medial margin of the repair.

Dissecting the Inguinal Canal

Most patients presenting with a recurrent inguinal hernia have had their previous repair performed with some variety of the Bassini technique; the spermatic cord thus remains in its normal location deep to the external oblique aponeurosis. In these cases, make an incision in the external oblique aponeurosis along the lines of its fibers aimed at the cephalad margin of the external inguinal ring, as described above. Perform a patient, meticulous dissection of the spermatic cord to avoid traumatizing the delicate spermatic veins. After mobilizing the spermatic cord, identify the hernial sac. In our experience the most common location of a recurrence is in the floor of Hesselbach's triangle medial to the deep inferior epigastric vessels. The previous surgeon probably did not identify the transversalis fascia and the aponeurosis of the transversus muscle. If this area is

virgin territory, repair the recurrent hernia by the classic Shouldice technique described in Chapter 87. This repair is also suitable in patients who have a recurrence of an indirect nature, as these patients almost always have considerable weakness of the inguinal canal. Of course, the indirect sac must be excised.

Repairing a Localized Defect in the Inguinal Floor

A number of patients with recurrent hernia suffer from a relatively small (≤2 cm) defect in the inguinal canal floor just medial to the pubic tubercle. Simple suturing of this defect produces excessive tension. Standard repair calls for an incision through the floor of the inguinal canal followed by a definitive Shouldice or McVay reconstruction. Mesh repair is an excellent alternative that avoids an extensive dissection. A plug of Marlex mesh is placed in the defect and sutured in place with one or two stitches of 2-0 Prolene as described for repair of a femoral hernia (see Fig. 92–7).

Prosthetic Mesh Repair

In most cases of recurrent hernia, after dissection of the inguinal canal the remaining tissues are simply not strong enough to ensure successful suturing of the hernial defect. By far the most common error made by surgeons repairing a recurrent hernia is to misjudge the strength of the tissues being sutured. Attenuated scar tissue sutured under tension *does not allow a successful long-term repair*. Do not hesitate to excise these weakened tissues. Make no attempt to close the defect by sutures; rather, insert prosthetic mesh, which can be inserted to replace the defect *without any tension at all*.

Complete the dissection of the inguinal canal through the layer of the transversalis fascia (see Figs. 87-3 to 87-12) so the peritoneum, Cooper's ligament, and the aponeurosis of the transversus muscle have all been exposed. Separate the peritoneum from the transversalis fascia for a distance of at least 3 cm around the perimeter of the inguinal defect. Trim away attenuated tissues. Now take a layer of Marlex or Prolene mesh and cut a patch in the shape of an ellipse whose diameter is 3–4 cm larger than that of the defect. Place the mesh behind the abdominal wall between the peritoneum and the transversalis fascia. Suture the mesh in place by means of 2-0 atraumatic Prolene stitches *through the entire abdominal wall* in a mattress fashion, as seen in **Figure 91–1a.** Continue to insert these interrupted mattress sutures around the perimeter of the defect and to penetrate the external oblique, internal oblique,

and transversus muscles and the transversalis fascia. Along the medial aspects of the hernial defect, the sutures penetrate the anterior rectus sheath, the rectus muscle, and the transversalis fascia. Along the lateral margin of the defect, suture the mesh to Cooper's ligament with interrupted or continuous 2-0 Prolene stitches going from the pubic tubercle laterally to the region of the femoral canal. Lateral to this point, suture the mesh to the femoral sheath and the shelving edge of Poupart's ligament. Cut a small section from the lateral portion of the mesh to avoid constricting the spermatic cord **(Fig. 91–1b).** *In most cases it is not possible to suture the layers of the abdominal wall together over the mesh without creating excessive tension.* After irrigating the operative area thoroughly with a dilute antibiotic solution, close Scarpa's fascia with 4-0 PG and close the skin with a continuous 4-0 PG subcuticular suture.

Abandoning the Anterior Approach

With rare recurrent inguinal hernias it may be apparent during dissection of the spermatic cord that there is such dense fibrosis as to endanger preservation of the cord. When these conditions are encountered, especially in young patients, simply abandon the anterior approach. Elevate the cephalad skin flap and make an incision through the abdominal wall down to the peritoneum, as described below for the preperitoneal approach to the repair of a recurrent hernia. Dissecting peritoneum away from the posterior wall of the inguinal canal via the preperitoneal approach does not endanger the spermatic cord because this dissection is carried out in territory free of scar tissue.

Preperitoneal Approach Using Mesh Prosthesis (Surgical Legacy Technique)

The technique described below is derived in many aspects from the contributions of Nyhus. It is described as used for a large right recurrent inguinal hernia.

Incision and Exposure

Enter the abdominal cavity by making a transverse incision in the lower quadrant at a level at least 3 cm above the upper margin of the hernial defect. Start the skin incision near the abdominal midline approximately two fingerbreadths above the pubic symphysis and proceed laterally for a distance of about 10 cm, aiming at a point just above the anterosuperior spine of the ilium. Expose the external

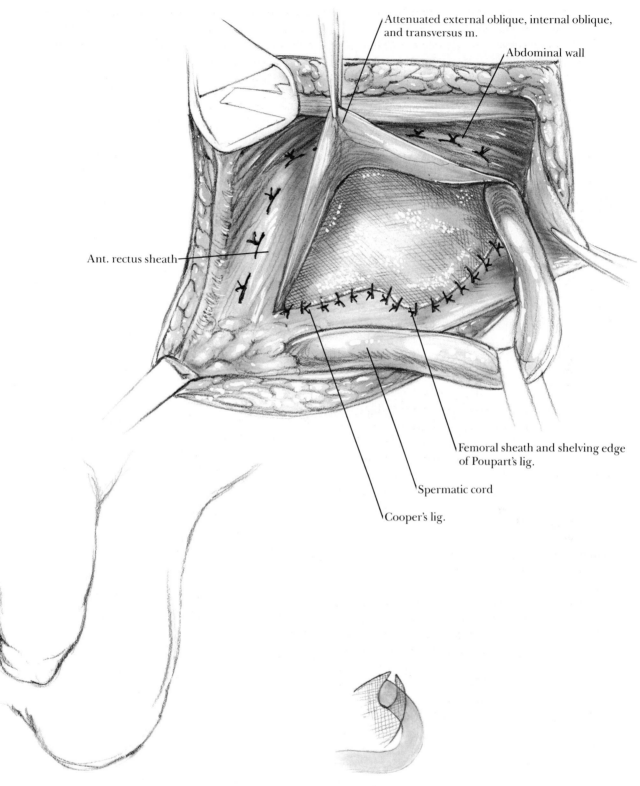

Fig. 91–1a

Fig. 91–1b

oblique aponeurosis and the artery. **Figure 91–2** illustrates the anatomy of structures encountered during this preperitoneal dissection on the *right* side of the patient.

Suturing the Mesh

Cut a square of Marlex or Prolene mesh sufficiently large to provide a layer of prosthesis that reaches from the abdominal incision (cephalad) to Cooper's ligament and to the iliopsoas fascia (caudad) and from the mid-rectus region medially to the anterosuperior iliac spine laterally.

For recurrent hernias repaired by this approach, do not attempt to close the hernial defect by suturing it because the tension would be excessive. Use 2-0 atraumatic Prolene swaged on a stout needle and take substantial bites of strong tissue to ensure that the mesh remains permanently in place. Do not ex-

pect that the ingrowth of fibrous tissue into the mesh will ensure fixation, as the polypropylene is relatively inert and substantial fibrous ingrowth does not *always* take place. Place the first suture in the ligamentous tissue adjacent to the pubic symphysis. Continue the suture line laterally, passing interrupted 2-0 atraumatic Prolene sutures through the layer of mesh deep into Cooper's ligament along the pubic ramus. At the femoral ring, suture the mesh to the femoral sheath and the shelving edge of the inguinal ligament. When the internal inguinal ring is reached, leave a space for the spermatic cord to exit from the abdominal cavity in the male patient. Lateral to the external iliac artery carry the suture line in a posterior direction and attach the mesh to the iliopsoas fascia proceeding laterally. Take deep bites into this fascia after identifying and protecting the femoral nerve, which runs just below the fascia. Continue the suture line in the iliopsoas fascia laterally

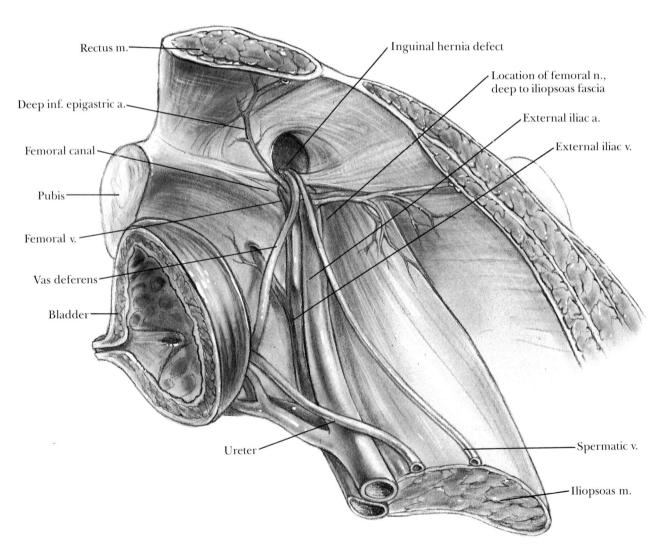

Fig. 91-2

toward the anterosuperior iliac spine until the lateral margin of the abdominal incision is reached. In the female patient, suturing the mesh to the femoral sheath and the iliopsoas fascia completely obliterates the internal inguinal ring, although this operation (using mesh to repair a large recurrent inguinal hernia) rarely is necessary in women.

Attach the medial margin of the layer of mesh to the medial portion of the rectus muscle by dissecting the subcutaneous fat off the anterior rectus sheath down to the pubis. Then insert 2-0 Prolene sutures by taking a bite first through the anterior rec-

tus sheath, next through the body of the rectus muscle, and then through the layer of mesh in the abdomen. Return the same suture as a mattress suture by taking a bite through the mesh, the body of the rectus muscle, and finally the anterior rectus sheath. After tying the stitch, the knot is on the anterior rectus sheath. Continue this suture line up to the level of the transverse abdominal incision. **Figure 91–3** depicts the appearance of the mesh sutured in place.

Intermittently during the operation irrigate the operative site with a dilute antibiotic solution. By this point in the operation, the mesh has been su-

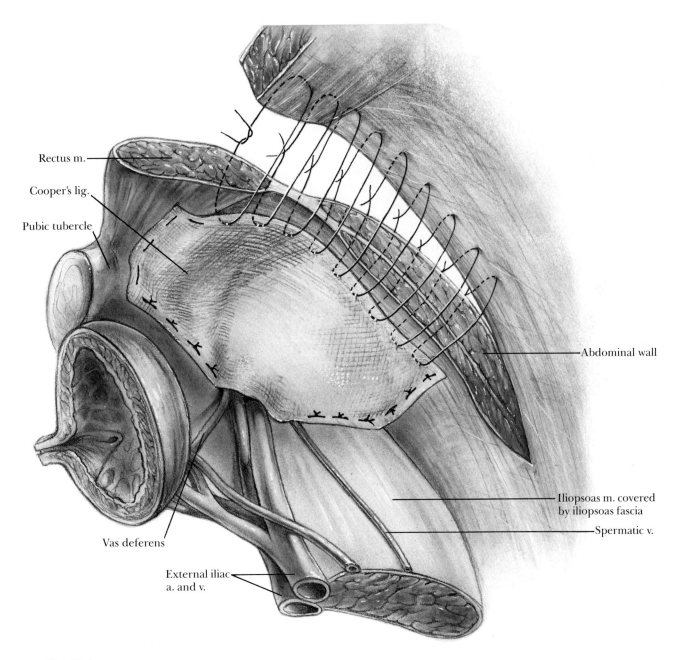

Rectus m.

Cooper's lig.

Pubic tubercle

Vas deferens

External iliac a. and v.

Abdominal wall

Iliopsoas m. covered by iliopsoas fascia

Spermatic v.

Fig. 91-3

tured into place medially, caudally, and laterally; only the cephalad margin is left unattached. Trim the mesh so this cephalad margin terminates evenly with the inferior margin of the transverse abdominal incision. Because of the irregular nature of the surface that has been covered by the flat patch of mesh, there is a surplus of mesh in the lateral portion of the incision. Correct this by making a vertical fold in the mesh, as necessary, to include the mesh in the closure of the abdominal incision. Prior to inserting many of the sutures, it is necessary to ligate and divide or to coagulate a number of blood vessels in the region of Cooper's ligament and the femoral sheath so inserting the sutures does not produce bleeding.

Closing the Abdominal Incision

Close the anterior rectus sheath with interrupted nonabsorbable sutures. Lateral to the rectus muscle close the abdominal incision using the Smead-Jones technique of interrupted 0 Prolene sutures that grasp a width of at least 1.5 cm of the abdominal wall including the external oblique aponeurosis, the internal oblique and transversus muscles, the transversalis fascia, and the *proximal edge of the mesh* in the caudal margin of the incision as well as the same layers on the cephalad margin except for the mesh. Close the skin with a continuous 4-0 PG subcuticular stitch. Figure 91–3 illustrates the completed incision sutureline.

POSTOPERATIVE CARE

Ambulate the patient the day of the operation.

COMPLICATIONS

Testicular swelling and/or atrophy.
Urinary retention in males.
Recurrence of hernia.
Wound hematoma.

Wound sepsis. When infection develops in patients who have undergone insertion of a mesh prosthesis, it is not always necessary to remove this foreign body to remedy the infection, as the mesh is made up of monofilament fibers. In most patients wide drainage of the skin incision accompanied by parenteral antibiotics with perhaps local antibiotic irrigation may prove effective. We have had no experience managing a pelvic infection after insertion of a mesh prosthesis in the pelvis by the preperitoneal route. If we encountered this problem, we would subject the patient to a trial of conservative therapy after opening the incision to explore the pelvis and to insert indwelling irrigating catheters and sump-suction drains.

REFERENCES

Abrahamson J. Etiology and pathophysiology of primary and recurrent groin hernia formation. Surg Clin North Am 1998;78:953.

Berliner S, Burson L, Katz P, et al. An anterior transversalis fascia repair for adult inguinal hernias. Am J Surg 1978;135:633.

Glassow F. Femoral hernia following inguinal herniorrhaphy. Can J Surg 1970;13:27.

Heifetz CJ. Resection of the spermatic cord in selected inguinal hernias. Arch Surg 1971;102:36.

Lichtenstein IL. A two-stitch repair of femoral and recurrent inguinal hernias by a "plug" technique. Contemp Surg 1982;20:35.

Lichtenstein IL, Shulman AG, Amid PK. The cause, prevention, and treatment of recurrent groin hernia. Surg Clin North Am 1993;73:529.

McVay CB, Halverson K. Inguinal and femoral hernias. In Beahrs OH, Beart RW (eds) General Surgery. Boston, Houghton Mifflin, 1980.

Nyhus LM. The preperitoneal approach and iliopubic tract repair of inguinal hernias. In Nyhus LM, Condon RE (eds) Hernia, 4th ed. Philadelphia, Lippincott, 1995, pp 153–177.

Nyhus LM. The recurrent groin hernia: therapeutic solutions. World J Surg 1989;13:541.

Shulman AG, Amid PK, Lichtenstein IL. The "plug" repair of 1,402 recurrent inguinal hernias. Arch Surg 1990;125:265.

92 Femoral Hernia Repair

INDICATIONS

As strangulation is common with femoral hernias, it is advisable to operate on all such patients unless their medical status is so precarious it contraindicates even an operation under local anesthesia.

PREOPERATIVE PREPARATION

If there are signs of intestinal obstruction, initiate nasogastric suction.

When a patient has symptoms suggestive of a femoral hernia but lacks definitive physical findings, request a sonogram of the groin. This study may reveal a small incarcerated femoral hernia. Sonography is also helpful for diagnosing symptomatic spigelian and other interstitial hernias of the abdominal wall.

PITFALLS AND DANGER POINTS

Injuring or constricting femoral vein

Transecting an aberrant obturator artery

OPERATIVE STRATEGY

Choose the operative approach (low groin, high inguinal, or preperitoneal) that best fits the situation. A low groin approach under local anesthesia is an excellent choice for the frail elderly patient (unless strangulated bowel is suspected). The preperitoneal approach offers the best access for bowel resection if strangulation has occurred. An inguinal approach allows any associated inguinal hernia to be repaired and gives adequate access for bowel resection, but it creates a defect in an otherwise intact inguinal floor. The low groin and preperitoneal approaches are described here.

Inguinal Approach

The inguinal approach is essentially identical to the McVay repair described in Chapter 88.

Low Groin Approach

For the low groin approach, after opening the sac and reducing its contents, amputate it. It is not necessary to close the neck of the sac with sutures (Ferguson). It is important, however, to clear the femoral canal of any fat or areolar tissue so the sutures can bring the inguinal ligament into direct contact with Cooper's ligament and the pectineus fascia. This maneuver obliterates the femoral canal but leaves an opening of 6-8 mm adjacent to the femoral vein. Equally good results can be obtained if the femoral canal is obliterated by inserting a plug of Marlex mesh. The technique avoids all tension on the suture line.

To reduce an incarcerated femoral hernia, an incision may be made to divide the constricting neck of the hernial sac. It should be done on the medial aspect of the hernial ring. Although we have never observed the phenomenon, a number of texts warn that an anomalous obturator artery may follow a course that brings it into contiguity with the neck of the hernial sac, making it vulnerable to injury when the constricted neck is incised. This accident *rarely* occurs if the neck of the sac is incised on its medial aspect. If hemorrhage is indeed encountered during this maneuver and the artery cannot be ligated from below, control the bleeding by finger pressure and rapidly expose the inner aspect of the pelvis by the Henry approach, which involves a midline incision from the umbilicus to the pubis, after which the peritoneum is swept in a cephalad direction to expose the femoral canal from above. With this exposure a bleeding obturator artery can be easily ligated. It should be emphasized that this complication is so rare it does not constitute a significant disadvantage of the low approach to femoral herniorrhaphy.

If the sutures drawing the inguinal ligament down to Cooper's ligament must be tied under excessive tension, abandon this technique. Then insert a plug of Martex mesh to obliterate the femoral canal, as described below.

OPERATIVE TECHNIQUE

Low Groin Approach for Left Femoral Hernia

Make an oblique incision about 6 cm in length along the groin skin crease curving down over the femoral hernia **(Fig. 92–1)**. Carry the incision down to the external oblique aponeurosis and the inferior aspect of the inguinal ligament. Identify the hernial sac as it emerges deep to the inguinal ligament in the space between the lacunar ligament and the common femoral vein **(Fig. 92–2)**. Dissect the sac down to its neck using Metzenbaum scissors.

Grasp the sac with two hemostats and incise with a scalpel. Often the peritoneum is covered by two or more layers of tissue, each of which may resemble a sac. They consist of preperitoneal tissues and fat. This situation is seen especially when intestine is incarcerated in the sac.

When the bowel or the omentum remains incarcerated after opening the sac, incise the hernial ring on its medial aspect by inserting a scalpel between the sac and the lacunar ligament **(Figs. 92–3, 92–4)**. After returning the bowel and the omentum to the abdominal cavity, amputate the sac at its neck. Although it is not necessary to ligate or suture the neck of the sac, this step may be performed if desired **(Fig. 92–5)**. Using a peanut sponge, push any remaining preperitoneal fat into the abdominal cavity, thereby clearing the femoral canal of all extraneous tissues.

Repair the hernial defect by suturing the inguinal ligament down to Cooper's ligament using interrupted 2-0 sutures of Prolene on a heavy Mayo needle. Often this can be accomplished if the inguinal ligament is pressed down and cephalad toward Cooper's ligament with the index finger. The nee-

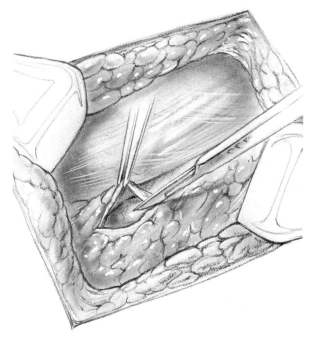

Fig. 92-2

dle is then passed through the inguinal ligament and through Cooper's ligament in one simultaneous motion. Cooper's ligament is indistinguishable from the periosteum overlying the cephalad aspect of the pubic ramus. An alternative method involves placing the stitch through the inguinal ligament and then positioning a narrow retractor in the femoral canal to take a bite of Cooper's ligament and pectineus fascia. No more than two or three sutures are generally necessary. Identify the common femoral vein where it emerges from underneath the inguinal ligament, and leave a gap of 4-6 mm between the femoral vein and the most lateral suture **(Fig. 92–6)**. Close the skin of the groin incision with either continuous 4-0 PG subcuticular sutures or interrupted 4-0 nylon sutures.

If strangulated bowel requiring resection is encountered after opening the hernial sac, make a second incision in the midline between the umbilicus

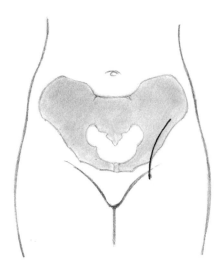

Fig. 92-1

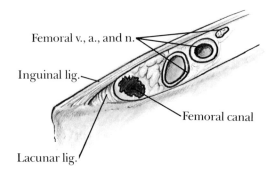

Femoral v., a., and n.

Inguinal lig.

Femoral canal

Lacunar lig.

Fig. 92-3

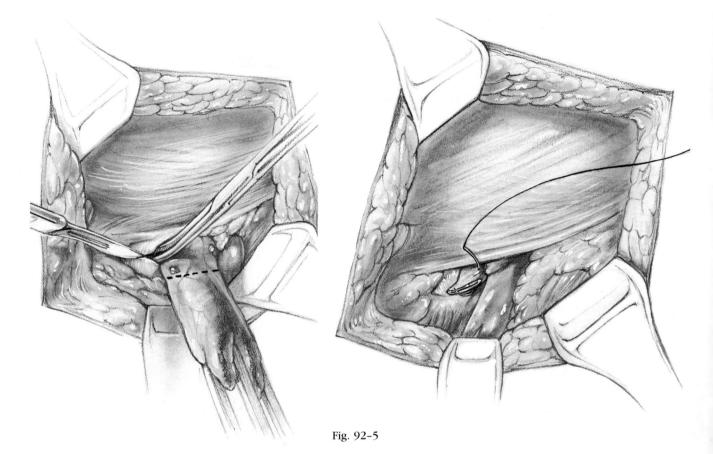

Fig. 92–5

Fig. 92–4

and the pubis. Separate the two rectus muscles and identify the peritoneum. Do not incise the peritoneum. Elevate the peritoneum from the pelvis by blunt dissection until the iliac vessels and the femoral hernial sac are identified. At this point, open the peritoneum just above the sac. Incise the constricting neck of the femoral canal on its medial aspect and reduce the strangulated bowel. After resecting the bowel, irrigate the femoral region with a dilute antibiotic solution and repair the femoral ring from below as already described. Irrigate the abdomen and close the abdominal incision in routine fashion.

Low Groin Approach Using Prosthetic Mesh "Plug"

Approximating the inguinal ligament to Cooper's ligament by sutures frequently requires excessive tension. Monro, who strongly favored the low groin approach, emphasized that the sutures should be tied loosely so they form a latticework of monofilament nylon. This technique serves to occlude the defect without producing tension.

The same end can be accomplished even more simply by inserting a rolled-up plug of Marlex mesh

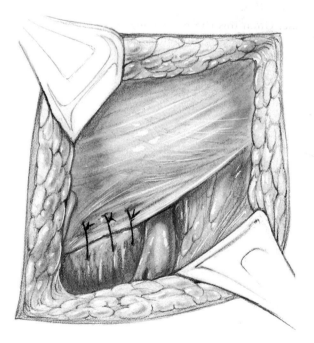

Fig. 92–6

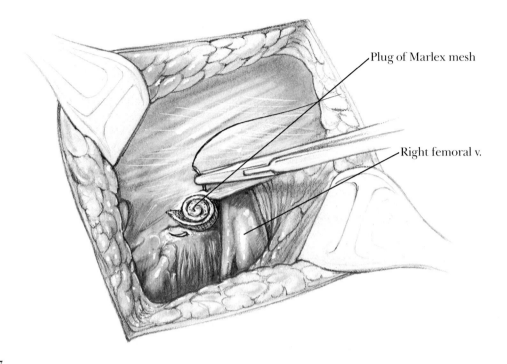

Plug of Marlex mesh

Right femoral v.

Fig. 92-7

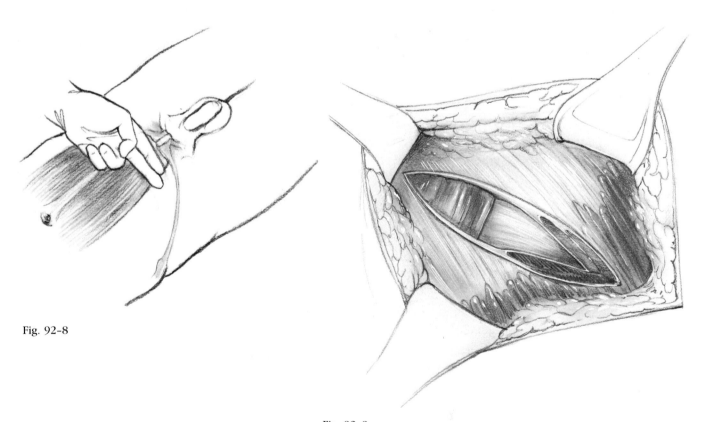

Fig. 92-8

Fig. 92-9

as advocated by Lichtenstein and Shore. *We believe this is the best method* for repairing a femoral hernia. Cut a strip of Marlex mesh about 2 × 10–12 cm. Roll the Marlex strip in the shape of a cigarette, 2 cm in length. After the hernial sac has been eliminated and all the fat has been cleared from the femoral canal, insert this Marlex plug into the femoral canal. The diameter of the plug may be adjusted by using a greater or lesser length of Marlex, as required. When the properly sized plug is snug in the femoral canal with about 0.3 cm of the plug protruding into the groin, fix the Marlex in place by inserting two sutures of 2-0 atraumatic Prolene **(Fig. 92–7)**. Insert the needle first through the inguinal ligament, then through the Marlex plug, and finally into the pectineal fascia or Cooper's ligament. After the two sutures have been tied, the plug should fit securely in the canal. After irrigating the wound with a dilute antibiotic solution, check for complete hemostasis and then close the skin incision without drainage. If the patient accumulates serum in the incision postoperatively, aspirate the fluid occasionally with a needle.

Preperitoneal Approach for Right Femoral Hernia (Nyhus)

Anesthesia

General or regional anesthesia with good muscle relaxation is required.

Incision

Start the skin incision at a point two fingerbreadths above the symphysis pubis **(Fig. 92–8)** and about 1.5 cm lateral to the abdominal midline. Carry the incision laterally for a distance of 8–10 cm and expose the anterior rectus sheath and the external oblique aponeurosis. Elevate the caudal skin flap sufficiently to expose the external inguinal ring.

Make a transverse incision in the anterior rectus sheath about 1.5 cm cephalad to the upper margin of the external inguinal ring for a distance of about 5 cm in a direction parallel to the inguinal canal **(Fig. 92–9)**. Retract the rectus muscle medially and deepen the incision through the full thickness of the internal oblique and transversus abdominis muscles, exposing the transversalis fascia. Carefully make a transverse incision in this layer but do not incise the peritoneum.

Apply a Richardson retractor against the lateral margin of the incised abdominal wall. Use blunt dissection to elevate the peritoneum out of the pelvis.

Mobilizing the Hernial Sac

If the femoral hernia is incarcerated, it is possible to mobilize the entire pelvic peritoneum except for that portion incarcerated in the femoral canal **(Fig. 92–10)**. If the hernia cannot be extracted by gentle blunt dissection around the femoral ring, incise the medial margin of the femoral ring and extract the

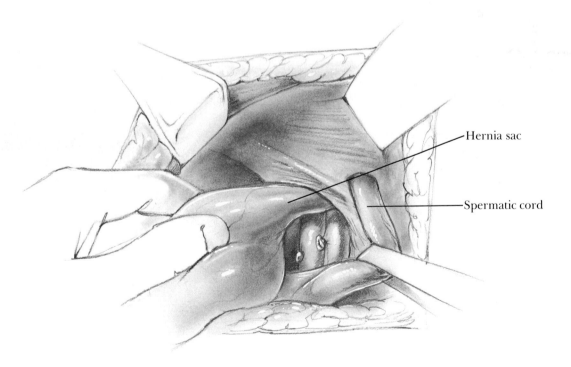

Hernia sac

Spermatic cord

Fig. 92-10

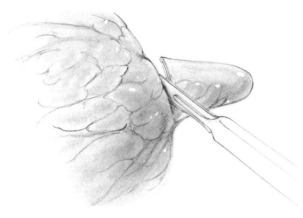

Fig. 92-11

hernial sac by combining traction plus external pressure against the sac in the groin. Although the presence of an aberrant obturator artery along the medial margin of the femoral ring is a rarity, there may be one or two small venous branches that require suture-ligation prior to incising the medial margin of the ring.

Open the sac **(Fig. 92–11)**. Evaluate the condition of the bowel. If strangulation mandates bowel resection, enlarge the incision enough so adequate exposure for a careful intestinal anastomosis may be guaranteed. If bowel has been resected, change gloves and instruments before initiating the repair. Irrigate the incision with a dilute antibiotic solution. Excise the peritoneal sac and close the peritoneal defect with continuous 3-0 PG.

Suturing the Hernial Ring

The superficial margin of the femoral ring consists of the iliopubic tract and the femoral sheath. These structures are just deep to the inguinal ligament. The deep margin of the femoral ring is Cooper's ligament, which represents the reinforced periosteum of the superior ramus of the pubis. When repairing the hernial defect, suture the strong tissue situated in the superficial margin of the femoral ring to Cooper's ligament with several interrupted sutures of 2-0 Tevdek of Prolene **(Figs. 92–12, 92–13)**. Whether the suture catching the superficial margin of the femoral ring contains only the iliopubic tract or it also catches a bite of inguinal ligament is immaterial so long as the tension is not excessive when the knot is tied. If closing the ring by approximat-

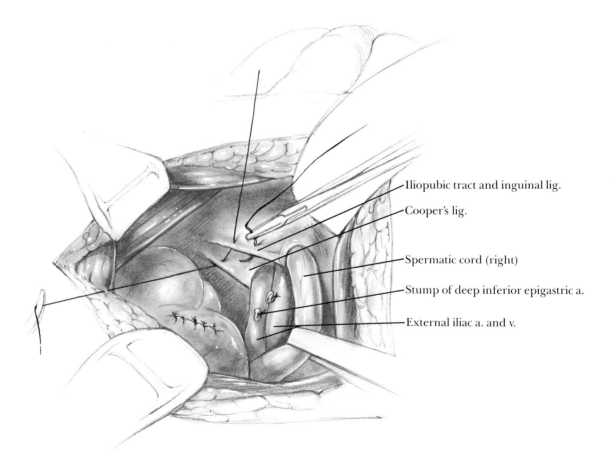

Iliopubic tract and inguinal lig.

Cooper's lig.

Spermatic cord (right)

Stump of deep inferior epigastric a.

External iliac a. and v.

Fig. 92-12

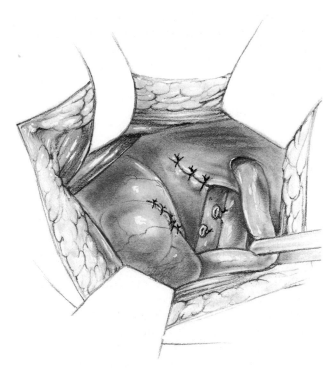

Fig. 92-13

ing strong tissues would result in tension, it is preferable to suture a small "cigarette" of Marlex into the femoral ring from the cephalad approach.

POSTOPERATIVE CARE

Early ambulation. Nonstrangulated femoral hernias are repaired in our ambulatory surgery unit.

Perioperative antibiotics are employed in patients with intestinal obstruction or those who have had bowel resection for strangulation. Use nasogastric suction in patients with intestinal obstruction or bowel resection.

COMPLICATIONS

Deep vein thrombosis has been reported secondary to constriction of the femoral vein by suturing.

Wound infections occur but are rare.

Ventral hernia may follow the preperitoneal approach to femoral hernia repair.

Recurrence is rare, although in some series it has ranged from 1% to 3%.

REFERENCES

Glassow F. Femoral hernias: review of 1143 consecutive repairs. Ann Surg 1966;163:227.

Lichtenstein IL, Shore JM. Simplified repair of femoral and recurrent inguinal hernia by a "plug" technique. Am J Surg 1974;128:439.

Monro A. In Nyhus LM, Harkins HN (eds) Hernia, 1st ed. Philadelphia, Lippincott, 1964.

Nyhus LM. Iliopubic tract repair of inguinal and femoral hernia: the posterior (preperitoneal) approach. Surg Clin North Am 1993;73:487.

Nyhus LM. The preperitoneal approach and iliopubic tract repair of femoral hernias. In Nyhus LM, Condon RE (eds) Hernia, 4th ed. Philadelphia, Lippincott, 1995, pp 178-187.

93 Operations for Large Ventral Hernia

INDICATIONS

Good-risk patients should undergo elective repair of a ventral hernia that has a defect of more than 1–2 cm. Early repair of the small hernia is a simple procedure. Nonoperative therapy is almost always followed by gradual enlargement of the hernial ring over time. Not only does this make the repair more difficult, but there is a significant incidence of incarceration.

PREOPERATIVE PREPARATION

Nasogastric tube prior to operation for large hernias

Perioperative antibiotics in patients with hernias large enough to require prosthetic mesh

PITFALLS AND DANGER POINTS

Excessive tension on the suture line

Sewing tissues that are too weak to hold sutures

Postoperative infection

Failure to achieve complete hemostasis

OPERATIVE STRATEGY

A thorough understanding of the factors that lead to incisional hernia formation is crucial. These same factors contribute to recurrence after repair.

Infection

Infection of the postoperative abdominal wound not uncommonly leads to an incisional hernia at a later date, especially if the infection was not detected and widely drained early during the course of its development. Strategies to minimize the incidence of wound infection during a contaminated abdominal operation are discussed in Chapter 7.

Occult Wound Dehiscence

When a large ventral hernia appears within the first few months after an abdominal operation, a likely cause of the hernia is contained dehiscence of the fascial and muscular layers of the abdominal wall during the early postoperative course in a patient whose skin incision has remained intact. Prevention of postoperative wound dehiscence is discussed in Chapter 3.

Making Too Large a Drain Wound

Postoperative hernias may occur at drain exit sites, particularly the large stab wounds used for Penrose drains. Generally, if the stab wound admits only one finger, a postoperative hernia is unlikely. When drainage of necrotic tissue (e.g., necrotizing pancreatitis) is required, large drainage wounds are appropriate and the risk of subsequent hernia formation is accepted. Closed-suction drains require smaller incisions and rarely become sites of hernia formation.

Failure to Close Laparoscopic Trocar Sites Adequately

In general, close the fascial defect after inserting any trocar larger than 5 mm in diameter.

Transverse Versus Vertical Incision

As discussed in Chapter 3, we have not detected an increased incidence of incisional hernia or wound dehiscence when comparing the midline vertical incision with transverse or oblique subcostal incisions, provided the midline incision has been closed with sutures that encompass large bites of abdominal wall, such as the Smead-Jones stitch.

Suturing Technique

Type of Suture Material

Closure with catgut results in a large number of wound dehiscences and incisional hernias and is no longer recommended. It is uncertain how the newer synthetic absorbable suture materials such as PDS performs, as long-term followup is lacking.

Size of Tissue Bites

The width of tissue included in each stitch is an important determinant of the incidence of wound dehiscence or incisional hernia, regardless of whether a continuous or interrupted technique is used. Sutures that contain small bites of tissue tend to cut through in response to muscle tension. We believe that *at least 2 cm* of musculofascial tissue on each side of the incision should be included in the stitch.

Tension with Which Suture Should Be Tied

When a stitch in an abdominal incision is tied with strangulating force, no matter how large a bite of tissue the stitch contains strangulation may cause the stitch to cut through the abdominal wall. This error manifests as a small hernia 1–2 cm lateral to the scar several months following operation. The hernial ring is often no more than 1.0–1.5 cm in diameter when first detected. This phenomenon is somewhat less likely to occur with synthetic monofilament sutures than with wire sutures because these sutures have a larger diameter than the equivalent-strength stainless steel suture.

It is easy to tie monofilament sutures too tightly because the knot has a tendency to slip. Resist the temptation to snug the knot down successively tighter with each throw. If the suture is tied with too much tension, it may cut through the necrotic tissue that results. Insist that the anesthesiologist provide adequate muscle relaxation at the time of closure, as it makes it easier to apply the proper tension to each suture.

Intercurrent Disease

Cirrhosis and ascites

Long-term high-dose steroid treatment

Marked obesity

Severe malnutrition

Abdominal wall defects secondary to tumor resection

Defects in the abdominal wall, secondary to resection for tumor, may be managed by inserting a prosthetic mesh as described below for ventral hernia repair provided adequate coverage of the mesh with viable skin and subcutaneous fat is possible. Otherwise, a full-thickness pedicle flap must be designed to cover the mesh.

Choice of Approach

This chapter describes several anterior approaches to large ventral hernias. They are applicable to virtually all incisional hernias. An emerging experience with laparoscopic ventral hernia repair makes it a potentially attractive option, especially for small defects. The technique is described in references listed at the end of the chapter. This method has not been in use long enough to accumulate data about recurrence rates, pitfalls, and problems.

Identifying Strong Tissues

Each ventral hernia is characterized by a defect, small or large, in the tissue of the abdominal wall. In the hope of facilitating approximation of the edges of the defect, the surgeon is often tempted to preserve, and insert sutures into, weak scar tissue instead of carrying the dissection beyond the edge of the hernial ring to expose the normal musculoaponeurotic tissue of the abdominal wall. Depending on scar tissue to hold sutures for repair of a hernia leads to a high recurrence rate. It is best to carry the dissection 2–3 cm beyond the perimeter of the hernial ring on all sides and clearly expose the anterior surface of the muscle fascia.

Often an obvious incisional hernia is accompanied by additional smaller hernias 3–5 cm away from the major defect. These secondary hernias occur because more than one suture, inserted at the previous closure, has cut through the tissue, leaving additional small defects. If the additional defects are close to the large hernial ring, incise the tissue bridges and convert the several defects into one large hernial ring.

Some surgeons advocate separating the abdominal wall into its component layers—peritoneum, muscle, fascia—and suture each layer separately. We believe that in most cases it is preferable to insert the suture by taking a large bite of the entire abdominal wall in each stitch, following the principle of the Smead-Jones technique, rather than splitting the abdominal wall and closing each layer separately. By the same token, we have not used relaxing incisions through the aponeurosis of the external oblique layer to expedite hernial closure because we have observed subsequent herniation through the area of the relaxing incision. Other surgeons have advocated creating a flap from the anterior rectus sheath on each side and then bridging the hernial defect by suturing one fascial flap to the other. Our experience suggests that this technique does not successfully repair an incisional hernia larger than a few centimeters in diameter.

Avoiding Tension During the Repair

By far the most dangerous threat to long-term success with hernial repair is *excessive tension on the suture line.* Although all surgeons agree with this principle, there is a wide variation in each surgeon's perception of what comprises "excessive" tension. We believe that *any degree of tension is "excessive"* because this judgment is always made with the patient under anesthesia. Even local anesthesia produces muscle relaxation in the area of anesthesia, so any degree of tension is magnified when the effects of anesthesia have disappeared.

In the case of *small* ventral hernias (< 3 cm in diameter) success may be anticipated if the weakened tissues are excised and the remaining defect in the abdominal wall is simply approximated with the Smead-Jones technique, just as one would close a primary abdominal incision (see Chapter 3). It is important to excise all of the attenuated tissues, but it is not necessary to remove the condensation of fibrous tissue that often forms a firm ring and separates the hernial defect from the normal tissues of the abdominal wall. Using the Smead-Jones stitch, simply insert the sutures 2–3 cm beyond the hernial ring through all layers of the abdominal wall including peritoneum. It may be preferable to close a circular defect in a transverse (rather than vertical) direction, but the main consideration is to select the direction that produces the least tension. Although it is sometimes possible to approximate abdominal wall defects 6–8 cm in width under anesthesia without appearing to have produced excessive tension, *many* of these patients return with recurrent hernias if they are followed 4–5 years or more.

Role of Prosthetic Mesh

If there is tension on the proposed suture line, do not close the defect at all. Rather, bridge the defect with one or two layers of a prosthetic mesh. No attempt is made to close the defect with this technique. The defect is thus *replaced* by the mesh, which is sutured in place by means of 2-0 or 0 Prolene mattress sutures that penetrate the full thickness of the abdominal wall.

The most serious complication following the use of prosthetic mesh arises when dense adhesions form between the small intestine and the fabric of the mesh. If intestinal obstruction in this situation requires subsequent laparotomy, it may prove impossible to separate the mesh from the bowel without extensive intestinal damage. Prolene mesh seems less prone to this complication than Marlex (Stone et al.). Although this complication is uncommon, it is important to take the precaution of interposing omentum between the mesh and the in-

testines whenever possible. When omentum is not available for this purpose, preserve the hernial sac and interpose this tissue between the intestines and the mesh, which is then sutured as an onlay patch over the defect. Although using an onlay patch mechanically does not result in as strong a repair as inserting stitches through the entire abdominal wall to fasten the mesh, it may be preferable to risk producing excessive intestinal adhesions.

Types of Mesh

There are three general types of prosthetic material in common use: absorbable PG mesh, monofilament polypropylene mesh, and expanded polytetrafluoroethylene (ePTFE). True long-term follow-up data are not available for many of these prosthetic materials.

Absorbable PG mesh is suitable for temporary closure of abdominal wall defects, particularly in the infected abdomen. Because the mesh absorbs, subsequent incisional hernia formation is inevitable. Absorbable mesh is not suitable for permanent repair of ventral hernias as described in this chapter.

Monofilament polypropylene meshes are available from several manufacturers, differing in chemical composition, stiffness (resistance to bending), and degree of stretch. As mentioned earlier, erosion into bowel and dense adhesion formation have been problems with these prosthetic materials. A major advantage of this mesh is its tolerance to infection. Because the mesh is composed of monofilament fibers, the patient often tolerates a wound infection without the need to remove the mesh. Opening the skin widely for drainage generally proves sufficient and in many cases avoids the need to remove the mesh.

Expanded PTFE is soft and pliable. Adhesion to bowel is much less of a problem than with the previously described meshes. Currently available ePTFE mesh does not tolerate infection well and is recommended for use only during clean procedures. If the operative field becomes contaminated during dissection (e.g., by inadvertent enterotomy or exposure of a buried chronic suture abscess), this mesh is not a good choice.

Myocutaneous Flap

Increased interest in the myocutaneous flap has resulted in the development of techniques that facilitate rotation of large flaps of muscle covered by skin and subcutaneous fat into defects of the abdominal wall with retention of an excellent blood supply to the flap. The tensor fasciae latae muscle is one example of such a myocutaneous flap that can be used to bridge defects in the abdomen. The exact role of this modality compared to prosthetic mesh for replacing abdominal defects is still under study. It should be emphasized, however, that a split-thickness skin graft cannot consistently be expected to survive if it is placed over a layer of prosthetic mesh, even if the mesh has been covered by healthy-appearing granulation tissue. In many cases the mesh must be covered by a pedicle flap of skin and subcutaneous tissue, or it must be replaced by a myocutaneous or microvascular free flap.

OPERATIVE TECHNIQUE

Elective Ventral Hernia Repair

Dissecting the Hernial Sac

Make an elliptical incision in the skin along the axis of the hernial ring and carry the incision down to the sac **(Figs. 93–1, 93–2)**. Dissect the skin away from the sac on each side until the area of the her-

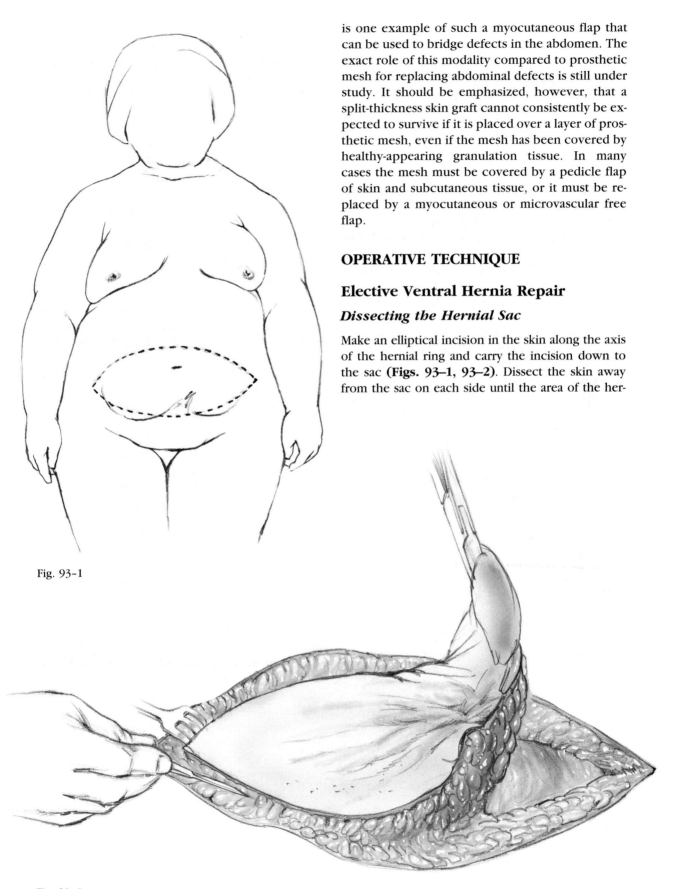

Fig. 93-1

Fig. 93-2

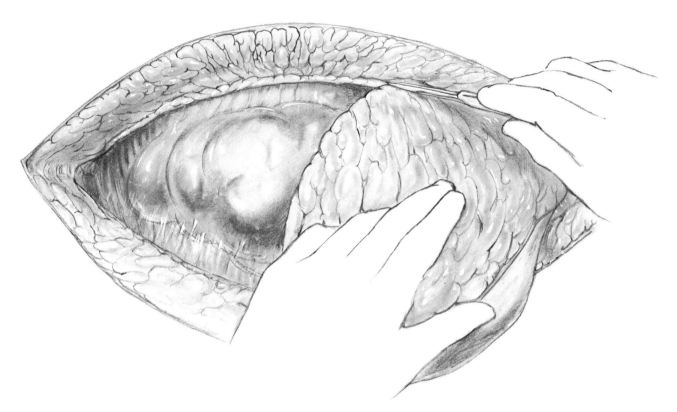

Fig. 93–3

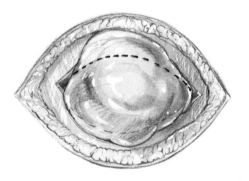

Fig. 93–4

nial ring itself has been exposed in its entire circumference **(Fig. 93–3)**. Retract the skin flap away from the sac and make a scalpel incision down to the anterior muscle fascia. Continue to dissect normal muscle fascia using a scalpel or Metzenbaum scissors until at least a 2 cm width of fascia has been exposed around the entire circumference of the hernial defect. This dissection generally leaves some residual subcutaneous fat attached to the area where the sac meets the hernial ring. Using scissors, remove this collar of fat from the base of the hernia.

Resecting the Hernial Sac

Make an incision along the apex of the hernial sac and divide all of the adhesions between the intestine and the sac **(Figs. 93–4, 93–5)**, reducing the intestines into the abdominal cavity **(Fig. 93–6)**. Expose the circumference of the hernial defect so the neck of the sac and a 2- to 3-cm width of peritoneum are freed of all adhesions around the entire circum-

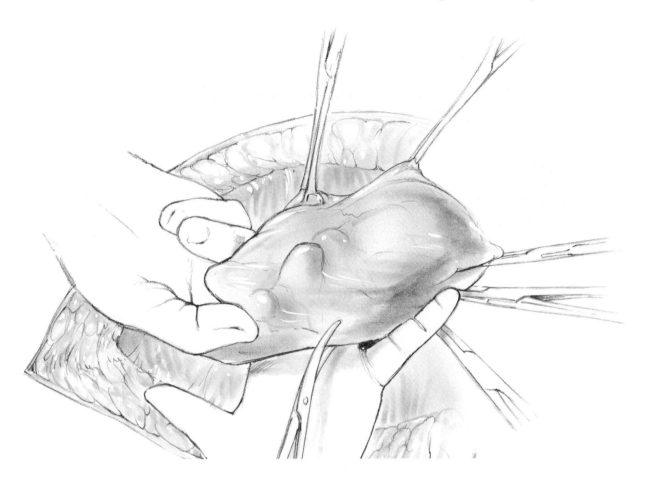

Fig. 93-5

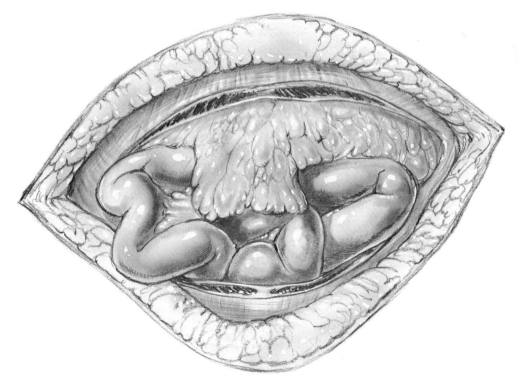

Fig. 93-6

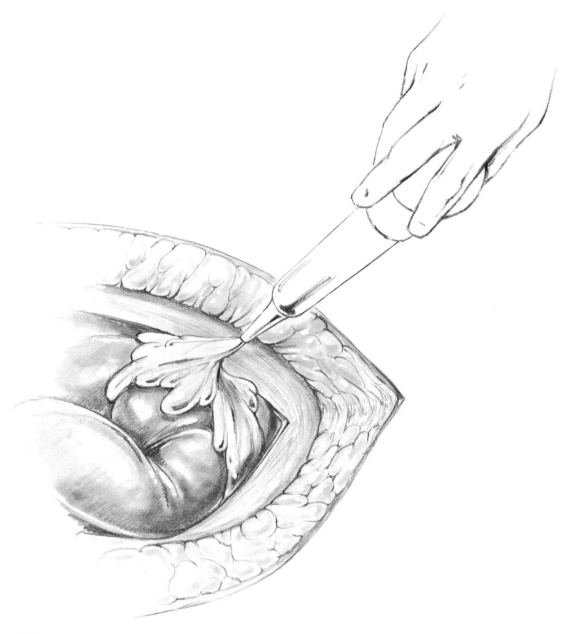

Fig. 93–7

ference of the hernia. Irrigate the wound with a dilute antibiotic solution intermittently **(Fig. 93–7)**.

Mesh Repair of Ventral Hernia

Sandwich Repair

The "sandwich repair" was first described by Usher. Two identical sheets of polypropylene mesh are cut from a large sheet. Each piece of mesh should be 2 cm larger than the hernial defect. One sheet is placed inside the abdominal cavity, and the other makes contact with the fascia around the hernial ring. The two sheets are held by sutures that go through the top sheet, then through the full thickness of the abdominal wall, and finally through the deep sheet of mesh. The stitch then returns as a mattress stitch penetrating the deep sheet of mesh, the full thickness of the abdominal wall, and finally the superficial sheet of mesh before being tied with a knot located in the subcutaneous layer **(Fig. 93–8)**. The deep layer of mesh should be separated from the bowel by the omentum. In the absence of a satisfactory layer of omentum, it may be preferable to omit the intraperitoneal layer of mesh and to preserve enough hernial sac so the sac, after being trimmed and sutured closed, can be retained as a

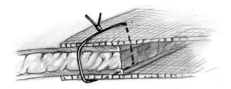

Fig. 93-8

protective layer to separate the intestines from the mesh, which is now used as an onlay patch, as described in the next section (see Fig. 93-13).

Application of the sandwich technique to a large recurrent ventral hernia in an obese patient is illustrated beginning with **Figure 93–9**. After the skin flaps have been elevated, which exposes healthy fascia around the entire circumference of the hernial defect, make certain there are no additional hernial defects above or below the major hernia. If there are additional hernias, combine them into one large defect by incising the bridge of tissue between them.

Excise the sac down to its point of attachment to the hernial ring and excise subcutaneous fat around the hernial ring. Then insert one sheet of mesh inside the abdominal cavity and the other over the rectus fascia. Place the mattress sutures through the mesh at a point about 2-3 cm away from the hernial ring to be certain the sutures engage normal abdominal muscle and aponeurosis. A horizontal mattress suture penetrates first the superficial layer of mesh, next the entire abdominal wall, and then the deep layer of mesh. When returning the suture, the width of the bite of mesh must be less than the width of the bite in the abdominal wall; otherwise the mesh tends to bunch together when the stitch is tied rather than lying flat. Therefore when returning the stitch through the deep layer of mesh, select a spot that encompasses only 7 mm of mesh while including a 1 cm width of abdominal wall. After penetrating the anterior rectus fascia, pass the needle through the anterior layer of mesh again at a point 7 mm away from the tail of the stitch. Tie the suture. We use the

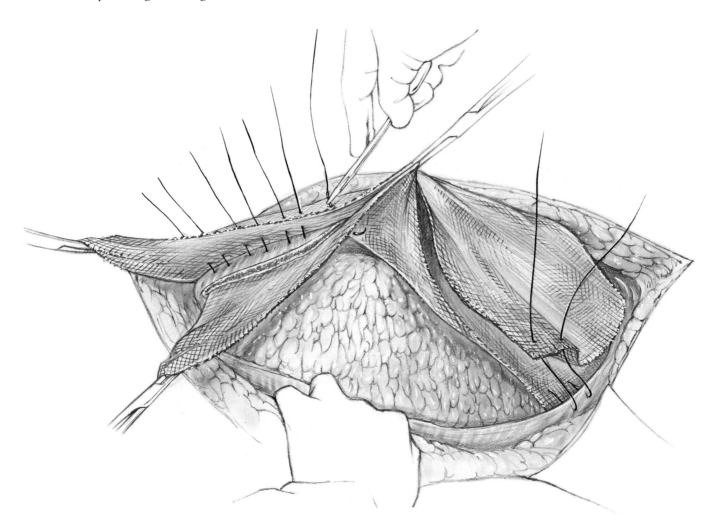

Fig. 93-9

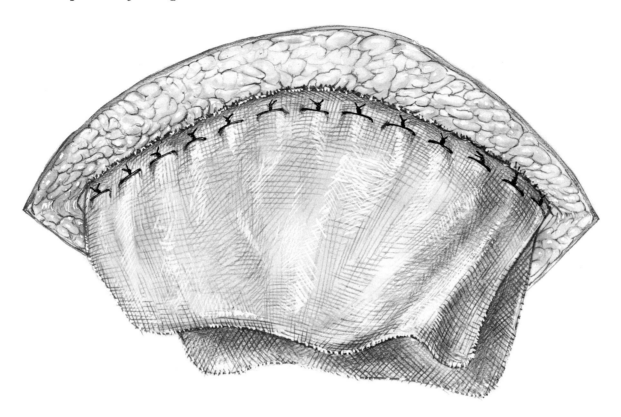

Fig. 93-10

3-1-2 knot (see Fig. 4-25), supplemented by a few additional throws. The suture material used is 2-0 Prolene on an atraumatic needle. Insert additional mattress sutures of the same material at intervals of about 1.0-1.5 cm until half of the sutures have been inserted and tied. Then insert the remaining sutures, but do not tie any of them until all have been properly inserted. After tying all the sutures, check for any possible defects in the repair **(Figs. 93–10, 93–11)**. When a hernial defect borders on the pubis, include the periosteum of the pubis in the sutures attaching the mesh to the margins of the defect.

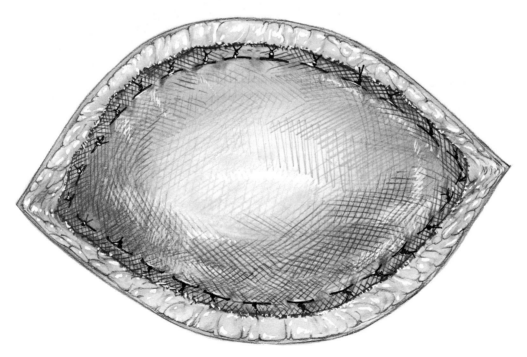

Fig. 93-11

Be certain to achieve complete hemostasis with electrocoagulation and fine PG ligatures. Insert a multiperforated closed-suction catheter through a small puncture wound in the skin. Lead the catheter across the superficial layer of the mesh and attach it to a Jackson-Pratt closed-suction device. Approximate the skin with interrupted nylon sutures. Apply a sterile pressure dressing.

Onlay Patch Mesh Repair

As mentioned above, the onlay patch mesh repair is suitable when there is no layer of omentum available to be interposed between the intestines and the mesh. Here the hernial sac is preserved. Trim away the excess sac, leaving enough tissue so it can be closed without tension by a continuous 2-0 atraumatic PG suture **(Fig. 93–12)**. This serves as a viable layer that hopefully will avoid the development of adhesions between the bowel and the mesh. The drawback to this technique is that its sutures, compared with those of the sandwich technique, are weaker because the bites of tissue are not equivalent to those of large mattress sutures, which penetrate the entire abdominal wall.

Only the peritoneum of the hernial sac is sutured to cover the defect with this method.

A piece of Prolene mesh is cut 2–3 cm larger on all sides than the diameter of the hernial defect. The first stitch of 0 Prolene starts at the caudal margin of the defect and catches the edge of the hernial ring. Tie the stitch and then proceed with a continuous stitch that fixes the mesh to the dense fibrous tissue at the margin of the hernial defect. When the cephalad edge of the hernial defect is reached, insert a second stitch and tie it. Anchor the first stitch by tying it to the tail of the second one. The second stitch runs in a continuous fashion along the opposite margin of the hernia and is terminated at the caudal edge of the hernial defect.

Using a similar technique, stitch the *edge* of the mesh to the anterior layer of muscle fascia in a continuous fashion using atraumatic 2-0 Prolene **(Fig. 93–13a, 93–13b)**. Insert a closed-suction catheter

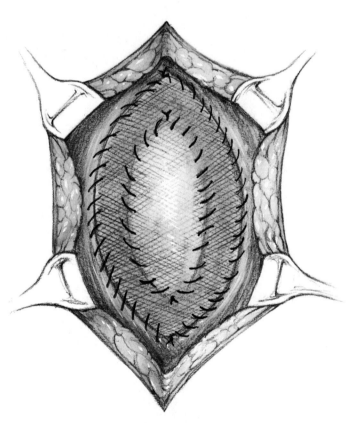

Fig. 93–13a

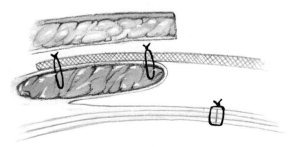

Fig. 93–13b

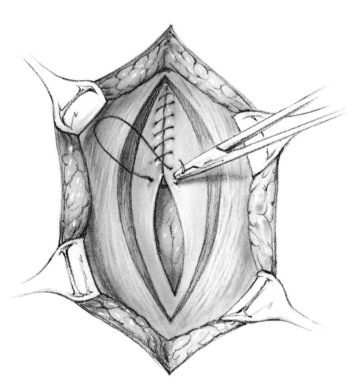

Fig. 93–12

through a puncture wound and close the skin in routine fashion.

POSTOPERATIVE CARE

Remove the suction drains 5–7 days following operation.

Give perioperative antibiotics.

Institute early ambulation promptly on recovery from anesthesia.

COMPLICATIONS

Wound Infection. With proper precautions wound infection should be rare following elective repair of a ventral hernia. If an infection of the subcutaneous wound does occur, it is not generally necessary to remove the mesh. Because of its monofilament nature, polypropylene mesh with monofilament Prolene sutures resists infection if the skin incision is promptly opened widely for drainage. Change the moist gauze packing daily until clean granulations have formed over the mesh. Then permit the skin to heal by secondary intention.

Hematoma. Most hematomas, unless large, can be treated expectantly.

REFERENCES

DeBord JR. The historical development of prosthetics in hernia surgery. Surg Clin North Am 1998;78:973.

DiBello JN Jr, Moore JH Jr. Sliding myofascial flap of the rectus abdominis muscles for the closure of recurrent ventral hernias. Plast Reconstr Surg 1996;98:464.

Heniford BT, Park A, Ramshaw BJ, Voeller G. Laparoscopic ventral and incisional hernia repair in 407 patients. J Am Coll Surg 2000;190:645.

Houston GC, Drew GS, Vazquez B, Given KS. The extended latissimus dorsi flap in repair of anterior abdominal wall defects. Plast Reconstr Surg 1988;81:917.

Larson GM. Laparoscopic repair of ventral hernia. In Scott-Conner CEH (ed) The SAGES Manual: Fundamentals of Laparoscopy and GI Endoscopy. New York, Springer-Verlag, 1999, pp 379–385.

Senoz O, Arifoglu K, Kocer U, et al. A new approach for the treatment of recurrent large abdominal hernias: the overlap flap. Plast Reconstr Surg 1997;99:2074.

Skandalakis JE, Gray SW, Mansberger AR Jr, Colborn GL, Skandalakis LJ. Hernia: Surgical Anatomy and Technique. New York, McGraw-Hill, 1989.

Stone HH, Fabian TC, Turkieson ML, et al. Management of acute full-thickness losses of the abdominal wall. Ann Surg 1981;193:612.

Usher FC. The surgeon at work: the repair of incisional and inguinal hernias. Surg Gynecol Obstet 1970;131:525.

Wantz GE. Atlas of Hernia Surgery. New York, Raven, 1991.

94 Operations for Infected Abdominal Wound Dehiscence and Necrotizing Fasciitis of the Abdominal Wall

INDICATIONS

Spreading infection of the anterior abdominal wall

Infected dehiscence, with or without evisceration

PREOPERATIVE PREPARATION

Administer therapeutic doses of systemic intravenous antibiotics effective against gram-negative rods, enterococci, and anaerobes, including clostridia, until definitive bacterial cultures and sensitivity studies are available. This requires an aminoglycoside, ampicillin or penicillin, and clindamycin (or metronidazole or chloramphenicol). Third- and fourth-generation cephalosporins may also prove effective in these cases.

Because intraabdominal sepsis is a frequent companion, if not the cause, of the necrotizing infection, many of these patients require total parenteral nutrition.

Perform abdominal computed tomography (CT) to identify any abdominal sepsis.

Establish nasogastric suction.

Insert a Foley catheter.

In the elderly and the critically ill patient, monitor fluid requirements and cardiorespiratory function by means of pulmonary arterial pressure measurements, cardiac output determinations, and frequent blood gas determinations.

PITFALLS AND DANGER POINTS

Inadequate débridement of devitalized tissue

Failure to identify and drain intraabdominal abscesses

OPERATIVE STRATEGY

Wide Débridement

Unhesitatingly cut away all devitalized tissue and continue the scalpel dissection until bleeding is encountered from the cut edge of the tissue. If even a small remnant of devitalized fat or other tissue is left, it is a haven in which bacteria can proliferate and destroy more of the abdominal wall.

Managing the Abdominal Wall Defect

Closure of even small abdominal wall defects in the setting of necrotizing infection is doomed to failure. The strategy that has evolved accepts the trade-off of a possible incisional hernia for a better chance of patient survival. Small defects (<4–6 cm in diameter) may be managed by Adaptic gauze covered with moist gauze packing. Larger defects require a patch of monofilament mesh, inserted by a rapid suture technique. Dressing changes and subsequent granulation tissue formation ultimately result in a surface that can be covered with a split-thickness skin graft. If an incisional hernia results, a delayed repair, possibly involving a musculocutaneous flap, is planned at a time remote from the life-threatening illness.

Repeat Laparotomy for Recurrence of Abdominal Sepsis

After successfully débriding an infected abdominal incision and repairing the defect with mesh, subsequent clinical observation may disclose the need to reexplore the abdomen for recurrent sepsis between the loops of small bowel, the pelvis, the subhepatic or subphrenic spaces, or elsewhere. If necessary, it is generally simple to make an incision through the mesh, perform the abdominal exploration, and then repair the mesh with a continuous 2-0 Prolene suture. Stone and associates noted that adhesions between bowel and Prolene mesh were much less marked than when Marlex mesh was used. For some cases in which Marlex has been used and a layer of omentum has not been interposed between the mesh and the intestines, dense adhesions have formed between the small bowel and the Marlex mesh. When a patient who suffers from this condition requires laparotomy, entering the abdomen in the vicinity of the Marlex mesh may prove impossible without *extensive* damage to the bowel. In some cases, placing the patient in a face-down position encourages drainage of abdominal infections through the pores of the mesh.

Management of Intestinal Stomas and Fistulas

When a patient who is taken to the operating room for débridement of an infected abdominal incision also requires exteriorization of an intestinal fistula or requires a colostomy, do not perform a loop colostomy or a loop enterostomy. This type of stoma is difficult to control, and secretions continuously contaminate the open abdominal wound. If possible, create matured end-stomas of the small bowel

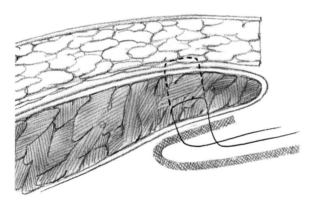

Fig. 94-1

or colon and bring them out at sites well away from the open abdominal wound.

Marsupialization and Open Abdomen Management

When complex collections with multiple loculations and necrotic tissue are encountered, the probability of recurrence is high. In the critically ill patient, consider leaving the abdomen open so daily explorations, débridements, irrigation, and packing can be done in the intensive care unit. Closure (generally using mesh) is performed once sepsis has been controlled.

OPERATIVE TECHNIQUE

During surgery for large abdominal defects that remain after wide débridement of infected abdominal incisions, we do not recommend the technique described in Chapter 93. To expedite the operation in these acutely ill patients, we prefer to use a single layer of Prolene mesh. For temporary closure, PG mesh is preferred. Cut the mesh so it is only 1 cm larger than the abdominal defect. Be certain that all intraabdominal abscesses have been evacuated. Attempt to place a layer of omentum between the mesh and the underlying bowel. In no case should a bowel *anastomosis* ever be left in contact with synthetic mesh. Then use atraumatic sutures of 2-0 Prolene to attach the cut end of the mcsh to the undersurface of the abdominal wall. In most cases continuous sutures are employed. The technique described by either Markgraf (**Fig. 94–1**) or Boyd (**Fig. 94–2**) may be used. For both techniques, take a larger bite of the abdominal wall than of the mesh; otherwise the mesh wrinkles. Apply slight tension to the mesh when inserting these sutures so it lies as flat as possible. Markgraf recommended that when inserting sutures into the abdominal wall below the

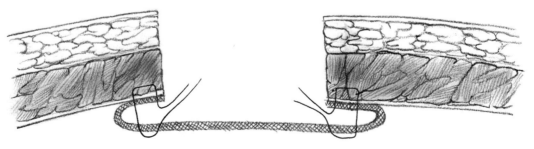

Fig. 94-2

semicircular line it is helpful to insert the suture through the entire thickness of the rectus muscle including the *anterior* rectus fascia; otherwise the muscle and peritoneum may have inadequate holding power.

After the mesh has been sutured in place, apply gauze packing moistened with isotonic saline. In some cases, it is appropriate to moisten the gauze with an antibiotic solution for the first 24 hours after débriding the wound.

POSTOPERATIVE CARE

Continue therapeutic dosages of appropriate antibiotics.

Change the gauze packing over the mesh every 8–12 hours until it is ascertained there has been no extension of the necrotizing infection.

Thereafter inspect the wound and change the dressing daily.

Observe the patient carefully for recurrent abdominal sepsis and take appropriate diagnostic, therapeutic, and surgical measures to correct this sepsis.

After the wound is clean and granulation has formed, if the defect is small it is possible that epithelialization may proceed spontaneously. In most cases, as abdominal distension disappears wrinkling of the mesh precludes spontaneous healing. In these cases, remove the mesh when the wound is clean and the patient's condition has stabilized, preferably around the 20th postoperative day. Then apply a split-thickness graft over the granulations covering the intestinal viscera. Delay definitive repair of a large abdominal hernia until a later date.

REFERENCES

Bilton BD, Zibari GB, McMillan RW, et al. Aggressive surgical management of necrotizing fasciitis serves to decrease mortality: a retrospective study. Am Surg 1998; 64:397.

Bosscha K, Hulstaert PF, Visser MR, van Vroonhoven TJ, van der Werken C. Open management of the abdomen and planned reoperations in severe bacterial peritonitis. Eur J Surg 2000;166:44.

Boyd WC. Use of Marlex mesh in acute loss of the abdominal wall due to infection. Surg Gynecol Obstet 1977;144:251.

Dellinger EP. Severe necrotizing soft-tissue infections: multiple disease entities requiring a common approach. JAMA 1981;246:1717.

Kingston D, Seal DV. Current hypotheses on synergistic microbial gangrene. Br J Surg 1990;77:260.

Markgraf WH. Abdominal wound dehiscence: a technique for repair with Marlex mesh. Arch Surg 1972;105:728.

Schein M. Planned reoperations and open management in critical intra-abdominal infections: prospective experience in 52 cases. World J Surg 1991;15:537.

Schein M, Saadia R, Decker GG. The open management of the septic abdomen. Surg Gynecol Obstet 1986;163:587.

Stone HH, Fabian TC, Turkelson ML, et al. Management of acute full-thickness losses of the abdominal wall. Ann Surg 1981;193:612.

Voyles CR, Richardson JD, Bland KI, et al. Emergency abdominal wall reconstruction with polypropylene mesh: short-term benefits versus long-term complications. Ann Surg 1981;194:219.

Wilson SE. A critical analysis of recent innovations in the treatment of intra-abdominal infection. Surg Gynecol Obstet 1993;177:11.

95 Drainage of Subphrenic and Other Abdominal Abscesses

SURGICAL LEGACY TECHNIQUE

INDICATIONS

Prompt drainage of a subphrenic abscess is indicated when it is diagnosed.

Only about two-thirds of patients with subphrenic abscesses demonstrate the typical clinical picture of fever, localized pain or tenderness, leukocytosis, and ipsilateral pleural effusion on the chest radiograph. Few of these manifestations may be present during the *early* stages. Consequently, recent advances in radiographic and other types of body imaging have been most welcome.

Although sonography has value for identifying subphrenic sepsis, computed tomography (CT) is by far the most accurate method for identifying an abdominal abscess. The accuracy of CT is so impressive it is cost-effective to perform this study on any patient who has an unexplained persistent fever following abdominal surgery.

Percutaneous drainage may be performed by the interventional radiologist if there is a well established fluid collection with a safe percutaneous access route. Occasionally a safe route cannot be planned, and operative drainage is required. Operative drainage is also needed when there are multiple abscesses or associated intraabdominal pathology that requires correction or when percutaneous drainage fails to eradicate the infection.

PREOPERATIVE PREPARATION

Therapeutic doses of appropriate antibiotics are administered. Until the culture report is available, we believe the patient should receive an aminoglycoside, clindamycin, and ampicillin intravenously because in most cases the causative organisms respond to these agents. Other antibiotic regimens that include various combinations of a third- or fourth-generation cephalosporin and metronidazole are also acceptable.

CT scanning is performed.

A nasogastric tube is placed.

PITFALLS AND DANGER POINTS

Failure to locate and adequately drain all loculations and multiple abscesses

Injuring the spleen, liver, or a hollow viscus

OPERATIVE STRATEGY

Classification of Spaces of the Upper Abdomen

For purposes of this discussion, we have adopted the classification of Boyd (for spaces of the upper abdomen) with a slight modification. On the right side there is a single suprahepatic subphrenic space and a right infrahepatic space. On the left there is a subphrenic space and a left infrahepatic space that can be divided into two spaces: (1) the posterior infrahepatic space, which constitutes the lesser sac; and (2) the left anterior infrahepatic space, which is situated anterior to the stomach.

Operative Approaches

Lateral and Subcostal Extraperitoneal Approach

DeCosse and associates modified the subcostal extraperitoneal approach by extending it in a lateral direction as far as the tip of the eleventh rib. The layers of the abdominal wall are divided down to the peritoneum. The surgeon's hand then dissects the peritoneum away from the diaphragm until the abscess is reached. The lateral extraperitoneal approach may also be used to treat a right posterior infrahepatic abscess. DeCosse and associates were successful in draining left subphrenic and left posterior infrahepatic abscesses in the lesser sac through the subcostal or lateral extraperitoneal approach. The lesser sac abscesses were reached by dissecting the peritoneum away from the upper pole of the kidney. The right suprahepatic subphrenic abscess is easily approached through an anterior (subcostal) extraperitoneal approach. An abscess in the left anterior infrahepatic space is best approached by performing a laparotomy.

Laparotomy

Although it is true that, thanks to modern antibiotics, there is no great risk of spreading the infection by draining an abscess transperitoneally instead of extraserously, no one can doubt that exploring the abdomen 2–3 weeks after major surgery is more difficult and more hazardous than is draining the abscess by an extraserous route. Before high-resolution CT scanning there was a considerable risk that the patient might have an abscess in more than one location. Under these conditions, an extraperitoneal operation might overlook the second or third abscess.

When a CT scan demonstrates a *solitary* right or left subphrenic abscess or a right posterior infrahepatic abscess, we prefer to attempt drainage by the extraserous approach because the operation is safe and relatively simple. If this procedure fails to eliminate the signs of sepsis, a laparotomy should be performed. However, this discussion may be hypothetic because almost all of the subphrenic abscesses in accessible locations such as the above are effectively managed by inserting percutaneous drainage catheters with CT guidance. Laparotomy is mandatory in patients suspected of having a lesser sac abscess, a peripancreatic or a left anterior infrahepatic abscess, or an anastomotic leak with multiple intermesenteric abscesses.

When the transperitoneal approach has been elected, we prefer a midline incision, especially if there is suspicion of an anastomotic leak or an abscess located within the folds or the small bowel mesentery. If exploration of the subphrenic, subhepatic, and lesser sac spaces does not reveal the source of the patient's sepsis, it may be necessary to free the entire small bowel and the pelvis to rule out an abdominal abscess.

Extraserous Approach

Dissection in the extraserous preperitoneal or retroperitoneal plane is generally simple if the surgeon enters the proper plane by incising the trans-

versalis fascia but not the peritoneum. The incision should be made long enough to admit the surgeon's hand. Blunt dissection then separates the peritoneum from the undersurface of the diaphragm until an area of induration is reached. This represents the abscess. Generally blunt dissection with a finger permits entry into the abscess. Intraoperative ultrasonography or aspiration with a long spinal needle helps establish the location with certainty in difficult cases. Although it is possible to drain abscesses in the posterior right subhepatic space and in the lesser sac by the extraserous approach, we usually prefer a laparotomy to drain these two spaces.

When an extraserous approach has failed to reveal an abscess, it is generally simple to lengthen the incision in the abdominal wall transversely, converting it to a subcostal incision. Then incise the peritoneum and continue the exploration for the abscess transperitoneally. Alternatively, make a second vertical midline incision for further exploration.

OPERATIVE TECHNIQUE

Extraserous Subcostal Drainage of Right Subphrenic Abscess

Incision and Exposure

Make a 10- to 12-cm incision, beginning near the tip of the right eleventh rib and continue medially parallel to the costal margin. Carry the incision through the external oblique muscle and aponeurosis **(Fig. 95–1)**. Generally, the internal oblique muscle **(Fig.**

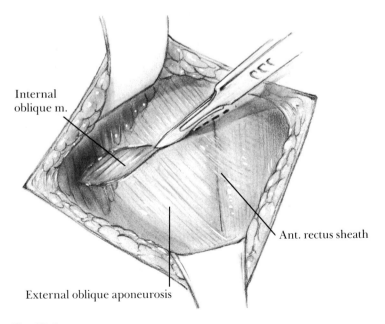

Internal oblique m.

Ant. rectus sheath

External oblique aponeurosis

Fig. 95–1

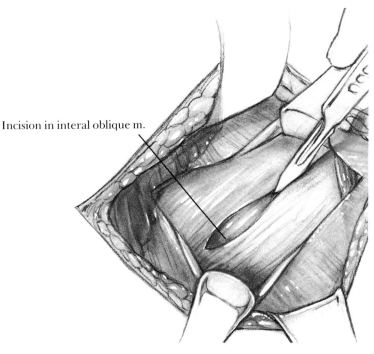

Incision in interal oblique m.

Fig. 95-2

Identify the transversalis fascia and carefully divide it with a scalpel **(Fig. 95–3)**, revealing the underlying peritoneal membrane. Use a gauze sponge on a sponge-holder to dissect the peritoneum away from the transversalis fascia. Continue the dissection upward by inserting the hand to separate the peritoneum further from the undersurface of the diaphragm until the dome of the liver is reached **(Fig. 95–4)**.

A right posterior infrahepatic abscess can be reached by the extraserous approach if the peritoneum is dissected laterally **(Fig. 95–5)** until the fat overlying Gerota's fascia is encountered, which is swept away from the posterolateral peritoneal envelope. The abscess is then encountered medial and superior to the upper pole of the right kidney. On the left side a posterior infrahepatic or lesser sac abscess can be approached in a similar fashion by dissecting the posterolateral peritoneum away from the fat over Gerota's capsule. The abscess is then encountered medial to the upper pole of the left kidney.

Drainage and Closure

After exposing an area of induration in one of the subphrenic spaces, enter the abscess by inserting a fingertip or the tip of a blunt Kelly hemostat. Open the abscess cavity widely and irrigate out the purulent material after obtaining a sample for routine and anaerobic cultures **(Fig. 95–6)**.

95–2) can be separated along the line of its fibers. It is usually necessary to divide the ninth intercostal nerve. Then transect the transversus muscle with electrocautery. If necessary, continue the incision through the lateral one-fourth of the rectus musclc.

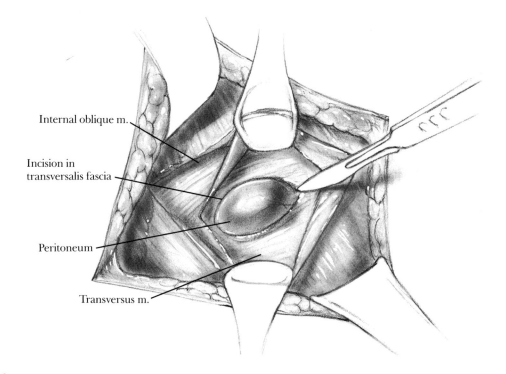

Internal oblique m.

Incision in
transversalis fascia

Peritoneum

Transversus m.

Fig. 95-3

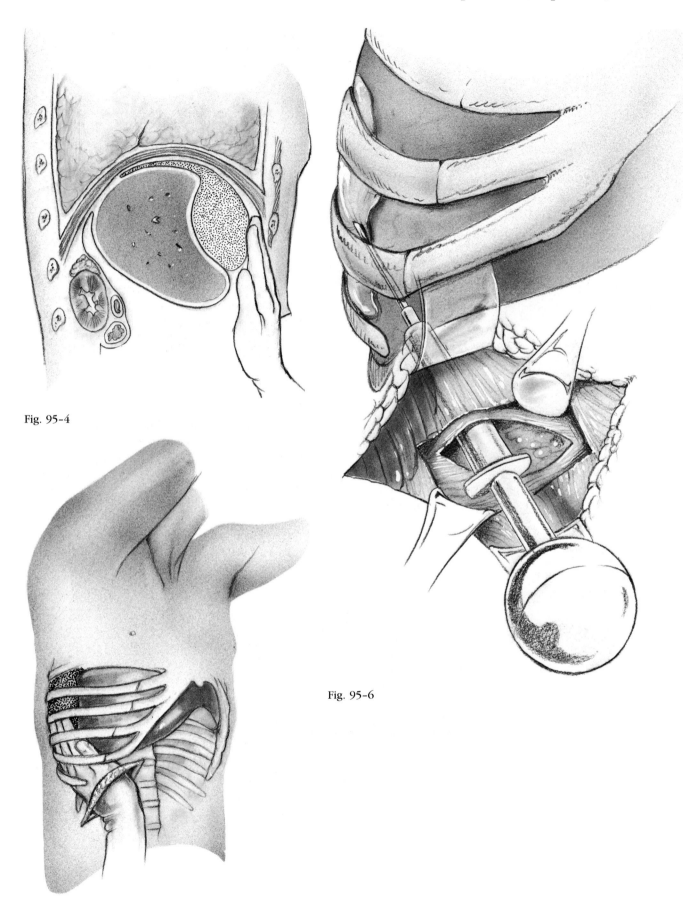

Fig. 95-4

Fig. 95-5

Fig. 95-6

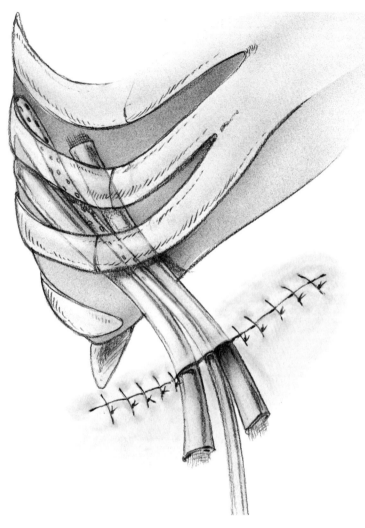

Fig. 95-7

If an abscess has been drained in its early stages, before its walls have become rigid, evacuating the pus permits the abscess cavity to collapse and disappear. In cases of this type it is necessary to insert only a single suction drain and a single large latex drain. These drains may be brought out through the incision **(Fig. 95–7)** (or through a stab wound). Close the remainder of the abdominal wall incision so one finger can be inserted into the abdominal cavity alongside the drains. Although many surgeons prefer to sew the skin closed after this operation, we believe that the skin and the subcutaneous tissue should be lightly packed with a strip of moistened gauze and left open. Several untied interrupted nylon skin sutures may be inserted, in anticipation of a delayed secondary closure at the bedside 4–7 days following operation. If the patient has a large subphrenic abscess with rigid walls that do not collapse after evacuating the pus, insert two suction drains and three or four large latex drains, antici-

pating that the drains may have to be left in for a number of weeks before the abscess cavity collapses or fills with granulation tissue.

Laparotomy for Subphrenic and Abdominal Abscesses

Incision and Exposure

When draining an accurately localized right infrahepatic abscess a right lateral subcostal incision is suitable. Left anterior infrahepatic and lesser sac abscesses, suprahepatic abscesses, and most other abdominal abscesses are better drained through midline incisions. If the patient has had a recent operation through a midline incision, try to enter the abdomen by extending the previous midline incision into a virginal area of the abdominal wall to minimize the chance of injuring densely adherent bowel. After the abdomen is opened, identify the falciform ligament and peritoneum. Dissect these two structures away from all the underlying bowel and omentum, first on the right side and then on the left. Then pass a hand over the liver to explore the suprahepatic and then the infrahepatic spaces.

Divide the avascular portion of the gastrohepatic ligament and enter the lesser sac behind the lesser curvature of the stomach. If this approach has been obliterated by previous surgery or adhesions, enter the lesser sac by dividing the omentum along the greater curvature and expose the posterior wall of the stomach and the anterior surface of the pancreas. Identify the right and left paracolic spaces and expose the pelvic cavity, as both are likely abscess sites, especially in patients suffering ruptured appendicitis or diverticulitis. Finally, if it is necessary to rule out the possibility of an interloop abscess, the surgeon must patiently free the entire length of small intestine and its mesentery. Perform a needle catheter jejunostomy in all patients not likely to resume oral nutrition early in the postoperative course.

Drainage and Closure

When a long midline incision has been used, bring drains out through suitable stab wounds. Although large sump drains are suitable for subphrenic abscesses, there is considerable risk of creating a colocutaneous or enterocutaneous fistula if a large plastic drain remains in contact with a segment of bowel for more than 2 weeks. Consequently, it may be preferable to use soft Silastic sump drains or latex Penrose drains rather than a more rigid drain.

Close the midline incision by the modified Smead-Jones technique (see Chapter 3) using No. 1 PDS sutures to the abdominal wall. Insert vertical mattress sutures of 3-0 interrupted nylon about 2 cm apart into the skin. Do not tie any of these sutures for 4–8 days.

POSTOPERATIVE CARE

Continue therapeutic doses of suitable antibiotics, guided by intraoperative Gram stains and bacterial culture results. Antibiotics are required for a minimum of 7–10 days in patients undergoing surgery for a subphrenic abscess.

If early feeding cannot be tolerated by the patient, initiate jejunostomy tube feeding.

If the abscess cavity was not rigid and its walls collapsed after the pus was evacuated, remove the drains after 10–14 days. If there is any question about a residual cavity, inject sterile Hypaque or other iodinated aqueous contrast medium through the sump drain to obtain a radiographic sinogram or CT scan. Leave at least one of the drains in place until the cavity has been eliminated.

If the patient has a large abscess cavity with rigid walls and thick pus, consider the advantages of irrigating the abscess daily through one of the sump catheters with a dilute antibiotic solution.

COMPLICATIONS

Residual or recurrent abscess
Overlooked abscess

Colocutaneous or enterocutaneous fistula

Hematoma secondary to hepatic or splenic operative trauma

REFERENCES

Boyd DP. The subphrenic spaces and the emperor's new robes. N Engl J Med 1966;275:911.

Crass JR, Maile CW, Frick MP. Catheter drainage of the left posterior subphrenic space: a reliable percutaneous approach. Gastrointest Radiol 1985;10:397.

DeCosse JJ, Poulin TL, Fox PS, et al. Subphrenic abscesses. Surg Gynecol Obstet 1974;138:841.

Johnson WC, Gerzof SG, Robbins AH, et al. Treatment of abdominal abscesses. Ann Surg 1981;194:510.

Levision MA. Percutaneous vs. open operative drainage of intraabdominal abscesses. Infect Dis Clin North Am 1992;6:525.

Mandel SR, Boyd D, Jaques PF, et al. Drainage of hepatic, intraabdominal, and mediastinal abscesses guided by computerized axial tomography; successful alternative to open drainage. Am J Surg 1983;145:120.

McNicholas MM, Mueller PR, Lee MJ, et al. Percutaneous drainage of subphrenic fluid collections that occur after splenectomy: efficacy and safety of transpleural versus extrapleural approach. AJR 1995;165:355.

Serrano A, Dahl EP, Rubin RM, et al. Eclectic drainage of subhepatic abscesses. Arch Surg 1984;119:942.

Van Gansbeke D, Matos C, Gelin M, et al. Percutaneous drainage of subphrenic abscesses. Br J Radiol 1989;62:127.

96 Concepts in Breast Surgery

Alison Estabrook

OPTIONS FOR BREAST BIOPSY

Noninvasive techniques such as fine-needle aspiration (FNA), core biopsy, and mammotome biopsy have almost completely replaced open techniques for diagnosing breast disease. Advantages include less trauma (both physical and mental) for the patient and lower cost [1]. Scheduling is generally faster for the percutaneous techniques than for a surgical biopsy, and the specimens are smaller; hence results are obtained more quickly. In breast centers, where a pathologist is readily available, the FNA can be interpreted in less than an hour. This enables the surgeon to discuss options with the patient in a more timely fashion. Patients who have a benign diagnosis may be followed at appropriate intervals by physical examination or ultrasonography, or elective surgery may be scheduled at a convenient time. For patients with a diagnosis of cancer, other advantages for the surgeon and the patient include not having to consider a large biopsy scar in the case of a mastectomy or biopsy cavity in the case of lumpectomy and the lack of a hematoma. Negative margins are more likely to be obtained at the first breast surgery if the diagnosis is known preoperatively [2]. Some data indicate that the sentinel node technique is more accurate if the cancer and its surrounding lymphatics are intact.

There are some limitations and pitfalls to these percutaneous techniques that must be clearly understood. Each is discussed in detail in the sections that follow.

Fine-Needle Aspiration

Fine-needle (20-25 gauge) aspiration is technically the easiest type of "biopsy" to perform. It is also the fastest and least expensive. It is generally used for palpable masses aided by ultrasound guidance when necessary. Although FNA was formerly used for stereotactic biopsy under mammographic guidance, it has largely been abandoned for core or mammotome biopsy.

Limitations and Pitfalls

Only a small number of cells are obtained with FNA, and often a specific diagnosis is elusive. A benign mass can be distinguished from a malignant one in more than 90% of cases, however. In the remaining small percentage a cytologic diagnosis or "suspicious" or "atypical" result may require a repeat FNA or a core biopsy with a 14- to 18-gauge needle) to obtain a definitive result. The sensitivity for FNA has varied from 68% to 93% and the specificity from 88% to 100% [3]. FNA is not an appropriate choice for mammographic microcalcifications, architectural distortion, or radial scars.

Cytology itself has some limitations. The cells obtained from a fibroadenoma are similar to those obtained from a phyllodes tumor, and therefore FNA cannot be used to differentiate between these two entities, nor can it reliably differentiate invasive ductal carcinoma from ductal carcinoma in situ or papilloma from papillary carcinoma. Because of the small cells of invasive lobular carcinoma and its diffuse appearance on mammography, this lesion is difficult to diagnose on FNA. Estrogen receptors (ERs), progesterone receptors (PRs), and *HER2 neu* status cannot be accurately obtained by FNA, and a core biopsy should be performed for patients in whom neoadjuvant chemotherapy is being considered. FNA requires a pathologist who has had specialized training in cytopathology.

The cytologic diagnosis must be correlated with the physical findings (in the case of palpable mass) and with the mammographic results [Breast Imaging Reporting and Data System (BIRADS) class] or ultrasonography results. If there is any discordance, a core biopsy should be performed.

Core and Mammotome Biopsy

Core biopsy needles range from 14 to 18 gauge and may be used for palpable or nonpalpable lesions. They require the use of local anesthesia and a small cut in the skin. They trap tissue in a notch in the trocar that is advanced into a lesion. A sharp cannula then advances over the trocar and its notch and shears off a piece of tissue, capturing it in the notch. The mammotome biopsy system uses a hollow 11-gauge needle and a vacuum system through which tissue is sucked out.

The stereotactic core and mammotome biopsies have several advantages over FNA.

A cytopathologist is not needed to interpret the specimen.

Insufficient tissue is rarely if ever a problem.

There are few false-negative results.

There have been no false-positive results reported.

Histologic evaluation can differentiate between in situ and invasive carcinomas.

It can be used for microcalcifications and in some cases of architectural distortion.

Upgrades from atypical ductal hyperplasia (ADH) to ductal carcinoma in situ (DCIS) or DCIS with intraductal carcinoma (IDC) with the initial 14-gauge core biopsy procedures were required in 50-55%; but with the 11-gauge sampling the upgrade rate was 11-25%. If ADH, atypical labor hyperplasia (ALH), or lobar carcinoma in situ (LCIS) is found on a core or mammotome specimen, the patient should be subjected to a needle localization biopsy and removal of the entire area of microcalcifications.

Incisional, Excisional, or Needle-Localized Biopsy

Incisional biopsy is rarely performed, as the core biopsy has almost completely replaced this technique. Incisional biopsy may be performed in patients with locally advanced breast cancer or those who have clinical inflammatory breast cancer. In these patients sufficient tissue is necessary for ER, PR, and *HER 2* assays; and a piece of overlying skin is needed to diagnose tumor in subdermal lymphatics (for definitively diagnosing inflammatory breast cancer).

Excisional biopsy is generally performed to remove a benign mass because the patient or the doctor is uncomfortable simply observing it for a period of time. The reason may be that the mass is enlarging or painful or that the exact pathology is unclear, such as with a papillary lesion or an atypical fibroadenoma that could be a phyllodes tumor.

Needle localization biopsy is used in two general instances: (1) when the lesion cannot be diagnosed by FNA or core biopsy because of technical problems; or (2) when the FNA or core or mammotome biopsy shows atypical cells or atypical hyperplasia or the pathology is not concordant with the pre-biopsy BIRADS classification. There may also be

technical problems associated with positioning the needle with particular breast-lesion geometries.

Needle localization biopsy is also used when pathology from the stereotactic core biopsy shows ADH, LDH, or LCIS, as 50% of those patients have demonstrated DCIS or invasive cancer on surgical excision [4,5]. Open biopsy should be used when the diagnosis of ADH is obtained on an 11-gauge mammotome biopsy specimen, as 11-25% of these lesions are upgraded to carcinoma [6].

The term "*needle localization lumpectomy*" applies when using a guidewire to remove a nonpalpable lesion that is a known cancer, usually diagnosed by FNA or core or mammotome biopsy.

EXCISION OF DUCTS

Duct excision is performed for spontaneous nipple discharge, the cause of which is usually intraductal papilloma. Other causes of spontaneous nipple discharge are intraductal carcinoma (8-14%) [7,8], duct ectasia, cystic disease, pregnancy, and some centrally acting medicines. Elicited nipple discharge is usually not of pathologic significance, as it comes from terminal ectatic ducts.

Nature of the Discharge

Spontaneous serous, bloody, or clear nipple discharge is most often caused by an intraductal papilloma, but a carcinoma is found in up to 14% of patients. Discharge that emanates from one duct on the nipple is more often a papilloma than a spontaneous nipple discharge that comes from several ducts (duct ectasia). Discharge that is thick and greenish is usually due to cystic disease or duct ectasia.

Preoperative Evaluation

It is important to identify the duct from which the discharge is emanating. The breast, especially the periareolar and subareolar areas, are checked for a mass. Papillomas generally measure 4-6 mm and often cannot be felt. If no mass is palpated, gentle palpation of the circumareolar region in a radial fashion often reveals a pressure point that produces the nipple discharge and localizes the duct containing the papilloma.

Occasionally when patients present with the complaint of nipple discharge, no mass can be felt and no pressure point elicits the discharge. For these patients repeat visits at 2-3 weeks are recommended to again check for the pressure point. An exploratory operation is not indicated. Cytology of the nipple discharge has been unrewarding.

Most *papillomas* are not visible by mammography, as they are small. On occasion they present as a fairly well circumscribed, lobulated mass. Some authors advocate ductography to evaluate nipple discharge, but this does not influence management, as cancers and intraductal papillomas are not distinguishable by ductography [9].

PARAAREOLAR ABSCESS OR FISTULA

Patients with a paraareolar abscess or fistula present with one or more inflammatory periareolar masses. These masses are often treated by incision, drainage, and antibiotics; but they always recur. Blockage of one of the terminal lactiferous ducts due to squamous metaplasia causes recurrent abscess and subsequent fistula formation [10]. Complete healing occurs only if the inflammatory tissues, including the fistula opening, inflammatory mass, involved duct, and terminal portions of the nipple, are totally excised [11].

BREAST ABSCESS

Breast abscess is most often seen in lactating women and is due to introduction of bacteria through the nipple into the ductal system. The abscess is treated by aspiration through a large (18 gauge) needle and antibiotics. it is important to chose antibiotics that do not harm the nursing infant. If the mother chooses not to nurse, she can use a breast pump until the infection has cleared. The pus obtained from the aspiration is sent for culture, and the antibiotics can then be changed to match the sensitivity of the organism cultured. On rare occasions incision and drainage with packing of the abscess is required. This is a painful procedure requiring removal of the packing and is indicated only if the patient is not responding to aspiration and antibiotics.

BREAST CANCER

Invasive Breast Cancer

At present the therapeutic alternatives for suitably selected patients with invasive breast cancer are lumpectomy followed by radiation therapy or total mastectomy. Each of these operations is followed by an axillary staging procedure. We offer this choice to patients based on our knowledge of several randomized trials that have shown that the overall survival for patients undergoing breast-conservation surgery (BCS) is the same as for patients undergoing mastectomy [12,13].

The addition of radiation therapy to breast-conserving surgery decreases the local recurrence rate from 8.8% to 0.3% at a median follow-up of 39 months for patients undergoing quadrantectomy [14] and from 35% to 10% at 12 years in patients undergoing lumpectomy [15].

Axillary Node Dissection and Sentinel Node Biopsy

Axillary node dissection (AND) is important for several reasons. The patient's prognosis and her treatment are based on the pathologic staging of the axillary nodes. Node dissection also significantly decreases the chance of an axillary recurrence. In addition there are some data that stage I patients treated with breast conservation without AND alone or in combination with irradiation or chemotherapy (or both) have poorer outcomes than do women with similarly staged lesions who undergo BCS plus AND alone or with adjuvant therapy [16]. The percentage of patients with involved axillary nodes increases with the size of the primary breast cancer; but even patients with cancers < 1 cm have a 7–26% chance of nodal involvement. Because this number is large and would change the indications for chemotherapy, we conclude that node dissection (or sentinel node biopsy) should be done in all patients who can withstand the surgery.

Sentinel node biopsy (SNB) is replacing level I–II node dissection for patients who have a clinically node-negative axilla. The sentinel node is the first node in the axilla to receive drainage from the cancer in the breast. If it is free of cancer, the other axillary nodes should be negative. The technique involves injection of lymphazurin blue dye or radioactive technetium 99m (^{99m}Tc) sulfur colloid. In the first case the injection is done minutes before the axillary incision, and a blue lymphatic terminating in a blue node is found by carefully dissecting the axilla. In the second case the ^{99m}Tc injection is done 30 minutes to 24 hours before surgery, and a hand-held gamma probe is used to localize the counts in the axilla (and sometimes elsewhere, such as the internal mammary nodes). The sentinel node is then removed by tracing the counts to it and dissecting it from the axilla.

Originally it was thought that there were several sentinel nodes, each draining a specific quadrant of the breast. Therefore to find the sentinel node, blue dye or technetium had to be injected specifically around the tumor. Many surgeons now think there is only one sentinel node that drains the entire breast, and to find it one need only inject the subareolar plexus of lymphatics. This change came about in an interesting way. Surgeons became interested in the lymphatic drainage of the breast, specifically in the significance of the subareolar lymphatic plexus. Two studies tested the hypothesis that the lymphatics of the overlying skin drain to the same axillary nodes as the underlying breast tissue [17,18]. In the first study, Brogstein et al. [17] used an intradermal injection of blue dye and an intraparenchymal injection of ^{99m}Tc and found 100% concordance in delineation of the sentinel node. Klimberg et al. [18] used intradermal subareolar injection of ^{99m}Tc and intraparenchymal blue dye and found that all the blue nodes were also radioactive. They concluded that subareolar injection of ^{99m}Tc is as accurate as peritumoral injection of blue dye. A central intradermal injection is easy and avoids the need for image-guided injection for nonpalpable tumors. It also reduces the problem of overlap of diffusion of radioactivity seen with injection of upper outer quadrant tumors and the axilla (shine-through effect).

There is a learning curve with this technique for both the surgeon and the nuclear radiologist performing the injection. In a multicenter trial, Krag et al. [19] found a false-negative rate that varied from 0% to 28.6% depending on the surgeon. It is advised that a surgeon have a lower than 5% false-negative rate before switching to SNB only. This means that the surgeon must perform 20 SNBs on node-positive patients followed by level I–II axillary node dissections and find only one patient to have a negative sentinel node. Guidelines are being discussed for credentialing surgeons by the American College of Surgeons (ACS).

If the sentinel mode contains cancer cells, the current guidelines are to continue with a full node dissection (if the metastases were discovered on frozen section) or to reoperate on the patient (if the node involvement was found on permanent section). The ACS has two randomized studies, one of which, Z11, randomized patients with involved sentinel nodes to further axillary node dissection (or not).

The advantages of SNB are numerous: less morbidity, no general anesthesia, no hospital stay, and most importantly more detailed pathologic examination of the node(s). The sentinel node is now serially sectioned and sent for immunohistochemical staining with cytokeratins. The importance of micrometastatic disease is being determined and appears to be significant [20,21].

See also Chapter 102.

Contraindications to BCS

The breast-conservation rate varies throughout the United States and ranges from about 50% to 80% of women with stage I–II breast cancer. The reasons for this variation are numerous. Some women prefer mastectomy to the necessary radiation treatments, and some are not candidates for breast conservation. Some of the contraindications to breast conservation are multifocal breast cancer, widespread microcalcifications that have been biopsied and were shown to be carcinoma, a history of irradiation, and active connective tissue disease (e.g., scleroderma or lupus). A relative contraindication is the tumor/breast size ratio, as a poor cosmetic outcome defeats the purpose of breast conservation.

Margins

When assessing a patient for breast conservation it is important to remember that not only must the palpable tumor be excised, the lumpectomy should have negative margins to decrease the local recurrence rate [22]. Margins are difficult to evaluate for the pathologist and have been reported in various ways. To summarize: in many studies the local recurrence rate increases if the margin is < 2 mm, if the margin is broadly positive rather than focally positive, if the patient is young (< 40 years old), if the patient is not treated with radiation or adjuvant therapy, and if the cancer has an extensive intraductal component. Ipsilateral breast tumor recurrence has been associated with a decrease in overall survival, but the association is controversial.

Skin-Sparing Mastectomy

Skin-sparing mastectomy refers to a technique where the only skin removed from the breast is the nipple areolar complex (NAC). This is done through a circumareolar incision that is extended from the lateral border of the NAC toward the axilla (a tennis racquet or lollipop incision) to open up the skin so all breast tissue, including the upper outer quadrant and tail of the breast, can easily be removed. The scar in the skin used for the biopsy is always excised separately; or if it is close to the NAC it is included in that periareolar incision. The defect is then filled in with tissue and the missing NAC with skin [transverse rectus abdominal myocutaneous (TRAM), or latissimus, flap]. The oncologic safety of this operation has been examined; and so long as margins are checked and there is no tumor involvement on any margin, it is considered safe [23,24].

Skin-sparing mastectomy with immediate breast reconstruction is popular and is often used in patients who have multifocal disease or who prefer mastectomy to breast conservation. It is also used in patients requesting prophylactic mastectomy. It should not be used in patients who have a breast cancer involving the skin.

Ductal Carcinoma in Situ

Ductal carcinoma in situ is defined as a proliferation of malignant cells within the breast ductal-lobular system. Once these cells break through the ductal basement membrane the cancer is termed "invasive or infiltrating."

It was once thought to be a multifocal disease, but detailed pathologic and radiologic studies have shown that DCIS is generally a unifocal, segmental disease [25]. Similar to invasive breast cancer, it can present as a small area or a large area. Magnification mammography is essential for the initial evaluating step.

It is generally diagnosed mammographically as microcalcifications, which are usually "the tip of the iceberg," representing only some of the DCIS. Careful pathologic evaluation of resected tissue is important for assessing the extent of the DCIS, the margin status, and the location of the microcalcifications (specifically whether the microcalcifications are associated only with the DCIS or are found in association with both DCIS and benign histology). Occasionally DCIS is detected clinically as a mass, as a spontaneous nipple discharge, or as Paget's disease of the nipple.

Local Therapy

As DCIS is confined to the breast, aggressive local therapy has been viewed to be more important for this disease than for invasive cancer, where the potential of metastatic disease, independent of local therapy, is higher. There are several possible local therapies: total mastectomy (TM), wide local excision (WLE), and wide local excision and radiation therapy (WLE/RT). Sentinel node biopsy is now being done in some women with DCIS [26] (see Chapter 102). Unlike the situation with invasive breast cancer, it is difficult to compare these three local therapies as no randomized studies have examined all three modalities.

Total mastectomy offers a cure rate in approximately 98% of women [27], and today it is generally used for DCIS, which is found as diffuse or scattered clusters of microcalcifications on mammography. If several highly suspicious clusters of microcalcifications are seen on mammography it is important to core (or mammotome) *each* cluster to be sure of the extent of the DCIS before recommending mastectomy as the treatment of choice. Often only one cluster is DCIS, and the others are benign.

As breast conservation for invasive breast cancer became more acceptable, women diagnosed with DCIS were more willing to enter studies that randomized them to WLE with or without RT. The crucial question here is whether in ipsilateral breast tumor recurrence (IBTR), especially an invasive one, decreases survival.

In Fisher et al.'s NSABP B-17 trial comparing WLE and WLE/RT for DCIS, there were 14 deaths due to breast cancer in 818 women followed for a mean of 90 months [28]. This is an overall survival rate of 94% for the women in the WLE group and 95% for women who received radiation ($p = 0.84$). Only three of these deaths occurred among the 151 patients who had an IBTR.

Although IBTR does not result in a decrease in overall survival, it is important to decrease the rate, as recurrence is disturbing to the patient, her family, and her doctors. In the B-17 trial the use of radiation decreased the incidence of IBTR from 13.4% to 3.9% ($p < 0.0001$) and the recurrence of DCIS from 13.4% to 8.2% ($p = 0.007$).

Criticisms of this sole randomized study looking at WLE with and without RT for DCIS are that margins were not uniformly evaluated, postoperative mammograms were not obtained to check for residual microcalcifications, and the nuclear grade was not taken into account. When these factors were examined in retrospect, at best as could be done, RT was shown to provide a benefit in all risk categories studied in the B-17 trial. There are several retrospective studies, however, showing that WLE alone among selected DCIS patients results in low recurrence rates [29,30].

Treatment Selection

Total mastectomy is the preferred treatment option for patients with widespread or multiple clusters of biopsy-proven DCIS. It is usually done as a skin-sparing mastectomy with immediate reconstruction.

Wide local excision is the preferred option for women with localized disease. B-17, the only randomized trial of WLE versus WLE/RT, has shown that there is no survival benefit associated with RT, but it decreases IBTR in all patients, although the magnitude of this benefit varies. Patients at high risk of IBTR are those with high-grade DCIS (lesions with comedo necrosis), a large area of DCIS, and a narrow margin. These women benefit from RT. Young women with a long life expectancy and women who are averse to any risk also benefit from irradiation. An excellent article outlining treatment choices, the rationale for these choices, and the use of tamoxifen for women with DCIS was written by Morrow and Schnitt in 2000 [31].

Lobular Carcinoma In Situ

In contrast to DCIS, LCIS is a marker for a generalized increase in breast cancer risk. DCIS requires excision with margins, whereas margin involvement is not important in LCIS because it is not considered a premalignant lesion per se.

Diagnosis and Treatment

Lobar carcinoma in situ is usually found incidentally during biopsy for a fibroadenoma or another benign palpable lesion. It may also be found on core biopsy or needle localization for microcalcifications. Often the microcalcifications are not associated with the LCIS, and LCIS has no specific mammographic features. If a core or a mammotome biopsy reveals LCIS, a needle localization procedure is performed to be certain no invasive carcinoma is found.

It is considered a marker lesion rather than a precursor lesion because several studies have shown that invasive cancer develops about equally in either breast at a rate of about 1% per year [32]. The type of cancer that develops may be lobular or ductal, the latter being the most common.

Although the pathologic distinction between DCIS and LCIS is usually not difficult, there are areas of overlap for these lesions [33]. Studies have shown that the cells of LCIS are characterized by loss of expression of the adhesion molecule E-cadherin, whereas the cells of DCIS consistently show strong immunostaining [34]. Estrogen receptor (ER) positivity is much higher in LCIS and noncomedo DCIS than in comedo-type DCIS.

Treatment of LCIS

There are four available options for the treatment of LCIS: close observation, tamoxifen, randomization into the NSABP Study of Tamoxifen and Raloxifene (STAR) trial, and bilateral mastectomy.

Close observation. This consists of a clinical examination every 6 months and yearly breast imaging. Breast imaging means mammography and possibly yearly ultrasonography. The physician is not looking for LCIS but rather for an early cancer, about half of which are invasive lobular carcinomas (ILCs). ILC is notoriously difficult to find on routine mammography, and ultrasonography may be of great help. Communication between the referring physician and the radiologist is extremely important.

Tamoxifen. The data from the NSABP Prevention Trial [35] showed that women with LCIS who took tamoxifen had a 65% decrease in the development of breast cancers compared with women on placebo. This may be due in part to the high frequency of ER positivity in LCIS.

STAR trial. This NSABP study randomizes high risk women, including those with LCIS, to either ta-

moxifen or raloxifene (Evista). Women with LCIS are excellent candidates for this trial.

Bilateral mastectomy. This operation was offered in the past because invasive breast cancer was as likely to develop in the contralateral breast as it was in the ipsilateral one. Breast imaging was not as accurate as it is now; and among patients who developed breast cancer 23% had involved nodes despite close observation. Although no specific studies on patients with LCIS undergoing close follow-up exist, a few studies have shown that women are diagnosed at an early stage [36]. Therefore bilateral mastectomy is rarely if ever recommended at present.

Prophylactic Mastectomy

Prophylactic mastectomy (PM) is used to decrease the risk of breast cancer in high risk women. These women fall into several categories: women who are *BRCA1/BRCA2* gene mutation carriers (bilateral PM); women with DCIS in one breast (contralateral PM); or women with a combination of risk factors, such as DCIS, ADH, or ALH, a family history of breast cancer, and mammograms that are difficult to interpret.

Bilateral PM decreases the risk of breast cancer in high risk women. Hartman et al. showed a 90% decrease in the incidence of breast cancer in high risk women undergoing prophylactic mastectomy and an 87% decrease in the death rate [37]. Working with a mathematic model, Schrag et al. determined that a woman with a *BRCA* mutation undergoing total mastectomy at age 30 could expect to gain 2.9–5.3 years of life [38].

Contralateral PM for patients with unilateral breast cancer has no survival benefits, and the survival duration is generally dictated by the first cancer that manifests clinically [39]. However contralateral PM does have potential benefits in terms of decreasing concerns over a future breast cancer and in terms of reconstruction. When using implants, better symmetry is achieved when performing bilateral reconstruction synchronously. TRAM flaps may be used to reconstruct both breasts if the need is known preoperatively. Otherwise once the TRAM is used to reconstruct one breast, it cannot be used again.

There are two mastectomy techniques: subcutaneous mastectomy and total mastectomy. *Subcutaneous mastectomy* is done through an inframammary incision and spares the nipple–areolar complex. *Total mastectomy* is done through an elliptical incision that includes the nipple–areolar complex. Both procedures can leave a small amount of breast tissue in the axilla and on the skin flaps, and a subcutaneous mastectomy definitely leaves a large amount of tissue under the nipple. For this reason, total (rather than subcutaneous) mastectomy is the preferred procedure.

Patient satisfaction with the procedure is not total. In one report the authors noted that 70% were satisfied, 11% were neutral, and 19% were dissatisfied [40]. Many women after surgery were dissatisfied with their sexual relationships, feelings of femininity, and body appearance. These negative findings must be weighed against the benefit of the generally improved psychological and social outcomes.

Male Breast Cancer

Only about 1% of all breast cancers occur in men. Risk factors for male breast cancer include age (the mean ages at diagnosis in the two studies cited here were 61.8 and 64.5 years, respectively, compared to 55.5 years for women), previous chest wall irradiation, family history of breast cancer in men or women, *BRCA1/BRCA2* mutations, and conditions of hyperestrogenism (testicular abnormalities, exogenous estrogens, Kleinfelter syndrome, obesity). Men who have a *BRCA2* mutation have a 6% risk of developing breast cancer. This represents a 100-fold increase over the general male population risk, matching the degree of risk seen in women.

The histology of these cancers is always ductal (invasive ductal or DCIS). Lobular carcinoma is rarely seen in men, as they do not have lobular tissue. The tumors are more likely to be ER$^+$ in men (87%) than in women (55%) [41]. Survival at 10 years is similar for men and women [42]. Because the location of the tumor is generally central and close to the nipple, and because men generally have little breast tissue, they usually undergo total mastectomy and sentinel node/axillary node dissection. Lumpectomy could be performed in selected patients with small tumors unattached to the nipple and large breasts.

Neoadjuvant or Induction Chemotherapy

Neoadjuvant or induction chemotherapy is chemotherapy given to a patient prior to surgery. It is generally used in those with stage III breast cancers but may be used in patients with large stage II cancers. The concept behind giving chemotherapy preoperatively is to evaluate the chemosensitivity of the cancer and to convert a patient needing a mastectomy to one in whom breast conservation is possible. To

date there has been no survival difference for neoadjuvant chemotherapy.

The advantage is that this approach enables the patient to receive treatment for systemic disease as soon as she is diagnosed. She need not wait until the surgery is performed and the incisions are healed. For women with stage III breast cancer this delay could be as long as 6 weeks if a mastectomy and flap reconstruction is planned. Neoadjuvant chemotherapy provides for an in vivo chemosensitivity test. If the cancer does not shrink after one or two cycles of chemotherapy, the regimen may be switched. Lastly, some patients may be able to undergo breast conservation. NSABPB-18 randomized 1,523 patients to pre- or postoperative chemotherapy [43]. The frequency of breast conservation therapy was greater in the preoperative group (60% vs. 66%; p = 0.002). This difference was greater in patients with tumors > 5 cm (8% in the postoperative group vs. 22% in the preoperative group).

Pitfalls of Neoadjuvant Therapy

Lumpectomy is sometimes performed in patients who have undergone neoadjuvant chemotherapy. In the NSABP B-18 trial, breast tumor size was reduced in 80% of patients after preoperative therapy, and 36% had a complete clinical response. When the primary tumor shrinks, it can do so in one of two ways: as a grape goes to a raisin or as a dandelion goes to seed. This poses a problem for the surgeon who must decide how much tissue to remove. Mammography, ultrasonography, and magnetic resonance imaging may be used to help evaluate residual disease, but they are not totally reliable. Many surgeons or radiologists are placing clips percutaneously around the tumor prior to administering chemotherapy. The clips are particularly important if there has been a complete clinical response. If clips have not been placed, the area that remains firm in the breast should be removed with margins of normal tissue. It may be necessary to remove skin during the resection, and it may require several resections after the pathologist checks the margins.

Sentinel node biopsy is not recommended in women who have undergone neoadjuvant chemotherapy even if the axilla was negative preoperatively. This is because preoperative evaluation by palpation is highly unreliable, and a positive sentinel node may now be sterilized by chemotherapy, leaving other axillary nodes still involved by tumor. Several centers (The John Wayne Cancer Center, Santa Monica, CA; Brigham and Women's Hospital, Boston, MA) intend to do a sentinel node biopsy for women with clinically negative axilla before they undergo neoadjuvant chemotherapy.

REFERENCES

1. Balch CM. The needle biopsy should replace open excisional biopsy . . . but will the surgeon's role in coordinating breast cancer treatment be diminished [editorial]? Ann Surg Oncol 1995;2:191.

2. Tartter PI, Kaplan J, Bleiweiss I, et al. Lumpectomy margins, reexcision, and local recurrence of breast cancer. Am J Surg. 2000;179:81.

3. NIH consensus meeting. September 9–10, 1996: the uniform approach to breast fine-needle aspiration biopsy. Am J Surg. 1997;174:371.

4. Dershaw DD, Morris EA, Liberman L, et al. Nondiagnostic stereotactic core biopsy: results or rebiopsy. Radiology 1996;198:232.

5. Dershaw DD, Liberman L. Stereotactic breast biopsy: indications and results. Oncology 1998;12:907.

6. Brem R, Behrndt VS, Sanow L, Gatewood OMB. Atypical ductal hyperplasia: histologic underestimation of carcinoma in tissue harvested from impalpable breast lesions using 11 gauge stereotactically guided directional vacuum-assisted biopsy. AJR 1999;172:1405.

7. Urban JA. Excision of the major duct system of the breast. Cancer 1963;16:516.

8. Haagensen CD. Diseases of the Breast. Philadelphia, 1971, Saunders, pp 250–291.

9. Kopans DB. Breast Imaging. Philadelphia, Lippincott, 1989, p 274.

10. Zuska JJ, Crile G Jr, Ayres WW. Fistulas of lactiferous ducts. Am J Surg 1951;81:312.

11. Anderson BB. Zuska's disease: obstructed mammary duct-related periareolar breast abscess. Contemp Surg 1995:47:324.

12. Veronesi U, Salvadori B, Luini A, et al. Conservative treatment of early breast cancer; long-term results of 1232 cases treated with quadrantectomy, axillary dissection, and radiotherapy. Ann Surg 1990;211:250.

13. Fisher B, Redmond C, Poisson R, et al. Eight-year results of a randomized clinical trial comparing total mastectomy and lumpectomy with or without irradiation in the treatment of breast cancer. N Engl J Med 1989;320:822.

14. Veronesi U, Luini A, Del Vecchio M, et al. Radiotherapy after breast-preserving surgery in women with localized cancer of the breast. N Engl J Med 1993;328:1587.

15. Fisher B, Anderson S, Redmond C, et al. Reanalysis and results after 12 years of follow-up in a randomized clinical trial comparing total mastectomy with lumpectomy with or without irradiation in the treatment of breast cancer. N Engl J Med 1995;333:1456.

16. Bland KI, Menck HR, Scott-Conner CE. The National Cancer Data Base 10-year survey of breast carcinoma treatment at hospitals in the United States. Cancer 1998;83:1262.

17. Borgstein PJ, Meijer S, Pijpers R. Intradermal blue dye to identify the sentinel lymph node in breast cancer. Lancet 1997;349:1668.

18. Klimberg VS, Rubio IT, Henry R, et al. Subareolar versus peritumoral injection for location of the sentinel lymph node. Ann Surg 1999;229:860.

19. Krag D, Weaver D, Takamaru A, et al. The sentinel node in breast cancer: a multicenter validation study. N Engl J Med 1998;339:941.

20. Cote RJ, Peterson, Chaiwun B, et al. Role of immunohistochemical detection of lymph-node metastases in management of breast cancer. Lancet 1999;354:896.

21. Dowlatshahi K, Fan M, Bloom KJ, et al. Occult metastases in the sentinel lymph nodes of patients with early stage breast carcinoma. Cancer 1999;86:990.

22. Fowble B. The significance of resection margin status in patients with early stage invasive cancer treated with breast conservation therapy. Breast J 1998;4:126.

23. Kroll SS, Schusterman MA, Tadjalli HE, et al. Risk of recurrence after treatment of early breast cancer with skin-sparing mastectomy. Ann Surg Oncol 1996;4:193.

24. Carlson GW, Bostwick J, Styblo TM, et al. Skin sparing mastectomy: oncologic and reconstructive considerations. Ann Surg 1997;225:570.

25. Holland R, Hendricks JH, Verbeek AL, et al. Extent, distribution and mammographic/histological correlations of breast ductal carcinoma in situ. Lancet 1990;335:519.

26. Pendas S, Dauway E, Giuliano R, et al. Sentinel node biopsy in ductal carcinoma in situ patients. Ann Surg Oncol 2000;7:15.

27. Kinne DW, Petrek JA, Osborne MP, et al. Breast carcinoma in situ. Arch Surg 1989;124:33.

28. Fisher B, Dignam J, Wolmark N, et al. Lumpectomy and radiation therapy for the treatment of intraductal breast cancer: findings from the National Surgical Adjuvant Breast and Bowel Project B-17. J Clin Oncol 1998;15:441.

29. Lagios MD, Margolin FR, Westdahl PR, et al. Mammographically detected duct carcinoma in situ: frequency of local recurrence following tylectomy and prognostic effect of nuclear grade on local recurrence. Cancer 1989;63:618.

30. Silverstein MJ. Van Nuys experience by treatment. In Silverstein MJ (ed) Ductal Carcinoma in Situ of the Breast. Baltimore, Williams & Wilkins, 1997, pp 443–447.

31. Morrow M, Schnitt SJ. Treatment selection in ductal carcinoma in situ. JAMA 2000;283:453.

32. Kinne DW. Lobular carcinoma in situ. Surg Oncol Clin North Am 1993;2:69.

33. Schnitt SJ, Morrow M. Lobular carcinoma in situ: current concepts and controversies. Semin Diagn Pathol 1999;16:209.

34. Jacobs TW, Pliss N, Kouria, Schnitt SJ. Carcinomas in situ (CIS) of the breast with indeterminate features: role of E-cadherin (e-cad) staining in categorization. Lab Invest 2000;80:23A.

35. Fisher B, Costantino JP, Wickerham DL, et al. Tamoxifen for prevention of breast cancer: report of the National Surgical Breast and Bowel Project P-1 Study. J Natl Cancer Inst 1991;90:1371.

36. Chart PL, Franssen E. Management of women at increased risk for breast cancer: preliminary results from a new program. Can Med Assoc J 1997;157:1235.

37. Hartman LC, Schaid DJ, Woods JE, et al. Efficacy of bilateral prophylactic mastectomy in women with a family history of breast cancer. N Engl J Med 1999;340:77.

38. Schrag D, Kuntz KM, Garber JE, et al. Decision analysis-effects of prophylactic mastectomy and oophorectomy on the life expectancy of women with BRCA1 or BRCA2 mutations. N Engl J Med 1997;336:1465.

39. Gajalakshmi CK, Shanta V, Hakama M. Survival from contralateral breast cancer. Breast Cancer Res Treat 1999;58:115.

40. Frost MH, Schaid DJ, Sellers TA, et al. Long term satisfaction and psychological and social function following bilateral prophylactic mastectomy. JAMA 2000;284:319.

41. Borgen PI, Senie RT, McKinnon WMP, et al. Carcinoma of the male breast: analysis of prognosis compared with matched females. Ann Surg Oncol 1997;4:385.

42. Vetto J, Jun S-Y, Padduch D, et al. Stages at presentation, prognostic factors, and outcome of breast cancer in males. Am J Surg 1999;177:379.

43. Fisher B, Brown A, Mamounas E, et al. Effect of preoperative chemotherapy on local-regional disease in women with operable breast cancer: findings from National Surgical Adjuvant Breast and Bowel Project B-18. J Clin Oncol 1997;15:2483.

97 Excision of Benign Palpable Breast Mass

INDICATIONS

See Chapter 96.

Fibroadenoma. Operation is indicated when a fibroadenoma enlarges or when the diagnosis is in doubt. Most fibroadenomas are small, round, freely movable, well encapsulated nodules that are easily diagnosed on physical examination. Occasionally carcinoma masquerades as a fibroadenoma.

Other well circumscribed benign palpable lesions.

PREOPERATIVE PREPARATION

Preoperative evaluation may include ultrasonography, fine-needle aspiration cytology, or mammography as individually appropriate.

OPERATIVE STRATEGY

Although most fibroadenomas are completely surrounded by a smooth fibrous capsule, the plane is not always well defined between the fibroadenoma and surrounding breast. Whenever this is the case,

include a narrow rim of normal adjacent breast in the specimen being excised; otherwise local recurrence of the tumor is possible. The strategy for biopsy or excision (lumpectomy) of a presumed malignant lesion is different (see Chapter 99).

Among the errors encountered during surgery for a palpable mass is failure to locate the lesion. This can occur when a deep-seated tumor is being excised under local anesthesia. Unless the tumor is easily palpable and superficial, it may not be easy to palpate, especially when the operation is being performed through a cosmetic circumareolar incision at a distance from the lesion.

A more important consideration, especially with large fibroadenomas, is the possibility of a phyllodes tumor, which resembles a large fibroadenoma on physical examination. The most important characteristic of both benign and malignant phyllodes tumors is a strong predilection for local recurrence. Therefore always include a 1 cm rim of normal breast tissue when excising a large fibroadenoma (> 4–5 cm in diameter) or one that has grown rapidly.

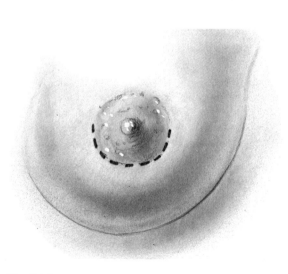

Fig. 97–1

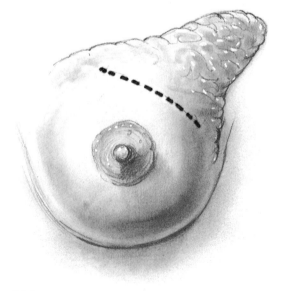

Fig. 97–2

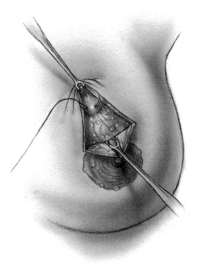

Fig. 97–3. Adapted with permission, from Scott-Conner CEH, Dawson DL. Operative Anatomy. Philadelphia, Lippincott, 1993.

OPERATIVE TECHNIQUE

Choice of Incision

Superior cosmetic results follow the use of a circumareolar incision **(Fig. 97–1)** or an incision made in the inframammary crease. However, it is not advisable to dissect through a large distance of breast when trying to extract a fibroadenoma via one of these incisions. For tumors more than 2–3 cm away from the areola, make an incision in the line of Langer directly over the tumor **(Fig. 97–2)**. These lines are essentially circular in nature in the skin overlying the breast, each circle being concentric with the areola.

Local Anesthesia

Raise a skin wheal along the line of the proposed incision using 1% xylocaine without epinephrine. (Epinephrine causes vasoconstriction, and delayed bleeding may result when the vasospasm relaxes). Infiltrate laterally in a fan-like pattern on all sides of the skin incision to anesthetize the skin and subcutaneous regions of the breast thoroughly. Do not inject directly into the area containing the mass; rather, inject in a circumferential manner *around* it. It may be necessary to inject *underneath* the mass as dissection progresses. Allow sufficient time for the anesthetic to work and use gentle technique. Sharp dissection is frequently better tolerated than electrocautery. Mild sedation may be beneficial.

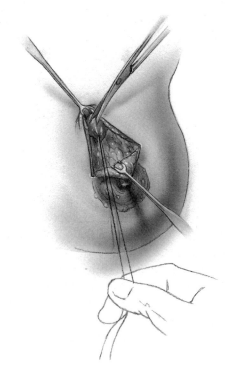

Fig. 97–4. Adapted with permission, from Scott-Conner CEH, Dawson DL. Operative Anatomy. Philadelphia, Lippincott, 1993.

Dissection

After opening the skin, use a scalpel to carry the incision through the subcutaneous fat down to breast tissue; then incise the breast tissue down to the lesion. Palpate to verify the location of the lesion as the dissection progresses. Electrocoagulate each bleeding point so the field remains bloodless.

Unless the lesion is quite superficial and the dissection is easy, a traction stitch facilitates subsequent dissection. Use 2-0 silk on a curved cutting needle to transfix the lesion or deep breast tissue just superficial to the mass **(Fig. 97–3)**. Place a figure-of-eight suture for security and use it to elevate and manipulate the lesion **(Fig. 97–4)**. When the capsule of the fibroadenoma appears, incise it with a scalpel. If the fibroadenoma then shells out with no further attachment, the capsule may be left behind. If there are any attachments between the fibroadenoma and the surrounding tissue, excise the capsule and a small rim of breast tissue with it.

Repair

Make no attempt to resuture the defect in the breast, as these sutures often create a mass at the site of the repair. During the months and years following surgery, evaluation of the patient's breast on physical

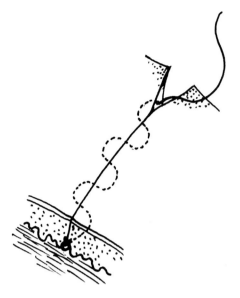

Fig. 97-5. Adapted with permission, from Scott-Conner CEH, Dawson DL. Operative Anatomy. Philadelphia, Lippincott, 1993.

examination can be made extremely difficult by the presence of a firm mass at the site of the previous excision. The defect in the breast will fill with fluid and serum and gradually be replaced by normal tissue.

Place several interrupted 3-0 PG sutures to approximate the subcutaneous layer just under the skin. Then close the skin with interrupted sutures of 5-0 nylon or a running subcuticular suture of 5-0 PDS **(Fig. 97–5)**. No drain is used.

POSTOPERATIVE CARE

To apply even pressure on the operative site, request that the patient wear a supportive brassiere over a bulky gauze dressing continuously for the first postoperative week.

COMPLICATIONS

Hematoma

Infection

Inadequate excision (missed lesion)

REFERENCE

Hughes LE. Fibroadenoma and related tumours. In Hughes LE, Mansel RE, Webster DJT (eds) Benign Disorders and Diseases of the Breast. Concepts and Clinical Management, 2nd ed. London, Saunders, 2000, pp 73-74.

98 Excision of Ducts, Operations for Breast Abscess

EXCISION OF DUCTS

Indications

Single duct discharge with or without palpable mass
Ductal ectasia

Preoperative Preparation

Perform mammography before operating on the ductal system.

Ultrasonography may demonstrate ductal pathology.

If single (rather than total) ductal excision is planned, localize the involved duct by the following methods.

Physical examination. Apply finger pressure at varying points along the outer margin of the areola to determine which segment of the breast contains the offending duct (the finger pressure induces discharge from this duct). If this is not accomplished at initial examination, apply collodion to the surface of the nipple to occlude all of the ducts temporarily and prevent any discharge. At subsequent examination a week later, remove the collodion and repeat the attempt to localize the offending duct. Also, collodion may be applied to the surface of the nipple 1 week prior to operation to cause distension of the diseased duct.

Ductography. Ductography may be performed by inserting a tiny catheter into the duct orifice and injecting a small amount of aqueous radiopaque medium.

Ductal endoscopy. This is an investigational technique that may prove useful.

Operative Strategy

Single Duct Excision Versus Total Duct Excision

When the indication for surgery is a bloody nipple discharge, the diagnosis is generally carcinoma or intraductal papilloma. Careful localization to a single duct allows precise excision, which is diagnostic in the case of carcinoma and therapeutic in the case of an intraductal papilloma. Single duct excision also provides better preservation of sensation in the nipple-areola complex and may permit breast feeding once healing has occurred. Multiple papillomas or ductal ectasia with recurrent subareolar abscesses may require complete ductal excision.

Prevention of Skin Necrosis

Total excision of the mammary ducts requires elevation of the entire areola, which may impair the vascularity of the distal tip of the skin flap unless careful dissection is performed. Do not make the circumareolar incision more than 40–50% of the circumference of the areola. Handle this skin flap delicately to avoid unnecessary trauma.

Operative Technique

Single Duct Excision

Incision

A single duct may be excised through a radial incision or an incision around the circumference of the areola. Use a sharp scalpel and obtain hemostasis with accurate electrocoagulation.

Identification and Excision

If a discharge is visible, cannulate the duct with a lacrimal duct probe and use it to guide dissection. If collodion has been used to occlude the surface of the nipple for a week prior to surgery, the diseased duct is by now distended. If it contains blood, the duct appears bluish. Gently dissect the duct from surrounding tissue. Divide it between hemostats at its junction with the nipple and dissect it out to a point about 1–2 cm beyond the circumareolar incision. Submit it for histologic examination.

If the duct cannot be clearly identified, it is necessary to excise an area of the ductal system beginning at the nipple and proceeding in a peripheral direction. Have the pathologist examine the specimen to ascertain that the pathology has indeed been excised.

Closure

In many cases it is necessary only to close the skin incision with interrupted 5-0 nylon sutures or a running subcuticular suture of 5-0 PDS. In some cases a few PG sutures may be placed if there is a significant defect in the underlying breast. If hemostasis is good, drainage is not necessary.

Total Duct Excision

Incision

Make an incision along the circumference of the areola at the exact margin between the areola and skin (see Fig. 97-1). The length of the incision should encompass no more than 50% of the areola's circumference. Insert sutures in the edge of the incised areola temporarily and apply a hemostat to each suture. These are used to apply traction while the areola is being dissected off the breast **(Fig. 98–1a 98–1,b)**. Use scalpel or scissors dissection to elevate the areola with a thin layer of fat. This dissection must be continued beyond the nipple so the entire skin of the areola has been elevated. Do not detach the nipple from its ducts at this stage of the operation.

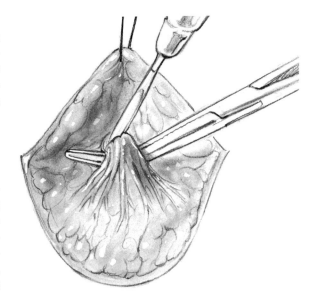

Fig. 98-2a

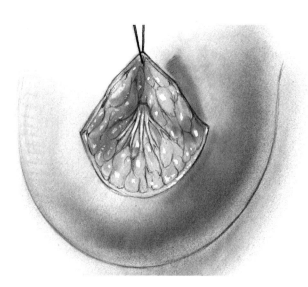

Fig. 98-1a

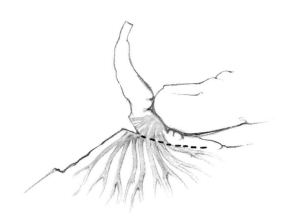

Fig. 98-2b

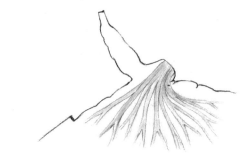

Fig. 98-1b

Excising the Ductal System

After the skin has been elevated, note that the approximately 12 ducts constitute the only attachment between the nipple and the underlying breast. Apply a ligature to these ducts and make an incision that detaches them flush with the nipple **(Fig. 98–2a, 98–2b)**.

Dissect the ducts for a distance of 3–5 cm. Using electrocautery, excise the circle of ducts and breast tissue **(Fig. 98–3a, 98–3b)**. The circular mass of tissue has a radius of 3–5 cm and a thickness of 1–2 cm. If any of the diseased ducts is dilated and extends beyond 5 cm, follow this duct and remove a further section until it disappears into the breast tissue. Occasionally a diseased duct involves a section of the nipple, which then appears inverted. In this case a tiny segment of nipple may be removed. Obtain complete hemostasis with electrocautery.

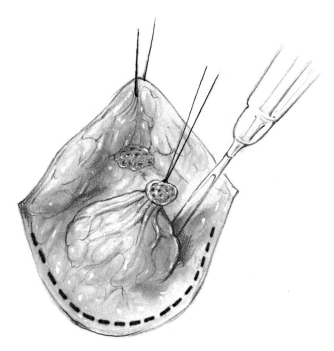

Fig. 98–3a

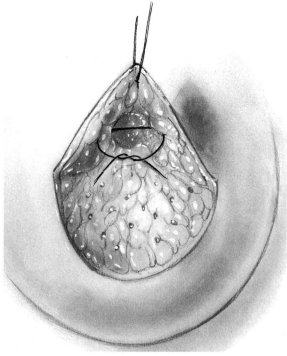

Fig. 98–4

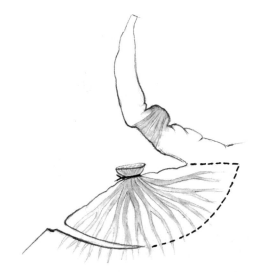

Fig. 98–3b

the nipple to invert, corrective measures must be taken. Before closing the skin incision, insert a 5-0 PG purse-string suture in the subcuticular tissues at the base of the nipple to maintain it in the erect position **(Fig. 98–4)**. Then close the skin incision with interrupted 5-0 nylon sutures **(Fig. 98–5)** or a subcuticular suture of 5-0 PDS.

Reconstruction

In the patient with a large breast, the resulting defect may be relatively shallow so the reconstructed areola rests on a solid base of breast tissue. In this case no further reconstruction is necessary. In many cases, however, there is a significant defect underneath the areola. Because the blood supply of the areola is somewhat tenuous, it requires a firm base of breast tissue for optimal healing. In this case close the defect in the breast in layers with interrupted small sutures of PG material.

If detaching the areola results in a tendency for

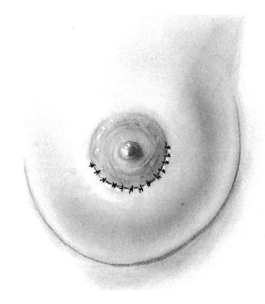

Fig. 98–5

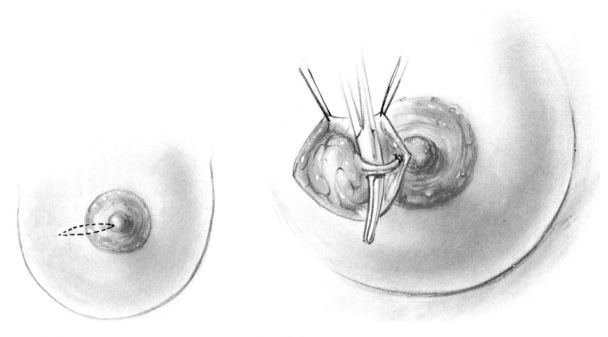

Fig. 98-6   Fig. 98-7

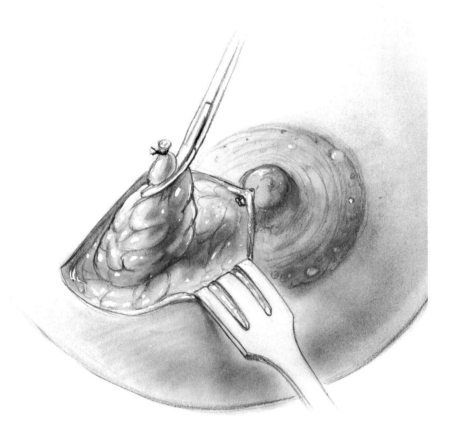

Fig. 98-8

Postoperative Care

Instruct the patient to wear a supportive brassiere over a moderately bulky dressing to apply even pressure for the first 7 days and nights after surgery.

Complications

Hematoma may appear.

Occasionally following total duct excision, elevation of the entire areola in a plane too close to the subcutis results in an area of *skin necrosis*.

BREAST ABSCESS

Breast abscesses are most often seen in nursing mothers. They are generally the result of bacteria being introduced via a break in the skin of the nipple. In the nonlactating woman, an abscess may appear with little surrounding inflammation and induration. In some of these cases, aspiration of pus under local anesthesia and treatment with antibiotics lead to rapid resolution. If pus is not obtained on aspiration or the abscess does not respond promptly, perform operative drainage with biopsy of the abscess wall. Evacuate the pus and loosely insert a gauze pack.

PARAAREOLAR ABSCESS OR FISTULA

An abscess in the region of the areola or just adjacent to the areola often originates in an obstructed mammary duct, termed duct ectasia. The latter may result in a recurring abscess at the same location or in a chronic draining fistula. In either case, proper treatment requires a radial elliptical incision **(Fig. 98–6)** overlying the duct, which can usually be palpated as a thickened cord running from the nipple toward the periphery of the breast. Remove a small ellipse of skin and surrounding breast tissue. Identify the duct **(Fig. 98–7)** and excise it together with the diseased tissue **(Fig. 98–8)**. If the incision has not been greatly contaminated, close the skin loosely around a drain. If the area *is* grossly contaminated, it may be wiser to insert skin sutures for delayed primary closure 4-6 days later. If the diseased duct is not removed, the abscess or fistula recurs.

REFERENCES

Cardenosa G, Doudna C, Eklund GW. Ductography of the breast: technique and findings. AJR 1994;162:1081.

Carty NJ, Mudan SS, Ravichandran D, et al. Prospective study of outcome in women presenting with nipple discharge. Ann R Coll Surg Engl 1994;76:387.

Dixon JM, Thompson AM. Effective surgical treatment for mammary duct fistula. Br J Surg 1991;78:1185.

Haagensen DD. Disease of the Breast. Philadelphia, Saunders, 1971.

Hughes LE. The duct ectasia/periductal mastitis complex. In Hughes LE, Mansel RE, Webster DJT (eds) Benign Disorders and Diseases of the Breast. Concepts and Clinical Management, 2nd ed. London, Saunders, 2000, pp 143-170.

Webster DJT. Nipple discharge. In Hughes LE, Mansel RE, Webster DJT (eds) Benign Disorders and Diseases of the Breast. Concepts and Clinical Management, 2nd ed. London, Saunders, 2000, pp 171-186.

99 Lumpectomy (Tylectomy) for Breast Cancer

INDICATIONS

Palpation of a suspicious breast mass or "dominant lump" even if the mammogram is normal

Detection of a suspicious shadow on mammography even if not palpable

Ductal carcinoma in situ (see Chapter 96)

Early-stage breast cancer in conjunction with axillary node dissection (see Chapter 103), as part of breast conservation

PITFALLS AND DANGER POINTS

Failure to include pathologic tissue in the biopsy specimen

OPERATIVE STRATEGY

Biopsy/Lumpectomy of Palpable Mass

In most cases, a diagnosis has been made by fine-needle aspiration (FNA). Make the incision directly over the mass and use the index finger of the nondominant hand to palpate the mass, retract it, and guide the dissection. In a thin-breasted woman a well localized mass is easily felt and removed. When the area is ill-defined, particularly if located in the axillary tail, it may be simpler to excise a segment of breast extending from the subcutaneous fat down to the pectoral fascia to be sure the cancer has been adequately resected.

Biopsy of Nonpalpable Breast Lesions

When mammography has detected a suspicious stellate mass or a suspicious cluster of microcalcifications in a breast where no mass is palpable, preoperative mammographic or ultrasonographic localization must be used to mark the lesion. In most of these cases, stereotactic core biopsy has provided a tissue diagnosis. A Kopans hooked guidewire inside a needle is placed in or close to the radiographically suspicious lesion by the radiologist, and the surgeon's task is then to locate and excise a mass of breast tissue around the tip of the wire. Because most of these nonpalpable lesions are relatively small, we endeavor to

excise the lesion completely together with normal breast tissue whenever possible. If no palpable lesion is encountered, we excise a liberal portion of breast from the area indicated by the needle. This is feasible because many patients with nonpalpable lesions have reasonably large breasts. It is frequently difficult to perform an accurate lumpectomy at a second stage following a guidewire-directed biopsy of this type. Care must be taken during dissection lest the wire be broken or dislodged. If the wire breaks, it is necessary to find and retrieve the broken end, a tedious process that may require use of a metal detector. The wire is unlikely to break if a scalpel or cutting cautery (rather than scissors) and gentle technique are used for the dissection.

Extent of Excision, Marking the Specimen, Closure

An adequate lumpectomy removes the cancer with a rim of surrounding normal tissue. Preserve the orientation of the specimen so positive margins can be identified and reexcised if necessary. We prefer to do this with two marking sutures, using the mnemonic "short stitch = *s*uperior margin, *l*ong stitch = *l*ateral margin."

After excising a segment of breast, do not attempt to close the defect by suturing the parenchyma of the breast together, as it would distort the shape of the breast and produce a mass lesion. Postoperatively, palpating a gap in the continuity of the breast tissue is easier to interpret than palpating a mass.

OPERATIVE TECHNIQUE

Lumpectomy for Palpable Mass
Incision

When performing a biopsy for a palpable mass, make the incision directly over the mass. The incision is made in the lines of Langer, which represent the natural skin creases and can be seen to run in a circular fashion, roughly parallel to the perimeter of the areola (see Fig. 97–2). For lesions located at the medial aspect of the breast, a horizontal incision along the 9 o'clock axis of the breast is acceptable. Elsewhere in the breast, curve the incision in a direction parallel to the areola. One should also consider that a mastectomy may be indicated subsequent to the biopsy. The biopsy site is preferably in a location that can be easily encompassed by the mastectomy incision.

The incision should be long enough to facilitate removal of the entire mass with a 1 cm shell of normal surrounding breast tissue without requiring excessive retraction of skin flaps. Local anesthesia may be used if concurrent axillary node dissection is not planned. If so, infiltrate as described in Chapter 97. Make the incision along the previous ink mark down into the subcutaneous layer using a scalpel. Elevate the skin flaps as necessary in the subcutaneous plane **(Fig. 99–1)**.

With the left index finger palpating the mass, carry the incision along one side of the tumor deep enough to palpate the deep aspect of the tumor. We prefer to use sharp dissection (or cutting electrocautery), avoiding the use of coagulating cautery to preserve the margins for histologic analysis.

Do not apply a tenaculum clamp to the tumor mass, as it would only make it more difficult to ascertain the outer margins of the tumor by tensing the tissues. Sometimes an accurately placed figure-of-eight suture in the tumor mass for retraction is of some benefit.

Initiate the dissection on the opposite side of the mass and carry the dissection down to a level of the breast deep to the mass, leaving a margin of normal breast tissue on the deep layer. Sometimes it is simpler to go down to the fascia of the pectoral muscle where there is a natural plane between the breast and the fascia **(Fig. 99–2)**. Under guidance of the index finger, excise the tumor. Obtain meticulous he-

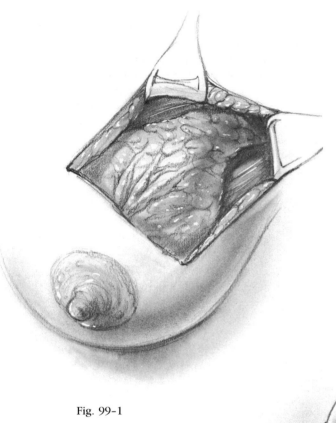

Fig. 99-1

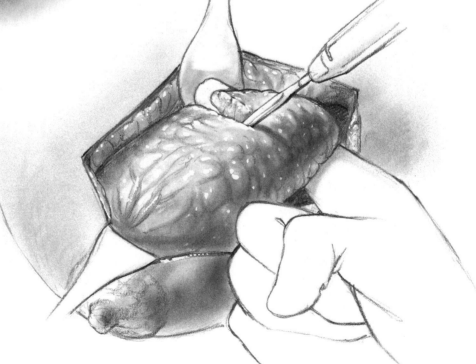

Fig. 99-2

mostasis utilizing the coagulating current of electrocautery. Because there will be a tissue defect in the breast, even minor bleeding produces a large postoperative hematoma, so hemostasis must be complete.

Closure

Do not attempt to close the defect in the breast parenchyma, and do not place a drain. Close the subcutaneous layer with three or four 3-0 PG sutures. Close the skin with a continuous subcuticular suture of 5-0 PDS.

Nonpalpable Lesion

In the case of nonpalpable lesions the patient is transferred from the radiography suite to the operating room with a Kopans hooked wire and needle inserted in the breast close to the suspicious radiographic shadow. Compare the localization radiographs with the original mammogram. Mentally extrapolate from the direction of the wire and its length and estimate the probable location of the tip. Gently palpate the breast in the region where the tip is thought to lie. Frequently the free end of the wire bobs when the tip is palpated, confirming the location.

If the area at the tip of the needle can be palpated or otherwise identified, make a curved incision in the skin crease overlying the tip of the needle and excise the breast tissue in that vicinity **(Fig. 99–3)**. If the tip is a considerable distance from the skin entry site, it may be preferable to place the incision halfway between the two. At a convenient time, gently draw the wire into the incision so it can be removed with the mass **(Fig. 99–4)**.

Unless the patient has a small breast, do not hesitate to excise a liberal quantity of tissue around the tip of the wire, perhaps $5 \times 3 \times 2$ cm. Submit the tissue with the wire in place to the radiography department where specimen mammography is performed and compared with the original studies to confirm that the lesion has been excised. Do not close the wound until confirmation that the suspicious shadow is located on the specimen mammogram. In the rare situation where the radiographic shadow was not included in the specimen, carefully palpate the entire area of dissection for any suspicious lesions. Excise such additional tissue and submit it for another specimen mammogram. If again no pathology can be detected, terminate the operation and subject the patient to a repeat mammogram in 2–3 months. If a suspicious lesion remains in the breast, perform another biopsy using the Kopans localizing procedure.

In cases where the tip of the Kopans device cannot be accurately localized, make the incision at the point where the needle enters the skin of the breast or midway along the estimated trajectory, as mentioned above. By measuring the wire external to the skin, calculate the length of wire that remains in the breast tissue. Dissect along the shaft of the wire. Remove a cylinder of breast tissue about 2 cm in diameter at the level of the incision and increase the diameter of the cylinder to 3–4 cm as one approaches the tip of the wire. Periodically palpate the tissue to ascertain that the wire has not been ex-

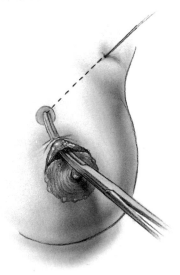

Fig. 99-3. Adapted, with permission, from Scott-Conner CEH, Dawson DL. Opreative Anatomy. Philadelphia, Lippincott, 1993.

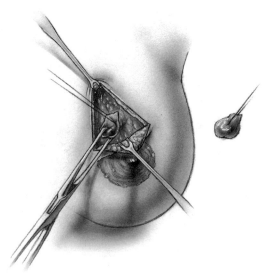

Fig. 99-4. Adapted, with permission, from Scott-Conner CEH, Dawson DL. Opreative Anatomy. Philadelphia, Lippincott, 1993.

posed during the dissection. When the proper depth has been reached, transect the cylinder of tissue and remove it together with the wire. Again, achieve complete hemostasis with electrocautery. Close the skin with a subcuticular or vertical mattress suture, as described above. Several fine Vicryl absorbable sutures may be placed in the subcutaneous layer if necessary.

Lumpectomy Following Previous Biopsy

The term "lumpectomy" refers to excision of a primary carcinoma of the breast with histologic confirmation that the entire malignancy has been enclosed in an envelope of normal breast tissue on all sides. In patients whose diagnosis of cancer has been confirmed by a needle biopsy, a lumpectomy is essentially the same procedure as that described above for excising a palpable mass.

In patients whose initial surgical biopsy resulted in histologic confirmation of the diagnosis of cancer but in whom no attempt was made at complete excision, a second operation for lumpectomy is indicated. In these cases, make an elliptical incision around the previous biopsy scar, with a 1 cm margin of normal skin on both sides. Thereafter use the scalpel to incise the breast tissue so the entire previous cavity left by the biopsy procedure is excised en bloc. If the deep margin of the biopsy cavity is close to the pectoral fascia, excise the pectoral fascia in this location together with the specimen. If excision of the amount of breast tissue required for lumpectomy produces a poor cosmetic result, lumpectomy is contraindicated and modified radical mastectomy followed by reconstruction of the breast is preferable. Achieve complete hemostasis with electrocoagulation and ligatures as necessary. After

hemostasis is complete, close the incision without drainage utilizing 4-0 Vicryl sutures to the subcutaneous fat and a subcuticular stitch of 4-0 PDS. Apply a gauze pressure dressing.

POSTOPERATIVE CARE

Apply a bulky gauze dressing over the area of dissection. Instruct the patient to wear her brassiere day and night for 7–10 days following surgery. The gauze dressing should be large enough that continuous pressure is applied to the defect created by the biopsy excision. This practice inhibits venous bleeding and controls the volume of serum that accumulates in this tissue defect.

COMPLICATIONS

Retained fragment of wire

Failure to identify and excise pathologic tissue in patients who have a breast cancer

Hematoma

Infection (should be seen in no more than 1–2% of patients)

REFERENCES

Harlow SP, Krag DN, Ames SE, Weaver DL. Intraoperative ultrasound localization to guide surgical excision of nonpalpable breast carcinoma. J Am Coll Surg 1999;189:241.

Luu HH, Otis CN, Reed WP Jr, Garb JL, Frank JL. The unsatisfactory margin in breast cancer surgery. Am J Surg 1999;178:362.

Margolese RG. Surgical considerations for invasive breast cancer. Surg Clin North Am 1999;79:1031.

100 Modified Radical Mastectomy, Simple (Total) Mastectomy

INDICATIONS

Modified radical mastectomy is the operation of choice for patients with an infiltrating carcinoma of the breast who are not eligible for breast conservation.

Simple (total) mastectomy is used for patients with ductal carcinoma in situ who are not candidates for breast conservation.

Simple mastectomy is occasionally performed as a salvage procedure when breast conservation fails.

PREOPERATIVE PREPARATION

Mammography

Additional staging studies guided by protocols and extent of disease

PITFALLS AND DANGER POINTS

Performing an inadequate biopsy that fails to detect the cancer

Ischemia of skin flaps

Injury to axillary vein or artery

Injury to brachial plexus

Injury to chest wall resulting in pneumothorax

Injury to lateral pectoral nerve resulting in atrophy of the major pectoral muscle

OPERATIVE STRATEGY

Establishing the Diagnosis

Most patients come to the operating room with an established histologic or cytologic diagnosis of malignancy. An occasional patient requires biopsy, frozen section, and then modified radical mastectomy as a single-stage procedure.

In this case, plan and orient the *biopsy* incision in such a manner that it can easily be excised at *mastectomy*. Perform an incisional biopsy of large tumors simply by excising a wedge of the tumor, leaving the bulk of the tumor behind. Otherwise, such a large defect is made in the breast that it is difficult to avoid entering the field of the biopsy procedure when performing the mastectomy. Small tumors (<3–4 cm) may be excised in their entirety. This has the theoretic advantage that manipulating the breast during the mastectomy does not dislodge additional tumor emboli into the lymphatic system and bloodstream.

Rapid and effective in accomplishing hemostasis during breast surgery, electrocautery nevertheless has one disadvantage. If excessive heat is applied to the breast tumor during excision, it may render the determination of estrogen receptors and histologic margins inaccurate. Consequently, use only the cutting current when incising the breast tissues surrounding the tumor, which does not result in excessive heat. When a bleeding point is encountered, use the electrocoagulating current only for the bleeding point. If the tumor is small, use electrocoagulation with great caution to avoid overheating the specimen.

Simple (Total) Versus Modified Radical Mastectomy

Simple mastectomy is used when axillary lymphadenectomy is not required. It can frequently be done through a small skin incision. Skin flaps are created in the same manner, and the dissection is terminated when the lateral border of the breast is reached. It is not uncommon for one or more lymph nodes to be included in the adipose tissue surrounding the axillary tail, but no effort is made to perform a lymphadenectomy.

Modified Radical Mastectomy

The term modified radical mastectomy as used currently is synonymous with total mastectomy and axillary node dissection. As originally described, modified radical mastectomy removed all of the breast tissue together with the underlying fascia of the major pectoral muscle in continuity with a total axillary lymphadenectomy. The minor pectoral muscle also was excised. Most surgeons currently simply retract the minor pectoral muscle, some divide it, and some remove it.

Axillary Lymph Node Anatomy for Breast Cancer Surgeons

Breast cancer surgeons conventionally divide the axillary lymph nodes into three levels. The minor pectoral muscle is the anatomic landmark that delimits the three levels. Level I nodes lie along the chest wall and under the lateral portion of the axillary neurovascular bundle. They include the external mammary group, the subscapular group, and the axillary vein group. The lateral border of the minor pectoral muscle forms the upper border of this node group. Level II nodes lie directly underneath (deep to) the minor pectoral muscle. Level III muscles are superomedial to the minor pectoral muscle. Thus the minor pectoral muscle, crossing the axillary neurovascular bundle, must be retracted, divided, or removed to perform a complete lymphadenectomy. Additional nodes, termed Rotter's nodes, are found between the major and minor pectoral muscles. Although most surgeons no longer divide or excise the minor pectoral muscle, there should be no hesitancy in doing so if exposure is poor.

Incision and Skin Flaps

Thickness of Skin Flap

The extremely thin skin flaps advocated as an integral part of the classic Halsted radical mastectomy were necessitated by the advanced stage of cancer common at that time. Furthermore, even thin flaps can be shown to harbor islands of glandular breast tissue.

How thin to make the skin flap depends on how much subcutaneous fat exists between the skin and the breast. There is frequently a relatively avascular cleavage plane between this fat and the fat of the breast. Obese patients may have 1–2 cm of subcutaneous fat, whereas thin patients may have only a few millimeters of fat in this location. The important strategy is to remove all of the grossly obvious breast tissue. Leaving behind a layer of subcutaneous fat on the skin flap helps ensure the viability of the flap and facilitates reconstruction of the breast at a subsequent operation for those patients who desire this procedure. It does not increase the risk of local recurrence. Cooper's ligaments extend from the breast to the subcutis and form a discontinuous layer of thin white fibrous tissue, visible against the background of yellow fat. Incising this fibrous layer where it joins the subcutaneous fat is a good method for ensuring complete removal of the breast tissue while at the same time preserving an even layer of subcutaneous fat. This technique is described below.

Alternative Incisions for Mastectomy

If immediate or delayed reconstruction is planned, allow the reconstructive surgeon to have input into the location, direction, and size of the scar. References at the end of the chapter describe skin-sparing mastectomy, an option for some women.

In general, placing the incision in a horizontal direction gives the best cosmetic result because the scar is not visible when the patient wears clothing with a low-cut neckline. Although the horizontal incision is easy to apply to tumors in the 3 and 9 o'clock positions **(Figs. 100–1, 100–2)**, some modifications are necessary for tumors in the upper or

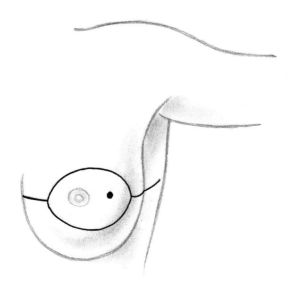

Fig. 100–1

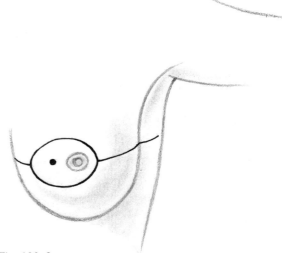

Fig. 100–2

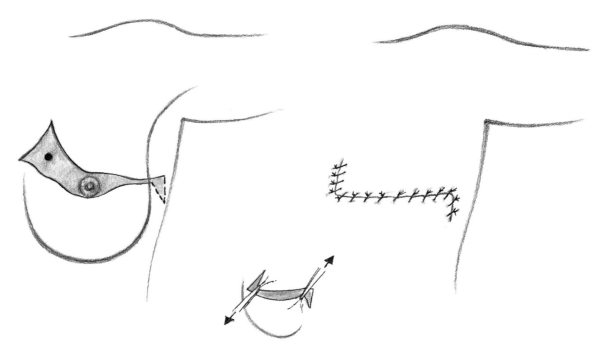

Fig. 100-3

lower portions of the breast. A good basic approach is to draw a circle around the tumor or biopsy incision, leaving a 3 cm margin on all sides. Plan the remainder of the incision so the entire areola is included in the specimen. If possible, accomplish this in a horizontal direction. After having drawn the circle around the tumor, preserve as much of the remaining skin as possible, as it avoids tension on the skin suture line. Excise the redundant skin after the specimen has been removed, or leave it in situ if subsequent reconstruction is planned.

There are a number of alternative incisions for tumors in various locations of the breast. **Figure 100–3** illustrates an incision tailored to encompass

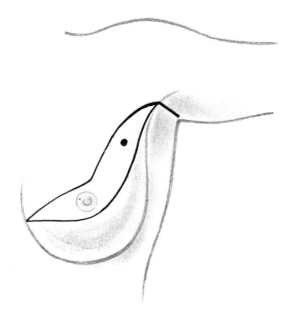

Fig. 100-4

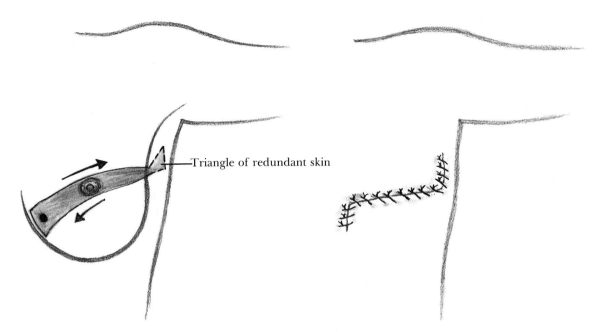

Triangle of redundant skin

Fig. 100-5

a lesion at 10 o'clock. Similarly, **Figure 100–4** shows an incision that accommodates a tumor in the upper outer quadrant of the breast yet is low medially where it is most likely to be visible.

Another cosmetic defect that should be avoided is the "dog-ear" deformity that can result at either end of the incision following mastectomy. This bunching together of skin is interpreted by many women as a residual tumor and is a cause for great anxiety. It is easily prevented by excising an additional triangle of skin until the incision lies flat on the chest wall **(Fig. 100–5)**.

OPERATIVE TECHNIQUE

Biopsy (If No Prior Diagnosis)

Determine the direction the mastectomy incision will take and make the biopsy incision directly over the tumor in the same direction as the anticipated mastectomy incision. If the tumor is 2–3 cm in diameter, make the biopsy incision 3–4 cm in length; then carry this incision through the subcutaneous fat down to the level of breast tissue. Apply rake retractors to the subcutaneous fat. Use the cutting current of electrocautery to dissect in the plane between the fat and the breast tissue until an area of breast about 3–4 cm in diameter has been exposed. If the tumor is easily identified, use the cutting current to incise the breast tissue around the perimeter of the tumor until the lesion has been removed. Pal-

pate the cavity and the excised mass to ensure that an adequate biopsy has been performed. Sometimes it is necessary to send additional material from the walls of the cavity to make a definitive diagnosis. Now use coagulating current to achieve complete hemostasis in the wound while the pathologist is performing a frozen section examination of the specimen. Be sure that a portion of the specimen is submitted for an estrogen receptor determination.

If the lesion is benign, close the skin with a subcuticular continuous suture of 4-0 PDS or interrupted 5-0 nylon sutures. If the specimen is reported to be malignant, close the incision with continuous heavy silk. Change gowns, gloves, and instruments, and redrape the patient.

Incision and Elevation of Skin Flaps

Position the patient so the arm is abducted 90° on an arm board and place a folded sheet, about 5 cm thick, underneath the patient's scapula and posterior hemithorax. Prepare the area of the breast, upper abdomen, shoulder, and upper arm with an iodophor solution. Enclose the entire arm in a double layer of sterile orthopedic stockinette to maintain sterility of the entire extremity because the arm must be flexed during dissection of the upper axilla. We prefer to place a sterile Mayo instrument stand over the patient's head. It is used for extra hemostats and gauze pads for the assistant and it supports the patient's arm during the period of the operation that requires it to be flexed.

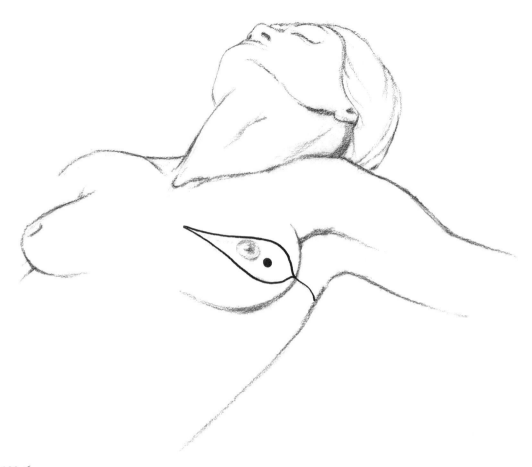

Fig. 100–6

Using a sterile marking pen, draw a circle 3 cm away from the perimeter of the primary tumor. Depending on the location of the tumor, mark the medial and lateral extensions of the incision as discussed above. In addition to the area of skin outlined by the circle drawn around the tumor, include the entire areola and nipple in the patch of skin left on the specimen (Fig. 100-1). If there is little or no risk of requiring a skin graft, make an elliptical incision **(Fig. 100–6)**. Then use a scalpel to make the incision through all layers of the skin. Attain hemostasis by applying electrocoagulation to each bleeding point.

Apply Adair clamps or rake retractors, about 2-3 cm apart, to the cut edge of the skin on the lower flap. Have the assistant elevate the skin flap by drawing the Adair clamps in an anterior direction. Apply countertraction by depressing the breast posteriorly. Then use the electrocautery set on a medium cutting current to incise Cooper's ligaments, which attach the subcutaneous tissues to the surface of the breast **(Fig. 100–7)**. Leave no visible breast tissue on the skin flap. When significant bleeding is encountered, simply switch to coagulating current to control the bleeding. This technique facilitates performing a mastectomy with minimal trauma and excellent hemostasis. Continue elevating the inferior skin flap until the dissection is beyond the breast. The medial margin for the dissection is the sternum. The lateral margin is the an-

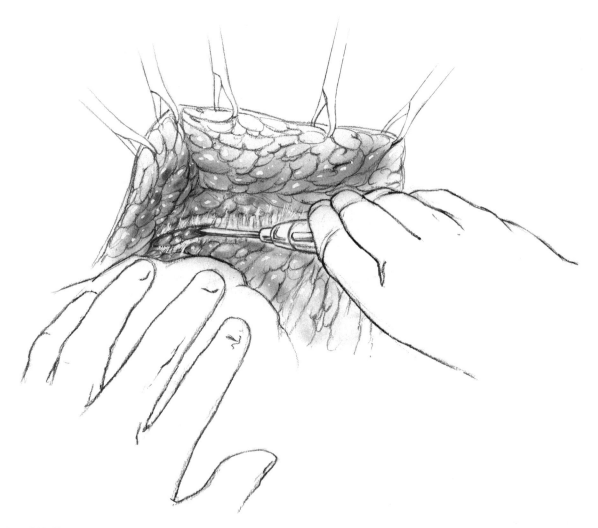

Fig. 100–7

terior border of the latissimus dorsi muscle, which is exposed for the first time during this phase of the operation. Apply a moist gauze pad to the operative site. Remove the Adair clamps from the lower skin flap and apply them now to the upper skin flap. Use the same technique to elevate the upper skin flap to a point about 3 cm below the clavicle. Whichever skin inci-

sion has been selected, it should permit wide exposure of the axillary contents from the clavicle to the point where the axillary vein crosses over the latissimus muscle. The final step in achieving exposure consists of clearing the fat from the anterior border of the latissimus muscle with a scalpel so the entire lateral margin of the dissection has been identified.

Clearing the Pectoral Fascia

After checking to ascertain that complete hemostasis has been achieved, use a scalpel to incise the fascia overlying the major pectoral muscle. Begin near the medial margin of this muscle and proceed with scalpel or electrocautery to dissect the fascia off the anterior surface of the major pectoral muscle from the sternum to the lateral margin **(Fig. 100–8)**. Simultaneous hemostasis is achieved if the first assistant electrocoagulates each of the branches of the mammary vessels as they are exposed or divided by the dissection. Whether using electrocautery or hemostats, exercise caution when pursuing a vessel that has retracted into the chest wall after being divided. We have on occasion, especially in thin patients, observed pneumothorax following this step. When the vessel is not easily controlled by electrocautery or a hemostat, simply apply a suture-ligature to control it.

When the lateral margin of the major pectoral muscle has been reached, use a combination of blunt and sharp dissection to elevate the edge of the pectoral muscle from its investing fascia. This maneuver maintains continuity between the breast, the pectoral fascia, and the lymph nodes of the axilla. If simple mastectomy is planned, terminate the dissection after removing the axillary tail of Spence.

Unroofing the Axillary Vein

Use a Richardson retractor to elevate the major pectoral muscle. Identify the minor pectoral muscle **(Fig. 100–9)**. Branches of the medial pectoral nerve are seen lateral to the origin of the minor pectoral muscle. They may be divided without serious consequence, but be sure to identify and preserve the major branch of the lateral pectoral nerve that emerges just *medial* to the origin of the minor pectoral muscle and travels along the undersurface of

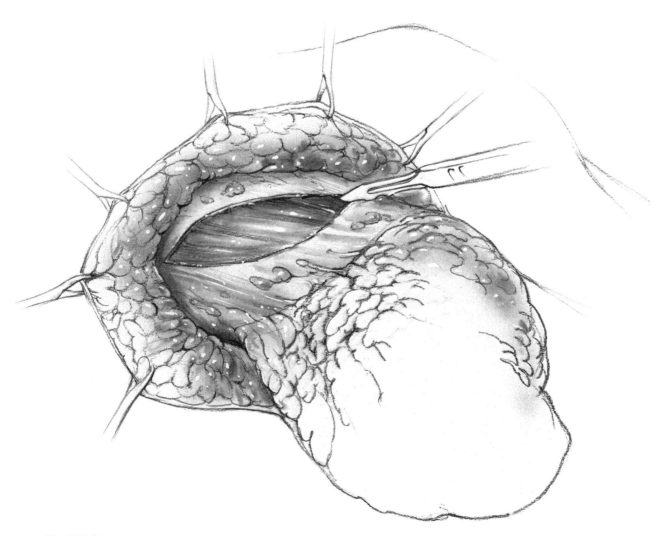

Fig. 100–8

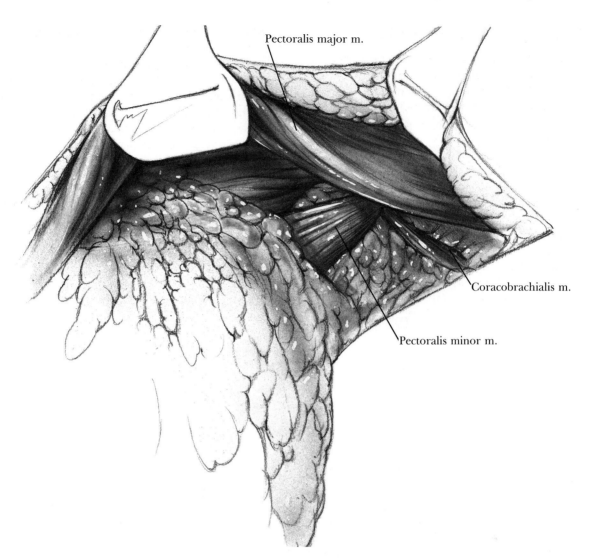

Pectoralis major m.

Coracobrachialis m.

Pectoralis minor m.

Fig. 100–9

the major pectoral muscle. Division of this nerve
may result in atrophy and contraction of the major
pectoral muscle. Dissect the fat and fascia off the an-
teroinferior edge of the coracobrachialis muscle using a scalpel. Directly inferior to this muscle is the
brachial plexus and the axillary vessels. Continuing
the dissection of the inferior border of the coracobrachialis in a medial direction leads to the coracoid
process, upon which the minor pectoral muscle inserts. Divide the minor pectoral muscle near its insertion using the electrocoagulator **(Fig. 100–10)**.
If you do not wish to excise level 3 lymph nodes,
do not divide the minor pectoral muscle; simply free
its posterior attachments and elevate it with a
Richardson retractor. Free up enough of the divided
muscle to provide complete exposure of the axillary
vein. Deep to the point where the minor pectoral
muscle was divided is a well defined fat pad overlying the junction of the cephalic and axillary veins.

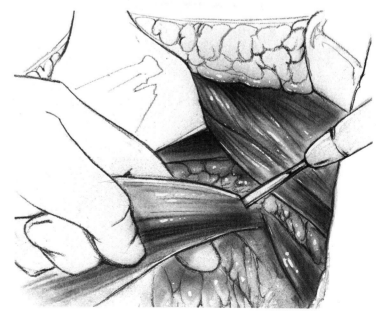

Fig. 100–10

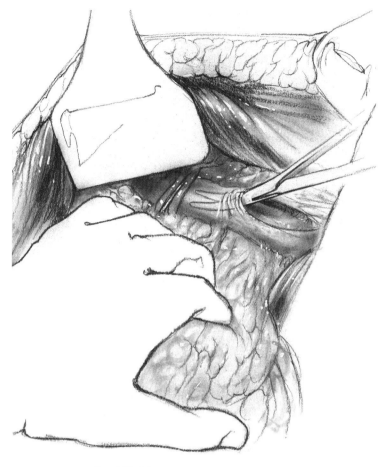

Fig. 100-11

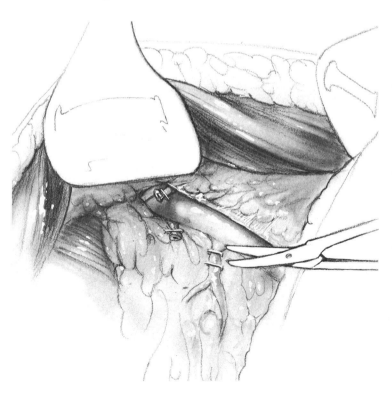

Fig. 100-12

Gentle blunt dissection generally succeeds in elevating this fat pad and drawing it in a caudal direction to expose the anterior surface of the axillary vein.

Now incise the adventitial sheath of the axillary vein **(Fig. 100–11)**. Although light dissection with the belly of the scalpel can accomplish this, most surgeons prefer to use Metzenbaum scissors. A few branches of the lateral anterior thoracic artery, vein, and nerve cross over the anterior wall of the axillary vein. Divide these branches between hemostatic clips. To complete division of the sheath of the axillary vein from the region of the latissimus muscle to the clavicle, it is necessary to flex the upper arm. This relaxes the major pectoral muscle, which is then elevated with a Richardson retractor.

Axillary Vein Dissection

Axillary lymphadenectomy aims at removing all of the lymph glands inferior to the axillary vein (levels I–III). Only when these glands are replaced by metastases does tumor spread to the nodes cephalad to the axillary vein and to the neck. Not only is it unnecessary to strip all of the fat from the brachial plexus, this maneuver produces lifelong painful neuritis in some patients.

Identify all the branches entering the axillary vein from below. Clear each of the branches of adventitia and divide each between hemoclips **(Fig. 100–12)**. Do not divide the subscapular vein, which enters the axillary vein from behind.

At this point it is essential to label the apex and the lateral margin of the axillary specimen. Many pathologists prefer that a third label be attached at the point where the minor pectoral muscle crosses the axillary specimen.

The upper boundary of the axillary dissection is the crossing of the clavicle over the axillary vein. Detach the lymphatic and areolar tissue at this point with the electrocoagulator. Now make a scalpel incision in the clavipectoral fascia on a line parallel to and 1 cm below the axillary vein. Do not retract the axillary vein in a cephalad direction, as it might expose the underlying axillary artery to injury during this step. If suspicious nodal tissue is identified cephalad to the axillary neurovascular bundle, biopsy it to document the extent of disease.

Dissect the areolar and lymphatic tissues off the intercostal muscles and ribs going from medial to lateral. When the minor pectoral muscle is encountered, divide it 2–3 cm from its origin with the electrocoagulator **(Fig. 100–13)** and leave the excised muscle attached to the specimen. If this muscle was not divided earlier in the operation, it is not necessary to resect it. Restore the arm to its previous position of 90° abduction. As the chest wall is cleared laterally, one or two intercostobrachial nerves are seen emerging from the intercostal muscle on their way to innervate the skin of the upper inner arm. Because these nerves penetrate the specimen, divide them even though it results in a sensory deficit in the upper inner arm **(Fig. 100–14)**. Use a sterile gauze pad to wipe the loose fat out of the subscapular space going from above downward. This maneuver exposes the long thoracic nerve that runs along the rib cage in the anterior axillary line in a vertical direction from above downward to innervate the anterior serratus muscle. The thoracodorsal nerve can be identified as it leaves the area of the subscapular vein and runs both laterally and downward together with the thoracodorsal artery and vein to innervate the latissimus dorsi muscle. Because these two nerves run close to the peripheral boundary of the dissection, they should be preserved when no metastatic lymph nodes are seen in their vicinity.

Detach the lymphatic tissue inferior to the portion of the axillary vein that crosses over the latissimus muscle. Preserving the long thoracic nerve is complicated by the fact that a number of small veins cross over the nerve in its distal portion. Circumvent this difficulty by moving the partly detached breast

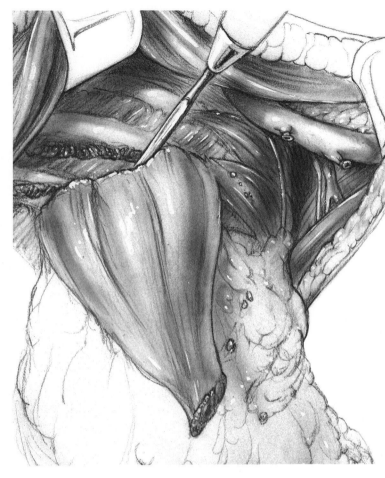

Fig. 100-13

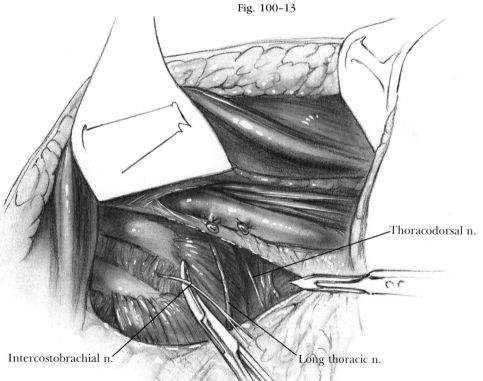

Intercostobrachial n.

Thoracodorsal n.

Long thoracic n.

Fig. 100–14

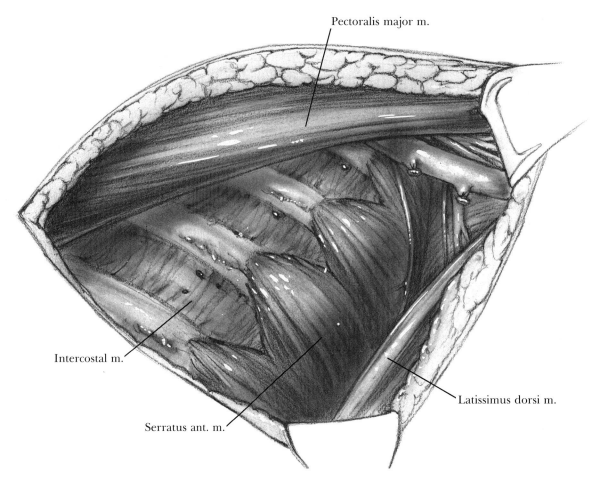

Pectoralis major m.

Intercostal m.

Latissimus dorsi m.

Serratus ant. m.

Fig. 100–15

in a medial direction so it rests on the patient's chest after freeing the specimen from the anterior border of the latissimus muscle. Then make an incision in the fascia of the serratus muscle 1 cm medial to the long thoracic nerve. Dissecting this fascia a few centimeters in a medial direction detaches the entire specimen from the chest wall **(Fig. 100–15)**.

Irrigation and Closure

Thoroughly irrigate the operative field. We use sterile water, which lyses not only clot and blood, making it easier to spot small bleeders, but also any spilled tumor cells that may have been dispersed into the operative field. Check the entire field to be sure *complete* hemostasis has been achieved.

Insert two large closed-suction drains through puncture wounds into the lower axilla. Bring one catheter deep to the axillary vein and the other catheter across the thoracic wall from the puncture wound to the region of the sternum. Suture each catheter to the skin at the site of the puncture wounds and attach to closed-suction drainage **(Fig. 100–16)**.

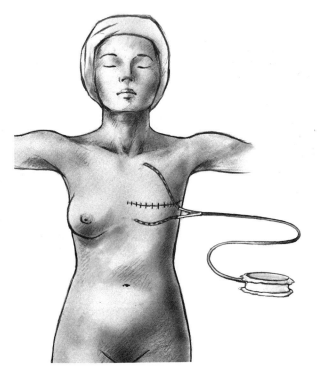

Fig. 100-16

Close the skin with subcuticular PDS, interrupted fine nylon sutures, or skin staples. Be certain there is no significant tension on the incision; otherwise postoperative necrosis of the skin flap may be anticipated. Often shifting the skin flaps in a medial or lateral direction relieves tension. Do not permit either of the skin flaps at the lateral margin of the incision to become bunched up in such a fashion that a "dog-ear" forms. Many patients are convinced that this represents residual tumor. The "dog-ear" deformity can be eliminated by excising a triangular wedge of skin as noted in Figures 100–3 and 100–5. When closed-suction drainage is used postoperatively, it is not necessary to apply a bulky pressure dressing.

POSTOPERATIVE CARE

Leave the two closed-suction drainage catheters in place until the daily drainage diminishes to 30–40 ml/day or about 7 days.

Encourage early ambulation but do not permit the patient to abduct the arm on the side of the operation for 5–7 days, as this activity prevents the skin flaps from adhering to the chest wall and encourages prolonged drainage of serum. Permit the patient to use this arm for ordinary activities not requiring abduction. We use a standardized series of graded physical exercises to ensure that the woman regains full mobility. Physical therapy is helpful in some cases.

Take appropriate steps throughout postoperative treatment to ensure the patient's emotional and physical rehabilitation.

Do not remove the skin staples or sutures for 2 weeks because the operation has separated the skin flaps from much of their blood supply, slowing the rate of healing.

Aspirate any significant collections of serum underneath the skin flaps with a sterile syringe and needle as necessary.

Refer the patient for adjuvant chemotherapy or for participation in one of many clinical trials.

Follow the patient for local recurrence or the development of cancer in the opposite breast.

Once the initial period of close follow-up is completed, we follow these patients annually for life.

Carefully inspect the arm for the development of lymphedema, which can become a disabling complication if not detected and treated early. Warn the patient to avoid trauma, including sunburn, to the arm and forearm of the operated side. If at any time the hand is traumatized or there is any evidence of infection in the hand or arm, prompt treatment with antibiotics (dicloxacillin) for 7–10 days, followed by application of a specially fitted elastic sleeve of the Jobst type, may prevent the development of permanent arm edema.

POSTOPERATIVE COMPLICATIONS

Ischemia of skin flap. This is a serious, partially preventable complication. Minimize its risk by avoiding tension on the suture line and excessive devascularization of the skin flaps. When ischemia is permitted to develop into gangrene of the skin, a process that takes 2 weeks or more, some degree of cellulitis invariably follows. This process occludes many residual collateral lymphatic channels through which the lymph fluid from the arm manages to return to the general circulation. Blocking these channels increases the incidence and severity of permanent lymphedema of the arm. Consequently, skin necrosis should be anticipated when purple discoloration appears in the skin flap on the 5th or 6th day following mastectomy. If this purple discoloration cannot be blanched by finger pressure, it represents devitalization of the skin; it is not cyanosis.

Once this skin change has been observed, the patient should be returned promptly to the operating room. With local anesthesia, excise the devitalized skin and replace it with a skin graft. At this early date infection has not yet ensued, and primary healing of the skin graft may be anticipated. This prompt action eliminates damage to the collateral lymphatic channels and weeks of morbidity. It is, of course, far preferable to prevent skin necrosis in the first place by utilizing a skin graft during the primary operation whenever excessive tension is observed during skin closure.

Wound infection. Wound infection is uncommon in the absence of skin necrosis.

Seromas. Collections of serum underneath the skin flap, seromas occur during the first few weeks following mastectomy when the skin flap has failed to adhere to the chest wall. This problem appears more commonly in obese patients. Treatment consists of aspirating the serum every 3–5 days. On rare occasions this process continues for several months. In such a case, it is preferable to make an incision under local anesthesia and insert a drain. Repeated aspiration over many weeks may result in infection of the seroma.

Lymphedema. Lymphedema of the arm is more common in obese patients, in those who have undergone axillary radiotherapy, and in those who have experienced skin necrosis, wound infection, or cellulitis of the arm. Treat cellulitis of the arm promptly with antibiotics. Lymphedema in the absence of any sign of infection is treated as soon as it is detected by applying a Jobst elastic sleeve, which applies a pressure of 50 mm Hg to the forearm and arm. These sleeves should be changed whenever they lose their elasticity, generally after 6 weeks. This treatment should be instituted whenever one detects an increase in circumference of the arm of 2 cm or more. Generally, elastic compression keeps the condition under control if it has not been long neglected. Once the edema has been permitted to remain for many months, subcutaneous fibrosis replaces the edema and makes it irreversible. Intermittent pneumatic compression has been recommended, but few patients tolerate the intermittent compression for the many hours a day necessary before significant progress is demonstrated with long-standing edema. Prompt treatment of the hand or arm with antibiotics and early application of elastic compression is helpful for preventing and controlling edema.

REFERENCES

Carlson GW, Bostwick J III, Styblo TM, et al. Skin-sparing mastectomy: oncologic and reconstructive considerations. Ann Surg 1997;225:570.

Hidalgo DA. Aesthetic refinement in breast reconstruction: complete skin-sparing mastectomy with autogenous tissue transfer. Plast Reconstr Surg 1998;102:63.

Kroll SS, Khoo A, Singletary SE, et al. Local recurrence risk after skin-sparing and conventional mastectomy: a 6 year followup. Plast Reconstr Surg 1999;104:421.

Margolese RG. Surgical considerations for invasive breast cancer. Surg Clin North Am 1999;79:1031.

Slavin AS, Schnitt SJ, Duda RB, et al. Skin-sparing mastectomy and immediate reconstruction: oncologic risks and aesthetic results in patients with early-stage breast cancer. Plast Reconstr Surg 1998;102:49.

101 Radical Mastectomy

Surgical Legacy Technique

INDICATIONS

Radical mastectomy is occasionally useful in highly selected patients for local control of advanced disease.

PREOPERATIVE PREPARATION

Same as for modified radical mastectomy (see Chapter 100)

PITFALLS AND DANGER POINTS

These are the same as for the modified radical mastectomy operation (see Chapter 100).

Pneumothorax may be produced by perforation in the chest cavity during attempts to control branches of the internal mammary artery.

OPERATIVE STRATEGY

After elevating the skin flaps by the usual technique, radical mastectomy can be accomplished in one of two sequences. With the technique described below, axillary lymphadenectomy precedes removal of the breast from the chest wall. It is also feasible to remove the breast and the major pectoral muscle from the chest wall prior to doing the axillary dissection, as described for modified radical mastectomy. Proponents of the latter sequence believe that it reduces the incidence of tumor emboli caused by traction applied to the specimen. When the breast is removed proceeding from medial to lateral, gravity provides sufficient retraction. No data are available comparing these two sequences, so the choice is based on personal preference.

OPERATIVE TECHNIQUE

Incision

The principles underlying the choice of incision for radical mastectomy **(Fig. 101–1)** are the same as those for modified radical mastectomy. Adequate ex-

cision of advanced disease may necessitate that considerable skin be excised and the resulting defect closed by a split-thickness skin graft.

Elevation of Skin Flaps

The same technique as for modified radical mastectomy is used to elevate the skin flaps (see Chapter 100).

Exposing the Axilla

To perform a complete axillary lymphadenectomy, it is not necessary to remove the portion of the major pectoral muscle that arises from the clavicle. Preservation of the clavicular head of this muscle im-

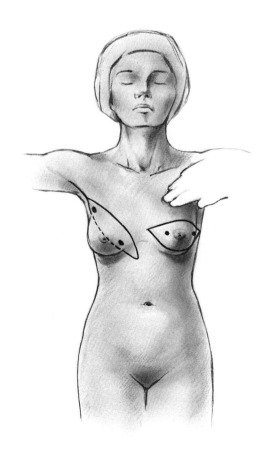

Fig. 101-1

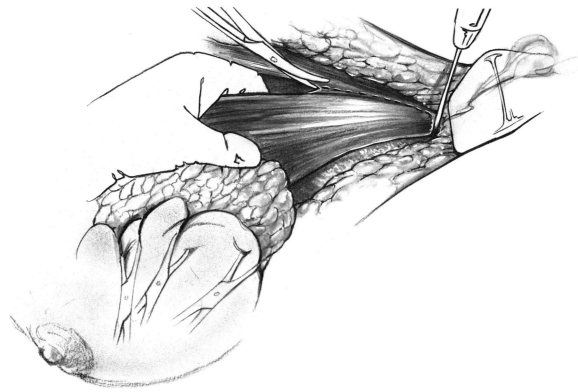

Fig. 101-2

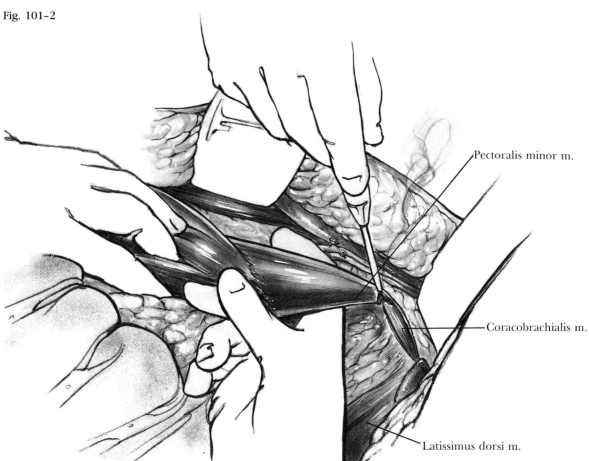

Pectoralis minor m.

Coracobrachialis m.

Latissimus dorsi m.

Fig. 101-3

proves the cosmetic appearance of the upper chest wall. Consequently, develop a line of separation by blunt dissection between the sternal and clavicular heads of the pectoral muscle. Continue this separation to the point where the major pectoral muscle inserts on the humerus. Place the left index finger underneath the sternal head of the muscle near its insertion and divide the muscle from its insertion with electrocoagulating current **(Fig. 101–2)**. Complete the line of division between the two heads of the muscle proceeding in a medial direction until the sternum is reached. A number of lateral anterior thoracic arteries, veins, and nerves are divided between hemoclips during this dissection. Also detach the upper 2-3 cm of the major pectoral muscle from the upper sternum.

Incise the areolar tissue and fascia over the surface of the coracobrachial muscle and continue in a medial direction until the coracoid process is reached. This move exposes the junction between the coracobrachial muscle and the insertion of the minor pectoral muscle **(Fig. 101–3)**. Just caudal to the coracobrachial muscle are the structures con-

tained in the axilla: the brachial plexus and the axillary artery and vein. They are covered not only by fat and lymphatic tissue but by a thin layer of costocoracoid fascia. Clearing the fascia away from the inferior border of the coracobrachial muscle serves to unroof the axilla and expose the insertion of the minor pectoral muscle. Detach this muscle from its insertion after isolating it by encircling it with the index finger; use the coagulating current to divide the muscle near the coracoid process (Fig. 101-3). A pad of fat overlying the axillary vein near the entrance of the cephalic branch can be swept downward by blunt dissection, exposing the axillary vein.

Dissecting the Axillary Vein

It is not necessary to clean the fat off the brachial plexus or to remove tissue cephalad to the axillary vein. Pick up the sheath of the axillary vein with Brown-Adson or DeBakey forceps and use Metzenbaum scissors to separate the adventitia from the underlying vein **(Fig. 101–4)**. Once the unopened scis-

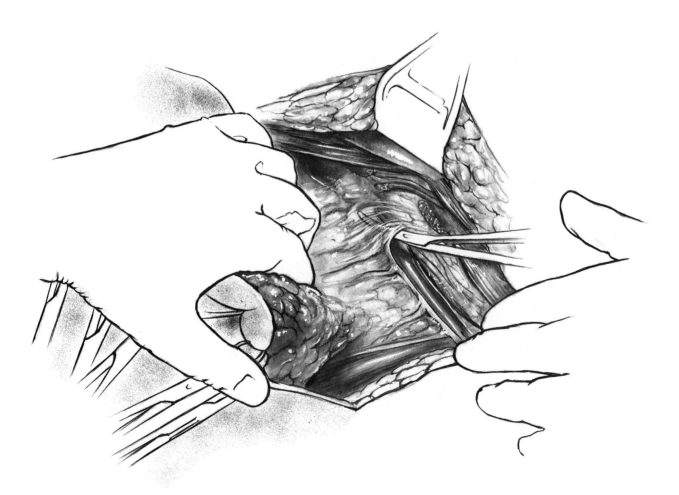

Fig. 101-4

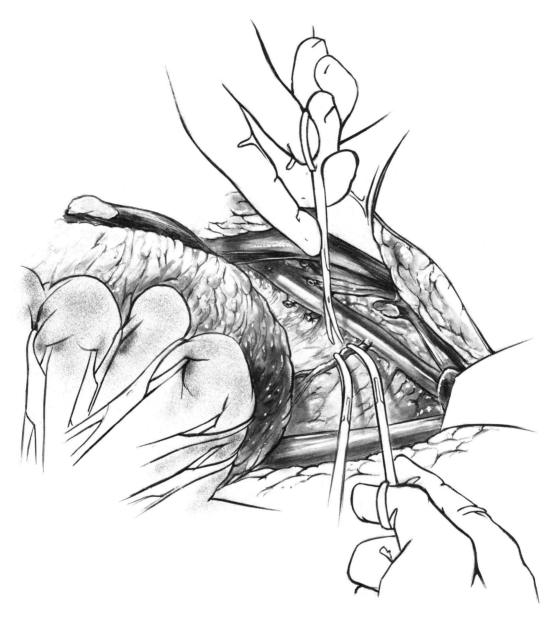

Fig. 101–5

sors have been inserted underneath the adventitia to establish the plane, remove the scissors and insert one blade of the scissors under this tissue. Close the scissors, dividing the adventitia. Continue this dissection along the anterior wall of the axillary vein from the region of the latissimus muscle to the clavicle. The only structures crossing anterior to the axillary vein are some thoracoacromial, lateral anterior thoracic, and pectoral blood vessels and nerves. Divide these structures between ligatures or hemoclips. At the conclusion of this step, the branches of the axillary vein have been fairly well skeletonized. Now divide each of the branches of the axillary vein

that comes from below using hemoclips or 3-0 PG ligatures **(Fig. 101–5)**. At this point use silk sutures to apply labels to mark the apex and the lateral portion of the lymphadenectomy specimen.

Dissecting the Chest Wall

Make a scalpel incision through the clavipectoral fascia just inferior to the medial portion of the axillary vein **(Fig. 101–6)**. This maneuver clears fat and lymphatic tissue from the upper chest wall. Continue this dissection laterally until the subscapular space has been reached; then clear the areolar tissue from

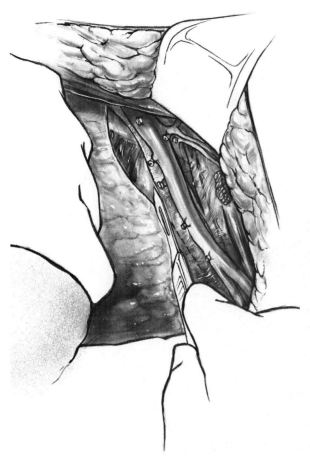

Fig. 101-6

the subscapular space using a gauze pad, bluntly dissecting from above downward. This maneuver reveals the location of the long thoracic nerve descending from the brachial plexus in apposition to the lateral aspect of the thoracic cage. Preserve this nerve. Identify the thoracodorsal nerve that crosses the subscapular vein and travels 2–3 cm laterally together with the artery and vein supplying the latissimus dorsi muscle **(Fig. 101–7)**. In the absence of obvious lymph node metastases in this area, dissect out the thoracodorsal nerve down to its junction with the latissimus dorsi muscle.

If the anterior border of the latissimus muscle has not yet been thoroughly exposed, complete this maneuver now. The entire lymphadenectomy specimen should be freed from the axillary vein, the upper anterior chest wall, and the anterior border of the latissimus muscle.

Detaching the Specimen

Keeping the long thoracic nerve in view, make an incision in the fascia of the anterior serratus muscle on a line parallel to and 1 cm medial to this nerve. Elevate the fascia by dissecting in a medial direction, exposing the underlying muscle until the interdigitations of the pectoral muscles are encountered

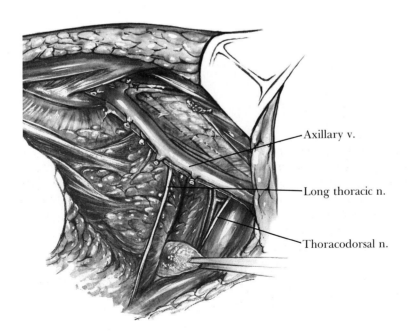

Axillary v.

Long thoracic n.

Thoracodorsal n.

Fig. 101-7

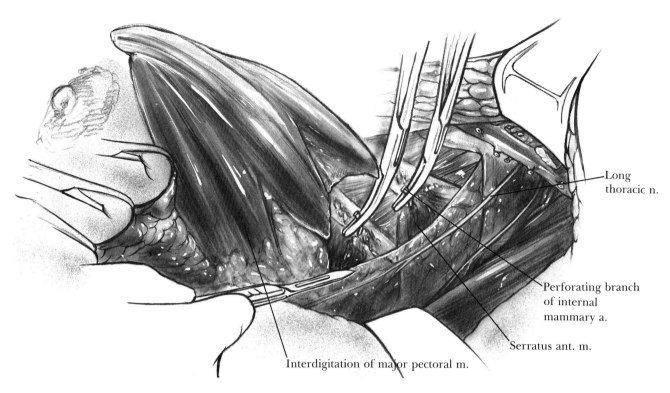

Long
thoracic n.

Perforating branch
of internal
mammary a.

Serratus ant. m.

Interdigitation of major pectoral m.

Fig. 101-8

(Fig. 101–8). Detach the pectoral muscles from their points of origin with electrocautery. Apply a small hemostat to each bleeding vessel. Try to avoid including any extraneous tissue in the hemostat other than the blood vessel. If this is accomplished, each of the blood vessels on the chest wall may be occluded by applying the coagulating current to each hemostat at the conclusion of the dissection. As the pectoral muscles are divided, leave about 0.5 cm of muscle tissue on the rib cage, as it facilitates applying hemostats to the perforating branches of the internal mammary vessel. If these are divided

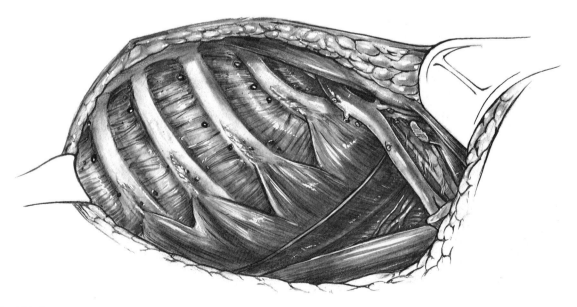

Fig. 101-9

flush with their point of emergence from the chest wall, they often retract into the chest, which makes hemostasis difficult and increases the risk of pneumothorax.

Continue the retraction medially in the direction of the pectoral muscles and the attached breast, proceeding until all of the internal mammary branches have been clamped and divided and the dissection has been completed at the border of the sternum. Remove the specimen and electrocoagulate each of the vessels. Ascertain that hemostasis is complete. Irrigate the entire operative field with sterile water in an attempt to wash out detached tissue and malignant cells **(Fig. 101–9)**.

Closure of Incision and Insertion of Drains

Closure and drainage procedures are the same as for the Patey operation **(Fig. 101–10)**.

Full-Thickness Skin Graft

Whenever an area of excessive tension is encountered while closing the skin wound by suturing, leave this portion of the incision unsutured. Measure the defect and determine if there is sufficient re-

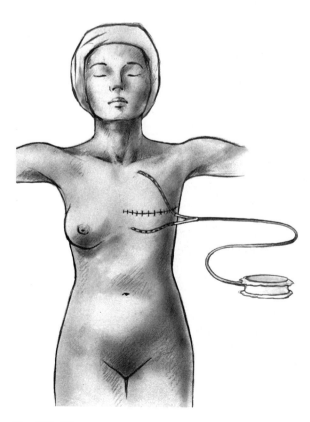

Fig. 101–10

dundant skin in other areas of the skin flaps that may be excised, defatted, and transplanted into the defect. To expedite the defatting of skin to be grafted, it is helpful to pin one edge of the skin patch down to a sterile board. Then grasp the fat with the forceps and use a large scalpel blade to dissect all of the fat off the skin. Sometimes a few remaining bits of fat are excised with curved Metzenbaum scissors. When a patch of skin has been sufficiently defatted to convert it into a full-thickness graft, the undersurface of the skin assumes a characteristic pitted appearance. Place the full-thickness skin graft into the defect and tailor its dimensions so there is mild tension on the graft after it is sutured into place.

First suture the edges of the skin down to the chest wall musculature with interrupted 3-0 silk: About six such sutures can stabilize the perimeter of the defect. Then insert a continuous over-and-over suture of atraumatic 5-0 nylon to attach the skin graft to the edges of the skin defect using small bites. Skin staples comprise another good method for fixing the graft in place.

Make multiple puncture wounds in the skin graft with a No. 10 scalpel blade to permit seepage of serum from the wound through the graft. Apply a single layer of iodophor gauze over the skin graft, and over this layer place a small mass of gauze fluffs. Tie the long ends of the previously placed silk sutures over the gauze stent to fix the skin graft in position with some pressure.

This step may be accelerated by omitting sutures entirely and fixing the skin graft in place with Steri-Strip adhesive tapes or skin staples. The gauze fluffs are then taped into place over the graft.

Split-Thickness Skin Graft

When there is no surplus of skin on the chest wall to be harvested for a skin graft, use a dermatome to obtain a split-thickness graft from the anterolateral portion of the upper thigh. After this area has been cleansed with soap and an iodophor solution has been applied, dry the area and apply a sterile lubricating solution of mineral oil. Have the assistants then stretch the skin by applying traction in opposite directions with wooden tongue depressors. Set the dermatome so the graft is 0.015 inch thick. Apply the dermatome to the surface of the skin with firm pressure and activate it. Maintain firm, even pressure while moving the dermatome cephalad. It may be helpful for the scrub nurse to pick up the cut edge of the graft with two forceps while the surgeon continues to operate the dermatome until an adequate patch of skin has been obtained. Place the skin graft in a normal saline solution temporarily. Apply a moist laparotomy pad to the donor site.

Dress the donor site with a semipermeable plastic adhesive skin covering followed by a dry sterile dressing. Suture the skin graft into the defect as described above.

POSTOPERATIVE CARE

Unless there are signs of infection, leave the gauze stent from the skin graft in place for 5-7 days. Afterward, leave the graft exposed or cover it with a loose, dry dressing.

Remove the gauze dressing from the donor site the day after surgery, but leave the plastic dressing intact until the site is healed (1-2 weeks). If blood or serum accumulates under the plastic dressing, aspirate it with a small sterile needle. This method of treating donor sites significantly reduces pain.

See also Chapter 100.

COMPLICATIONS

See Chapter 100.

With reference to the skin graft, complications include *infection* of the grafted area and occasionally of the donor site. *Failure of a complete "take"* is generally due to hematoma or serum collecting underneath the graft and separating it from its bed. It can be prevented by careful hemostasis at the time of surgery and by making several perforations with a scalpel blade to permit seepage of serum.

REFERENCE

Bijker N, Rutgers EJ, Peterse JL, et al. Low risk of locoregional recurrence of primary breast carcinoma after treatment with a modification of the Halsted radical mastectomy and selective use of radiotherapy. Cancer 1999;85:1773.

Part XII
Lymph Nodes

102 Concepts in Lymphadenectomy

Stephen B. Edge

John F. Gibbs

Lymphadenectomy is most commonly performed for breast cancer, melanoma, gynecologic malignancies, and occasionally other cancers. The role of lymph node dissection is evolving with increased awareness of the systemic nature of many cancers, improved means of defining prognosis without node dissection, and improved and potentially less toxic systemic therapies. In most situations, lymph node dissection provides important prognostic information and affects the choice of adjuvant systemic therapy. In general, lymph node surgery is "therapeutic" only in cases where there is clinically evident disease in the nodes. The therapeutic benefit is the prevention of painful, bulky cancer growth in the node basin. For breast cancer with clinically negative nodes, the data overwhelmingly indicate that node dissection has no impact on survival from breast cancer. For melanoma, there may be specific circumstances where node dissection improves survival.

The principles of lymph node surgery are the same regardless of the disease and the area dissected. Lymph node-bearing tissue within defined anatomic boundaries is removed, and the pathologist searches the tissue to identify individual nodes for histologic examination. The anatomic boundaries of the dissection may vary depending on the cancer type, affected node basin, and the extent of node involvement.

Lymph node dissection is generally a safe operation. In both axilla and groin, injury to cutaneous nerves leads to transient or permanent numbness and paresthesias. This is particularly disturbing after axillary dissection with numbness on the inner and posterior portion of the upper arm. There is also risk of injury to the motor nerves innervating the serratus anterior and latissimus dorsi muscles. Injury to the long thoracic nerve causes instability of the shoulder girdle, with protrusion, or "winging," of the scapula.

The most significant complication of lymph node dissection is interruption of a portion of the lymphatic flow from the extremity. This leaves the extremity at risk of developing swelling called lymph-edema. This occurs in a mild form in up to 30–40% of patients and is severe in 10–20%. It is more common and severe in the lower extremity. Lymph-edema may develop soon after surgery, or it may appear after many years. The risk of lymphedema of the upper extremity may be minimized by efforts to minimize skeletonization of the axillary vein during surgery. However, the patient who has undergone node dissection is at lifelong risk of developing lymph-edema. Once it occurs, lymphedema is permanent. Therapy includes manual lymphatic drainage and the use of compression garments that help reduce the degree of edema.

An alternative to surgery to determine lymph node status without the morbidity of complete dissection would be attractive. Nonsurgical techniques that have been studied include anatomic imaging with ultrasonography, computed tomography, magnetic resonance imaging, and functional imaging including fluorodeoxyglucose positron emission tomography and sestamibi nuclear imaging. None of these techniques provides sufficient sensitivity or specificity, and surgery remains the only accurate method for identifying the presence of node metastases.

A surgical alternative to complete dissection of the nodes is mapping the specific drainage pattern from a given cancer to identify the specific first node or nodes to which the cancer spreads. Mapping the lymphatic drainage from a cancer has been used for years to define the nodal drainage of melanoma. Most commonly used for truncal melanomas, lymphoscintigraphy with radiolabeled colloids can determine if a melanoma in a watershed area between nodal basins drains to the axilla, the groin, or both. Morton and colleagues in Los Angeles proposed that lymphatic mapping could identify the first node or nodes in the drainage basin, the so-called sentinel nodes [1]. The concept is that if these sentinel nodes do not contain cancer the entire nodal basin is free of node metastases, making removal of the remaining nodes unnecessary. First proposed and validated in melanoma patients, sentinel lymph node biopsy

(SLNB) has been tested and has proved highly accurate in breast cancer patients. It is being investigated for gastrointestinal cancers, head and neck tumors, and gynecologic malignancies [2]. SLNB reduces the short- and long-term risks of lymph node surgery [3].

The technique for SLNB includes preoperatively injecting a colloidal material around the melanoma, in breast tissue around the cancer, or at a prior biopsy site. The axillary or inguinal space is then explored for lymph nodes to which the colloid has traveled by following the blue tracks to blue-stained nodes using a hand-held gamma detector to find nodes concentrating the radiolabeled colloid, or both. Only these nodes are removed for pathologic examination. The colloids used are the colloidal dye isosulfan blue and radiolabeled colloids. The most widely tested radiolabeled colloid is technetium 99m (^{99m}Tc) sulfur colloid. Infrequently epitrochlear and popliteal nodal basins require dissection for melanoma. Additionally, update of the radiocolloid may occur at in-transit sites requiring resection.

The indications for lymph node surgery and the factors that may change these indications in the future in breast cancer and melanoma are discussed below.

BREAST CANCER

In general, full axillary dissection is the best treatment for clinically involved nodes. The need for axillary surgery with clinically negative nodes is influenced by the risk of node metastases and the extent to which nodal status influences the choice of adjuvant systemic therapy. With clinically negative nodes, the risk of cancer recurrence in the axilla is low even without axillary dissection. In one series of 92 cases treated with standard breast tangential radiation without axillary dissection, there was no axillary recurrence [4]. Although the evidence is overwhelming that axillary lymph node dissection does not itself improve survival from breast cancer, axillary lymph node status is the single most important prognostic factor. Axillary staging remains a key element of breast cancer treatment [5].

Axillary dissection entails removing the axillary contents in so-called levels I and II (excluding the tissue medial to the minor pectoral muscle). The number of nodes harvested by a level I/II dissection depends on the extent of surgery and the diligence of the pathologist in identifying nodes (average 15 nodes). If fewer than 10 lymph nodes are regularly obtained in an axillary dissection specimen, the techniques of the surgeon and pathologist should be reviewed.

Sentinel lymph node biopsy has proved highly accurate in breast cancer patients [2]. Overall, a sentinel node is identified in more than 90% of cases. There is a risk of a false-negative sentinel node (defined as the number of patients with a negative sentinel node among those with any positive axillary node) ranging in reports from 0% to 15% (average 5%). It appears that the rate of false-negative SLNBs is lower with increased surgeon experience. Most experts believe the false-negative rate with sentinel nodes is low enough to accept the report of a negative sentinel node and omit full axillary dissection.

The issues of SLNB are being addressed by two large-scale national clinical trials that opened in 1999 addressing the role of SLNB in breast cancer [6]. The NSABP B-32 trial randomized women with clinically negative nodes between axillary node dissection and SLNB without dissection to determine if there is any survival advantage to axillary dissection. The American College of Surgeons Oncology Group (ACOSOG) Z0010 and Z0011 trials are testing whether axillary dissection is necessary for women with a positive sentinel node by randomizing women with a positive sentinel node to complete dissection or no further surgery.

The use of axillary surgery in specific clinical situations for women with clinically negative nodes is discussed below.

Ductal carcinoma in situ (DCIS). With DCIS, the incidence of node involvement is extremely low ($\leq 1\%$). Lesions with positive nodes are generally larger and likely to be high grade or have comedo histology; and they probably harbor a component of invasive cancer that was not present or recognized on the pathology sections. The long-term survival of women with DCIS is excellent regardless of grade and histologic subtype. High grade and comedo histology are not themselves indications for axillary surgery. There is generally no indication for axillary dissection with DCIS.

It is appropriate to include low axillary nodes when mastectomy is necessary for DCIS because these nodes are entwined with the breast tissue in the axillary tail. The use of SLNB with mastectomy for DCIS is a questionable practice because mastectomy is required only for large and multicentric lesions for which sentinel mapping may be less accurate, and level I nodes are removed anyway.

Reports of SLNB with DCIS have demonstrated rates of node involvement as high as 8%. Most of these involved nodes contained micrometastases identified by cytokeratin immunohistochemistry (IH). The clinical significance of this finding is unknown. The use of SLNB with DCIS is investigational.

Microscopic invasion. Microinvasion (defined as invasive cancer <1 mm) may be identified in conjunction with DCIS. The incidence of node metastases with microinvasion is extremely low. It is not necessary to subject all women with microinvasion to axillary surgery and its complications.

T1a and T1b breast cancer (0.1–1.0 cm). For T1a and T1b cancer with clinically negative nodes, the rate of positive nodes is as high as 20%. No tumor factors can define a subset with such a low risk of node involvement as to preclude axillary staging [7]. With negative nodes, the risk of subsequent distant metastases without systemic therapy for tumors <1 cm is less than 10%, and there is little benefit to chemotherapy. If the nodes are positive, the risk of distant disease may be 50% or more, and chemotherapy should be considered as for any woman with stage II disease. Therefore it is for tumors 0.1–1.0 cm that axillary staging has the most impact on the choice of adjuvant therapy and axillary staging is generally indicated.

T1c (1.1–2.0 cm) and T2 (2.1–5.0) cancers. The incidence of positive nodes is 20–30% with T1c cancer and higher with T2 lesions. The risk of distant metastases is 30–40% even with negative nodes. Hence chemotherapy is usually administered, especially to young patients. More intensive chemotherapy may be used if nodes are positive (e.g., addition of a taxane). Therefore axillary staging is generally performed with T1c and T2 cancers.

Older women. Almost half of the women with breast cancer are over age 65. Breast cancer treatment should not be limited simply because of age, as healthy older women have an excellent life expectancy. However, it is reasonable to consider age when making treatment decisions. The major purpose of axillary staging is to assist with the choice of adjuvant systemic therapy. Although chemotherapy is generally well tolerated by women in their seventies, the proportional reduction in the risk of recurrence from chemotherapy is lower for older women than for young women. Adding chemotherapy to tamoxifen in older women may provide only minimal benefit. Many women age 70+ choose tamoxifen alone and omit chemotherapy even with positive nodes. If the nodes are not removed, there is a risk of axillary recurrence, but it is quite low. In one large series of women over age 70 with T1 and T2 cancer treated with excision plus tamoxifen without irradiation or axillary dissection, the rate of axillary failure and death from breast cancer was 5% at 7 years [8]. Defining a specific age where axillary staging can be omitted is difficult, but omitting axillary surgery with small tumors is a reasonable practice in older women with clinically negative nodes in situations where node status does not affect the choice of adjuvant therapy.

Serious co-morbid conditions. Axillary surgery may be omitted if life expectancy is shortened by serious co-morbid conditions or when the use of chemotherapy is limited by other illnesses.

OTHER ISSUES IN AXILLARY SURGERY FOR BREAST CANCER

Indications for Use of Sentinel Node Biopsy

The SLNB is appropriate for invasive cancer with clinically negative nodes in the hands of an experienced sentinel node surgeon and team. SLNB is not appropriate with clinically positive nodes. Most authors recommend full axillary dissection with larger T2 lesions because the incidence of node metastases is 40% or more and the accuracy of sentinel node mapping may be lower with a large tumor. SLNB is generally not performed with mastectomy because the latter includes the level I nodes and it is usually performed for large or multicentric cancers. If mastectomy is performed for small cancers because of patient choice (e.g., in women with inherited susceptibility who choose mastectomy), SLNB may be reasonable.

Extent of Axillary Dissection

In general, axillary dissection is limited to levels I and II. The risk of node involvement in level III (nodal tissue medial to the minor pectoral muscle) is low in the absence of clinically apparent involvement at levels I and II. Performing a level III dissection may require division of the insertion of the minor pectoral muscle from the coracoid process and may increase the long-term risk of lymphedema. Level III dissection is usually performed only when there is clinically apparent node disease.

Axillary Irradiation

Irradiation of the axilla may be used to supplement or in place of axillary surgery. For clinically involved nodes, irradiation controls the local disease in 60–80% of cases without surgery and may be appropriate in women with co-morbidity that precludes surgery or in those with metastatic disease. Radiation to the axilla and supraclavicular fossa may be warranted after axillary dissection in patients with extensive lymph node involvement. Irradiation itself may cause lymphedema. Axillary or supraclavicular irradiation alone can cause lymphedema. The combination of irradiation and axillary dissection markedly increases the risk of lymphedema. Axillary irradiation should not be used after a negative SLNB.

Internal Mammary Node Biopsy

In a small number of cases lymphatic drainage of the breast is to the ipsilateral internal mammary chain. Although internal mammary node dissection was abandoned during the 1970s, the presence of internal mammary node metastases probably has the same prognostic significance as axillary metastases. SLNB has led to renewed interest in internal mammary node staging. Lymphoscintigraphy and intraoperative mapping with the gamma detector can identify drainage to the internal mammary chain. If internal mammary drainage is identified during SLNB, an incision can be made over the appropriate interspace and the sentinel node removed with minimal morbidity. This is an appropriate practice in experienced hands.

Bone Marrow Aspiration as a Prognostic Factor to Replace Axillary Surgery

Bone marrow micrometastases are present at the time of diagnosis in many women with early-stage breast cancer. An increasing literature suggests that bone marrow micrometastasis is a more powerful independent prognostic factor than lymph node involvement [9]. It is possible in the future that bone marrow aspiration to detect micrometastases will be used routinely to complement or even replace axillary surgery for staging breast cancer. Bone marrow aspiration is currently under evaluation as part of the ACOSOG Z0010 trial of the sentinel node biopsy.

MELANOMA

Regional lymph node status remains the most powerful predictor of outcome in patients with melanoma [10]. In addition, lymphadenectomy in the regional nodal basin draining the site of the primary tumor may improve locoregional control and prolong survival. Lymphadenectomy in these nodal basins is a therapeutic lymph node dissection (TLND) for clinically evident disease and elective lymph node dissection (ELND) with clinically negative nodes.

A cloud of controversy has surrounded the importance of early detection of nodal micrometastasis. The prognosis of patients with micrometastatic nodal involvement is distinctly different from that of patients with gross nodal disease, with 5-year survivals averaging 50–60% versus 15–20%, respectively [11]. The benefit of ELND has not been proven in prospective randomized trials outside of controversial subsets of patients. A multiinstitutional prospective randomized trial showed no difference in overall survival for patients with intermediate-thickness melanoma (1–4 mm) who underwent excision alone compared to those who underwent excision plus ELND [12]. A recent update of this trial demon-

strated a possible trend in 10-year overall survival (ELND 77%, nodal observation 73%; $p = 0.12$) [13].

The SLNB has been demonstrated to be a simple, minimally invasive, accurate method by which to diagnose microscopic regional metastases in patients without clinically palpable disease [14]. The SLNB allows physicians to apply regional lymphadenectomy more selectively and to avoid potential long-term morbidity associated with the procedure in patients who prove not to harbor regional disease. A number of important issues regarding the use of SLNB and the management of lymph node disease with melanoma are discussed below.

Indications for SLNB

Indications for SLNB with primary cutaneous melanoma are Breslow thickness of >1 mm, lesions < 1 mm with invasion of the reticular dermis to Clark's level IV, or lesions exhibiting known poor prognostic indicators such as regression, ulceration, or lymphovascular space invasion. Patients with microscopic disease identified by SLNB generally undergo completion nodal dissection, resulting in selective lymph node dissection (SLND) only for those with nodal involvement. A low rate of regional failure after SLNB with SLND has been observed, supporting the accuracy of the sentinel node technique for predicting the status of the regional nodal basin [15]. Although any survival advantage has been argued to be secondary to lead time bias, identification of patients with micrometastases may also allow a more rational application of emerging adjuvant biologic therapies. Several multicenter trials are evaluating these and other aspects of the role of sentinel lymph node biopsy in melanoma.

Pathologic Assessment of the Sentinel Node

The permanent hematoxylin and eosin (H&E) section is considered to be the gold standard for pathologic evaluation of the lymph nodes. H&E evaluation is highly sensitive when the lymph node is prepared with multiple serial sections and examined by a pathologist experienced in diagnosing malignant melanoma. However, a 14–29% false-negative incidence has been demonstrated when only H&E sections are examined. Immunohistochemical (IH) analysis with S-100 and HMB-45 may detect small foci of malignant melanoma within the sentinel lymph node not noted initially on H&E sections. However, these small deposits of malignant melanoma can usually be identified on the initial H&E sections retrospectively. Therefore it is recommended that routine assessment of the sentinel node in melanoma patients include H&E on six to eight levels of each sentinel node, supplemented by IH with S-100 with or without HMB45 on all H&E-negative SLNBs [16].

Frozen Section

Because of the difficulty assessing melanoma on frozen section and the need for multilevel sectioning and IH, frozen section analysis of the sentinel lymph node to detect small metastatic deposits in the hope of proceeding with a SLND under one anesthetic has not proved useful [16]. We evaluated the accuracy of intraoperative frozen sections compared to permanent H&E sections, deeper H&E sections, and IH. Of 69 patients (20%) treated at Roswell Park Cancer Institute, 14 were found to have positive SLNs. Seventy-nine percent of patients in our series had melanoma micrometastatic deposits measuring < 2 mm. Only six patients were diagnosed with positive or suspicious SLNs by original frozen section analysis.

Molecular Diagnostics for Sentinel Node Evaluation

Examination of the sentinel node by the polymerase chain reaction (PCR) reverse transcription (RT) of tyrosinase or other melanoma-associated antigens may improve detection of lymph node metastases. There is preliminary evidence suggesting that the risk of recurrence is higher for patients with nodes with RT-PCR-only detected disease compared to negative nodes [17]. Molecular analysis of the SLN must be viewed as investigational and complementary to complete architectural evaluation with permanent H&E sections and IH.

Nodal Failure after Lymphadenectomy

The melanoma recurrence rate in a previously dissected lymph node basin ranges from 9% to 52% [18]. The risk of recurrence is related to the burden of disease in the initially dissected lymph node station. It is higher with palpable adenopathy, multiple involved nodes, and extranodal or extracapsular disease. It is clear that the biology of the melanoma, not the extent of the surgical procedure, governs outcome. We reviewed our 26-year experience with regional lymphadenectomy for melanoma in a surgical population that did not undergo postoperative irradiation to evaluate risk factors for nodal failure in patients who initially displayed microscopic lymph node involvement or palpable lymph node metastases [19]. Of 2,455 patients, 338 (14%) were found to have nodal metastases following ELND ($n = 85$) or TLND ($n = 253$) for malignant melanoma. The most important factors associated with nodal recur-

rence were the number of positive nodes, gross versus microscopic disease, and the presence of extranodal extension.

The prognosis of patients who suffer a recurrence in a previously dissected basin is poor. Eighty-seven percent of patients who relapsed regionally had synchronous metastatic disease or developed metastatic disease on follow-up [19]. This translated to a 10-year disease-specific survival of 10% for those whose lesion recurred compared to 45% for those whose lesion did not. Only 8 of 84 patients (10%) who developed isolated nodal recurrence without evidence of distant disease were amenable to re-resection. A local surgical approach may be warranted in patients with combined systemic and bulky regional disease to prevent difficult wound management problems, patient discomfort, or bleeding.

Adjuvant Radiotherapy

Despite the significant incidence of regional failure after node dissection for melanoma, few studies have addressed alternative or adjunctive means to improve regional control. Because of the dismal prognosis associated with nodal basin failure, attempts to prevent initial failure should be prioritized [20]. Adjuvant radiation therapy has been shown in single institution trials to achieve nodal basin control in 87–95% of patients. The addition of radiation therapy, however, has failed to translate into a survival advantage. The National Comprehensive Cancer Network recommends the use of irradiation in high-risk patients (those with multiple involved nodes or extranodal disease, especially in the head and neck region [21].

Current Recommendations

Every attempt should be made to control nodal disease accompanying malignant melanoma when it is microscopic. Therefore lymphatic mapping and SLNB is indicated for most patients with primary melanoma, with TLND for those with positive nodes by H&E or IH. Adjuvant radiation therapy should be considered for patients with four or more positive nodes or extra capsule extension (ECE) because the consequences of nodal recurrence are severe.

SENTINEL LYMPH NODE DISSECTION FOR OTHER MALIGNANCIES

Regional nodal metastasis for many solid organ cancers has significant prognostic implications. Traditionally, regional nodal dissection has been recommended for staging the extent of disease, and it provides regional tumor control. Information concerning micrometastases in clinically uninvolved lymph nodes may have additional diagnostic and therapeutic value for other solid organ malignancies as well. Sentinel lymph node dissection has been reported for solid tumors including nonmelanoma cutaneous malignancies, thyroid cancer, colorectal cancer, penile carcinoma, and vulva cancer [22].

Although regional nodal dissection to identify the SLN can be easily performed, peritumoral injection of the primary site with vital blue dye (e.g., 1% isosulfan blue) or a radiopharmaceutical agent (e.g., technetium 99-sulfur colloid) alone or in combination must be defined for each malignancy. Peritumoral injection into the dermis of epithelial cancers (e.g., Merkel cell, penile carcinoma, vulva cancer), the adjacent parenchyma for breast cancer, or intratumorally for thyroid cancer illustrates this point. In addition, peritumoral injection of the gastrointestinal tract (e.g., esophageal or colorectal cancers) with isosulfan blue is performed through the serosa into the submucosa. We have applied this technique to hepatic malignancies [23]. Subcapsular injection of isosulfan blue dye in the segment of the liver harboring the tumor has allowed us to identify nonpredicted periportal draining lymph nodes. Although sentinel lymph dissection is technically feasible for other solid organ tumors, the implications of micrometastases must be defined.

REFERENCES

1. Morton DL, Wen DR, Wong JH, et al. Technical details of intraoperative lymphatic mapping for early stage melanoma. Arch Surg 1992;127:392.

2. Ollila DW, Brennan MB, Giuliano AE. The role of intraoperative lymphatic mapping and sentinel lymphadenectomy in the management of patients with breast cancer. Adv Surg 1999;32:349.

3. Schrenk P, Rieger R, Shamiyeh A, et al. Morbidity following sentinel lymph node biopsy versus axillary lymph node dissection for patients with breast carcinoma. Cancer 2000;88:608.

4. Wong JS, Recht A, Beard CJ, et al. Treatment outcome after tangential radiation therapy without axillary dissection in patients with early-stage breast cancer and clinically negative axillary nodes. Int J Radiat Oncol Biol Phys 1997;39:915.

5. Recht A, Houlihan MJ. Axillary lymph nodes and breast cancer: a review. Cancer 1995;76:1491.

6. Edge SB, Hurd TC. Sentinel node update: breast cancer. Oncology 1999;13:11A.

7. Gann PH, Colilla SA, Gapstur SM, et al. Factors associated with axillary lymph node metastasis from breast carcinoma: descriptive and predictive analysis. Cancer 1999;86:1511.

8. Martelli G, DePalo G, Rossi N, et al. Long-term follow-up of elderly patients with operable breast cancer treated with surgery without axillary dissection plus adjuvant tamoxifen. Br J Cancer 1995;72:1251.

9. Braun S, Pantel K, Muller P, et al. Cytokeratin-positive cells in the bone marrow and survival of patients with stage I, II or III breast cancer. N Engl J Med 2000;342:525.

10. Coit DG, Rogatko A, Brennan MF. Prognostic factors in patients with melanoma metastatic to axillary or inguinal lymph nodes: a multivariate analysis. Ann Surg 1991;214:627.

11. Reintgen D. Melanoma nodal mets: biologic significance and therapeutic considerations. Surg Oncol Clin North Am 1995;5:104.

12. Balch CM, Soong SJ, Bartolucci AA, et al. Efficacy of an elective regional lymph node dissection of 1 to 4 mm thick melanomas for patients 60 years of age and younger. Ann Surg 1996;224:25.

13. Balch CM, Soong SJ, Ross MI, et al. Long term results of a multi-institutional randomized trial comparing prognostic factor and surgical results for intermediate thickness melanomas (1.0 to 4.0 mm). Ann Surg Oncol 2000;7:87.

14. Sabel MS, Gibbs JF, Cheney R, et al. Evolution of sentinel lymph node biopsy for melanoma at an NCI designated cancer center. Surgery 2000;128:556.

15. Gershenwald JE, Colome MI, Lee JE, et al. Patterns of recurrence following a negative sentinel lymph node biopsy in 243 patients with stage I or II melanoma. J Clin Oncol 1998;16:2253.

16. Gibbs JE, Huang PP, Zhang PJ, Kraybill WG, Cheney R. Accuracy of pathologic techniques for the diagnosis of metastatic melanoma in sentinel lymph nodes. Ann Surg Oncol 1999;6:699.

17. Shivers SC, Wang W, Li W, et al. Molecular staging of malignant melanoma: correlation with clinical outcome. JAMA 1998;280:1410.

18. Gadd MA, Coit DG. Recurrence patterns and outcome in 1019 patients undergoing axillary or inguinal lymphadenectomy for melanoma. Arch Surg 1992;127:1412.

19. Pidhorecky I, Lee RJ, Kollmorgen DR, et al. Risk factors for nodal recurrence after lymphadenectomy for melanoma. Ann Surg Oncol (in press).

20. Lee RJ, Gibbs JF, Proulx GM, et al. Nodal basin recurrence following lymph node dissection for melanoma: implications for adjuvant radiotherapy. Int J Radiat Oncol Biol Phys 2000;46:467.

21. Houghton A, Coit D, Bloomer W, et al. NCCN melanoma practice guidelines: National Comprehensive Cancer Network. Oncology 1998;12(7A):153.

22. Haigh PI, Giuliano AE. A critical evaluation of sentinel lymph node dissection in malignancy. Principles Practice Oncol Updates 2000;14:1.

23. Kahlenberg MS, Kane JM, Kanter PM, et al. Hepatic lymphatic mapping: a pilot study for sentinel node identification. Cancer Invest (in press).

103 Axillary Lymphadenectomy

INDICATIONS

After lumpectomy for breast cancer (see Chapter 99), axillary lymphadenectomy indicated for therapy and staging

Malignant melanoma (see Chapter 102)

Palpable lymph node metastases from other primary malignancies involving the skin of the upper extremity and shoulder, breast, and upper trunk

PREOPERATIVE PREPARATION

Obtain a positive biopsy for malignancy.

Perform staging studies such as computed tomography (CT) of the chest or abdomen, as indicated for the particular malignancy.

PITFALLS AND DANGER POINTS

Nerve injury (lateral pectoral, long thoracic, or thoracodorsal nerve; brachial plexus)

Injury to axillary vein

OPERATIVE STRATEGY

Fundamentally, axillary lymphadenectomy employs the same strategy as that used for the modified radical mastectomy. Adipose and lymphatic tissues inferior to the axillary vein are excised en bloc from the clavicle to the anterior border of the latissimus muscle. Adequate exposure requires that the arm be flexed on the trunk to relax the major pectoral muscle during the medial part of the dissection. The levels of the axilla from level I (the lowest) to level III (the highest) are discussed in Chapter 100. Optimal access to level III nodes requires division and sometimes even removal of the minor pectoral muscle. The long thoracic and thoracodorsal nerves may be preserved if they are not involved with tumor.

OPERATIVE TECHNIQUE

See Chapter 100.

Incision

The skin incision, in a general way, follows the course of the axillary vein. Start the incision at the lateral border of the major pectoral muscle and continue laterally across the axilla to the level of the latissimus muscle. The line of the incision is shown in **Figure 103–1**. Frequently the incision can be made much shorter and confined to the area directly below the hair-bearing area of the axilla. An alternate skin incision, preferred by some surgeons, can be made parallel to the edge of the major pectoral muscle and slightly lateral to it. Elevate both the superior and inferior skin flaps, leaving no more than 8 mm of fat on the skin over the area indicated by the dotted lines in Figure 103-1. The superior dissection exposes the anterior surface of the major pectoral muscle in its medial aspect, the fat overlying the axillary vein and brachial plexus in the middle, and the coracobrachialis and latissimus muscles

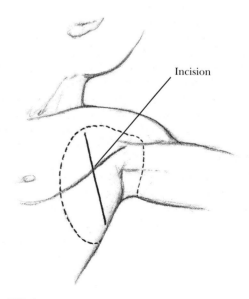

Incision

Fig. 103-1

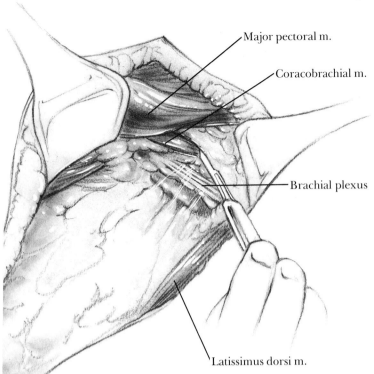

Major pectoral m.

Coracobrachial m.

Brachial plexus

Latissimus dorsi m.

Fig. 103–2

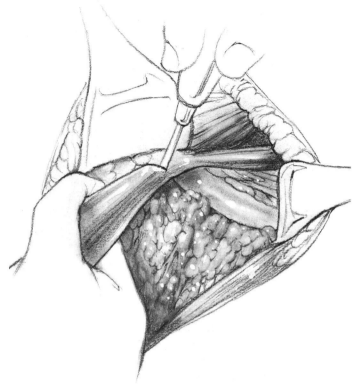

Fig. 103–3

laterally **(Fig. 103–2)**. Dissect the lower flap for a distance of 8 cm.

Exposing the Axillary Contents

Incise the fascia overlying the lateral border of the major pectoral muscle, and dissect it away from the undersurface of the muscle. Insert a Richardson retractor underneath the pectoral muscle and expose the coracobrachial muscle. Dissect fat and fascia off the inferior surface of the coracobrachial muscle and continue this dissection toward the coracoid process where the coracobrachial meets the minor pectoral muscle. Encircle the minor pectoral muscle with the index finger and divide it near its insertion using electrocautery **(Fig. 103–3)** if level III lymph nodes are to be excised. Branches of the medial pectoral nerve are seen entering the minor pectoral muscle near its *lateral* border. Divide these nerves, but take care to *protect the pectoral nerve, which emerges along the medial margin of the minor pectoral muscle* because this nerve largely constitutes the innervation of the major pectoral muscle. Freeing the minor pectoral muscle from the chest wall improves exposure for the axillary dissection. Incise the fat along the anterior border of the latissimus muscle to identify the lateral boundary of the lymphadenectomy.

Incise the thin layer of costocoracoid ligament at a level calculated to be just cephalad to the course

of axillary vein. Do not skeletonize the nerves of the brachial plexus as it may produce a permanent painful neuritis. After dividing this ligament, sweeping the loose fat in a caudal direction generally exposes the axillary vein.

Clearing the Axillary Vein

Identify the axillary vein in the lateral portion of the axilla. Elevate its adventitia with a Brown-Adson or DeBakey forceps and incise it with Metzenbaum scis-

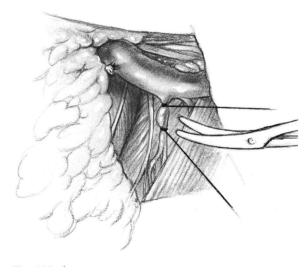

Fig. 103–4

sors. Continue this division of the adventitia in a medial direction until the clavicle is reached. Several branches of the lateral anterior thoracic and thoracoacromial nerves and blood vessels are encountered crossing over the axillary vein. Divide each between hemostatic clips.

Dissect the adventitia in a caudal direction exposing the various branches of the axillary vein coming from below. Divide and ligate or clip each of the branches that enters the axillary vein on its inferior surface **(Fig. 103–4)**. Preserve the subscapular vein, which enters the posterior wall of the axillary vein.

Dissecting the Chest Wall

Incise the clavipectoral fascia on a line parallel and just caudal to the axillary vein beginning at the level of the clavicle and continuing to the subscapular space. Suture a label to the lymph nodes at the apex of the dissection (near the clavicle). Make a vertical incision in the fascia from the apex of the dissection downward for 4-6 cm parallel to the sternum. Now sweep the lymphatic and adipose tissue, leaving its proximal half attached to the thorax. Divide the intercostobrachial nerve that emerges from the second intercostal space and enters the specimen. At this point in the dissection the anterior and inferior portions of the axillary vein have been cleared along the upper 6-10 cm of the anterior chest wall.

Subscapular Space

In the subscapular space, use a gauze pad to dissect the loose fat and areolar tissue bluntly from above downward to clear the space between the scapula and the lateral chest wall. This step exposes the long thoracic nerve, which tends to hug the thoracic cage. Identify the thoracodorsal nerve, which crosses the subscapular vein and moves laterally together with the vessels supplying the latissimus muscle **(Fig. 103–5)**.

If the anterior border of latissimus muscle was not dissected free during the first step in this operation, liberate this muscle now, preserving the thoracodorsal nerve. Dissect the specimen free of the chest wall after dissecting out and preserving the long thoracic nerve. Label the lateral margin of the lymph node dissection to orient the pathologist.

Drainage and Closure

Make a puncture wound in the anterior axillary line about 10 cm below the armpit and pass a closed-suction catheter into the apex of the axillary dissection near the point where the axillary vein goes under the clavicle. It may be necessary to suture the catheter in place with fine absorbable suture material.

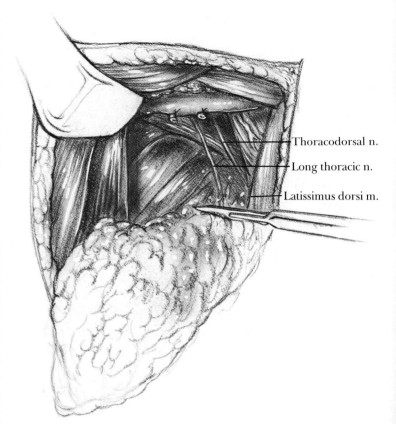

Thoracodorsal n.
Long thoracic n.
Latissimus dorsi m.

Fig. 103-5

Close the skin incision with interrupted 4-0 nylon sutures or skin staples. Attach the catheter to a closed-suction drainage device **(Fig. 103–6)**.

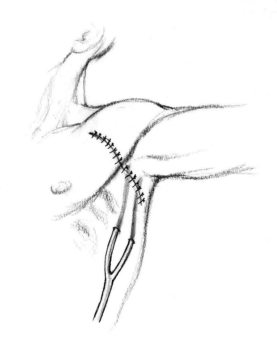

Fig. 103-6

POSTOPERATIVE CARE

Maintain suction on the catheter until the drainage is less than 30 ml/day, and then remove the catheter.

Limit abduction of the arm during the first postoperative week, but thereafter encourage the patient to exercise the shoulder joint through its entire range of motion.

Encourage the patient to achieve full ambulation on the day after the operation.

A seroma may develop under the skin flap later in the postoperative course. If so, aspirate the fluid once or twice weekly as necessary.

COMPLICATIONS

Hematoma or seroma

Wound infection

Lymphedema (see Chapter 100)

REFERENCES

Cox CE, Bass SS, Ku NN, et al. Sentinel lymphadenectomy: a safe answer to less axillary surgery? Recent Results Cancer Res 1998;152:170.

Luini A, Zurrida S, Galimberti V, Andreoni G. Axillary dissection in breast cancer. Crit Rev Oncol Hematol 1999; 30:63.

McNeil C. Endoscopy removal of axillary nodes gains ground abroad, toehold in U.S. J Nat Cancer Inst 1999; 91:582.

Moore MM, Nguyen DH, Spotnitz WD. Fibrin sealant reduces serous drainage and allows for earlier drain removal after axillary dissection: a randomized prospective trial. Am Surg 1997;63:97.

Reintgen DS, McCarty KS, Woodard B, et al. Metastatic malignant melanoma with an unknown primary. Surg Gynecol Obstet 1983;156:335.

Roses D, Harris M, Hidalgo D, et al. Primary melanoma thickness correlated with regional lymph node metastases. Arch Surg 1982;117:921.

104 Inguinal and Pelvic Lymphadenectomy

INDICATIONS

Metastatic involvement of inguinal lymph nodes secondary to malignant melanoma or epidermoid carcinoma of the skin of the lower extremity, lower trunk, or external genitalia (see Chapter 102)

PREOPERATIVE PREPARATION

Prescribe perioperative systemic antibiotics.

Prior to hospitalization, have the patient's lower extremity measured for a fitted elastic stocking to cover the area from the toes to the upper thigh (e.g., Jobst).

Evaluate the extent of disease (computed tomography, magnetic resonance imaging, position emission tomography).

PITFALLS AND DANGER POINTS

Impairing the viability of the skin flaps

Injuring the iliofemoral artery or vein

Injuring the femoral nerve and its branches

OPERATIVE STRATEGY

Preserving Skin Viability

Traditionally, surgeons have used a vertical elliptical incision centered on the femoral vessels and have emphasized wide dissection of thin skin flaps. This practice often leads to areas of necrosis in the dissected skin. Delayed healing by secondary intention then causes some degree of subacute cellulitis and occlusion of collateral lymphatic pathways, increasing the incidence or severity of postoperative lymphedema of the extremity.

It is not necessary to dissect the skin flaps beyond the confines of the femoral triangle. The less extensive the dissection, the less impairment there is of the blood supply to the skin flaps. A primarily oblique skin incision along the inguinal crease is less apt to cause loss of viability than is the vertical incision.

Extent of Lymphadenectomy

Two lymph node groups are accessible and may be removed during a groin dissection: inguinal and pelvic lymph nodes. The inguinal (or superficial) nodes are located in the femoral triangle based on the inguinal ligament, with its apex formed by the crossing of the adductor longus and the sartorius muscles. The pelvic (or deep) component of the dissection includes the lymph nodes in a triangular area whose apex is formed by the bifurcation of the common iliac artery and whose base is essentially the fascia over the obturator foramen. The extent of lymphadenectomy is determined by the nature of the pathology. For example, extensive involvement of the inguinal nodes by melanoma of the lower extremity is generally considered an indication to remove the pelvic nodes. In such a case, the dissection generally begins with the superficial component and then progresses more deeply.

Exposing the Iliac Region

When exposing the region of the iliac vessels for a pelvic lymphadenectomy, two approaches have commonly been employed. One involves vertical division of the inguinal ligament along the line of the iliofemoral vein with later resuturing of this ligament and the floor of the inguinal canal. In some patients this suture line is insecure, resulting in a hernia. Moreover, patients in whom this approach is employed appear to have an increased number of skin complications. An alternative approach to the pelvis for iliac lymphadenectomy is to place a second incision in the lower abdomen parallel to and about 3–4 cm cephalad to the inguinal ligament. After this incision has been carried through the transversalis fascia, the peritoneal sac is retracted upward to expose the iliac vessels and their adjacent fat and lymph nodes. Exposure by this approach is adequate, and closing the incision is simple.

OPERATIVE TECHNIQUE

Incision and Exposure

Position the lower extremity so the thigh is mildly abducted and flexed as well as being externally rotated. Support the leg in this position by a firm pillow or sandbag.

Start the incision 2-3 cm cephalad and medial to the anterosuperior spine of the ilium. Continue caudally to a point 1-2 cm below the inguinal crease. Continue along the inguinal crease in a medial direction until the femoral vein has been reached. At this point curve the incision gently in a caudal direction for about 5 cm, as noted in **Figure 104-1**. Elevate the cephalad skin flap with rake retractors. Use electrocautery with a low cutting current or a scalpel to dissect the skin flap in a superior direction in a plane that leaves 4-5 mm of subcutaneous fat on the skin. In obese patients we make the plane of dissection somewhat deeper than 4-5 mm. As the skin flap is dissected toward the outer margin of the operative field, increase the thickness of the flap in a tapered fashion so the base of the flap is thicker than its apex. The cephalad margin of the dissection should be 5-6 cm above the inguinal ligament. Now dissect the inferior skin flap in a similar fashion. Remember that it is not necessary to elevate this skin flap beyond the lower boundaries of the femoral triangle. The lateral boundary consists of the medial border of the sartorius muscle, and the lateral aspect of the adductor longus muscle is the medial boundary. The apex of the femoral triangle constitutes the point where the sartorious muscle meets the adductor longus. Dissecting the skin beyond the femoral triangle has no therapeutic value and may impair blood supply to the skin.

Exposing the Femoral Triangle

Initiate the dissection along a line parallel and 5-6 cm cephalad to the inguinal ligament. Incise the fat down to the aponeurosis of the external oblique muscle. Using a scalpel, dissect the abdominal fat off this aponeurosis down to and beyond the inguinal ligament. In men, identify and preserve the spermatic cord as it emerges from the external inguinal ring **(Fig. 104-2)**.

Use a scalpel or Metzenbaum scissors to incise the fat overlying the adductor longus muscle just below the inguinal ligament, about 2 cm medial to the pubic tubercle. Expose the muscle fibers of the adductor muscle and use a scalpel to dissect the fat and fascia down along the lateral boarder of this muscle. Continue the dissection along this muscle in a caudal direction to a point where the sartorius muscle crosses the lateral margin of the adductor longus muscle. Sweep the muscle fascia, fat, and lymph nodes in a medial direction **(Fig. 104-3)**. At the apex of the femoral triangle, identify, ligate, and divide the internal saphenous vein. Then incise the fascia overlying the sartorius muscle beginning at the apex of the femoral triangle and continuing in a cephalad direction up to the origin of the sartorius muscle at the iliac bone. Sweep the fat, lymphatic tissue, and fascia overlying the sartorius muscle by dissecting in a medial direction.

Dissecting the Femoral Artery, Vein, and Nerve

Identify the femoral artery and vein near the apex of the femoral triangle. Using Metzenbaum scissors dissection, elevate the areolar tissue and fat from the anterior surfaces of the femoral vessels proceeding in a cephalad direction (Fig. 104-3). Dissect the specimen from the medial border of the femoral triangle in a lateral direction to expose the medial aspect of the femoral vein. There are no branches on this side of the vein. Identify the entrance of the internal saphenous vein into the anterior surface of the femoral vein. Ligate and divide the saphenous vein. This dissection has exposed the pectineus muscle deep to the femoral vein and medial to the adductor

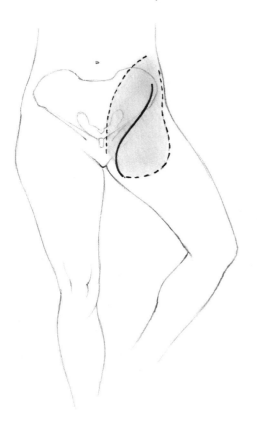

Fig. 104-1

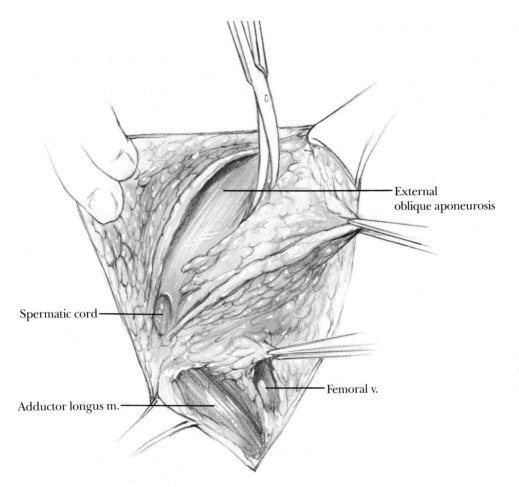

Fig. 104-2

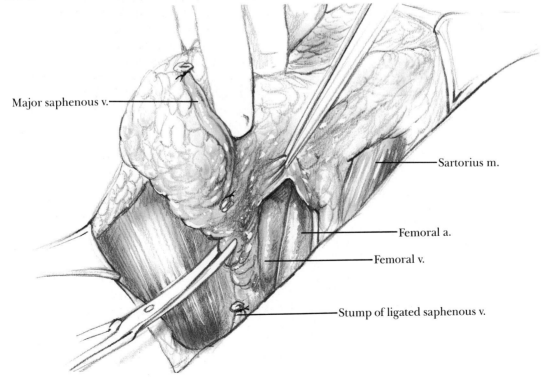

Fig. 104-3

longus muscle. The femoral canal is located deep to the inguinal ligament just medial to the femoral vein. Remove and identify the cephalad lymph node situated in this triangle, and label it for the pathologist. Continue to dissect the specimen laterally, exposing the length of the femoral artery. Several small arterial branches going to the specimen must be divided and ligated before the specimen can be separated from this vessel. Note that the femoral nerve, situated just lateral to the femoral artery, is covered by a thin fibrous layer of the femoral sheath. Carefully incise this layer at a point below the inguinal ligament and lateral to the femoral artery. Identify and preserve the branches of the femoral nerve as the nerve passes deep to the sartorius muscle. After this step, detach the specimen.

Irrigate the operative field and achieve complete hemostasis by means of PG ligatures and electro-

cautery. This step concludes the inguinal (superficial) groin dissection. The appearance of the operative field is illustrated in **Figure 104–4**.

Transposing Sartorius Muscle

Necrosis of the skin overlying the femoral vessels occurs in some patients and endangers the viability of these structures. To protect the femoral artery and vein from the consequences of a possible slough, transpose the sartorius muscle in a medial direction so it lies over the femoral vessels **(Fig. 104–5)**. Transect the sartorius muscle at its insertion with the electrocoagulating device **(Fig. 104–6)**. Free the proximal 6–7 cm of this muscle from underlying attachments and transpose it in a medial direction so it is now situated in a vertical line overlying the femoral vessels. Suture the cut end of the sartorius

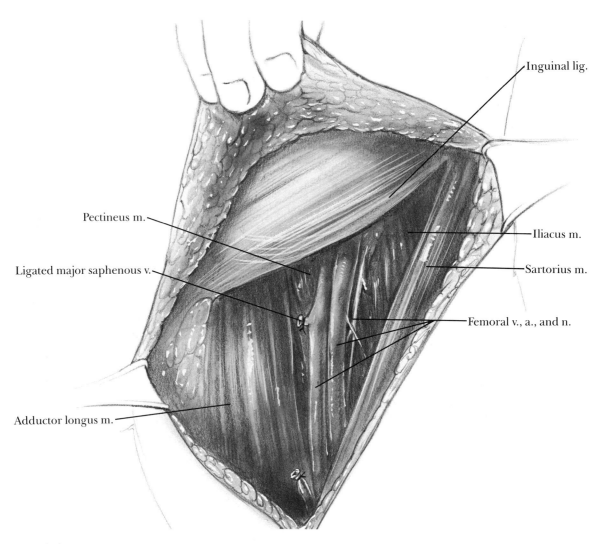

Pectineus m.

Ligated major saphenous v.

Adductor longus m.

Inguinal lig.

Iliacus m.

Sartorius m.

Femoral v., a., and n.

Fig. 104-4

muscle to the inguinal ligament using interrupted 3-0 Tevdek sutures **(Fig. 104–7)** prior to closing the skin.

Pelvic Lymphadenectomy

Make an incision with the scalpel in the direction of the fibers of the external oblique aponeurosis at a level about 3–4 cm above the inguinal ligament from the region above the external inguinal ring to the anterosuperior spine (Fig. 104-7). Divide the underlying internal oblique muscle with the electrocoagulator, carrying the incision through the transversus muscle together with the underlying transversalis fascia but not through the peritoneum. This procedure is similar to that used in Chapter 88 for the exposure required during a Cooper's ligament repair of an inguinal or femoral hernia. Identify the deep inferior epigastric artery and vein arising just above the inguinal ligament from the external iliac artery and vein. Ligate and divide the deep inferior epigastric vessels. Use gauze dissection to sweep the peritoneum together with the abdominal contents in a cephalad direction. Insert a moist gauze pad and a wide, deep retractor to elevate these structures out of the pelvic cavity. *Identify and preserve* the ureter, which generally remains adherent to the peritoneal layer and has been elevated together with the abdominal structures behind the retractor.

The area to be dissected is that contained between the external iliac and the internal iliac vessels

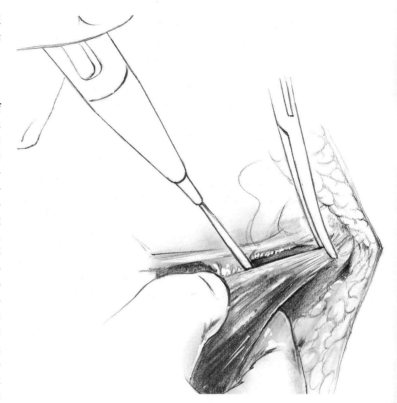

Fig. 104-6

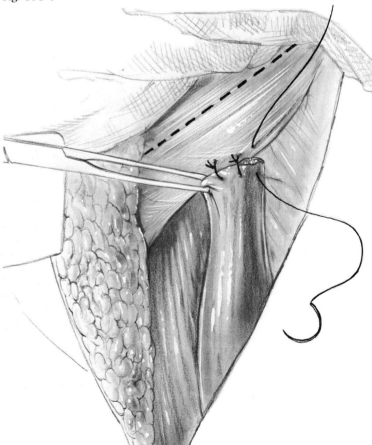

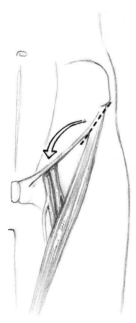

Fig. 104-5

Fig. 104-7

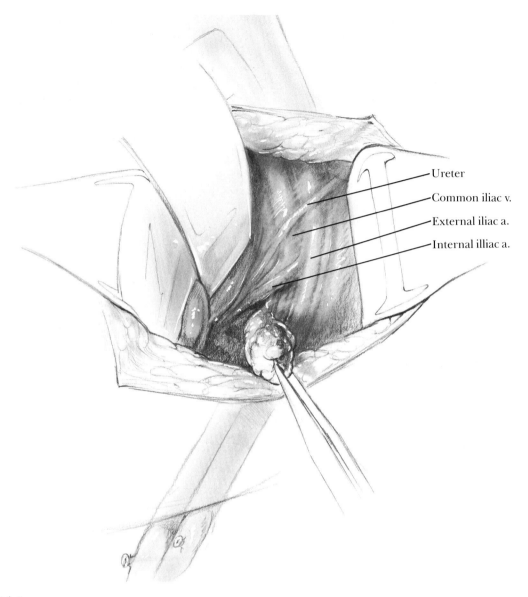

Ureter
Common iliac v.
External iliac a.
Internal illiac a.

Fig. 104–8

down to the obturator membrane overlying the obturator foramen **(Fig. 104–8)**. Initiate the mobilization by dissecting the lymph nodes and fat overlying the external iliac artery and vein beginning at the inguinal ligament and proceeding in a cephalad direction to the junction with the internal iliac vessels. Be careful when clearing fat and lymphatic tissue from the iliac vein, as this structure is quite fragile. Lacerations of the vein produce considerable hemorrhage that is difficult to control. After sweeping the fat and lymphatic tissues from the apex of the dissection in a downward direction, identify and preserve the obturator artery and vein. Terminate the dissection at this point and remove the specimen. Hemostasis is achieved during this dissection primarily by careful application of hemoclips and lig-

atures. After hemostasis is ensured, irrigate the pelvis with a dilute antibiotic solution.

Close the incision of the lower abdomen in layers by inserting interrupted 2-0 silk sutures into the transversalis fascia and the overlying aponeurosis of the transversus muscle, then into the internal oblique muscle, and finally into the external oblique aponeurosis. Close the defect in the femoral canal by suturing the inguinal ligament down to Cooper's ligament or the pectineus fascia from below. No drains are placed in the pelvis.

Skin Closure and Drainage

Drain the area of the femoral triangle by passing two perforated plastic catheters (3.0 mm in internal diameter) through puncture wounds in the area of the inguinal lymphadenectomy. Attach the catheters to a closed-suction drainage device. Irrigate the operative field again with a dilute antibiotic solution. Trim away any portion of the skin that seems devitalized. Close the skin with interrupted sutures of 4-0 nylon.

POSTOPERATIVE CARE

Prescribe perioperative antibiotics.

Continue closed-suction drainage until the volume is less than 40 ml/day.

In the operating room, apply the elastic stocking that was ordered preoperatively to fit this patient's lower extremity.

Keep the patient at bed rest with the extremity elevated for no more than 2–3 days. Thereafter, although patients are permitted to walk, they should spend only a short time sitting in a chair. Rather, much of the day should be spent in bed with the leg

elevated. After discharge from the hospital, patients should continue to wear a snug elastic stocking up to the upper thigh for at least 6 months. For the first 6–8 weeks they should lie down with the leg elevated for 1 hour three times daily; otherwise permanent lymphedema of the extremity is likely.

COMPLICATIONS

Skin necrosis is preventable if care is taken when preparing the skin flaps and if unnecessarily extensive dissection of the skin flaps is avoided.

REFERENCES

Karakousis CP. Therapeutic node dissections in malignant melanoma. Ann Surg Oncol 1998;5:473.

Pearlman NW, Robinsom WA, Dreiling LK, et al. Modified ilioinguinal node dissection for metastatic melanoma. Am J Surg 1995;170:647.

Part XIII
Head and Neck

105 Concepts in Head and Neck Surgery

Jade Hiramoto
Jeffrey A. Norton

PAROTID GLAND

Indications for Parotidectomy

Benign Neoplasms

Approximately 80% of parotid tumors are benign, the most common type being the pleomorphic adenoma [1]. Parotid neoplasms usually occur in the tail of the gland. Fine-needle aspiration (FNA) is the study of choice for diagnosis. Tumors are usually palpable, although ultrasonography may help with needle placement. Other imaging studies are not indicated for evaluating benign parotid tumors. Computed tomography (CT) and magnetic resonance imaging (MRI) are used when assessing malignant or recurrent neoplasms, large tumors, or those involving adjacent or deep structures.

Most pleomorphic adenomas (90%) are superficial to the facial nerve, and the rest are deep lobe tumors or parapharyngeal space tumors. Treatment requires complete excision with negative margins, as 30–50% of cases recur after simple enucleation. Tumors superficial to the facial nerve require superficial parotidectomy. Those posterior to the nerve are resected after superficial parotidectomy and identification of the facial nerve.

Warthin's tumor, or papillary cystadenoma lymphomatosum, is the second most common benign parotid tumor (6–10% of all parotid tumors). They most commonly occur in men and are associated with tobacco smoking and exposure to ionizing radiation. The tumor usually occurs in the tail of the parotid gland. Approximately 10% are bilateral. Malignant degeneration is rare. The surgical treatment is complete excision by enucleation or superficial parotidectomy.

Malignant Neoplasms

Most malignant parotid tumors occur during the fifth and sixth decades of life. Like benign tumors, malignant tumors usually present as a painless slow-growing mass. The presence of pain, facial nerve involvement, or fixation of the mass to adjacent structures indicates a more advanced stage with a worse prognosis. FNA is the initial step in the evaluation, followed by CT or MRI if the lesion is large or involves the deep lobe.

Mucoepidermoid carcinoma is the most common malignant tumor of the parotid gland (15% of parotid tumors) [2]. Treatment consists of superficial parotidectomy with preservation of the facial nerve unless it is directly involved. Other malignant neoplasms, including adenoid cystic carcinoma, malignant mixed tumor, acinic cell carcinoma, and adenocarcinoma, require superficial parotidectomy. Total parotidectomy is reserved for tumors emanating from the deep lobe, superficial lobe tumors with extension to the deep lobe, high grade malignancies, parotid lesions involving the parapharyngeal space, or recurrent pleomorphic adenoma [3].

Facial Nerve

The facial nerve runs between the superficial and deep lobes of the parotid gland and should be preserved unless involved by tumor [4]. All branches of the nerve should be identified. When performing a total parotidectomy, the branches of the facial nerve can be visualized on the lateral surface of the deep lobe after the superficial lobe is removed. The facial nerve branches are elevated off the deep lobe, which is then dissected away from the masseter and other muscles.

Most malignant tumors of the deep lobe of the parotid gland require facial nerve resection. If the facial nerve is inadvertently transected, it must be repaired; and when it is sacrificed because of tumor involvement, reinnervation is attempted. An interposition nerve graft can be placed if the distal branches of the facial nerve are preserved. The most commonly used donor nerve is the great auricular nerve, followed by the sural nerve. An advantage of using the sural nerve is its length, as up to 35 cm can be obtained. The ansa hypolossi and the medial antebrachial cutaneous nerves can also serve as donors.

If the distal branches of the facial nerve or mimetic musculature are sacrificed during the resection, reconstruction should be performed with transfer of an innervated, vascularized muscle. Regional muscles such as the temporalis or masseter can be used. A distant muscle such as the gracilis can also be used for a microneurovascular free tissue transfer.

Frey Syndrome

Frey syndrome, or gustatory sweating and flushing, occurs after the parasympathetic fibers of the auriculotemporal nerve are sectioned [5]. Aberrant regeneration to the vessels and sweat glands of the overlying skin in the region of parotidectomy results in local vasodilation and sweating during eating. The incidence of clinical Frey syndrome is 40–50% after parotidectomy, rising to 80% when objective tests are used. The incidence can be reduced by placing an implant [e.g., polytetrafluoroethylene (PTFE)] in the wound to cover the parotid bed or by using the superficial musculoaponeurotic system flap technique.

THYROID

Indications for Thyroidectomy

Hyperthyroidism

Hyperthyroidism is the constellation of symptoms and signs that result from excessive secretion of thyroid hormone [6]. The diagnosis is based on elevated serum levels of thyroxine (T_4) and triiodothyronine (T_3) and a decreased serum level of thyroid-stimulating hormone (TSH). Long-term definitive treatment for hyperthyroidism is radioactive iodine or total thyroidectomy. Thyroidectomy is indicated when patients opt for surgical treatment, are pregnant, or have severe ophthalmopathy. Initial management is primarily medical including propylthiouracil (PTU) or methimazole to decrease serum T_4 and T_3 levels to the normal range. β-Blockers such as propranol are used to control the cardiac effects of excessive thyroid hormone secretion. The pulse is regulated at approximately 80 beats per minute. Lugol's solution or supersaturated potassium iodide is instituted approximately 7–14 days before surgery to decrease the vasularity of the thyroid tissue. These medications are used to attain a euthyroid state preoperatively and minimize the risk of thyroid storm.

Total thyroidectomy is recommended because lesser procedures are associated with a high likelihood of recurrent disease. Furthermore, reports suggest that patients with ophthalmopathy have im-

proved visual function and less eye protuberance with total thyroidectomy [7]. In poorly prepared patients surgery may precipitate thyroid storm. Treatment includes PTU and cortisol to block the peripheral conversion of T_4 to T_3, intravenous or oral iodine to block the uptake of iodine, and β-blockers. The patient should be monitored closely in the intensive care unit. Supportive therapy with intravenous fluids, oxygen, cooling blankets, and hemodynamic support should also be provided. Complications of surgery include hypoparathyroidism and recurrent laryngeal nerve injury. Patients with hyperthyroidism often have osteoporosis and bone hunger that requires calcitriol (dihydocholecalciferol) and calcium administration postoperatively even with measurable parathyroid hormone (PTH) secretion. Furthermore, with total thyroidectomy postoperative hypothyroidism occurs approximately 1 week postoperatively, and thyroxine replacement therapy is indicated.

Goiter

A goiter is defined as enlargement of one or both lobes of the thyroid gland [6]. The enlargement can present as a single nodule, a diffuse swelling of one or both lobes, or multiple nodules. Goiters most frequently result from iodine deficiency. Indications for surgery of nontoxic goiters include suspicious or malignant cytology and related symptoms including difficulty breathing and dysphagia. In preparation for surgery, patients with deviation or compression of the trachea from a large goiter or who display inspiratory stridor and hoarseness should undergo laryngoscopy and awake intubation. Postoperatively, these patients should be followed closely in the recovery room for signs of respiratory distress. Thyroid lobectomy with resection of the isthmus is indicated for a nontoxic, unilobar goiter; and near-total thyroidectomy is indicated for a bilateral goiter. Studies have demonstrated that total thyroidectomy is associated with a decreased occurrence of recurrent goiter and a similar incidence of complications.

Thyroid Nodule

Thyroid nodules are common: 100,000 new patients each year in the United States develop a thyroid nodule [8]. Nodules affect approximately 5–10% of the general population, but fewer than 5% are malignant. The major issue is how to select malignant nodules for surgery and avoid surgery for benign nodules. Thyroid nodules are classified as solitary, dominant, and multiple. Although each type of nodule may be cancerous, the solitary and dominant ones have a higher probability of malignancy.

Evaluation begins with a thorough history and

physical examination. Factors that increase the risk of malignancy include male gender, age (children and the elderly are more likely to have malignant disease), and exposure to irradiation. A positive family history for thyroid or endocrine disease raises the possibility of medullary thyroid carcinoma (MTC). Papillary thyroid cancer is associated with radiation exposure. Hard and fixed nodules, cervical lymphadenopathy, and recurrent laryngeal nerve palsy are suggestive of malignancy.

Laboratory studies include measurement of thyroid function via serum T_4 and TSH levels. Some nodules autonomously produce excessive thyroid hormone and are best treated by surgery after appropriate preoperative preparation, as described previously. If serum hormone levels are normal, FNA is performed for cytology. When nodules with benign cytology are observed, a repeat FNA is performed yearly. Approximately 40–60% of patients have benign cells on cytology, and surgery can be safely avoided. Nodules with malignant or suspicious cytology require surgery.

Papillary Thyroid Cancer

Papillary thyroid cancer (PTC) is the most common thyroid malignancy [9], accounting for approximately 80% of all thyroid cancers. Clinically mixed PTC/follicular lesions behave like PTC. PTC is associated with radiation exposure, and in these patients it is commonly multifocal and bilateral. Small tumors (< 1 cm in diameter) without multifocality or grossly involved nodes and extracapsular thyroid extension are treated by ipsilateral thyroid lobectomy. Otherwise, total thyroidectomy is the treatment of choice. Total thyroidectomy, radioactive iodine, and thyroxine to suppress serum levels of TSH have each been shown to decrease the probability of recurrence. Following treatment, serum thyroglobulin assays, physical examination, and thyroid scans are used to detect recurrence. The 10-year survival of patients with PTC is approximately 90%. Older age (> 50 years), male gender, extrathyroidal invasion, distant metastases, and a tall-cell variant of PTC each portends a poorer prognosis.

Follicular Carcinoma

Follicular carcinoma is the second most common thyroid malignancy and accounts for 10% of thyroid cancers. Hurthle cell tumors comprise a subtype of follicular carcinoma and should be treated as such. FNA that suggests follicular or Hurthle cells on cytology dictates that thyroid lobectomy be done to diagnose malignancy, which is based on histologic evidence of capsular or vascular invasion. Total thy-roidectomy is performed if carcinoma is diagnosed. There are more deaths caused by follicular thyroid carcinoma than any other type. The 10-year survival is 80%, as these tumors more commonly spread to distant sites. Treatment includes total thyroidectomy, radioactive iodine, and thyroxine to suppress serum TSH levels.

Medullary Thyroid Carcinoma

Medullary carcinoma of the thyroid occurs sporadically, but it is also associated with three autosomal dominant inherited familial syndromes: multiple endocrine neoplasia types IIa and IIb (MEN-IIa, MEN-IIb) and familial MTC. Each of these syndromes is caused by a missense mutation of the transmembrane RET gene on chromosome 10. MEN-IIa and MEN-IIb are also associated with pheochromocytomas that must be excluded prior to surgery for MTC. MTC is always bilateral in the familial forms and unilateral in the sporadic form. It is a tumor of calcitonin secreting c-cells that occur at the junction of the superior and middle third of the thyroid. Serum calcitonin levels serve as a marker for MTC. Treatment consists of total thyroidectomy with central lymph node dissection. The familial forms can be detected by genetic testing of peripheral blood leukocytes for RET gene mutation. When present, total thyroidectomy is recommended before other clinical signs of MTC. With early detection, the familial forms are usually curable. The sporadic form typically presents as a palpable mass and has a 5-year survival of 50%. Surgery is the only effective treatment and is recommended for primary tumors and localized recurrent disease.

Anaplastic Carcinoma of the Thyroid

Anaplastic thyroid carcinoma is rare, representing only 1–2% of thyroid cancers. Patients typically present with locally advanced disease that is diagnosed by FNA or cutting needle biopsy. Thyroidectomy is not recommended, as the median survival is only 6 months. Doxorubicin and hyperfractionated radiation therapy usually prove local control of tumor, and patients die from distant metastases.

Complications of Thyroidectomy

The two major complications of thyroidectomy include hypoparathyroidism and recurrent laryngeal nerve injury. The incidence of each is approximately 1–2%. Permanent hypoparathyroidism can be avoided by transplantation of any ischemic-appearing parathyroid tissue into the sternocleidomastoid muscle. Experienced thyroid surgeons do this in approxi-

hypercalcemia that is detected on laboratory screening studies [15]. Some have symptoms that include bone pain, kidney stones, altered mental status, abdominal pain, and weakness. The diagnosis is ascertained by measuring the serum calcium and intact PTH levels, which are elevated. About 85% of patients with HPT have a single abnormal gland or adenoma as the cause. 12% have hyperplasia, 1–2% have a double adenoma, and 1% have carcinoma. The indications for surgery are bone disease, muscle weakness, nephrocalcinosis, kidney stones, severe hypercalcemia and hypercalciuria, and young age [16].

Hypercalcemia

Patients with severe hypercalcemia may have altered mental status and may be in a comatose state. Prompt reduction in serum calcium levels is required in the patient whose level is > 13 mg/dl. The patient is initially treated with intravenous volume expansion using isotonic saline, which increases the glomerular filtration rate and calcium excretion. Once adequate urine output is observed, a loop diuretic (furosemide) is given. Calcitonin and diphosphanates are then added to further decrease the serum calcium levels. In patients with end-stage renal disease, dialysis is indicated to reduce the serum calcium level prior to surgery [17].

Hypocalcemia

After most successful parathyroid surgery there is some degree of postoperative hypocalcemia. The magnitude depends on the age of the patient, the severity of disease, and the size and amount of parathyroid tissue removed. Symptomatic hypocalcemia (circumoral paresthesias, tetany, Chvostek's or Trousseau's sign) or profound hypocalcemia (serum calcium level < 8 mg/dl) should be treated with intravenous calcium followed by oral calcium. Calcitriol (vitamin D_3) is reserved for patients who have persistent symptoms or who develop hyperphosphatemia. Follow-up serum calcium and phosphorus levels should be monitored and the dosages adjusted.

CRICOTHYROIDOTOMY

Cricothyroidotomy may be a life-saving procedure. The primary *indication* is an inability to intubate the trachea. Circumstances include facial trauma, where tracheal intubation may not be possible, and an unstable fractured cervical spine that limits neck extension.

Complications of cricothyroidotomy include injury to the larynx, tracheal stenosis, and bleeding.

mately 20–40% of cases. Treatment of postoperative hypocalcemia requires intravenous or oral calcium supplementation. If hyperphosphatemia occurs, calcitriol is added. Because permanent hypoparathyroidism is rare after thyroid surgery, calcium and calcitriol supplementation can usually be discontinued after 2–3 weeks.

Injury to the recurrent laryngeal nerve presents as hoarseness of the voice. It is diagnosed by indirect or direct laryngoscopy. The right vocal cord is more commonly affected than the left vocal cord because of the more oblique course of the right recurrent laryngeal nerve. It is usually a paresis rather than a paralysis and is the result of a stretch or contusion of the nerve. In these instances complete recovery occurs in approximately 3–6 months. If paralysis persists, the quality of the voice may be improved by Teflon injection of the vocal cord to displace it medially. Bilateral recurrent laryngeal nerve injury is a more significant complication. It presents with postoperative stridor that must be managed by tracheostomy to allow adequate ventilation.

PARATHYROID

Localization Studies

Most experienced surgeons do not recommend parathyroid imaging in a previously unoperated patient, as surgery is successful about 95% of the time without it. However, there has been recent enthusiasm for a minimally invasive approach and unilateral neck exploration [10–14]. A unilateral approach could reduce the risk of recurrent laryngeal nerve injury, decrease the likelihood of postoperative hypoparathyroidism, and shorten hospital costs and stay. With this less invasive approach, preoperative localization studies are essential. Udelsman et al. reported successful parathyroid surgery using a less invasive surgical procedure based on preoperative localization with sestamibi scan and intraoperative PTH assay [14].

It is essential to have accurate localization studies in the reoperative setting. The most sensitive technique is the sestamibi scan. This radionuclide is selectively retained in abnormal parathyroid glands and is imaged with single-photon emission tomography (SPECT). If sestamibi is unsuccessful, ultrasonography, CT, or MRI can be performed followed by angiography and venous sampling.

Primary Hyperparathyroidism

Primary hyperparathyroidism (HPT) is a common condition, with an incidence of 5 per 100,000 in the population. Most patients have apparently asymptomatic

TRACHEOSTOMY

Cricothyroidotomy is the best procedure for emergency situations. Avoid performing a tracheostomy under these conditions, as it would clearly increase the complication rate. When possible, an adequate airway is first secured with an endotracheal tube; and the appropriate surgical instruments, lighting, and suction are obtained. It is best to perform this procedure in the operating room.

The *indications* for tracheostomy include upper airway obstruction (infection, neoplasm, foreign body) and long-term ventilator dependence. It is also used as an adjunct for major head/neck/chest surgery where prolonged ventilation or ventilatory problems are anticipated, in emergency situations when intubation and cricothyroidotomy have failed, in the presence of extensive maxillofacial trauma, and for bilateral recurrent nerve injury.

Complications of tracheostomy include bleeding, infection, tracheoesophageal fistula, tracheoinnominate fistula, tracheal stenosis, and tube decannulation/obstruction [18].

REFERENCES

1. Califano J, Eisele DW. Benign salivary gland neoplasms. Otolaryngol Clin North Am 1999;32:861.
2. Rice DH. Malignant salivary gland neoplasms. Otolaryngol Clin North Am 1999;32:875.
3. Sinha UK, Ng M. Surgery of the salivary glands. Otolaryngol Clin North Am 1999;32:887.
4. Shindo M. Management of facial nerve paralysis. Otolaryngol Clin North Am 1999;32:945.
5. Dulguerov P, Quinodoz D, Cosendai G, et al. Prevention of Frey syndrome during parotidectomy. Arch Otolaryngol Head Neck Surg 1999;125:833.
6. Mack E. Nontoxic goiters. In Cameron JL (ed) Current Surgical Therapy. St. Louis, Mosby, 1998, pp 587–593.
7. Alsanea O, Clark OH. Treatment of Graves' disease: the advantages of surgery. Endocrinol Metab Clin North Am 2000;29:321.
8. Wong CKM, Wheeler MH. Thyroid nodules: rational management. World J Surg 2000;24:934.
9. Udelsman R, Chen H. The current management of thyroid cancer. Adv Surg 1999;33:1.
10. Neumann DR, Esselstyn CB, Madera AM. Sestamibi/iodine subtraction single photon emission computed tomography in reoperative secondary hyperparathyroidism. Surgery 2000;128:22.
11. Moka D, Voth E, Dietlein M, et al. Technetium 99m-MIBI-SPECT: a highly sensitive diagnostic tool for localization of parathyroid adenomas. Surgery 2000;128:29.
12. Mitchell BK, Merrell RC, Kinder BK. Localization studies in patients with hyperparathyroidism. Surg Clin North Am 1995;75:483.
13. Reeve TS, Babidge WJ, Parkyn RF, et al. Minimally invasive surgery for primary hyperparathyroidism. Arch Surg 2000;135:481.
14. Udelsman R, Donovan PI, Sokoll LJ. One hundred consecutive minimally invasive parathyroid explorations. Ann Surg 2000;212:331.
15. Centers for Disease Control Panel. Diagnosis and management of asymptomatic primary hyperparathyroidism: consensus development conference statement. Ann Intern Med 1991;114:593.
16. Kinder BK. Primary hyperparathyroidism. In Cameron JL (ed) Current Surgical Therapy. St. Louis, Mosby, 1998, pp 606–611.
17. Packman KS, Demeure MJ. Indications for parathyroidectomy and extent of treatment for patients with secondary hyperparathyroidism. Surg Clin North Am 1995;75:465.
18. Goldenberg D, Ari EG, Golz A, et al. Tracheostomy complications: a retrospective study of 1130 cases. Otolaryngol Head Neck Surg 2000;123:495.

106 Parotidectomy

INDICATIONS

Tumors of the parotid gland

Chronic sialadenitis or calculi of the parotid ducts

PITFALLS AND DANGER POINTS

Damage to facial nerve and its branches

Failure to excise a mixed tumor with a sufficient margin of normal parotid tissue

OPERATIVE STRATEGY

Extent of Resection

Although the parotid gland is not anatomically a truly bilobed structure, the surgeon may visualize it as having a superficial lobe and a deep lobe, with the branches of the facial nerve passing between these two structures. Consequently, it is feasible to excise the superficial lobe with preservation of the branches of the facial nerve. This dissection is indicated for most patients who have mixed tumors of the parotid gland. A few mixed tumors arise in the deep lobe of the gland. In these cases, perform a superficial parotid lobectomy to identify each of the facial nerve branches. Then, with preservation of the facial nerve, remove the deep lobe.

Occasional small benign tumors require dissection of the facial nerve only in the region of the tumor. The tumor may then be resected with a good margin of parotid tissue by doing a partial superficial lobectomy.

Malignant tumors of the parotid gland, unless unusually small, should be removed by total parotidectomy with excision of that portion of the facial nerve lying within the tumor. Microsurgical techniques allow the nerve to be reconstructed with a graft, which is often taken from the auriculotemporal nerve.

Locating and Preserving the Facial Nerve

There are two methods for identifying and dissecting the facial nerve. Some surgeons prefer to locate the major trunk of the facial nerve by first identifying a peripheral branch, such as the marginal mandibular branch. They then trace this nerve backward toward its junction with the cervical facial branch and finally

to the main facial trunk. We prefer the more common technique of first identifying the main trunk of the facial nerve posterior to the parotid gland. Before it enters the parotid gland, the main facial nerve is a large structure, often measuring 2 mm in diameter. Once this main trunk is identified, the key to the dissection technique is to use either fine, blunt-tipped Jones scissors or a mosquito hemostat. The closed hemostat tip is inserted in the plane immediately anterior to the nerve. After the surgeon gently opens the hemostat, the assistant cuts the loose fibrous tissue that attaches the nerve to the overlying parotid gland. Never divide any parotid tissue before identifying the facial nerve and its branches.

If the proper plane of dissection is maintained, bleeding is rarely a problem. Most bleeding arises from small veins, and it generally stops with application of gauze pressure. An important part of the dissection technique is for the surgeon to apply pressure on the tissue posterior to the nerve with gauze while the assistant applies tension to the superficial lobe of the parotid gland using Allis clamps or small retractors. An occasional small vein must be clamped with a small mosquito hemostat and tied with a fine absorbable ligature. Electrocautery may be used for hemostasis in areas of the dissection away from the facial nerve and its branches.

The surgeon should have sufficient familiarity with the appearance of the facial nerve to make a positive visual identification. Occasionally, some fibers of questionable nature attach to the facial nerve branches. They may be tested by gently pinching or stimulating the fiber and then looking at the cheek for muscle twitching. This test, of course, requires that the entire cheek and the corner of the eye be exposed when the surgical field is draped.

The key to successful nerve preservation is early identification of the main facial trunk. The facial nerve emerges from the skull through the stylomastoid foramen, which is situated just anterior to the mastoid process and just below the external auditory canal. Beahrs emphasized that if the surgeon places the tip of the index finger over the mastoid process with the fingertip aimed toward the nose the middle of this finger is pointing to the facial trunk, which emerges about 0.5 cm anterior to the center of the fingertip and perhaps 1 cm deep to the external surface of the mastoid process. An idea of the depth at which the nerve emerges can be gained by identifying the posterior digastric muscle and tracing it toward its insertion deep to the mastoid process. The nerve crosses at a level equivalent to the surface of the digastric muscle. In other words, dissect along the anterior surface of the sternomastoid muscle and the mastoid process posterior to the parotid gland. There are no vital structures in this plane crossing superficial to the main trunk of the facial nerve.

There is a tiny arterial branch (posterior auricular artery) crossing just superficial to the facial trunk. If the exposure is not adequate for accurate clamping and ligating, simple pressure stops bleeding from this vessel if it has been transected. Consequently, focus intense attention on an area about 1 cm in diameter just anterior to the mastoid process and about 1 cm deep to its surface. This is where the facial trunk is found unless a tumor in the deep portion of the parotid gland has displaced the nerve to a more superficial plane. The cephalad margin of this 1 cm area of intense attention may be considered to be the fissure between the external auditory canal and the superior portion of the mastoid process.

One should be cautious while elevating the skin flap along the inferior border of the parotid to avoid nerve damage. Avoid elevating the caudal portion of the flap beyond the anterior edge of the parotid gland before the facial nerve dissection because the marginal mandibular branch of the facial nerve emerges from the parotid gland together with the posterior facial vein with which the nerve may be in contact. This is the smallest branch of the facial nerve and the easiest to injure because it is quite superficial at this point. Damage to this nerve causes weakness in the area of the lateral portion of the lower lip.

OPERATIVE TECHNIQUE

Incision and Exposure

Although many incisions have been devised for this operation, we prefer the one illustrated in **Figure 106–1**. It starts in a skin crease just anterior to the tragus and continues in the form of a Y, as shown. Continue the posterior limb of the incision over the mastoid process in a caudal direction roughly parallel to the underlying sternomastoid muscle down to a point about 1 cm below the angle of the mandible. Do not make the angle of the Y too acute. Carry the incision through the platysma muscle. Obtain hemostasis with accurate electrocautery. Apply small rake retractors to the anterior skin flap and strongly elevate the tissue in the plane just deep to the platysma. As soon as the surface of the parotid gland is exposed, continue the dissection with small Metzenbaum scissors. Some of the fibrous tissue attaching the parotid

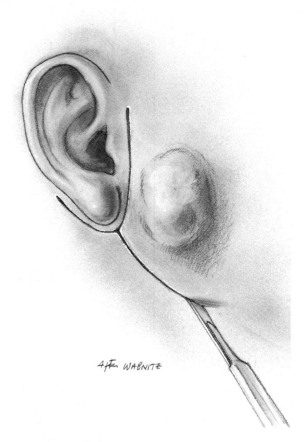

Fig. 106–1

gland to the overlying tissue resembles tiny nerve fibers. There are no facial nerve fibers superficial to the parotid gland. Therefore each of these fibers may be rapidly divided. If a total superficial lobectomy is planned, continue the dissection in a cephalad direction to the level of the zygomatic process and anteriorly to the anterior margin of the parotid gland. Do not continue the dissection beyond the anterior and inferior margins of the gland, as the small facial nerve branches may inadvertently be injured if this is done before identifying the facial nerve.

Elevate the skin flaps and the lobe of the ear in a cephalad posterior direction to expose the underlying sternomastoid muscle, mastoid process, and cartilage of the external auditory canal. Elevate the posterior flap to expose 1–2 cm of underlying sternomastoid muscle. Obtain complete hemostasis. Some surgeons prefer to place a few sutures to attach the skin flaps temporarily to the underlying cheek, maintaining exposure of the gland.

Exposing the Posterior Margin of the Parotid Gland

Identify the great auricular nerve overlying the surface of the sternomastoid muscle about 3–4 cm caudal to the mastoid process. Divide the branch of the

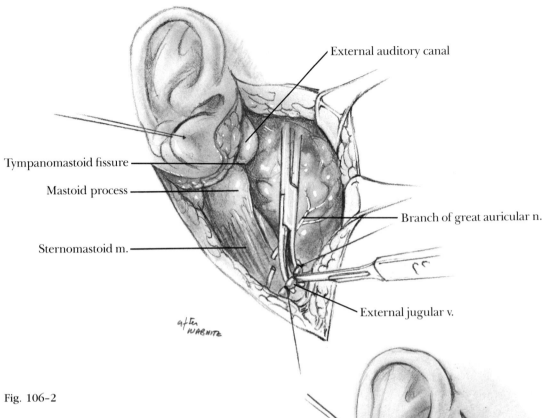

Fig. 106-2

great auricular nerve that enters the parotid gland. Adjacent to this nerve is found the external jugular vein, which is generally also divided and ligated posterior to the parotid gland **(Fig. 106–2)**. Expose the anterior border of the sternomastoid muscle and continue this dissection in a cephalad direction toward the mastoid process. When dissecting the tissues away from the anterior surface of the mastoid process there may be some bleeding from branches of the superficial temporal vessels. It can be controlled by accurate clamping or electrocautery.

Locating the Facial Nerve

Running from the tympanomastoid fissure to the parotid gland is a fairly dense layer of temporoparotid fascia. Elevate this layer of fascia with a small hemostat or right-angle clamp and divide it **(Fig. 106–3)**. Continue the dissection deep along the anterior surface of the mastoid process. Remember that the main trunk of the facial nerve is located in a 1 cm area anterior to the tympanomastoid fissure and the upper half of the mastoid process at 0.5-1.0 cm depth. Try to identify the small arterial branch of the posterior auricular artery in this area. Divide and ligate it. If it has been inadvertently divided and accurate clamping cannot be achieved, simply apply pressure for a few minutes to stop the bleeding. Continue the blunt dissection using a hemostat until the posterior portion of the parotid gland can be retracted away from the mastoid

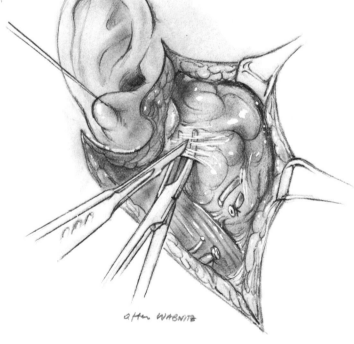

Fig. 106-3

process. Continuing to separate and divide the fibrous tissue in this area uncovers the main trunk of the facial nerve. Although the nerve usually runs in a transverse direction from the mastoid process toward the gland, it sometimes can run obliquely from the upper left portion of the operative field toward the right lower portion as it enters the parotid gland. Some idea of how deep the dissection must be carried to expose the facial nerve can be obtained by observing the

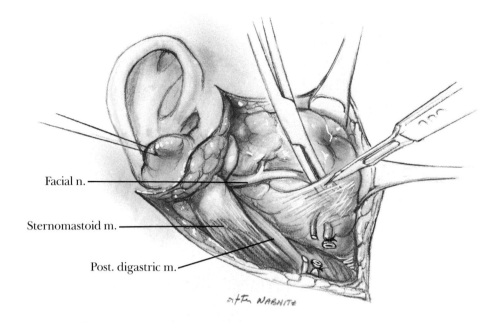

Fig. 106-4

depth of the surface of the posterior digastric muscle as it reaches its origin behind the mastoid process. The nerve is at or just superficial to this vessel **(Fig. 106–4)**.

Dissecting Facial Nerve Branches

Apply traction to the superficial lobe of the parotid using several Allis clamps or retractors. Insert a small hemostat in the plane *just superficial* to the facial nerve. Ask the assistant to divide the fibrous tissue being elevated by the hemostat (Fig. 106-4). Continue the dissection in this plane until each of the branches of the facial nerve has been separated from the overlying parotid tissue. Pay special attention to the cervical division and its marginal mandibular branch, as it permits elevation of the lowermost portion of the parotid gland. As the dissection reaches the anterior margin of the parotid gland, identify Stensen's duct. Ligate with 3-0 PG and divide the duct **(Fig. 106–5)**. After all of the nerve

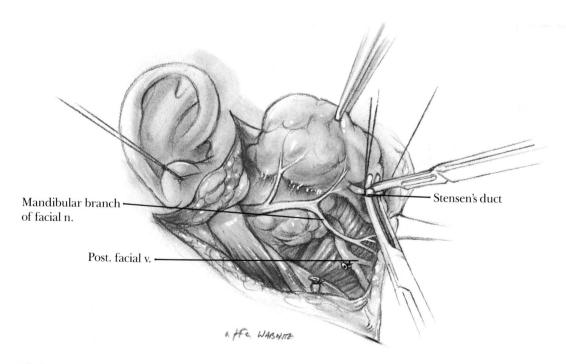

Fig. 106-5

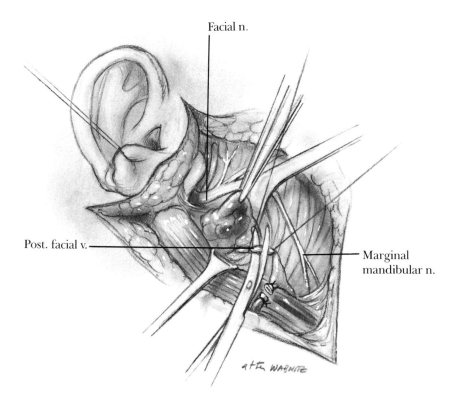

Fig. 106-6

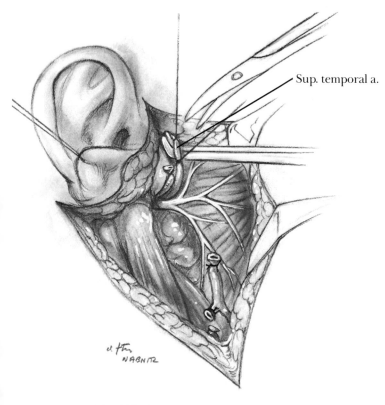

Fig. 106-7

branches have been identified and the duct has been divided, remove the superficial lobe of the gland.

Hemostasis during the nerve dissection can generally be achieved by gauze pressure. At this point in the dissection, carefully identify each bleeding point and clamp it with a mosquito hemostat. Ligate with 4-0 or 5-0 PG. Do not use electrocautery in areas close to the nerve.

Removing Deep Lobe of Parotid Gland (When Indicated)

To remove the deep lobe of the parotid gland, first excise the superficial lobe of the parotid as described above; then carefully free the lower division of the facial nerve from the underlying tissue. By retracting one or more of these divisions, one can begin to mobilize the deep lobe.

Identify the posterior facial vein. Separate the marginal mandibular nerve branch from the vein; then divide and ligate the posterior facial vein with 4-0 PG as in **Figure 106–6**. Now divide the superficial temporal artery and vein as in **Figure 106–7**. Elevate the lower border of the gland and divide and ligate the external carotid artery; then divide and ligate the internal maxillary and the transverse facial arteries at the anterior border of the gland. The deep lobe may now be removed. The appearance of the

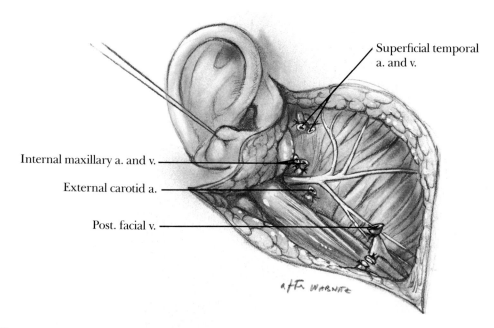

Superficial temporal a. and v.

Internal maxillary a. and v.

External carotid a.

Post. facial v.

after WARNITE

Fig. 106–8

operative field after removing the deep lobe is seen in **Figure 106–8**.

Drainage and Closure

Place a small Silastic closed-suction drain through a puncture wound posterior to the incision. Close the incision using interrupted 5-0 PG sutures to the platysma and subcutaneous fat. Close the skin with interrupted 5-0 nylon sutures.

POSTOPERATIVE CARE

Leave the closed suction drain in place until the drainage has essentially ceased (3–4 days).

COMPLICATIONS

Facial weakness due to nerve damage.

Hematoma.

Infection.

Gustatory sweating. Otherwise known as Frey syndrome, it manifests as almost painful sweating in the skin of the operative area while eating. It occurs to some extent in as many as 25% of patients. This is believed to be due to the regrowth of parasympathetic motor nerve fibers of the auriculotemporal nerve into cutaneous nerve fibers of the skin flap.

Such crossed innervation of the sweat glands produces uncomfortable gustatory sweating. Loré stated that it may be prevented by removing a section of the auriculotemporal nerve during surgery of the parotid gland.

Salivary fistula. This may appear when a significant portion of the parotid gland has been left intact. It generally corrects itself with expectant treatment.

REFERENCES

Beahrs OH. Parotidectomy. Surg Clin North Am 1977;57: 477.

Califano J, Eisele DW. Benign salivary gland neoplasms. Otolaryngol Clin North Am 1999;32:861.

Christensen NR, Jacobsen SD. Parotidectomy: preserving the posterior branch of the great auricular nerve. J Laryngol Otol 1997;111:556.

Dulguerov P, Quinodoz D, Cosendai G, et al. Prevention of Frey syndrome during parotidectomy. Arch Otolaryngol Head Neck Surg 1999;125:833.

Loré JM. An Atlas of Head and Neck Surgery. Philadelphia, Saunders, 1962.

Rice DH. Malignant salivary gland neoplasms. Otolaryngol Clin North Am 1999;32:875.

Terrell JE, Kileny PR, Yian C, et al. Clinical outcome of continuous facial nerve monitoring during primary parotidectomy. Arch Otolaryngol Head Neck Surg 1997;123:1081.

107 Thyroidectomy

INDICATIONS

Goiter

Hyperthyroidism

Selected solitary thyroid nodules

Thyroid carcinoma

See Chapter 105

PREOPERATIVE PREPARATION

Patients with hyperthyroidism require careful preoperative preparation to decrease the vascularity of the thyroid and the risk of thyroid storm. Agents commonly used are propranolol, antithyroid medications, and iodine. Because of the long half-life of thyroxine (T₄), treatment with propranolol must be continued for 7–10 days postoperatively.

Workup of a solitary thyroid nodule may include any or all of the following:

Ultrasonography

Fine-needle aspiration cytology

Radionuclide scan

Thyroid suppression therapy

A patient suspected of having medullary carcinoma of the thyroid should undergo preoperative studies to detect a pheochromocytoma or a parathyroid adenoma, which commonly coexist.

PITFALLS AND DANGER POINTS

Trauma to or inadvertent excision of parathyroid glands

Trauma to recurrent laryngeal or superior laryngeal nerves

Inadequate preoperative preparation of the toxic patient resulting in postoperative thyroid storm

Inadequate surgery for thyroid cancer

OPERATIVE STRATEGY

Preserving Parathyroid Glands

Preventing damage to the parathyroid glands requires the surgeon to achieve thorough familiarity with the anatomic location and appearance of these structures. Wearing telescopic lenses with about 2.5× magnification can be helpful for identifying both the parathyroid glands and the recurrent nerve. The surgeon who takes the time to identify the parathyroid glands during every thyroid operation soon finds that this maneuver can be accomplished with progressively more efficiency. The inferior parathyroid gland is frequently found in the fat that surrounds the inferior thyroid artery at the point where it divides into several branches (**Fig. 107–1**). Normally, the inferior gland is anteromedial to the recurrent laryngeal nerve, and the superior parathyroid is posterolateral to the nerve (**Fig. 107–2**). With the thyroid gland retracted anteriorly, both parathyroids may assume an anteromedial position relative to the nerve (**Fig. 107–3**). The superior gland is generally situated on the posterior surface of the upper third of the thyroid gland, fairly close to the cricoid cartilage. Frequently, the parathyroids are loosely surrounded by fat and are red-brown. Measuring only about 5–8 mm in maximum diameter, the average gland weighs about 30 mg.

One method for protecting the parathyroid glands is to preserve the posterior capsule of the thyroid gland by incising the thyroid along the line sketched in Figure 107–11. Also, divide the branches of the inferior thyroid artery at a point distal to the origin of the blood supply to the parathyroids. Some surgeons believe that ligating the inferior thyroid artery lateral to the thyroid gland impairs the blood supply to the parathyroid glands, but this contention has never been proved.

When a total lobectomy is performed, the only means of ensuring preservation of the parathyroid glands is to identify the inferior and superior glands positively. Then dissect each gland carefully away from the thyroid without impairing its blood supply.

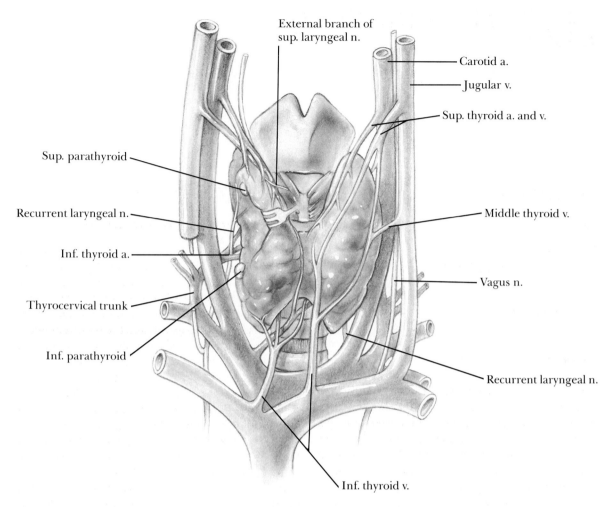

External branch of
sup. laryngeal n.

Carotid a.

Jugular v.

Sup. thyroid a. and v.

Sup. parathyroid

Middle thyroid v.

Recurrent laryngeal n.

Inf. thyroid a.

Vagus n.

Thyrocervical trunk

Inf. parathyroid

Recurrent laryngeal n.

Inf. thyroid v.

Fig. 107-1

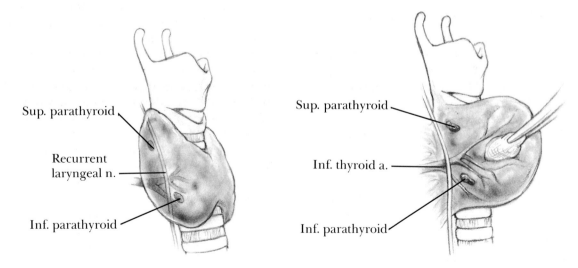

Sup. parathyroid

Recurrent
laryngeal n.

Inf. parathyroid

Sup. parathyroid

Inf. thyroid a.

Inf. parathyroid

Fig. 107-2

Fig. 107-3

If a parathyroid gland has been inadvertently excised, and this error is recognized during the operation, it is possible to slice the gland into particles measuring 1×1 mm and then transplant these fragments into pockets made in the muscles of the neck or the forearm (Wells et al.).

Preserving the Recurrent Laryngeal Nerve

The recurrent laryngeal nerve ascends slightly lateral to the tracheoesophageal groove. At the level of the inferior thyroid artery, the nerve almost always makes contact with this vessel, passing directly under or over the artery. Sometimes the nerve passes between the branches of the inferior thyroid vessel. Above the level of the artery, the nerve ascends to enter the larynx between the cricoid cartilage and the inferior cornu of the thyroid cartilage. In this area the nerve lies in close proximity to the posterior capsule of the thyroid gland. It may divide into two or more branches prior to entering the larynx. On rare occasions the recurrent nerve does not recur but travels from the vagus directly medially to enter the larynx near the superior thyroid vessels or at a slightly lower level relative to the thyroid gland.

For most surgeons the best way to locate the recurrent laryngeal nerve is to trace the inferior thyroid artery from the point where it emerges behind the carotid artery to the point where it crosses over or under the recurrent nerve. Using the inferior thyroid artery as a guide, locate the recurrent nerve immediately deep to or superficial to this artery and carefully dissect the nerve in a cephalad direction until it reaches the cricothyroid membrane just below the inferior cornu of the thyroid cartilage. Remember that the nerve may divide into two or more branches in the area cephalad to the inferior thyroid artery. Once the nerve has been exposed throughout its course behind the thyroid gland, it is a simple matter to avoid damaging it.

Preserving the Superior Laryngeal Nerve

The internal branch of the superior laryngeal nerve penetrates the thyrohyoid membrane and is the sensory nerve of the larynx; the external branch controls the cricothyroid muscle. Although it is possible to damage both branches of the superior laryngeal nerve by passing a mass ligature around the superior thyroid artery and vein above the superior pole of the thyroid, the external branch is the one most often injured. Transection of the external branch impairs the patient's ability to voice high-pitched sounds. Because the external branch may be intertwined with branches of the superior thyroid artery and vein (Fig. 107-1), avoiding damage to this nerve requires that each branch of the superior thyroid vessels be isolated, ligated, and divided individually at the point where it enters the thyroid gland. If the superior thyroid artery and vein are dissected *above* the superior pole of the thyroid, it is necessary to identify and preserve the superior laryngeal nerve and its branches. This step is not necessary if the terminal branches of the superior thyroid vessels are individually isolated and ligated.

OPERATIVE TECHNIQUE

Incision and Exposure

Place a small pillow or other support underneath the patient's shoulders to extend the head and neck. It is helpful to elevate the upper half of the operating table so the patient assumes a semisitting position. Make a slightly curved incision transversely in the neck at a level two to three fingerbreadths above the sternal notch **(Fig. 107–4)**. The incision should extend just beyond the anterior border of the sternomastoid muscle on each side. A longer incision is necessary in patients with large goiters. Carry the incision down to the platysma muscle. This muscle is easier to identify in the lateral portions of the incision. When the longitudinal fibers of this muscle are seen, transect them with precision because the upper flap will be dissected in a plane along the deep aspect of the platysma. There is a thin layer of fat deep to this muscle. If the plane of dissection is carried down to the cervical fascia, a number of veins are encountered that produce unnecessary bleeding. Leaving a thin layer of fat on these veins avoids this problem. Continue the dissection along the deep surface of the platysma muscle in a cephalad direction using both sharp and blunt maneuvers until a point 1-2 cm above the notch of the thyroid cartilage has been reached in the midline of the dissection **(Fig. 107–5)**. Now elevate the lateral portions of the flap. Adequate exposure requires wide dissection of this musculocutaneous flap. Achieve hemostasis, primarily with electrocautery. Elevate the inferior flap for a distance of about 2 cm.

Palpate the prominence of the thyroid cartilage to identify the midline. Make an incision through the cervical fascia in the midline **(Fig. 107–6)** and extend the incision in the fascia to expose the full length of the strap muscles. Elevate the sternohyoid muscle in the midline; then elevate the sternothyroid muscle and dissect the thyroid capsule away from it on both sides. This permits adequate digital

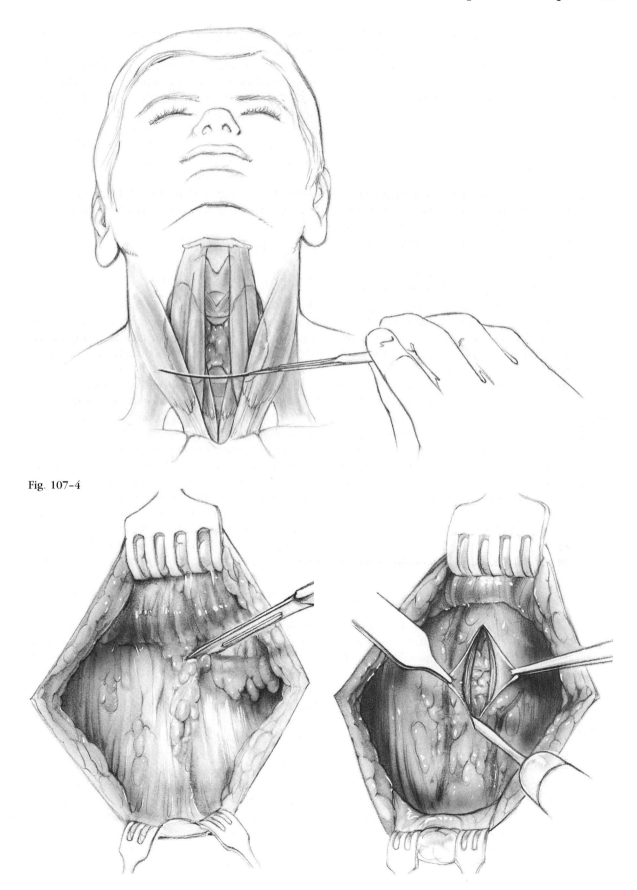

Fig. 107-4

Fig. 107-5

Fig. 107-6

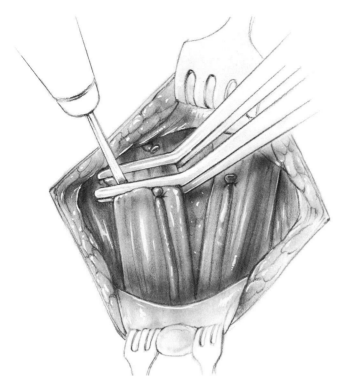

Fig. 107-7

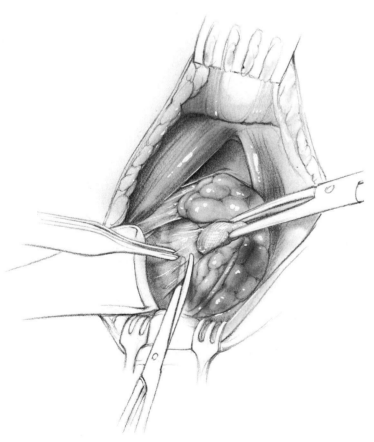

Fig. 107-8

exploration of the entire thyroid gland. In most cases retracting the strap muscles laterally while the thyroid lobe is retracted in the opposite direction provides good exposure for thyroidectomy. If the gland is unusually large or the exposure is inadequate, do not hesitate to transect the sternohyoid and sternothyroid muscles. Transect them in their upper thirds **(Fig. 107–7)**, as their innervation enters from below.

Identifying the Inferior Thyroid Artery, Recurrent Laryngeal Nerve, and Inferior Parathyroid Gland

Retract the strap muscles firmly with a small Richardson retractor while forcefully drawing the thyroid gland in a medial direction using a peanut sponge **(Fig. 107–8)** or a gauze square held in the assistant's fingers. A layer of thin fibrous and areolar tissue is now divided in layers by Metzenbaum scissors or by dissecting bluntly with a hemostat. A variable distribution of one or more middle thyroid veins may be encountered along the anterolateral margin of the thyroid. Divide these veins between ligatures **(Fig. 107–9)**, thereby permitting further elevation of the lower portion of the thyroid lobe.

Identify the carotid artery. Carry the dissection through the fibrous tissue along the medial surface of the carotid artery down to the level of the prevertebral fascia. Now retract the carotid artery laterally. Dissection medial to this vessel reveals the inferior thyroid artery passing deep to the carotid toward the junction of the middle and lower thirds of the thyroid gland **(Fig. 107–10)**. Once the inferior thyroid artery has been identified, encircle it with a Silastic loop. Apply mild traction to the artery and follow the anterior surface of this structure in a medial direction by blunt dissection with Metzenbaum scissors.

Before this vessel enters the thyroid gland, it passes directly underneath or crosses directly over the recurrent laryngeal nerve. Make use of the inferior thyroid artery as a guide to the nerve. If the nerve is not seen immediately, dissect the loose fibrous tissue at a point just inferior to the artery near the groove between the trachea and the esophagus to identify the recurrent nerve. Once the nerve is identified, use a small hemostat to delineate the plane just superficial to the nerve. Continue this plane of dissection in a cephalad direction up to the inferior cornu of the thyroid cartilage, the point near which the nerve enters the larynx. Be aware that the nerve may divide into two or more branches along its course from the level of the inferior thyroid artery to that of the larynx.

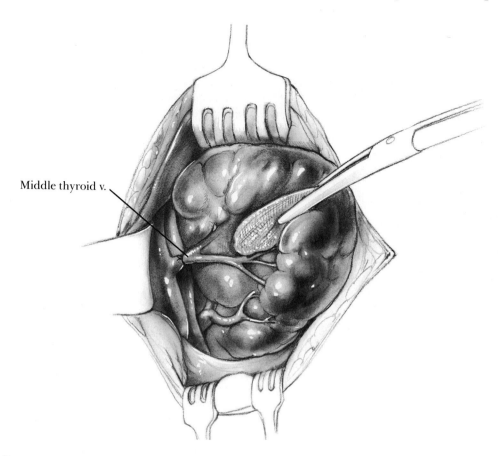

Middle thyroid v.

Fig. 107-9

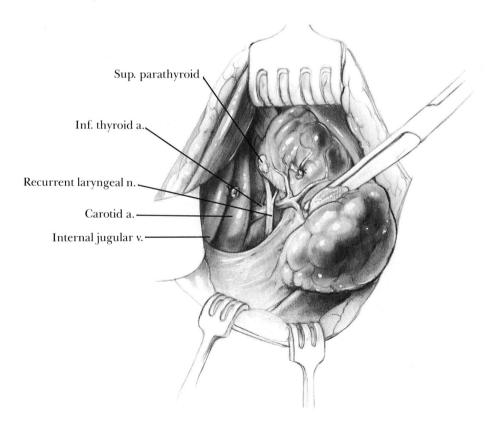

Sup. parathyroid

Inf. thyroid a.

Recurrent laryngeal n.

Carotid a.

Internal jugular v.

Fig. 107-10

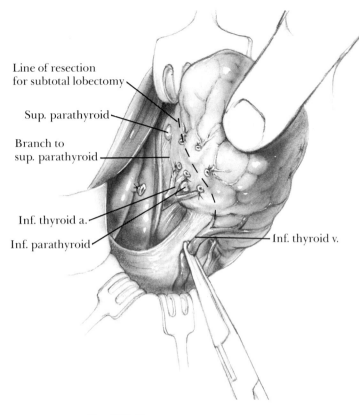

Line of resection
for subtotal lobectomy

Sup. parathyroid

Branch to
sup. parathyroid

Inf. thyroid a.

Inf. parathyroid

Inf. thyroid v.

Fig. 107-11

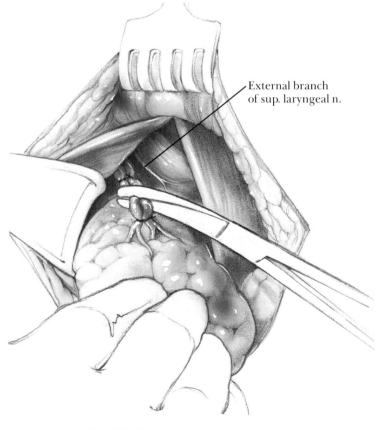

External branch
of sup. laryngeal n.

Fig. 107-12

Identify the inferior parathyroid gland, generally located close to the point at which the inferior thyroid artery divides into its branches (**Fig. 107–11**). Divide each of these branches of the inferior thyroid artery between ligatures on a line medial to the parathyroid gland so the blood supply to the parathyroid is not impaired.

Once the recurrent nerve has been identified, proceed to dissect out the lower pole of the thyroid lobe. One or more inferior thyroid veins are encountered in this location. Divide and ligate each of these veins and liberate the inferior pole.

Dissecting the Superior Pole and Superior Parathyroid Gland

Identify the upper portion of the thyroid isthmus. If a finger-like projection of thyroid tissue can be identified extending from the region of the isthmus in a cephalad direction, it represents the pyramidal lobe of the thyroid. If a thyroidectomy is being performed for Graves' disease, it is important to remove the pyramidal lobe. Otherwise, postoperatively it may become markedly hypertrophied and cause a serious cosmetic deformity overlying the thyroid cartilage.

With a retractor drawing the upper portion of the strap muscles in a cephalad direction, use a peanut sponge dissector to sweep the upper pole of the thyroid away from the larynx. This maneuver separates the upper pole from the external branch of the superior laryngeal nerve, which is closely applied to the cricothyroid muscle at this level. Also free the lateral portion of the superior pole by blunt dissection. One or two small veins may be entering the posterior portion of the upper pole. Be careful to identify and ligate these branches if encountered. Then identify the terminal branches of the superior thyroid artery and vein. Ligate each of these vessels with two 2-0 Vicryl ligatures and divide each of them between the ligatures (**Fig. 107–12**). After they have been ligated and divided, the superior pole of the thyroid is completely liberated and can be lifted out of the neck. Now search along the posterior surface of the upper third of the thyroid lobe for the superior parathyroid gland. Its usual location is sketched in Figure 107-11. Dissect the gland away from the thyroid into the neck.

If any difficulty is encountered when exposing the recurrent laryngeal nerve, the inferior thyroid artery, or the inferior parathyroid gland, do not hesitate to perform the superior pole dissection earlier in the operation to improve exposure of the posterior aspect of the thyroid gland.

At this point the surgeon must decide whether to

perform a subtotal or total thyroid lobectomy. Generally, if the patient has what obviously appears to be a localized benign tumor, perform a subtotal thyroid lobectomy and obtain an immediate frozen section analysis if possible. If the frozen section should prove to be malignant, total lobectomy is indicated, as discussed above. For large tumors suspected to be malignant, perform a total thyroid lobectomy.

Subtotal Thyroid Lobectomy

If subtotal resection of the lobe is the operation elected, free the upper pole completely and divide the lobe along the line of resection as outlined in Figure 107-11. At this level of the dissection both parathyroid glands and the recurrent nerve, all of which have been previously identified, may be left in their normal locations. Divide the remaining gland between hemostats until the anterior surface of the trachea has been reached. At this point transect the isthmus as described below. Some surgeons believe that the lateral margin of the residual segment of thyroid should be sutured to the trachea, but this step is not essential. For patients undergoing bilateral

subtotal thyroidectomy for Graves' disease, leave no more than 2-4 g of thyroid tissue on each side.

Total Thyroid Lobectomy

Before considering total lobectomy, be certain you have positively identified the recurrent nerve and the superior and inferior parathyroid glands. After these structures have been dissected away from the thyroid, proceed with the total lobectomy. The gland is firmly attached to the two upper tracheal rings by dense fibrous tissue that constitutes the ligament of Berry **(Fig. 107-13)**. The upper portion of the recurrent laryngeal nerve passes close to the point where this ligament attaches to the trachea. Moreover, often there is a small artery passing close to the recurrent nerve in this ligament. Be careful to control this vessel without injuring the nerve before dividing the ligament. After this ligament has been freed, the thyroid lobe can easily be liberated from the trachea by clamping and dividing several small blood vessels until the isthmus has been elevated. The isthmus may be divided serially between hemostats or by a single application of the 55/3.5 mm

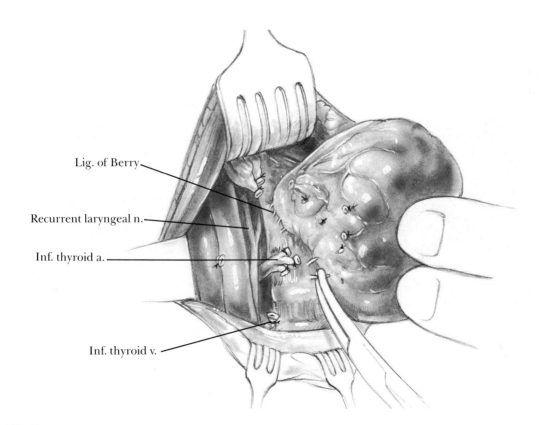

Lig. of Berry

Recurrent laryngeal n.

Inf. thyroid a.

Inf. thyroid v.

Fig. 107-13

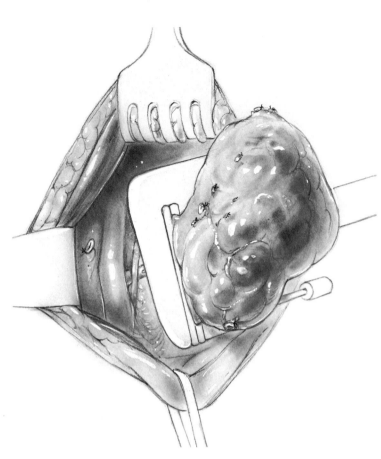

Fig. 107-14

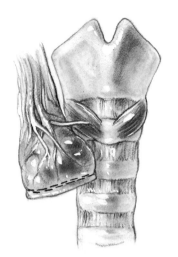

Fig. 107-16

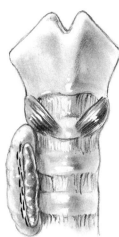

Fig. 107-17

linear stapling device, as seen in **Figure 107–14**. Then divide the isthmus with a scalpel leaving the left lobe of the thyroid in place, as seen in **Figure 107–15**.

Irrigate the operative field with saline and obtain *complete* hemostasis by ligatures and electrocautery. Always keep the recurrent nerve and the parathyroid glands in view while taking these steps.

Partial Thyroid Lobectomy

On some occasions what appears to be an obviously benign lesion occupies a small portion of the

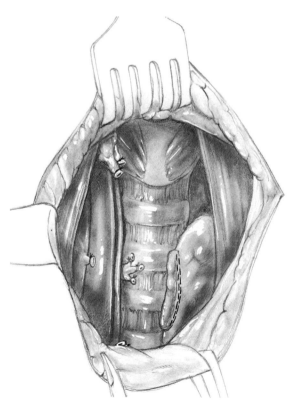

Fig. 107-15

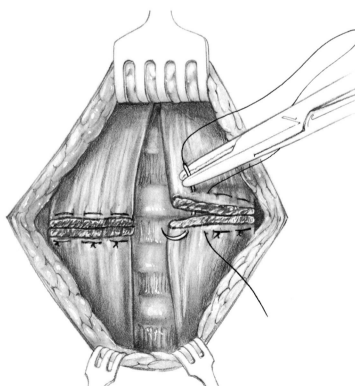

Fig. 107-18

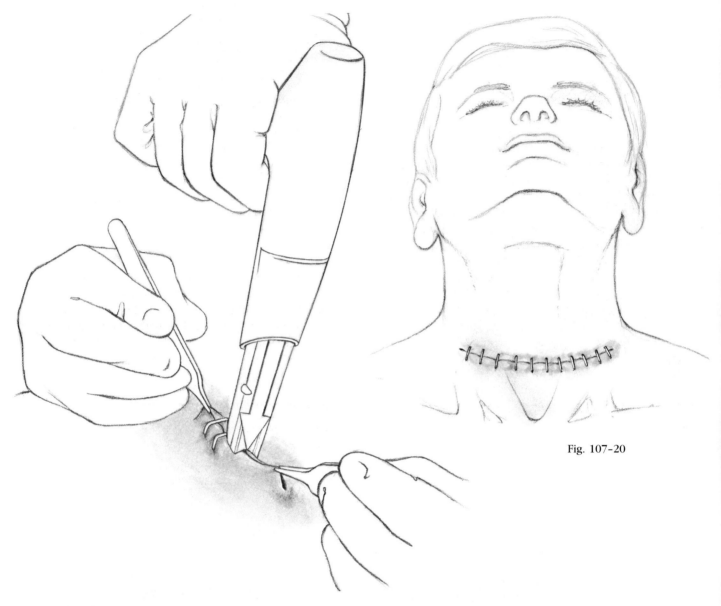

Fig. 107–20

Fig. 107–19

thyroid gland. Under these conditions, local excision or partial lobectomy may be indicated. The stapling device is sometimes useful under these conditions. **Figure 107–16** illustrates removal of the lower half of the right thyroid lobe, a stapling device having been used first to close and control bleeding from the remaining segment of thyroid. Remember that *identification and preservation* of the recurrent nerve must be achieved early in the dissection. If the gland is fairly thick, use 4.8 mm staples.

For benign lesions of the isthmus, dissect the isthmus away from the trachea. Then apply the stapling device to the junction between the isthmus and the adjacent thyroid lobes **(Fig. 107–17)**.

Closure

In the unusual situation where the strap muscles have been transected, resuture these two muscles by means of interrupted mattress sutures of 2-0 PG, as illustrated in **Figure 107–18**. In other cases simply suture the right and left strap muscles together loosely with interrupted 4-0 PG sutures. We rarely place drains in thyroidectomy cases. Hemostasis should be *perfect* before the operation is terminated. It is not safe to depend on a drain to evacuate blood clots.

After the strap muscles have been reapproximated, suture the divided platysma muscle together using interrupted 5-0 PG stitches. Close the skin by means of carefully applied skin staples **(Figs. 107–19, 107–20)** or interrupted fine nylon.

POSTOPERATIVE CARE

In patients with Graves' disease, carefully monitor vital signs to detect early evidence of *thyroid storm*. Patients who were prepared for operation with propranolol require treatment with this medication for 7–10 days following the operation.

Carefully observe the patient's neck for signs of swelling or ecchymosis. Active *bleeding* in the bed of the excised thyroid gland can rapidly compress the trachea and cause respiratory obstruction, especially if the bleeding is due to a major artery. Under rare circumstances it is necessary to remove all sutures in the skin and strap muscles to release the blood clot at the patient's bedside. In most cases, evacuate the blood clot in the operating room. After removing a large goiter, occasionally there is gradual swelling of the tissues of the neck due to slow venous bleeding that infiltrates the tissues. It may produce respiratory distress due to laryngeal edema. This patient requires orotracheal intubation and evacuation of the clot in the operating room. It is rare that exploration or a tracheostomy must be done at the patient's bedside.

Following bilateral thyroid lobectomy, check for *hypocalcemia* by measuring the serum calcium level until the patient is discharged. Observe for signs of paresthesia of the extremities or face, symptoms that generally appear when the calcium level drops below 7–8 mg/dl. Treat the symptoms with intravenous calcium gluconate (1 g of a 10% solution several times a day). Give oral calcium carbonate tablets (2–4 g/day) as required to maintain the serum calcium level. If calcium administration alone does not control the symptoms, administer vitamin D (50,000–100,000 units a day by mouth). The milder form of hypocalcemia following thyroid surgery is usually transient because it is caused by minor trauma to the parathyroid glands. Severe postoperative hypoparathyroidism is often permanent.

The patient who has undergone trauma to both recurrent laryngeal nerves may develop complete *airway obstruction* requiring prompt endotracheal intubation and then tracheostomy. This complication is rare.

COMPLICATIONS

Hematoma with possible tracheal compression and respiratory distress may occur.

There may be *injury to the recurrent laryngeal nerve*. If the injury is unilateral, it generally produces some degree of hoarseness and weakness of the voice. As mentioned above, bilateral recurrent nerve

damage causes bilateral vocal cord paralysis and marked narrowing of the glottis with respiratory obstruction, which often requires immediate tracheostomy. The airway may later be improved by an arytenoidectomy. Postoperative hoarseness may be also due to transient vocal cord edema or vocal cord injury caused by the endotracheal tube used for anesthesia.

Superior laryngeal nerve injury may result in the patient being unable to utter high-pitched sounds.

Hypoparathyroidism, transient or permanent, results from inadvertent removal of or trauma to several of the parathyroid glands. If during operation it is noted that one or more parathyroid glands have been removed, slice them into segments 1 × 1 mm each. Then transplant them into a muscle of the forearm or the neck. If the fragments are sufficiently small, satisfactory function may develop. Transient hypoparathyroidism lasting as long as several months may result from manipulation of the parathyroid glands without permanent damage.

Thyroid storm may develop following thyroidectomy for Graves' disease, especially if the preoperative preparation has not been adequate. This condition is characterized by fever, severe tachycardia, mental confusion, delirium, and restlessness. Rarely seen today, thyroid storm may be treated by adequate doses of propylthiouracil and intravenous sodium iodide; it may also be treated with propranolol, 2 mg IV with electrocardiographic control followed by 10–40 mg PO several times a day. A hypothermia blanket may be required to manage the high fever.

Hypothyroidism may follow bilateral subtotal thyroidectomy. Although many surgeons believe that after an interval of 1–2 years following thyroidectomy thyroid hormone secretion continues at a stable rate, others contend that, like radioactive iodine, thyroidectomy may induce hypothyroidism many years after operation. Consequently, these patients should be checked for thyroid function at intervals of 1–2 years for an indefinite period of time.

REFERENCES

Block MA. Surgery of thyroid nodules and malignancy. Curr Probl Surg 1983;20:137.

Katz AD, Nemiroff P. Anastamoses and bifurcations of the recurrent laryngeal nerve: report of 1177 nerves visualized. Am Surg 1993;54:188.

Lekacos NL, Tzardis PJ, Sfikakis PG, Patoulis SD, Restos SD. Course of the recurrent laryngeal nerve relative to the inferior thyroid artery and the suspensory ligament of Berry. Int Surg 1992;77:287.

Levin KE, Clark AH, Duh Q-Y, et al. Reoperative thyroid surgery. Surgery 1992;111:604.

Schwartz AE, Friedman EW. Preservation of the parathyroid glands in total thyroidectomy. Surg Gynecol Obstet 1987;165:327.

Soh EY, Clark OH. Surgical considerations and approach to thyroid cancer. Endocrinol Metab Clin North Am 1996;25:115.

Wells SA Jr, Ross AJ, Dale JK, et al. Transplantation of the parathyroid glands: current status. Surg Clin North Am 1979;59:167.

108 Parathyroidectomy

Nelson J. Gurll

INDICATIONS

Primary hyperparathyroidism is a common disease. Parathyroidectomy is required in most patients with primary hyperparathyroidism to prevent the osseous and renal complications and relieve symptoms of this disease because there is no effective nonoperative treatment. Some patients with mild hypercalcemia (serum calcium <1 mg/dl or 0.25 mmol/L higher than the upper range of normal) and no renal, bone, gastrointestinal, psychiatric, or neuromuscular symptoms can be treated nonoperatively. The diagnosis is made by finding persistent hypercalcemia and an elevated serum parathyroid hormone (PTH) concentration. The double site assay for intact PTH is more reliable than previous assays [1]. Other causes of hypercalcemia are ruled out by the history, particularly the use of lithium and thiazide diuretics. A 24-hour urine collection is valuable for documenting the extent of hypercalciuria and to rule out familial hypocalciuric hypercalcemia (FHH). Preoperative localization studies are not needed before the initial neck exploration for primary hyperparathyroidism by an experienced parathyroid surgeon but are mandatory before reoperation. The sestamibi scan is the most reliable of the localization techniques but is still not as reliable as an experienced parathyroid surgeon.

The cause for primary hyperparathyroidism in most patients is unknown. It can be induced by irradiation, or it may be familial in origin. Hyperparathyroidism occurs in at least 90% of patients with multiple endocrine neoplasia type I (MEN-I), 10–40% of patients with MEN-IIA, and rarely in those with MEN-IIB.

An NIH consensus conference [2] defined accepted indications for parathyroidectomy in primary hyperparathyroidism as the following.

Hypercalcemic crisis (serum calcium >14.5 mg/dl or 3.62 mmol/L)

Kidney stone

Bone pain

Age < 50 years

Urine calcium excretion > 400 mg/day (100 mmol/day)

Serum calcium concentration >1.0–1.6 mg/dl (0.25–0.40 mmol/L) higher than upper limit of normal

Bone mass > 2 standard deviations below age-, gender-, and race-matched controls

Creatinine clearance reduced by 30% compared with age-matched subjects

Consistent follow-up unlikely

Coexistent illness complicating nonoperative management

Secondary hyperparathyroidism results from chronic renal failure (CRF) or malabsorption and is characterized by hypocalcemia and hyperphosphatemia. It is common in patients with CRF and usually responds to treatment with phosphate binders, calcium, and vitamin D. About 5–10% of these patients require parathyroidectomy because of metabolic complications or symptoms. Some patients with CRF develop tertiary hyperparathyroidism with autonomous parathyroid function resulting in hypercalcemia despite removal of the stimulus (for hyperparathyroidism) by dialysis or renal transplantation. Clark [3] defined indications for surgery in patients with secondary and tertiary hyperparathyroidism as the following.

Bone pain

Spontaneous bone fractures

Ca × PO$_4$ solubility product > 70

Ectopic or vascular calcifications

Calciphylaxis

Serum calcium > 12 mg/dl (3 mmol/L)

Pruritus

Psychoneurologic symptoms

Conjunctivitis

Persistent hypercalcemia > 11.5 mg/dl (2.88 mmol/L) (more than 6 months) after successful renal transplantation

Recurrent hypercalcemia and increasing alkaline phosphatase after renal transplantation.

PREOPERATIVE PREPARATION

Laryngoscopy, either indirect or direct fiberoptic

Serum calcium and potassium day before operation

Dialysis with regional heparinization the day before operation for secondary hyperparathyroidism

PITFALLS AND DANGER POINTS

The major pitfall is failing to cure the disease because of missing multiglandular disease or failing to find the offending adenoma.

Injury to the recurrent laryngeal nerve is possible with resultant change in voice, aspiration of liquids, failure to protect the airway, and possible upper airway obstruction. Damage to the motor branch of the superior laryngeal nerve is less common and produces only minor changes in the voice.

Recurrence of hypercalcemia is low after excision of a solitary parathyroid adenoma but higher with hyperplasia or adenomatosis due to familial disease or secondary hyperparathyroidism. Removal of too much parathyroid tissue is also possible, especially if everything found at operation is biopsied or excised.

OPERATIVE STRATEGY

Curing the Disease

Do a careful bilateral neck exploration in all patients. This avoids missing multiglandular disease, including double adenomas and hyperplasia. The role of a pathologist is mostly supportive. They can tell us that we removed or biopsied parathyroid tissue and the weight of the material. The decision about what to do is based on the gross findings.

The sine qua non of parathyroid surgery is a bloodless field. The presence of blood around a lymph node or a bit of fat make it look like a parathyroid gland. It is for this reason that we perform sharp dissection with scalpels utilizing an electrical current or heat for cauterization. We do not use electrocautery close to the recurrent laryngeal nerve to avoid injuring it by local spread of the electrical current.

A subtotal parathyroidectomy or a total parathyroidectomy with autotransplantation (of fresh or cryopreserved tissue) is performed for hyperplasia, MEN-I, MEN-IIA, and secondary hyperparathyroidism. The choice of which procedure to use depends on the findings at operation, the relative risks of hypocalcemia and recurrent hypercalcemia, the availability of cryopreservation, and patient reliability. Subtotal parathyroidectomy is used in patients with secondary hy-

perparathyroidism who can be relied on to take calcium and vitamin D to prevent the parathyroid remnant from growing. We agree with Clark [3] that a total parathyroidectomy with autotransplantation is advised for unreliable patients.

The cervical thymus is removed from patients with primary or secondary hyperplasia because of the 15–25% incidence of supernumerary parathyroids (many of which are in the thymus) in these conditions [4].

Preserving the Recurrent Laryngeal Nerve

The superior parathyroids are lateral and posterior to the nerve, and the inferior parathyroids are generally anterior and medial to the nerve (see Fig. 107–2). The recurrent laryngeal nerve inserts into the larynx just caudad to the caudad edge of the cricothyroideus muscle, so the superior pole of thyroid can be mobilized cephalad to this muscle without worrying about damage to this nerve **(Fig. 108–1)**. Even a nonrecurrent recurrent laryngeal nerve, which occurs on the right side with an incidence of only 1%, still inserts into the larynx caudad to the cricothyroideus muscle. The nerve can bifurcate, but generally it does so within about 1 cm of its insertion into the larynx. Gross identification of the nerve is aided by the presence of a vaso vasorum that looks like a "red racing stripe" on the anterior surface of the nerve. The nerve runs slightly obliquely in the tracheoesophageal groove. Structures running along this course are not the inferior thyroid artery (which is a misnomer). This artery actually corresponds in position to the middle thyroid vein. Unfortunately, the nomenclature suggests to the novice that the artery should be running from an inferior location cephalad to the thyroid, whereas it runs transversely in the neck. The recurrent laryngeal nerve is most commonly injured at the ligament of Berry, as

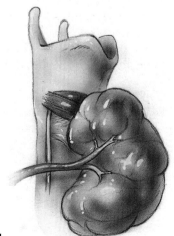

Fig. 108–1

the nerve can be closely adherent to or even run through the substance of the ligament.

Preserving the Superior Laryngeal Nerve

The motor branch of the superior laryngeal nerve may descend low and anterior to, interdigitate with branches of, or be enveloped in the same fascial sheath as the superior thyroid artery **(Fig. 108–2)**. This makes injury to the nerve possible particularly during thyroid lobectomy. It is less of a problem during parathyroidectomy but still must be borne in mind. Some surgeons verify the position of this nerve on the basis of electrical stimulation to see movement of the cricothyroideus muscle.

Preserving Normal Parathyroid Tissue

The neck should be explored on both sides before excising or biopsying tissue. Parathyroids that are normal grossly should not be excised. We tend to be conservative in our operations, preferring to excise only abnormally enlarged parathyroids and biopsy the next largest normal parathyroid. Gross identification of the parathyroids is adequate if the surgeon is experienced.

OPERATIVE TECHNIQUE

Incision and Exposure

Mark a line (a skin crease or one of Langer's lines) using a suture at the base of the neck with the pa-

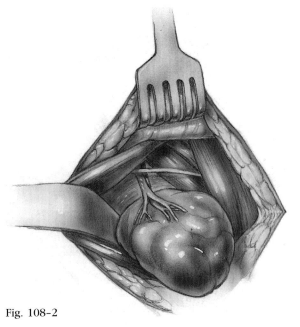

Fig. 108-2

tient sitting in a comfortable position (with arms folded in the lap) to achieve the best cosmetic result. Lightly scratch the mark with a Keith needle, and wipe the mark with an alcohol sponge to elicit Lewis' triple response. To wait until the patient is supine and then mark the incision belies the fact that most people see the patient erect. The shift in the skin line when they do become supine varies two to three fingerbreadths above the sternal notch, and the depth of the sternal notch varies from patient to patient, making the incision line variable in its ultimate location.

Place a folded sheet longitudinally along the thoracic spine to allow the shoulders to roll laterally. Extend the neck gently with a rolled towel underneath the neck and the patient's head in a donut or padded support. Move the patient to the barber chair position with arms at the side and flexion at the hips and the knees.

Make a skin incision 7-8 cm long with a No. 15 blade (see Fig. 107-4). Divide the subcutaneous tissues and platysma muscle transversely. Elevate subplatysmal skin flaps cephalad to the notch of the thyroid cartilage and caudad to the sternal notch (see Fig. 107-5). Incise the investing layer of the deep cervical fascia in the midline from notch to notch (see Fig. 107-6). Separate the strap muscles from each other and from their contralateral partners. Divide the areolar tissue between the thyroid and the strap muscles. Dividing the strap muscles transversely is not required.

Identify Crossing of the Inferior Thyroid Artery and the Recurrent Laryngeal Nerve

Mobilize the thyroid lobe medially to separate it from the carotid sheath (see Fig. 107-8). The middle thyroid vein need not be divided, especially as subsequent localization for a missed adenoma by angiography and venous sampling for the PTH assay is helped by being able to sample this vein. The recurrent laryngeal nerve runs posterior (most commonly) or anterior to the inferior thyroid artery and sometimes even interdigitates with branches of the artery. The relation of the inferior thyroid artery and recurrent laryngeal nerve is important because we locate the parathyroids relative to the crossing of the nerve and the artery.

Find the nerve low in the neck and trace it cephalad by careful blunt dissection anterior to the nerve. This generally allows you to find and preserve the bifurcation and avoid injury to the nerve at the ligament of Berry.

Identifying Inferior and Superior Parathyroids

The two parathyroids on each side are often surprisingly close to each other. The superior parathyroids are usually juxtacricoidal, and the inferior parathyroids are usually within a 2 cm radius of the inferior pole of the thyroid. Inspect the posterior capsule of the thyroid and the areas posterior and lateral to the thyroid. A reddish-brown color is the visual clue to an adenoma. It is different in appearance from the thyroid, bits of fat, or lymph nodes. The normal parathyroid is yellow-brown and generally tongue-shaped, although it can have other shapes. Gently palpate these areas to detect masses. Follow the course of the recurrent laryngeal nerve. Inspect and palpate both sides of the neck to determine if you are dealing with a solitary adenoma or multiglandular disease. It may be necessary to mobilize the superior pole of the thyroid to find the superior parathyroid.

Resecting the Adenoma

Mobilize the adenoma from surrounding tissues sharply with the electrocautery unit, making sure you have preserved the recurrent laryngeal nerve. Divide the hilar blood supply to the adenoma between clamps and ties of fine permanent sutures. Do not grasp the adenoma with forceps, which would increase the chance of breaking the capsule, leading to implantation of parathyroid tissue and recurrent hypercalcemia.

Biopsying Normal Parathyroid

Biopsy the next largest parathyroid gland. Place a gauze sponge around the parathyroid to adsorb any parathyroid cells dropped from the biopsy **(Fig. 108–3)**. Mobilize the antihilar one-third to one-fourth of the parathyroid sharply and excise it as a

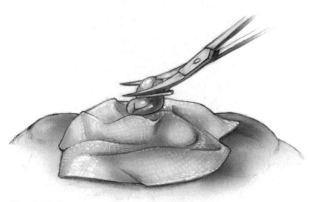

Fig. 108–3

biopsy. The cut edge of a parathyroid typically bleeds uniformly, which helps with its identification. Control the bleeding with a hemostatic clip, which also marks the position of this gland. Remove and discard the sponge after it has sopped up serum and free cells. Irrigate the area with sterile water to lyse any loose parathyroid cells.

Subtotal Parathyroidectomy

The term "three and a half gland parathyroidectomy" is imprecise and should be abandoned. First fashion a well vascularized remnant of the most normal-looking parathyroid away from the recurrent laryngeal nerve. Excise tissue sharply from the antihilar end until the remnant is about 50 mg ($5 \times 3 \times 2$ mm). Mobilize and excise each of the other parathyroids sequentially, looking back to confirm the viability of the original remnant before excising the next gland. If this remnant is not viable, fashion another well vascularized remnant from one of the remaining glands. This practice provides four opportunities to obtain a well vascularized remnant. Cryopreserve all parathyroid tissue removed and not given to the pathologist.

Total Parathyroidectomy with Autotransplantation

Remove all four parathyroids. Set aside parathyroid tissue for autotransplantation immediately (on ice) or after cryopreservation (slow freezing).

Make a longitudinal incision in the volar aspect of the nondominant forearm. Sharply divide subcutaneous tissues down to the fascia of the forearm musculature. Create 12–15 pockets in the volar aspect of the forearm musculature using the electrocautery unit for the fascia and careful blunt dissection in the direction of the muscle fibers to avoid eschar and hematoma formation, respectively. Mince a parathyroid into $1 \times 1 \times 1$ mm pieces. Place each piece in an individual muscle pocket, and close it over with a fine permanent suture; mark it with a hemoclip. Close the skin with absorbable subcuticular sutures and adhesive skin strips.

Sequence for an Unfound Adenoma

Explore for the adenoma in all the usual locations. Follow the branches of the inferior thyroid artery, which can be a clue to its location. Gently pull on an enlarged branch of the inferior thyroid artery going to a suspected adenoma after you have found three normal parathyroids. Incise the thyroid capsule over any area of discoloration that might be due

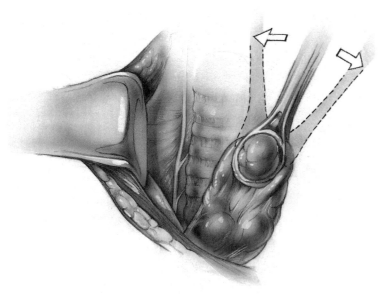

Fig. 108-4

to devascularization of an intrathyroidal parathyroid. Mobilize the thyrothymic ligament to help mobilize the cervical thymus to search for an intrathymic parathyroid adenoma. Inspect and palpate behind the pharynx and esophagus. Open the carotid sheath to inspect for parathyroids associated with the vagus nerve. Inspect and palpate again along the embryologic course of the parathyroids from the hyoid bone to the aortic arch.

Perform a thyroid lobectomy on the side of a missing superior parathyroid adenoma. The technique is similar to that shown in Chapter 107.

Perform a cervical thymectomy for a missing inferior parathyroid adenoma. Grasp thyrothymic fat and thymus with ring forceps. Sharply mobilize the adenoma off the trachea between the recurrent laryngeal nerves as far caudad as you can reach. Bluntly mobilize it from underneath the manubrium aided by a rocking, back-and-fourth motion of the ring forceps grasping the tissue (**Fig. 108–4**). Excise this tissue.

Closure

Achieve hemostasis using a hot scalpel or by fine suture-ligatures for bleeding close to the recurrent laryngeal nerve. Close the strap muscles in layers with interrupted absorbable sutures and the investing layer of the deep cervical fascia with a running absorbable suture. Close the platysma muscle with interrupted absorbable sutures, and approximate the skin edges with Michel clips or subcuticular absorbable sutures and adhesive skin strips.

Reoperation

Reoperation may be indicated if the patient does not achieve normocalcemia and has significant disease. Localization studies are required. If the suspected adenoma is localized to one side, incise the investing layer of deep cervical fascia between the strap muscles and the sternocleidomastoid muscle on that side (**Fig. 108–5**). Dissect down to the carotid sheath. Divide or mobilize and retract the omohyoid muscle. Find the recurrent laryngeal nerve. Approach the thyroid from its lateral aspect, avoiding scars from the previous operation. If the suspected adenoma has not been localized, reexploration on both sides is necessary. Do this in a systematic way, exploring the usual locations first, as the missing adenoma is usually there.

A partial or full median sternotomy is almost never done at the initial exploration but may be necessary if the suspected adenoma is in the chest. Incise the skin vertically in the midline from the midpoint of the low collar incision to the third intercostal space or to the xiphoid process. Place a finger behind the sternum. Cut the manubrium and the sternum with a vibrating saw in the midline after dividing the muscles. Retract the sternum. The sternum should be closed with wire sutures.

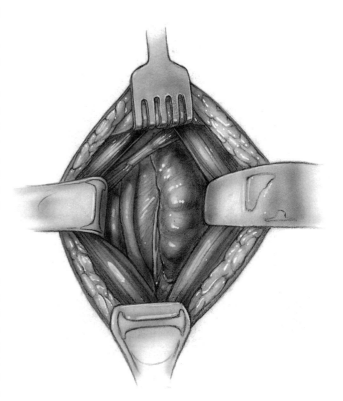

Fig. 108-5

POSTOPERATIVE CARE

Cover the incision with a dry sterile dressing. Give clear liquids the night of the operation, and advance some patients to a regular diet if tolerated. Check them closely for upper airway obstruction and signs of damage to the parathyroids or laryngeal nerves. Check the serum calcium level daily. Incisional pain is tolerable and responds to acetaminophen with or without codeine.

Dialyze patients with secondary hyperparathyroidism 1–2 days after operation using regional heparinization. Check the serum potassium and calcium levels the evening of the operation and daily thereafter in these patients.

COMPLICATIONS

Bleeding is a possibility after any neck exploration and is of vital concern when it causes tracheal compression and respiratory compromise. It usually manifests the evening of operation as dyspnea and is managed by evacuating the hematoma emergently using a sterile clamp that has been taped to the bed for just this possibility. Take the patient to the operating room to explore the neck. Usually no single bleeding point is found.

There are several causes of *upper airway obstruction* in addition to hematoma. The most common is soft tissues, usually the tongue, falling posteriorly. This complication typically occurs in the recovery room and is usually reversed by the chin lift or jaw thrust maneuver. *Laryngospasm* is also possible particularly early after operation and is often relieved by the same maneuvers but may require reintubation. *Recurrent laryngeal nerve palsy*, particularly bilaterally, can cause upper airway obstruction. It is typically seen right after operation but may be delayed because of swelling, causing paresis of the nerve 1–2 days postoperatively. It may require reintubation or tracheostomy. *Tracheomalacia* can also cause upper airway obstruction. It is due to softening of the trachea owing to the presence of a long-standing goiter; it is not common with hyperparathyroidism. Finally, *laryngeal tetany* can cause

upper airway obstruction because of hypocalcemia from hypoparathyroidism. It responds quickly to parenteral calcium.

Recurrent laryngeal nerve palsy can arise simply from dissecting the nerve (without a direct injury). Identifying the recurrent laryngeal nerve at operation may increase the chance of temporary palsy but probably decreases the chance of permanent palsy. A nerve transection during neck exploration should be repaired using magnification, microsurgical instruments, and fine permanent sutures to approximate the neurilemmal sheath.

Superior laryngeal nerve palsy is uncommon— or perhaps it is uncommonly detected. It should be a problem only to patients who use their voice professionally, such as the opera star Amelita Galli-Curci, whose career was cut short by injury to this nerve at thyroidectomy.

Patients may develop *hypocalcemia* as the disease reverses itself after successful parathyroidectomy. It is usually temporary and responds to parenteral and oral calcium. Give calcium chloride or calcium gluconate 1 g IV and then calcium carbonate 1.5 g PO qid. For significant hypocalcemia, I usually add Rocaltrol 0.25–0.50 μg PO qd. If the serum calcium is normal 1–2 weeks postoperatively on oral calcium alone, the calcium dose can usually be tapered and stopped or reduced to replacement doses given for optimal bone health.

REFERENCES

1. Nussbaum SR, Zahrachnik RJ, Lavigne JR, et al. Highly sensitive two-site immunoradiometric assay of parathyrin and its clinical utility in evaluating patients with hypercalcemia. Clin Chem 1987;33:1364.

2. NIH Conference. Diagnosis and management of asymptomatic primary hyperparathyroidism: consensus development conference statement. Ann Intern Med 1991;114:593.

3. Clark OH. Secondary hyperparathyroidism. In Clark OH (ed) Endocrine Surgery of the Thyroid and Parathyroid Glands. St. Louis, Mosby, 1985, pp 241–255.

4. Edis AJ, Levitt MD. Supernumerary parathyroid glands: implications for the surgical treatment of secondary hyperparathyroidism. World J Surg 1987;11:398.

109 Cricothyroidotomy

INDICATIONS

Establishing an emergency airway when oral or nasal endotracheal intubation cannot be achieved

PREOPERATIVE PREPARATION

Like tracheotomy, cricothyroidotomy is simpler to perform in a patient who has already been orally intubated, but many cricothyroidotomy procedures are performed under emergency conditions where no preoperative preparation is possible.

PITFALLS AND DANGER POINTS

Erroneous incision in thyrohyoid membrane. A dangerous error, occasionally incurred by a neophyte under conditions of excitement, is to make the incision *above* the thyroid cartilage in the thyrohyoid membrane instead of *below* it in the cricothyroid region. This mistake may cause serious damage to the structures of the larynx. When learning to do this

operation, remember that the incision is made at the lower border of the thyroid cartilage between the thyroid and the cricoid cartilages.

Failure to control subcutaneous bleeding. Occasionally a vein in the subcutaneous space is transected. The veins should be ligated or electrocauterized to avoid postoperative bleeding. In the emergency setting, venous bleeding may be temporarily controlled by pressure or packing. Definitive hemostasis can then be obtained after the patient is stabilized.

OPERATIVE STRATEGY

Because cricothyroidotomy is often performed in an emergency situation, local infiltration of the anesthetic into the skin over the cricothyroid membrane is usually employed. In desperate situations, of course, no anesthesia is necessary.

Because the most dangerous error is making the incision in the wrong place, avoid this problem by grasping the lateral margins of the thyroid cartilage between the thumb and the middle finger of the left hand us-

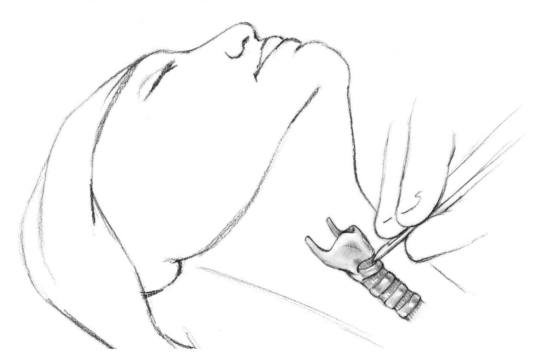

Fig. 109-1

912

ing the tip of the index finger to palpate the space between the lower margin of the thyroid cartilage and the upper margin of the cricoid. With this maneuver, one can accurately pinpoint the proper site for the incision. Under conditions of desperate emergency in the field without instruments, it is possible to perform this procedure with a sharp penknife by inserting the tip of the blade through the skin and the cricothyroid membrane with one motion. Then twist the blade 70°-90° to provide a temporary airway until some type of tube can be inserted into the trachea.

OPERATIVE TECHNIQUE

Place a folded sheet under the patient's shoulders to elevate them 4-8 cm above table level. This extends the neck somewhat. After the usual skin preparation, grasp the lateral margin of the thyroid cartilage between the thumb and the middle finger of the left hand. Palpate the cricothyroid space accurately with the tip of the index finger; then infiltrate the line of the incision with local anesthesia. Make a 2 cm long transverse incision in the cricothyroid space. Carry the incision down to the cricothyroid membrane. Occlude any bleeding points with ligatures or electrocoagulation. Use a scalpel with a No. 15 blade to stab the cricothyroid membrane **(Figs. 109–1, 109–2)**. Enlarge the stab wound with a small hemostat or a Trousseau dilator, if available. Then insert heavy Mayo scissors into the incision and spread the tissues transversely **(Fig. 109–3)** until the open-

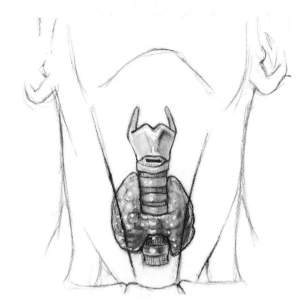

Fig. 109-2

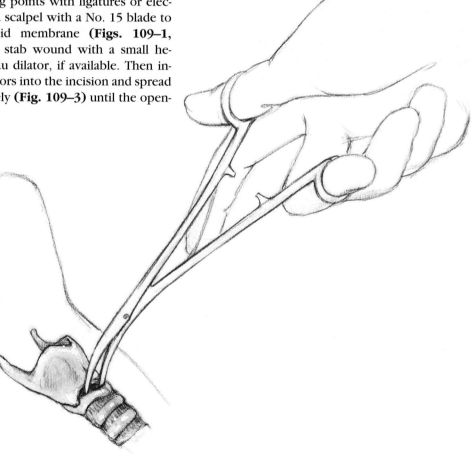

Fig. 109-3

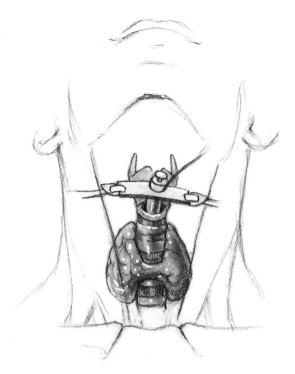

Fig. 109-4

ing is sufficiently large to insert a low-pressure cuff tracheostomy tube, generally 8 mm in diameter **(Fig. 109–4)**. Fix the tube in place and maintain it in the same manner as employed for intubation through the traditional tracheostomy incision. Closure of the skin wound is generally not necessary.

POSTOPERATIVE CARE

See Chapter 110.

COMPLICATIONS

Peristomal bleeding

Transient hoarseness

Infection, cellulitis

Subglottic stenosis has not been seen unless the patient had undergone preoperative endotracheal intubation for more than 7 days or had an inflammatory condition of the larynx prior to operation.

REFERENCES

American College of Surgeons. Advanced Trauma Life Support Manual, 6th ed. 1997, pp 93–95.

Boyd AD, Romita M, Conlan A, et al. A clinical evaluation of cricothyroidotomy. Surg Gynecol Obstet 1979;149: 365.

Brantigan CO, Grow JB. Subglottic stenosis after cricothyroidotomy. Surgery 1982;91:217.

110 Tracheostomy

INDICATIONS

Upper airway obstruction

Radical oropharyngeal or thyroid surgery

Severe laryngeal trauma

Long-term ventilatory support

PREOPERATIVE PREPARATION

Pass an oral or nasal endotracheal tube preoperatively whenever possible.

PITFALLS AND DANGER POINTS

Injury to the cricoid or first tracheal ring during surgery

Inadequate hemostasis

Asphyxia

OPERATIVE STRATEGY

Because most tracheostomy operations are performed with an orotracheal or nasotracheal tube in place, local or general anesthesia may be used. With an indwelling endotracheal tube in place, the risk of anoxia during tracheostomy is virtually eliminated. If for some reason an endotracheal tube is not in place, be certain hemostasis is adequate before opening the trachea. Otherwise, blood may pour into the tracheal stoma, obstructing the airway. Always have an adequate suction apparatus available during tracheostomy. This is one reason a cricothyroidotomy is a better operation during an emergency situation when an endotracheal tube has not been passed.

If the incision in the trachea is made in the area of the first ring or the cricoid cartilage, there is a high risk of subglottic stenosis after the tracheostomy tube has been removed. It should be rec-

ognized that the opening in the trachea made by the tracheostomy tube heals by cicatrization, incurring the risk of mild narrowing of the trachea at the site of the tracheostomy. If this occurs in the subglottic region, corrective therapy is extremely difficult. For this reason, take every precaution to avoid incising or injuring the first ring or cricoid cartilage.

A low tracheostomy incision (e.g., in the fourth) may also entail unnecessary risk for the patient. Pressure exerted by the tip or cuff of the tube may erode into the innominate artery, resulting in massive hemorrhage into the trachea with prompt asphyxiation of the patient. This risk is especially applicable in children, where the innominate artery is relatively close to the tracheostomy site.

OPERATIVE TECHNIQUE

Endotracheal Tube

Virtually all patients should have an endotracheal tube in place prior to undergoing tracheostomy.

Incision and Exposure

Position the patient with a folded sheet underneath the shoulders so the neck is extended. Although some surgeons believe that a horizontal skin incision produces a better scar, the generally preferred incision is a vertical one beginning at the level of the cricoid and continuing in a caudal direction for about 4-5 cm. This incision gives better exposure and access. Carry the incision through the subcutaneous fat and the platysma muscle directly over the midline of the trachea, exposing the sternohyoid muscles. Achieve complete hemostasis with electrocautery and PG ligatures. Now elevate the strap muscles and make a vertical incision down the midline separating these two muscles. Carry the incision down to the upper trachea and expose and divide the capsule of the thyroid gland. Clamp, divide, and ligate all veins in this vicinity. Identify the thyroid

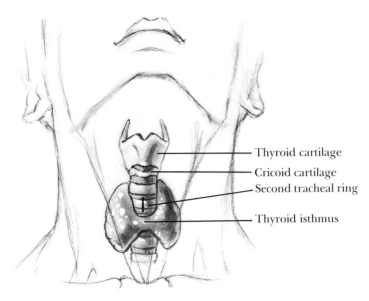

Fig. 110-1

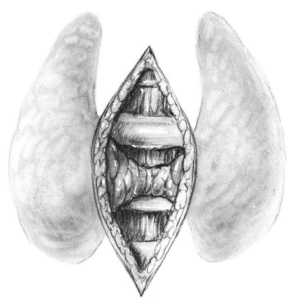

Fig. 110-2

isthmus. This bridge of tissue crosses the trachea generally in the vicinity of the third tracheal ring (**Figs. 110–1, 110–2**).

Identifying the Tracheal Rings

Clearly visualize the cricoid cartilage and the first tracheal ring. Preserve these two structures from injury. Occasionally, it is possible to retract the thyroid isthmus in a cephalad direction to expose the second and third tracheal rings. In most cases, it is necessary to free the thyroid isthmus from the trachea by sliding Metzenbaum scissors underneath the isthmus and elevating it. Then divide the isthmus between clamps and insert suture-ligatures to maintain complete hemostasis. This maneuver clearly reveals the identity of the second and third tracheal rings (**Fig. 110–3**).

Opening the Trachea

Ensure that hemostasis is complete. Also check the tracheostomy tube and cuff and that the suction apparatus is functioning.

In some cases incising only the second ring provides an adequate tracheostomy opening, but generally it is necessary to incise both the second and third rings. This procedure is facilitated by inserting a single hook retractor to elevate the upper portion of the second ring. Insert a scalpel with a No. 15 blade to incise the membrane transversely just above the second ring. Then divide the second ring with the scalpel (Fig. 110-3) and the third ring if necessary. Never divide the first ring or the cricoid cartilage.

Inserting Tracheostomy Tube

Retract the edges of the trachea by inserting a hemostat, two small hook retractors, or a Trousseau three-pronged retractor (**Fig. 110–4**). Because most tracheostomy operations require insertion of a tube with a large balloon cuff for mechanical ventilation, be certain to apply a water-soluble lubricant to the tip of the tracheostomy tube and cuff; then insert the tube into the tracheal incision (**Fig. 110–5**) while the anesthesiologist extracts the nasotracheal tube.

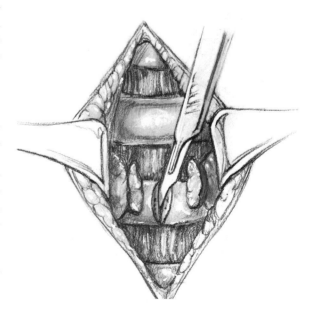

Fig. 110-3

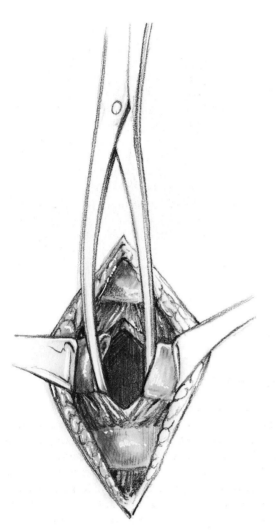

Fig. 110-4

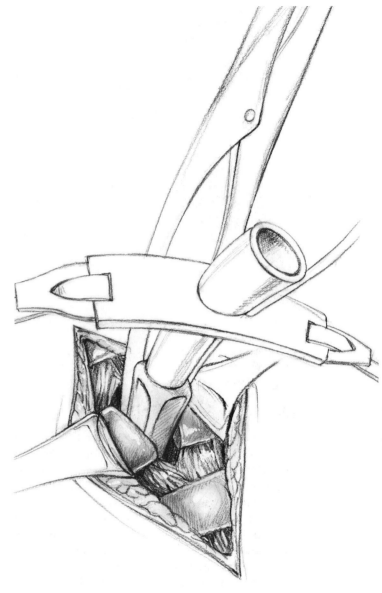

Fig. 110-5

Insert a suction catheter into the tracheostomy tube and aspirate mucus from the bronchial tree. Attach an oxygen line to the tracheostomy tube if necessary.

Closure

Some surgeons routinely place one or two sutures through the tracheal incision and leave them long, protruding from the wound. If the tracheostomy tube is dislodged prematurely, these sutures greatly facilitate reinsertion.

Reapproximate the sternohyoid muscles in the midline with interrupted 4-0 PG sutures. Insert several additional sutures to reapproximate the platysma muscle; then close the skin *loosely* with interrupted 4-0 nylon sutures. Suture the tracheostomy tube to the skin in two places. As soon as is practicable, tie the cotton tapes together at the back of the patient's neck to guarantee fixation of the tracheostomy tube.

POSTOPERATIVE CARE

Humidified air is necessary to prevent crusting of secretions and eventual obstruction of the tracheostomy tube. Use lightweight swivel connectors to attach the tracheostomy tube to the ventilator to avoid unnecessary pressure on the trachea at the stoma.

If the tracheostomy tube must be changed within the first one or two postoperative weeks, be certain to have instruments available for instant endotracheal intubation or emergency cricothyroidotomy if difficulty is encountered when reinserting a tracheostomy tube. Remember, the track between the skin and the tracheal stoma is not established for a variable number of days after the operation. After premature decannulation, the tracheal stoma typically retracts deep into the neck, where it is extremely difficult to find. This procedure must not be performed by the inexperienced.

When it is necessary to change the tracheostomy tube, first place the patient in a recumbent position with a sheet or sandbag underneath the shoulders. This maneuver extends the head and neck, bringing the tracheal stoma closer to the skin incision. Only with the patient in this position and with good light and suction at hand should the old tracheostomy tube be removed and replaced. Never attempt this maneuver during the first two postoperative weeks with the patient in a sitting position.

COMPLICATIONS

Hemorrhage following tracheostomy may occur as a result of the surgeon's having failed to ligate the bleeding points in the wound. The problem manifests as bleeding around the tracheostomy tube. A far more serious type of hemorrhage may occur late in the postoperative period, the result of the tip of the tracheostomy tube or the balloon cuff eroding through the anterior wall or the trachea into the innominate artery. This is a life-threatening complication manifested by arterial bleeding into the trachea. Emergency management of this condition depends on temporarily controlling the bleeding by inflating the balloon cuff. If inflating the cuff around the tracheostomy tube does not promptly control the bleeding, remove it and immediately insert an orotracheal tube. Secure immediate control of the bleeding by passing an index finger into the tracheostomy stoma and occluding the bleeding site against the underside of the sternum. Sometimes inflating the cuff of the orotracheal tube is sufficient to control the bleeding temporarily. Emergency resection of the innominate artery with suture of both ends may be necessary for definitive repair of the fistula, with

resection also of the damaged trachea in some cases. Subcutaneous emphysema may be avoided if the tissues are not sutured too snugly against the tracheostomy tube. There may be some air leakage between the trachea and the tracheostomy tube. If this air has access to the outside, subcutaneous emphysema does not occur.

Stenosis may occur sometime after the tracheostomy tube has been removed. The stenosis may be at the tracheal stoma or in the area of the trachea occluded by the balloon cuff. *Strictures* at the stoma level may be minimized by making the incision in the trachea as small as possible. Constrictions lower in the trachea have been virtually eliminated by large-volume, low-pressure balloon cuffs. If a patient who has undergone a period of mechanical ventilation with a tracheal tube ever develops signs of an upper airway obstruction (stridor, wheezing, shortness of breath), a stricture of the trachea should be strongly suspected. A lateral radiograph of the neck can disclose an *upper tracheal stricture*, and an oblique chest radiograph should identify *lower tracheal lesions*. Computed tomography or magnetic resonance imaging provide better imaging details. Tracheal resection and anastomosis may be necessary for serious strictures. A granuloma may be resected through a bronchoscope utilizing the laser in some cases.

Wound infection, pneumothorax (rare), and *accidental displacement of the tracheostomy tube* may also occur.

REFERENCES

Berrouschot J, Oeken J, Steiniger L, Schneider D. Perioperative complications of percutaneous dilational tracheotomy. Laryngoscope 1997;107:1538.

Dulguerov P, Gysin C, Perneger TV, Chevrolet JC. Percutaneous or surgical tracheostomy: a meta-analysis. Crit Care Med 1999;27:1617.

Powell DM, Prive PD, Forrest LA. Review of percutaneous tracheostomy. Laryngoscope 1998;108:170.

Part XIV
Appendix

Illustrated Glossary of Surgical Instruments

Jamal Hoballah

Instruments used during open surgery are shown first, followed by instruments used during laparoscopic surgery.

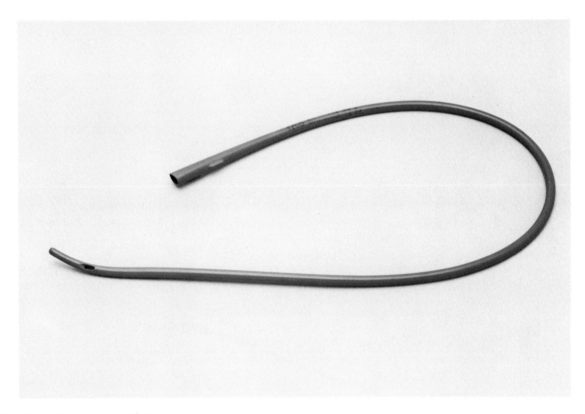

Fig. G-1. Catheter, Coudé tip.

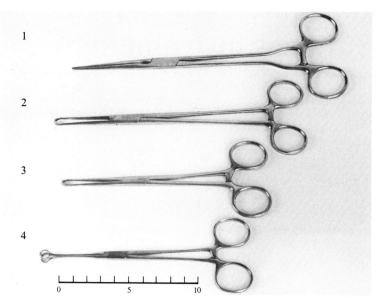

Fig. G-2.   Clamps: Allen (1); Allis (2, 3); Babcock (4).

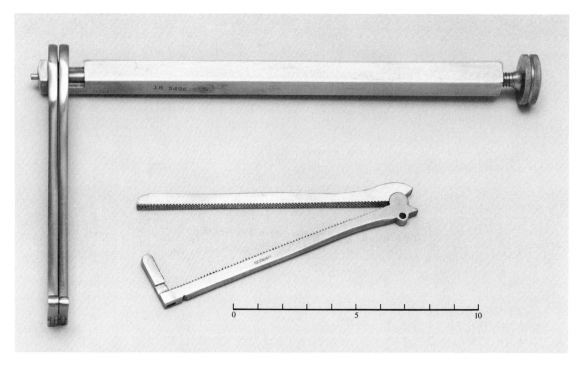

Fig. G-3.   Clamp: DeMartel (surgical legacy instrument).

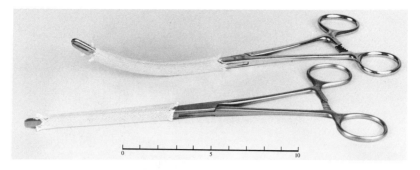

Fig. G–4.   Clamps: Doyen noncrushing intestinal, linen-shod.

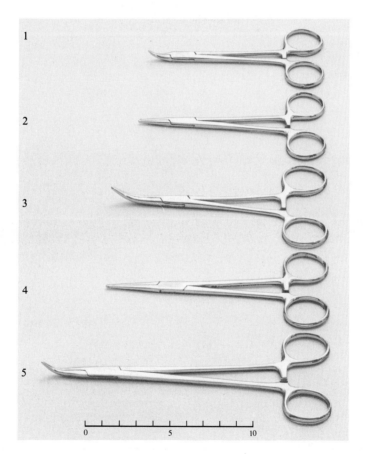

Fig. G–5.   Clamps, hemostatic: Halsted (1, 2); Crile (3, 4); Adson (tonsil) (5).

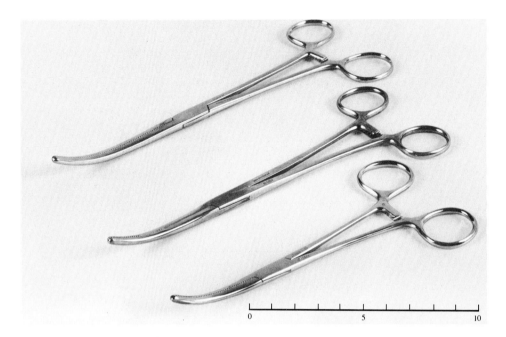

Fig. G-6.   Clamps, hemostatic: Kelly.

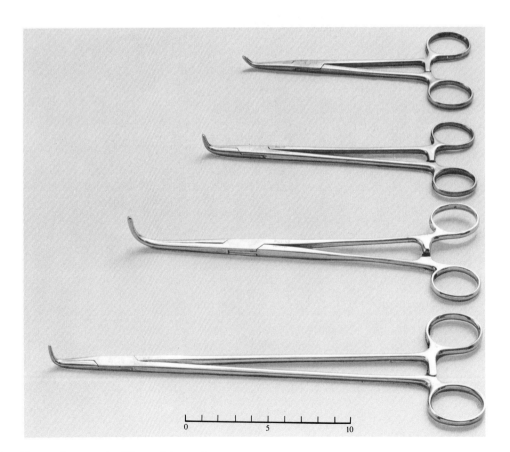

Fig. G-7.   Clamps, hemostatic: Mixter right angle.

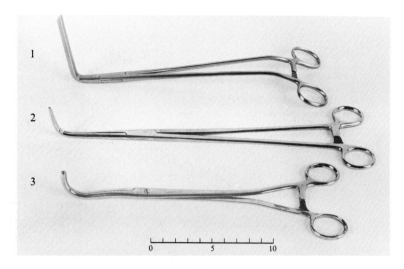

Fig. G-8. Clamps: kidney, right angle (1); bronchus (2); Moynihan (3).

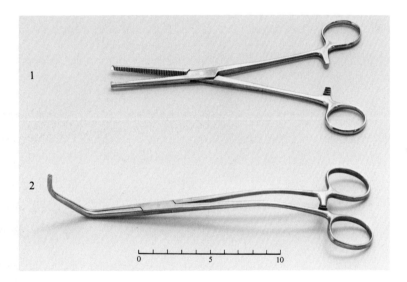

Fig. G-9. Clamps: Kocher (1); Satinsky (2).

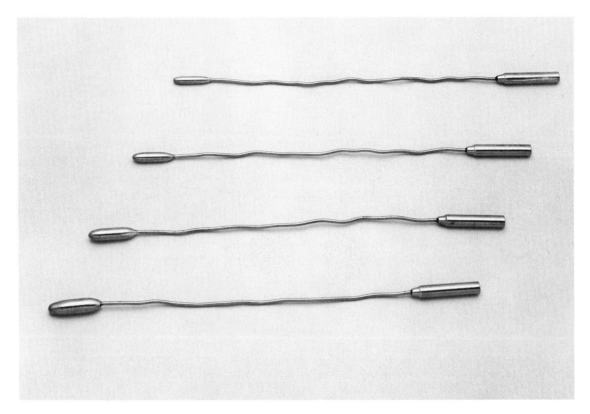

Fig. G–10.   Dilators, Bakes (surgical legacy instruments).

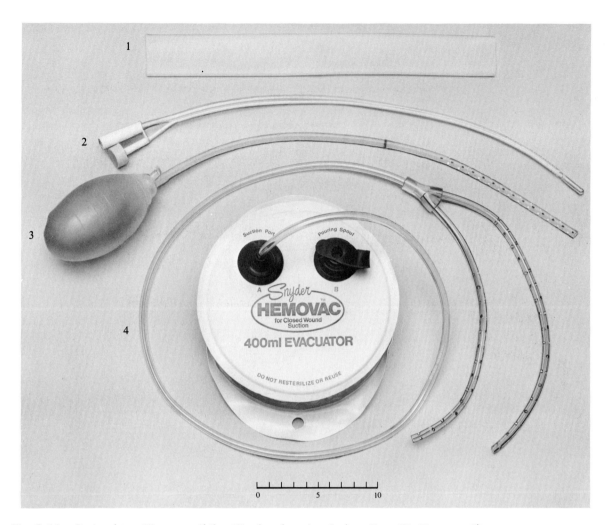

Fig. G-11.   Drains: latex (1); sump, Shiley (2); closed-suction, Jackson-Pratt (3); Hemovac (4).

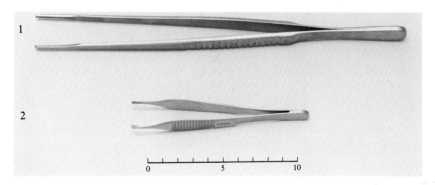

Fig. G-12.   Forceps: Debakey (1); Brown-Adson (2).

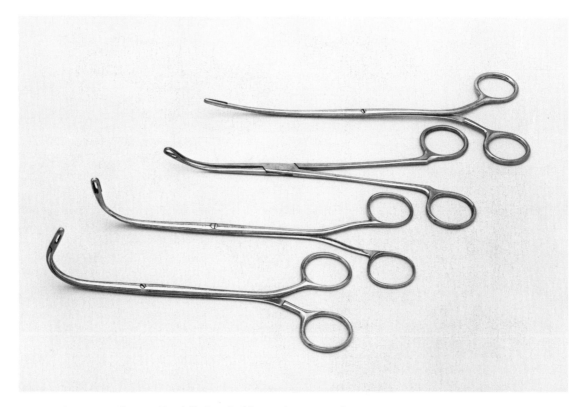

Fig. G-13.   Forceps: gallstone (Randall) (surgical legacy instruments).

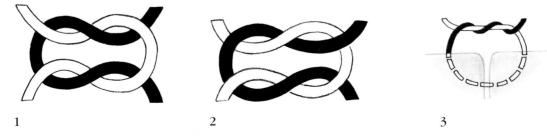

1   2   3

Fig. G-14.   Knots: square (1); granny (2); surgeon's (3).

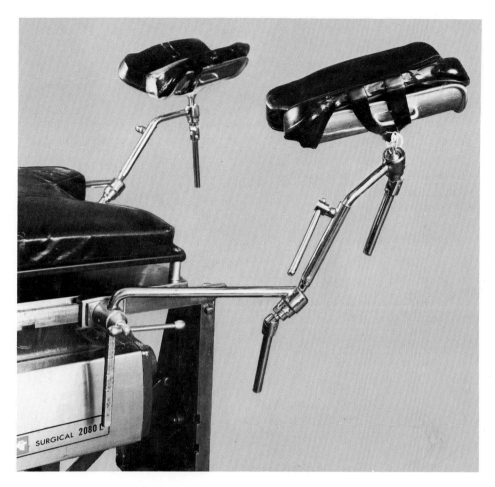

Fig. G-15.   Lloyd-Davies leg rests.

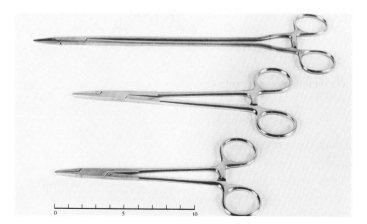

Fig. G-16.   Needle-holders, straight.

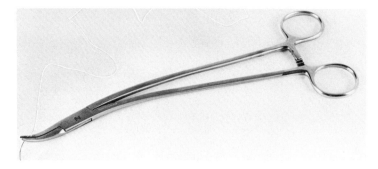

Fig. G–17.   Needle-holder, Stratte.

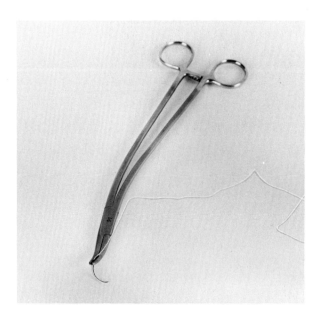

Fig. G–18.   Needle-holder, Stratte, grasping an atraumatic suture.

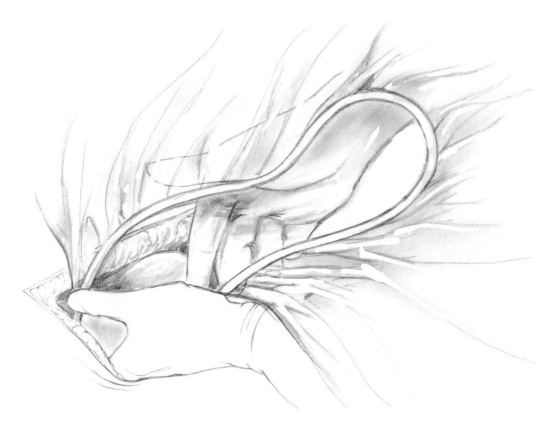

Fig. G-19.   Plastic drape being inserted.

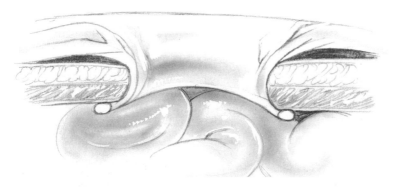

Fig. G-20.   Plastic drape in place.

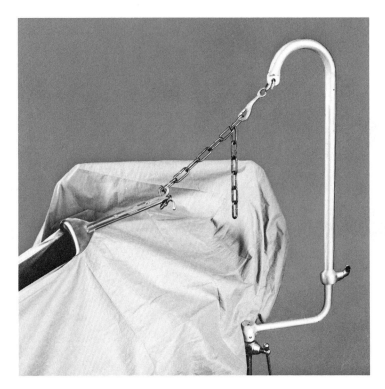

Fig. G-21.   Retractor: "chain."

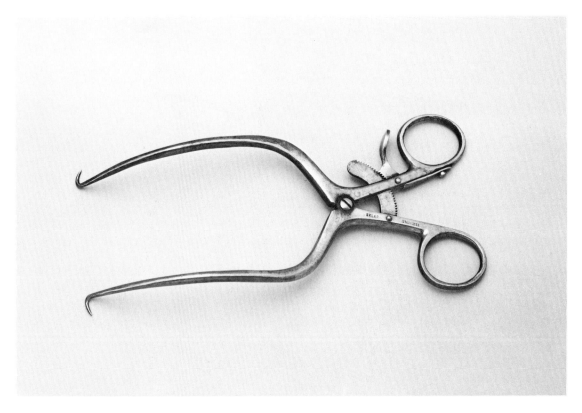

Fig. G-22.   Retractor, Gelpi.

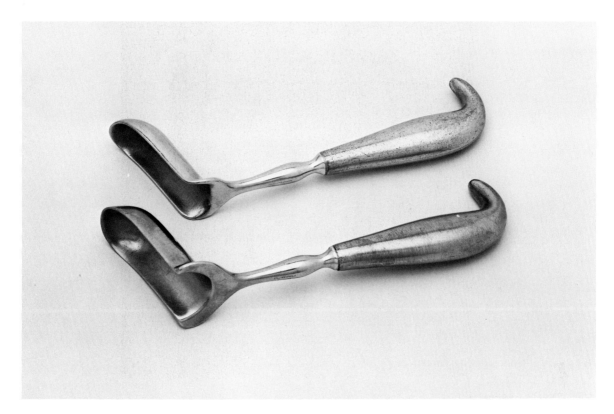

Fig. G-23.   Retractors, Hill-Ferguson.

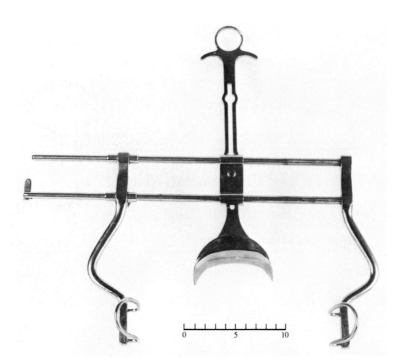

Fig. G-24.   Retractor, self-retaining: Balfour.

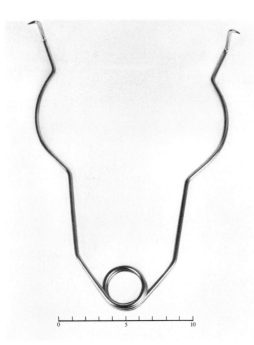

Fig. G–25.   Retractor, self-retaining: Farr.

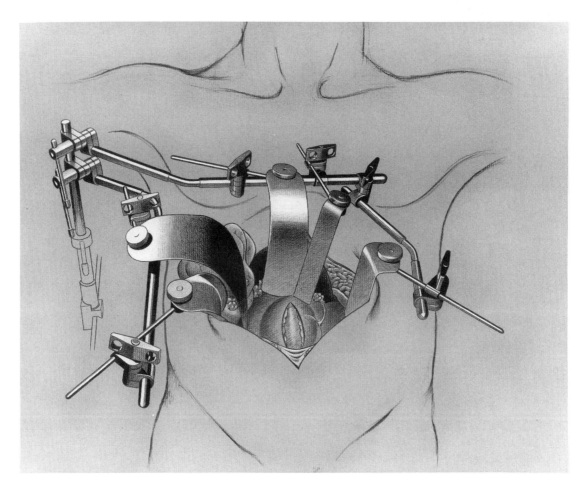

Fig. G–26.   Retractor, Thompson.

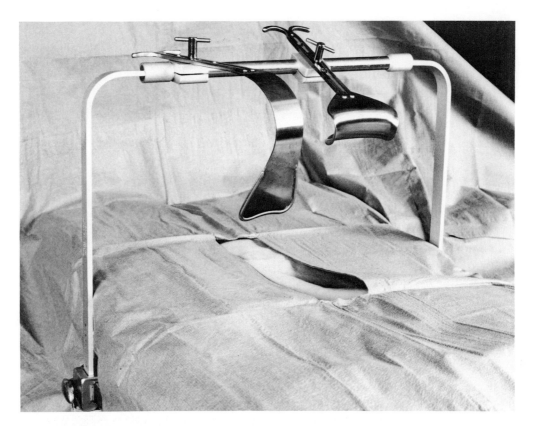

Fig. G-27. Retractor, Upper Hand.

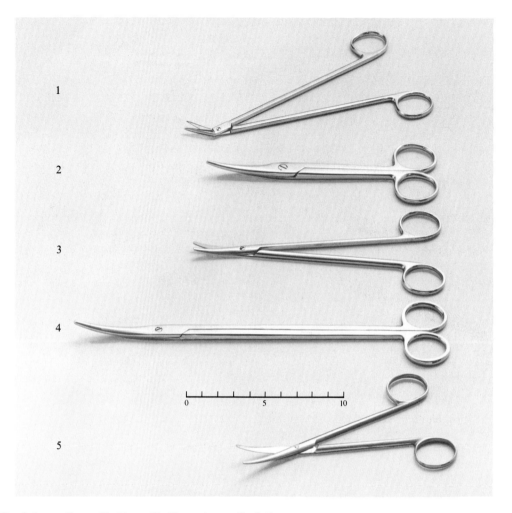

Fig. G-28.   Scissors: Potts (1); Mayo (2); Metzenbaum (3, 4, 5).

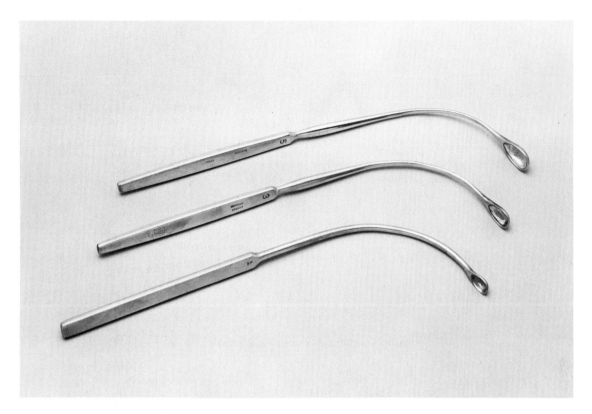

Fig. G-29.   Scoops, pituitary (surgical legacy instrument).

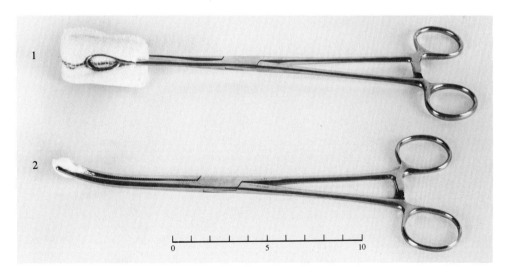

Fig. G-30.   Sponge-holder with 10 × 10 cm gauze square (1); peanut sponge (Kuttner) dissector (2).

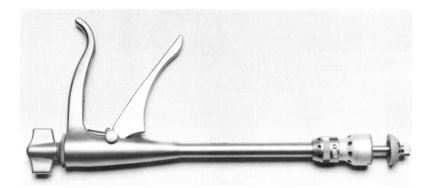

Fig. G-31.   Stapler, circular.

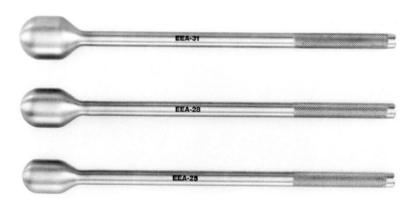

Fig. G-32.   Stapler, circular, sizers.

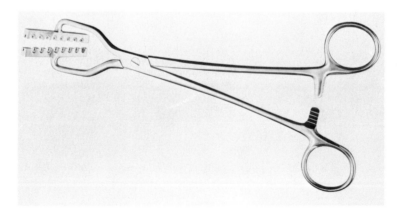

Fig. G-33.   Stapler, purse-string instrument for circular stapler.

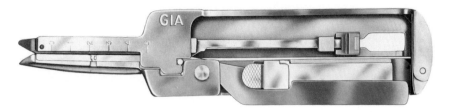

Fig. G-34. Stapler, linear cutting.

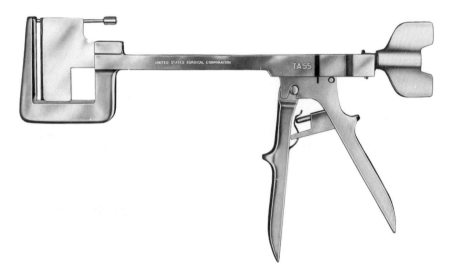

Fig. G-35. Stapler, linear (55 mm).

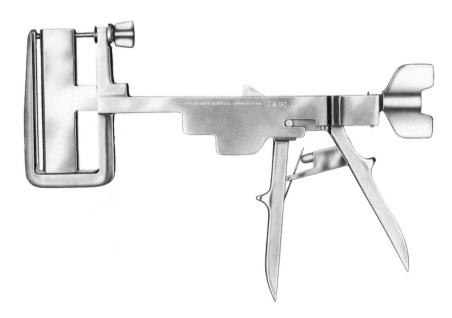

Fig. G-36. Stapler, linear (90 mm).

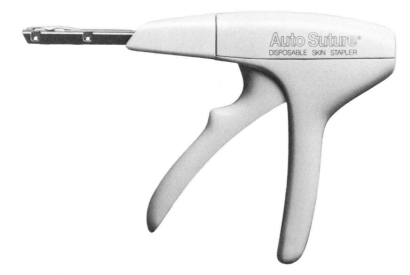

Fig. G-37.   Stapler, skin.

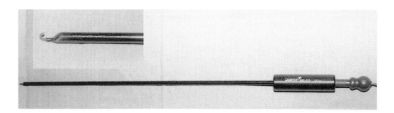

Fig. G-38.   Electrocautery, hook tip.

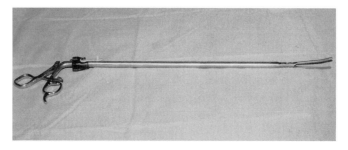

Fig. G-39.   Grasper, atraumatic.

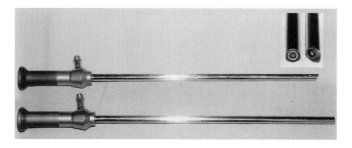

Fig. G-40.   Laparoscopes, straight and angled.

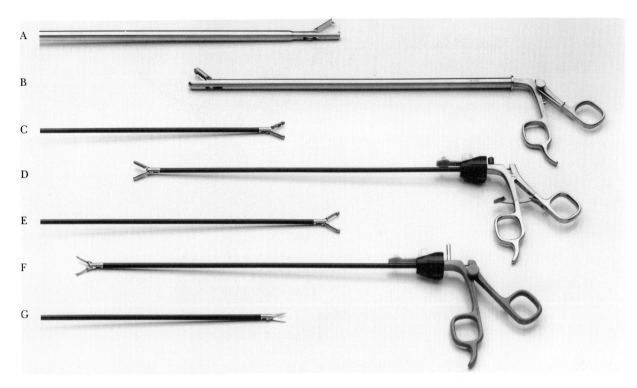

Fig. G-41. Laparoscopic cholecystectomy instruments. A. Claw to grasp and remove gallbladder from the abdominal cavity. B. Large-mouth stone forceps. C-G. Various shapes of grasping and dissecting forceps.

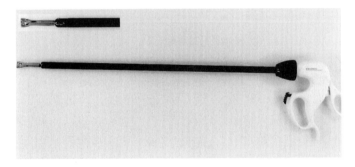

Fig. G-42. Laparoscopic clamp, Babcock.

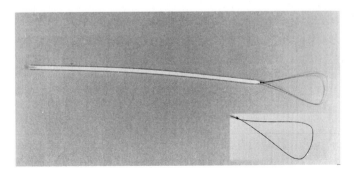

Fig. G-43. Pretied suture ligature.

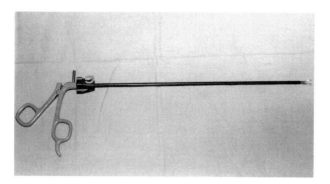

Fig. G-44.   Scissors, curved tip.

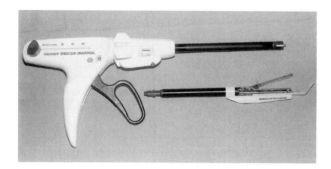

Fig. G-45.   Stapler, linear, cutting.

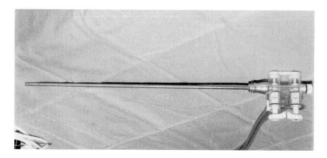

Fig. G-46.   Suction-irrigator.

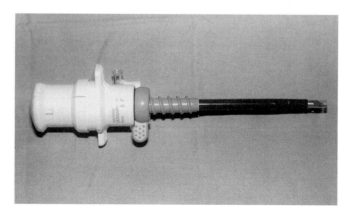

Fig. G-47.   Trocar, disposable, assembled.

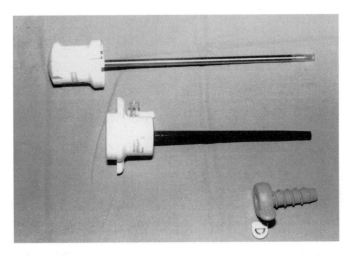

Fig. G–48.   Trocar, disposable, disassembled to show parts. The central trocar has a plastic safety sheath. The outer cannula has a port for insufflation. The grip screws into the skin and subtaneous tissue to anchor the trocar.

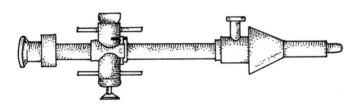

Fig. G–49.   Trocar, Hassan. (Reproduced, by permission, from Scott-Conner CEH (ed) The SAGES Manual: Fundamentals of Laparoscopy and GI Endoscopy. New York, Springer-Verlag, 1999.)

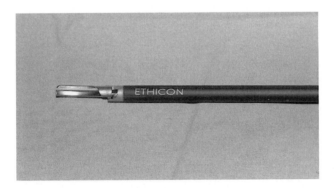

Fig. G–50.   Ultrasonic shears, tip.

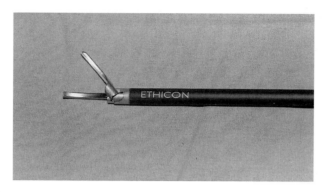

Fig. G-51.   Ultrasonic shears, tip. The fixed blade is the active blade and becomes hot during use.

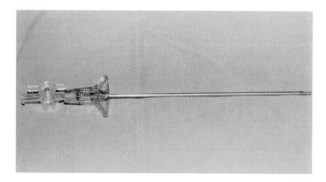

Fig. G-52.   Veress needle.

Index

Note: Page numbers followed by *f* indicate figures.

surgical management of,
668–670
exocrine insufficiency and, 666
gastrectomy and, 281
pancreatectomy and, 714
postoperative, 608
Pancreatoduodenectomy
partial
complications of, 695
contraindications to, 673
indications for, 673
operative strategy for, 673–675
operative technique for,
675–694
pitfalls related to, 673
postoperative care, 694–695
preoperative preparation for,
673
total
complications of, 708
contraindications to, 696
indications for, 696
operative strategy for, 696–697
operative technique for,
697–706
postoperative care, 706, 708
Papillary cystadenoma
lymphomatosum, 883
Papillary thyroid cancer, 885
Papillomas, 820, 821
Paraareolar abscess, 821, 835
Paraesophageal hernia. *See* Hernia
Parathyroid gland
biopsy of, 909
dissection of, 900–901
identification of, 898–900, 909
preservation of, 894, 895f, 896
Parathyroid imaging, 886
Parathyroid tissue, preservation of,
908
Parathyroidectomy
complications of, 911
indications for, 906
operative strategy for, 907–908
operative technique for, 908–910
pitfalls related to, 907
postoperative care, 910–911
Parotid tumors, 883
Parotidectomy
complications of, 893
indications for, 883, 888
operative strategy for, 888–889
operative technique for, 889–893
pitfalls related to, 888
postoperative care, 893
Partial pancreatoduodenectomy. *See*
Pancreatoduodenectomy
Partial thyroid lobectomy, 902–903
Patient
body position during surgery, 52
perioperative parenteral
antibiotics to, 48
position during surgery, 53f
preparation, 54
resuscitation of, 47–48
risk assessment of, 47

Peanut sponge, 26
Peanut sponge (Kuttner) dissector,
937f
Pelvic floor
intestinal obstruction and, 451
management of, 458–461
Pelvic hemostasis, 431, 453
Pelvic lymphadenectomy. *See*
Lymphadenectomy
Pelvic sepsis, 448–449
Pelvirectal superalevator abscess,
539–540
Peptic ulcer
duodenal ulcer and, 226–227
gastrectomy for
complications of, 281–283
operative strategy for, 258–259
operative technique for,
259–281
postoperative care, 281
gastric ulcer and, 225–226
gastrostomy for, 227
perforated
complications of, 285–286
indications for treating, 284
operative strategy for treating,
284
operative technique for
treating, 284–285
postoperative care, 285
preoperative preparation for,
284
surgery for, 225
Percutaneous endoscopic
gastrostomy, 227
Percutaneous transhepatic
cholangiography (PTC), 662
Perforated duodenal ulcer. *See*
Duodenal ulcer
Perianal abscess, 523, 537–538
Perineal dissection, 455–458
Perineal incision, 486–488
Perineal infections, 519
Perineal pain, Thiersch operation
and, 555
Perineum
closure of, 451–452
dissection of, 452
Perioperative antibiotics, 48
Peripheral vasoconstriction, 47
Peristomal sepsis
cecostomy and, 497
transverse colostomy and, 500
Peritoneal dissection, 503
Peritoneal lavage, peptic ulcer and,
285
Pfannenstiel incision, 30
Pharyngoesophageal diverticulum,
75–76
complications of, 204
indications for treating, 200
operative strategy for treating, 200
operative technique for treating,
200–204
postoperative care, 204
preoperative preparation for, 200

Pilonidal disease
management of, 524
operations for
complications of, 560–561
indications for, 556
operative strategy for, 556
operative technique for,
556–560
pitfall related to, 556
postoperative care, 560
Plain catgut material, 34
Planes. *See* Anatomic planes
Plastic drape, 931f
Pleomorphic adenomas, 883
Plication technique
Baker tube stitchless, 342–343
laparoscopic
complications of, 290
operative strategy for, 287
operative technique for,
287–289
pitfalls related to, 287
postoperative care, 289–290
preoperative preparation for,
287
for peptic ulcer, 284–285
Pneumoperitoneum
Hasson cannula for creating,
56–57
Veress needle technique for
creating, 55–56
Pneumothorax, 138
Polyethylene drain, 63
Polyglycolic synthetic sutures, 34–35
Polyps
management of, 366–367
synchronous, 367–368
Port placement, 58–59
Portal vein dissection, 676–679
Posterior gastropexy (Hill repair)
complications of, 180
indications for, 173
operative strategy for, 173–174
operative technique for, 174–180
pitfalls related to, 173
postoperative care, 180
Postoperative feeding, colorectal
cancer and, 377
Postoperative obstruction, 336,
340
Posttraumatic hernia. *See* Hernia
Pouchitis, management of, 378–379
Pregnancy, cholecystectomy during,
567
Presacral dissection
abdominoperineal resection and,
453
prevention of hemorrhage and,
423–424
procedure, 428–431
Ripstein operation and, 511
Pretied suture ligature, 941f
Primary hyperparathyroidism (HPT),
886, 906
Proctectomy, 365
Proctocolectomy, 364, 365

ISBN 0-387-95204-7